Principles and Practice of Pharmaceutical Medicine

EDITED BY

Lionel D. Edwards

President Pharma Pro Plus Inc. New Jersey, and Adjunct Professor,
Temple University, School of Pharmacy, Philadelphia, USA

Anthony W. Fox

EBD Group Inc., California, USA and Munich, Germany, and Adjunct Associate Professor,
Skaggs SPPS, University of California, San Diego, USA

Peter D. Stonier

School of Biomedical & Health Sciences, King's College London, UK

THIRD EDITION

WILEY-BLACKWELL

A John Wiley & Sons, Ltd., Publication

This edition first published 2011, © 2011 by Blackwell Publishing Ltd.

Blackwell Publishing was acquired by John Wiley & Sons in February 2007. Blackwell's publishing program has been merged with Wiley's global Scientific, Technical and Medical business to form Wiley-Blackwell.

Registered office: John Wiley & Sons Ltd, The Atrium, Southern Gate, Chichester, West Sussex, PO19 8SQ, UK

Editorial offices: 9600 Garsington Road, Oxford, OX4 2DQ, UK
The Atrium, Southern Gate, Chichester, West Sussex, PO19 8SQ, UK
111 River Street, Hoboken, NJ 07030-5774, USA

For details of our global editorial offices, for customer services and for information about how to apply for permission to reuse the copyright material in this book please see our website at www.wiley.com/wiley-blackwell

Library of Congress Cataloging-in-Publication Data

Principles and practice of pharmaceutical medicine / edited by Lionel D. Edwards, Anthony W. Fox, Peter D. Stonier. – 3rd ed.
  p. ; cm.
  Includes bibliographical references and index.
  ISBN 978-1-4051-9472-3
  1. Drug development.   2. Drugs–Research.   3. Pharmacology.   I. Edwards, Lionel D.   II. Fox, Anthony W., 1956-   III. Stonier, P. D.
  [DNLM: 1. Drug Evaluation.   2. Drug Industry–organization & administration.   QV 736]
  RM301.25.P75   2010
  615'.19–dc22

                                                                          2010027197

A catalogue record for this book is available from the British Library.

Set in 9/12pt Meridien by Aptara® Inc., New Delhi, India

1   2011

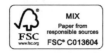

Contents

Contributors

Anbar, Dan
DANA Pharmaceutical Consulting, Inc., NJ, USA
Email: dananbar@verizon.net

Armstrong, Edward
Pharmacy Practice and Science, College of Pharmacy,
University of Arizona, USA

Barrett, Jane
Gawsworth, Cheshire, UK
Email: janebarrett@doctors.org.uk

Belsey, Jonathan
JB Medical Ltd, Sudbury, Suffolk, UK
Email: jbelsey@jbmedical.com

Boyer, J. Gregory
Accreditation Council for Pharmacy Education,
Chicago, ILL, USA

Chaponis, Robert J.
Novartis, Parsippany, NJ, USA
Email: robert.chaponis@novartis.com

Choi, Han W.
Oracle Investment Management, Inc., Greenwich, CT, USA
Email: HChoi@oraclepartners.com

Cobb, Ronald R.
RiverWood BioConsulting Inc., Gainesville, FL, USA
Email: rcobb@rtix.com

Croft, Sarah
Shook, Hardy and Bacon International LLP, London, UK
Email: scroft@shb.com

Curry, Stephen, H.
University of Rochester, Rochester, NY, USA
Email: stephenhcurry@earthlink.net

DeCory, Helen H.
Bausch and Lomb Inc.,Rochester, NY, USA

Drucker, R.
Technomark Life Sciences LLP, Durham, NC, USA

Dziewanowska, Zofia
New Drug Associates, Inc., La Jolla, CA, USA
Email: zofia@mindspring.com

Fletcher, Andrew J.
Temple University School of Pharmacy, PHARM-QA/RA,
Philadelphia, PA, USA
Email: andrew.fletcher@temple.edu

Freidank-Mueschenborn, Edda
Bungalowsiedlung 1 B, D-17406 Rankwitz, Germany

Gabrielsson, Johan
AstraZeneca AB, Gothenburg, Sweden

Geba, Gregory P.
Clinical Development, MedImmune, LLC, Gaithersburg, MD
Email: gebag@medimmune.com

Griffin, John P.
Asklepieion Consultancy Ltd, Welwyn, Hertfordshire, UK
Email: JQmans5@aol.com

Sheila Gwizdak
Pfizer Inc., New London, CT, USA

Hanson-Divers, Christine
AstraZeneca, Cary, NC, USA

Hattemer-Apostel, Rita
Verdandi AG, 8049 Zurich, Switzerland
Email: rha@verdandi.ch

Hoxie, Thomas
Hoxie & Associates LLC, Millburn, NJ, USA

Husson, Jean-Marc
Paris, France

Hughes, R. Graham
Consultant in Pharmaceutical Development, Merlimont,
France

Johnson-Pratt, Lisa R.
Bryn Mawr, PA, USA
Email: lisa_johnsonpratt_md@merck.com

Kennedy, William

König, Anja
Engelhard Arzneimittel AG, Niederdorfelden, Germany

Kulkarni, Darshan
The Kulkarni Law Firm, Philadelphia, PA, USA
Email: Darshan@conformlaw.com

Labbé, Etienne
UCB S.A., Brussels, Belgium

Lee, Jae Hong
Morrison & Foerster LLP, San Diego, CA, USA
Email: JaeHongLee@mofo.com

Lee, T.Y.
Clinical Development and Asian Ventures, Kendle
International Inc.,Cincinnati, OH, USA

Lopez, Gabriel
Basking Ridge, NJ, USA
Email: lopezg4@yahoo.com

Malone, Daniel
Pharmacy Practice and Science, College of Pharmacy,
University of Arizona, USA

van Manen, Robbert
Health Economics and Clinical Outcomes Research, Medical
Affairs, Centocor Inc., Horsham, PA, USA

Mann, Ronald
University of Southampton, Hants, UK
Email: ronmann@professormann.com

Marks, Peter
Pfizer Limited, Sandwich, Kent, UK
Email: Peter.Marks@pfizer.com

Métry, Jean-Michel (Deceased)

Minor, Michael
Clinical Development and Asian Ventures, Kendle
International Inc., Cincinnati, OH, USA

Miskin, Barry
Department of Surgery, Nova Southeastern University,
College of Osteopathic Medicine, Fort Lauderdale – Davie,
Florida, USA
Email: miskinmd@aol.com

Molony, Leslie J.
Transgeneron Therapeutics, Inc., Gainesville, FL, USA
Email: Leslie@transgeneron.com

Morimoto, Bruce H.
Allon Therapeutics Inc., Redwood City, CA, USA
Email: bmorimoto@allontherapeutics.com

Naito, C.
Teikyo University, Tokyo, Japan

Osterhaus, Jane T.
Wasatch Health Outcomes, Park City, UT, USA
Email: jtosterhaus@mindspring.com

Packard, Linda
American Academy of Pharmaceutical Physicians, Research
Triangle Park, NC, USA

Papaluca Amati, Marisa
European Agency for the Evaluation of Medicinal Products,
London, UK

Rahman, Mirza I.
Health Economics and Reimbursement, Evidence Based
Medicine, Ortho-Clinical Diagnostics, Inc., Rochester,
NY, USA
Email: MRahman7@its.jnj.com

Reno, Fred (retired)
Merritt Island, FL, USA

Roy, Douglas
Division of Pathway Medicine, Medical School, University of
Edinburgh, Edinburgh, UK

Sands, Robert
Sanofi-aventis, Cambridge, MA, USA
Email: rob.sands@sanofi-aventis.com

Shapiro, David A.
Intercept Pharmaceuticals, San Diego, CA, USA
Email: dshapiro@interceptpharma.com

Spilker, Bert
Bert Spilker Associates, Bethesda, MD, USA
Email: bspilker@comcast.net

Starkey, Paul W.
Merck Consumer Care, Whitehouse Station, NJ, USA
Email: pgvstar@aol.com

Starkey, Yan Yan Li
GlaxoSmithKline Consumer Healthcare, Parsippany, NJ, USA
Email: Listarkey@aol.com

Tabusso, Giuliana
Milan, Italy
Email: giulianatabusso@libero.it

Tilson, Hugh H.
School of Public Health, University of North Carolina,
Chapel Hill, NC, USA
Email: hugh_tilson@unc.edu

Townsend, Raymond J.
Elan Pharmaceuticals, San Diego, CA, USA
Email: raytownsend@elan.com

van Troostenburg, Anne-Ruth
Takeda Group R&D, London, UK
Email: ar.vantroostenburg@tgrd.com

Vogel, John
John R. Vogel Associates Inc., Kihei, HI, USA
Email: john@jrvogel.com

Walker, Stuart
Centre for Medicines Research, International Institute for
Regulatory Science, London UK
Email: swalker@cmr.org

Wells, Marilyn J.
East Stroudsburg University, East Stroudsburg, PA, USA

Williams, Roger L.
US Pharmacopia, Rockville, MD, USA

Wood, Katie P.J.
Foster City, CA, USA
Email: kpjwood@gmail.com

Yasurhara, H.
Teikyo University, Tokyo, Japan

Young, Michael
MDY Associates, Philadelphia, PA, USA
Email: MichaelDYoungMD@aol.com

Preface to the First Edition

Pharmaceutical medicine is a relatively new, but rapidly growing, academic discipline. As these trends continue into the 21st century, pharmaceutical physicians are increasingly regarding consultancy work and contract research organization (CRO) affiliation as good career opportunities, and now recognize the need for continuing education and training in this broad spectrum discipline.

As editors, we would like to thank our contributors for their expertise, their dedication, and their vision. We would like to thank and acknowledge the work and counsel of our colleague Robert Bell, MD, PhC, who helped us greatly during the early part of this project. We would also like to thank and acknowledge the enormous help, encouragement, and patience of the team at John Wiley & Sons, Ltd, UK, with whom we have worked closely over these past few years, among whom we have particularly stressed (!) Michael Davis, Deborah Reece, Hannah Bradley, Lewis Derrick, and Hilary Rowe.

Lastly, we would like to thank our families, and friends, who have withstood the frequent telephone calls, e-mails, and meetings, often late into the night. Indeed, to all who made this project possible, both authors and non-authors, we thank you. We are certain that this specialty, and our patients, even though we may help them vicariously, will benefit because of your contributions.

Andrew Fletcher
Lionel Edwards
Tony Fox
Peter Stonier

Preface to the Second Edition

Since the first edition of this book, pharmaceutical medicine has only become more diverse and has also become widely accepted as a recognized medical specialty, for example, with its first graduates of specialist training in the United Kingdom, to add to those of Switzerland and Mexico. This has been accompanied by pharmaceutical medicine's rapid progress toward specialty recognition within the European Community, and many changes in the pharmaceutical environment. So, we have taken this book further with this second edition. There are new chapters on European regulations, risk management, the Middle East, Asia, and other topical subjects in pharmaceutical medicine. Those chapters that did appear in the first edition have all been brought up to date.

But this book is for all those working in pharmaceutical medicine, regardless of their degrees, titles, or affiliations. Although it comprehensively covers the internationally harmonized syllabus for the Diplomas in Pharmaceutical Medicine that are awarded in Belgium, Switzerland, and the United Kingdom, this book will also usefully serve those teaching other types of certificates and (usually Master's) degrees in this field, as well as being a *vade mecum* for those who are not undertaking academic courses.

We would again like to thank the team at John Wiley and Sons, Ltd, Chichester (UK). Hannah Bradley got this second edition started, but then went off on a tour around the world; the editors strenuously deny that they are the reason why. Lucy Sayer and Juliet Booker have since piloted the ship to the dock-side, successfully cajoling us into getting this edition done before its second decade. Not least, we would like to thank you, the reader, for your continued support and suggestions. So here is our second edition, it is more than a simple update, and it is even less US-centric than before.

Lionel Edwards
Andrew Fletcher
Tony Fox
Peter Stonier

Preface to the Third Edition

Pharmaceutical medicine is now practiced by people with a wider range of backgrounds than ever before. Clinical trials now demand the skills of ethicists, clinical pharmacologists, dental surgeons, medical practitioners, nurses, psychologists, regulators, and many others who will have attended diverse types of graduate and medical schools. This book is for all of them.

Pharmaceutical medicine is a discipline that is also spreading geographically. Not only are clinical trials now being conducted on a global scale, but also academic rigor in pharmaceutical medicine is being pursued in more and more countries. For example, we anticipate that during the currency of this edition the Diploma in Pharmaceutical Medicine, which began in the United Kingdom, either has already been or will have become established in Belgium, India, Mexico, South Africa, and Switzerland. In addition, there are well-established Master of Science degrees, covering much of the same syllabus, in most of the developed world. We have aimed this textbook to support all these academic endeavors.

Like the discipline itself, perseverance with our particular brand of editing has spread geographically during this third edition. We began with Lucy Sayer, who was bravely willing to take us on, yet again, from Portsmouth, UK. Then, one previously unpublished consequence of the merger of John Wiley and Sons with Blackwell Publishing was that Adam Gilbert, Robyn Lyons, and Gill Whitley accepted the awkward role of joining an ongoing project, while blissfully unaware of the cantankerous editors that came with it. But pressure is load divided by the area receiving it, and our load now is borne across a broad arc extending from Oxford, via London, to Normandy. We hope that this spreading of the load has reduced the megaPascals that we have created.

Other people deserve our thanks because this third edition would never have appeared without them. As before, these include Rob Bell MD, PhC and Andrew Fletcher MB BChir, MSc, DipPharmMedRCP, FFPM, both of whom were seminal to this project. Our families, too, are big indirect contributors.

But the reason that we have done this, now for the third time in a decade, is because of you, the reader, and through you, even if it is vicariously, for your patients.

Lionel Edwards
Tony Fox
Peter Stonier

About the Editors

Lionel D. Edwards, MB, BS, LRCP, MRCS, Dip COG, FFPM, is President of Pharma Pro Plus Inc., a drug development consulting company. Dr Edwards has been involved in all aspects of clinical trials for over 37 years on many different research drug and devices in 10 therapeutic areas. Previously, he was Senior Director at Novartis, a managing consultant at PA consulting, Vice President of Clinical Research at Bio-Technology Pharmaceutical Corporation, a small biotechnology firm operating both in the United States and internationally. Prior to this, he worked at Noven Inc., a small Skin Patch Technology firm with large International licensed partners: CIBA and Rhone Poulenc Rorer. He was Assistant Vice President, International Clinical Research at Hoffman-La Roche, Senior Director of Schering-Plough International Research, and Director of US Domestic Gastrointestinal, Hormonal, and OTC Research Departments. Dr Edwards chaired the PMA (PhRMA) Special Populations Committee, and also sat on the Institute of Medicine Committee for Research in Women, through the US National Institutes of Health. He also served on the Efficacy subcommittee Topic 5 (Acceptability of Foreign Clinical Data) for the International Committee on Harmonization (ICH) and contributed to the working paper on E Topic 1 (Research in Geriatric Patients). Dr Edwards is a Fellow of the Faculty of Pharmaceutical Medicine and an Adjunct Professor at Temple University Graduate School of Pharmacology. He has taught for the Pharmaceutical Education & Research Institute for over 12 years and was on the teaching faculty of the National Association of Physicians. He is a Founder member of the American Academy of Pharmaceutical Physicians now part of the Association of Clinical Research Professionals (ACRP). Dr Edwards has homes in New Jersey and Florida.

Anthony ("Tony") W. Fox, BSc, MBBS, FFPM, FRCP, MD(Lond), DipPharmMedRCP, CBiol FIBiol is President of EBD Consulting, and one of four Managing Directors of FGK Representative Services (Munich, Germany and Zug, Switzerland). From The (now Royal) London Hospital, after general clinical training, he was Rotary International Fellow at Emory University (Atlanta, Georgia), and CIBA-Geigy Fellow at Harvard. Industrial positions with Procter and Gamble, Glaxo Inc (Research Triangle Park, North Carolina), and a small company called Cypros Pharmaceuticals (Carlsbad, California) came next. From time to time, he serves as Chief Medical Officer for small companies (currently Conatus Pharmaceuticals and Zogenix Inc., both in San Diego, California). Tony was a Charter Member, and sometime Vice-President and Trustee, of the American Academy of Pharmaceutical Physicians; he is also a founder, Secretary, and Treasurer of the Southern California Pharmaceutical Medicine Group. He is a liveryman *guardant* of the Society of Apothecaries of London, and is a voluntary Associate Clinical Professor at the University of California, San Diego. His publications span several areas of pharmaceutical medicine, including regulation, pharmacology, clinical trial methodology, pharmacovigilance, migraine, and analgesics, with occasional excursions into toxicology and human metabolism. He is a named inventor on several patents. Tony is currently one of the six editors of *Int J Clin Pharmacol Ther*, and the Consulting Editor for *Pharmaceutical Medicine*. Proud to be an Essex man (!), he researches the history of that county, and is a Fellow of the Royal Geographical Society, the Royal Numismatic

Society, and the Royal Society for the Encouragement of Arts, Manufactures, and Commerce (FRSA).

Peter D. Stonier, BA, BSc, PhD, MBChB, MRCPsych, FRCP, FRCPE, FFPM has over 30 years experience in pharmaceutical medicine. He is a graduate of Manchester Medical school, qualifying in 1974, following a BSc degree in Physiology (University of Birmingham) and a PhD in protein chemistry (inborn errors of metabolism, University of Sheffield). He is a pharmaceutical physician and was Medical Adviser with the UK Hoechst Group of companies from 1977, serving as Medical Director and Board Director until 2000. He is Group Medical Director of the pharmaceutical company Amdipharm plc. Formerly he was President of the International Federation of Associations of Pharmaceutical Physicians (IFAPP) and Chairman of the British Association of Pharmaceutical Physicians (BrAPP). He is a founder Board member and Past President of the Faculty of Pharmaceutical Medicine (FPM), Royal Colleges of Physicians, UK,

and is currently Director of Education & Training of the Faculty.

He is Visiting Professor in Pharmaceutical Medicine at King's College London, School of Biomedical & Health Sciences. In 1993, while Visiting Professor in Pharmaceutical Medicine at the University of Surrey, the first Masters programme (MSc) in Pharmaceutical Medicine was introduced under his co-direction.

His publications include texts in pharmaceutical medicine and edited works in human psychopharmacology, clinical research and paediatric clinical research, medical marketing, and careers with the pharmaceutical industry. In 2002 he became Honorary Member of the Belgian College of Pharmaceutical Medicine. He is a member of the Council for Education in Pharmaceutical Medicine (CEPM/IFAPP). In 2006 he received the Lifetime Achievement Award of the Academy of Pharmaceutical Physicians and Investigators (APPI/ACRP) for distinguished contributions and leadership in the field of pharmaceutical medicine.

SECTION I
Overview of Pharmaceutical Medicine

CHAPTER 1

The Practice and Practitioners of Pharmaceutical Medicine

Anthony W. Fox

EBD Group Inc., Carlsbad, CA, USA and Munich, Germany, and Skaggs SPPS, University of California, San Diego, USA

Pharmaceutical medicine is unquestionably a young specialty, formalized within the past forty years or so, and its diversity is probably greater than most medical specialties. It is also a specialty that is frequently misunderstood by those outside it.

The diversity of pharmaceutical medicine

Elements of what we regard today as pharmaceutical medicine have resided in the specialties of general and/or internal medicine for a long time. Some of these may be found in the chapters that follow, but obvious examples include Lind's clinical trial (see the index) and Withering's bit of pharmacognosy when he identified *Digitalis purpurea* as a treatment for what was then called dropsy. Moreover, every prescription written is a clinical trial of some sort, where $n = 1$, because human beings are anisogenetic.

Pharmaceutical medicine is also a discipline that overlaps with many others: Techniques shared with the fields of epidemiology and public health are obvious. Moreover, like orthopedics or dental surgery, there are borrowings from as far afield as the discipline of engineering (e.g., adaptive clinical trials designs, and some aspects of pharmaceutics). Ever since the need to demonstrate efficacy, tolerability, and purity in drug products (and their

equivalents in diagnostics and devices), pharmaceutical medicine has been evidence-based. It is interesting that only lately have the more venerable medical specialties adopted an interest in evidence-based approaches to clinical practice, slowly catching up with pharmaceutical physicians!

The diversity of the practitioners

It is therefore unsurprising that the diverse discipline of pharmaceutical medicine is populated by people with varied educational backgrounds. There can be no doubt that clinical experience is always a good prelude to a career in pharmaceutical medicine. But this experience can be found among dental surgeons, medical practitioners, nurses, pharmacists, physical therapists, psychologists, and many other members of the allied health professions; satisfying careers in pharmaceutical medicine, and international distinction, are available to people with all these sorts of early training. For those with a lifelong thirst to learn on a cross-disciplinary basis, it is this breadth of intellectual interaction that forms one of the greatest attractors to the specialty.

As a generalization, one difference between pharmaceutical medicine and other medical specialties is the sizes of the teams that one works within. General practitioners, for example, probably work with six (or so) other types of professional (perhaps nurses, health visitors, administrators, their hospital colleagues, social workers, and, doubtless from time to time, the judiciary).

Principles and Practice of Pharmaceutical Medicine, 3rd edition.
Edited by L.D. Edwards, A.W. Fox, P.D. Stonier.
© 2011 Blackwell Publishing Ltd.

Radiologists might add radiographers and physicists to this list and delete health visitors and social workers. But in comparison, the following list of nouns comprises pharmaceutical medicine, all of which have their own specialists (in no particular order): ethics, chemistry, pharmacology, computational modeling, pharmaceutics, project planning, toxicology, regulatory affairs, logistics, quality control engineering, biostatistics, pharmacogenomics, clinical trials, politics, economics, public relations, teaching, pharmacovigilance, marketing, finance, pharmacokinetics, technical writing, data automation, actuarial analysis, pharmacoeconomics, information science, publishing, public health, international aid and development, intellectual property, and other forms of law; and this is not an exhaustive list. Conversance, if not advanced capability, with these specialists should be an early goal of any career in pharmaceutical medicine.

Surely, there is no other industry where as many diverse professionals all have the sick patient as their ultimate concern?

Problem-solving in the pharmaceutical enterprise is often by teamwork. For physicians and pharmacists, the greatest difference between this specialty and all others is the value placed on their versatility and adaptability. Moreover, these specialists must learn that in pharmaceutical medicine they are unlikely to be as dominant in decision-making as in ordinary clinical practice. Knowing when to lead, when to follow, and when to get out of the way, rather than presuming a leadership role in all situations, will always be valued.

Organizations and educational systems

There is no need to embark on international disputes about who got where first. For more than thirty years, most countries in the developed world have had one or more national societies or academies devoted to the specialty of pharmaceutical medicine. All hold education and training as central to their mission, whereas some societies engage in the regulatory or political debates over particular issues.

In the European Economic Area (the European Union plus Iceland, Norway, and Lichtenstein) together with Switzerland, pharmaceutical medicine is becoming recognized as a specialty deserving of its own program of specialist training with accredited certification, through a Certificate of Completion of Training (CCT) or equivalent. To date, the United Kingdom, Ireland, Belgium and Switzerland are European countries that have formally recognized the specialty of pharmaceutical medicine.

These higher qualifications are attained after obtaining a more general knowledge base for the specialty. The latter has been examined by the Royal Colleges of Physicians (RCP) in the United Kingdom for more than thirty years and its Diploma in Pharmaceutical Medicine (DipPharmMedRCP) qualifies the holder as a Member of the Faculty of Pharmaceutical Medicine (MFPM) within those colleges. The Belgian Academy of Pharmaceutical Medicine and the Basel, Switzerland-based European Centre for Pharmaceutical Medicine (ECPM) with three associated Universities (EUCOR) have diplomas that are recognized reciprocally with the DipPharmMedRCP. Mexico has also recognized the specialty of pharmaceutical medicine. Progress towards an analogous goal ("Board certification") is being made in North America. The international compatibility and recognition of these qualifications would seem essential in a world where drug development is being increasingly globalized, drug regulation has become increasingly harmonized, and many employment opportunities are in companies that are now international conglomerates.

This is not to say, however, that qualifications in pharmaceutical medicine are uniquely enabling to the practitioner. All of the long list of sub-specializations mentioned above have their own diplomas and degrees. Human resources departments have to be well-informed about the diversity of formal recognitions held by the many specialists who can contribute to the work of the industry and its regulators.

Finally, in pursuit of evidence for all the optimism above, it should be noted that in the year

2000, in the (then) American Academy of Pharmaceutical Physicians (AAPP), more than 90% of members indicated satisfaction with their choice of specialty. This was unlike the results of similar surveys conducted within other medical subspecialties. What is now the Academy of Pharmaceutical Physicians and Investigators (APPI), and the Association of Clinical Research Professionals (ACRP) thrive, and have transatlantic activities.

Further reading

Smethurst D. Pharmaceutical medicine: making the leap. *Student BMJ* 2004; **12**:45–58.

Stonier PD (ed.). *Careers with the Pharmaceutical Industry.* John Wiley & Sons Ltd: Chichester UK, 2003, second edition. ISBN 0-470-84328-4.

Useful websites include: www.fpm.org.uk and www. acrpnet.org (both accessed April 20, 2010).

CHAPTER 2

Pharmaceutical Medicine as a Medical Specialty

Michael D. Young[1] & Peter D. Stonier[2]
[1] MDY Associates, Philadelphia, PA, USA
[2] School of Biomedical & Health Sciences, King's College London, UK

Medicine is an art that has been practiced since time immemorial. The use of herbs and natural medicaments to relieve pain or to aid the sick in coping with their afflictions has been part of all societies. In the Western world, medicine has developed at least since the time of the Greeks and Romans—the Hippocratic oath reminds us of this nearly 2500-year history. However, the progress of medicine has been very different from that of many other arts within society. It has come of age after an incredibly long maturation period. As a function capable of offering a successful treatment for a human ailment, medicine is very much a development of the last 100–150 years. Indeed, the major advances have come in the last 50–75 years.

The role of physicians in society has changed over the centuries. It may have reached its nadir during the early renaissance, when the general attitude was, as Shakespeare said, "Trust not the physician; his antidotes are poison." From the 19th century onwards, with their growing diagnostic understanding and their therapeutic agents becoming increasingly effective, physicians have come to be increasingly valued. Today, much of the practice of medicine in all its subspecialties is based on a physician's diagnosis and treatment with drugs, devices, or surgery. This radical change to an era of focused treatments, after aeons of using homespun remedies and then watching hopefully for the crisis

or the fever to pass, has accompanied the recent revolutions in the understanding of biological processes and in technical and biotechnical capabilities. These developments have allowed us to produce pure therapeutic agents and establish their safe and effective use.

The exponential growth in scientific knowledge, particularly over the last 100 years, has brought about a paradigm shift in our approach to pharmaceuticals. Until the 20th century, the sale and use of medicines and medical devices was almost entirely unregulated by governments. It was a case of *caveat emptor*, with only the drug taker's common sense to protect against the dangers of the so-called patent medicines and "snake oils." The obvious abuses in these situations eventually led to government intervention, professional regulation, and requirements that drugs be pure and unadulterated. With advances in science and in the ability to define and establish drug efficacy came a requirement to demonstrate that drugs were also safe. Finally, as late as the second half of the 20th century, came the legal requirement to establish that pharmaceuticals were effective before they were marketed. These legal requirements reflected changes in social attitudes and expectations grounded in the questions that the development of biological and basic sciences had made it possible to ask and answer. The response to these changes led to the development of the specialty of pharmaceutical medicine.

Pharmaceutical medicine can be defined as "the discipline of medicine that is devoted to the discovery, research, development, and support of

Principles and Practice of Pharmaceutical Medicine, 3rd edition.
Edited by L.D. Edwards, A.W. Fox, P.D. Stonier.
© 2011 Blackwell Publishing Ltd.

ethical promotion and safe use of pharmaceuticals, vaccines, medical devices, and diagnostics" (bylaws of the Academy of Pharmaceutical Physicians and Investigators, APPI). Pharmaceutical medicine covers all medically active agents from neutraceuticals, through cosmeceuticals and over-the-counter (OTC) pharmaceuticals, to prescription drugs. Furthermore, the specialty is not confined to those physicians working within what is classically considered the pharmaceutical industry but includes those involved in the clinical management or regulation of all healthcare products. It is the basic specialty for physicians within the cosmetics and nutrition industry, for those in the device industry, and for those in not-for-profit companies, such as those responsible for the national blood supplies and/or for specialized blood products. Furthermore, it is the fundamental discipline for physicians who are in government health ministries, insurance companies, National Health Trusts or HMO management, drug regulatory agencies, or any other oversight or regulatory function for healthcare.

In the early part of this half-century, for a medicine to be adopted and to sell, it was sufficient that science could conceive of a new treatment, that technology could deliver that treatment, and that clinical research could prove it effective and safe for the physician to use. This is no longer the case.

Over the past three decades, we have seen the emergence of two major influences in decisions about new advances in healthcare: the payer—providers and the patient—consumers. Their role in the decision-making process has increased rapidly in the last 25 years, as can be seen in Figure 2.1.

With an increasing proportion of society's healthcare budget spent on pharmaceuticals, even

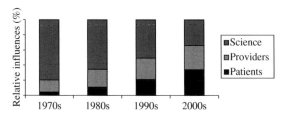

Figure 2.1 The influencers of healthcare provision.

a growth in the percentage of the gross national product that governments are willing to allocate to healthcare has been unable to meet the demands of unbridled development. This has made the payer–provider a major determiner of the use of pharmaceuticals. All possible treatments cannot be freely available to all and a cost-to-benefit consideration has to be introduced. This, in turn, has ensured that pharmaceutical medicine involves pharmacoeconomics training and even media training to deal with what, for some, may be seen as the rationing and/or means-testing of access to the totality of healthcare options. These are significant ethical and social issues, and physicians within the pharmaceutical industry or the health regulatory agencies will inevitably be required to provide a perspective, both internally and to those outside.

The second new decision-maker in the provision of healthcare has arrived even more recently as a crucial component. This is the end-user or patient groups. The rising status of the physician since the 19th century had encouraged a paternalistic doctor–patient relationship, with the physician clearly in the lead. In recent times, the nature of this relationship has come under question. The advent of holistic medical concepts focused on the whole patient, and taking into account the entirety of an individual patient's life has forced changes in the focusing of any therapeutic interaction. The general increase in educational standards within the developed world and the massive increase in available information culminating today with the electronic media and the Internet have inevitably produced a more informed patient. This has empowered the patient and led to the formation of all kinds of public interest and patient groups. Furthermore, the ability in this century to think in terms of the maintenance of good health and even of the abolition of disease (e.g., smallpox and polio) has changed the patient's and society's attitudes to what they can and should expect of physicians. Today, we are very much moving towards a balance in the therapeutic interaction, if not to a patient–doctor relationship. This change is a seminal one for the delivery of healthcare and for the development of new therapeutic agents.

For prescription drugs, the major factor bringing about the involvement of patient groups was probably the revolution in the new drug evaluation process caused by the AIDS epidemic. This terrible affliction occurred at a time when groups within society were forming to fight for their recognition and/or rights quite independent of the occurrence of a life-threatening disease. Nonetheless, within the Western world, it is clear that these groups rapidly came to form a vanguard for patients' rights with respect to AIDS. They challenged the paternalism within medicine and insisted on access and full disclosure of what was going on in pharmaceutical medicine and within academic medical politics. Without this openness such patients would have lost confidence in pharmaceutical companies, academia, and the medical and regulatory establishments. Having forced a re-evaluation and a greater respect for patients' needs, AIDS Coalition To Unleash Power (ACTUP) and others have brought patient representatives into the drug development process. Such educated and involved patients have, in their turn, come to understand the scientific methodology and the requirement for the adequate testing of new drugs. Indeed, the requirements have consequently become much more acceptable to patients in general. Nevertheless, there is no doubt that these proactive patient representative groups have forever changed the role of the patient in the development of therapeutics and of healthcare within society.

Pharmaceutical medicine is the discipline that specializes within medicine in overseeing the process of developing new therapeutics to improve the standard of health and the quality of life within society. Inevitably, then, it was one of the first medical specialties to feel this change in patients' view of the quality of their care. An integral part of all progress in healthcare is evaluating the needs of patients and society and the gaps in the present provisions for those needs. To oversee this progress, pharmaceutical medicine involves the combination of the following: first, the medical sciences to evaluate disease; second, the economic sciences to evaluate the value with respect to costs; and third, the ethical and social sciences to evaluate the utility of any new drug to patients and to society as a whole.

Table 2.1 Controlling factors in the adoption of new therapeutic agents

Influences	Controllers/"gatekeepers"
Medical science	Regulatory agencies
	Physicians
	Health professionals
Healthcare providers	Politicians
	National Health Services/HMOs
	Insurance companies
Consumers	Patient groups
	Pharmacists
	Media

As with all products, truly successful therapeutic agents are those that meet all the customers' needs. In today's and tomorrow's world, the concept that all that is needed is for medicines to meet the scientific requirements of being effective and safe is essentially outdated. It is not just the scientific factors and customers that must be satisfied. Table 2.1 shows that the two other critical factors or influences outlined in Figure 2.1 produce many more customers to be served.

As members of the public become generally more and more informed, it is inevitable that they will want to take more of a role in deciding on their own health and how any disease that they might have is to be treated. It is important to realize that this is likely to change the demand for healthcare. Some of the focus will shift to areas not classically considered as diseases or to health areas considered today as an inevitability of life or a condition for which the patient should "just take charge." Typical examples will be, on the one hand, an increased focus on the quality of life or on the effects of ageing (such as cognitive dysfunction, menopause, osteoporosis, and waning immunological function, with consequent increase in vulnerability to disease), and, on the other hand, disorders such as obesity, attention deficit, hyperactivity, and even anorexia/bulimia. As the patients or their representatives respond and "take charge," we should not be surprised to see a change in what are considered therapeutic modalities and how they are made available. We might expect a demand for products that do not need prescriptions (e.g., minerals,

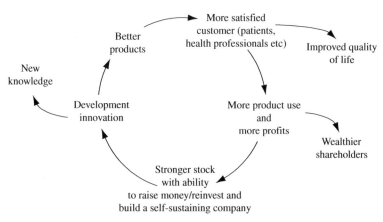

Figure 2.2 The cycle that drives the pharmaceutical industry.

neutraceuticals, and cosmeceuticals) or for patients to be able to self-diagnose and use prescription drugs moved to a "pharmacy only" or full OTC status. Some of these moves may well fit within one or more governments' desire to reduce the national pharmaceutical bill and hence may be something that has both patient and provider endorsement.

Those seeking to develop therapeutic products will need to understand these dynamic interactions and the consequent potential changes in one or more of society's approaches to its healthcare. Indeed, this is another opportunity for pharmaceutical medicine to expand. The specialty should cover all pharmacologically active treatments, all disease preventions, and all health maintenance modalities. The objective is to maximize patient benefits and extend product life cycles, as well as company sales. Clearly, pharmaceutical medicine requires an ability to read the direction that society is taking and an understanding that, on a global basis, various societies can take different attitudes to how they will regulate and/or classify a therapeutic agent. However they are classified or regulated, new therapeutic agents will continue to be needed, health benefits to deliver now, and to be potentially significant revenue generators for a business, allowing investment in future therapeutics. This is the basic cycle (see Figure 2.2) driving the pharmaceutical industry.

The R&D process is moving forward as biomedical science progresses and disease processes are bet-

ter understood. The process of developing a therapeutic agent is much more than a better understanding of a disease leading to a new approach to its management. The process includes the following: first, state-of-the-art technical manufacturing sciences to ensure a drug substance is pure; second, appropriate and innovative pre-clinical science to ensure that a new chemical entity is as safe as possible before being used by humans; third, the most sophisticated clinical evaluation methodology, which must establish the efficacy and safety of a new treatment in humans and include a multidisciplinary approach to medical, social, and economic issues of quality of life and cost–benefit. Finally, the process includes the business management of social and political issues inherent in establishing, communicating, and assuring the value of the new drug within a global economy.

The amount spent on R&D by the pharmaceutical industry has grown exponentially over the past few decades, and now the industry outspends the National Institutes of Health in the United States.

Similar growth in R&D investment has been seen outside United States, for example in the United Kingdom. With such a massive R&D effort, the process has inevitably become subdivided into several functional sections, the following being the most obvious:

- *Basic chemical or structural research*: Exploring the genetic basis of a disease or the microstructure of a receptor or enzyme active site, and from that, developing tailored molecules to provide specific interactions and potential therapeutic outcomes.

• *Pre-clinical research and development*: Using biological systems, up to and including animal models, to explore the causes of diseases and the potential safety and efficacy of new therapeutic agents.

• *Clinical development*: Using humans, both the healthy and those with a disease, to evaluate the safety and efficacy of a new drug. This section is itself, by convention, subdivided into three phases.

• *Regulatory and societal development*: Ensuring that the entire development of each new therapeutic is seen in the context of its need to meet governmental requirements and that the appropriate value-added components (e.g., quality of life, cost–benefit, evidence-based medicine, relative competitive positioning) over and above the basic demonstration of safety and efficacy are integrated into the product's database.

• *Post-market approval medical affairs*: This involves the promotion of each product by marketing and sales functions and the oversight of this process by pharmaceutical physicians. Two other critical post-marketing components are as follows: first, continued learning about the safety and efficacy of the product in normal medical practice, as opposed to clinical trials; and second, the development of new or improved uses of the product as more is learned about it and as medical science progresses.

So, the whole process of developing a new drug is extremely expensive and time-consuming. It is also a very difficult and risky process. Indeed, the majority of initial new product leads never reach the level of being tested on humans, and over 80% of the products that are tested on humans never become licensed drugs. Of course, all the many failed research and development efforts must be paid for, as well as the relatively few successful projects. This can only be done from the earnings on the new treatments that are developed. This and the need to return to shareholders a profit on their long-term investment in the R&D process are the basic factors in the cost of new drug. A major role of pharmaceutical medicine is to ensure that the value of new therapies is clearly demonstrated so that society can see the cost–benefit of new medicines.

Overall, the process of moving from a research concept through development to a marketed drug and then further refining the drug's value throughout what marketers would call the product's life cycle involves many disciplines, as can be seen in Figure 2.3. The basic responsibility for establishing and maintaining the safety and efficacy of a drug involves knowing where all of these differing functions can have an effect on the risks and the benefits of medicines for patients.

In the 1950s and 1960s, random screening and serendipity was the basis of the approach to new drug discovery. The structure–activity relationships were rudimentary and used simplistic pharmacophores and animal "models of diseases." This approach had essentially thousands of chemicals chasing a few models to find (it was hoped) a new drug. The 1970s and 1980s saw the impact of receptor science, and the development of protein chemistry and elucidation of many enzymes and cell surface structures. The 1990s witnessed the impact of enabling biomolecular technologies, such as combinatorial chemistry, genomics and high-throughput screening, and computer-assisted drug design, and so we have basic pharmaceutical discovery being carried out at the molecular and disease mechanism

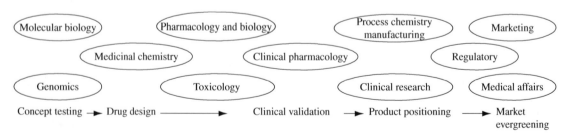

Figure 2.3 Integrated drug discovery and development.

level. As such, we now have many models to evaluate and have probably reversed the development paradigm to one that Dr Stanley Crooke, the Chief Executive Officer of Isis Inc., Carlsbad, California, has described as "target-rich [but] chemical-poor."

Inevitably, in today's world, where science seems to be producing amazing advances almost weekly, the focus is on R&D and further improvements in healthcare in the future. This should not cause us to take our eye off the needs of today and the ability of today's medicines to be used most effectively. The value of a new therapeutic agent is not maximal at the time of its first approval. Much can be done after market approval to ensure that a new drug's utility is both fully understood and actually realized. The physicians within pharmaceutical medicine need to oversee and lead this process, which requires that they are trained in economics and business as well as medicine. Indeed, some may well go on to specialized courses in those areas leading to diplomas and even university degrees.

The rapid advances in the biosciences and our gains in the understanding of diseases offer the opportunity of new benefits or uses for drugs to be developed after they have been marketed. Consequently, there is a real and ongoing role for those in pharmaceutical medicine to follow the advances of medical sciences and improve the value of the drugs of today within the medical and healthcare practices of tomorrow. This "ever-greening" process is analogous to physicians in their practice learning about a therapy and, as they come to know more about the use of the treatment and their practice dynamics change, modifying the use of that therapy to the maximum benefit of patients.

The management of a drug on the market is a professional challenge for which no medical school trains its physicians. The overall process and skill is an important part of the training within the specialty of pharmaceutical medicine. This effort may include the issues of quality-of-life evaluations, together with the appropriate development of evidence-based medicine, outcomes research, and cost–utility sciences. All these are techniques needed within pharmaceutical medicine. Used appropriately, they can help not only to establish

the curative value of a new medicine but also to ensure that the therapy gets delivered optimally.

Just as with one's personal practice of medicine, there is no more rewarding experience than the optimal use of a treatment modality in a complex clinical case with a successful outcome and a happy patient; there is an equivalent reward in pharmaceutical medicine for a physician who positions a product to deliver the best benefit for all patients, convinces all those delivering the care to use the product, and sees a consequent real improvement in society's level of healthcare. In the past, many good therapeutic agents have not been used as or when they should have been. This was not because patients in trials have not been benefited, but rather because the value message had not been positioned adequately for the care providers and/or for those who have to manage the healthcare resources of our societies. Even when well-developed and used appropriately for their approved indication, many drugs take on a new lease of life as medical sciences change and new therapeutic uses become possible; for example, lidocaine was a very well-known local anesthetic and was in use for decades when it found a new role as an anti-arrhythmic within the new context of cardiac resuscitation and coronary care units.

By the same token, as medicine progresses the acceptability and safety of a drug can change. It is a basic axiom of pharmaceutical medicine that no drug can ever be considered completely safe. This is true no matter how much human-use data are available. For example, PhisoHex (hexachlorophene) gained broad usage as a skin wash and scrub to combat the spread of infection. It was used in pediatric and neonatal units in hospitals, by nurses and surgeons, as a scrub and was even sold over the counter as a teenage acne remedy. Notwithstanding all this, it became a safety issue. This was because, as medical science advanced, more and more premature babies were able to survive. The skin of these babies was more permeable than that of full-term babies, children, or adults. There was therefore a new potentially "at-risk" group. Hexachlorophene toxicity in humans was considered to have resulted, and this led to the product being modified or removed in many markets worldwide.

The scale of the response to this issue provides a case history that highlights another skill and training required within pharmaceutical medicine, namely crisis management. This is a very important technique that is critical in addressing substantive health issues. In a relatively recent history of healthcare, there have been several such issues, for example, Zomax, Oraflex, Tylenol tampering, toxic shock syndrome, Reye's syndrome, the Dalcon shield, contaminated blood supply, silicon implants, and the so-called "generic drug scandal," to mention but a few.

Today, as much as being a leader in R&D, it is part of the role of a pharmaceutical physician to recognize new opportunities and to be alert for any emerging evidence of potential added benefits and/or new safety issues, as products and those of competitors are used more broadly outside the confines of clinical trials.

Many of the areas of expertise needed in pharmaceutical medicine overlap with the expertise of other medical disciplines. The most obvious overlap perhaps seems to be with clinical pharmacology. Indeed, clinical pharmacologists have a real interest in the R&D of the pharmaceutical industry and their training is good for entry into the industry. However, clinical pharmacology is by no means the entirety of pharmaceutical medicine. Indeed, some pharmaceutical physicians will work in even more basic and theoretical science settings, whereas others will work in more commercial settings. Of course, many within the specialty can and do focus on the development of disease models and the evaluation of new chemical entities in these diseases. The most modern methods in such areas are vital to the successful development of new drugs, and the continued and continuous interaction between the industry and academia is absolutely necessary.

Indeed, the distinction between academia and pharmaceutical medicine is becoming blurred. The pharmaceutical industry R&D effort is now leading to Nobel prizes being awarded to those in the industry for pioneering work on subjects as diverse as prostaglandins, anti-infectives, immuno-suppression and pharmacological receptors such as the histamine and the β-adrenergic receptor. The direct interaction within a company between those involved in basic research on receptors, active sites, or genetic code reading sites, those synthesizing new molecules, and those testing them in the clinic, leads to the potential for a very fruitful research effort.

Naturally, the industry as a prime inventor has the opportunity to carry out seminal work with entirely unique concepts, even if many of them do not become therapies for humans. The human is a unique animal that can, and does, exhibit unique responses to a new chemical entity. No pre-clinical work can be entirely predictive of a successful response in the clinic, and there can, in the end, be no substitute for human testing. Some products fail because of safety problems specific to humans and some because the early promise of efficacy in model systems is not realized in humans.

Those who join this new specialty may come from many medical backgrounds and can well spend much of their time doing things other than pharmacology. In a very real way, those in pharmaceutical medicine are practicing medicine. They are responsible for the products of the pharmaceutical industry that are in use today. As such, they are influencing the health of far more people globally than they ever could in the context of their own individual clinical practice.

Any discussion of the discipline of pharmaceutical medicine today would be incomplete without a comment on the impact of biotechnology and the burgeoning biotechnology revolution. This is a revolution that is driven in a very different way than that in which the pharmaceutical industry has classically been run. The prime drivers are a multitude of small venture capital companies, which are espousing the very cutting edges of research in biologics, genetics, and technology. They are largely managed by a combination of bioscientists and financiers. In this context, the role of pharmaceutical medicine takes on its most extreme variants. At one end are physicians/scientists, who are the research brain of the venture, and at the other end are physicians/businesspeople, who are the money-raising voice of the venture. In either of these settings, pharmaceutical medicine is needed and the specialist will apply all of the training components that, as already indicated, compose this new discipline.

The biotechnology industry is carrying forward some of the best and brightest projects of the world's leading academic institutions. It is moving pure research concepts through applied research into development and finally to the production of remarkable new therapeutic products. This industry has already created three new companies of substance, with sales of over US$1 billion per year and a capitalization measured in billions. More than these obvious and huge successes, the industry has spawned literally thousands of venture capital efforts and new companies developing drugs, devices, diagnostics, and all manner of medical technologies. Amazingly, this is an industry that has come into being only in the last decade or two. Like the PC and software industry, it is revolutionizing society's approach to new product development and even to what a new therapeutic agent actually is. Already, companies are finding that the major transition points in the therapeutic product development process, from molecular to biochemical system, to cellular system, to organ model, to intact organism, to mammalian model, to humans, are all real watersheds. Pharmaceutical medicine provides the required understanding of each of these processes and particularly of the transition points. In a very real sense, the success of these emerging companies will be determined by the quality of their pharmaceutical medicine efforts.

Pharmaceutical medicine is a discipline that has only very recently become recognized in its own right as a specialty within medicine. Indeed, the Faculty of Pharmaceutical Medicine of the Royal Colleges of Physicians was only founded in 1989 in the United Kingdom and the Academy in the United States even more recently in 1993. Like many new ventures, this new medical specialty is not seen by all today as one of the premiere medical roles. However, there is a growing involvement of academics within the pharmaceutical industry and Nobel prize-winning work is being done within the

industry (v.s.). Furthermore, there is a growing understanding within academia that in the past someone else was capitalizing on their intellectual endeavors, so we are seeing more medical and bioscience academics patenting their discoveries and going into business. As this progress continues, the two disciplines of research and business are coming to realize that neither can do the other's work. Pharmaceutical medicine is the natural common pathway and the integrating specialty that will fill this need and deliver the healthcare advances of the future. If this is so, pharmaceutical medicine will become a leadership medical function throughout this century. The specialty lies at the conjunction of changing societal needs for healthcare, the burgeoning biosciences, and the understandings of how to provide improved quality of life and cost–utility for patients today. The expertise it contains and provides includes basic sciences, such as chemistry and mathematics, applied sciences, such as engineering, economics, and business, biological sciences, such as pharmacology and toxicology, and the medical sciences from pediatrics to geriatrics and from family medicine to the individual subspecialties. As such, pharmaceutical medicine is one of the most challenging, exciting, and rewarding areas of medicine. It is a career for those who wish to be in the vanguard of research on multiple fronts.

Education and training in pharmaceutical medicine

Doctors working with the pharmaceutical industry as pharmaceutical physicians are encouraged to undertake training in pharmaceutical medicine, which is the medical discipline or specialty that encompasses their work in medical departments of the pharmaceutical and related healthcare companies, in clinical research units, and in regulatory bodies. Courses covering general and specialized aspects of pharmaceutical medicine have been established for many years in a number of European countries and elsewhere around the world.

Some background to pharmaceutical physician education and training

Training opportunities currently available and recommended for pharmaceutical physicians in the international field of pharmaceutical medicine in a global industry have increased enormously in recent years and space is not available here to cover them all. A recommended source of specific training opportunities originates from the professional bodies that support pharmaceutical physician training. Many commercial training companies run competitive alternatives, and trainees are advised to consider all the options that are appropriate to their individual training needs as well as evaluating the experience of others.

The desire to learn through continuous improvement is matched by the desire to improve through continuous learning. Adequate education and training can fulfill these needs, but it is important to apply rules of measurement and evaluation. Only by evaluation of training through competency assessment can the trainee be nurtured into a position of excellence.

The résumé or CV offers a simple way to keep track of training received, but a more detailed record should be kept by trainees themselves to illustrate specific examples of how the skills and knowledge gained from training have been implemented. With this information, individuals can identify outstanding training needs and, more significantly, highlight achieved goals, thus increasing their career opportunities.

All trainees should become aware of the expected learning cycle and their training needs with the scope of career options. Proactive trainees should insist on an induction program when starting with a new company whatever their status and experience.

The term "trainee" may seem pejorative to those doctors who embark on industry careers with high levels of educational and professional qualifications, experience, and expertise, and who have gained their positions through competitive selection and with expectations of making an immediate effective contribution. The term is used first, however, because there is no ready alternative and second because in the context of the rapidly changing technological, managerial, and organizational industrial setting, continuing education and training are an inherent career-long learning process, regardless of seniority, longevity, or trajectory: we are all trainees now.

The learning cycle

A simple cycle of events can be assessed continually as part of an active career plan. Continuing professional development (CPD) demands that, at whatever level, training is reviewed and acted upon. There will never be a situation when there are no training needs, and this is a worthwhile exercise to apply to all activities when considering training opportunities.

Relating the essential components of acquisition of knowledge, skills, and behaviours to the learning outcomes, and the learning cycle of experience, reflection, and deliberate testing, can help clarify training needs within career objectives. Therefore, identify learning needs, analyze training needs, set learning objectives, design and implement training, and evaluate training.

The evaluation of training, set against the original objectives, should allow a competency level to be assigned. This may be set by the manager or the employer, and if not, it is worthwhile to include a grade in a personal development plan (e.g., basic, competent, distinguished, expert). Personal development plans should feature a combination of performance assessment, career plan, and business need.

Induction

Following an analysis of training needs, built around experience, résumé, and job description, an induction program for a new post or role can be developed. Whether trainee, trainer, or manager, it is worthwhile applying a simple template to ensure that key information is understood and all new staff are benchmarked to accepted quality standards. Review of training needs will highlight unfamiliar tasks that must be taken onboard quickly and efficiently and are of benefit to all parties.

A knowledge and skills profile offers the best headlines for an induction template. It is important that the extension of knowledge and skills goes beyond the simple "doing of the job." There are five main characteristics to cover:

- General knowledge at the corporate level, for example:
    - pharmaceutical business (local and global);
    - organization of company (national and international);
    - product portfolio.
- Job-specific roles and responsibilities, for example:
    - sales techniques;
    - clinical research practices;
    - regulatory requirements.
- Therapeutic and product knowledge, for example:
    - indication and related disorders;
    - physiology and pharmacology;
    - formulations and competitors.
- Other technical requirements, for example:
    - marketing plans;
    - medical responsibilities;
    - statistics, pharmacokinetics.
- Transferable skills, for example:
    - presentation and communication skills;
    - time management;
    - team building, leadership.

Such an induction cannot be immediate unless the company organizes a full 2–4-week induction program prior to starting the job. It is essential that the many topics to be covered are prioritized by setting key objectives. Other aspects to consider are resources, including budget and specialized needs. Self-development may well be essential, when resources are limited, but care must be taken to be efficient with training opportunities and not cause conflict with active roles and responsibilities. Development of competency comes with time and experience.

Appraisal and personal development

Following induction, the individual and sponsor company have a joint responsibility for ensuring personal development. The benefits to both parties may be obvious, and yet progress must be monitored continually to guarantee that both parties are satisfied with agreed goals and targets. In the event

of dissatisfaction, continual review allows prompt action and reassessment of goals. Measurement of training needs is usually performed at appraisal, and the individual should expect appraisals to be stretching and challenging, if performed properly. Appraisals should decide a career plan based on knowledge, skills, and performance to date: that is, recorded competencies.

The sponsor company will consider training to be an investment. It does not wish to train the individual to take a career step out of the company but must take the risk that this may occur. Appraisal will measure the adequacy of training for the role or for the future role of the appraisee. A sponsor company will want to be sure that the training has a clear link with corporate business needs, that training is the most effective solution to a learning need, and through continued appraisal, realize that benefits of training are evaluated beyond course satisfaction.

The usual appraiser will be the line manager of the appraisee, although it is important that a relationship exists between these two and the sponsor company departments of human resources and training. A company template for appraisal and subsequent training plans—a career plan—is likely to be in place to enable consistency and efficient measurement across individuals, teams, and departments. If working individually without a career plan, it may be worth using such an example as a guide.

Whether appraiser or appraisee, the first training to be undertaken may well be a short course ensuring that everyone uses the appraisal process in the same manner.

The appraisal will cover many more areas than training and development needs, for example, performance output and relationships, yet ultimately outcomes from appraisal will focus around the career plan and what has to be done to achieve agreed goals. The training cycle remains the same, and the five categories listed above under induction may also be used to cover more focused training needs. At appraisal, it is important to recognise that not only the appraisee is being measured. Appraisal is an opportunity to record and assess support and performance of the appraiser, other staff, and the training personnel, perhaps through use of multi-source feedback (360° assessment).

Continuing professional development

A personal "curriculum" will develop through frequent appraisals leading to a CPD program. When this begins to include acquired further qualifications and formally evaluated course work, it may be called a CPD plan or Personal Development Plan (PDP). Many supporting professional bodies in pharmaceutical medicine provide extensive literature on PDPs, some of which are mandatory.

A PDP is a useful tool for identifying and measuring lifelong learning; in other words, it can be described as the data that supports the résumé and gives direction to the career plan.

A PDP allows for:
• planning short-term learning needs;
• recognising previously unseen learning opportunities;
• involving the employer to match personal needs with business needs;
• collating a portfolio of evidence to demonstrate competencies;
• keeping up to date with the chosen profession;
• collating a portable record of progress and achievement;
• increasing awareness of potential career options;
• analysing strengths and weaknesses;
• reflecting on learning and promoting self-awareness and motivation;
• focusing on development needs and career ambitions.

Regulations and training records

Aside from personal development needs and the business requirements of corporate progress, the pharmaceutical industry is one of the most highly regulated in the world. The strict regulation extends to matters concerning training and development, and the majority of disciplines will find themselves governed by formal guidelines and legal requirements for the quality and quantity of training before and during the specific function. In the scientific areas, these are usually referred to as GxPs, such as Good Laboratory Practice (GLP) or Good Clinical Practice (GCP), whereas sales and marketing personnel have to adhere strictly to Codes of Practice, and regulatory staff must be completely aware of and work within all aspects across the regulatory and legal framework.

The medical profession is incorporating CPDs and PDPs into plans for demonstrating continuing competency to practice, based on annual appraisals and, for example in the United Kingdom, a proposed 5-yearly assessment for revalidation in order for a practitioner to remain on the general and specialist medical registers and be relicensed and certified to practice. Everyone should undertake a professional and ethical obligation to remain up to date with best practice standards in the role performed.

Apart from direct observation, which must also be undertaken, the sponsor company management, sponsor company auditors, and external inspection units can only be sure of correct adherence to formal training requirements by correct and meticulous record keeping. All training and development in the pharmaceutical industry must be recorded and records maintained.

The responsibility for keeping the training logs of staff varies from company to company, being held by the human resources or training departments or by the manager of the department to which the individual belongs. However, it is recommended that individuals keep a copy of their own records where they can; this can form part of their personal PDP and is inherently part of the information supporting their résumé. It is important to be able to verify the effectiveness of the training undertaken. The simplest form of record, which details only title, date, and attendees, does not inform an inspector, of any kind, whether the training was of value or not.

The most usual way of tracking value is by comparing the training data against the actual performance changes at appraisal. Again, this may be viewed as purely a top-level assessment and can raise more questions than it answers. It is recommended to introduce a direct competency measurement to the evaluation of training. Here, a manager, coach, or trainer will identify the training need prior to training, and through witnessing the trainees "put into practice" what they have learnt, be able to verify through dated signature the success or failure of the training. It is important, however, that the training records are not made too complex, leading to a maze of information, which serves to confuse rather than to clarify.

Training sources

Whether self-supporting or with the aid of a "training-aware" sponsor company, the ambitious trainee has a number of options available in order to satisfy the identified training needs. Most of the larger sponsor companies run consolidated in-house courses covering a vast array of topics from specific skills training, for example GxPs, therapy areas, and IT, to challenging transferable skills, for example problem solving, time management, and cultural communication.

In addition, their training programs will be indexed to competency assessment and appraisal. In smaller companies and as individuals, such in-house programs may not be available. This need not be a disadvantage. A greater spectrum of training experience may give greater value to a personal portfolio and offer a wider outlook of the bigger picture. The marketplace offering commercial courses to support any of the training needs for all the disciplines within pharmaceutical medicine is huge.

Commercial courses are not usually inexpensive, and a considered decision must be made based on previous experience or advice from another source when applying to become a delegate.

As has been highlighted, networking in the industry is essential. Training may be competitive between the commercial companies themselves, but information on "good" and "bad" courses is usually shared across sponsor companies. Human resources or heads of specific departments are good sources of relevant information. The most effective commercial training companies are often those that can tailor their training material to the needs of the trainees, and this material can be customized to specific sponsor company requirements when a group or team is involved. Clearly, the best source of specific training comes from the professional bodies supporting pharmaceutical medicine. In the majority of cases, their primary objective is

education based in order to maintain the highest possible standards for their profession.

Education and training programs in pharmaceutical medicine

In recent years, a common syllabus has become established through the International Federation of Associations of Pharmaceutical Physicians (IFAPP) from which core curricula for courses have been derived and form the basis for examinations for diplomas and degrees where these have been established. The syllabus in pharmaceutical medicine covers drug discovery, medicines regulations, clinical pharmacology, statistics and data management, clinical development, healthcare marketplace, drug safety and surveillance, and pharmacotherapeutics.

The first postgraduate course in pharmaceutical medicine was inaugurated in 1975 in the United Kingdom by AMAPI (now BrAPP) and was transferred to the University of Cardiff in 1978. Since that time several similar courses have been founded in European universities, most from a close cooperation between pharmaceutical physicians, often represented by the national association of pharmaceutical physicians and academia.

Although there are national variations, to undertake training where there is an outcome by examination to obtain a diploma or degree, doctors must be registered in their country of medical qualification, must have undertaken a prescribed number of years of approved clinical training prior to taking a post in pharmaceutical medicine, and must have spent a prescribed amount of time working in pharmaceutical medicine prior to obtaining the diploma or degree.

More recently, pharmaceutical medicine has been recognized and listed as a medical specialty in four countries, Switzerland, Mexico, United Kingdom, and Ireland, resulting in accreditation of the physician specialists as the outcome of their training.

It might be expected that the content of courses following the syllabus in pharmaceutical medicine would be quite similar. However, cultural differences and local academic standards and practices have induced major differences in the structure of courses and the techniques of assessment and examination. It is in the interest of pharmaceutical medicine in general, and pharmaceutical physicians in particular working in the international field of medicines development and maintenance, that there should be mutual recognition between countries of the diplomas in pharmaceutical medicine given by awarding bodies, and therefore a process of harmonization and approval of courses has been established by the IFAPP.

In 2002, the Council for Education in Pharmaceutical Medicine (CEPM) was inaugurated by the IFAPP with the objectives, inter alia, of contributing to the harmonization of existing postgraduate courses in pharmaceutical medicine and promoting mutual recognition of equivalent educational qualifications between countries.

The CEPM has approved diploma courses in pharmaceutical medicine in United Kingdom (2), Switzerland, Belgium, Spain (2), Sweden, and Germany. The Faculty of Pharmaceutical Medicine (London) has recognized two diplomas, in Belgium and Switzerland, as being equivalent to that of the United Kingdom.

United Kingdom

The Diploma in Pharmaceutical Medicine was established in 1976 by the three Royal Colleges of Physicians (RCP) of the United Kingdom. The diploma is awarded by examination once a year by the RCP's Faculty of Pharmaceutical Medicine. The examination is knowledge-based and comprises MCQs, short-answer questions, essays, and a critical review of a research paper.

In 2002, pharmaceutical medicine became a listed medical specialty in the United Kingdom, and the specialist training program was established to become the basis of accredited education and training in pharmaceutical medicine for physicians. This is a competency-based in-work program over four years, which incorporates the Diploma in Pharmaceutical Medicine as the specialty knowledge base and six practical modules: medicines regulation, clinical pharmacology, statistics and data management, clinical development, healthcare marketplace, and drug safety surveillance. A generic module provides interpersonal and management skills and working to the principles of Good Medical Practice, as laid down by the General Medical Council, ensuring that pharmaceutical physicians practice to high standards of competency, care, and conduct in their work, common to the ethics and professionalism of all doctors.

The supervised in-work program is complemented by module- and topic-based courses. Progress and achievement is ensured through in-work and course-based assessments, regular educational and performance appraisal, and an Annual Review of Competence Progression (ARCP) by the RCP and Faculty of Pharmaceutical Medicine. The outcome is the Certificate of Completion of Training, a recognized European credential of specialist training common to all medical specialties.

Switzerland

Pharmaceutical medicine is a recognized medical specialty (since 1999) by the FMH, the Swiss Association of Medical Doctors. The European Center of Pharmaceutical Medicine (ECPM) offers a Diploma in Advanced Studies in Pharmaceutical Medicine, through the University of Basel. The diploma examination comprises written papers, MCQ, and oral. The diploma is recognized by the Faculty of Pharmaceutical Medicine as equivalent to that in the United Kingdom.

The EUCOR Medical Schools of the Universities of Basel, Freiburg (in Germany), and Strasbourg (in France) award the title of "University Professional in Pharmaceutical Medicine" to those who complete successfully a course cycle and pass the diploma examination.

For physicians, the University Professional title covers the theoretical part required for the FMH specialty title in pharmaceutical medicine as defined by the Swiss Society for Pharmaceutical Medicine (SGPM). The Swiss Association of Pharmaceutical Professionals (SwAPP) offers an equivalent title for PhDs and other pharmaceutical professionals. The specialist title is a postgraduate qualification of theoretical and practical training in pharmaceutical medicine. To qualify, physicians must have full membership of SwAPP and provide documentary evidence of five years supervised post-graduate training, two years of which must be in relevant professional activity and three years in pharmaceutical medicine, including two years in clinical development and one year in drug safety, medical-scientific information, and registration.

Belgium

The Free University of Brussels (ULB) has offered the Diploma in Pharmaceutical Medicine since 1992 in conjunction with ABEMEP, the national association of pharmaceutical physicians. This is a non-residential course consisting of eight modules. All modules are taught each year, but students can spread their training over 1–3 years. Each of the modules takes one full week every month between November and June, leading to 280 hours of teaching.

Oral and written examinations are organized at least once a year; it is not required to follow the course to register for the examination, provided the candidate has adequate experience in pharmaceutical medicine.

Physicians passing the examinations are awarded the Diploma in Pharmaceutical Medicine, which is recognized by the Belgian College of Pharmaceutical medicine, established in 2000 by two Belgian Royal Academies of Medicine. Holders are added to a specialist register held by the Belgian College of Pharmaceutical Medicine.

The diploma is recognized by the Faculty of Pharmaceutical Medicine (London) as being equivalent to that of the United Kingdom.

Ireland

The Association of Pharmaceutical Physicians in Ireland (APPI) is the leading force in establishing Higher Medical Training in Ireland. The APPI gained acceptance for pharmaceutical medicine as a specialty from the Irish Committee for Higher Medical Training (ICHMT) of the Royal College of Physicians of Ireland. This was accepted by the Irish Medical Council in 2004, and the medical specialty was approved by the Ministry of Health in 2005. The APPI is working with other new specialties on the practicalities of establishing the new specialty, and it has constructed the curriculum and will work through the ICHMT on the necessary training requirements for specialist accreditation for pharmaceutical physicians.

France

The EUDIPHARM program was established in 1999 based at the University of Lyon with funding from the European Union. The program involves the participation of 14 universities in 11 countries of the EU. There is an international teaching faculty involving many from the United Kingdom, Sweden, Germany, and Italy. The course is at variance with other courses in pharmaceutical medicine in that during the first year, all students attend three residential seminars of 3-weeks duration, representing a basic training module with 18 submodules.

In the second year, students elect to specialize in one of the series of subspecialty options, namely drug development, regulatory affairs, postmarketing monitoring, and medical marketing, attending three to four modules, each of 2-weeks duration. In the first year, all courses are at the University of Lyon, but in the second year, students move around the various participating universities. To obtain the diploma, the candidate sits written and oral examinations and submits a dissertation. There is a total of 325 teaching hours.

Spain

The University of Barcelona offers a 2-year non-residential course consisting of 14 modules between 4–30 hours depending on the subject. Courses are taught at the university one day per week from January to June each year, representing a total of 222 hours of teaching. Written examinations are conducted twice a year. Successful candidates receive a Diploma in Pharmaceutical Medicine.

The University of Madrid offers a 2-year non-residential course, which consists of 14 modules from October to June; a total of 300 hours of teaching at the university. Examinations, written and oral, are conducted once a year; to register for the examinations, students must have attended at least 75% of the courses. Successful candidates receive a Diploma in Pharmaceutical Medicine.

Portugal

The University of Lisbon has, since 1999, offered a 6-month non-residential course in pharmaceutical medicine taught every year from January till June. The course has 11 modules with two 2-day sessions per month, representing a total of 176 hours of teaching. Assessments are made at the end of each module, and only those students who have passed the 11 assessments and have attended 100% of the course are allowed to submit a dissertation of 20,000 words at the end of the course. Successful candidates receive a Diploma in Pharmaceutical Medicine recognized by the Portuguese National Board of Physicians, where the Pharmaceutical Industry is listed as a postgraduate competence (*capacidade*).

Sweden

There is a 2-year diploma course in pharmaceutical medicine given at the Karolinska Institute and the Medical Products Agency, Stockholm, organized for pharmaceutical physicians in conjunction with the Swedish Board of Pharmaceutical Medicine.

Germany

There is a Diploma in Pharmaceutical Medicine in Germany that is provided by the DGPharMed (German Society for Pharmaceutical Medicine). Since 2005, the University of Essen-Duisburg has offered a 2-year course leading to a Master of Science in pharmaceutical medicine. The course has 450 hours of teaching in 18 modules and a further 1350 hours are planned for homework. The last six months are needed for the preparation of a thesis, its presentation, and oral examination. This course has a long heritage, having being transferred from the University of Witten-Herdecke, which since 1997 offered a course leading to a Diploma in Pharmaceutical Medicine.

Italy

In pharmaceutical medicine, efforts are being made to establish a diploma course at the University of Pisa supported by the Italian Association of Pharmaceutical Physicians (SSFA).

Innovative Medicines Initiative (IMI)

As part of the IMI—a joint undertaking by the European Commission and a consortium of EFPIA pharmaceutical companies, universities, and pharmaceutical professional, training, and standard-setting bodies—a proposed Pharmaceutical Medicine training program, "PharmaTrain," is being developed to provide for education and training in integrated drug development for all medical and scientific professionals involved across the healthcare industries. The programs will be tailored towards greatly enhancing the skillsets and competencies of all key contributors in the drug development and regulatory processes. Teaching and training methods will be based on the latest scientific approaches using the impact of pathophysiology, safety and risk-awareness, patient and population-based benefit, as well as methods to make the drug development process faster. It is hoped that this will help to make R&D in Europe more economical and more competitive with other parts of the world than until now.

PharmaTrain is to be a pan-European multi-modular training program at the postgraduate Masters level: Master of Advanced Studies in Pharmaceutical Medicine/Drug Development Sciences (MDDS). To harmonize this European initiative, the program will comply with the Bologna credit and title system, and will be well-structured, blended with distance e-learning, self-sustaining, and underpinned by a quality management system. The proposed program of pan-European accredited courses in Pharmaceutical Medicine/Drug Development Sciences will facilitate exchange between the pharmaceutical industry, regulatory authorities, and academia thereby, it is hoped, remove some of the previous barriers to effective drug development. Furthermore, the modular program with increased distance e-learning capability will support mobility of staff throughout Europe: a PharmaTrain module will be a true European "currency." This, combined with an extension program, will provide the same high level of training and education throughout the EU. This creates the opportunity to fulfill many of the requirements and needs for an individual's PDP for effective work-related professional education and training, and CPD, mentioned earlier.

Mexico

Mexico granted pharmaceutical medicine specialty status in 1999. There is a 2-year specialist training program organized by the National Polytechnic Institute, Faculty of Medicine, Postgraduate Studies Section, leading to a specialist qualification in Pharmaceutical Medicine. There is an entry examination to the program, which then includes 17 subjects (84 credits) over four semesters. There are practical rotations through pharmaceutical industry departments in the fourth semester.

Argentina

The University of Buenos Aires offers a postgraduate education program in pharmaceutical medicine, comprising 420 teaching hours and 240 practice hours.

Brazil

The Federal University of Sao Paulo offers a postgraduate course in pharmaceutical medicine comprising 200 teaching hours and 160 practice hours.

References

Centre for Medicines Research. *UK Pharmaceutical R&D Expenditure 1982–1986*. Monograph, CMR: London, UK, 1996.

Ernst & Young. *Biotechnology Annual Report*. 2001. www.ey.com; accessed March 27, 2010.

Further reading

Pharmaceutical Research Manufacturers Association. *PhRMA Annual Report 1999–2000*. Monograph. PhRMA: Washington, DC, USA, 1997. www.phrma.org: accessed March 27, 2010.

Stonier PD (ed.). *Careers with the Pharmaceutical Industry*, John Wiley & Sons Ltd: Chichester, UK, 2003, second edition.

CHAPTER 3

Clinical Research Education and Training for Biopharmaceutical Staff

Peter Marks[1] & Sheila Gwizdak[2]
[1]Pfizer Limited, Sandwich, Kent, UK
[2]Pfizer Inc., New London, CT, USA

Introduction

The biopharmaceutical industry is a highly regulated industry, in which many of the activities and tasks performed by company staff are defined by regulations and guidelines issued by international regulatory authorities. The training requirements for the clinical staff of pharmaceutical companies or sponsors can be relatively well defined.

The International Conference on Harmonization (ICH) Guideline for Good Clinical Practices (GCP), for example, describes a minimum standard for the ethical and scientific standards for designing, conducting, and reporting clinical research. The ICH GCP Guideline is the unified standard for the European Union (EU), Japan, and the United States to facilitate mutual acceptance of clinical data. The ICH GCP Guideline, together with other ICH Guidelines, provides operational definitions of the core competencies needed by clinical staff to conduct world-class clinical research.

One of the principles of ICH GCP is that "each individual involved in conducting a trial should be qualified by education, training and experience to perform his or her respective task(s)." Specifically, regarding the selection and qualifications of monitors, the ICH GCP Guideline states that "monitors should be appropriately trained and should have the scientific and/or clinical knowl-

edge needed to monitor the trial adequately." Most major pharmaceutical firms have always had varying degrees of in-house education and training for staff, supplemented (as appropriate) by external workshops, courses, and training meetings. The ICH GCP Guidelines help to formalize the desired elements of education programs to comply with current GCP requirements.

What is a competency-based training program?

Few people come to the pharmaceutical industry from academia and health-related positions with the requisite knowledge and skills necessary to plan, conduct, and report clinical research to regulatory authority standards. This knowledge and skill usually need to be provided by sponsors to all levels of new staff through in-house training.

One approach to education and training in the industry is what is called "competency-based training." A competency is a skill, knowledge, or behavior required to undertake effectively the tasks and responsibilities for which an individual is responsible.

A competency-based education and training system (CBETS) details the essential knowledge and skills needed by the sponsor's staff to complete the requirements of GCP. The concept of a CBETS is different to traditional educational and training approaches. Traditional approaches tend to address the training needs of individuals based on their job descriptions. For example, within a sponsor

Principles and Practice of Pharmaceutical Medicine, 3rd edition.
Edited by L.D. Edwards, A.W. Fox, P.D. Stonier.
© 2011 Blackwell Publishing Ltd.

company, a monitor will receive training on how to monitor a clinical trial and a physician will receive training in protocol development. In this traditional education and training model, the required tasks are functionally defined. The monitor may not learn much about preparing protocols and the physician may not learn much about monitoring. However, each may be intimately involved in both tasks.

The CBETS asks what tasks the sponsor needs to do to meet its drug development goals. The primary tasks of clinical research and good clinical practice can be described rather precisely. Once one knows what the major tasks are and what activities are needed to accomplish these tasks, one can then ask what knowledge and skills are needed by staff for the tasks and, finally, what education and training should be provided to communicate the knowledge and skills. A CBETS only asks who is going to do these tasks. Only when the tasks and activities are fully defined is it necessary to ask who is going to do it and how competent they need to be to complete the tasks. In the example provided above, it is useful for the physician to have a fundamental knowledge of the monitoring process even though he or she will not be performing the tasks. The physician may, however, be supervising the monitors. It is appropriate for monitors to receive advanced training in the requirements of monitoring because this is one of their major functions. In terms of protocol development, the physician and monitor each need competencies to perform the tasks of developing the protocol. The CBETS is applicable to behavioral and management training, as well as technical training.

Education and training programs in the pharmaceutical industry should be designed to provide the competencies necessary to prevent or remove obstacles to staff performance.

Competency-based training program for staff associated with conducting clinical trials

The following is a description of the typical knowledge and competencies needed to plan, conduct, and report clinical research in a regulated environment. Each competency is described along with the knowledge and skills a sponsor's representative would need to be successful in completing the task.

General clinical competencies

Understanding the drug development process

New clinical staff need to understand the overall drug development process. Before new investigational products can be given to the public, extensive preclinical and toxicological studies are performed. Staff who will be responsible for the clinical portion of investigational product development need to have an understanding of the work that has been undertaken to progress the compound through to the clinical phases. Many clinical investigators are also involved in basic research and often will expect the sponsor's representative to be able to discuss the total background on the investigational product.

This includes understanding the vision, mission, and objectives of the sponsor. Most sponsors have a company-specific clinical development strategy and product development system. Individuals new to the industry should understand the strategy and function of the major departments comprising the development process, as well as the decision-making approach of the sponsor's management bodies.

To gain this knowledge, new staff members should attend appropriate orientation programs on drug development and, if recommended, Pharmaceutical Education and Research Institute, Inc. (PERI), Drug Information Association (DIA) overview courses on investigational drug development or equivalent international courses. There is considerable literature available that discusses the drug development process such as the *Guide to Clinical Trials* (Spilker, 1991) and *Multinational Drug* Companies (Spilker, 1989). Many regulatory authorities also provide useful literature and guidelines on registration expectations. New staff should carefully review and discuss with experienced sponsor management and have internal documentation explaining the company's systems and processes. Senior-level staff can also attend the noted and advanced course on international investigational product development and regulatory issues sponsored by Tufts University at the Tufts Center for the Study of Drug Development.

Understanding good clinical practices

Understanding the responsibilities and obligations of sponsors in terms of good clinical practices is fundamental knowledge essential to conduct clinical research. Currently, most pharmaceutical firms reference the ICH GCP Guideline as the minimum standard for conducting clinical trials. There are excellent PERI or DIA overview courses covering good clinical practices.

The responsibilities and obligations include knowledge of the elements of informed consent, the role and responsibilities of Institutional Review Boards/Independent Ethics Committees (IRB/IEC), and the importance of Clinical Study Quality Assurance.

Understanding the regulations of the countries in which drug development will occur

Although historically the US Food and Drug Administration (FDA) has been the dominant regulatory authority in the world, in recent years other regions (e.g., the EU and Japan) have emerged to challenge that dominance. As multinational companies consider conducting a larger proportion of trials outside the United States, knowledge of global regulations has become increasingly important.

An understanding of the regulatory structure, operations, and functions is very important to individuals new to the pharmaceutical industry or new to clinical development.

Knowledge and skills are required for communication with the regulatory agencies, covering, for example, End-of-Phase II Meetings, Investigational New Drug (IND)/Clinical Trial Application (CTA) Annual Report, Advisory Committee Meetings, Pre-New Drug Application (NDA)/Biologics License Application (BLA)/Marketing Authorization Application (MAA) Meetings, Clinical Hold, IND/CTA Termination, and regulatory inspections.

Competencies associated with planning clinical development

Conceptualization and development of clinical development plans (CDPs)

Developing an international CDP to answer questions defined by the investigational product target profile is a key activity of senior-level industry personnel. This competency requires an understanding of toxicology and clinical pharmacology to identify clinical target profile criteria. The CDP defines the critical path for the clinical program and the clinical budget. The CDP also defines investigational drug development assessment and decision points, and the project resource (personnel and budget) estimates.

CDPs will cover the following issues:
- draft labeling or target product profile;
- preparing the clinical section of IND/CTA submission;
- preparing clinical reports needed to support IND/CTA submissions;
- clinical research and scientific methodology;
- exploratory INDs (in the United States)/pilot efficacy studies;
- Phase I studies;
- Phase II studies;
- Phase III studies;
- Phase IV studies;
- pharmacokinetic and bioavailability studies;
- dose-ranging studies;
- dose-titration studies;
- marketing and safety surveillance studies;
- studies supporting over-the-counter switches (see Chapter 15).

The goal of these plans is to provide a lean, efficient NDA/BLA/MAA with the minimum studies needed for registration and approval in the world markets. The medical, scientific, regulatory, and marketing opinions must be weighed and balanced in the plans.

Understanding and conceptualizing clinical study design

To create a CDP successfully, the individual must know the basic concepts of research design and statistics, the concepts of clinical research, and investigational drug development; possess an in-depth understanding of the concepts of clinical pharmacology, pharmacokinetics, pharmacodynamics, toxicology, state-of-the-art therapeutic medicine and methodology, FDA/EU/ICH therapeutic research guidelines and regulatory issues; and understand basic concepts of project planning and scheduling. Knowledge of new methodology (e.g., better use of PK/PD modeling/simulations and computer-assisted trial design), "right-sizing" trials, and alternative statistical designs (e.g., futility analyses, adaptive designs) are becoming essential as companies look to improve efficiency and reduce costs of the clinical development process.

Preparation of the investigator's brochure (IB)

The IB is a compilation of clinical and preclinical data on the investigational product that is relevant to the study of the investigational product in human subjects and the investigator's assessment of risk in participating in the study. The sponsor compiles clinical information for the preparation of the IB.

Clinical staff or a medical writing group may perform the preparation of an IB. The activities included in preparing the IB include the following:
• coordination of the compilation of clinical and preclinical data from contributing departments (e.g., Clinical Pharmacology, Toxicology);
• describing the physical, chemical, and pharmaceutical properties and formulation;
• preparing a clear, concise summary of the information relating to the safety and effectiveness of the investigational product;
• providing a detailed description of possible risks and benefits of the investigational product;
• defining a clear rationale for the dosage and dosing interval.

To prepare an IB, the sponsor's representative must understand the fundamental purpose and uses of the IB, the basic format and content of sponsor IBs, the clinical pharmacology and toxicology findings, the investigational product–disease relationships, the international regulatory requirements governing IBs, and the indications and safety profile of the investigational product.

Design and preparation of clinical protocols

The clinical protocol describes the objectives, design, methodology, statistical considerations, and organization of the trial. The sponsor is usually responsible for developing the protocol in industry-sponsored clinical trials. However, internal and external content experts (e.g., specialists, key opinion leaders) are frequently consulted. Protocols must be written ensuring medical soundness and clinical practicality.

Frequently, the sponsor uses a template to complete the sections of the protocol. The tasks of developing a protocol include the following:
• defining clear protocol objectives;
• identifying primary efficacy and safety parameters;
• determining appropriate subject selection criteria;
• identifying correct dosages and route.

This could be a two-step process where the protocol summary containing all the key elements is prepared and approved, triggering key operational activities such as case report form (CRF) and database design, manufacturing, and packaging of investigational product supply. While these activities are being carried out, the full protocol text can be refined to meet regulatory requirements and investigator needs.

To prepare appropriate protocols, staff must understand research design and statistical inference for clinical research, state-of-the-art research designs (e.g., adaptive designs, futility analyses) and trials, therapeutic area guidelines, good clinical practice, regulatory requirements, guidelines and country-specific issues, national and international medical practices, sponsor protocol review and approval procedures, and possess in-depth investigational product–disease knowledge.

Clinical protocols are the building blocks of the CDP and the NDA/BLA/MAA. Protocols specify the conditions that permit and lead to meaningful and credible results in clinical programs. Operationally, protocols provide a written agreement between the sponsor and the investigator on how the trial is going to be conducted. This agreement allows the sponsor to ensure that the study will be done to the highest ethical and medical standards and

Table 3.1 Elements of clinical protocols

Background and rationale
Study objectives
Experimental design and methods
Schedule of assessments
Subject selection criteria
Trial procedures (screening, trial period, follow-up, assessments)

Adverse event reporting
Trial medication
Premature withdrawal
Subject replacement policy
Criteria for excluding data
Data analysis/statistical methods
Quality control/assurance
Data handling and record keeping
Ethics (e.g., IRB/IEC approval)
Definition of end of trial
Sponsor discontinuation criteria
Signatures

that the quality of the data can be relied upon as credible and accurate.

All clinical protocols and supporting documents are reviewed and approved internally by a group of senior Clinical Research & Development managers. This group assesses the overall study design and ability of the study to meet its objectives, as well as the quantity and quality of the data. In addition, the group reviews the procedures for the safety and welfare of the subjects to ensure compliance to good clinical practices and ethical principles.

The quality of a clinical protocol can be assessed by how well the elements of the protocol are prepared. The elements of clinical protocols are described in Table 3.1.

The extent of a Background section will vary with the drug's stage of development. New clinical data not already included in the IB should be emphasized. The Rationale provides a concise statement of the reasons for conducting the study and the basis for the dosage selection and duration that will be used in the trial. Quality protocols should target relevant information in the Background and convincing Rationale for the study.

Every protocol must state a primary, quantifiable study objective. Secondary objectives should be limited in scope and related to the primary

question. Objectives must be specific and capable of answering a key clinical question required by the CDP.

The study design is an important element in assessment of quality protocols. The overall purpose of the study design is to reduce the variability or bias inherent in all research. Good study design will always address control methods that reduce experimental bias. These control methods will often include treatment blinding, randomization, and between- or within-patient study designs. The Schedule of Assessments describes a schedule of time and events and provides a complete profile of the overall trial design. Good quality Schedule of Assessments sections also include acceptable time windows around the variables being collected that can minimize protocol deviations.

The inclusion and exclusion criteria are described in the Subject Selection part of the protocol. To a large extent, the success or failure of a particular clinical trial can often be traced back to how well these criteria were developed. Good protocol authors strive to include the most appropriate patient population to satisfy the study objective and still include those kinds of patients who will ultimately receive the drug. Therefore, selection criteria can be unreasonable and unnecessary in some cases and vague and not specific in other cases. The management of concomitant medications is particularly problematic. The protocol must attempt to define those medications that are permitted for intercurrent illnesses and those that are prohibited because they will interfere with the interpretation of the test medication. Although there are no easy answers, quality protocols are able to justify with some precision the rationale for each inclusion and criteria. How these criteria are applied is handled in the Screening for Study Entry section.

The efficacy and safety parameters describe how and when the variables are going to be recorded, usually in relation to drug administration and follow-up periods. How adverse events are managed and recorded are particularly important to the sponsor and to regulatory authorities. Protocol authors should ensure that the study defines the criteria for success or failure of treatment. Endpoints should be clear and defined. As many clinical phenomena are open to interpretation, protocols should provide definitions of variables and time windows for their collection. If the assessments are purely subjective, provision for observer alignment must be provided. Addressing these issues will improve the quality and meaningfulness of the results of the study. Training on such assessments at investigator meetings before the trial starts proves a valuable investment.

The description of the management of trial medication is often a source of confusion. Protocols must include clear directions for dosing intervals and adjustments. Because patients will never follow a protocol precisely in all cases, provisions for missing doses or "what if" situations should be anticipated. Good protocols always include, in addition, adequate compliance checks of drug consumption by the subjects of the study.

Protocols should predetermine how subjects will be replaced following dropping out of the study. This is important because the means by which subjects are replaced can adversely affect the statistical analysis. Similarly, a decision concerning the conditions under which a subject would not be evaluable must be stated explicitly before the study starts. This is intended to minimize intentional or unintentional data manipulation.

The Quality Control/Assurance section addresses the sponsor's conduct of periodic monitoring visits to ensure that the protocol and GCPs are being followed. The sponsor's representatives (monitors or Clinical Research Associates; CRAs) will review source documents to confirm that the data recorded on CRFs are accurate: this is a fundamental requirement of quality clinical research. This section also alerts the investigator and clinical institution that the sponsor's representatives (for monitoring and/or audit purposes) and possibly appropriate regulatory authorities (for inspections) will require direct access to source documents to perform this verification. It is important that the investigator(s) and relevant personnel are available during the monitoring visits and possible audits or inspections, and that sufficient time is devoted to the process.

The Data Handling and Record Retention section of the protocol will address the requirement to maintain data (whether on a paper CRF or using an electronic data collection tool (DCT)) of each trial subject. It will address expectations of ownership of the completed CRF data, and the investigator's responsibility to ensure accuracy and completeness of data recording. This section will also address the requirements for retention of records at the trial site in accordance with relevant guidelines and regulatory requirements.

The Ethics section of the protocol deals with the fundamental requirement for prospective IRB/IEC approval of the trial protocol, protocol amendments, informed consent forms, and other relevant documents (e.g., subject recruitment advertisements). The section also details the requirements for obtaining informed consent from trial subjects.

For trials conducted in the EU, the protocol must include a definition of the end to the trial (in an EU member state or in all participating countries).

The Sponsor Discontinuation section of the protocol provides a reminder to the investigator that the trial may be terminated prematurely as a result of a regulatory authority decision, a change in opinion of the IRB/IEC, drug safety problems, or at the discretion of the sponsor. In addition, most sponsors will reserve the right to discontinue development of the investigational product at any time.

Design of the format and content of CRFs

The CRF is the document used to record all of the protocol-specified data to describe individual subject results. Many sponsors use standard modules to prepare the CRF and are increasingly using electronic data capture technology.

To prepare successful CRFs, the sponsor's staff must know typical clinical practices, therapeutic conventions, investigator and staff needs, data management and analysis plans, project-specific definitions and procedures, CRF completion problem areas, remote data/electronic entry, and review and approval procedures for CRFs. Ideally, CRFs should be pretested with internal and external experts (e.g., investigational sites).

The quality of a clinical trial can be influenced by how well the CRF is designed. If the investigator's staff cannot enter the protocol data as required, the sponsor will have a considerable challenge in trying to interpret the results. There are a number of design principles that facilitate the use of CRFs in clinical trials. These principles include the concepts of standardization and minimization. The sponsor standardizes the design of CRFs in one consistent international format. This permits uniform databases, consistency in collection, and more rapid data entry/capture. In addition, standardization facilitates the monitoring process and therefore increases accuracy of the data. Although efficiency is an important variable in the design process, the systems must also be sufficiently flexible to account for the variances between projects. Finally, an important principle of both protocol and CRF design is to collect only the data needed to satisfy the objectives of the protocol. The inherent temptation to collect more data must be resisted.

There are several CRF design characteristics that define quality CRFs, including
- limiting the amount of space or blank fields for free text;
- providing instructions on the CRF or within the electronic tool for its completion;
- consistent layout of information within the CRF;
- simple, unambiguous language, particularly for multinational trials;
- collecting only raw data, letting the computer do transformation calculations;
- intensive monitor training in the use of the CRFs.

High-quality CRF design is probably the cheapest investment in big returns on a clinical trial.

Packaging and labeling of investigational product

The investigational product is the active ingredient or placebo being tested in a clinical trial. Forecasting investigational drug supplies is important in that it must be done well in advance of the start date of the clinical trial. To make this forecast, it is necessary to estimate, from the CDP, the bulk investigational product supply needs. Often, the protocol summary provides the trigger to begin packaging and labeling of investigational supplies for the trial.

To handle drug supplies successfully, the sponsor's representative must know the following information:
- procedures for ordering bulk investigational product supplies;
- models for bulk investigational product quantity estimation;

- investigational product packaging time frames;
- protocol-specific and country-specific requirements for packaging and shipping investigational product supplies;
- procedures for packaging international investigational product supplies;
- investigational product supply tracking systems;
- investigational product ordering and packaging processes;
- general investigational product formulation and packaging processes and configurations;
- protocol design;
- randomization procedures;
- investigational product dispensing and accountability.

Identification and selection of clinical investigators for study placement and conducting pre-study evaluation visits

Selecting investigators

The proper selection of clinical investigators is one of the key success factors for any clinical program. The investigator (sometimes referred to as the principal investigator) has the primary responsibility for the success of the trial. His or her leadership and direction of subinvestigators and study staff are critical in performing the requirements of today's trials. Time spent in learning who the best investigators are is well spent and pays significant dividends in the end.

To identify and select clinical investigators successfully, the sponsor's representatives need to carry out the following: identify internal and external sources of potential investigators; define investigator selection criteria, protocol requirements, expected cost of the study, and investigator and facility qualifications; interview potential investigators; and schedule and conduct pre-study site evaluation visits.

The International Clinical Team (ICT) has an important role in determining the quality selection of clinical investigators. Selection criteria will be based upon the needs of the CDP and the individual protocols. Quality investigators can be identified by the following items:
- previous clinical research experience;
- previous performance on sponsor and other company trials;

Table 3.2 Sources of quality investigators

Clinical leaders/therapeutic area heads
Country company heads/medical directors
Consultants
Colleague recommendations
Investigator recommendations
Scientific and medical literature
Physician directories
Speakers at professional meetings

Table 3.3 Pre-study visit questions

How will the protocol specifically operate at the prospective center?
How will informed consent be obtained? By whom?
How will source documents be managed?
How will adverse events be handled and followed up? Serious and nonserious events?
How many studies is the investigator conducting currently?

- reputation among peers and the quality of their publications;
- experience and training of their support staff;
- quality and reputation of their research facilities.

Potential sources of quality investigators are shown in Table 3.2.

Many physicians may need to be considered before the best investigators can be identified. Preliminary contact should be done by telephone. Only those investigators who satisfy the primary selection criteria need to be visited.

Pre-study visits

The purpose of the pre-study visit is to evaluate the investigator's interest and ability to conduct the study to the required sponsor standards. Normally, the monitor or CRA conducts this visit. Special attention is paid to the quality of the investigator's staff and facilities, as well as to the availability of the required patient population. In conducting the pre-study site evaluation visit, the sponsor's representative determines whether or not the investigator is qualified by training and experience to conduct the trial.

The pre-study visit is a professional exchange of information. The investigator is informed of the preclinical and clinical background of the drug. Of primary importance to the investigator is the rationale for use of the drug and the expected safety profile. Much can be inferred from the investigator's preparation and questions about the investigational drug. The protocol should be explained, including the requirements for the patient population, the study design, and a description of the safety and efficacy variables.

Other aspects of the study are also discussed with the investigator, such as the completion of the CRF,

access to source documents, and management of drug supplies. The nature and form of informed consent are reviewed. In these discussions, the sponsor's representative is attempting to identify aspects of the study that present difficulties or problems for the investigator. Quality investigators usually have a clear understanding and strategy for the above activities. Examples of the questions that require answering during pre-study visits are shown in Table 3.3.

Some objective measure of the availability of the correct patient population is important during a pre-study visit. The sponsor's representative can often best accomplish this through a chart or hospital census review.

The time spent doing this aspect of a clinical trial will invariably result in better and more timely results in clinical programs.

Assuming that the outcome of the pre-study visit(s) is successful, the sponsor's representative will need to develop and negotiate study contracts and secure essential documents.

Competencies associated with conducting clinical research

Investigator meeting

Sponsors now try to conduct many initiation activities via an investigator meeting. Such meetings (which may be in person or use videoconferencing or Internet technology) can be used to orient all investigators to the fundamental practical requirements of the protocol and trial (CRF completion, investigational product handling, discussion of audits/inspections, etc.). These meetings provide an opportunity to ensure common understanding of issues, subjective grading systems, and so on.

However, investigator meetings tend not to be attended by all the staff who will be involved in the conduct of the trial at the institution. Inevitably, this means that the sponsor's representative has to conduct study initiation activities at the institution with some key staff.

Conducting study initiation

The study initiation visit is sometimes confused with the pre-study visit. The purpose of the study initiation visit is to orient the study staff (subinvestigators, study coordinators, etc.) to the requirements of the protocol. At the point of the study initiation visit, the study site should be fully ready to begin all aspects of the trial. The monitor must ensure that the study medication and materials are available at the site. In addition, all essential documentation must be completed and available. Key study documentation is shown in Table 3.4.

All study staff who will have direct involvement in the trial should participate in the study initiation visit or investigator meeting. This usually includes the investigator and subinvestigator(s), the study coordinator or research nurse, pharmacist, and laboratory personnel or specialists as needed.

During the meeting, all major points and requirements of the protocol are reviewed and discussed. Procedures for subject enrollment are particularly important because this is the area that may cause most of the problems for the site. During the presentation, participants may raise important medical or logistical issues that have or have not been anticipated by the protocol authors. It is important to note these concerns and communicate them to the protocol authors, as appropriate.

Table 3.4 Key study documentation

Approved protocol and CRF
Informed Consent Form and Subject Information Sheet
Investigator's résumé
Written IRB/IEC approval
Local regulatory approval
Signed study contract
Laboratory ranges and accreditation

The sponsor's representative should be more than merely competent in the basic medical and scientific issues of the investigational product and protocol, know the target disease or symptoms, be able to train the investigative staff on the conduct of the study, confirm facility capabilities, conduct the site initiation meeting, describe adverse event reporting requirements, and be able to resolve protocol issues during and after meeting.

Conducting clinical trial monitoring

Clinical trial monitoring includes those activities that ensure that the study is being conducted according to the protocol. Monitoring permits an in-process assessment of the quality of the data being collected. The first alert to safety issues is often revealed during the process of monitoring the clinical trial.

Monitoring clinical studies involves the act of overseeing the progress of a clinical trial. Monitors ensure that the study is conducted, recorded, and reported in accordance with the protocol. This is accomplished by the review of paper CRFs or paper copies of electronic DCTs on-site for possible errors, inconsistencies, and omissions. The monitor identifies errors and discrepancies that require discussion with the investigator or staff and any safety questions or issues. The monitor compares CRFs with source documents (source document verification or SDV), confirming that source data are consistent with CRF entries, identifies all serious adverse events (SAEs), resolves previous and current data queries, and confirms completeness of investigator records and files.

To be a successful monitor, the sponsor representative should know how to interpret hospital/clinic records and charts, laboratory tests and interpretations, query resolution procedures, protocol and CRF data requirements, medical nomenclature, SAE procedures, and health authority requirements. In addition, a monitor needs to have excellent interpersonal communication and problem-solving skills.

Clinical monitoring requires clinical, interpretive, and administrative skills. The monitor needs to confirm subject selection and patient enrollment compliance. Quality monitoring will always include and confirm the following activities:

- properly obtained informed consent;
- adherence to the protocol procedures and inclusion/exclusion criteria;
- transcription of data from source documents to the CRF that is both consistent and logical;
- identification of any safety issues including SAEs;
- proper accountability and reconciliation of drug supplies;
- continued adequacy of facilities and staffing.

The frequency of clinical monitoring depends on the actual accrual rate of the subjects. Complex studies may need to be visited more frequently depending on the accrual rate of subjects, the amount of data, and the number of visits. Generally, most investigators should be monitored every four to six weeks. The monitors should anticipate sufficient time for good monitoring practices.

Following a monitoring visit, the monitor will prepare a monitoring report for sponsor records and follow-up correspondence to the trial site.

The monitor may need to plan intervention and possible replacement of nonperforming or non-compliant trial centers.

Managing drug accountability

The sponsor is responsible for providing the investigator with investigational product. Both the sponsor and investigator have a role in drug accountability.

The sponsor's representative inspects storage of investigational product supplies, checks study site investigational product dispensing records, checks randomization and blinding, and maintains records of investigational product shipments.

The monitor reconciles investigational product shipped, dispensed, and returned, arranges for shipment of investigational product to core country or investigative sites, checks investigational product supplies at site against enrollment and withdrawals, maintains investigational product accountability records, resolves investigational product inventory problems, implements tracking system for investigational product management on a study and project level, arranges for the return and/or destruction of unused or expired investigational product supplies, and ensures final reconciliation of investigational product supplies.

Good clinical practices require sponsors to be able to account for the drug supplies prepared and shipped to the investigator, the investigator's use of those supplies, and the return and destruction of remaining drug supplies. Planning drug supplies is a detailed and complex activity. Bulk and formulated drug requests must be made at least six months in advance of the need for those supplies, in order to account for the ordering of intermediates or finished drug, purchasing of comparator agents, and for quality control testing.

Drug packaging needs to follow as consistent a format as possible within a project, and must be identical within multicenter trials. Regulatory documents required for investigational drug use in the core countries must be anticipated and made available when needed: for example, methods/certificates of analysis, stability data, and customs declarations.

The typical requirements for drug labels are described in Table 3.5.

Once the study is underway, the investigator's staff must account for the use of the investigational drug. Subjects should return unused medication and empty containers to the investigator. The amount of drug dispensed and the amount used by the patients are compared for discrepancies, which provides a measure of compliance by the study subjects. Monitors must also check that drug supplies are being kept under the required storage conditions.

Table 3.5 Typical labeling requirements for investigational drug

Local language	Route of administration
Name of investigator	Dosage
Study number	Dosage form
Bottle number	Quantity or volume
Lot number	Storage precautions
Drug name or code	Directions for use
Manufacturer name	Note: "For Clinical Trial"
Manufacturer address	Caution statement
Local affiliate name	Expiry date

Study drug must be dispensed according to the randomization schedule. Failure to do so can result in some of the data having to be discarded during statistical analysis. This issue can prove to be problematic when a single site is studying patients at different locations. Finally, the double-blind code must not be broken except when essential for the management of adverse events. The breaking of treatment codes can make that patient's data unusable for efficacy analyses.

Handling adverse drug events (ADEs)

Safety concerns are present throughout the drug development process. From the filing of INDs/CTAs through the conduct of clinical trials to the approval process of the NDA/BLA/MAA and the marketing of the drug, safety is the primary concern of any clinical program.

Management of safety is a principal responsibility of the sponsor monitor. The monitor has responsibility for informing the investigator about the safety requirements of the study. This will include a discussion of expected and unexpected adverse events, how to report adverse events if they occur, and how to characterize the adverse events in terms of project-specific definitions.

Monitors are expected to review CRFs and source documents with particular attention to potential safety problems. On the CRF, the adverse event section and laboratory result section are reviewed for important findings. Often, the investigator makes relevant notes in the comment section of the CRF. In source documents, safety issues may be uncovered in the progress notes of hospital charts or the interpretative reports of various diagnostic tests, for example, chest X-rays and EKGs. Safety problems can manifest themselves in many ways. Monitors must be alert to exaggerated changes from baseline with expected pharmacological effects, acute and chronic effects, and multiple drug treatment reactions.

Monitors are often the first company representatives to learn about an adverse event. The timeliness of reporting the event to sponsor safety group is important in satisfying regulatory reporting requirements. In general, the expectation is that the sponsor will learn of the event within 24 hours of its occurrence. The monitor should immediately notify appropriate safety staff of serious ADEs that are unexpectedly discovered. These strict timelines are designed to keep us in compliance with the regulatory authorities. Failure to adhere to the reporting timelines required for regulatory authorities is evidence of negligence on the part of the sponsor. The sponsor monitor is responsible for ensuring adherence to reporting systems for managing SAEs and for ensuring that the investigator's staff is aware of these requirements of being in compliance with the regulatory authorities.

The sponsor monitor is responsible for the timely follow-up of all SAEs. The cases must be followed to completion. The monitor needs to collect all required follow-up information on ADEs.

To be successful, monitors need to be competent in

- basic medicine and therapeutics;
- recognizing clinical signs and symptoms;
- interpretation of laboratory findings;
- medical practice, nomenclature, and terminology;
- relevant regulatory requirements;
- protocol requirements.

The sponsor needs to provide ongoing review of safety data for investigational products.

Closing down the center

Closing down a study is important because it may represent the sponsor's last best chance to obtain the data required in the trial. The study closedown (closeout) visit usually occurs after the last subject has completed the trial including any posttreatment follow-up visits. Drug supplies need to be reconciled, and the integrity of the double-blind treatment codes should be confirmed. Any outstanding queries need to be resolved and documented.

Arrangements for retaining source data should be confirmed with the investigator. In addition, the investigator needs to notify the IRB/IEC of the completion of the study. When the final draft of the clinical study report is available, it should be given to the investigator for signature. In multicenter trials, a single lead investigator may sign a pooled study report.

Reviewing, editing, and verifying in-house case report data and databases

Although the goal of monitoring is to provide "clean" CRFs, it is necessary to review CRFs for consistency and unrecognized errors once they are received in-house. The use of computer edit and logic checks supports this effort, where computer output is verified against CRF data. Discrepancies are identified and CRF queries are generated for resolution.

The goal of managing CRFs is to get the data from the CRFs to a clean database in the fastest time possible while maintaining the highest level of quality. To accomplish this task, CRFs must be ready for data entry at the site. CRFs must be cleaned on an ongoing basis during the study. To do this, efficient systems must be incorporated to simplify the query process. The approach used by some sponsors permits electronic exchange of CRF data between the investigator, monitor, and data entry personnel. SDV is still a fundamental requirement even when using electronic data capture and exchange. Computerized checking programs and edit checks make the process more value-added for the monitors.

Clinical teams should design databases before the trial begins, reduce the amount of data collected, use standardized CRFs, and complete the review process on an ongoing basis. The philosophy is "do it right, first time" at the source.

To be successful, the staff must know how to prepare CRFs for data entry, be able to verify database consistency with original records and CRFs, and ensure that queries are handled effectively.

Competencies associated with reporting clinical research

Preparing clinical study reports

The requirements for reporting clinical trials to international regulatory authorities are similar in intent but differ in detail. Sponsors approach preparation of NDA/BLA/MAA documentation in a modular format. Each module satisfies a specific documentation need. The modules are generally organized as follows:

- *Module I*: Includes a basic summary of the study not unlike a publication, including study rationale, objectives, methods, results, and conclusions. Module I also has a large appendix that includes a list of investigators, drug lot numbers, concomitant diseases and medications, intent-to-treat analysis, patient listings of adverse events, and relevant laboratory abnormalities, and publications on the study.
- *Module II*: Includes the protocol and any modifications, CRF, detailed methodology, and the glossary of original terminology and preferred terms.
- *Module III*: Presents the detailed efficacy findings including the intent-to-treat analysis population and the efficacy data listings.
- *Module IV*: Presents the detailed safety findings including the intent-to-treat analysis population and the safety data listings.
- *Module V*: Includes individual center summary reports, quality assurance measures, statistical methods, and analyses and randomization lists.

The skills necessary to prepare a clinical study report include the following:
- advanced research design, methodology, and statistics;
- preparation and review of study tabulations;
- ability to confirm that study tabulations conform to protocol design;
- ability to verify study tabulations against computer data listings;
- clarification of outstanding issues regarding data analysis and presentation;
- drafting of assigned study report sections according to the clinical study report prototype;
- interpretation of adverse events;
- interpretation of laboratory findings;
- interpretation of efficacy findings;
- ability to ensure that the conclusions are supported by the data;
- ability to ensure that reports satisfy regulatory requirements;
- developing clear, simple graphs, tables, and figures to illustrate and support findings;

• ability to write a clear, concise report that accurately summarizes and interprets the results.

Preparing annual safety reports

Sponsors are required to submit annually to regulatory authorities a summary of safety findings of investigational products. This process involves verification of adverse event tabulations against computer data listings and the preparation of safety tables. The current findings are reviewed and compared with AE data from the past reporting period.

The sponsor's representatives must be able to clarify any outstanding issues regarding safety interpretation and presentation of the data. As this information is of critical importance to the regulatory authorities, the annual report must be written in a clear, concise manner that accurately summarizes and interprets the safety results. The annual report need to provide clear, simple graphs, tables, and figures to illustrate and support safety findings.

Following the submission of the annual report, safety findings are usually integrated into an updated version of the IB.

To be able to prepare annual reports, the sponsor's representative should know how the reports satisfy regulatory authority requirements. The clinical representative should be able to interpret clinical safety and laboratory findings. The ability to understand computer-generated clinical output and the organization and structure of the NDA/BLA/MAA safety database is important.

The annual report and NDA/BLA/MAA safety update review and approval procedures must be understood, as well as the procedures for the preparation of the IB.

Preparing clinical sections of NDA/BLA/MAA

The knowledge and skill needed to prepare an NDA/BLA/MAA include the ability to
• verify individual study tabulations against overall summary computer listings;
• prepare brief descriptions of the studies;
• interpret critical clinical safety and efficacy results;
• interpret laboratory findings;

• develop clear tables and figures to illustrate and support clinical findings;
• summarize, interpret, and integrate the overall safety and efficacy results;
• prepare NDA/BLA/MAA clinical study summaries, benefit/risk summary, expert reports, and Package Insert.

In addition, an understanding of electronic NDA/BLA/MAAs and regulatory authority data presentation requirements are useful.

The expert report usually generates considerable discussion within a project. The sponsor often prepares this document under the guidance of an external expert. Although internal experts are acceptable, it should be remembered that the regulatory authorities are looking for an individual who knows the drug thoroughly and can express an unbiased opinion of its medical importance. The expert report is not only a summary, but also a critical assessment of the clinical evaluation of the drug. The expert report provides an independent assessment of the risk-to-benefit ratio of the drug and its use. The text is limited to 25 pages, but may include an "unlimited" number of attachments. Many companies have been creative in font size and two-sided preparation of the document.

Certain trends and directions can be recognized in the preparation of NDA/BLA/MAAs. The ICH has the long-term goal of harmonizing the content of European, US, and Japanese NDA/BLA/MAAs. EU registration dossiers are becoming more detailed in the process, and are expected to include integrated summaries in the future. The US FDA will accept more non-US data for drug approval as common high standards for clinical trials become well established in the world. Electronic NDA/BLA/MAAs will become the norm and are already required in the United States.

How and where are competencies taught?

Quite apart from established in-house training programs, there is a wide selection of vendors offering competency-based training. The format of their programs may include:
• workshops, seminars, and lectures;
• self-instructional manuals;
• computer-based training systems;

- videotape libraries;
- job aids;
- preceptorships and mentoring programs;
- educational organizations such as PERI and DIA;
- professional meetings and conferences.

Most vendors advertise widely in the trade journals, and many of their courses are tailored to meet the several certifications that are now available in clinical research or regulatory affairs.

References

Spilker B. *Guide to Clinical Trials*. Raven: New York, USA, 1991.

Spilker B. *Multinational Drug Companies: Issues in drug discovery and development*. Raven: New York, USA, 1989.

SECTION II
Drug Discovery and Development

With a very low probability, a chemical can sometimes be transformed into a medicine. What governs this process forms the central theme of the chapters in this section of the book. This theme could also be named the "pre-marketing" stage of the drug life-cycle.

A limitation is that these chapters have had to be designed to describe the general case. For example, preclinical pharmacology is almost always product-specific, and so only the broadest of generalities from that subspecialty can be included here. Similarly, if to a relatively lesser extent, almost no drug passes through the stereotypical toxicology process described here: Results from these typical studies usually lead to additional investigations with specialized designs to address specific issues for particular drugs.

Regulatory affairs is so central to the entire life-cycle of a drug that it deserves its own section in this book (Section V). The drug lifecycle is really a continuum, and especially in drug regulation, dividing that continuum into phases or stages is especially artificial. For the same reason, much of the content within this section overlaps from phase-to-phase and also applies to Phase IV drug development. These overlaps are intentional and pursue the notion of taking an integrated approach to drug development.

CHAPTER 4

Drug Discovery: Design and Development

Ronald R. Cobb[1] & Leslie J. Molony[2]
[1]RiverWood BioConsulting Inc., Gainesville, FL, USA
[2]Transgeneron Therapeutics Inc., Gainesville, FL, USA

Introduction

How is it that medicines are discovered? In ancient times, and even today, tribal people knew the healing or hallucinogenic properties of indigenous plants and animals. The knowledge was accumulated through generations, recorded by chant and living memory, and derived largely from human experience. Although many of the drugs in use today were discovered by chance, most drug discovery scientists engage in directed research, based on a series of steps, each requiring substantial scientific input. Although available facilities, resources, technology focus, or even corporate culture can define the procedures followed by researchers at particular institutions, there are some obvious, generally applicable milestones in this process that facilitate the discovery of therapeutics.

Targeted medicines and their implications

The understanding and use of medicines by physicians and healers have evolved significantly, keeping in step with technological and biological breakthroughs. From the use of herbal remedies to toxic chemotherapeutic substances (*Vinca* alkaloids being an example of both!), today's ideal case is a medicine directed at an identified pathological process, and/or specific receptors controlling these pathologies. Well-targeted medicines are often substantially safer, and are likely to have fewer adverse events (side effects) in a larger patient population than those with multiple pharmacological properties. Research and development leading to a new, well-targeted pharmaceutical product is a long, complex, and expensive process. Historically, the cost of a new drug has been escalating by close to US$100,000,000 every five years. In 2005, the estimated cost of bringing a new drug from the laboratory bench into the marketplace was US$800,000,000 (about €670,000,000 or £450,000,000). Average development time is 7–10 years, although some "blockbuster" drugs have taken 20 years. Of all commercial products, these are among the longest of all development cycles, permitting patent exploitation among the shortest periods. Hence, the drug discovery and development process is a two-part exercise in mitigating the economic punishment to product sponsors while maximizing the probability that something that can be developed successfully is actually found. As few as 1% of promising lead molecules will be tested in human beings; fewer than one-third of those tested will become marketed products, and among those only about a half will produce financial returns that are disproportionately higher than their costs of development.

Despite the high risk and escalating costs of developing new medicines, the benefits of pharmaceuticals to human healthcare provide both

Principles and Practice of Pharmaceutical Medicine, 3rd edition.
Edited by L.D. Edwards, A.W. Fox, P.D. Stonier.
© 2011 Blackwell Publishing Ltd.

financial and humanitarian motivations to pharmaceutical companies and to the individual drug discovery.

Designing a drug discovery project

Chance favors the prepared mind.

– Anon.

All drug discovery projects depend on luck to be successful, but research and careful planning can improve the chances of success and lower the cost. Project teams can streamline the discovery process by using the tools that can lead to a discovery most directly. These tools are drawn from the repertoires of modern biology, chemistry, robotics, and computer simulations. In comparison with older processes of *in vivo* screening of huge numbers of molecules, however, these innovations have not been associated with shortening the development time of 7–10 years (see Figure 4.1). Some think that modern biology as well as other fields have only increased the number of "hits" overall, whereas others think that an increase in speed of discovery has compensated for an increase in regulatory stringency during the last two decades.

The "unmet clinical need" as a market niche

Usually, scientists are directed to research new targets in specific therapeutic areas based on unmet clinical needs and market opportunities that are foreseen in the medium-to-long term. Both medical and business considerations are weighed. Larger companies will rarely fund internal research for drug discovery of orphan drug products (or products targeting diseases with few patients). On the other hand, small market niche needs are often sufficient for smaller companies (often researching in biotechnology).

When a medical need and market niche are identified, and a particular therapeutic area chosen, the biological research begins. It is during this first stage of drug discovery that anecdotal clinical observations, empirical outcomes, and "data" from folk medicine are often employed, if only as direction-finding tools.

Once a direction is chosen, it must be validated scientifically, within a defined biological system. Human disease or pathology is usually multifactorial, and the first task of the researcher is to narrow down the search by defining the molecular mechanisms better; optimally this will be a small number

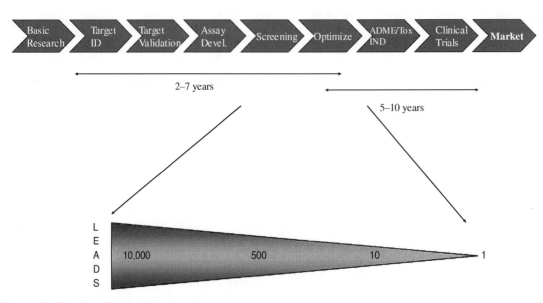

Figure 4.1 The drug discovery process.

of pathophysiologically observable processes, for example, the pinpointing of one or two types of cells that are etiological.

From that cellular stage, the researcher next defines specific molecular targets, such as receptors on or specific iso enzymes in those cells, which create the destructive phenotype. Is there an anomaly in a cell derived from a tumor, to use a cancer example, which renders that tumor cell unique from normal cells derived from the same tissue? If the difference is significant and can be reproducibly observed in the laboratory, it can be exploited for drug discovery. In other diseases, the cell that is identified can be normal but activated to a destructive state by stimulation with disease pathogens. In rheumatoid arthritis, for example, the normal T lymphocyte is stimulated to react to antigens present in the joint, thus developing a destructive phenotype.

The wider effects of inhibiting, modifying, or eliminating this new molecular target on the organism must also be considered. An enzyme that is essential to life is a "no-hoper" from the point of view of the drug developer. The perfect target is organ-, tissue-, or cell-specific, thereby limiting effects to the system involved in the disease. The choice of a target for a disease will be critical to the outcome and performance of the drug, and determines what organs or tissues will be susceptible to side effects. The ideal molecular drug target is also one that is proprietary, whether having been discovered in-house or in-licensed.

At this stage, an assessment is made as to whether the medicine that could result is likely to be palliative or "disease-modifying." Disease modifying drugs (DMD) are those that directly and beneficially deflect the natural history of the disease. Non-steroidal anti-inflammatory drugs and methotrexate are examples of each of these in patients with rheumatoid arthritis. Then, the probability of one or the other can alter economic assessments of the research program, and lead to a go-no-go decision in some cases.

Combining basic and applied research

Molecular targets are not always obvious, even though cellular and histological disease pathologies have been well described in the literature. At this point, the researcher returns to the laboratory bench to design critical experiments (see Figure 4.2).

The design and use of highly specific, monoclonal antibodies (MAs) to proteins (or receptors) derived from diseased tissue is a common approach to probing for the correct molecular target. One refinement of this approach is to use a variety of these MAs to screen hybridoma supernatants for activity in preventing a cellular manifestation of the disease of interest. Taking cancer as an example, malignant cells often contain overexpressed, mutated, or absent "oncogenes" (i.e., genes that code for particular proteins or receptors in normal cells, but are mutated, and thus cause pathological overactivity or underactivity of those gene products in tumor cells). Two well-known examples of oncogenes are the *RAS* and *SRC* oncogenes, which code for the production of RAS and SRC proteins, respectively. Normal RAS protein regulates cellular division and coordinates the nuclear changes to alterations in the cellular architecture required for mitosis (cytoskeleton and cell motility). Meanwhile, SRC protein is a key signaling molecule, which alters cell growth by modulating the activation of the epidermal growth factor (EGF) receptor by its ligand. Many drug discovery efforts have, therefore, targeted SRC, RAS, the EGF receptor, or any of their associated enzymes. Thus, for example, RAS inhibitor discovery projects include prevention of the enzymatic event which allows translocation of RAS from the cytosol to the plasma membrane in cancer cells as one way to prevent the effects of RAS.

Taking another example, consider the case of a novel approach to treating inflammatory disease. In 1997, a cell or molecular biologist beginning such a research program might have found reports in the literature of transgenic mice which, when genetically engineered to cause monocytes to express constant levels of the cytokine (TNF), develop arthritis, as well as some of the early clinical trials using anti-tumor necrosis factor (TNF) antibodies in human rheumatoid arthritis. There would also have been a lot of data available concerning cellular infiltrates in joint effusions, with monocytes

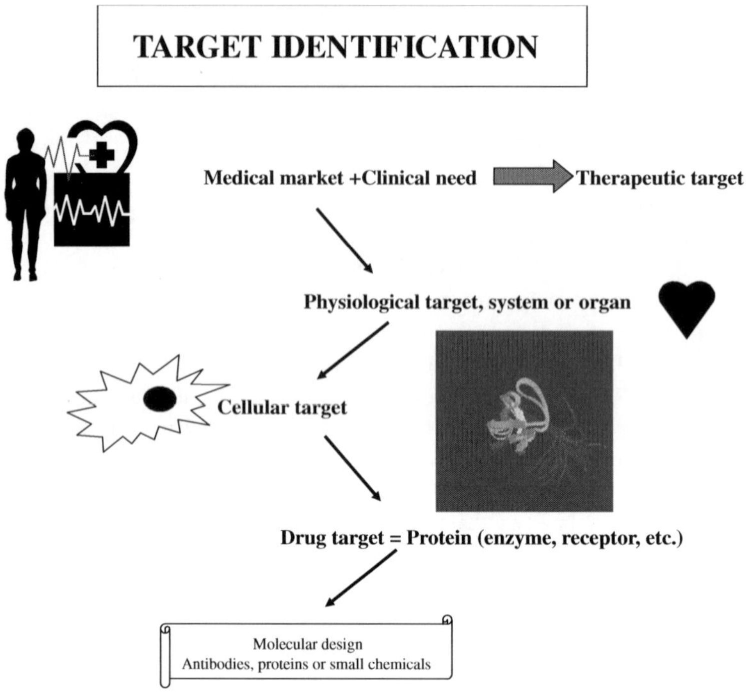

Figure 4.2 Target identification.

and T-lymphocytes being the most prevalent. High concentrations of other mediators of inflammation, such as interleukin-1β, leukotrienes, and phospholipases had also been reported in rheumatoid joints. The scientist might then conclude that inhibitors of TNF receptor activations, rather than antibodies to the ligand (TNF) itself, could also benefit inflammatory arthropathy. A range of ways in which this might be accomplished would then present themselves: irreversible antagonism of the TNF receptor, interruption of that receptor's transduction mechanism, or prevention of the expression of either TNF itself, or its TNF receptor, in the nucleus or ribosome.

The investigator might then seek the counsel of marketing experts and physicians regarding the use of the antibodies, and again review the clinical trial data available through the literature on the anti-TNF antibodies. Such antibodies will be competing products for a long time in the future, given that it is difficult to obtain regulatory approval for "generic" biotechnology products, regardless of

the patent situation. But the antibodies are also unattractive drugs. They are not orally available, and they elicit immune responses after several doses (anti-anti-TNF antibody humoral response). Thus, these criteria would then be applied when sorting through the alternative modes of attack on the TNF receptor. An orally bioavailable, nonpeptide drug might become the goal.

The next question to be answered is whether *a priori* the receptor itself, or one of the associated regulatory enzymes, is likely to be specifically targetable using an oral, non-peptide drug. Little literature on this subject was available in 1997, and no competitor seems to have taken this approach. The company's laboratories are then set to work.

Each individual laboratory (lab) working on TNF as a therapeutic target approaches the problem from a different direction. For example, one lab may seek to inhibit transcription factor activation by phosphorylation or proteolysis, and to examine the sorts of compound that may be capable of this. Another group might seek to interfere with the

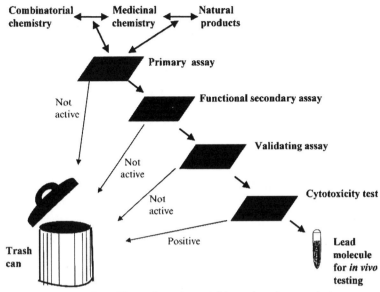

Figure 4.3 Drug screening flowchart.

binding of the transcription regulatory complex to DNA.

A key decision in each lab is when to incur the expense and time to clone the molecular target and set up the robotized *in vitro* assays that can screen compounds with a high rate of throughput. The best assays are those that relate directly to cellular events, which allow screening of huge numbers of chemical compounds and which predict *in vivo* responses. Other assays during this exploratory stage may be used as secondary screens for candidates identified by the first one, if at rather slower throughput.

Genomics and molecular biological approaches

The Human Genome Project has had a significant effect on target identification. One by-product was that gene expression profiling technologies were invented that allowed for direct comparisons of mRNA levels in normal and diseased cells (e.g., "gene microarrays" or "gene chips"; Clarke *et al.*, 2001; Cunningham *et al.*, 2000). Technologies such as these allow the pharmaceutical researcher to compare the expression levels of nearly all the

genes in the genome in one experiment, and in an automated fashion. Gene expression profiling is useful not only in target identification as described here but also in finding significant use in later stages of drug development such as toxicology, surrogate marker generation, and mechanism of action studies (see Figure 4.3).

"Antisense oligonucleotides" are short, single-stranded DNA molecules that are complementary to a target mRNA (Baker and Monia, 1999; Crooke, 1999; Koller *et al.*, 2000). Once bound to the mRNA of interest, it is targeted for cleavage and degradation resulting in a loss of protein expression. There are several naturally occurring catalytic RNAs including "hammerhead," "hairpin," and "hepatitis delta virus" introns, and the RNA subunit of RNAase P (Khan and Lal, 2003). Catalogues exist in which the researcher can simply look up which genes a particular antisense sequence will map to, and the use of fluorescent tags can then be used to probe the location of disease-producing mutants.

But the pharmaceutical researcher should not rely entirely on gene expression profiling for target identification, even though the technology is very powerful. Gene expression does not automatically lead to predictable protein synthesis. Protein activity and abundance does not always correlate with mRNA levels (Chen *et al.*, 2002; Gygi, Rist, Gerber *et al.*, 1999; Gygi, Rochon, Franza, Aebersold, 1999).

The "one-gene-one-protein" hypothesis is now well and truly dead. Proteins hugely outnumber genes in all mammals. The term *proteomics* has been coined to describe the analogous study of proteins within particular cells or tissues (Figeys, 2003; Petricoin *et al.*, 2002; Tyers and Mann, 2003; Zhu and Snyder, 2003). Moreover, many proteins are modified after translation in ways that are crucial in regulating their function. Thus, the application of proteomics also extends far beyond the target identification stage in drug development.

Further exploitation of this genomic and proteinomic can be obtained by making comparisons of these data with epidemiological observations in human populations. Patterns of familial disease, with mapping to differences between individuals in terms of DNA or mRNA, can identify which of many genetic variations is the etiology. This is known as "linkage analysis," and ultimately, the precise chromosomal location, relative to the location of other known genes, can be found using a technique known as "positional cloning." An example of new target identification using these methods was the identification of ApoE as a causative factor in Alzheimer's disease (Pericak-Vance, 1991).

Mutations that cause disease can arise spontaneously. Genetic mapping methods using positional cloning can help identify disease-causative genes and their proteins in animals that have spontaneously developed diseases similar to those of humans. An example of this type of technology is the ob/ob genetic mouse, which is obese and has mutations in a gene for a peptide hormone known as leptin. A similar mouse, the Agouti strain, is also obese and has defects in melanocortin receptors, which develops type II diabetes, and therefore can be used as an animal model of that disease in humans. Of course, human disease is rarely as simple as a single genetic defect, and so these models must be used with some caution when testing drugs or when identifying the causative genes. Pathophysiological studies of organisms that have been engineered to contain (transgenic "splice in"), or to be free from ("knock out"), the identified gene is an extension of this concept (see also below).

The sequencing of genes does not directly identify new molecular targets for disease. But it does permit the rapid identification of target proteins, because their codes are known. Usually, only a few trial peptides need then be synthesized, shaving months off of the discovery process. In turn, this allows rapid identification and cloning of new targets for assay development.

Whole tissue studies

Pharmacologists are often able to develop tissue and whole animal models of human disease. In some instances, studies on isolated tissues, such as blood vessels, heart muscle, or brain slices, will allow a tissue- or organ-specific understanding of the effects of potential new drugs. Cardiovascular pharmacologists often study isolated arteries, which are maintained in a physiological salt solution. Electric stimulation can induce contraction of the vascular smooth muscle, and the effects of hypertensive drugs on vascular contraction can then be measured. Historically, these systems were often used as primary drug screening tools. Because these methods are much less direct than molecular screening, they are now relegated to secondary or tertiary roles as validation of the targets or drugs discovered, using assays that directly employ the molecular or cellular targets. Whole animal models are often seen as critical decision-making points for a newly discovered drug.

Human pathology is inevitably more varied than that of rats and mice. Thus, it is often necessary to induce a pathological state by introduction of a pathogen or stimulant directly into a healthy animal. The development of new animal models is a time-consuming process and must be overseen by the appropriate ethics committees and expert veterinarian advice.

Why are *in vivo* (whole animal) studies still important to drug discovery? All the new technology, as well as mathematical modeling using computers, has reduced but not eliminated the need for animal experimentation. Computer models still cannot accurately predict the effects of chemical compounds on the cell, let alone in systems with higher orders of complexity—that is, whole tissues, organs, and organisms—with their emergent properties that define the discipline of complex systems biology. *In vivo* cells operate in a dynamic and communicative environment, where an effect of a drug in one place may well lead to corresponding or compensatory changes elsewhere. The summation of these innumerable responses often defeats the predictions of high-throughput screens and three-dimensional drug-receptor "design the key for the lock" calculations.

In vivo target validation also still requires the use of animal models. It is now possible to monitor multiple targets within the same cells by intercrossing independently derived strains of mice that have been engineered to express different target genes and/or to lack one or more target genes. These models provide a powerful genetic approach for determining specific events and signaling networks that are involved in the disease process.

Other sources of compounds

Pharmacognosy is the science of identifying potential drugs that are naturally formed within plants or animals. One large pharmaceutical company has concluded an agreement with a Central American country to preserve its entire flora and give the company exclusive rights to any pharmacophores within it.

Combinatorial chemistry

The breakthroughs in technology that have allowed sequencing of genes "on a chip" and high-throughput screening of compounds in microtiter plate format have also caused a revolution in chemical synthesis, known as combinatorial chemistry.

Biological therapeutics

Chapter 24 on biotechnology drugs enlarges on this subject in more detail, but suffice it to say here that vaccines, antibodies, proteins, peptides, and gene therapies all now exist. These biological drugs bring with them specific, regulatory, clinical trials, and manufacturing difficulties. Gene therapy, in particular, carries human safety risks that do not apply to other classes of therapy, for example, the infective nature of some types of vector that are employed, and the potential for incorporation of the test genetic material into the genome in males, leading to expression of gene products in offspring.

New uses for old drugs

Opportunities still exist for astute clinicians to find new uses for old drugs, and for these newly discovered uses to lead to new and unexpected drugs. The recent approval of bupropion as a smoking cessation agent is a good example of a chance observation, while the drug was being used for its initial indication as an antidepressant. This has led to realization of the influence of nicotine on depression, and investigational drugs of a new class, based on this alkaloid molecule, are now being designed. Viagra is another good example of a drug that was originally designed for one therapeutic action (lowering blood pressure) and wound up becoming a blockbuster drug in another therapeutic area (erectile dysfunction).

Summary

This chapter began with a survey of the modern methods of drug discovery. Pharmaceutical physicians should be aware of some of the techniques employed and the rapid rate at which genetic information is becoming available. It should be noted that this modern revolution has not quite completely swept away the occasional new drug found by serendipity or astute clinical observation.

References

Baker BF, Monia BP. Novel mechanisms for antisense-mediated regulation of gene expression. *Biochim Biophys Acta* 1999; **1489**(1):3–18.

Chen G, Gharib TG, Huang CC, Taylor JM, Misek DE, Kardia SL, Giordano TJ, Iannettoni MD, Orringer MB, Hanash SM, Beer DG. Discordant protein and mRNA expression in lung adenocarcinomas. *Mol Cell Proteomics* 2002; **1**(4):304–313

Clarke PA, te Poele R, Wooster R, Workman P. Gene expression microarray analysis in cancer biology, pharmacology, and drug development: progress and potential. *Biochem Pharmacol* 2001; **62**(10):1311–1336.

Crooke ST. Molecular mechanisms of action of antisense drugs. *Biochim Biophys Acta* 1999; **1489**(1):31–44.

Cunningham MJ, Liang S, Fuhrman S, Seilhamer JJ, Somogyi R. Gene expression microarray data analysis for toxicology profiling. *Ann N Y Acad Sci* 2000; **919**: 52–67.

Figeys D. Novel approaches to map protein interactions. *Curr Opin Biotechnol* 2003; **14**(1):119–125.

Gygi SP, Rist B, Gerber SA, Turecek F, Gelb MH, Aebersold R. Quantitative analysis of complex protein mixtures using isotope-coded affinity tags. *Nat Biotechnol* 1999; **17**(10):994–999.

Gygi SP, Rochon Y, Franza BR, Aebersold R. Correlation between protein and mRNA abundance in yeast. *Mol Cell Biol* 1999; **19**(3):1720–1730.

Khan AU, Lal SK. Ribozymes: a modern tool in medicine. *J Biomed Sci* 2003; **10**(5):457–467.

Koller E, Gaarde WA, Monia BP. Elucidating cell signaling mechanisms using antisense technology. *Trends Pharmacol Sci* 2000; **21**(4):142–148.

Pericak-Vance MA, Bebout JL, Gaskell PC, *et al.* Linkage studies in familial Alzheimer disease: evidence for chromosome 19 linkage. *Am J Hum Genet* 1991; **48**:1034–1050.

Petricoin EF, Zoon KC, Kohn EC, Barrett JC, Liotta LA. Clinical proteomics: translating benchside promise into bedside reality. *Nat Rev Drug Discov* 2002; **1**(9):683–695.

Tyers M, Mann M. From genomics to proteomics. *Nature* 2003; **422**(6928):193–197.

Zhu H, Snyder M. Protein chip technology. *Curr Opin Chem Biol* 2003; **7**(1):55–63.

Further reading

Amersham Life Science. Brochure on scintillation. Drug Discovery proximity assays. Publication No. S 593/657/4/93/09, 1993, Amersham International.

Beeley LJ, Duckworth DM. The impact of genomics on drug design. *Drug Discov Today* 1996; **1**(11):474–480.

Bugrim A, Nikolskaya T, Nikolsky Y. *Drug Discov Today* 2004; **9**:127–135.

Chapman D. The measurement of molecular diversity: A three dimensional approach. *J Comput-Aided Mol Des* 1996; **10**:501–512.

Downward J. Targeting RAS signaling pathways in cancer therapy. *Nat Rev Cancer* 2002; **3**:11–21.

Goffeau A, *et al.* Life with 6000 genes. *Science* 1996; **274**:546–567.

Kozlowski MR. Problem solving in laboratory automation. *Drug Discov Today* 1996; **1**(11):481–488.

Lipinski CA, *et al.* Experimental and computational approaches to estimate solubility and permeability in drug discovery and development settings. *Adv Drug Deliv Rev* 1997; **23**:3–29.

Lipper RA. How can we optimize selection of drug development candidates from many compounds at the discovery stage? *Mod Drug Discov* 1999; **2**(1):55–60.

Schuler GD, *et al.* A gene map of the human genome. *Science* 1996; **274**:540–546.

Van Drie JH. Strategies for the determination of pharmacophoric 3D database queries. *J Comput-Aided Mol Des* 1997; **11**:39–52.

CHAPTER 5

Translational Medicine, Pharmaceutical Physicians, Patients, and Payers

Robert Sands[1] & Douglas Roy[2]
[1]Sanofi-aventis, Cambridge, MA, USA
[2]Division of Pathway Medicine, University of Edinburgh, Edinburgh, UK

Introduction

Translational medicine is a rapidly emerging discipline focused on bridging technologies and discoveries in the laboratory with their application in clinical research, drug discovery, and development. This vision of translational medicine is central to the role and mission of a pharmaceutical physician. The Faculty of Pharmaceutical Medicine in the UK has as its stated aim: "To advance the science and practice of pharmaceutical medicine by working to develop and maintain competence, ethics and integrity and the highest professional standards for the benefit of patients."

Given the overlap in the objectives of translational and pharmaceutical medicine, their respective agendas and shared interests are set to converge and evolve further together. It is no coincidence that the home page of the UK Faculty of Pharmaceutical Medicine website contains a reference and a plea for government to work in partnership with healthcare professionals and the pharmaceutical industry to ensure that patients have access to innovative and life-enhancing medicines and interventions. This spirit of collaborative working is a central theme running throughout this chapter.

There is no single definition of "translational medicine" and the term is being used to convey how new scientific advances, interdisciplinary approaches, and restructuring and re-organization of research collaborations is being promoted to narrow the gap between basic and clinical science, maximize the potential of science in healthcare, and facilitate bidirectional flows of knowledge and information from "bench to bedside, petri dish to patient or human to molecule." It is also a way forward to address the Research and Development (R&D) productivity challenges facing pharmaceutical companies and importantly provides a framework that can promote effective collaborative working practice of all the stakeholders involved in addressing unmet medical needs.

The scope of translational medicine is broad and no single discipline or organization is equipped on its own to exploit its full potential. As hinted in the title, the *raison d'être* of this approach is the ability to translate insights across disciplines and organizations to the ultimate benefit of patients. By implication, if executed correctly, this process should translate into more productivity and reduce redundancy, and hence resonate with the two underpinning principles of healthcare: namely improved effectiveness and efficiency. It is therefore understandable why the term translation medicine is referred to in many and varying contexts.

Principles and Practice of Pharmaceutical Medicine, 3rd edition.
Edited by L.D. Edwards, A.W. Fox, P.D. Stonier.
© 2011 Blackwell Publishing Ltd.

Pharmaceutical medicine and the R&D productivity gap

Pharmaceutical medicine is the medical scientific discipline concerned with the discovery, development, evaluation, registration, monitoring, and medical aspects of the marketing of drugs for the benefit of patients and the health of the community. The fact that there has been a decline in the number of new drugs suggests a failure to translate the opportunities of recent scientific and clinical innovations, and pharmaceutical physicians have to take some responsibility for this poor productivity and translation of scientific insights into everyday practice. This failure is compounded by an unsustainable increase in operational costs, the pharmaceutical equivalent of "the perfect storm."

It is now well established that despite R&D investment increasing two to three fold, there has been no associated increase in the number of new drugs. This unsustainable model is further compounded by the fact that many of the widely prescribed medicines that have funded this record R&D investment are at the end of their patent life, with the inevitable generic substitution occurring sooner due to constrained healthcare budgets. The profitability of this industry is further threatened by the implementation of cost containment measures through managed healthcare delivery, as governments try to contain ever spiraling health costs by targeting the more defined drug expenditure.

Strategies to ensure a viable future for the pharmaceutical industry have been implemented at various levels. At a macroeconomic perspective, there has been a drive to be less reliant on the North American and European markets, which are experiencing a more significant slow down in growth, with more focus being placed on the emerging markets such as Brazil, Russia, India, China, and Mexico. A caveat of this shift in investment is that many of these markets approach intellectual property law differently, and hence the need for bespoke business models with greater emphasis on generics. Another approach has been to look for alternative sources of income through diversifying into all forms of the healthcare industry, rather than focusing only on the prescription-only

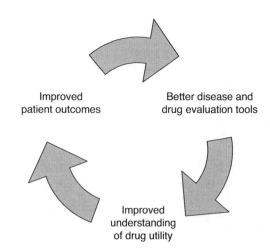

Figure 5.1 Insights from translational medicine will improve patient outcomes.

medicine business. This strategic shift should bring more stability because these other revenue streams are not subject to the same patent expiration issues.

Innovation has been synonymous with this industry and it too has come under scrutiny. Translational medicine has the potential to play an important role in reviving the fortunes of the pharmaceutical industry. It is a novel approach to harnessing the innovation of science and technology for the ultimate benefit of patients (see Figure 5.1).

Translation of science—an overview

The past several decades have seen an explosion in our understanding of the molecular basis of biological processes. Following on from the global genome sequencing efforts, there have been rapid developments in functional genomic technologies for high-throughput and global analysis at the genomic, transcriptomic, and increasingly, proteomic levels. This leap forward is being driven by the development and application of platform technologies and sophisticated analytical systems to enable global and parallel molecular, biochemical, and cellular analyses. There now exists an extensive functional genomic toolbox available to researchers to address the challenges of scale, complexity, and diversity within biological systems. Increasingly, there is a move towards the development of miniaturized readout platforms, which reflect advances in microfluidics and micro-engineering coupled with advanced bioassays for sophisticated multiplexed and multi-parameter detection systems (Fan *et al.*, 2008; Schulze *et al.*, 2009).

DNA microarrays provide a powerful example of the utility of platform technologies for genome-wide analysis of transcriptional activity, DNA sequencing, mutational analysis, and structural genomics (Brown and Botstein, 1999). The generation of RNA transcriptional signature profiles using DNA microarrays coupled with genotyping information is providing important new insights for the elucidation of pathways and networks in disease and development. In addition, the functional genomic toolbox is being used to unravel new areas of biology such as the role of micro RNA in biological control (Drakai and Iliopoulos, 2009). Coupled with the advent of next-generation DNA sequencing technologies for genome wide mutational scanning, these approaches will link the genetic basis of disease with functional pathways and networks (Hanash, 2004; Wang *et al.*, 2007; Zhang *et al.*, 2009).

Proteomic analysis via mass spectroscopy is advancing rapidly and moving towards higher throughput sampling and analysis methods, which will be required to address the complexity of the proteome. Interactome studies using yeast-2-hybrid screening approaches are defining extensive protein–protein interaction networks, which can then be validated in situ using established cellular, molecular, and biochemical readouts (Aebersold and Mann, 2003; Azad *et al.*, 2006; Hanash, 2003).

Central to these post-genomic developments is the critical role for computational and bioinformatic inputs for the handling, analysis, and visualization of the often huge datasets produced. In this way, biomedical research is becoming increasingly data-driven where large scale datasets are required to be "mined" by computational and bioinformatics approaches to ensure that interpretable information is derived. The ability to analyze globally the activity of genomic and proteomic com-

ponents is the key starting point for the representation and analysis of biological pathways and networks (Raza *et al.*, 2008; Rho *et al.*, 2008). However, sophisticated understanding of the systems involved is not automatically derived and huge challenges remain in identifying pathways and interactions using computational and bioinformatic techniques from data-driven studies. Indeed, established hypothesis-driven research remains of paramount importance because this provides the contextual and focused readouts to validate high-throughput studies.

The most sophisticated application of the functional genomics toolbox has been with model organisms such as *E. coli*, yeast, and *Drosophila*, which are experimentally tractable and have powerful genetic and biochemical systems. There is now a sophisticated understanding of the molecular components and their genetic and physiological control in these organisms (Collins *et al.*, 2009). This is crucial to informing our understanding of the fundamental processes underlying biological systems that are conserved throughout evolution.

The ultimate challenge of course is to translate these rapid technological advances into an improved understanding of disease mechanisms and to facilitate the identification and development of new diagnostics, therapeutics, and interventions. The underlying biology of human disease is massively complex, spanning a hierarchy from the molecular to whole body. Only by understanding the complexities of the underlying biology and physiology, can we obtain a full understanding of the cause and progression of disease.

The full armory of molecular and clinical techniques is being applied to elucidate the causes and pathogenesis of human disease. Genome wide mutational scanning is being extensively employed in case control and cohort studies to analyze the genetic basis of disease (Wellcome Trust Case Control Consortium, 2007). This is particularly important for unraveling the genetic basis of multifactorial disease. Coupled with transcriptomic and proteomic studies, this approach is beginning to reveal the underlying pathways and networks in human disease (Chin and Gray, 2008). Next-generation sequencing methods, which will allow rapid sequencing of human genomes and their transcriptional activity, are moving the era of personalized medicine ever closer (Ansorge, 2009; Shendure and Ji, 2008).

A key component of the translational research effort is focused on the identification and evaluation of biomarkers which represent surrogate markers for the monitoring of disease progression or the activity and response to drugs and therapies. The use of functional genomic readouts is of central importance for the identification of suitable biomarkers in translational research (Bhattacharya and Mariana, 2009; Mendrick and Schnackenberg, 2009) and will complement established clinical or biochemical readouts.

Biomedical and clinical research advances must be coupled to maximize the potential for successful disease research and the testing of drugs. Along with advances in analytical systems for *in vivo* and *ex vivo* analysis is the adoption of increasingly sophisticated technological approaches for high-throughput screening of chemical libraries and advances in cheminformatic applications for the design and modeling of drugs and drug-target interactions. Again, central to these advances is computational and bioinformatic approaches for target identification, *in silico* analysis and interactive drug design and selection. The characterization of candidate drugs is benefiting from the development of advanced cell screening systems which offer high-throughput and multi-parameter screening (Butcher *et al.*, 2004; Oprea *et al.*, 2007; Schneider and Fechner, 2005).

Translational medicine is an interdisciplinary activity requiring the input and interaction of multiple lines of investigation and activity. Multiple scientific and clinical inputs are critical but must ultimately be combined to provide a fundamental understanding of the underlying biology and how it relates to the triggers and pathogenesis of disease. The expectation is that this will lead to improvements in the identification of drug targets and the identification of other innovative therapeutic approaches. In the following decades it is likely that comprehensive cataloging of the components of the disease hierarchy and an improved understanding of how these components operate together will provide a sound basis for the development of a more personalized approach to diagnostics and therapeutic interventions based on an improved understanding of the underlying pathways and networks and the genetic basis and control. This requires the challenging prospect of understanding disease at the systems level.

The concept of systems medicine encapsulates this and requires the integration of multiple different molecular and clinical readouts and datasets to allow robust system level definition (Ahn *et al.*, 2006; Auffray *et al.*, 2009; Deisboeck, 2009; Hood and Perlmutter, 2004). Integration at this level requires the application of computational, mathematical, and bioinformatics approaches in order to analyze and model differential inputs. Systems level modeling of human development and disease is hugely challenging, but there is significant momentum in this direction particularly via the formation of interdisciplinary centers of systems biology and systems medicine. A key aim is that systems medicine will be important for the identification of biomarkers for pre-symptomatic disease diagnosis (Hood *et al.*, 2004). Systems level approaches will be needed to dissect the complexities of multifactorial disease in particular, but will also become increasingly valuable for translational advances in disease monitoring and drug discovery and development

Translation of genomics into clinical practice

Information from the human genome sequence is set to alter many aspects of clinical practice. In the near term, knowledge of the genome will have a significant impact on the diagnostic capability of clinical genetics laboratories because molecular phenotyping using genetic and genomic information will allow for more timely and accurate prediction and diagnosis of disease and disease progression. This will provide the opportunity for medicine to become more focused on disease prevention, rather than the current model where the entire therapeutic endeavor is focused on the late stages of the disease.

Improving the therapeutic ratio of a given drug through enhancing efficacy and reducing toxicity are two of the most important goals of genomics and genetics in clinical practice. Translating the recent genetic insights into infectious diseases, cancer, asthma, and cardiovascular disease, for example, will create a new approach to clinical practice with many benefits to patients. In infectious diseases such as Hepatitis C and HIV, viral load or disease resistance can be rapidly and efficiently measured to inform and guide therapy early in the course of the disease caused by these persistent viruses. Furthermore, mutation screening can help to provide molecular profiling of drug resistance. Many non-infectious diseases will also benefit from the synergy of diagnostics and therapeutics. It is anticipated that new tools will allow identification of patients at risk in the presymptomatic phase of a disease such as BRCA gene-associated breast cancers. Personalized therapy will also be made possible by insights into individual pathophysiology and their responsiveness to therapy.

Common diseases are typically mechanistically heterogeneous as a result of interplay of multiple mutations, secondary genetic, and environmental factors. It is however possible that genetic disease-related polymorphisms could be used in conjunction with other factors to define population and individual risk. The first chip-based diagnostics are now available for predicting cytochrome P450 metabolism. As this enzyme is responsible for the oxidative metabolism of many drugs, it is a useful indicator of therapeutic response. It may also be possible to predict drug non-responders on the basis of polymorphisms in drug targets and pathways. This information may guide targeting of treatment with obvious cost-effectiveness benefits.

Diagnostic medicine that includes predisposition testing, early detection, stratified therapy, and therapeutic monitoring has not been systematically taught or applied in drug development to date.

The molecular targeted approach is currently being incorporated and validated in cancer care. For two of the three DNA-microarray multigene tests that are available, large prospective randomized trials are in progress in the management of early breast cancer. The TAILORx (Sparano, 2006) is validating the 16-gene signature marketed as Oncotype DX and the MINDACT (Mook, 2007) is validating the 70-gene signature marketed as MammaPrint. Diagnostic tests have traditionally been thought of as low-cost items in the healthcare chain, however, the new generation of molecular diagnostic tests will be similar in their impact to that of drugs in the management of patients.

The increased expenditure on molecular diagnostics could be off-set by the reduction in drug use, improved efficacy, reduced morbidity, minimized complications, and their management costs. Furthermore, these tests will assist in identifying patients who stand to gain most from a targeted therapy. Increasingly, drugs will be developed in conjunction with dedicated companion molecular diagnostic tests. At a superficial level this approach may seem threatening and unattractive to the pharmaceutical companies by reducing the size of the market. On the contrary, however, this approach improves the cost-effectiveness of a drug and expands market access. It may also reveal commonalities across tumors, for example, and potentially expand a drug's indications. The co-registration and approval of a drug and diagnostic test also expands the intellectual property of a patent and serves as a further hurdle to biosimilars (see Figure 5.2).

Translational medicine and drug development

The failure of R&D to deliver new medicines despite running more trials than ever before, testing more compounds than ever before, and spending more money than ever before, led the United States Food and Drug Administration (FDA) to undertake a comprehensive review referred to in the Challenge and Opportunity on the Critical Path to New Medical Products (http://www.fda.gov/oc/initiatives/criticalpath). Furthermore, this disappointment in productivity is despite the important recent advances in biomedical science just described. This report made reference to the importance and opportunities provided by translational medicine to improving

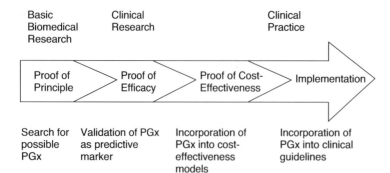

Figure 5.2 Clinical implementation of pharmacogenomics (PGx).

efficiency and effectiveness (early termination of a project) of the R&D process. Similarly, in the UK the report by Sir David Cooksey also refers to the opportunity provided by translational medicine.

Advances in technology have provided the opportunity for several translational approaches in drug development as described in the following three sections.

Phase 0 studies

One innovative approach to overcoming the stagnation in the critical path of drug development is the introduction of exploratory investigational new drug studies. These studies are performed early in Phase I and referred to as Phase 0 studies or microdosing studies. Their purpose is to assist in the go versus no-go decision-making process of a drug's fate earlier in the development process, using relevant human models rather than relying on animal data. This approach also assists to confirm important endpoints such as mechanism of action, pharmacology, bioavailability, pharmacodynamics, and metabolic microdose assessments. These studies of novel agents expose a small number of patients (<15) to a limited duration (<8 days) and dose range of single doses 100th of the predicted pharmacological dose given to healthy volunteers which are also less than 100 mg per day. Accelerator Mass Spectrometry (AMS) is used to generate PK information on these low doses.

There are important considerations before initiating a Phase 0, study such as having insight into the mechanism of action when evaluating pharmacodynamic effects, in order avoid misleading data. It is also important to have a biomarker when evaluat-

ing a drug target effect. The biomarker must be easy to measure and be validated. Microdosing studies are limited by the fact that because microdoses do not saturate metabolic pathways, microdosing data may not be truly predictive of pharmacokinetics at pharmacological doses. The use of AMS in mass balance, metabolite, and absolute bioavailability studies earlier in the development process provides the advantages of requiring smaller toxicological and stability packages, providing data to inform the choice of animal species for long-tem toxicology studies, obtaining absolute bioavailability for poorly soluble compounds, and improving safety for human volunteers.

Non-invasive imaging using tracer doses of imaging probes can be ideally applied in the Phase 0 setting. Imaging provides the opportunity to monitor effects in the whole body, whereas a biopsy looks only at a tiny sample. It also provides the opportunity to monitor the effects over time. There are several Phase 0 studies underway at the National Cancer Institute using positron emission tomography or single-photon emission computed tomography imaging modalities coupled with highly selective radiolabel probe molecules.

The design of a Phase 0 study should guide the endpoints in the subsequent studies and the information gathered in real time should be used to guide subsequent intervention studies. To enable this requires a multidisciplinary team of biostatisticians, clinicians, and basic and translational scientists. This is exemplified in the team who managed the Phase 0 trial of the novel oral Poly(ADP-Ribose) Polymerase inhibitor (Kummar *et al.*, 2009). Using information from the Phase 0 studies the compound was moved expeditiously into combination trials, and thereby bypassing the traditional monotherapy Phase I clinical trial. Phase 0 studies will make a contribution to more effective drug development.

Adaptive trial designs

Inefficiencies in clinical trials result from the high attrition rate of compounds due either to a failure to meet the efficacy criteria or because of excessive safety risks. The traditional model applied to clinical trial design is referred to as the frequentist model, has three distinct phases, and presupposes the following development steps: safety, optimal dose exploration, and finally efficacy assessment. This rigid approach is further limited by setting a hypothesis, performing a power calculation based on an effect size and its variability, and having to adhere to these assumptions until the trial is completed. One way round this problem is to use interim analysis, but this does come at a statistical cost with requirements to adjust the p value. So, typically in clinical trials, once the study has started there are no opportunities to review and modify agreed protocols until the completion of the study. Sample sizes and clinical endpoints are fixed before the study starts and one final analysis of efficacy and safety is made at the end of the study.

A more flexible model, also referred to as adaptive trial design, is defined as "a multistage study design that uses accumulating data to decide how to modify aspects of the study without undermining the validity and integrity of the trial." This approach may incorporate elements of the Bayesian statistical methods and computational analyses with complex numerical algorithms. Bayesian statistical approaches have also been applied to evaluate results that contradict prior evidence (Miksad, 2009). The advantages include the opportunity to make changes to a study in response to accumulating data while maintaining the trial's integrity and validity. Other potential advantages include the opportunity to maximize the study outcome, whether that is to stop the study early for positive or negative reasons or refine the study population with obvious time and costs saving benefits. Adaptive trial design allows

information gathering during the initial period of the trial (this could inform other related studies), which may lead to amendments to the protocol and statistical plan (see also pp. 114–117).

Adaptive trial designs are not a remedy for poor planning or even unforeseen difficulties, but instead a means of controlling the type 1 error and that early termination will reduce the totality of the evidence. They present many advantages over the traditional model such as improved decision-making, more comprehensive exploration of dose-response relationships, increased patient exposure to doses that are to be developed further, reduced cost, adjustment of ongoing trials that may be heading towards failure, and earlier termination of futile trials. The advances in technology that allow for real time access to clinical data (eCRF, patient diary, PK/PD data, etc.) make this approach a reality. The ever-decreasing pool of patients for clinical trials may be the ultimate driver for this approach to be incorporated in clinical development.

Biomarkers

The so called personalized or stratified evolution of medical practice is dependent on recognizing patient specific characteristics. Biomarkers have the potential to play an important role in diagnosis and in the identification of patients that could benefit from a targeted therapy. They also serve as markers of drug efficacy, and can be used to monitor treatment effectiveness, drug toxicity, and the development of drug resistance. The utility of a pharmacogenomic biomarker is best represented by the testing for Her-2/ERB2 over-expression in patients with breast cancer. Implementing biomarkers in clinical trials is a major aspect of translational medicine and will improve decision-making in clinical drug development. Biomarker development should follow the different stages of clinical trial development. For the early stages biomarkers can confirm molecular targets and help optimize dose schedules that may correlate with clinical benefit. In the later stages of clinical development, identified markers could be used to select the patients most likely to respond to the targeted agent. Any biomarker used as a basis for patient selection must demonstrate excellent sensitivity and specificity.

Biomarkers that act as surrogates for clinical benefits have the potential to be used as endpoints in clinical trials. Furthermore, biomarkers that correlate drug with outcome are of predictive value and have important cost-effectiveness benefits.

It is important that biomarkers are qualified and validated with the level of qualification dependent on the context of the biomarker's intended use. The FDA has proposed a path for qualification of preclinical safety biomarkers. Biomarkers are being employed in the pharmaceutical industry to facilitate go/no-go decision-making in Phase I and II clinical trials. The overarching role played by biomarkers in translational discovery and development is shown in Figure 5.3.

Translation of innovation and interdisciplinary skills

Interdisciplinary approaches are critical to the successful practice of translational medicine. It determines the way in which teams work and "how" becomes as important as "what" is achieved to exploit translational processes for therapeutic advances. Since translational medicine requires the successful integration of a number of different

scientific disciplines, competencies, and skills sets, the concept of interdisciplinary working is vital. The situation can be contrasted with multidisciplinary research in which each discipline works in a self-contained manner and there is little cross-fertilization between the disciplines.

The interdisciplinary approach uses the competencies from established disciplines, rather than the disciplines themselves, to solve new research questions. Two broad categories of interdisciplinary research have been described namely "problem" and "academically orientated" interactions. The former tackles the research question at a fundamental level and contributes towards the development of the discipline whereas the latter is typically more short term and directed at specific clinical problems. In the context of collaboration with academic medical institutions, generally interdisciplinary research is critical for overall success. It is noteworthy that medical charities are increasingly expecting an interdisciplinary approach because the integration of disciplines may provide new insights to tackle research questions that individual disciplines are unable to solve. Translational medicine approaches are being widely adopted by the pharmaceutical industry, leading to various levels of restructuring and reorganization.

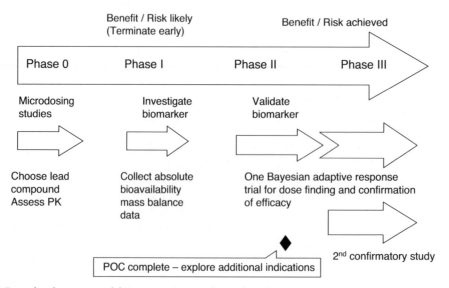

Figure 5.3 Drug development model incorporating translational medicine.

From a philosophical perspective it is important to be mindful of the limitations of the multidisciplinary approach to research, because it is constrained by the competencies and methodological approaches of the given disciplines, which to some degree dictate the outcomes to the research question. With the interdisciplinary approach the framework is less well defined. Systems Biology is an example of interdisciplinary working in practice because it uses bioinformatic tools and requires the competencies of biologists as well as mathematicians and computer scientists to develop in-silico models of biological systems.

Translational medicine encourages the application of interdisciplinary competencies and various institutions to progress important medical research questions. It promotes the translation from the reductionist approach to research questions, which focus on components (disease driven, additive), to that of systems science concentrating on interactions and dynamics, and spends less time studying the individual components (multidimensional, time sensitive, space sensitive, synergistic).

Training for translational medicine

For translational medicine to be truly successful, it requires practitioners who can work at the interface of an interdisciplinary system that integrates science, medicine, regulatory, and socio-economic sectors. We are now facing a pressing need for training that will enable successful cross-sector collaboration.

The UK has begun to address this requirement via a variety of clinical-scientist training schemes, which include the NIHR translational research schemes and those offered by the MRC and Wellcome Trust, the latter having extensive interaction with the pharmaceutical industry (http://www.wellcome.ac.uk/Funding/Biomedical-science/Grants/PhD-programmes-and-student ships/WTD027975.htm).

In the US, a number of clinician/physician-scientist training schemes provide multidisciplinary career development training programs at various levels and are frequently associated with General Clinical Research Centers and other interdisciplinary biomedical research organizations (http://nihroadmap.nih.gov/clinicalresearch/overview-training.asp).

The increased funding for translational medicine research in the UK and US will have the knock-on effect of enhancing the training of postdoctoral scientists in interdisciplinary biomedical research. However, additional schemes will be required to provide more specific training for those working at the translational interface.

The MSc in Translational Medicine offered by the University of Edinburgh (www.transmed.ed.ac.uk) is one program that has been specifically designed to address these needs because it delivers comprehensive training in the interacting scientific, medical, and regulatory facets required of translational medicine. This unique program is delivered wholly online and brings together working professionals from around the world engaged in medical, scientific, and regulatory sectors in academia, government, and industry.

Conclusion

The industrial revolution followed the application of much and varied innovation in engineering to the ultimate benefit of society. The bioscience sector has undergone significant advances in innovation over the last decade and it behoves pharmaceutical physicians to work effectively with other interdisciplinary colleagues to translate these advances to the ultimate benefit of patients. The pharmaceutical industry should therefore become more effective and efficient as a result of this revolution in the biosciences.

Those readers who are not convinced of the compelling argument for embracing translational medicine should be reminded of the investigation conducted in 1923 that followed various reports suggesting that brighter lighting may improve productivity. The study conducted in Western Electric's Hawthorne plant in Illinois revealed that when light levels were increased there was indeed an increase in productivity. Paradoxically, when light levels were reduced, an increase in productivity also followed. This phenomenon, in which simply the focus of increased attention, be it a trial or audit, results in an increased performance or recovery from illness, has now become known as the *Hawthorne Effect*. The traditional pharmaceutical business model needs to change and as Nye Bevan founder of the National Health Service in the UK stated, "we know what happens to people who stand in the middle of the road. They get run over."

Acknowledgement

The authors are grateful to members of the Translational Medicine Development Team at the University of Edinburgh for helpful advice and comments during the preparation of this chapter.

References

(Note: all websites cited in the text were accessed April 20, 2010.)

Aebersold R, Mann M. Mass spectrometry-based proteomics. *Nature* 2003; **422**:198–207.

Ahn AC, Tewari M, Poon C-S, *et al.*, The clinical applications of a systems approach. *PLoS Medicine* 2006; **3**:0956–0960.

Ansorge WJ. Next-generation DNA sequencing technologies. *New Biotechnology* 2009; **25**:195–203.

Auffray C, Chen Z, Hood L. Systems medicine: the future of medical genomics and healthcare. *Genome Medicine* 2009; **1**: doi:10.1186/gm2.

Azad SA, Rasool N, Annunziata CM, *et al.* Proteomics in clinical trials and practice. *Molecular and cellular Proteomics* 2006; **5**:1819–1829.

Bhattacharya S, Mariani TJ. Array of hope: expression profiling identifies disease biomarkers and mechanism. *Biochem Soc Trans* 2009; **37**:855–862.

Brown PO, Botstein D. Exploring the new world of the genome with DNA microarrays. *Nature Genetics Supplements* 1999; **21**:33–37.

Butcher EC, Berg EL, Kunkel EJ. Systems biology in drug discovery. *Nature Biotechnology* 2004; **22**:1253–1259.

Chin L, Gray JW. Translating insights from the cancer genome into clinical practice. *Nature* 2008; **452**:553–563.

Collins SR, Weissman JS, Krogan NJ. From information to knowledge: new technologies for defining gene function. *Nature Methods* 2009; **6**:721–723.

Deisboeck TS. Personalising medicine: a systems biology perspective. *Molecular Systems Biology* 2009; **5**: doi:10.1038/msb.2009.8.

Drakai A, Iliopoulos D. MicroRNA networks in oncognesis. *Curr Genomics* 2009; **10**(1):35–41.

Fan R, Vermesh O, Srivastava A, *et al.* Integrated barcode chips for rapid, multiplexed analysis of proteins in microliter quantities of blood. *Nature Biotechnology* 2008; **26**:1373–1378.

Hanash S. Disease proteomics. *Nature* 2003; **422**:226–232.

Hanash S. Integrated global profiling of cancer. *Nature Reviews Cancer* 2004; **4**:638–643.

Hood L, Heath JR, Phelps ME, *et al.* Systems biology and new technologies enable predictive and preventative medicine. *Science* 2004; **306**:640–643.

Hood L, Perlmutter RM. The impact of systems approaches on biological problems in drug discovery. *Nature biotechnology* 2004; **22**:1215–1217.

Kummar S, Kinders R, Gutierrez ME, *et al.* Phase 0 clinical trial of the poly (ADP-ribose) polymerase inhibitor ABT-888 in patients with advanced malignancies. *J Clin Oncol* 2009; **1**:27(16):2705–2711.

Mendrick DL, Schnackenberg L. Genomic and metabolomic advances in the identification of disease and adverse event biomarkers. *Biomarkers Med* 2009; **3**:605–615.

Miksad RA, Gonen M, Lynch TJ, *et al.* Interpreting trial results in light of conflicting evidence: a Bayesian analysis of adjuvant chemotherapy for non-small-cell lung cancer *J Clin Oncol* 2009; **27**:2245–2252.

Mook S. Individualisation of therapy using Mammoprint: from development to the MINDACT Trial. *Cancer Genomics Proteomics* 2007; **4**:147–155.

Oprea TI, Tropsha A, Faulon J-L, *et al.* Systems chemical biology. *Nature Chemical Biology* 2007; **3**:447–450.

Raza S, Robertson KA, Lacaze PA, *et al.* A logic-based diagram of signalling pathways central to macrophage activation. *Bmc Systems Biology* 2008; **2**.

Rho S, You S, Kim Y, *et al.* From proteomics toward systems biology: integration of different types of proteomics data into network models. *BMB Reports* 2008; **41**:184–193.

Sparono JA. TAILORx: trial assigning individualised options for treatment (Rx). *Clin Breast Cancer* 2006; **7**:347–350.

Schneider G, Fechner U Computer-based de novo design of drug-like molecules. *Nature Reviews Drug Discovery* 2005; **4**:649–663.

Schulze H, Giraud G, Crain J, *et al.* Multiplexed optical pathogen detection with lab-on-a-chip devices. *Biophotonics* 2009; **2**:199–211.

Shendure J, Ji H. Next-generation DNA sequencing. *Nature Biotechnology* 2008; 1135–1145.

Wang E, Lenferink A, O'Connor-McCourt O. Cancer systems biology: exploring cancer-associated genes on cellular networks. *Cell Mol Life Sci* 2007; **64**:1752–1762.

Wellcome Trust Case Control Consortium. Genome-wide association study of 14,000 cases of seven common diseases and 3,000 shared controls. *Nature* 2007; **447**: doi:10.1038/nature05911.

Zhang DY, Ye F, Gao L, *et al.* Proteomics, pathway array and signalling network-based medicine in cancer. *Cell Division* 2009; **4**:20: doi:10.1186/1747-1028-4-20.

CHAPTER 6

Pharmaceutics

Anthony W. Fox

EBD Group Inc., Carlsbad, CA, USA and Munich, Germany, and Skaggs SPPS, University of California, San Diego, USA

Introduction

It is a triumph of modern pharmaceutics that most of us give no thought to the difference between a white powder and a tablet, and think that "a drug is a drug is a drug." This huge presumption is doubtless because we no longer make pharmaceutical (or Gallenical) formulations ourselves, and precious few of us have even observed that complicated process. Nevertheless, it is important to understand some elements of this science for the following reasons:

• Packaged white powders are probably not marketable, and overcoming Gallenical problems is a *sine qua non* for product success.

• A suitable formulation permits the conduct of clinical trials.

• Formulations constrain clinical trial design. Among other things, likely bioavailability must be reconciled with toxicology coverage, well-matched placebos may or may not be available, and special procedures may be required (e.g., masking colored intravenous infusions).

• Product storage and stability (or lack thereof) can bias clinical trials results, and dictate shelf life in labeling.

• Formulation can strongly influence patient acceptability and compliance.

For all these reasons, and more, marketing and clinical input on suitable formulations should be included in the earliest considerations of project

Principles and Practice of Pharmaceutical Medicine, 3rd edition.
Edited by L.D. Edwards, A.W. Fox, P.D. Stonier.
© 2011 Blackwell Publishing Ltd.

feasibility, and it behooves the clinical researcher to be able to provide such input in an informed manner. Equally, we should understand the constraints, difficulties, and regulatory ramifications that all of our colleagues experience, including those in the research pharmacy. At the end of the day, product licenses are awarded and New Drug Applications (NDAs) are approved typically after the resolution of at least as many questions about "chemistry, manufacturing, and controls" (for which read "pharmaceutics") as about clinical efficacy and safety.

The constituents of a medicine

"A drug is not a drug is not a drug" because, when administered to a human being, in the general case, it contains the following:

• active compound at a dose that is precise and within a limited tolerance (sometimes as a racemate);

• manufacturing impurities;

• one or more excipients;

• degradants of the active compound;

• degradants of the impurities;

• degradants of the excipients.

Impurities

An *impurity* is defined as a compound that is the byproduct of the manufacturing process used for the active compound and has not been removed prior to formulation. Impurities can have their own toxic potential, and control of impurity content is therefore a highly important feature in any NDA.

Excipients

An *excipient* is defined as a material that is deliberately incorporated into the formulation to aid some physicochemical process. For example, excipients can enhance tablet integrity, dissolution, bioavailability, or taste. Excipients are typically chosen from among many compounds without pharmacological properties (e.g., lactose), although there are examples where pharmacokinetics change with the excipient used. There are specialized examples of excipients; for example, *propellants* are excipients that assist in the delivery of inhaled drugs to the respiratory tract. For intravenous infusions or ophthalmic products, the excipients are usually pH buffers or preservatives, and for dermatological products they may include emollients and solvents.

Degradants

A *degradant* is defined as a compound that cumulates during the storage of bulk drug or finished formulation. For example, the vinegar-like odor of old aspirin tablets is due to acetic acid, which is a degradant due to the hydrolysis of acetylsalicylate, which is an organic ester.

Formulation-associated intolerability

Many tablets carry printed identification markings or are color-coated; dyestuffs are special excipients, and allergies to them have been documented. Formulations also have more subtle, but nonetheless differential, characteristics, such as whether the tablet was compressed at a higher or lower pressure. Finally, differential efficacy exists among differently colored placebos, and this should therefore also be expected for active formulations.

Impurities and degradants can possess their own toxicological properties. Early in development, the structures of these impurities and degradants may be poorly characterized. Typically, both bulk drug and finished product become more refined as clinical development proceeds. Thus, in order to preclude any new toxicology problems developing later during clinical development, it is common practice to use the *less pure* bulk drug for toxicology studies. This is commonly accomplished by using drug removed from the production process before the last step, for example, before the last recrystallization. This usually guarantees that a lower purity, i.e., mixture with greater molecular diversity than the clinical supplies, will have been tested toxicologically than that to which patients will actually be exposed. The research clinician should always check the qualitative and quantitative impurity profiles of the batches used in the toxicology studies, as well as reviewing the allometrically-scaled proposed human experimental dose size.

The evasion of formulation and toxicological testing by "herbal medicine" manufacturers is completely illogical in this context. For example, the Butterbur (or Bog Rhubarb; *Petasites hybridus*) contains well-characterized carcinogens. Butterbur extract tablets are sold as chronic oral therapies for bladder dysfunction and migraine prevention, and are claimed to be innocuous on grounds of chemical purity, but without much biological, toxicological testing. Similarly, oral melatonin has an absolute bioavailability of about 15% maximum, and was eventually withdrawn in the United Kingdom and Japan after safety concerns arose (DeMuro *et al.*, 2000). The types and amounts of degradants and impurities in these products is unknown.

Formulation choice

The formulation chosen for particular drugs is not random, but the degree to which it is critical varies from drug to drug. For example, hydrocortisone is available in at least seven formulations: tablets, various creams and ointments, intraocular solutions, suppositories, intra-rectal foams, injections, and eardrops. Even newer drugs, with fewer indications than hydrocortisone, seek greater market acceptability by providing a variety of alternative formulations (e.g., sumatriptan is available as an injection, intranasal spray, suppository, and tablets).

One commonly used principle is to target drug delivery to the organ where beneficial effects are likely to occur. This can achieve

- relatively fast onset of effect;
- locally high drug concentrations;
- relatively low systemic drug concentration, avoiding toxicity.

Probably the most common applications of this principle are the administration of beta-adrenergic agonists bronchodilators by inhalation, and the use of topical hydrocortisone creams.

Formulation characterization

Various physicochemical properties of bulk drug can be measured. Some will be reasonably familiar from college biochemistry, for example, the one or more pK values for active drug or excipients, or the pH of drug solutions in specified aqueous solutions. Log P is a measure of *lipophilicity*, usually being measured as the octanol/water distribution coefficient when the aqueous phase is buffered at pH = 7.4. *Powder density* is the ratio of weight to volume occupied by a powder; some powder particles pack together more efficiently. A comparison between table salt and talcum powder is an illustration, the latter being less dense. *Particle size* and distribution is often measured using an infrared devices. *Maximum solubility* (x mg/ml) in various solvents is also often helpful not only to those whose task is to make drugs into prescribable pharmaceutical formulations, but also to toxicologists estimating a maximum feasible dose in a given species by a particular route of administration. *Hygroscopicity* is a measure of the capability of a drug to absorb water from the atmosphere; such drugs gain weight with time, and are often less stable than drugs lacking this property, and may predicate an aluminum foil packaging. Standard manuals such as *Merck Index* provide many of these data.

Specific formulations

Oral formulations include tablets, syrups, wafers, and suspensions depending upon the excipients. *Binders* are used to hold the various components together, and examples would be starch or polyvinylpyrrolidine (to which dogs exhibit a species-specific allergy). *Bulking agents* (sometimes called dilutants, or confusingly for a solid formulation, diluents) include lactose and cellulose; these increase tablet weight, which can improve production uniformity. Silica and starch can also be used to improve the flow of powder in mass production, when they are

known as *pro-glidants*. Stearic acid salts are used to enable tablets to escape from the press when finished, this being an unusual use of the term *lubricant*. *Coatings* are often sugars or cellulose and may be employed when a drug tastes foul. Particular color schemes can be created with dyestuffs or iron oxide.

Most wafer formulations dissolve in the mouth and are actually converted into a solution for swallowing and gastrointestinal absorption (e.g., rizatriptan-wafer). Benzocaine lozenges are intended for the same purpose but to dissolve more slowly, thus bathing the oesophagus as a symptomatic treatment (for example) for radiation oesophagitis; a similar approach is used with antifungal drugs.

Bioequivalence and generic products

Exemption from demonstration of efficacy for generic products is obtained only after bioequivalence with a prototype, approved product has been demonstrated. There is no regulatory requirement for innovative and generic drugs to have identical excipients.

The standards for bioequivalence are similar worldwide, but as a specimen we can use the *Code of Federal Regulations*, Title 21 (21CFR), parts 320.1–320.63 in the United States. The regulation states that bioequivalence is "…demonstrated if the product's rate and extent of absorption, as determined by comparison of measured parameters, e.g., concentration of active drug ingredient in the blood, urinary excretion rates, or pharmacological effects, do not indicate a significant difference from the reference material's rate and extent of absorption."

Traditionally, the data that have been most persuasive for demonstrating the bioequivalence of two formulations have been a pharmacokinetic comparison of the generic and reference drugs in humans. The most common study design is to compare two oral formulations with the following optimal design features (21CFR 320.26):

- Normal volunteers in the fasting state.
- Single-dose, randomized, crossover with well-defined reference material.

- Collection of blood samples for at least three half-times of elimination, and at a frequency that captures distribution phase, C_{max} and T_{max}, all at identical times post-dose for each formulation being compared.
- When there are major metabolites, collections should accommodate at least three half-times of their elimination.

In this case, the T_{max}, C_{max}, AUC, and half-time of elimination for parent drug and principal metabolites become the endpoints of the study. For combination therapies, these endpoints have to be measured and fulfilled for all active components, and they should not be administered separately.

The regulation does not define what a significant difference might be, although a commonly applied standard seems to be a formulation whose mean T_{max}, C_{max}, and AUC is within 20% of the reference material, and is also within the 95% confidence interval. However, these limits are tightened when

- the therapeutic ratio of the drug is low;
- the drug has solubility <5 mg/ml;
- tablet dissolution *in vitro* is slower than 50% in 30 minutes;
- the absolute bioavailability is <50%;
- there is extensive first pass metabolism that makes rate of absorption, as well as extent, a factor governing exposure;
- there are special physicochemical constraints such as chelation, complex formation, or crystallization to consider (see 21CFR 320.33).

There are also alternative ways to demonstrate bioequivalence. It may be possible to demonstrate bioequivalence using well-validated *in vitro* or animal methods, and these appear at 21CFR 320.24 (ii)–(iii). For example, two oral formulations can be compared with an intravenous dose of equal or unequal size. For drugs that are concentrated in the urine, but have negligible plasma concentrations (e.g., nitrofurantoin antibiotics), urine sampling with a frequency that matches the blood samples could be employed. Multiple dose bioequivalence study designs are also available. Rarely, the testing of bioequivalence at steady-state in patients is needed because normal volunteers would face an undue hazard, and patients cannot ethically be withdrawn from therapy (anti-retroviral agents are

one example). Chronopharmacological effect can also be exploited, that is, using pharmacodynamic data with a frequency and timing of endpoints in much the same way as for the blood samples described above. This can be useful for drugs that are not intended to be absorbed systemically, for example, the rate of onset and offset of local anesthesia to a standardized experimental injury.

Biological methods to demonstrate bioequivalence are not new: insulin batches have been standardized in this way for many years. At the time of writing (summer 2009), the United States Food and Drug Administration (FDA) is about to approve a generic antibiotic on the basis of tablet dissolution and *in vitro* bactericidal concentrations. These sorts of tactics will surely become more common as "follow-on biological" products find their regulatory pathway.

The Clinical Trials Directive now requires the filing of a clinical trial application for bioequivalence studies in normal volunteers or patients. In the United States, an Investigational New Drug (IND) application is always needed if the generic drug is without an approved innovator in the USA, is radioactive, or is a cytotoxic. However, when single- or multiple-dose studies in normal volunteers do not exceed the approved clinical dose sizes, and when retention samples will be available for inspection, there can be exemption from the need to file an IND. An IND is needed for a multiple dose bioequivalence study, when a single-dose study has not preceded it. The usual protections for human subjects are required, and, of course, these include an Institutional Review Board approval. Note that this is unlike the situation in Europe where the European Medicines Agency (EMA) guidance is that all active comparators (including those in bioequivalence studies) should be treated as investigational agents for regulatory purposes.

Sustained release oral formulations

By definition, sustained release formulations differ pharmaceutically and pharmacokinetically from the innovator drug. The excipients and particle sizes (usually larger) of the formulation are designed to dissolve more slowly, and these are almost always drugs for chronic diseases. The common advantages are reduction in dose frequency (and thus, hopefully, improved patient compliance; see Chapter 30), or reduction of C_{max} for a standard AUC, which can improve tolerability when adverse events are plasma concentration-related ("Type A" adverse events). Regulatory approval of these formulations usually hinges on the following factors (see 21CFR320.25(f)):

• Equivalence of area under the time–plasma concentration curve AUC to the prototype "rapid release" drug.
• Steady-state plasma concentrations that do not exceed, and are usually within a narrower range than, the prototype.
• Absence of any chance of "dose dumping," because the gross weight of active drug in a single slow-release capsule will always exceed that of a single dose of the prototype.
• Consistency of performance from dose to dose.

There are various formulation tactics. Active drug granules of larger size have smaller surface area to volume ratios and dissolve more slowly. These granules can also be coated with different thicknesses of polymer, and mixtures of these can be contained within a single capsule. Osmotically driven tablets slowly release drug through a small aperture during the entire traverse of the small bowel. Tablets can be compacted with layers that have different rates of dissolution, and can also be designed to release their contents only in relatively alkaline environments (i.e., beyond the ampulla of Vater). It is illogical to seek sustained release formulations for drugs with relatively long half-times of elimination (amiodarone, frovatriptan). Note that these are not generic compounds and have their own place in the US statutes at the *Food, Drugs and Cosmetics Act*, as currently amended 2007, section 505(b)2.

Oral transmucosal formulations

The best drugs for oral transmucosal administration are those that have high potency, good lipophilicity, and do not taste bad. For example, among opioids, the two drugs that have been successfully developed using this type of formulation are buprenorphine and fentanyl. The formulations and excipients include sublingual pellets, chewable gums, and sugary solids held on a stick, somewhat like a lollipop. Drugs that do not cross the oral mucosa readily can do so if held in place with an excipient that acts as a bioadhesive (see References/Further reading sections at the end of this chapter).

Gases

The physics of gases and the partial pressure at which they can achieve anesthesia is beyond the scope of this chapter. For one thing, this huge subject begs the question of how the state of anesthesia can be measured, and this is one of the more difficult clinical trial endpoints. One wit, a famous British cardiothoracic anesthesiologist, has commented: "If you can tell me what consciousness is, then I will tell you what anesthesia is!"

Gases are usually administered either "pure" (i.e., with limits on impurities) or in combination with excipients, for example, oxygen, air, or helium in the gas stream that is vaporizing a liquid halogenated hydrocarbon (validated vaporizers, usually designated for use with a single active compound, are required). When the route of administration includes mechanical ventilator (including a hand-squeezed bag), drug economy, occupational exposure of the staff, carbon dioxide scrubbing, and other pharmacokinetic problems emerge that are rarely encountered elsewhere. Gas flow can be measured with various devices, and exhaled gas concentrations (including carbon dioxide) can now be measured instantaneously. A rare adverse event, malignant hyperthermia, is associated with inhalation of halogenated hydrocarbons (as well as some depolarizing neuromuscular junction blocking drugs), and this can be treated with intravenous dantrolene (Strazis and Fox, 1993).

There are some uses for gaseous drugs outside of surgery. Nitrous oxide and oxygen mixtures are sometimes used as analgesics during labor, or when transferring patients in pain by road or helicopter. In very cold weather, nitrous oxide can liquify, reducing the delivered dose; shaking the container helps.

Helium/oxygen mixtures are used to improve oxygenation in patients with sub-total airways obstruction, exploiting the superior flow (pro-glidant) properties of the lighter gas. The use of this mixture, as prophylaxis against nitrogen narcosis at high inspired pressures (deep sea divers), or to minimize fire hazard is also well-described. Fire hazard due to oxygen (arguably a gaseous drug under some circumstances) is important. Patients are often burned when on oxygen therapy for lung disease that they are encouraging with an illicit cigarette. The disastrous fire inside the command capsule of Apollo 3, during a launch rehearsal on Pad 39B at Cape Kennedy, started in a pure oxygen, normal pressure, atmosphere. Reduction in total atmospheric pressure and adding excipient nitrogen has since been employed in all pressurized American space vehicles, but they still contain supra-atmospheric partial pressures of oxygen, and fire has broken out in the Russian-American Space Station.

Metered dose inhalers and nebulized drugs

In general, and with a few rare exceptions (see below), the inhaled route of administration is the most difficult that is commonly encountered. Metered dose inhalers and nebulizers are considered together here because they are both aerosols of drug solution.

In textbooks for a general audience, it is customary to insert, at this point, a graph that relates aerosol particle size to the penetration by drugs of various levels of the airway. Particles >10 μm are stated to impact in the pharynx, <5 μm are assumed to be ideal for alveolar delivery, and particles <0.05 μm are said not to impact at all, being liable to be exhaled. This is an oversimplification.

Inhaled particle deposition is actually dependent on a large number of factors, attested to by a vast literature in the fields of respiratory medicine, pulmonary physiology, and industrial hygiene. These factors include (with example studies) the following:
- coughing (Camner *et al.*, 1979);
- mucociliary action (Lippmann *et al.*, 1980);
- exercise and minute ventilation (Bennett *et al.*, 1985);
- mucous production and ability to expectorate (Agnew *et al.*, 1985);
- apnoeic pause at the end of inhalation (Legath *et al.*, 1988);
- whether or not the patient is actually having an asthma attack (Patel *et al.*, 1990);
- breathing pattern, airway calibre, device spacers, and reservoirs (Bennett, 1991);
- the physicochemical properties of the drug(s) (Zanen *et al.*, 1996);
- lung morphometry (Hoffmann, 1996);
- sampling techniques, on which exposure calculations are based (Cherrie and Aitken, 1999).

The reality is that it is impossible to measure accurately the lung deposition of inhaled drugs in humans.

Much vaunted *in vitro* studies actually use apparati that do not model well the anatomy of a human respiratory tree, let alone one that is diseased. The British Association for Lung Research has recognized this complexity and issued a consensus statement (Snell and Ganderton, 1998), which recommends, at a minimum, a 5-stage collection apparatus, examination of a range of particle sizes 0.05–5 μm, a range of flow rates and patterns to mimic the various physiological states, the development of an apparatus modeled on the shape of the human pharynx, regional lung assessments in three dimensions, the concomitant use of swallowed activated charcoal in to minimize systemic absorption of drug that was swallowed after impacting on the oropharynx, and further development of better statistics for analyzing the data.

The metered-dose inhaler has been in use for about 50 years and doubtless forms the mainstay for the treatment of asthma, as well as patients with chronic bronchitis with a reversible component. Great technical challenge has been experienced in the last few years due to the need to change excipients (propellants) in metered-dose inhalers, so as to avoid non-fluorohydrocarbon materials. In comparison with domestic refrigerators, industrial refrigeration plants, and cattle-generated methane, this contribution to protecting the atmospheric ozone layer must be negligible. Nonetheless, huge drug re-development costs were borne by health care systems worldwide in the late 1990s in anticipation of the unavailability of freons. In this case, although a bioequivalence approach has been taken when changing the propellant, the clinical studies have mostly relied on efficacy parameters (acute bronchodilation measured by spirometry), because not only of the inability to quantitate lung deposition, but also the irrelevance of systemic drug absorption (except from a safety point of view). Inhaled insulin is being studied on the basis of both pharmacodynamic and pharmacokinetic parameters.

A wide variety of nebulizers are now available. They all have their own physicochemical properties. In the absence of the ability to quantitate lung deposition, most modern product labeling specifies the combination of the drug with a particular nebulizer device (the labeling for alpha-dornase was the first to exhibit this change in regulatory policy). The corollary is that product development plans should decide, as early as possible, which nebulizer is intended for the market place, and that device should be used in all inhalational toxicology studies and subsequent clinical trials.

Intranasal formulations

The absorptive capacity of the nasal mucosa has been known for centuries: nicotine (Victorians using snuff) and cocaine (aboriginal peoples since time immemorial) are two historical examples of systemic drug absorption via the nose. The opposite pharmacokinetic aspiration is illustrated by anti-allergy and decongestant drugs, which are now administered to the noses of the developed world literally by the tonne: here the intent is to treat local symptoms and avoid significant systemic exposure of drugs with varied pharmacology such as alpha-adrenergic agonists, antihistamines, and corticosteroids. These products also contain buffers and preservatives that can cope with the acid-base problems of a normal nose (pH = about 5.5) or one with a cold (pH = about 7.4).

There is particular interest in the nasal mucosa because it can provide systemic absorption of drugs that otherwise must be administered by injection. These are often polypeptide drugs. Calcitonin and vasopressin-like drugs (nonapeptides) for diabetes insipidus in patients with panhypopituitarism are examples; the former benefits from lipisomal packaging (Chen *et al.*, 2009).

There is a specific guidance document from the International Conference on Harmonization that discusses the demonstration of bioequivalence for nasal sprays and aerosols. Although the intention of this guideline is to facilitate the development of generic products for use by this route of administration, it has been challenged on several scientific and technical grounds (e.g., Harrison, 2000).

Transdermal and topical formulations

The principal distinction between transdermal and topical drugs is that the former are intended for systemic drug delivery whereas the latter are not. Both drugs are subject to the same skin irritancy testing prior to human exposures; pre-clinical and clinical skin irritancy testing is reasonably stereotypical and commodity priced.

Biologically, the skin is designed to be a barrier. Evading this barrier is not easy, because drugs must traverse both live dermis and dead epidermis. Lipophilic drugs tends to form a reservoir in the former, even after traversing the hydrophobic latter. As in oral transmucosal administration, potent drugs with modest requirements for mass absorbed and reasonable lipophilicity are the best candidates for transdermal delivery: fentanyl, nicotine, and scopolamine are good examples.

Novel excipients for transdermal drug delivery include anodes and cathodes (*electroporators*). Under certain circumstances, the electric current that is thereby created (on the order of milliamps) can enhance the absorption of hydrophilic drugs across the skin (e.g., Pierce *et al.*, 2009). Under ideal circumstances, plasma concentration–time curves looking like slow intravenous infusions can be created.

Suppositories are probably the clearest illustration of cross-cultural differences in pharmaceuticals. A surgeon on a famous ocean liner has commented that: "Part of the problem stocking one's pharmacy is that one needs three times as many products as when working on land: Tablets for the Brits, shots (injectables) for the Yanks, and suppositories for the French!"

However, this route of administration is eminently logical, in several circumstances. For the acute treatment of migraine, oral drugs are often vomited (sumatriptan). For treating acute asthma, children often cannot use an inhalational device properly (theophyliine). For peri-operative antibiotics, patients are often nil by mouth (metronidazole). For inflammatory bowel disease, and proctitis, this is simply a topical administration.

Diazepam and paraldehyde administered rectally are effective for terminating a seizure, especially in children, without the need to find a vein. Use a glass syringe for the paraldehyde. The venous drainage of the lower part of the rectum is systemic, not portal, and thus first-pass clearance can also be evaded by this route.

Vaginal pessaries are suppositories designed for a more acidic environment (pH = about 5.5) than that found in the rectum (neutral pH). Topical uses include treatments for *Candida albicans* and *Trichomonas* infections, as well as for preparation of the cervix prior to induction of labor. Contraceptive devices are outside of the scope of a chapter on pharmaceutics, although the nonoxyl containing sponge pessary is a unique formulation, and there is also a polymer ring that releases estragens slowly for contraception after systemic absorption.

Injectates (s.c., i.m, i.v.)

The solubility of a drug, and the compatibility of a particular solvent with the site of injection, are inter-related factors governing the suitability of this route of administration, and the pharmaceutical formulation that is employed. The route of administration may also be governed by tolerability aspects associated with the formulation. If a drug cannot be dissolved in a concentrated manner in a suitable vehicle, the dose size must often increase. For example, intravenous injections of penicillin-type antibiotics are much more comfortable than when the same dose is administered intramuscularly.

Intravenous formulations are probably the least demanding of all injectates; the human vein is quite robust, although venous irritancy is often encountered in clinical trials. A surprising example of this robustness is seen when inducing anesthesia with thiopental sodium (sodium thiopentone). The upper limb veins tolerate these alkaline solutions with impunity, but they are very damaging when

occasionally and iatrogenically administered into the cubital fossa; a solution at pH = 9 can cause serious injury to the structures at the elbow, including the median nerve.

Organic solvents are often used to enhance the rate of absorption from subcutaneous or intramuscular sites of administration. For example, benzyl alcohol and sodium benzoate are used to dissolve diazepam, and extravasation of this formulation is not as serious a problem as for thiopental.

Water-soluble drugs are usually also hygroscopic. If not shipped and stored as solutions, an anhydrous environment is needed for product stability. This is most easily achieved as a lyophilized powder in an evacuated and sealed glass vial. This can be reconstituted with water or saline immediately prior to injection. Lyophilizates in stoppered vials can also be subjected to gamma irradiation to ensure sterility. Stability studies should include not only the range of temperatures and humidities (see below) but also with the vials inverted.

Rarely, adverse events are reported when an apparently innocuous formulation is administered by the wrong route. Usually these problems arise because of excipients in which the typical physician takes little interest. As one example, intravenous remifentanil is formulated with glycine, and hence it is not well-suited for epidural administration. The intravenous administration of liquid enteral diets is occasionally achieved, in spite of all precautions with non-Luer equipped tubing and prominent labeling; profound metabolic acidosis is the result.

The development of an injectate is often one tactic used for obtaining a patent. Even though a composition of matter patent (i.e., the structure of the drug molecule itself) may be old, the development of a non-obvious injectate, and its method of use for a new indication, may be sufficient to obtain a further patent and thus extend effective proprietary coverage. Such patents are usually stronger in the United States than in European jurisdictions.

Packaging

The selection of an inert package is an essential part of the pharmaceutical development of a drug. There are many standard stoppers, plastic and glass bottles, and so on with which regulatory authorities are very familiar, and for which drug master files are already in place. Stability studies must be conducted, of course, in the same sorts of packaging.

Packaging nonetheless degrades, and over a period of months or years an apparently impervious material may permit the ingress of water. Foil wraps are generally available for all tablets and are usually the most impervious of all materials; however, these can be inconvenient for arthritic hands. PVC blister packs are at the other end of the spectrum: Padfield (1985) has provided one example where a 0.8% increase in tablet weight within a PVC package occurred within 12 weeks.

Drugs, both investigational and prescription, are today transported over great distances. Airlines often advertise their cargo holds as being pressurized and temperature-controlled, but even so require special arrangements for the conveyance of livestock. The potential for condensation during unloading at a warm, humid airport, or degradation because the pallet sat for several hours on the unshaded tarmac in Dakar, is great.

Stability testing

Stability testing of drugs is its own sub-specialty. In brief, it is the research pharmacist's duty to stress-test drugs in storage using factorial combinations of
• low and high temperatures;
• low and high humidity;
• exceeding the labeled drug shelf-life;
• in contact with all feasible components of the packaging (e.g., both the glass and the stopper of a vial, the latter by inverted storage);
• exposure to bright and subdued light (in some case clear and amber glass bottles).

It is these data that justify the approval and continued marketing of a drug that complies with the "quality" criterion of the oft-quoted triad "safety, efficacy, quality." This is usually not a trivial exercise.

Innovation in pharmaceutics

Innovation has always been a very visible activity in pharmaceutics. As noted above, we very rarely administer powders out of paper cones today.

Particular drugs have driven innovation, even though the new formations later find broader use. For example, the dry-powder inhaler was initially devised for sodium cromoglycate (which is almost insoluble), but has now also helped to solve the hydrofluorocarbon propellant problem with metered-dose inhalers. The intravenous emulsion of propofol was unique, again being invented out of necessity, but is now also used for antifungal agents. There are several other examples of unique formulations or routes of administration that we may expect to be further exploited in the future. AIDS-associated infective retinitis is treated with a drug administered by intraocular injection, and the current parlous state of retinal detachment treatments suggests that this route of administration may find wider use.

What are we likely to see in the future? Novel pharmaceutical formulations seem to fall into two groups: those being used for gene therapy and those being used elsewhere.

Investigational gene therapies are comprised of two components: the DNA itself (the "construct") and usually a method of delivery (the "vector"). Naked DNA can be injected but its expression is inefficient. Vectors may include viruses. However, such viruses have to be human, and their attenuation sometimes is lost after administration, leading to very serious adverse events. Nonviral vectors can include targeted liposomes, microspheres, and emulsions.

Needleless injectors have been available for decades, and yet they still seem to be underused (the needleless injector used by Dr "Bones" McCoy of the *USS Enterprise* is clockwork, develops several thousand pounds pressure per square inch, and feels like a mild middle-finger percussion when used over the deltoid). A needle-free formulation of subcutaneous sumatriptan was approved in the United States during the summer of 2009 (Linn *et al.*, 2007).

Summary

The objective of this chapter has been to provide some appreciation of the complexity of pharmaceutical development. Conversance with the research pharmacist's terminology will help participation in team meetings where pharmaceutical and clinical development must be coordinated. A chapter on this scale will never equip the generalist to conduct pharmaceutical development. But, at the very least, it should now be clear that a drug is not a drug is not a drug.

References

Agnew JE, Pavia D, Clarke SW. Factors affecting the "alveolar deposition" of 5 microns inhaled particles in healthy subjects. *Clin Phys Physiol Meas* 1985; **6**: 27–36.

Bennett WD. Aerosolized drug delivery: fractional deposition of inhaled particles. *J Aerosol Med* 1991; **4**:223–227.

Bennett WD, Messina MS, Smaldone GC. Effect of exercise on deposition and subsequent retention of inhaled particles. *J Appl Physiol* 1985; **59**:1046–1054.

Camner P, Mossberg B, Philipson K, Strandberg K. Elimination of test particles from the human tracheobronchial tract by voluntary coughing. *Scand J Resp Dis* 1979; **60**:56–62.

Chen M, Li XR, Zhou YX, Yang KW, Chen XW, Deng Q, Liu Y, Ren LJ. Improved absorption of salmon calcitonin by ultraflexible lipisomes through intranasal delivery. *Peptides* 2009; **30**:1288–1295.

Cherrie JW, Aitken RJ. Measurement of human exposure to biologically relevant fractions of inhaled aerosols. *Occup Environ Med* 1999; **56**:747–752.

DeMuro RL, Nafziger AN, Blask DE, Menhinick AM, Bertino JS. The absolute bioavailability of oral melatonin. *J Clin Pharmacol* 2000; **40**:781–784.

Harrison LI. Commentary on the FDA draft guidance for bioequivalence studies for nasal aerosols and nasal sprays for local action: An industry view. *J Clin Pharmacol* 2000; **40**:701–707.

Hoffmann W. Modeling techniques for inhaled particle deposition: the state of the art. *J Aerosol Med* 1996; **9**:369–388.

Legath L, Naus A, Halik J. Determining the basic characteristics of aerosols suitable for studies of deposition in the respiratory tract. *J Hyg Epidemiol Microbiol Immunol* 1988; **32**:287–297.

Linn L, Boyd B, Iontchev H, King T, Farr SJ. The effects of system parameters on *in vivo* injection performance of a needle-free injector in human volunteers. *Pharm Res* 2007; **24**:1501–1507.

Lippmann M, Yeates DB, Albert RE. Deposition, retention, and clearance of inhaled particles. *Br J Industr Med* 1980; **37**:337–362.

Padfield JM. Making drugs into medicines. In *Pharmaceutical Medicine*, Burley DM, Binns TB (eds). Arnold: London, UK, and New York, USA, 1985, 51.

Patel P, Mukai D, Wilson AF. Dose-response effects of two sizes of monodisperse isoproterenol in mild asthma. *Am Rev Resp Dis* 1990; **141**:357–360.

Pierce M, Marbury T, O'Neill C, Siegel S, Du W, Sebree T. Zelrix: a novel transdermal forumation of sumatriptan. *Headache* 2009; **49**:817–825.

Snell NJ, Ganderton D. Assessing lung deposition of inhaled medications. Consensus statement from a workshop of the British Association for Lung Research, held at the Institute of Biology, London, UK, April 17, 1998. *Resp Med* 1999; **93**:123–133.

Strazis KP, Fox AW. Malignant hyperthermia: A review of published cases. *Anesth Analg* 1993; **77**:297–304.

Zanen P, Go LT, Lammers JW. Optimal particle size for beta 2 agonist and anticholinergic aerosols in patients with severe airflow obstruction. *Thorax* 1996; **51**:977–980.

Further reading

Madhav NV, Shakya AK, Shakya P, Singh K. Orotransmucosal drug delivery systems: a review. *J Control Release* 2009; **140**(1):2–11.

Sudhakar Y, Kuotsu K, Bandyopadhyay AK. Buccal bioadhesive drug delivery – a promising option for orally less efficient drugs. *J Control Release* 2006; **114**:15–40.

Zhang H, Zhang J, Streisand JB. Oral mucosal drug delivery: clinical pharmacokinetics and therapeutic applications. *Clin Pharmacokinet* 2002; **41**:661–680.

CHAPTER 7

Nonclinical Toxicology

Frederick Reno
Merritt Island, FL, USA

The evaluation of the safety of new pharmaceutical agents through nonclinical studies is a critical aspect of any development program. Usually in the discovery stage, or what can be considered the "research" phase of research and development, either *in vivo* or *in vitro* studies have established the pharmacological profile of the new drug and a rationale for its potential clinical efficacy. At this stage, the potential agent can be considered a new chemical entity (NCE) or perhaps an analog or metabolite of an existing one. Preliminary studies are also made with respect to drug absorption, metabolism, and excretion. In many companies, drug metabolism is a separate entity from the toxicology function but, for the sake of completeness of this chapter, a discussion of this important research area will be included. At some point, a decision is made to move the agent into the "development" phase, and the initiation of nonclinical toxicology studies necessary to establish safety for initial clinical trials is begun.

Historically, regulatory authorities in the USA, Europe, and Japan established their own guidelines for the types and extent of preclinical studies needed to support human research. Although often quite detailed, these jurisdictions were rarely similar; designing a nonclinical toxicology program that would be universally accepted was difficult, if not impossible. The International Conference on Harmonization (ICH), a tripartite group that consists of regulators and pharmaceutical company representatives from the three geographical areas, has now met for several years and harmonized many aspects of the drug development process, including preclinical toxicology. These guidelines (whether draft or final) will be identified throughout this chapter. In addition, all nonclinical toxicology studies that are intended to support clinical trials or marketing applications must be conducted in compliance with good laboratory practices (GLP; *Federal Register*, December, 1978). The volume edited by Williams and Hottenderf (1997) provides more information on the subjects that are discussed below.

Considerations related to the clinical development plan

The nature, timing, and extent of the initial nonclinical toxicology program depend on the clinical development plan that it must support. The ICH guidelines specify the extent and duration of nonclinical studies that are required to initiate or continue clinical studies (*Federal Register*, November 1997, and see below). Therefore, it is important that the clinical development plan, at least the initial stages, be clearly delineated.

Initial clinical studies
Usually, the initial clinical goals are to study tolerability and to provide initial animal pharmacokinetic assessments. These studies may only involve single doses of the drug administered to normal volunteers. Such a clinical study would require a restricted set of toxicity studies to support the safe use of the drug in this situation. On the other hand, some companies achieve economies by having the initial toxicology program be sufficient to support

Principles and Practice of Pharmaceutical Medicine, 3rd edition.
Edited by L.D. Edwards, A.W. Fox, P.D. Stonier.
© 2011 Blackwell Publishing Ltd.

not only initial clinical studies but also Phase II. The toxicology studies may then involve repeated doses over a period of weeks. Thus, the initial clinical studies must be determined before the nonclinical program can be designed.

Initial proof of principle

In most cases, a proof of principle (i.e., initial indication of clinical efficacy) during early Phase II clinical studies will require clinical treatment for some period of time, ranging from days (diagnostic agents, etc.) to weeks or months (for other types of drug). Since exposure of patients in clinical trials (in most cases) cannot last beyond the duration of the animal studies, careful consideration of the development schedule must be made, so that no delays are caused through lack of toxicological coverage. This requires that the appropriate preclinical reports are available prior to the planned initiation of the clinical trial.

Enrollment of women

Most regulatory agencies now request that women be enrolled into the clinical studies as early in Phase II as possible. Since the thalidomide tragedy, reproduction and teratology studies have been required prior to enrollment of large numbers of women in clinical studies. In some cases, depending upon the proposed indication for the drug, postmenopausal or otherwise reproductively incapable women can be used. However, the timing of the enrollment of women needs to be understood well in advance so that the lack of appropriate nonclinical reports does not hinder clinical development.

Consideration of regulatory strategy

Before the EU clinical trials directive (2001/20, implemented 2004–2005), it was common for American companies to carry out initial Phase I studies in Europe. This was because Phase I studies could often be initiated in The Netherlands or the UK, with little regulatory involvement, and with safety considerations being reviewed by an Institutional Review Board (IRB) or ethics committee, and

the company accepted the entire responsibility for any hazards or risks to the study subjects. This had the effect of allowing Phase I studies to be initiated more rapidly and thus obtaining information on preliminary safety and pharmacokinetic data earlier. This is no longer the case.

Initial nonclinical considerations

Of equal importance to the successful initiation of a nonclinical program are several factors that can have a great impact on the rapidity with which a program can be implemented. Experience has shown that overlooking the importance of these factors can result in unanticipated delays, costing time and money, and they are almost regardless of the regulatory constraints.

Formulation aspects

It is desirable for the pivotal nonclinical studies to be carried out using the proposed clinical route of administration, and with a formulation that either best approximates that anticipated for initial clinical usage, or if that is not possible, a formulation that is definitely *less* pure than that which will reach the clinic. Of course, this is unlikely to be the formulation that is eventually marketed should the program be successful. Scale-up of manufacturing processes can result in bulk drug with different impurities, and adverse effects may be due to parent drug, metabolites or impurities; hence, if the preclinical active pharmaceutical ingredient (API) is "dirty" (e.g., being removed from the production process before a final crystallization), it is more likely that the impurity profile in the clinic will have been exceeded, and that the animal toxicology will cover whatever the result of scale-up might be.

Furthermore, tablets or capsules cannot be given to most animal species, and the nonclinical studies are therefore carried out using dosing solutions or suspensions. The type of formulation can affect the pharmacokinetics of the drug, thus altering the toxicological profile, making comparison of animal and human pharmacokinetics, in the context of the formulations used, into a critical element in the evaluation of human safety.

Impurities/stability

Early-stage small-scale synthesis methods will often create a different profile of impurities or degradants than drug supplies produced by scaled-up processes. Every batch of drug used in nonclinical studies must have a certificate of analysis that clearly specifies the purity levels and the quantities of impurities (which may include residual solvents, unreacted starting materials, or degradants). The impurities must be reviewed in terms of the potential contribution that they can make to toxic effects that may be manifested in the nonclinical studies. There are ICH guidelines that pertain to impurities, and the extent to which additional toxicity studies need to be performed in impurities (*Federal Register*, January 4, 1996, March 19, 1996).

Of equal importance is the stability of the drug in the nonclinical formulation. This can determine whether the nonclinical formulations must be prepared daily or can be prepared weekly. If drugs are to be given orally, it is obvious that they must be resistant to degradation of gastric acids and must be stable in the formulation itself (water, carboxymethylcellulose suspensions, etc.). As will be discussed in more detail later, this requires the availability of an analytical method at the earliest stages of development.

Drug requirements

The amount of bulk drug that is typically required to carry out the nonclinical studies may be literally a "big" surprise. It is usually more than that needed for initial clinical studies. While many biologically derived drugs may require relatively small quantities, due to the potency of the material or the limited number of nonclinical studies that are possible (see below), a typical program need for "first time in humans" drugs that are relatively nontoxic may require 2–3 kg of active drug. For many companies, this can be difficult from either a manufacturing standpoint (small quantities synthesized prior to scale-up) or cost.

Analytical methods for dose and plasma determinations

GLP regulations require confirmation of the potency of all formulations used in nonclinical studies. Furthermore, current ICH guidelines also require toxicokinetic data (i.e., animal pharmacokinetics determined at one or more time points during a nonclinical toxicology study). Both the potency and toxicokinetic assays require an analytical method for the determination of parent drug (and possible major metabolites) in solvents and plasma, usually validated for multiple nonclinical species. This is not always a waste because cross-validating to biological matrices is usually easier when a GLP assay is already available.

Appropriate species

In the early stages of the development of any drug, there is little, if any, information on which to make a scientific judgment relative to the most appropriate animal species for nonclinical studies that will best predict responses in the human. In these cases, regulatory agencies generally require the use of the following:

• both a rodent and a non-rodent species (the typical approach would be to use rat and dog for the toxicity studies);
• mice or rabbits for reproductive toxicology;
• mice or rats for *in vivo* genotoxicology.

Primates may be needed when the background data suggest human-ididosyncratic properties among wanted and unwanted drug target receptors, whether in terms of hematology (e.g., rhesus antigen), blood chemistry (e.g., monoamine oxidase-A elimination), or histopathology (e.g., hepatitis C virus liver injury). Topical formulations are another special case, and the rabbit is commonly employed. The selection of the animal species for the nonclinical program is therefore often not straightforward.

When candidate drugs are proteins (e.g., animal-derived monoclonal antibodies), antibody formation may be major issue and this again may dictate the choice of species. For example, it may be known that only the chimpanzee does not develop neutralizing antibodies to the drug, which would lead one to select that species as the nonclinical model.

Toxicological support pre-IND and for Phase I clinical studies

The preliminary evaluation of the safety assessment of any Investigational New Drug (IND) requires multiple studies, some of which evaluate general and multiple endpoints (such as toxicity studies). Other studies evaluate more specific and defined endpoints (such as mutagenicity studies and safety pharmacology studies). Drugs that are derived from a biological origin, such as proteins, monoclonal antibodies, or drugs produced by biological vectors (or what are generally referred to as "biotechnology products"), present additional problems that require a significantly modified approach. The ICH guidelines recognize that unique approaches may be needed (and addresses this issue in a further guideline (ICH, 1997)), which poses additional problems for the toxicologist (Terrell and Green, 1994). This section will elaborate on those studies needed to support the safety of a typical xenobiotic agent, although the same general principles follow for biotechnology products, often being necessary but not sufficient. There are two types of guidelines that must be considered in initiating the nonclinical program. The first relates to the types of studies required; the second relates to protocol requirements for the studies themselves.

The types of studies needed are dictated by national regulatory requirement, although the ICH has promulgated a international guideline (*Federal Register*, November 25, 1997; ICH M3 second revision). These studies, outlined in Tables 7.1 and 7.2, vary somewhat by the phase of the clinical trial, and may still vary among countries where the trial is being conducted. The US Food and Drug Administration (FDA) has also published guidelines that outline the requirements necessary to initiate initial clinical studies (FDA, 1995; ICH S4). This latter document focuses more on the extent of study documentation required than the study types, and allows for data to be submitted that is not in final report form. The special case of QT prolongation (ICH S7B) is covered in Chapter 23.

The following sections briefly describe the studies that would typically be performed to support initial studies in humana. Additional specialized studies

Table 7.1 Duration of repeated-dose toxicity studies to support Phase I and II clinical trials in the EU, and Phase I, II, and III clinical trials in the USA and Japan[a]

Duration of clinical trial	Minimum duration of repeated-dose toxicity studies	
	Rodents	Non-rodents
Single dose	2–4 weeks[b]	2 weeks
≤ 2 weeks	2–4 weeks[b]	2 weeks
≤ 1 month	1 month	1 month
≤ 3 months	3 months	3 months
≤ 6 months	6 months	6 months[c]
> 6 months	6 months	chronic[c]

[a] In Japan, if there are no Phase II clinical trials of equivalent duration to the proposed Phase III trials, nonclinical toxicology studies of the durations shown in Table 6.2 should be considered.
[b] In the EU and USA, 2-week studies are the minimum duration. In Japan, 2-week non-rodent and 4-week rodent studies are needed. In the USA, with FDA concurrence, single-dose toxicity studies with extended examinations can support single-dose human exposures.
[c] Data from 6 months of administration in non-rodents should be available before clinical exposures of more than 3 months. Alternatively, if applicable, data from a 9-month non-rodent study should be available before clinical treatment duration exceeds that supported by other toxicology studies.

Table 7.2 Duration of repeated-dose toxicity studies to support Phase III clinical trials in the EU, and product marketing in all jurisdictions[a]

Duration of clinical trial	Minimum duration of repeated-dose toxicity studies	
	Rodents	Non-rodents
≤ 2 weeks	1 month	1 month
≤ 1 month	3 months	3 months
≤ 3 months	6 months	3 months
> 3 months	6 months	Chronic

[a] The table reflects the marketing recommendations in all three ICH regions, except that a chronic non-rodent study is recommended for clinical use >1 month in Japan.

might be needed in order to study the potential for an effect that may be characteristic of drugs in the particular class in question (e.g., antibody determinations for some biological products, neurotoxicity studies for drugs acting on the central nervous system, etc.).

Acute toxicity studies

Single-dose studies in animals are an important first step in establishing a safety profile. Note, however, that the calculation of an LD_{50} is no longer required or scientifically necessary. The aim of single-dose studies is to explore a range of doses. Identification of doses without drug-related effects, a dose that produces some level of exaggerated effect (not necessarily death) that helps identify potential side effects, and other doses in between helps all further toxicological (and clinical) tolerability assessments. These studies can be designed using "up-and-down" (Dixon Design) dose regimens or other tactics to reduce the time and number of animals required. These studies may then guide dose selection for the first repeated-dose studies. Various guidelines for the performance of these studies are available, and the ICH has also published its own guideline (see *Federal Register*, August 26, 1996).

Repeated-dose toxicity studies

Repeated-dose studies are designed to identify safe levels of the drug following treatment regimens that are designed to provide continuous exposure of the animals to the test drug for a defined interval. Ideally, the route of administration should mimic that planned in humans, and the animal studies should involve longer durations of exposure and higher doses than those planned clinically. The type and duration of specific studies, and which ones are needed relative to different stages of clinical development, were mentioned previously (*Federal Register*, November 25, 1997; ICH M3 second revision). Protocols must specify the number of animals per group, numbers of groups and experimental procedures to be carried out, and standard versions of these have been available for some time. In general, for initial repeated-dose studies, protocols require the use of three dose groups plus a control, and a minimum of ten rodents and three non-

rodents per sex per group. Doses must be selected that will allow for the identification of toxic effects at the highest dose as well as a no-effect level at the middle or lowest dose.

Usual experimental procedures include the determination of body weights and food consumption on at least a weekly basis, evaluation of hematology and blood chemistry parameters during the treatment period, ophthalmoscopic examinations, the recording of macroscopic examinations at necropsy, and the determination of organ weights. A complete histopathological examination of tissues from animals is required. In rodent studies, this can take the form of examination of all high-dose and control animals and the examination of target organs at the two lower doses. In non-rodent studies, it is typical to examine tissues from all animals in the study.

It is crucial that plasma concentrations of drug are measured in these studies to allow for determination of effects on the basis of exposure ("toxicokinetics"). Frequently this is a more appropriate measure of comparing effects in animals and humans, because rates of absorption, distribution, and excretion can vary extensively between these species. An ICH guideline (*Federal Register*, March 1, 1995) specifies minimum requirements in terms of the number of time-points examined, number of animals per time-point, and the requirements for calculation of various pharmacokinetic parameters such as C_{max}, AUC, and so on. These will become important for comparison with human data as they become available later.

Mutagenicity studies

There are multiple hereditary components in both somatic and germinal cells that may be affected by drugs, and mutagenicity studies are highly specialized (ICH S2A). During the 1970s, it was thought (somewhat naïvely) that these studies may be replacements for the long and costly carcinogenicity studies that are required for many drugs (see ICH S1B and S1C, revised). Although this goal was never realized, mutagenicity studies nonetheless provide useful indications of the ability of a drug to alter genetic material, which may later be manifested in studies of carcinogenic or teratogenic effects (Kowalski, 2001). Genotoxicity studies are relatively inexpensive and may also serve, early in the drug development process, to assure drug developers and regulators that no obvious risk of such adverse effects exists, albeit knowing that more definitive studies to evaluate teratogenic and carcinogenic effects will not come until later.

An exhaustive review of the various components of a mutagenicity evaluation will not be attempted here: Multiple guidelines are available. Those issued by the ICH include general guidelines (*Federal Register*, April 24, 1996; ICH S2A) and specifics related to the core battery of studies required (*Federal Register*, April 3, 1997). Tennant *et al.* (1986) have summarized the correlation between the results of a battery of mutagenicity assays and the probability of the material producing a positive carcinogenic response in long-term rodent studies. Obviously, mutagenicity studies cannot address issues of non-genetic carcinogenicity or teratogenicity (e.g., sex steroids).

Positive results in one or more mutagenicity assays do not necessarily translate into human risks. Mechanistic studies may show that such responses would not occur in the human cell population, or the concentrations at which positive responses occurred may far exceed any concentration of drug that may occur in the clinical setting. Many drugs are on the market today that have produced some type of positive response in these studies and yet it has been concluded that no human risk is present or the potential risk is not known (e.g., aspirin causes chromosomal breaks). A fairly standard, worked example is provided by Fox *et al.* (1996).

Pharmacokinetic studies

In the early stages of drug development, it is crucial to identify important parameters that relate to the absorption and excretion pathways for the drug. In the later stages of development, studies on the extent of tissue distribution and the identification of metabolites become important. Another reason why this is important is that it assists the investigator in knowing that the appropriate species has been selected for the nonclinical toxicology program. It is vital to human safety evaluation that

the nonclinical models chosen are representative of the metabolism of the drug in humans. Therefore, it is necessary to have pharmacokinetic information early in the program, so that it can be compared to the data generated in the early clinical studies.

Drug metabolism is another specialized field, and its sophistication is increasing all the time. A relatively new technique that is available to the preclinical investigator is the use of *in vitro* methods to establish and confirm similar mechanisms in drug metabolism between animals and humans (see Chapter 9). These procedures involve the use of liver slices and/or liver hepatocyte homogenates and can be done in human and animal cultures at the earliest stages of drug development.

Toxicokinetic data is generally obtained from repeated-dose toxicity studies, and generally determines whether: (a) the plasma concentrations of the drug increase in a linear fashion over the range of the increasing doses used in the studies; (b) plasma concentrations increase over time, suggesting an accumulation of the drug in plasma or tissues; (c) there is a relationship between the plasma concentrations of the drug (or metabolites) and the toxicity associated with higher levels of the drug; and (d) the effects are more closely related to peak concentrations or to overall exposure (measured by the area under the concentration time curve, AUC).

Toxicokinetic data are generally collected on the first day of dosing in a repeated-dose study, and near the last day of dosing, that is during the last week and at steady-state of a 90 day toxicity study. In rodent studies, satellite groups of animals may be required due to the blood volumes needed for assay. For larger non-rodents, the main study animals can usually provide the samples. Guidelines have been made available covering most aspects of the collection and analysis of these data (*Federal Register*, March 1, 1995).

Finally, pharmacokinetic assessment requires tissue distribution studies in nonclinical models to determine the extent of localization of the drug in tissues. In some situations, where single-dose tissue distribution studies suggest drug localization, a tissue distribution study following repeated dosing may be indicated. The conditions under which such studies may be necessary have been delineated in an ICH guideline (*Federal Register*, March 1, 1997; ICH S3A).

Safety pharmacology

Studies related to safety pharmacology (sometimes confusingly termed "general pharmacology" studies) tend now also to be performed earlier in the drug development process than was previously the case. Although in some respects considered an aspect of the discipline of pharmacology, the purpose of safety pharmacology is to evaluate the potential pharmacological properties that may be unrelated to the intended indication for the drug. An example of this would be significant effects of a drug on the cardiovascular system that may in fact be under development for the treatment of gastric ulcers.

Most major developed countries have stated guidelines indicating that safety pharmacology studies are required. Table 7.3 lists the guidelines from major countries. As can be seen from these guidelines, it is not always clear when such studies are required. All of the major organ systems need to be evaluated, and therefore studies need to be performed that would identify potential effects on the central nervous, cardiovascular, and gastrointestinal systems, as well as an evaluation of renal function and possibly immunogenicity (see US FDA Draft Guidance for Industry *Immunotoxicology Evaluation of Investigational New Drugs*, April 2001).

Like many other disciplines, there are a multitude of protocols and procedures that can be followed for each pharmacology study, and a comprehensive review of all of them is beyond the scope of this discussion. Those pertaining to QT prolongation are described in more detail in Chapter 23.

Nonclinical summary documents

Prior to starting initial studies in humans, it is important that all the nonclinical information available is formed into an integrated summary. This information must be included in the clinical investigators' brochure so that the clinical protocol can be modified to include relevant biochemical or other markers to minimize human risk. The regulatory authority and ethics committees are further target audiences, and the company may wish to use this for formal internal proceedings to justify the decision to proceed with initial human exposure.

Toxicological support for Phase II and III studies

Nonclinical toxicology studies required to support Phase II and III stages of the program depend upon

Table 7.3 International regulatory guidelines for safety pharmacology studies (excerpts from international regulatory documents)

USA: "Studies that otherwise define the pharmacological properties of the drug or are pertinent to possible adverse effects" (21CFR314.50, para 2).

EU: "A general pharmacological characterization of the substance, with special reference to collateral effects" (EC Directive 91/507/EEC).

UK: "A general pharmacological profile of the substance is required, with special reference to collateral effects ... the aim should be to establish a pattern of pharmacological activity within major physiological systems using a variety of experimental models" (MAL2, p. A3F-1).

Canada: "Secondary actions—studies related to secondary pharmacological actions of the new drug which may be relevant to expected use or to adverse effects of the new drug" (Canada RA5, exhibit 2, p. 21).

Australia: "Studies should reveal potentially useful and harmful properties of the drug in a quantitative manner, which will permit an assessment of the therapeutic risk ... Investigations of the general pharmacological profile should be carried out" (Guidelines under the Clinical Trial Exemption Scheme, pp. 12, 15)

Nordic countries: New drugs should be studied in a biological screening program so as to define any action over and above that which is desirable for the therapeutic use of the product.

Japan: "The objective of general pharmacological studies is to examine extensively the kind and potency of actions other than the primary pharmacological actions, predict potential adverse effects likely to manifest in clinical practice..." (Japanese Guidelines, 29 January 1991).

---

a variety of factors. First, as shown in Tables 7.1 and 7.2, the ultimate clinical regimen, that is, duration of therapy or treatment, determines the ultimate duration of the animal studies. For example, a diagnostic agent or a drug with a 3–4 day regimen (as might be the case in general anesthesia, or for disease or trauma situations that are handled in the intensive care unit) may require little in the way of additional repeated-dose toxicity studies. In comparison, a new antihypertensive agent may require all of the longer-term studies.

Second, the drug development strategy established by the company may call for the availability of proof of absorption and perhaps even preliminary proof of efficacy (sometimes called "proof of principle") before expending resources for the longer and more expensive studies. On the other hand, the company may have determined that the drug in question is on a "fast track," and is willing to expend resources early and at risk, in the hopes of getting an earlier marketing approval. The following sections summarize the areas that need to be addressed in the usual cases.

Chronic toxicity studies

As discussed above, the extent of additional repeated-dose studies are generally outlined in Table 7.2. The maximum duration of chronic studies is generally 6 months, except for carcinogenicity testing (see below). The ICH guidelines describe situations where studies of 9–12 months duration in a non-rodent species may be necessary, particularly for the US FDA for product approval, and note how these differ from those needed for the conduct of clinical trials (ICH M3 second revision).

Protocols for these studies are similar to those for studies of shorter duration. A minimum of 10–15 rodents/group and four non-rodents/sex/group are usually required, thus being somewhat larger than in the earlier toxicology studies. Toxicokinetic measurements are still required. The usual in-life and post-mortem observations are performed, as described above.

Reproductive and teratology studies

The thalidomide tragedy demonstrated the need to evaluate new drugs in reproductive toxicol-

ogy studies. Some of the earliest guidelines were issued by the US FDA (the "Goldenthal guidelines"). An ICH guideline now covers the performance of these studies (*Federal Register*, September 22, 1994; ICH S5 second revision), as amended in 1995 to address possible effects on male reproduction.

In general, there are three phases of the reproductive process that are evaluated. The first phase (historically referred to as "Segment I study," and now under ICH as "Stage A") evaluates the effect of the new drug on fertility and the early implantation stages of embryogenesis. In these studies, breeding animals of one species (usually rats or rabbits) of both sexes are treated for 2 or more weeks prior to mating, and then the females are further dosed until day 6 of gestation. The second stage of testing (historically "Segment II studies," now "ICH Stage B studies") is the teratology study (sometimes termed "the developmental toxicity study") and is done in both of the same two species. The third stage ("Segment III" or "ICH Stage C") evaluates treatment during late gestation, parturition, and lactation. Behavioral and neurodevelopmental assessments in the offspring are often made in Segment III studies. In some cases, two of the studies can be combined and still satisfy the ICH guideline.

The period in the drug development process at which results of these studies are required varies somewhat from country to country, and is discussed in the ICH guideline. Hoyer (2001) reviews the current situation, and provides additional perspective.

Carcinogenicity studies

Carcinogenicity studies involve the treatment of rodents for long periods of time (18 months to 2 years) in order to determine whether the material possesses the capability to initiate or promote the development of tumors. The relevance of these models to the human situation has been debated for many years. Carcinogenicity studies have been required for all drugs where clinical therapy may extend for 6 months or longer, and some regulatory authorities demand them even for shorter clinical ratment courses. Although the scientific debate about relevance of these studies continues, they remain required by regulation.

Several different ICH guidelines have been issued that address the various aspects of the carcinogenicity testing of drugs, including when studies are needed (duration of clinical therapy; *Federal Register*, March 1, 1996; ICH S1C, revised). Other features of the new drug may mandate carcinogenicity testing, such as structure–activity similarities to known carcinogens, evidence of preneoplastic lesions in repeated-dose nonclinical studies, or long-term tissue sequestration of the drug. Another guideline (ICH S1C) addresses the complex issue of the selection of doses for these studies; this responds to much criticism of the prior recommendation to use the maximum tolerated dose (which had been suggested by the National Toxicology Program; Haseman and Lockhart, 1994). The current ICH guideline recommends a high dose causing up to a 25-fold greater plasma AUC in rodents compared to the AUC in humans at steady state. A subsequent amendment to this guideline (*Federal Register*, December 4, 1997; ICH S1C revised) adds a further proviso that the highest dose in a carcinogenicity study need not exceed 1500 mg/kg/day when (a) there is no evidence of genotoxicity and (b) the maximum recommended human dose is no bigger than 500 mg/day. The basis for species selection, circumstances needing mechanistic studies, and exploitation of pharmacokinetic information in carcinogenicity testing is described in yet another guideline (*Federal Register*, August 21, 1996; ICH S1B).

Modern protocols for carcinogenicity studies have changed little since first established in the early 1970s. In recent years, the use of mice (historically the second of the two required species in addition to rats) has come under scrutiny because they may be inappropriate models, with unusual sensitivity to certain classes of chlorinated hydrocarbons. The most recent ICH guideline (*Federal Register*, August 21, 1996; ICH S1B) allows for the option of using transgenic mice and study designs of somewhat shorter duration.

Of growing importance is the interaction of factors that are critical to a successful toxicology program. For example, if a transgenic mouse model is selected, the choice of strain is important and may depend upon whether the drug is non-genotoxic (TG.AC model, ras*H*2 or genotoxic p53 model). Metabolic and pharmacokinetic data are important to ensure that the selected models handle and metabolize the drug in a fashion at least reasonably similar to humans, and may vary for the same drug according to the toxic effect of interest. Perhaps the most important factor is the relevance of the doses selected to those in humans. A recent review of the status of carcinogenicity testing (Reno, 1997) addresses the many factors that should be considered in a carcinogenicity program.

Special studies

It is not uncommon in drug development programs for specific toxicities to be uncovered. In most cases, additional studies are then carried out that will attempt to elucidate additional information with regard to the mechanism of the effect. For example, the identification of a non-specific behavioral effect (e.g., tremors and/or convulsions) may trigger the performance of a neurotoxicity study, which includes an exhaustive evaluation of the potential effects on central and peripheral nervous tissues. The identification of an effect on reproduction may warrant the performance of detailed studies to identify the specific mechanism or phase of the reproductive cycle that is affected. In-depth metabolic studies may prove that the effect is related to a metabolite in animals that has no relevance to humans, and prevent the abandonment of an otherwise promising drug. It is rare that a drug development program does not involve some type of special study.

NDA requirements

Format and content of the application

The FDA, in what was referred to as the "New Drug Application (NDA) Rewrite," issued guidelines for how a nonclinical section of an NDA should be organized (the guideline contains not only requirements on what is required, but also a basic table of contents for this document); its electronic construction is intricate but beyond the scope of this chapter. But within the NDA, the integrated pharmacology and toxicology summary is crucial. This document contains an overview of all studies that were conducted, how the pharmacology, pharmacokinetic, and toxicology study information is interrelated (Peck *et al.*, 1992), and what significance the data have to human safety. A well-written integrated summary can be beneficial not only to the regulator, but also to the NDA sponsor. Some of the information in this summary will also be needed for the package insert. Crucially, it should include comparisons between effects seen in animals and the likelihood that such findings would be expected in clinical usage. These comparisons are often quantitative, and must be made both on a mg/kg and a surface area (mg/m^2) basis (Voisin *et al.*, 1990).

CANDA requirements

The Computer Assisted NDA (CANDA) refers to the submission of data to the FDA in machine-readable form. At the present time, it is required that, at a minimum, the data from the carcinogenicity studies be submitted to the agency in a specified format that is available from the FDA. This allows the agency to apply its own criteria and statistics to the data and independently confirm the sponsor's conclusions. This agency review is then submitted to the FDA's Carcinogenicity Assessment Committee for final review and conclusions.

Expert reports

The European Community, and other countries, require several expert reports in each dossier, one of which examines the nonclinical toxicology of the new drug. These documents are typically about 20–30 pages long and summarize all the toxicology data, as well as the clinical implications.

Much material from the US integrated summary (if any) described above may be reused in this report, with the exception of the expert, who must personally sign the report. Expert reports contain the expert's résumé, and part of the regulatory review process is to evaluate whether the expert is actually qualified for this role. The choice

of expert is important, and his or her independence is crucial because the role is that of a reviewer, not of a sponsor. Experts may nonetheless be drawn from within the sponsoring company with appropriate protections, although those from outside may carry more credibility in some jurisdictions.

Summary

The obvious advice to any clinical trialist is to get the toxicologist in and do so early on the project. The scale and timing of the studies are rarely automatic, and must be designed so as to always be ahead of the needs of the clinical trial program. The complexities about dose size, species choice, and duration of exposure, together with the toxicology study endpoints, have been outlined above, but are not decisions for the inexperienced. Finally, in spite of ICH, there are still differences in practice between regulatory authorities in this field, and toxicology is often a useful subject for discussion at scientific advice meetings in Europe and their equivalent in Canada and the USA.

References

(Note: all references for US FDA guidelines (draft or final) and ICH guidances can be found at www.fda.gov (accessed April 20, 2010.)

Fox AW, Yang X, Murli H, Lawlor TE, Cifone MA, Reno FE. Absence of mutagenic effects of sodium dichloroacetate. *Fund Appl Tox* 1996; **32**:87–95.

Hoyer PB. Reproductive toxicology: current and future directions. *Biochem Pharmacol* 2001; **62**:1557–1564.

Kowalski LA. In vitro carcinogenicity testing: present and future perspectives in pharmaceutical development. *Cure Opin Drug Discov Devel* 2001; **4**:29–35.

Peck CC, Barr WH, Benet LZ, *et al.* Opportunities for integration of pharmacokinetics, Pharmacodynamics, and toxicokinetics in rational drug development. *Clin Pharmacol Ther* 1992; **51**:465–473.

Reno FE. Carcinogenicity studies. In *Comprehensive Toxicology Vol 2: Toxicological Testing and Evaluation*, Williams PD, Hottendorf GH (eds). Elsevier: London, UK, 1997, 121–131.

Tennant RW, Stasiewicz S, Spalding JW. Comparison of Multiple parameters of rodent carcinogenicity and in vitro genetic toxicity *Environ Mutagen* 1986;**8**:205–227.

Terrell TG, Green JD. Issues with biotechnology products in toxicologic pathology. *Toxicol Pathol* 1994; **22**:187–193.

Voisin EM, Ruthsatz M, Collins JM, Hoyle PC. Extrapolation of animal toxicity to humans: interspecies comparisons in drug development. *Regulat Toxicol Pharmacol* 1990; **12**:107–116.

Williams PD, Hottendof GH (eds). *Comprehensive Toxicology Vol.2: Toxicological testing & Evaluation*. Elsevier: London, 1997.

CHAPTER 8

Informed Consent

Anthony W. Fox

EBD Group Inc., Carlsbad, CA, USA and Munich, Germany, and Skaggs SPPS, University of California, San Diego, USA

Introduction

There is a tendency to assume that the principles of informed consent are self-evident. In fact, evidence that this is not the case comes from many sources. Ethics committees are frequently dissatisfied with proposed informed consent documents. Sophisticated Western governments, from time to time, have conducted clinical trials without it (e.g., the Tuskeegee travesty). A recent gene therapy accident in an eminent university in the United States led to the death of the participant; the subsequent litigation centered not around whether the clinical trial was unduly hazardous, but rather on whether the consent that the patient gave was truly and fully informed. Unless stated, this chapter envisions informed consent in the testing of investigational medicinal products.

Codification of informed consent began with the Declaration of Helsinki, and in response to the atrocities of the Second World War. The principles of informed consent have been under continuous review and discussion ever since. This is to be expected when reasonable standards of informed consent are dependent not only upon the design of a particular study, but also on environmental factors, the current state of medicine, and particular local characteristics of clinical trials populations, all of which are themselves continuously changing.

Principles and Practice of Pharmaceutical Medicine, 3rd edition.
Edited by L.D. Edwards, A.W. Fox, P.D. Stonier.
© 2011 Blackwell Publishing Ltd.

Ethical basis

Although enlarged upon elsewhere in this book, the two ethical principles guiding informed consent are those of *autonomy* and *equipoise*. *Autonomy* is the concept that the patient is an individual under no duress, whether subtle or obvious, actual or inferred, who is competent to make a choice according to his or her free will. Clinical trials conducted on persons in custody, or on subordinate soldiers, may both be violations of the patient's autonomy. *Equipoise* is the concept that the investigator, and those sponsoring the trial, are truly uncertain as to the outcome of the study. In practical terms, equipoise guarantees that the patient will not be disadvantaged by unfavorable randomization because the treatment options are known to have equivalent risk-benefit assessment.

Written informed consent

The large majority of clinical trials use a written informed consent document. In the absence of any special circumstances, the essential elements of such a document are as follows:
- A clear statement that the study is a research procedure.
- A clear statement that participation is voluntary and that there will be no repercussions either in the patient's relationship with the investigator, or with the patient's other care-givers, if the patient decides not to take part in the study.
- A description of the scope and aims of the research, and whether or not there may be benefits to patients exposed to the test medications.

The foreseeable risks and discomforts should also be disclosed. The possibility of placebo treatment, and the probability of being treated with each test therapy, should be stated.

• Clear descriptions of alternative therapies or standard therapies or procedures (if any), in order that the patient can judge whether to enter the study.

• The methods for compensation that may be available in the case of injury (these vary greatly from country to country).

• Name and telephone number of persons that the patient may contact in case of any difficulty during the study. Also the identity of the person(s) of whom the patient may ask questions during the day-to-day conduct of the study, and an expression of willingness on the part of the investigator to provide answers to any questions that the patient may have.

• A confidentiality statement. This should include the degree to which the patient's identity could be revealed to an inspecting regulatory authority or patient registry, and whether information from the clinical study will automatically be communicated to the patient's primary care or referring physician. In any case, there should be an assurance that no patient identity information will be made public.

• A statement of the circumstances under which the patient will be withdrawn from the study (e.g., noncompliance with test procedures).

• A clear statement that the patient may withdraw from the study at any time and for any reason, again without repercussions to his or her relationship with any clinical care-giver.

• A statement that the patient is responsible for giving a full and accurate clinical and treatment history on study entry and periodically thereafter (according to the study design).

• Assurance that any new information that arises (e.g., in other studies) and which may alter the assessment of hazard of study participation will be communicated to the patient without delay.

• A statement about the number of patients taking part in the study, and a brief summary of how many patients in the past have been exposed to the test medication.

Written informed consent documents should be signed by both the patient and the investigator, and ideally the patient should sign before an impartial witness. Informed consent documents should be written in a language that is understandable to the patient, and ideally at a level of complexity that could be understood by a young adolescent of average intelligence from the same community as the patient. All written informed consent documents should be approved by an ethics committee or an institutional review board (IRB).

Importantly, the patient should have adequate time to review the document. Good study sites might see the patient weekly, provide the informed consent document, and perhaps allow a week before the patient returns for the initial study screening procedures.

Unwritten Informed Consent

Informed consent, in law, must be informed, but need not be written. In very rare clinical situations, ethics committees and IRBs may sanction specific methods for the documentation of oral informed consent. Often these are in association with tests of emergency therapies.

Surrogate informed consent

Some patients are incapable of providing informed consent, whether written or not. Children, various types of neurological disease (e.g., Alzheimer's disease), the mentally handicapped, and emergency patients (e.g., unconscious head injury, stroke, multiple trauma, etc.) are good examples. Many of these patients have a poor prognosis, and epitomize the concept of unmet medical need. Consequently, these are patients for whom there is also encouragement to the pharmaceutical industry by governments, activists, and others for greater clinical research. For these patients, clinical research would be impossible if written informed consent was an essential pre-requisite.

For children, most ethics committees agree that provision of written informed consent by a parent or guardian is acceptable. If the child is of sufficient age, his or her concurrence may also be sought;

although this is not sufficient evidence of informed consent, the refusal to provide concurrence by a child who is likely to be competent to understand the clinical trial conditions should be sufficient to exclude the child from a study.

In the case of studies in incompetent adults, again most ethical committees will accept a legal guardian or custodian *in lieu* of the patient himself or herself. In that case, there must also be sufficient evidence that the custodian has a *bona fide* and independent interest in the patient's welfare. Again, forms of concurrence can be employed when possible. Note that a Court Order for a patient to take part in a clinical trial would usually be a form of duress, violating the concept of autonomy described above.

When informed consent is impossible

Emergency patients have as much right to take part in clinical research as any other type of patient. For example, patients with acute head injury and a low Glasgow Coma Score have a dismal prognosis, and therapeutic interventions (if ever likely to be successful) must be instituted quickly. Under these conditions there is often not even the time to find relatives to provide surrogate informed consent. Even if relatives can be found quickly enough, their emotional state may not be suited to becoming truly informed before giving consent.

Experiments are now under way to investigate whether some substitute for informed consent may be used. One set of guidelines suggests that such clinical trials can be conducted when the following apply:
• There is clinical and public agreement that the disease merits clinical investigation with the investigational therapy.
• There has been advertising and publicity in the likely catchment area of suitable patients that such a study is being undertaken.
• The ethics committee or IRB has approved, in detail, the methods used in pursuit of local publicity.
• An independent, clinically-experienced individual confirms that the patient is a member of the well-defined population that is the subject of the

clinical research, and that it is not unreasonable to include the patient in the study for any other reason.
• No relative (if any is available in a timely fashion) objects.

It is likely that these guidelines will be refined, possibly on an international basis, in the near future.

Responsibility of parties to informed consent

It is the responsibility of all parties to the informed consent that they all remain within its ethical and practical constraints. The informed consent document is essentially an agreement between ethics committee, investigator, and patient. However, for example, an investigator is responsible for the patient's role in the informed consent: if the investigator suspects that the patient is not truly informed, even in the absence of any deficiency on the part of the investigator, the investigator should nonetheless police the patient's autonomy. This is entirely different from the notion of a contract, where each party to the contract is responsible only for fulfilling its own commitments.

Audit of some of the elements listed above may also form part of the duty of a regulatory authority. For example, in the United States, the Food and Drug Administration (FDA) will audit IRBs and issue citations if the IRB is not ensuring that written informed consent documents are complete and appropriate. The FDA will also audit study sites, and discipline investigators (including prosecution), who do not ensure that appropriate informed consent procedures are being followed. Some FDA reviewing divisions will ask for, and require changes to, informed consent document prior to allowing an Investigational New Drug (IND) to become active.

Although under law it is not the primary responsibility of the typical pharmaceutical company, it nonetheless behooves study sponsors to ensure that appropriate informed consent is being obtained in all company-sponsored studies. Many companies recognize this within their own Standard Operating

Procedures and creation of patient ("central" or "IND-inspection") files that require a copy of the signed informed consent. Investigators are often grateful if the company will draft an informed consent document that complies with the guidelines, which the investigator can then review, approve, and submit to the ethics committee or IRB.

Unsettled issues

Informed consent as it applies to human tissues brings complications that were previously unimagined. Concepts of tissue ownership were never even considered when the great pathology museums were being built up, and in some countries there has never been a concept of property title in specimens from biopsies, surgery, or autopsy. However, with modern technology things are no longer so simple.

Perhaps the most vitriolic controversy in this area at present is the use of human embryonic stem cells (HESCs). These are cultured from the embryos created during *in vitro* fertilization procedures. In the United States, using the terminology of this chapter and cutting through much of the tangential argument that has accreted, there is a cultural view among a large number of the general public that use of such HESCs is wrong because it violates *the embryo's autonomy* (and that this is an extension of the violation of the autonomy of a fetus during elective abortion). This view holds (among other things) that the parents therefore have no right to sign informed consent for the use of an embryo for making HESCs. The counter-arguments are that either an embryo is too immature to be accorded possession of autonomy, or, as a practical matter, even if such autonomy existed, these embryos were created in excess and when the appropriate number of pregnancies had been achieved, they would have been destroyed.

The cross-cultural aspects of this argument are currently resolving differently in different parts of the United States. Federal research funding may only be applied to 12 longstanding stem cell lines, established several years ago, whereas research

funding by the state of California can be applied to any newly created HESC line as well.

Another aspect of how informed consent impinges on human tissues was exemplified by the Human Tissue Act (2004) in the United Kingdom (implemented in September 2006), which replaced several earlier Acts concerning human tissues. The Act establishes the Human Tissue Authority (HTA), which is a national competent authority ensuring compliance with the over-arching EU Tissues and Cells Directive (2007). Under the Act, it is illegal to carry out research involving human tissues, organs, or bodily fluids without proof of appropriate informed consent. There are exceptions: tissues held since before 2006; "residual tissue from living beings" in anonymized research studies with ethics board approval; tissues or cadavers with donor's consent and ethics committee approval in the country of donation; and specimens more than 100 years old of any type. Licensing (and periodic inspection) releases research institutions from further research ethics committee review. This practice contrasts with the United States, where all human subjects research requires IRB approval. Guidance for international studies (where US funding may be used in European studies) is being developed (see http://www.niaid.nih.gov/ncn/grants/int/insights/uk-human.htm; accessed April 20, 2010).

Turning to the tissue bank itself (including blood sample storage), increasingly large libraries of indefinitely stored samples of blood and other tissues from clinical trials are being collected. These are intended (either now or in the future) to support genomics research as part of the drive towards personalized medicine. These create problems of assurance of anonymity rather than with informed consent *per se*. Patterns of single nucleotide polymorphisms in the nuclear and/or mitochondrial genomes can identify an individual; a single white blood cell, theoretically at least, can now defeat the anonymized sample labeling that might have been approved by ethics committees at the time of collection. If these libraries have been developed with a promise of eternal anonymity included in the donor's informed consent, what if that can be abrogated at some remote date in the future?

Marketed products

A recent innovation has been the used of informed consent when particularly hazardous marketed products are prescribed. This is one tactic among many for managing risk for such hazardous products. For example, in the United States, this is common when prescribing isotretinoin or thalidomide. In Europe, however, informed consent for prescribable products is more likely to be objected to on the grounds of duress (i.e., taking away the patient's autonomy): no informed consent means no treatment, and the patient knows it. Please see Chapter 45 on Risk Management, where this topic is enlarged upon.

Further reading

Angell E, Tarrant C, Dixon-Woods M. Research involving storage and use of human tissues: how did the Human Tissues Act affect decisions by research ethics committees? *J Clin Pathol* 2009; **62**:825–829.

Applebaum PS, Lidz CW, Meisel A. *Informed Consent: Legal theory and clinical practice.* Oxford University Press: New York, USA, 1987.

Brandon AR, Shivakumar G, Lee SC, Inrig SJ, Sadler JZ. Ethical issues in perinatal mental health research. *Curr Opin Psychiatr* 2009; **22**(6):601–606.

Manson NC, O'Neill O. *Rethinking Informed Consent in Bioethics.* Cambridge University Press: Cambridge, UK, 2007. ISBN 0-521-87458-8.

Marsh BT. Informed consent. *J Roy Soc Med* 1990; **83**:603–606.

Meisel A, Kuczewski M. Legal and ethical myths about informed consent. *Arch Int Med* 1996; **156**:2521–2526.

CHAPTER 9

Phase I: The First Opportunity for Extrapolation from Animal Data to Human Exposure

Stephen H. Curry[1], Helen H. DeCory[2], & Johan Gabrielsson[3]
[1]University of Rochester, NY, USA
[2]Bausch and Lomb Inc., Rochester, NY, USA
[3]AstraZeneca AB, Gothenburg, Sweden

There is a need to make reliable and rapid predictions of human responses from animal data. Although drug discovery is primarily designed to find compounds with desired efficacy, most research-orientated pharmaceutical companies also use data on absorption, metabolism, and pharmacokinetics in the decision-making process (Welling and Tse, 1995). Usually, the strategy is to use all available data to choose one or two candidates from a whole pharmacological class of new drugs for Phase I testing (Welling and Tse, 1995). Thus, compounds are chosen on the basis of animal data, partly because of suitable bioavailability, half-life, and tissue penetration characteristics. The possibility of multiphasic plasma level decay patterns following intravenous doses is an important element in this selection process.

Data for chosen compounds will commonly also have been subjected to simultaneous modeling of pharmacokinetic and pharmacodynamic data from animals, again in an effort to optimize the chances that the drugs chosen will have the properties in humans specified in a pre-discovery product profile. The pharmacodynamic information available typically includes data from receptor-binding studies, *in vitro* functional assays, and *in vivo* phar-

macological screening experiments. Pharmacokinetic studies, related when possible to observed drug effects, are powerful and critical elements of the pivotal step from animal research to human research in the drug development process. For many drug researchers, Phase I is an endpoint in itself, as both the end of the research and discovery process and the beginning of the clinical process, and none can doubt that the first-in-human study, and achieving an active Clinical Trials Exemption (CTX) or Investigational New Drug (IND) (or equivalent regulatory permissions in other countries), are important milestones in the history of a drug. The essence of this crucial step of drug development is the making of valid predictions of *in vivo* drug effects from *in vitro* data.

The collection of *in vitro* data from animal materials and extrapolation—(i) from physical properties to *in vitro* data; (ii) from *in vitro* data to non-human *in vivo* data; and (iii) from non-human *in vivo* data to clinical *in vivo* responses—can be done more efficiently using online analysis and simulations. This chapter seeks to show how rapid progression may be achieved for new chemical entities through this process, using *in vitro* and *in vivo* data and advanced modeling procedures. This must be seen in the context of the entire drug discovery process, which on a larger scale is designed to find potent, safe drugs (in humans), based on animal data (see Figure 9.1). We anticipate a time when *in vitro*

Principles and Practice of Pharmaceutical Medicine, 3rd edition.
Edited by L.D. Edwards, A.W. Fox, P.D. Stonier.
© 2011 Blackwell Publishing Ltd.

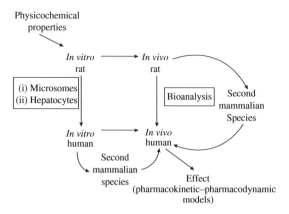

Figure 9.1 General scheme showing the pharmacokinetic prediction pathway from physicochemical properties to human drug response via *in vitro* and *in vivo* studies in laboratory animals.

pharmacodynamic data will be routinely combined with *in vitro* drug metabolism data in a rational prediction of drug responses in healthy human volunteers, with consequent acceleration of the drug discovery effort, and therefore a general trend for more efficient use of resources in early clinical development.

The *in vitro/in vivo* prediction

The challenge is to predict systemic clearance, volume of distribution, and oral bioavailability in humans from a combination of *in vitro* and *in vivo* preclinical data. If this prediction can become reliable, Phase I studies become more confirmatory. The use of human hepatocytes and isolated enzymes can form a critical part of the *in vitro* database.

Clearance of almost all drugs is by renal, metabolic, and/or biliary mechanisms. There are rare exceptions, such as anesthetic gases that are exhaled unchanged. However, here we shall concentrate on the typical situation.

Physicochemical properties, especially lipophilicity, frequently govern the clearance route; lipophilicity is commonly measured as log $D_{7.4}$, where this variable equals $\log_{10}$ ([drug in octanol]/[drug in buffer]) at pH = 7.4, in a closed system at equilibrium. Generally, compounds with a log

$D_{7.4}$ value below 0 have significant renal clearance values, whereas compounds with log $D_{7.4}$ values above 0 will principally undergo metabolism (Smith *et al.*, 1996). Molecular size also has some effect on these clearance routes. For example, compounds with molecular weights greater than 400 Da are often eliminated through the bile unchanged, while smaller lipophilic compounds will generally be metabolized.

Elementary aspects of clearance

The common, clinical measurement of drug clearance involves taking serial venous blood samples. As time passes after dosing, drug concentrations are seen to decline: this is in fact merely the modeling of drug disappearance, and is essentially a descriptive process, requiring actual human exposures.

First-order elimination, after equilibrium in the circulating compartment, has a constant (k) with units of h^{-1}, and plasma concentration (C) and is modeled by equations of the general form

$$C = Ae^{-kt}$$

where A is the concentration of drug at time (t) = 0, assuming that there was instantaneous and homogenous equilibration of the dose into the circulating compartment. As the number of compartments increases, so do the number of terms of the form shown on the right-hand side of the equation shown above. The *elimination rate* always has units of (mass/time) for any elimination process. For first-order processes, the elimination rate is represented by a tangent to the elimination curve.

Note that first-order elimination curves are routinely analyzed as semi-logarithmic plots (which linearizes the curve). These semi-log plots are so common that the literature is sometimes ambiguous in its use of the term "linear data," and authors often presume the semi-logarithmic transformation is to be taken as read, leading to "linear elimination" (or other loose terminology).

In contrast, *zero-order elimination* processes are occasionally encountered. These usually represent saturation by the drug of the elimination mechanism(s). These "drug disappearance" curves are straight, and thus described simply, by

$$C = A - bt$$

where the elimination rate (b) does not change with time or drug concentration. If followed for long enough, most drugs that are subject to zero-order elimination eventually fall to such low concentrations that the elimination mechanism becomes unsaturated, and first-order elimination then supervenes; good examples include ethanol and sodium dichloroacetate (Hawkins and Kalant, 1972; Curry et al., 1985; Fox et al., 1996).

The elimination rate for zero-order processes may also be treated as a maximal rate of reaction (V_{max}), and thus this type of data may be subject to ordinary Michaelis–Menten analysis (see further, below).

When the elimination rate is known, clearance (Cl; L/h) is defined simply as

Cl = elimination rate/C

where C is again drug concentration. Note that in first-order elimination processes, the elimination rate of the drug (with units of mass/time) changes with time (and drug concentration), and thus only instantaneous elimination rates, specifying time or drug concentration, can be stated. But perhaps counter-intuitively, clearance remains constant during first-order processes because the elimination rate (g/h) declines with plasma concentration (g/L) with the mass terms canceling to find clearance. However, the clearance increases continuously during zero-order elimination.

Urinary clearance, obviously, may only partly explain the rate of drug disappearance from plasma. In any case, the urinary clearance of an agent may be found from the familiar equation:

Cl = (U × V)/P

where U is the urinary concentration, V is the volume of urine excreted during a specified time period, and P is the average plasma concentration during that time period. Clinicians will remember that for inulin and sodium iothalamate, but not for creatinine or urea, the urinary clearance is a good estimate of glomerular filtration rate.

These elementary aspects of clearance may be revised in any textbook (e.g., Curry, 1980; Benet et al., 1996; Curry and Whelpton, 2010). The purpose of the remainder of this section is to show how much more informative the concept of clearance may be, and to provide an illustration of its use.

Prediction of human drug clearance

For those compounds predominantly cleared by metabolism, human blood clearance can be predicted using simple enzyme kinetic data (Houston, 1994; Ashforth et al., 1995; Iwatsubo et al., 1996; Obach, 1996a). These predictions may be strengthened by comparing preclinical in vivo data with the predictions made from in vitro data using tissues from the same preclinical species (Rane et al., 1977). As an illustration, consider a novel compound, at one time under development as a neuroprotective agent, identified as Compound X (Bialobok et al., 1999). This compound has a molecular weight less than 400, and a log $D_{7.4}$ value of approximately 0.5, suggesting that it could undergo both renal and hepatic clearance. Preclinical in vivo studies indicate that Compound X is eliminated largely unchanged in the urine in the rat (~90%). Several oxidative biotransformation pathways have nonetheless been identified. In common with studies of Compound X clearance in humans, simple in vitro enzyme kinetic studies were used in conjunction with knowledge from rat in vivo data. The general strategy for prediction of kinetic studies, is shown in Figure 9.2.

Using liver microsomes from different species, the intrinsic clearance (Cl'_{int}) for each species can be determined, and then scaled to hepatic clearance.

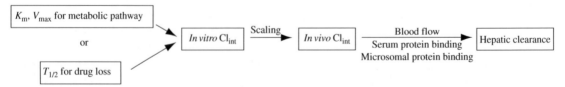

Figure 9.2 Strategy for the *in vitro–in vivo* scaling of hepatic clearance (see for example Iwatsubo et al., 1996).

This is typically done by first determining *in vitro* K_m (the Michaelis–Menten constant) and V_{max} (the maximal rate of metabolism) for each metabolic reaction, using substrate saturation plots (using the familiar algebra and, because of enzyme saturation, finding that $Cl'_{int} = V_{max}/K_m$). However, for Compound X, the situation is more complicated because we know that the Cl'_{int} (drug disappearance) actually is due to several combined biotransformation pathways (i.e., $Cl'_{int}(\text{total}) = Cl'_{int1} + Cl'_{int2} + Cl'_{int3} + \ldots$), thus complicating any K_m and V_{max} determinations from a simple substrate saturation plot.

To determine the Cl'_{int} of Compound X, we are able to use the *in vitro* half-life method, which is simpler than finding all the component Cl'_{int} values. When the substrate concentration is much smaller than the K_m, the Michaelis–Menten equation simplifies from velocity $(V) = V_{max}([S])/(K_m + [S])$, because ($[S]$ is substrate concentration) becomes negligible. Furthermore, under these conditions the *in vitro* half-life ($T_{1/2} = 0.693/K_{el}$) can be measured, and this in turn is related to the Michaelis–Menten equation through the relationship velocity $(V) = $ volume $\times K_{el}$ (where volume is standardized for the volume containing 1 mg of microsomal protein). When both V and V_{max} are known, the K_m is also found. Although simpler than finding a complicated Cl'_{int}, one caveat of the *in vitro* half-life method is that one assumes that the substrate concentration is much smaller than the K_m. It may be necessary to repeat the half-life determinations at several substrate concentrations, and even model the asymptote of this relationship, because very low substrate concentrations that are beneath biochemical detection may be needed to fulfill the assumptions needed to simplify the Michaelis–Menten equation.

Note that in this *in vitro* application, intrinsic clearance, like all conventional mathematical evaluation of clearances, has units of volume $\times$ time^{-1}. It is obtained from V_{max} and K_m measurements, where V_{max} has units of mass $\times$ time^{-1}. The definition of intrinsic clearance as $V_{max} \times K_m^{-1}$ should not be confused with the historically prevalent calculation of k_{el} (the first-order rate constant of decay of concentration in plasma), calculated from $k_{el} = V_{max} \times K_m^{-1}$, where V_{max} is the zero order rate of plasma concentration decay seen at high concentrations, and K_m is the concentration is plasma at half-maximal rate of plasma level decay.

Once the *in vitro* intrinsic clearance has been determined, the next step, scaling *in vitro* intrinsic clearance to the whole liver, proceeds as follows:

In vivo $Cl'_{int} = $ *in vitro* Cl'_{int}

$\times$ weight microsomal protein/g liver

$\times$ weight liver/kg body weight

The amount of microsomal protein/g liver is constant across species (45 mg g^{-1} liver). Thus, the only species-dependent variable is the weight of liver tissue/kg body weight.

In vivo, hepatic clearance is determined by factoring in the hepatic blood flow (Q), the fraction of drug unbound in the blood (fu), and the fraction of drug unbound in the microsomal incubations ($fu_{(inc)}$), against the intrinsic clearance of the drug by the whole liver (the *in vivo* Cl'_{int}). The fu and $fu_{(inc)}$ are included when the drug shows considerable plasma or microsomal protein binding (Obach, 1996b). Several models are available for scaling *in vivo* intrinsic clearance to hepatic clearance, including the parallel tube model or sinusoidal perfusion model, the well-stirred model or venous equilibration model, and the distributed sinusoidal perfusion model (Wilkinson, 1987).

Thus far, for Compound X, we have obtained good results in this context with the simplest of these, the well-stirred model (see Table 9.1 for the equations, with and without significant plasma and/or microsomal protein binding). Using this well-stirred model, it has proved possible to predict the hepatic clearance from *in vitro* intrinsic clearance rates in rat, dog, and human (see Table 9.2). The hepatic clearance value for the rat (0.972 ml $\cdot$ min^{-1} $\cdot$ mg protein^{-1}) was approximately one-tenth the actual clearance found *in vivo*; well in agreement with the observation that *in vivo* Compound X was eliminated by the rat, largely unchanged, by the kidneys ($\sim$90%).

To predict hepatic clearance of Compound X in humans, human *in vitro* intrinsic clearance could then be scaled to hepatic clearance, using a technique that had been validated in the rat

Table 9.1 Equations for predicting hepatic clearance using the well-stirred model

In the absence of plasma or microsomal protein binding	In the presence of significant plasma protein binding	In the presence of both plasma and microsomal protein binding
$Cl_{hepatic} = \dfrac{Q \times Cl'_{int}}{Q + Cl'_{int}}$	$Cl_{hepatic} = \dfrac{Q \times f_u \times Cl'_{int}}{Q + f_u \times Cl'_{int}}$	$Cl_{hepatic} = \dfrac{Q \times f_u \times Cl'_{int} \times f_{u(inc)}}{Q + f_u \times Cl'_{int} \times f_{u(inc)}}$

(Ashforth *et al.*, 1995). Renal clearance is subject to an allometric relationship and can generally be scaled across species (see below). The predicted *in vivo* renal *Cl* for the rat (observed to be the predicted hepatic *Cl* × 9) may be scaled allometrically to obtain a prediction for human *in vivo* renal clearance. Total or systemic *Cl* in humans can then be estimated by adding the two clearance parameters (hepatic and renal) together; in practice, for Compound X, later first-in-human data revealed an actual *in vivo* *Cl* nearly identical to the predicted total *Cl* (2.15 vs. 1.87–2.45 ml min^{-1}mg^{-1}, respectively; see Table 9.2). Here, then, is a real-world example of, first, how rat *in vitro* and *in vivo* preclinical data were used to develop and validate a scaling method for Compound X in the rat; and second, how the scaling method successfully predicted *in vivo* overall drug clearance in humans.

However, if the same methods are used for Compound X in the dog, things initially appear to be different. Scaling the *in vitro* intrinsic clearance to hepatic *Cl* using the rat-validated method, in conjunction with allometric scaling of renal *Cl*, resulted in a five-fold underprediction of total or systemic clearance *in vivo*. However, further metabolism

studies in the dog *in vivo* revealed that Compound X undergoes significant additional biotransformation, particularly *N*-methylation, which is almost unique (as far as we are aware) to this species, and invalidates some of our *in vitro* assumptions. This canine biotransformation pathway was not detected by our initial microsomal studies because there are no *N*-methyl transferases in microsomes. Thus, although we did not successfully predict dog systemic clearance for Compound X, our scaling tactics did eventually teach us about a new clearance mechanism, and how important this was for the systemic clearance of Compound X in the dog.

This is an example of how *in vitro* studies can be combined with *in vivo* preclinical data, leading to useful prediction of human systemic drug clearance. Nonetheless, several caveats are encountered in such scaling exercises, which warrant restating.

The first caveat is that all clearance pathways (hepatic, renal, biliary, or other) must be taken into consideration. If a compound undergoes a high level of hepatic clearance, *in vitro–in vivo* scaling may be used to predict the fraction of systemic clearance expected from this pathway. If a compound undergoes a high level of renal elimination,

Table 9.2 Comparison of the predicted *in vivo* hepatic clearance and the actual clearance values for Compound X

	Predicted *in vivo* hepatic *Cl* (ml min^{-1} kg^{-1})	Predicted *in vivo* renal *Cl* (ml min^{-1} kg^{-1})	Predicted *in vivo* total *Cl* (ml min^{-1}kg^{-1})	Actual *in vivo* *Cl* (ml min^{-1} kg^{-1})
Rat	0.972	8.75	9.72	8.17–10.7
Human	0.223	1.93	2.15	1.87–2.45
Dog	0.463	3.74	4.20	21.2–22.5

Predicted values were scaled from *in vitro* half-life data using liver microsomes and the well-stirred model of hepatic extraction. Hepatic *Cl* predictions were corrected for plasma and microsomal protein binding. Predicted total *Cl* was obtained by adding in renal *Cl* estimates which were, in turn, scaled allometrically ($Y = aW^{0.75}$)

allometric scaling may be also used to predict the clearance attributed to this pathway.

The second caveat is that, in order to predict accurately hepatic clearance, the correct *in vitro* system must be chosen. If the candidate drug is primarily oxidatively metabolized, liver microsomes will be sufficient. However, if the potential for non-microsomal biotransformation exists, a different *in vitro* system, such as hepatocyte suspensions, should be used. In the illustration above, it turned out, as far as clearance of Compound X is concerned, humans are specifically like rats, and unlike dogs.

The third caveat is that one must consider the variability in the expression of metabolizing enzymes between individuals. Oxidative metabolism (seen *in vivo* and in microsomal enzymes), and especially cytochrome P$_{450}$s, vary tremendously between human individuals (Meyer, 1994; Shimada *et al.*, 1994). Had we used a single donor microsomal sample, rather than pooled liver microsomes (a pool consisting of at least eight individual donors), to scale *in vitro* data to *in vivo* hepatic clearance, we might have made greatly misleading predictions (note that oxidative, initial drug metabolism is sometimes called "Phase I metabolism" in the literature, causing ambiguity with the stage of drug development or type of clinical trial).

Volumes of distribution

Review of elementary concepts
Volume of distribution is a theoretical concept that may or may not correspond to the anatomical compartment(s) that drugs or metabolites may access after dosing. When size of the dose (*D*) is known, and when drug concentration (*C*) may be found by sampling biological fluids, then, in the simplest case, the volume of distribution (*VD*) is

$$VD = D/C$$

Clinical protocols can usually only prescribe the sampling of a subset of compartments when a drug is known to distribute widely in the body. For example, a lipophilic drug may penetrate lipophilic organs such as brain, and obviously, brain sampling simply for pharmacokinetic purposes is usually possible only in animals. In such cases, blood concentrations fall far lower than if the dose had distributed solely into the circulating compartment; *C* becomes very small, and *VD* becomes correspondingly very large. The opposite effect would require the drug to be restricted to a fraction of the compartment that is sampled, essentially suggesting that too few compartments have been postulated, and is almost never encountered. Again, see Curry (1980), Curry and Whelpton (2010), or Benet *et al.* (1996) for expansion of these elementary aspects of volume of distribution.

Prediction of human volumes of distribution
The free (not plasma protein-bound) volume of distribution of experimental drugs is generally considered to be constant for all species. Thus, the volume of distribution in humans can easily be predicted through a simple proportionality between *in vitro* plasma protein binding data in humans and in a preclinical species, and *in vivo* volume of distribution in that same preclinical species (where *fu* is the proportion unbound):

$$VD_{\text{human}} = \frac{VD_{\text{preclinical species}} \times fu_{\text{human}}}{fu_{\text{preclinical species}}}$$

Table 9.3 shows the predicted volume of distribution of a single intravenous bolus dose of Compound X in humans; this is found by using the above equation, an *in vitro* estimate of protein binding data for rat and dog plasma, and the observed volumes of distribution for these two species *in vivo*. For humans, VD_{human} was predicted

Table 9.3 *In vitro* plasma protein binding, *in vivo* volume of distribution and predicted volume of distribution in humans

	Fraction of Compound X unbound in the plasma (*f*$_u$)	*In vivo* volume of distribution (l kg)	Predicted volume of distribution in humans (l kg)
Rat	0.45	3.02–3.97	3.48–4.59
Human	0.52	–	–
Dog	0.66	3.82–6.43	3.01–5.06

to be $3.48\text{–}4.591\,\text{kg}^{-1}$ using the rat data and $3.01\text{–}5.061\,\text{kg}^{-1}$ using the dog data.

Elementary aspects of oral bioavailability

The oral bioavailability (F) of a drug is dependent on (i) the absorption of the drug from the gastrointestinal (GI) tract, and (ii) the capability of the gut wall and liver to clear the drug during its first pass through the portal venous system. Oral bioavailability may be described as the fraction of the total oral dose for which systemic exposure is achieved. It is a measurement of *extent* of exposure, and contrasts with the *rates* of absorption or elimination discussed above.

Clinically, F is found by comparing the systemic exposures that result after intravenous and oral doses of the same drug. Note that this comparison need not be for doses of the same size (importantly useful for tolerability of the intravenous (IV) dose in normal volunteer protocols). It is, in fact, preferable to achieve concentrations in the same range from the two doses. Typically, $C_{\max}$ for a standard dose is going to be higher after bolus intravenous dosing than after oral administration (PO), and adverse effects of new agents are likely to be concentration-dependent. The relevant equation is

$$F(\%) = [(AUC_{\text{PO}} \times Dose_{\text{IV}})/(AUC_{\text{IV}} \times Dose_{\text{PO}})]$$
$$\times\ 100$$

where AUC (mg h^{-1}) is the area under the time–plasma concentration curve after each of the respective administrations (the dose terms cancel when equally sized doses are administered by both routes of administration). A residual of less than 15% (sometimes 10%) of the total AUC is a commonly-used standard for timing the last plasma sample. These studies are usually conducted under standard conditions, and using crossover protocols, although, occasionally, a double-label study may be used to measure F instantaneously. Comparison of generic with innovator's formulations, and slow-release with rapidly absorbed formulations, may be compared using equations of the same form. Similarly, subcutaneous and intravenous injections can be compared. The intravenous administration

of a dose is assumed to be 100% bioavailable (very rare exceptions include some very short-acting drugs, e.g., some arachidonate derivatives, remifentanil, esmolol, and adenosine, which may be metabolized during their first return circulation after intravenous administration, and still not achieve 100% "bioavailability"). Also, the concept is not applicable to topically-acting drugs. However, assessing the bioavailability of these drugs by any other route of administration is usually pointless, unless there is some highly specialized issue, e.g., absorption after intrathecal administration or potential for drug abuse.

Fluctuation of plasma drug concentration is an important aspect of the bioavailability of slow release formulations, which almost always have lower $C_{\max}$ values for a standard dose size than, but a similar AUC to, a more rapidly absorbed tablet of equal dose size. Assuming that the assay can handle the inevitably lower plasma concentrations, a useful measure of fluctuation, after the initial absorption phase of the curve, and during the next four half-lives of elimination, is

$$(C_{\max} - C_{\min})/C_{\text{avg}}$$

where C_{avg} is the average concentration during the specified time period; whether to use the arithmetic or geometric average is a controversy, with respected protagonists on both sides. Some authorities prefer $(C_{\max} - C_{\min})/C_{\max}$, or even equations using AUC measurements.

Prediction of oral bioavailability

Oral bioavailability can be predicted using the following equation:

$$F = Fa \cdot (1 - Cl/Q)$$

where Fa represents the fraction of drug absorbed through the intestinal lining, Cl is the hepatic clearance (predicted from *in vitro* studies, see the earlier section), and Q is the hepatic blood flow in humans (see, for example, Rane *et al.*, 1977). Octanol/water partitioning has traditionally been used to predict the fraction absorbed through the intestinal lining. Recently, Caco-2 cell permeability studies have replaced the use of octanol/buffer partitioning studies. Yee (1997) established a relationship between

Fa and Caco-2 cell permeability, expressed as the apparent permeability constant (P_{app}), as follows:

$P_{app} < 10^{-6}$ cm/s, then $Fa = 0 - 20\%$

$1 \leq P_{app} \leq 10 \times 10^{-6}$ cm/s, then $Fa = 20 - 70\%$

$P_{app} > 10^{-5}$ cm/s, then $Fa => 70\%$

The use of Caco-2 cell permeability studies has resulted in more accurate oral bioavailability predictions. Using the predicted hepatic clearance for Compound X in humans (see above), estimating Fa by extrapolation from the Caco-2 cell P_{app}, and an assumed hepatic blood flow for humans (see, for example, Rane $et\ al.$, 1977) of 20 ml min^{-1} kg^{-1}, the human oral bioavailability of 69–98% for Compound X is predicted. This compares well with the known oral bioavailability of this compound in rats and dogs (83% and 72%, respectively).

Prediction from animals to humans *in vivo*

Elementary aspects

Allometric scaling is an empirical method for predicting physiological, anatomical, and pharmacokinetic measures across species in relation to time and size (Boxenbaum 1982; Ings, 1990; Boxenbaum and DiLea, 1995). Allometric scaling is based on similarities among species in their physiology, anatomy, and biochemistry, coupled with the observation that smaller animals perform physiological functions that are similar to larger animals, but at a faster rate. The allometric equation is $Y = aW^b$, and a log transformation of this formula yields the straight line:

$$\log\ Y = b\ \log\ W + \log\ a$$

where Y is the pharmacokinetic or physiological variable of interest, a is the allometric coefficient (and log a is the intercept of the line), W is body weight, and b is allometric exponent (slope of the line).

One of the first applications of allometric scaling was the use of the toxicity of anticancer agents in animals to predict toxicity in humans. It was observed that the toxic dose of a drug is similar among species when the dose is com-

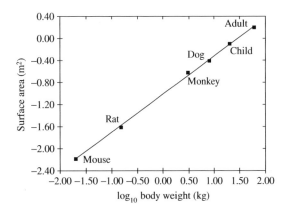

Figure 9.3 Allometric relationship between body surface area and species body weight on a log versus log plot.

pared on the basis of body surface area (Freireich $et\ al.$, 1966). For most vertebrate species, the body weight/volume ratio varies very little, but the surface area/volume ratio reduces as species become bigger, and as individual animals grow. Allometric correction of dose multiples in toxicology (compared with proposed human doses) is thus important, especially when small rodents provide the principal toxicology coverage.

Body surface area (Y) is related to body weight (W, in kg) by the formula

$$Y = 0.1\ W^{0.67}$$

This allometric relationship between body surface area and species body weight then allows for a simple conversion of drug doses across species (see Figure 9.3), and allometrically equivalent doses of drugs (mg kg^{-1}) can be calculated for any species (see Table 9.4). The conversion factor (km is simply the body weight divided by the body surface area. Thus, by using the km factors, the dose in Species 1 (in mg kg^{-1}) is equivalent to ($km_{species2}/km_{species1}$) times the dose in Species 2 (in mg kg^{-1}). For example, a 50 mg kg^{-1} dose of drug in mouse would be equivalent to a 4.1 mg kg^{-1} dose in humans, that is, approximately one-twelfth of the dose (see Table 9.4). Likewise, the conversion factor can be used to calculate equivalent doses between any species. An equivalent dose in mg kg^{-1} in rat would be twice that for the mouse.

Species	Body weight (kg)	Body surface area (kg m^{-2})	Factor* (k_m)	Approximate human dose equivalent
Mouse	0.02	0.0067	3.0	1/12
Rat	0.100	0.0192	5.2	1/7
Dog	8.0	0.400	20	1/2
Monkey	2.5	0.217	11.5	1/3
Human	60	1.62	37	N/A

Table 9.4 Equivalent surface area dosage conversion factors

*Dose in species 1 (mg kg^{-1}) = dose in species 2 (mg kg^{-1}).

Allometric approaches to drug discovery

Using limited data, allometric scaling may be used as a part of drug discovery. To do this we assume that, for the formula $Y = aW^b$, the value of the power function "b" (or slope of the line from a log vs. log plot) is drug-independent, unlike the intercept "a," which is drug-dependent. By doing this we can use data from a single species (the rat) to successfully predict the pharmacokinetics of Compound X in larger animals and humans. This method could be expected to save time and money in the drug discovery process by enabling us to the following:

1. Select the correct dose in an animal model of disease. These studies are expensive and time-consuming. The selection of the wrong dose in an animal model, especially in a model in a larger species such as cat, could lead to invalid results, either through toxicity (if the dose is too high) or inactivity (if the dose is too low).

2. Provide confidence that the pharmacological model will predict efficacy in humans. If a drug is effective in therapeutic models using different species and these animals receive equivalent exposures (as measured by the maximum plasma concentration, C_{max}, or area under the plasma concentration curve, AUC), the clinician can choose a dose for trials with confidence.

3. Eliminate unnecessary doses and plasma samples in the first trials in humans.

The discovery process for Compound X, which is efficacious in a number of *in vivo* models, is again an illustration of how allometric considerations can enhance the development process. The whole brain concentrations of this compound are in equilibrium with plasma concentrations within 5 min after dosing, and it is also eliminated from the brain in equilibrium with the declining plasma concentration. We also know that Compound X is ~80% orally bioavailable in rats and dogs (see above), and has linear (first-order elimination) and predictable pharmacokinetics in animals.

Next, this compound was tested in a model of excitotoxicity, in which the neurotoxin malonate was injected into the striatum of rats. A subcutaneous injection of Compound X at 9 mg kg^{-1} caused an 80% reduction in the lesion activity produced by malonate. The C_{max} plasma levels of Compound X at this dose would be about 1500 ng ml^{-1}.

In a study using spontaneously hypertensive rats, a dose of 12 mg kg^{-1} of Compound X was also neuroprotective (these rats were subjected to 2 h of focal ischemia by occlusion of the right middle cerebral artery (MCA), followed by 22 h of reperfusion). With the assumption of 100% systemic absorption, the expected plasma C_{max} at this dose was 2000 ng ml^{-1}. In this model, there was a significant reduction (greater than 30%) in cortical infarct volume, compared with saline controls, when the drug was given at the time of occlusion and at 0, 0.5, 1, and 1.5 h post-MCA occlusion.

Using the data from the neuroprotection models from rats, we then scaled a dose to the cat that was expected to achieve a neuroprotective plasma concentration of 1500 ng ml^{-1}. To do this, we predicted the volume of distribution (V_{1cat}) using data collected from the volume of distribution in rat (V_{1rat}). For our calculations we used a value of 0.938 for the power function b (see Ings, 1990, Table 2).

In doing this we made the standard assumption that in the formula $Y = aW^b$ the value of the power function b was compound-independent and that the function a was compound-dependent (Ings observed that the power function b is reasonably constant for each pharmacokinetic parameter). Substituting into the allometric formula, $\log (V_{1cat}) = b \log W + \log a$, we found

$$\log 0.426 \text{ liters} = 0.938 \log 0.3 \text{ kg} + \log a$$

Thus:

$$\log a = 0.120$$

By substituting back into the formula and using a cat weight of 4 kg, we found

$$V_{1cat} = 4.8 \text{ l or } 1.21 \text{ l kg}^{-1}$$

Our formula for calculating the dose to be administered was

$$Dose_{cat} = Dose_{rat}(V_{1cat}/V_{1rat})$$

The formula for predicting the plasma half-life was

$$T_{1/2cat} = T_{1/2rat}(W_{cat}/W_{rat})^{y-x}$$

in which y is as defined earlier and x is a clearance parameter (Boxenbaum and Ronfeld, 1983). The measured plasma half-life in the rat was 4.53 h. Filling in the formula (Boxenbaum and Ronfeld, 1983), we predicted a plasma half-life in the cat of 7.3 h ($= 4.53 \times (4/0.3)^{0.938-0.75}$). The measured plasma half-life in the cat was 6 h. We knew from data collected in the rat that a dose of 3.06 mg kg^{-1} administered over 15 min would give a plasma C_{max} of 1500 ng ml^{-1} of plasma. This equated to a dose in the cat of 2.6 mg kg^{-1} over 15 min or 175 µg kg^{-1}min^{-1} for 15 min.

When we performed studies to determine the C_{max} in cats following a dose of 2.6 mg kg^{-1} administered over 15 min, our predicted values were very close to the actual values, with a measured C_{max} of 1240 ± 100 ng ml^{-1}.

Data from the rat can also be used to predict the pharmacokinetics of Compound X in humans. As with the cat we made our predictions prospectively, by assuming, as stated earlier, that for the formula $Y = aW^b$, the value of the power function b (or

slope of the line from a log vs. log plot) was drug-independent, and that the intercept function a was drug-dependent. We assigned values of 0.75, 0.938, and 0.25 for clearance, volume of distribution, and plasma half-life, respectively, using data taken from the literature and discussed above. The intercept function a was then determined for each parameter by substituting the pharmacokinetic data from rats, that is, clearance = 0.54 l h^{-1} kg^{-1}, V_1 = 1.421 kg^{-1}, V_{dss} = 3.33 l kg^{-1}. We estimated the pharmacokinetic parameters for humans by substituting the calculated intercept function back into the formula and solving for Y for a 70-kg human. The prediction of the plasma half-life in humans was determined by three separate methods. For our predictions, we also assumed that the protein binding was the same in rats and in humans and that the metabolism of Compound X was similar in both species. Clearly, approaches like this could be a routine part of drug discovery.

The values estimated by allometric scaling were compared with those observed in the single-dose human volunteer study (see Table 9.5). We predicted that for Compound X in humans the plasma half-life would be 14.5 h, the plasma clearance would be 0.138 l h^{-1}kg^{-1}, and the V_1, V_{dss}, and $V_{d\beta}$ would be 1.01, 2.37, and 2.56 l kg^{-1}, respectively. The predictions using rat data were within 15% of the actual mean values in human volunteers. A complex Dedrick plot of the rat and human data showed nearly superimposable concentration–time curves, (Figure 9.4).

Table 9.5 Predicted and actual pharmacokinetic parameters for humans

Pharmacokinetic parameter	Predicted	Actual
Clearance	0.138 l/h/kg	0.123
Half-life[a]	14.5 h	13.6 h
V_1	1.01 l/kg	1.02 l/kg
V_{dss}	2.4 l/kg	2.1 l/kg

[a]Plasma half-life is the average from three values by three different methods: (a) $T_{1/2 \text{ human}} = (0.693 \times V_d)/Cl_p$; (b) $T_{1/2 \text{ human}} = T_{1/2 \text{ rat}} (W_{\text{human}}/W_{\text{rat}})^{x-y}$; and (c) $\log T_{1/2 \text{ human}} = \log a + b \log W_{\text{human}}$.

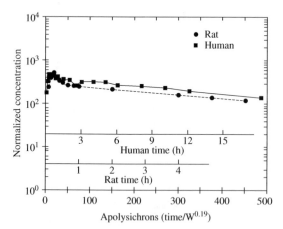

Figure 9.4 Complex Dedrick plot of rat and human data for Compound X again showing very good scaling between rat and human.

This illustrates how allometric scaling is a useful part of the drug discovery process: we avoided studying irrelevant doses and saved time. Ideally, allometric scaling should be done using pharmacokinetic data from at least four species, even though accurate predictions can be made using data from a single species. If possible, information about differences in metabolism among species should be considered when making predictions.

Pharmacokinetic/pharmacodynamic models

Elementary aspects

The possibility that time since dose changes the relationship between pharmacological effect size and drug concentrations in plasma has been known for a long time (Levy, 1964, 1966; Levy and Nelson, 1965; Wagner, 1968; Curry, 1980). The pioneering work was done by Levy and his colleagues in the 1960s on single dose–plasma level–effect relationships, and on the duration of action of drugs as a function of dose. Brodie and colleagues had shown even earlier how complicated the relationships are when drugs with multicompartment distribution are studied in this context (e.g., Brodie, 1967). Lasagna and colleagues, using diuretics, found that

depending on whether a cumulative effect (24 h urine production) or an "instant" effect (rate of urine flow at a particular time) were measured, different relationships of response were possible (Murphy *et al.*, 1961). Nagashima *et al.* (1969) demonstrated the relative time courses of anticoagulant concentration and effect. Thus, the relationship between effect size and concentration of drug in plasma should not be expected to be constant or simple, and can vary with time.

The objectives of modern analysis of drug action are to delineate the chemical or physical interactions between drug and target cell and to characterize the full sequence and scope of actions of each drug (Ross, 1996). Preclinical models describing the relationship between the concentration of drug in blood or plasma, and drug receptor occupancy or functional response, provide clinically useful tools regarding *potency*, *efficacy*, and the time course of effect.

Potency is an expression of the activity of a compound, in terms of either the concentration or amount needed to produce a defined effect. E_{max} is the maximal drug-induced effect. EC_{50} is the concentration of an agonist that produces 50% of the maximal possible response. An EC_{50} can be described for drug concentrations using *in vitro* assays, or as a plasma concentration *in vivo*. IC_{50} is the concentration of an antagonist that reduces a specified response to 50% of its former value.

A measure of the tendency of a ligand and its receptor to bind to each other is expressed as K_d in receptor occupancy studies. K_d is the equilibrium constant for the two processes of drug–receptor combination and dissociation. K_d may be found for both agonists and antagonists, although sometimes the former poses more technical challenge, due to alterations to the conformation of the binding site. In contrast, *efficacy* is a relative measure, among different agonists, describing response size for a standard degree of receptor occupation (Jenkinson *et al.*, 1995). When an agonist must occupy 100% of available receptors to cause E_{max}, its efficacy may be said to be unity. If occupation of all receptors achieves a response that is less than E_{max}, the agonist's efficacy is less than one, and equal to the ratio of observed maximal effect/maximal effect for an agonist with efficacy = 1 (we call these *partial agonists* or *agonist–antagonists*). Some agonists need occupy only a subset of the available receptors, in order to achieve E_{max}, and these have efficacy greater than unity. In the latter case, the concentration–response curve lies to the left of the concentration–receptor occupancy curve (e.g., Minneman *et al.*, 1983). Drugs with efficacy ≥ 1 are also called *full agonists*.

Below, we present some model relationships between observed concentration and effect size, as examples from a considerable volume of literature. The reader is referred to key texts for comprehensive coverage of this topic (e.g., Smolen, 1971; Gibaldi and Perrier, 1982; Dayneka *et al.*, 1993; Levy, 1993; Lesko and Williams, 1994; Colburn, 1995; Derendorf and Hochhaus, 1995; Gabrielsson and Weiner, 1997; Sharma and Jusko 1997).

Pharmacokinetic–Pharmacodynamic (PK/PD) modeling

Single-compartment, time-independent PK/PD models

The simplest model is where: (i) the drug distributes into a single compartment, represented by plasma; and (ii) the effect is an instantaneous, direct function of the concentration in that compartment. In this situation, the relationship between drug concentration (C) and a pharmacological effect (E) can be simply described by the linear function

$$E = S \times C$$

where S is a slope parameter. If the measured effect has some baseline value (E_0), when drug is absent (e.g., physiological, diastolic blood pressure, or resting tension on the tissue in an organ bath), the model may be expressed as

$$E = E_0 + S \times C$$

The parameters of this model, S and E_0, may be estimated by linear regression. This model does not contain any information about efficacy and potency, cannot identify the maximum effect, and thus cannot be used to find EC_{50}.

When effect can be measured for a wide concentration range, the relationship between effect and concentration is often observed to be curvilinear. A semi-logarithmic plot of effect versus log concentration commonly linearizes these data within the approximate range 20–80% of maximal effect. This log-transformation of the concentration axis facilitates a graphical estimation of the *slope* of the apparently linear segment of the curve:

$$E = m \times \ln(C + C_0)$$

where m and C_0 are the slope and the hypothetical baseline concentration (usually zero, but not for experiments of add-on therapy or when administering molecules that are also present endogenously), respectively. In this equation, the pharmacological effect may be expressed, when the drug concentration is zero, as

$$E_0 = m \times \ln(C_0)$$

As mentioned earlier, for functional data based on biophase, plasma, or tissue measurements, we often represent potency as EC_{50}, and when two compounds are compared with respect to potency, the one with the lowest EC_{50} value has the highest potency. A general expression for observed effect, by analogy with the Michaelis–Menten equation (above) is

$$E = \frac{E_{max}C}{EC_{50} + C}$$

There are various forms of this function for agonist (stimulatory) and antagonist (inhibitory) effects. For example, if there is a baseline effect (E_0), this may be added to the right-hand side of the equation:

$$E = E_0 + \frac{E_{max}C}{EC_{50} + C}$$

Alternatively, the relationship between concentration and effect for an antagonist, including a baseline value, is

$$E = E_0 - \frac{I_{max}C}{IC_{50} + C}$$

In the E_{max} model above, plasma concentration and EC_{50} are raised to the power of n (Hill factor) equal to 1. A more general form of the equation is the sigmoid curve:

$$E = \frac{E_{max}C^n}{EC_{50}^n + C^n}$$

where, by addition of a single parameter (n) to the E_{max} model, it is possible to account for curves that are both shallower and steeper than when $n = 1$ (i.e., unlike the ordinary E_{max} models). Note that the sigmoidicity parameter (n) does not necessarily have a direct biological interpretation and should be viewed as an extension of the original E_{max} model to account for curvature.

The larger the value of the exponent, the more curved (steeper, concave downwards) is the line. A very high exponent can be viewed as indicating an all-or-none effect (e.g., the development of an action potential in a nerve). Within a narrow concentration range the observed effect goes from all to nothing, or *vice versa*. An exponent less than unity (<1) sometimes indicates active metabolites and/or multiple receptor sites.

The corresponding inhibitory sigmoid E_{max} model is functionally described as follows:

$$E = E_0 - \frac{I_{max}C^n}{IC_{50}^n + C^n}$$

In vivo, these models, analogous to the classical dose or log dose–response curves of *in vitro* pharmacology, are limited to direct effects in single compartment systems. These models make no allowance for time-dependent events in drug response.

Complex PK/PD and time-dependent models

The most common approach to *in vivo* pharmacokinetic and pharmacodynamic modeling involves sequential analysis of the concentration versus time and effect versus time data, such that the kinetic model provides an independent variable, such as concentration, *driving* the dynamics. Only in limited situations could it be anticipated that the effect influences the kinetics, for example, effects on blood flow or drug clearance itself.

Levy (1964), Jusko (1971), and Smolen (1971, 1976) described the analysis of dose–response time data. They developed a theoretical basis for the performance of this analysis from data obtained from the observation of the time course of pharmacological response, after a single dose of drug, by any route of administration. Smolen (1976) extended the analysis to application of dose–response time data for bioequivalence testing.

In dose–response time models the underlying assumption is that pharmacodynamic data gives us information on the kinetics of drug in the *biophase* (i.e., the tissue or compartment precisely where the drug exhibits its effect). In other words, apparent half-life, bioavailability, and potency can be obtained simultaneously from dose–response–time data. Considering such a model, assuming (i) first-order input/output processes and (ii) extravascular dosing, the kinetic model then drives the inhibition function of the dynamic model. It is the *dynamic behavior* that is described by the response model. A zero-order input and first-order output governs the *turnover* of the response. This permits us to consider situations where the plasma concentration represents delivery of the drug to an effect compartment; the time course of drug concentration and of effect (both in the biophase) is different from that simply observed in plasma concentrations.

The amount of drug in a single hypothetical compartment after an IV dose is usually modeled with mono-exponential decline, and is analogous to the "plasma disappearance" curve (above):

$$X_{IV} = D_{IV}e^{-Kt}$$

The amount of drug in a single hypothetical compartment after an extravascular dose is then modeled with first-order input/output kinetics:

$$X_{po} = \frac{K_a F D_{po}}{K_a - K}[e^{-K(t-t_{lag})} - e^{K_a(t-t_{lag})}]$$

Concentration–time effect modeling is illustrated by the example that follows. This example was chosen to illustrate a single dose of drug causing the reversal of a symptom (pain). Many other types of examples exist.

The plasma kinetics of the analgesic were describable by the following expression after the intravenous bolus dose, with $C_0 = 45.0$ and $K = 0.50$ h^{-1}:

$$C = 45.0e^{-0.50t}$$

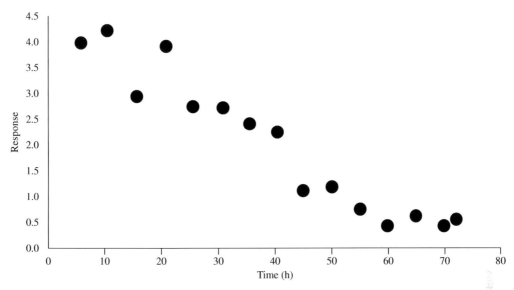

Figure 9.5 Observed effect-time data for an analgesic.

In the same study, effect measurements were recorded during 80 min, as shown in Figure 9.5.

Often, drug effects do not parallel changes in plasma concentration. This can result from distribution phenomena, such as when the effect occurs outside the plasma compartment (e.g., the sedative effect of a dose of benzodiazepine, which occurs in the brain), or when the effect recorded reflects, for example, a chain of biochemical events triggered by the presence of drug (e.g., the aborting of a migraine attack by a serotoninergic drug). In relation to the first of these possibilities, a model sometimes called a "link model" (also called the "effect-compartment" or the "effect-distribution" model) allows estimation of the *in vivo* pharmacodynamic effect from non-steady-state effect (*E*) versus time and concentration (*C*) versus time data, within which potential exists for observed *E* and *C* to display temporal displacement with respect to each other (Segre 1968; Wagner 1968; Dahlstrom et al., 1978; Sheiner et al., 1979). The rate of change of drug amount (A_e) in a hypothetical effect compartment can be expressed as:

$$\frac{\mathrm{d}A_e}{\mathrm{d}t} = k_{le} A_1 - k_{e0} A_e$$

where *A* is the amount of drug in the central compartment of a pharmacokinetic model, linked to the effect compartment, with first-order rate constants k_{le} and k_{e0}. The corresponding expression for the amount of drug in the effect compartment, for a one-compartment model with bolus input of dose (*D*), is:

$$A_e = \frac{k_{le} D}{k_{e0} - K} [e^{-Kt} - e^{-k_{e0}t}]$$

where *K* is the elimination rate constant. The concentration of drug in the effect compartment, C_e, is obtained by dividing A_e by the effect compartment volume, V_e:

$$C_e = \frac{k_{le} D}{V_e(k_{e0} - K)} [e^{-Kt} - e^{k_{e0}t}]$$

At equilibrium, the rates of drug transfer between the central and effect compartments are equal:

$$k_{le} A = k_{e0} A_e$$
$$k_{le} V_c C = k_{e0} V_e C_e$$

If the partition coefficient, K_p, equals C_e/C at equilibrium (steady-state), we can rearrange the above equation:

$$V_e = \frac{k_{le} V_1}{K_p k_{e0}}$$

Substituting for V_e in the above equation (i.e., $k_{le} = k_{e0}$) yields:

$$C_e = \frac{k_{e0} D K_p}{V_1 (k_{e0} - K)} [e^{-Kt} - e^{-k_{e0}t}]$$

At equilibrium, C will be equal to C_e/K_p by definition, and thus:

$$C_e = \frac{k_{e0} D}{V_1 (k_{e0} - K)} [e^{-Kt} - e^{-k_{e0}t}]$$

This is how the link-model relates the kinetics in plasma to the kinetics of drug in the effect compartment. When used together with the E_{max} model for estimation of the maximal drug-induced effect, the concentration at half-maximal effect (apparent EC_{50}), and the rate constant of the disappearance of the effect (k_{e0}):

$$E = \frac{E_{max} C_e^n}{EC_{50}^n + C_e^n}$$

Computer fitting of the equations to the effect data and estimation of the rate constant for the disappearance of the effect, k_{e0}, EC_{50}, and E_{max} follows, assuming the sigmoidicity factor (n) to be equal to unity.

At steady-state, C_e is directly proportional to the plasma concentration (C), since $C_e = K_p C$. Consequently, the potency (EC_{50}) obtained by regressing the last two equations, represents the steady-state plasma concentration producing 50% of E_{max}.

Note that the effect equilibration rate constant (k_{e0}) may be viewed as a first-order distribution rate constant. It can also be thought of in terms of the rate of presentation of a drug to a specific tissue, determined by, for example, tissue perfusion rate, apparent volume of the tissue, and eventual diffusion into the tissue. The results of the data fitting in this exercise with the analgesic are: E_{max} 4.5; EC_{50} 0.61 ng $\times$ ml^{-1} and k_{e0} 0.07 h^{-1}.

Effect compartment or link models are limited by their applicability to situations in which the equilibrium between plasma and response is due

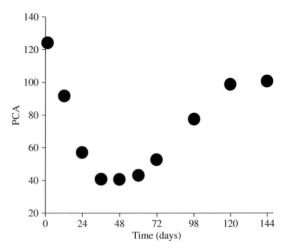

Figure 9.6 Observed Prothrombin Complex Activity time course following the administration of an intravenous bolus dose of warfarin.

to distributional phenomena. In reality, there is often a delay between occurrence of maximum drug concentration in the effect compartment and maximum intensity of effect caused by slow development of the effect, rather than by slow distribution to the site of action. In this situation, indirect or "physiological substance" models are more appropriate (Dayneka *et al.*, 1993; Levy, 1994; Sharma and Jusko, 1997). Warfarin is a good example, where this drug inhibits the prothrombin complex activity (PCA) (inhibition of production of effect). This is illustrated by the following example, which relates changes in (s)-warfarin concentration to observed PCA. The dose was intravenous. The change in PCA is shown in Figure 9.6.

The plasma kinetics of (s)-warfarin were described by the following mono-exponential expression:

$$C_{w(s)} = 1.05 e^{-0.0228t}$$

and the equation for the turnover of clotting factor [P] was:

$$\frac{dP}{dt} = k_d \left[\frac{P_0}{1 + \left[\frac{C_{w(s)}}{IC_{50s}} \right]^n} - P \right]$$

In this equation, k_d is the apparent first-order degradation rate constant (also called k_{out}). This constant can be obtained experimentally from the slope of a ln (P) versus time plot, after administration of a synthesis-blocking dose of coumarin anticoagulant (Nagashima et al., 1969; Pitsui et al., 1993). P_0 is the baseline value of the prothrombin time, $C_{w(s)}$ the concentration of (s)-warfarin, and IC_{50S} concentration of warfarin at 50% of maximal blocking effect. It was also possible to estimate the half-life of the apparent first-order degradation.

An alternative model, including a lag-time to allow for distributional effects embedded in the observed time delay of the onset of the effect after warfarin administration, was published by Pitsui et al. (1993). Setting the baseline value of clotting factor activity in the absence of warfarin (P_0) to a fixed mean of three predose measurements, the program can estimate that parameter.

The model equations are as follows:

$$\frac{dPCA}{dt} = \frac{K_{in}}{I(C_{w(s)})} - k_d \times P$$

where $I(C_{w(s)})$ is the inhibition function of warfarin (see next equation). It is appropriate to substitute K_{in} with $k_d \times P_0$. Inhibition of synthesis (rate in) has an impact upon the peak (trough) level rather than the time to the peak. This is similar to a constant-rate of drug infusion into a one-compartment system. The time to steady state is only governed by the elimination-rate constant and not the rate of infusion. At steady state:

$$\frac{dR}{dt} = \frac{K_{in}}{I(C_{w(s)})} - k_{out}P = 0$$

If the baseline condition for PCA with no inhibition of drug is

$$PCA = P_0$$

then the steady-state condition for the pharmacological response (PCA_{ss}) with drug present becomes:

$$PCA_{ss} = \frac{P_0}{I(C)} = P_0 \frac{1}{1 + \left[\dfrac{C_{w(s)}}{IC_{50S}}\right]^n}$$

and where $I(C_{w(s)})$ is a function of $C_{w(s)}$, n, and IC_{50S}, then:

$$I(C_{w(s)}) = 1 + \left[\frac{C_{w(s)}}{IC_{50S}}\right]^n$$

As stated before, the intensity of a pharmacological response may not be due to a direct effect of the drug on the receptor. Rather, it may be the net result of several processes only one of which is influenced by the drug. The process that is influenced by the drug must be identified and an attempt made to relate plasma drug concentration to changes in that process. Warfarin provides a good example of this, because the anticoagulant (hypothrombinemic) effect is an inhibition of the synthesis of certain vitamin K-dependent clotting factors.

Initial parameter estimates were obtained from the PCA versus time data. The baseline value (120 s) was obtained from the intercept on the effect axis. This value is the ratio K_{in}/k_d. From the intercept and slope, K_{in} was calculated to be 3.5 s h^{-1}. The plasma concentration at the time of the trough of the effect corresponded approximately with the EC_{50} value. Thus, $IC_{50} = 0.35$ mg $\cdot$ l^{-1}, $k_d = 0.3\,h^{-1}$, $n = 3.5$, $P_0 = 130\,s$, and $t_{lag} = 0\,h$. The computer fitting gave 0.262 ± 9.46 for the IC_{50}, 0.033 ± 17.9 for k_d, 2.68 ± 39.6 for n, and 121 ± 58 for P_0 (limits are CV%) with no lag time. Precision increased when a finite lag time was included in the fitting.

As stated earlier, these are two of many examples that can be chosen to illustrate principles. These two cases, however, are especially relevant to the relationship between animal work and Phase I studies in which only the simplest effects, such as counteraction of a painful stimulus, or raising/lowering of a physiological parameter such as PCA, are likely to be commonly measured. The reader is again referred to standard texts for more thorough treatment of models of this kind (Sharma and Jusko, 1997).

Commentary

Readers should note the emergence in recent years of a new modern term: "translational science." The distinction between translational science and Phase I is important, because both are concerned with the transition from preclinical work to clinical work, from animals to humans, from the bench to the

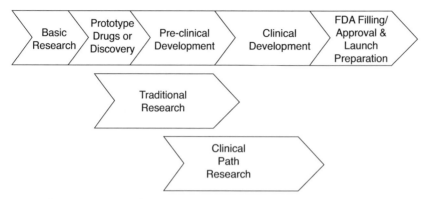

Figure 9.7 Translation science as defined by the FDA.

bedside. Translational science defines a phase of the drug discovery process starting in the relatively late stages of preclinical work, and ending in the early stages of product development in the clinic (see Figure 9.7). Thus Phase I is a section of translational science, but on the face of it, nothing has been changed by the application of this new terminology. However, the concept of translational science can be traced back some 15 years, mainly in oncology literature, and this modern use of the term has emerged as the result of a desire within the National Institutes of Health (NIH) and Food and Drug Administration (FDA) to provide funding to enable the products of discoveries made in academia and research institutes to be at least partially developed into commercially viable pharmaceuticals within such institutions. It is to be hoped that this will make the new drug discovery process faster and more scientifically rigorous.

Translational science should lead to the use of better predictions of the desired human properties of candidate drugs. Indeed, it has been suggested that the application of project management methods, such as the use of "target product profile," should be used to define in advance the desired properties in humans of a proposed new drug destined to reach Phase I, and then to use the scaling techniques described in this chapter to back-predict the desired properties that should be sought in the preclinical research phase in laboratory animals. In other words, we would change the paradigm from "discovery of the perfect drug for the healthy rat, hoping that it is good in humans" to "define

the perfect drug for the diseased human, and then determine the properties to be sought in the healthy rat that would lead to the discovery of that drug" (Curry, 2008). This would involve improvement in our methods of conduct of preclinical work, including the prediction of drug interactions.

One of the most exciting developments in this field in recent years has been the emergence of human microdosing. Scientifically, it means that doses below the threshold for any conceivable toxicity can be used in human studies with minimal interest from regulators and with quite limited preclinical safety work completed. The ultrasensitive methods of analysis used permit the study of very small doses, allowing for example, the early detection of deviations from pharmacokinetic linearity, and most important of all, the comparison of multiple compounds in early human testing, thus making the human, rather than the rat, the primary test species. This is sometimes termed "Phase 0," or it can be considered as an early stage of Phase I. Secondary consequences of this approach are lessened use of animals, the ability to study IV and oral doses in humans with all candidate drugs, often in the same investigation, improvement in the quality of data available when planning Phase II, and lesser need for early CMC and preformulation work.

We have not sought here to describe Phase I studies as such. This is a postgraduate textbook, and we wish to convey how *in vitro* and *in vivo* data of various kinds may be used to help extrapolate observed drug effects from simple experimental

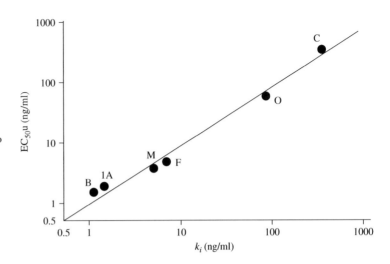

Figure 9.8 Correlation ($r = 0.993$, $p < 0.001$) between benzodiazepine free drug concentrations EC_{50} units producing 50% of the maximal EEG effect (change in amplitudes in the β frequency band, as determined by aperiodic EEG analysis) and affinity to the GABA–benzodiazepine receptor complex (K_i). Binding to the benzodiazepine receptor was determined on basis of displacement of [^{3}H]flumazenil in washed brain homogenate at 37°C. (Reproduced with permission from Danhof and Mandema, 1995).

systems to more complex situation. The ultimate need is to obtain useful predictions of response in healthy human subjects (Phase I studies) from observed drug effects in animals or in the test tube.

What are the strengths and weaknesses of these approaches? The use of intrinsic clearance *in vitro* permits predictions between species for the particular enzyme/route of metabolism concerned. If humans have qualitatively different routes of metabolism for any particular compound, this will weaken the predictive value of the *in vitro* observation. Similarly, allometric scaling works best for compounds with a high component of non-enzymatic elimination, such as our model compound with approximately 90% excretion as unchanged drug. This prediction weakens as variations in rates of enzymatic reactions become more important. The pharmacokinetic–pharmacodynamic modeling approaches use existing *in vivo* data to calculate constants that can be applied to other *in vivo* data, but does not, in its present form, link *in vitro* and *in vivo* data.

Significantly, none of these approaches uses drug–receptor binding data. Although K_d values are generated during initial screening of the scores of compounds emerging from medicinal chemistry laboratories, it has been a traditional problem that relative efficacy remains unknown (this does not detract from their value in chemical, structure–activity analyses). Neither do any

of these approaches use results of *in vitro* functional assays which emerge from screening of the compounds in biochemistry laboratories. It should be added that there are exceptions, however: drug–receptor binding constants and EC_{50} values from *in vivo* studies in animals were used by Danhof and Mandema (1995) to model drug effects at benzodiazepine receptors and effects on EEG (see Figure 9.8). Rowley *et al.* (1997) have taken a similar approach with NMDA antagonists.

Prospectus

In the future, models will exist that will link constants for *in vitro* binding to cloned human receptors (K_d), data from *in vitro* functional assays (IC_{50}), and animal and human *in vivo* EC_{50} values. A composite prediction matrix will be applied rapidly and accurately to the process of synthesis of new compounds for Phase I testing.

In the shorter term, what can we now do to expedite the drug selection process? Figure 9.9 represents a flow chart illustrating one form of metabolism/pharmacokinetics input into the drug discovery process. Arrows (indicating the flow of work and communication) pointing to the right represent perceived progress, whereas arrows pointing to the left represent "disappointments" (and other feedback) leading to corrections

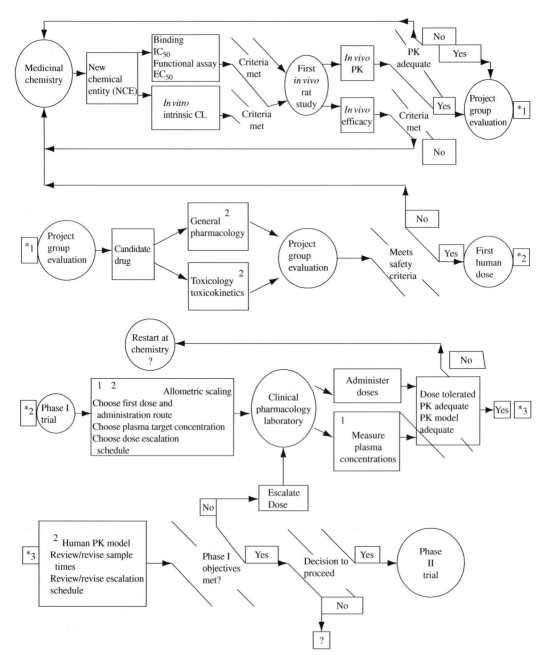

Figure 9.9 Flow diagram for involvement of pharmacokinetic and pharmacodynamic mode/computer-generated feedback into the iterative process of drug discovery from medicinal chemistry to the decision to enter Phase II trials. This is not a comprehensive flow diagram for all aspects of drug discovery—it is restricted to the components of the process discussed in this chapter. This flow diagram emphasizes efficient involvement of *in vitro* and *in vivo* experimental science and computer modeling, in review of data obtained in Phase I studies, in the decisions related to selection of the best compound for patient studies.

and revisions. The numbered asterisks indicate continuations. The "flow of time" is from left to right, and from the top panel to the bottom panel. The rectangles indicate tasks that are to be completed, and rectangles in a column within a panel represent work done by different departments, which may be simultaneous or not simultaneous but does not require much interaction between the investigators involved. Unlike the flow chart of a computer program, after which the diagram is modeled, most of the decisions are made in discussions among committee members, and may not necessarily be based on hard and fast criteria. Also, unlike a computer flow chart, the decision concerning a particular drug will usually be based in part on the results of work with other compounds that have the same indication.

In the boxes representing tasks to complete in the Phase I study in humans, we have used the symbol 1 to represent work that can be expedited by good validated preclinical data. The symbol 2 represents the tasks that can be expedited by online pharmacokinetic modeling. Among the pharmacokinetic questions that will be asked online in the Phase I trial are the following:

1. As the doses are escalated, do the kinetics of the drug appear to be linear or nonlinear over the dose range?

2. With repeated dosing, is there any evidence of a change in kinetics, e.g., a higher elimination rate that might be indicative of autoinduction?

3. Does the drug accumulate in tissues more than predicted with repeated dosing?

4. If preclinical work identified metabolite(s) to measure in humans, are the pharmacokinetics of metabolite(s) linear and as predicted?

5. Does the relationship between concentration and effect change with dose, time, and duration of treatment?

We expect that the task lists represented by some of the boxes will increase. For example, within the box including "*in vitro* intrinsic clearance," there may be *in vitro* predictors of oral availability, and measures of potentially toxic metabolites. The "*in vivo* pharmacokinetics" in rats may include an increasing number of compartments whose concentrations are measured by microdialysis, and

may include measures of a few selected metabolite concentrations.

This diagram is *not* a comprehensive guide to drug discovery. However, it does show that the chemists discover new chemical entities with desirable properties. *In vitro* biochemistry is followed by initial *in vivo* work in the rat, which is conducted with pharmacokinetic support and *in vitro* drug metabolism in parallel. Compounds meeting pre-arranged criteria proceed through pharmacological screening to general pharmacology and toxicology, all with pharmacokinetic support, which involves the development of pharmacokinetic and pharmacodynamic models. As a chemical series develops, correlations such as that in Figure 9.6 are developed. Eventually, a compound or compounds is/are chosen for Phase I studies.

In this scheme, Phase I is influenced by pharmacokinetic and pharmacodynamic modeling. This modeling is used to refine the Phase I protocol, providing advice on sampling times, doses, and warning signs of difficulty if they occur, as well as permitting comparison of, for example, EC_{50} data from humans with EC_{50} data from animals, and *in vitro/in vivo* comparisons. The objective is expeditious choice of the best compound, with the ever-present limitations on information available. Note that this scheme can involve feedback from Phase I to renewed chemical synthesis, as well as choice of a second or third compound for human testing.

Currently, Phase I studies themselves tend to be quite straightforward and focus on single compounds. Typically, after adequate preclinical characterization of a candidate drug and 14 day and/or 3 month multiple-dose toxicology studies in two mammalian species, a very low dose is chosen for the first human exposure to the drug. In later exposures, the dose is escalated according to some pre-arranged criteria until the drug concentrations in plasma associated with undesirable properties in animals are reached, and/or until some other limiting response is threatened or observed in the human volunteers. Doses may be single or short multiple-dose series. Simple physiological and biochemical measurements are routinely made in order to monitor for safety. If possible, responses to the drug are also measured when relevant to the intended therapeutic use. A drug successfully passes to Phase II if, with appropriate plasma levels, responses are predictable, reversible, related to the known pharmacological mechanisms of the drug, and there is a viewpoint among the investigators concerned that the drug could safely be given in initial studies to patients from its target population. Hopefully, all or most of what is observed in Phase I is in line with predictions based on the pharmacokinetic and pharmacodynamic properties of the drug in animals.

Once Phase I is complete, the human becomes the first-choice test species, under all but the most specialized of circumstances (e.g., effects on reproduction). In this context, Phase I serves as the interface between preclinical research and clinical development, and the validity of the predictions from animals to humans involved is of paramount importance.

We believe that with enhanced integrated study of animals and humans, and with data feedback based on computer models, the process of drug discovery from synthesis to proof of safety in humans could be dramatically improved in its efficiency. This is beyond what has traditionally been expected from departments of drug metabolism and pharmacokinetics (Welling and Tse, 1995). The time saved could be used to permit a larger number of compounds with better prospects, from a single research program, to be compared in Phase I studies. Consequently, the extremely costly testing programs in patients that follow Phase I could be started sooner and conducted better.

References

Ashforth EIL, Carlile DJ, Chenery R, Houston JB. Prediction of *in vivo* disposition from *in vitro* systems: clearance of phenytoin and tolbutamide using rat hepatic microsomal and hepatocyte data. *J Pharmacol Exp Ther* 1995; **274**:761–766.

Benet LZ, Kroetz DL, Sheiner LB. Pharmacokinetics: The dynamics of drug absorption, distribution and elimination. In *Goodman and Gilman's Pharmacological Basis of Therapeutics*, ninth edition, Hardman JG et al. (eds). McGraw-Hill: New York, USA, 1996, 3–28.

Bialobok P, Cregan EF, Sydserff SG, Eisman MS, Miller JA, Cross AJ, Simmons R, Gendron P, McCarthy DJ, Palmer GC. Efficacy of AR-R15896AR in the rat monofilament model of transient middle cerebral artery occlusion. *J Stroke Cerebrovasc Dis* 1999; **8**:388–397.

Boxenbaum H. Interspecies scaling, allometry, physiological time and the ground plan for pharmacokinetics. *J Pharmacokin Biopharm* 1982; **10**:201–227.

Boxenbaum H, DiLea C. First-time-in-human dose selection: allometric thoughts and perspectives. *J Clin Pharmacol* 1995; **35**:957.

Boxenbaum H, Ronfeld R. Interspecies pharmacokinetic scaling and the Dedrick plots. *Am J Physiol* 1983; **245**:R768–774.

Brodie BB. Physical and biochemical aspects of pharmacology. *J Am Med Assoc* 1967; **202**:600–609.

Colburn WA. Clinical markers and endpoints in bioequivalence assessment. *Drug Inf J* 1995; **29**:917.

Curry SH. *Drug Disposition and Pharmacokinetics*, third edition. Blackwell Scientific: Oxford, UK, 1980.

Curry SH and Whelpton R. *Drug Disposition and Pharmacokinetics*. John Wiley & Sons Ltd: Chichester, UK, 2010.

Curry SH. Translational science: past, present and future. *Biotechniques for Preclinical Development* 2008; **44**:ii–viii.

Curry SH, Chu P, Baumgartner TG, Stacpoole PW. Plasma concentrations and metabolic effects of intravenous sodium dichloroacetate. *Clin Pharmacol Ther* 1985; **37**:89–93.

Dahlstrom B, Paalzow LK, Segre G et al. Relation between morphine pharmacokinetics and analgesia. *J Pharmacokin Biopharm* 1978; **6**:41.

Danhof M, Mandema JW. Modeling of relationships between pharmacokinetics and pharmacodynamics. In *Pharmacokinetics: Regulatory—Industrial—Academic Perspectives*, second edition, Welling PG, Tse FLS (eds). Marcel Dekker: New York, USA, 1995, 139–194.

Dayneka NL, Garg V, Jusko W. Comparison of four basic models of indirect pharmacodynamic responses. *J Pharmacokin Biopharm* 1993; **21**:457.

Derendorf H, Hochhaus G (eds). *Pharmacokinetic/ Pharmacodynamic Correlation*. CRC Press: Boca Raton, FL, USA, 1995.

Fox AW, Sullivan BW, Buffini JD, *et al.* Reduction of serum lactate by sodium dichloroacetate, and human pharmacokinetic–pharmacodynamic relationships. *J Pharmacol Exp Ther* 1996; **279**:686–693.

Freireich EJ, Gehan EA, Rall DP, *et al.* Quantitative comparison of toxicity of anticancer agents in mouse, rat, hamster, dog, monkey and man. *Cancer Chemother Rep* 1966; **50**:219–240.

Gabrielsson J, Weiner D. *Pharmacokinetic and Pharmaco-dynamic Data Analysis: Concepts and Applications*, second edition. Apotekarsocieteten: Stockholm, Sweden, 1997.

Gibaldi M, Perrier D. *Pharmacokinetics*, second edition. Marcel Dekker: New York, USA, 1982, 231–232.

Hawkins RD, Kalant H. The metabolism of ethanol and its metabolic effects. *Pharmacol Rev* 1972; **24**:242–249.

Houston JB. Utility of *in vitro* drug metabolism data in predicting *in vivo* metabolic clearance. *Biochem Pharmacol* 1994; **47**:1469–1479.

Ings RMJ. Interspecies scaling and comparisons in drug development and toxicokinetics. *Xenobiotica* 1990; **20**:1201–1231.

Iwatsubo T, Hirota N, Ooie T, *et al.* Prediction of *in vivo* drug disposition from *in vitro* data based on physiological pharmacokinetics. *Biopharmaceut Drug Disposit* 1996; **17**:273–310.

Jenkinson DH, Barnard EA, Hoyer D, *et al.* International union of pharmacology committee on receptor nomenclature and drug classification. IX. Recommendations on terms and symbols in quantitative pharmacology. *Pharmacol Rev* 1995; **47**:225.

Jusko WJ. Pharmacodynamics of chemotherapeutic effects: dose–time response relationships for phase-non-specific agents. *J Pharm Sci* 1971; **60**:892.

Lesko LJ, Williams RL. Regulatory perspectives: The role of pharmacokinetics and pharmacodynamics. In *Pharmacodynamics and Drug Development: Perspectives in Clinical Pharmacology*, Cutler NR, Sramek JJ, Narang PK (eds). John Wiley & Sons Ltd: Chichester, UK, 1994.

Levy G. Relationship between elimination rate of drugs and rate of decline of their pharmacologic effects. *J Pharm Sci* 1964; **53**:342.

Levy G. Kinetics of pharmacological effects. *Clin Pharmacol Ther* 1966; **7**:362.

Levy G. The case for preclinical pharmacodynamics. In *Integration of Pharmacokinetics, Pharmacodynamics, and Toxicokinetics in Rational Drug Development*, Yacobi A, Shah VP, Skelley JP, Benet LZ (eds). Plenum: New York, USA, 1993.

Levy G. Mechanism-based pharmacodynamic modeling. *Clin Pharmacol Ther* 1994; **56**:356.

Levy G, Nelson E. Theoretical relationship between dose, elimination rate and duration of pharmacological effect of drugs. *J Pharm Sci* 1965; **54**:872.

Meyer UA. The molecular basis of genetic polymorphisms of drug metabolism. *J Pharm Pharmacol* 1994; **46**(suppl 1): 409–415.

Minneman KP, Fox AW, Abel PA. Occupancy of α-adrenergic receptors and contraction of rat vas deferens. *Mol Pharmacol* 1983; **23**:359–368.

Murphy J, Casey W, Lasagna L. The effect of dosing regimen on the diuretic efficacy of chlorothiazide in human subjects. *J Pharmacol Exp Ther* 1961; **134**:286.

Nagashima R, O'Reilly RA, Levy G. Kinetics of pharmacologic effects in man: the anticoagulant action of warfarin. *Clin Pharmacol Ther* 1969; **10**:22.

Obach RS. Prediction of human pharmacokinetics using *in vitro–in vivo* correlations. In *Pharmacokinetic/ Pharmacodynamic Analysis: Accelerating Drug Discovery and Development*, Schlegel J (ed.). Biomedical Library Series. International Business Communications: Southborough, MA, USA, 1996a.

Obach RS. The importance of nonspecific binding *in vitro* matrices, its impact on kinetic studies of drug metabolism reactions, and implications for *in vitro–in vivo* correlations. *Drug Metab Disposit* 1996b; **24**:1047–1049.

Pitsui M, Parker E, Aarons L, Rowland M. Population pharmacokinetics and pharmacodynamics of warfarin in healthy young adults. *Eur J Pharm Sci* 1993; **1**: 151.

Rane A, Wilkinson G, Shand D. Prediction of hepatic extraction from *in vitro* measurement of intrinsic clearance. *J Pharmacol Exp Ther* 1977; **200**:420–424.

Ross EM. Pharmacodynamics: mechanisms of drug action and the relationship between drug concentration and effect. In *Goodman and Gilman's Pharmacological Basis of Therapeutics*, tenth edition. Hardman JG et al. (eds). Pergamon: New York, USA, 1996.

Rowley M, Kulagowski JJ, Walt AP, *et al.* Effect of plasma protein binding on *in vivo* activity and brain penetration of glycine/NMDA receptor antagonists. *J Med Chem* 1997; **40**:4053–4068.

Segre G. Kinetics of interaction between drugs and biological systems. *Il Farmaco* 1968; **23**:907.

Sharma A, Jusko WJ. Characterization of four basic models of indirect pharmacological responses. *J Pharmacokin Biopharmaceut* 1997; **24**:611–635.

Sheiner LB, Stanski DR, Vozeh S, *et al.* Simultaneous modelling of pharmacokinetics and pharmacodynamics: application to D-tubocurarine. *Clin Pharmacol Ther* 1979; **25**:358.

Shimada T, Yamazaki H, Minura M, *et al.* Inter-individual variations in human liver cytochrome P450 enzymes involved in the oxidation of drugs, carcinogens, and toxic chemicals: studies with liver microsomes of 30 Japanese and 30 Caucasians. *J Pharmacol Exp Ther* 1994; **270**:414–423.

Smith DA, Jones BC, Walker DK. Design of drugs involving the concepts and theories of drug metabolism and pharmacokinetics. *Med Res Rev* 1996; **16**:243–266.

Smolen VF. Quantitative determination of drug bioavailability and biokinetic behavior from pharmacological data for ophthalmic and oral administration of a mydriatic drug. *J Pharm Sci* 1971; **60**:354.

Smolen VF. Theoretical and computational basis for drug bioavailability determinations using pharmacological data I: general considerations and procedures. *J Pharmacokin Biopharm* 1976; **4**:337.

Wagner JG. Kinetics of pharmacological response: I. Proposed relationships between response and drug concentration in the intact animal and man. *J Theoret Biol* 1968; **20**:173.

Welling PG, Tse FLS (eds). *Pharmacokinetics: Regulatory–Industrial–Academic Perspectives*, section edition. Marcel Dekker: New York, USA, 1995.

Wilkinson GR. Clearance approaches in pharmacology. *Pharmacol Rev* 1987; **39**:1–47.

Yee S. *In vitro* permeability across Caco-2 cells (colonic) can predict *in vivo* (small intestinal) absorption in man—fact or myth. *Pharm Res* 1997; **14**:763–766.

Further reading

Gabrielsson J, Dolgos H, Gillberg P-G, Bradberg U, Benthem B, Duker G. Early integration of pharmacokinetic and dynamic reasoning is essential for optimal development of lead compounds: strategic considerations. *Drug Discovery Today* 2009; **14**:358–372.

Gabrielsson J, Green AR. Quantitative pharmacology or pharmacokinetic pharmacodynamic integration should be a vital component in integrative pharmacology. *The Journal of Pharmacology and Experimental Theurapeutics* 2009; **331**: 767–774.

Van der Graaf PH, Gabrielsson J. Pharmacokinetic-pharmacodynamic reasoning in drug discovery and early development. *Future Med Chem* 2010, in press.

CHAPTER 10

Phase II and Phase III Clinical Studies

Anthony W. Fox

EBD Group Inc., Carlsbad, CA, USA and Munich, Germany, and Skaggs SPPS, University of California, San Diego, USA

The phases of drug development: an obsolete model?

In former times, it was assumed that developmental drugs proceeded in step-wise fashion from Phase I, through Phase II, to Phase III, prior to filing a Product Licensing Agreement (PLA) or New Drug Application (NDA). Phase I was conducted in "normal volunteers" (although some medical students might hardly characterize this term!). Phase II trials were initial studies in selected patients, and Phase III was seen as wide-scale studies in broader patient populations. After approval, certain studies to find new indications, address special patient subpopulations, for marketing purposes, or to otherwise broaden product labeling might or might not be conducted. All post-approval studies were termed Phase IV.

In modern practice, the distinctions between Phases I, II, III, and IV are very often blurred. Three principal, and interlocking, pressures have caused this blurring: time, finance, and an evolving regulatory environment.

Of these three pressures, the most important is time. Strategies such as the overlapping of development "phases," as well as the use of early dose-ranging studies as pivotal, and choosing doses based on surrogate endpoints, are technical responses to this challenge.

Financial pressures, even for the largest pharmaceutical companies, are generally much greater than in the past. The technical response is to maximize resources, avoiding any and all redundant clinical studies (see Chapters 53 and 57).

The regulatory pressures come both from the regulatory authorities and from within the pharmaceutical companies themselves. Regulatory authorities have increased in their scientific sophistication during the last thirty years. The questions that are now asked of companies, and the earlier stages of drug development when these questions are asked, have driven change in clinical study design. Increasingly sophisticated data are now developed at earlier and earlier stages of drug development.

In the later stages of the development of successful drugs, the interval between PLA or NDA filing and product launch is not wasted. The term "Phase IIIb" has been invented for the conduct of Phase IV-type studies during the pre-approval period. Furthermore, in some companies, the old "Phase IV", is now divided into Phases IV and V, without any generally agreed definitions except, perhaps, that the studies are run by different teams.

Quite apart from these general trends blurring the distinctions between Phases I, II, and III, there are (and always have been) sound medical or pharmacological reasons for doing so. Good examples might be the following:

- It would be unreasonable to study the pharmacokinetics of relatively toxic agents, at potentially therapeutic doses, in normal volunteers due to the near-certainty of the adverse events. Typically, this information can be gained in patients with diseases potentially responsive to these agents. Thus the first-in-human studies in this case are "Phase II," using the classic nomenclature. Cytotoxic and anti-viral drugs are two important classes of agent where this is commonly the case.

Principles and Practice of Pharmaceutical Medicine, 3rd edition.
Edited by L.D. Edwards, A.W. Fox, P.D. Stonier.

• There is little point in testing the tolerability of drugs in normal volunteers, when only patients with the disease of interest are able to demonstrate a relevant pharmacodynamic effect. The doses at which tolerability must be confirmed are unknown until the exposure of patients can indicate the doses that may be effective. The development of potent opioids such as alfentanil, sufentanil, and remifentanil, as anesthetic agents, are one example.

• There are some diseases that have no animal model, or relevant pharmacodynamic or surrogate endpoint in normal volunteers. Such diseases may also alter the pharmacokinetics of the drug, thus invalidating anything that might be learned from normal volunteers. An example is the migraine syndrome. No animal species has migraine, and normal volunteers cannot report an anti-migraine effect. Nausea, vomiting, and gastric stasis are common during migraine attacks and may be expected to alter the pharmacokinetics and effectiveness of oral therapies.

There is nonetheless little hope that the Phase I, II, III aphorism will die. Nevertheless, it is quite wrong to assume that these "classical" terms and definitions still apply to how drugs are developed according to modern practice. The classical four-phase strategy of drug development is far too stereotyped, simplistic, and pedestrian to have survived into the modern era of drug development. None of today's successful companies actually use such a strategy. We are simply shackled with an outmoded terminology.

Concepts of bias and statistical necessities

Bias is a general consideration in clinical trial design, regardless of the type of trial being conducted. It is considered here as an overarching issue, to be applied to the systematic description of the types of study design considered below.

The word bias has many definitions, but in this context it is best described as a distortion of, or prejudice towards, observed effects that may or may not truly be due to the action of the test drug(s). Many things can distort the true measure-ment of drug action, and bias is the trialist's most unremitting enemy. This enemy comes from many quarters (see Table 10.1). The clinical trialist must be sufficiently humble to realize that he or she, himself or herself, may be a source of bias.

The clinical trialist may not be expected to be a specialist statistician, and statistics are not the subject of this chapter. However, the ability to talk to and understand statisticians is absolutely essential. *Sine qua non: involve a good statistician from the moment a clinical trial is contemplated.* Furthermore, the clinical trialist should be confident of a sound understanding of the concepts of type I and type II error, and the probabilities α and β (e.g., Freiman *et al.*, 1978). This is one of the best defenses against bias.

Prospective definitions: the only way to interpret what you measure

It does not require a training in advanced statistics to hold a common-sense and accurate approach to creating clinical hypotheses, translate them into the precise quantities of a measured endpoint, and then interpret the results. Although the finer points of statistics are presented in Chapter 28, it is common sense that the only way to interpret what you measure is to define this whole process *before* the experiment starts.

Thinking carefully about what might actually constitute an observed response *before* you measure it, removes at least one important source of bias: the clinical trialist him- or herself. There has been too little emphasis in recent years on the funda-mentals of endpoints, their variability, and how they are measured. Furthermore the relationship between what is measured and its clinical relevance is always debatable: the tendency is to measure something that *can* be measured, rather than some-thing that *needs validation as clinically relevant*. Good examples include rheumatological studies: counts of inflamed joints before and after therapy may be reported, but do not reveal whether the exper-imental treatment or the corresponding placebo caused some of the patients to recover the ability

Table 10.1 Some example sources of bias in clinical trials

Poorly matched placebos
Subtle or obvious non-randomization of patients
Failure of double-blinding, e.g., when pharmacodynamic effects cannot be controlled
Prompting of prejudiced subjective responses
Nonuniform medical monitoring
Protocol amendments with unequal effects on treatment groups
Peculiarities of the study site itself (e.g., psychotropic drug effects in psychiatric institutions that fail to predict effects in out-patients)

Differing medical definitions across languages, dialects, or countries (e.g., "mania")
CRF with leading questions, either toward or away from adverse event reporting
Informal, "break the blind" games played at study sites
Selective rigor in collection and storage of biological samples
Selectively incomplete datasets for each patient
Inappropriate use of parametric or nonparametric statistical techniques
Failure adequately to define endpoints prospectively, and retrospective "data dredging"
Acceptance of correlation as evidence of causation
Averaging of proportionate responses from nonhomogenous treatment groups, also known as Simpson's paradox; see Spilker (1991)

Unskeptically accepting anecdotal reports
Tendency to publish only positive results

CRF: case report form; the term "controlled" is used in its technical sense, as used in this chapter)

to write or others the ability to walk (Chaput de Saintonge and Vere, 1982). Chapter 26 addresses some similar issues.

Most clinical trialists experience the urge, especially in early studies, to collect every piece of data that they possibly can, before and after every drug exposure. This urge comes from natural scientific curiosity, as well as a proper ethical concern because the hazard associated with clinical trials is never zero. It behooves us to maximize the amount of information gained in return for the risk that the patient takes, and for medicine in general.

Consequently, large numbers of variables are typically measured before and after drug (or placebo) administration. These variables all exhibit biological variation. Many of these variations have familiar, unimodal, symmetrical distributions, which are supposed to resemble Gaussian (Normal), Chi-squared, f, binomial, and so on, probability density functions. An intrinsic property of biological variables is that when measured one hundred times, then, on the average and if Normally distributed, 5% of those measurements will be more than ± 2 standard deviations from the

mean (there are corollaries for the other probability density functions). This meets a typical, prospective "$P < 0.05$, and therefore it is significant" mantra. It is also true that if you measure one hundred different variables, on two occasions only, before and after administration of the test material, then, on the average, 5% of those variables are going to be significantly different after treatment (this masquerades sometimes in findings among "selected secondary endpoints"). A sound interpretation, of course, is based upon only those endpoints that were selected before the experiment began, and comparing these with those for which no such statistical differences were found.

Historical clinical trials

There is a single clinical trial in ancient literature, with the date being somewhere between the 2nd and 6th centuries BCE. Daniel was one of a group of selected youths who were sent to Babylon because they were thought that they could benefit from the education that was available at the King's court. Wanting to maintain their religion in this heathen land, Daniel and a few of his companions persuaded the officers of the court to allow them their kosher diet, instead of insisting that they ate the usual palace food. The trial period was ten days. At the end of those ten days, the court officers judged the Israelites to be in better health than the rest of the group who had continued to eat "the King's meat" (*Book of Daniel*, 1:8–16). This open-label, parallel-group study, with an unrandomized, age-matched control group, had an endpoint (healthy appearance) and, evidently to the surprise of the King's officers, an accepted alternative hypothesis (kosher diet apparently more healthy than "the King's meat"). A humanistic endpoint was that it reinforced the faith of Daniel and his friends, who had turned away from the *a priori* temptations of the largesse of the Court; a clear example of patient outcome benefit resulting from clinical trial participation. We do not know whether this clinical trial finding was used to adapt the court diet more generally thereafter (and can probably safely assume not). In spite of some anachronisms in recent fiction, there is no other evidence that the ancient world or the medieval Arabs carried out prospective clinical studies, nor that there were any controlled experiments in animal husbandry or plant domestication during those eras.

The next known clinical trialist is probably Sir John Elwes, a famous 18th century miser, of Marcham Manor, Berkshire, England (now The Denman College of the Womens' Institute). Apothecaries were the general practitioners of the time, and Elwes had suffered burns to both his legs. So the apothecary's fee was gambled on his professional treatment of one leg, while Elwes would treat his other leg being left to his own devices. The apothecary duly lost his fee because the professionally-treated leg took two weeks longer to heal. The precise date of this $n = 1$ clinical trial is uncertain, but it must have been close to what is generally accepted as the earliest clinical trial, conducted by Lt. James Lind, RN.

Scurvy was rampant in the Royal Navy during the 18th and 19th centuries, often literally decimating ships' crews. Thomas (1997) has pointed out that sailing men-of-war frequently went many months without docking (for example, Nelson spent 24 unbroken months on *HMS Victory* while blockading French ports, and it is said that Collingwood once went 22 months without even dropping anchor). Sailors survived on the poor diets carried aboard for these long periods, with water-weevils and biscuit-maggots constituting important dietary protein! Even before Lind's time, the Dutch had already learned to treat scurvy by replenishing their ships at sea with fresh fruit and vegetables.

Lind had been pressed into the Royal Navy, as a Surgeon's Mate, in 1739, and with some experience as an apprentice surgeon in Edinburgh. It is a nice irony that the first prospective clinical study with $n > 1$ was actually conducted by a surgeon!

The clinical trial was held at a single site, *HMS Salisbury*, a frigate in the English Channel during the early summer of 1747 (Lind, 1753; Frey 1969; Thomas, 1997). The experimental controls included that all twelve patients met the same inclusion criteria (putrid gums, spots on the skin, lassitude, and weakness of the knees). All patients received the same diet except for the test materials. All treatments were administered simultaneously (parallel-group). Compliance with therapy was confirmed by direct observation in all cases. The trial had six parallel groups, with $n = 2$ patients per group. The test medications were (daily dose size): a) cider (1 quart); b) elixir of vitriol (25 drops); c) vinegar (two spoonfuls plus vinegar added to the diet and used as a gargle); d) sea water ("a course"); e) citrus fruit (two oranges, plus one lemon when it could be spared); and f) nutmeg (a "bigness"). Lind noted, with some disdain, that this last treatment was tested only because it was recommended by a surgeon on land. The famous result was that within 6 days only 2 of the 12 patients had improved, both in the citrus fruit group, one of whom became fit for duty and the other at least fit enough to nurse the remaining ten patients.

We should note the absence of dose-standardization and probably of randomization because Lind's two sea-water patients were noted to have "tendons in the ham rigid," unlike the others. However, the result had been crudely replicated by using $n = 2$ in each group. If we accept that the hypothesis was that the citrus-treated patients alone would improve (Lind was certainly skeptical of the anecdotal support for the other five alternative treatments), then using a binomial probability distribution, the result has $p = 0.0075$. But statistics had hardly been invented, and Lind had no need of them to interpret the clinical significance of this brilliant clinical trial.

Lind was not quick to publish his most famous treatise reporting this clinical trial (Lind, 1753). Indeed, in 1748, his Edinburgh MD thesis was on an entirely unrelated subject. Subsequently, Lind was Treasurer of the Royal College of Surgeons of Edinburgh, and then appointed physician to the Royal Naval Hospital, Haslar (a fifth of his first 6000-odd admissions were for scurvy). He subsequently developed a large private practice, but little fame amongst his peers, and was buried at Gosport in 1794. The Royal Navy was even slower to act on his findings, only instituting citrus juice into sailors' diets the year after Lind's death, following much administrative resistance but no scientific controversy (Bardolph and Taylor, 1997).

The British, especially those in the Royal Navy, are still known as "limeys." This is the unique example of a national nickname based on a therapy proven by clinical trial.

Thus, Lind illustrates some other aspects of clinical trials. First, he had little academic kudos, although he was clearly qualified by experience and training (a requirement of trialists by law in the United States). Second, he did not publish his results rapidly. Third, his results were not implemented promptly in the interests of the public health. It is important to realize that these undesirable aspects of clinical trials persist to this day.

Limitations of controlled clinical trials

Modern clinical trials are therefore not necessarily the holy grail of therapeutic progress. Chance observations have historically led to huge advances. Today's three most commonly used cardiovascular drugs are good examples: digoxin is a component of digitalis (famously reported by Withering after observing the treatment of a dropsical lady by a gypsy), aspirin is derived from the willow tree bark first reported by the Rev. Edmund Brown to treat his own malarious fevers, and warfarin is the result of a University of Wisconsin investigation into a hemorrhagic disease of cattle. Lest we forget, Jenner's experiments would be ethically impossible today: they included deliberate exposure to small pox. Moreover, aspirin is a drug that would doubtless fail during modern preclinical toxicology due to chromosomal breaks and the gastrointestinal adverse effects in rodents which are due to systemic, not local, exposure. Thus, major advances in therapeutics have not always arisen from controlled clinical trials.

Statistical theory must also be held not only with respect but also healthy skepticism (although this is really the subject of Chapter 28). It should be remembered that the development of statistics, as they have come to be applied to clinical trials, has arisen from a variety of non-mammalian biological sources. Experimental agriculture stimulated the early giants (Drs Fisher, Yates) to explore probability density functions. While epidemiological studies have confirmed much that is similar in human populations, it is unknown whether these probability density functions apply uniformly to all disease states. Any statistical test that we employ makes assumptions that are usually not stated.

The clinical development plan

It is impossible to consider clinical trial protocol design in isolation. All clinical protocols should be written after a clinical development plan and target product profile have been agreed by the diverse membership of the clinical development team. The clinical development plan should itself follow the construction of a hypothetical drug label (see Chapter 43). The goals of such a plan might be as limited as to provide for the start of Phase II, or as complex as mapping an entire route from first-in-human studies to product registration. The path from the present status to the overall goal can then be understood. It may be added that, within a large company, this is also a good way for clinical and marketing departments to communicate.

Protocols, case-report forms, and investigators' brochures

Chapters 34, 35 and 37 describe the regulatory governance of clinical trials, and little needs to be added here. These clinical trial documents are central to these processes. Equally the regulatory requirements (which still vary from country to country), and the documents needed to support them, must be taken into account when constructing the clinical development plan.

Objectives and pre-requisites of Phase II studies

Gallenical forms

Most regulatory authorities will want reassurance that the pharmacokinetic properties of the marketed product closely resemble those in which the pivotal studies are carried out. Easiest is when pivotal clinical trials for registration purposes are conducted with the same formulation and manufacturing process that is proposed to be taken to market. The alternative is to "bridge" a Phase III study to the marketed formulation by the demonstration, for example, that two different tablets have the same pharmacokinetic (PK) profile. However, the risk is that different formulations will not turn out to possess the same PK profile, and then either new pivotal studies have to be conducted with the new formulation, or registration be delayed until the new formulation is adapted, and a repeat "bridging study" is successful. For inhaled drugs, where it is not possible to measure deposition fraction in humans, this is especially difficult. It is a risky gamble to leave development of the final formulation until the end of a clinical development plan.

Informed consent

This is considered in detail in Chapter 8. The clinical trialist should remember, however, that he or she ultimately carries the ethical responsibility for this document, regardless of what corporate lawyers and others may wish to do with it. Typically, Institutional Review Boards in the US are more likely to be tolerant of long forms than ethics committees in Europe.

Anticipating tolerability issues

Toxicological coverage is covered in more detail in Chapter 7. However, the clinical trialist is encouraged to consider this for every protocol. A useful method is to start with the general case: What is the relationship between duration and dose size(s) in prior animal studies and the clinical protocol-specified dose size and duration? This exercise ought to be conducted using methods that standardize both for body weight and body surface area across species. Close review of all the prior human exposure to the test drug is also recommended. Does this, or other aspects of the known pharmacology of the investigational drug, suggest any particular tolerability issues for which special monitoring methods are needed? Is the disease under study likely to bring additional hazard in comparison to what has been observed before? And *think laterally*.

For example, what is likely to be the adverse effects of a potassium channel-blocking drug being investigated for a central nervous system indication? The answer may lie in all the excitable tissues that contain potassium channels. Is there is any preclinical evidence that the drug discriminates between potassium channels in different tissues? Was a hERG study done? Are there changes in the EEG or ECG in the non-human database or among prior human exposures to the test agent, which escaped being reported because "not thought to be clinically significant" ? Would it be more appropriate to do a human thorough QT study before conducting this clinical trial in (say) patients with epilepsy?

Common Phase II/III study designs

Many initial studies are conducted in an uncontrolled fashion. Eminent professors will treat a few of their patients with a test medication (perhaps under an Investigators' Investigational New Drug (IND) in the United States) and form opinions about the worth (or otherwise) of a new therapy. Although this may be grist for the mill of press releases and fund-raising for small companies, these uncontrolled observations often mistakenly

Table 10.2 Basic trial designs and the factors that are suited and unsuited to each

Trial type	Factors suited	Factors unsuited
Parallel-group, single treatment	Episodic disease Imperfect placebo matching Blinding difficult (e.g., surgical procedures, psychtropic drugs)	Rare disease
Parallel-group, chronic treatment	Stable disease state	Unethical to use active comparator or placebo
Crossover with washout	Stable disease state Ethical to use placebo after active	Untreated washout not ethical
Sequential	Rare disease Homogenous disease state Urgent need to save life	Complicated tolerability profile Many concomitant disease factors
"N of 1"	Stable disease state	Few or no feasible alternative therapies
"Large simple"	Very common disease Easily measured endpoints Well-understood drug	Tolerability issues not closely related to efficacy variable
Open label	Tolerability issues only	Spontaneous adverse event frequency high.
Within-patient dose ranging	Stable disease state Intolerable high initial dose	Drug tolerance
Combination therapy	*A priori* reason to expect favorable drug interaction.	Unethical to use single therapy

become a false, yet cast-iron credo for the sponsoring company. An observed effect, any effect, is viewed as better than none, and the relative lack of scientific controls permits large biases to arise.

The first risk from this haphazard start to clinical development is that potentially good options for a test compound may be needlessly rejected. The professor's patient population may not include a disease state or disease subtype for which the new drug is actually well-suited. Equally, efficacy, and tolerability may be dose-dependent, and this can only be assessed when studied in a systematic fashion. Finally, most drugs are just one of a series of compounds that share closely related properties in preclinical testing. It is impossible to know which of these is the most promising, when only one has been tested.

Assuming that reasonable tolerability, reasonable understanding of pharmacokinetics, and (preferably) a relevant pharmacodynamic effect has been observed in normal volunteers (see Chapter 2.07),

the first task is to reassess all of these in a relevant disease state. This is slower and needs more patients than small, uncontrolled observations. But at the end of a small number of such small studies there ought to be good information about the feasibility of a pivotal clinical trials program, and if not, then what the feasible course corrections might be (e.g., alternative indications). Note that one such course correction may be ceasing to develop the drug, and switching to another member in the series. "Killing" drugs at the earliest appropriate moment can be the most valuable thing that a Phase II program can accomplish, allowing finite resources of time and money to be diverted to something more promising.

When choosing a clinical trial design (see Table 10.2), economic factors include numbers of patients, time that will elapse, drug supply, and total cost. Although these economies are important and relevant in all design choices, they should also be factored against the endpoints that may or will be measured. The relevance of an endpoint, and its sensitivity to detect a drug-related effect, may be primarily dependent upon the duration of patient exposure. For example, a short period of observation is unlikely to detect a difference in time to next seizure in a study of anti-epileptic drug with an add-on design in patients who are only moderately disabled by epilepsy. On the other hand, the identification of a PK interaction between a new and an established therapy in the same population may only require very short observation periods.

There are several common classes of study design. These classes apply to almost all phases of drug development. No list of trial designs can be exhaustive, because almost all clinical trials are different. What follows is an attempt to review briefly the classes of clinical trial design that will encompass a large majority of studies, and to comment on their economy and endpoint possibilities.

Parallel-group studies are typically thought of as the most straightforward design case. In fact, a bewildering array of variations exist within this class.

In the simplest case of parallel-group study, a group of patients presenting sequentially are randomized to one of two equally-sized treatment groups, until a prospectively determined total number of patients has been recruited. All these patients are followed for a pre-determined period of time, or until some endpoint is achieved. The database is quality assured and locked before the randomization code is broken. The patients are then sorted according to their treatment, the endpoint measurements are subjected to a statistical test, and an interpretation of the effect (or absence thereof) of the drug is made. What could possibly go wrong?

The answer is that little can go wrong when there are ample patients, plenty of drug available, the choice of dose-size has been perfect, the endpoints are incontrovertible, the measurements are possible using a rational or absolute scale, there is ample toxicological coverage for all the dose sizes employed, and the trialist has unlimited time and budget! This utopian combination of conditions never exists.

The *ascending dose-ranging cohort* design is one variant within the parallel-group class. It is best suited when there is no cast-iron assurance of tolerability for all the dose sizes of interest. Patients are randomized in cohorts to either active- or placebo-treatment; frequently there are fewer placebo-treated patients in each cohort.

The objective is to cumulate tolerability experience as dose size gradually increases. If the treatments in the first cohort prove to be well-tolerated, the next cohort is randomized in the same way except that the active-treated patients receive a larger dose size. Note that this judgment can be made without breaking the blind. A comparable number of placebo-treated patients to any single active-treatment group can be cumulated across several cohorts, each cohort having fewer placebo- than active-treated patients. This economizes on patient numbers in comparison to randomizing each cohort in a 1:1 fashion, and may also economize on both drug and patients if two doses are found to be similarly effective and well-tolerated, albeit not the highest dose that was projected.

Sequential cohorts do not usually economize on time. Treatment codes can be broken at the end of each cohort (and not introduce bias into observations of succeeding cohorts). Sometimes this can lead to early closure of the study when the desired pharmacodynamic effect is observed at a lower dose than the maximum projected by the study or when unreasonable intolerability is shown to be associated with active treatment. However, the deliberations of safety committees at the end of each cohort can often be time-consuming.

Within patient dose titration designs may be conceptualized as the application of an ascending dose cohort design within a single patient. The advantages of such designs are when immediate high-dose therapy is contraindicated for tolerability reasons, and when there is likely to be large variations *between patients* in the tolerability and efficacy of the test drug.

Patients are reviewed during and after completion of a course of therapy, which may include programmed changes in dose size. If the drug was well-tolerated they may progress to a course of therapy at higher dose. A prospective limit on dosing and the number of courses of treatment is made (for example, according to toxicology coverage). Dosing may be curtailed at any time when either there is unreasonable intolerance of the drug, or when acceptable efficacy and simultaneous tolerability has been observed. This is not unlike the approach to therapy under ordinary clinical circumstances. For example, patients with epilepsy are often treated by dose alterations. Another advantage of this design is that at the end of the study, the range of tolerated and efficacious doses can be examined among all treated patients in comparison to demographic factors, disease subtypes, and so on.

The greatest difficulty with ascending-dose, within-patient designs is usually in treatment-masking. Double-blind requirements have to take into account a wide variety of dose sizes, and that contemporaneous placebo formulations will be needed. Some studies of this type are hybridized with a crossover strategy (see the next section). Dose-tailing at the end of the study may be viewed as the same procedure in reverse, although may be conducted open-label and more rapidly (guided by suitable PK information) than when therapy is being introduced.

Sources of bias in this study design arise from the exposure of patients to lower doses first. Patients obligatorily must tolerate, and fail to respond to, lower doses before being exposed to higher doses. Any degree of treatment familiarization, tachyphylaxis, or patient withdrawal rate biases dose–response curves to the right (i.e., tends to overestimate the ED50) in comparison to a parallel-group study in the same patients with the same endpoints.

Crossover studies

Generally, crossover studies are more complicated than parallel-group designs. Patients are exposed to more than one test medication, in sequential treatment periods, perhaps with periods of no therapy intervening between those of active therapy ("washout"). Active therapies may be different drugs, or different doses of the same drug, or in complicated studies, both.

The most famous problem is eliminating carry-over effects (inadequate "washout"). Ideally, end-points should be measured and unambiguously attributable to one of the test regimens. This requires no residual effects of the previous regimen(s) (see Laska *et al.*, 1983). If this involves intervening placebo-treatment periods in between test medications, then clearly this approach is not possible when placebos are ethically unjustifiable.

Usually, patients are randomized to a particular treatment order, and all patients are eventually exposed to the same variety of treatments. Large numbers of treatment periods, assigned using a Latin square, have been reported; however, the logistics and patient retention in such studies is usually difficult, and these ideal designs are likely to be successful only when treatment periods are short; ideal designs are most common for normal volunteer studies (e.g., Amin *et al.*, 1995).

In later phase studies, if there are still numerous treatments or dose sizes that need to be tested, "partial crossover" designs can be used. These expose patients to a random subset of all the study treatments, again in a random order. "Partial crossover" designs necessarily require the availability of large numbers of patients. However, there can be economies of the amounts of test drug needed, and in the time needed to conduct the study, in comparison to an equivalent, complete, crossover design. Shorter durations of patient participation are also usually associated with less missing data and fewer patients lost for administrative reasons. Overall patient recruitment is more efficient.

Clinical trialists should be wary of using randomized, crossover designs when there is likely to be appreciable numbers of patients who are withdrawn before completing the study. This can cause serious imbalance among treatment groups and seriously jeopardize the likelihood of achieving a statistically robust result. Crossover studies with three or more periods have a substantial advantage over two-period designs, when the amount of missing data is likely to be large, and statistical salvage is necessary (Ebbutt, 1984).

Minimization trials

Less common are trial designs that specifically and adaptively minimize the number of patients needed, while preserving design integrity for appropriate statistical analysis. Early "evolutionary" designs are now being succeeded by independent treatment allocation, in pursuit of this goal. All

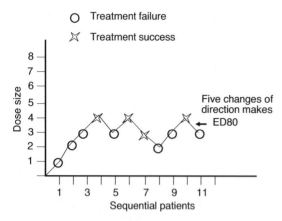

Figure 10.1 The Dixon up-down ("adaptive") clinical trial design. Patients are recruited sequentially into the study, at a rate where each one reaches the study endpoint before the dose for the next one is selected. The study begins at the lowest dose. If there is no response (circle) then the next patient gets the next higher dose. In the event that a patient responds to therapy, or unacceptable toxicity is encountered (star), the next patient receives the previous (lower) dose. The study is complete after the plot has changed directions five times.

minimization designs involve arduous statistical planning and the clinical trialist should seek expert help from the outset.

Evolutionary designs were introduced by Dixon and Armitage. Although the statistical analysis is rather different, they have the same objective, which is to detect a treatment effect at the earliest moment possible, using the fewest possible patients, while retaining statistical robustness. Both types are suited for exploratory clinical research, and both types are suited for diseases that are rare.

The *Dixon "Up-Down"* technique was first described in the statistical literature in 1947. It is designed to estimate an ED50 in clinical trials or toxicological tests, when a quantal response is measured (see Figure 10.1). However, it should be remembered that continuous responses can be converted into quantal responses with appropriate, prospective efficacy criteria. For example, blood pressure is a continuous variable, but a drug may be deemed effective or ineffective by stating prospectively that a desired response is quantal positive after a 15 mmHg fall in diastolic blood pressure

within 60 days of commencing therapy. Theoretically, this strategy can be implemented with groups of patients treated in the same way instead of individuals. Sometimes this technique is termed an "adaptive" trial design, because dose size is adapted according to the response of the previous patient or group of patients.

The *Armitage technique* or "sequential analysis" was originally employed in the testing of explosive ordnance. Patients or groups of patients are paired, and then treated with alternative therapies. A control chart is developed that records the result of each comparison with time, and crossing a boundary on the chart, after an unpredictable number of paired comparisons, gives the trial result. For a trial of a new therapy that can both benefit and harm the patient, a typical probability control chart forms a "double-triangle" pattern, as shown in Figure 10.2.

The original methods have been extended in many ways. The design of control charts is always prospective, and their shape depends upon the *a priori* expectations of the development team. For example, when it is important to test only the tolerability of a compound, the chart can have an "open top": this is when it is important to the development team to detect drug toxicity early, but not efficacy. Similarly, depending upon the hypotheses under test, control charts can be rhomboidal, parallelogram, or many other shapes. Whitehead (1999) is the best entry to the literature on this specialized topic.

Contemporaneous independent treatment allocation

Taves (1974) has described a study design that requires an independent coordinator who allocates each patient, as he or she is recruited, to one or other treatment group. The independent coordinator allocates each patient so as to minimize the difference between the two treatment groups according to prospectively defined patient characteristics, for example, age, sex, genotype, disease state or stage, or concomitant therapy. This allocation is therefore also based upon the cumulating characteristics of the treatment groups as has developed

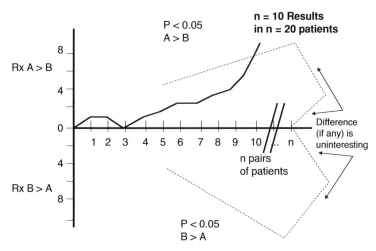

Figure 10.2 The Armitage ("sequential analysis") clinical trial design. Patients are recruited sequentially and randomized 1:1 to either treatment A or B in pairs. When both members of the pair of patients have reached the study endpoint, it is determined which of the pair of patients had the better outcome. If the patient receiving treatment A did best, the control chart plots its next point upwards; if the patient receiving Treatment B did best, it plots downwards, and if the outcome was the same, it plots horizontally. A probability model can be plotted as a mask on the chart (broken line), and when the control plot beaks one or other edge of the mask, the trial outcome is final. In this example, Treatment A was superior to Treatment B, and 10 pairs of patients were needed to demonstrate that treatment effect.

during the study to date. Patients are therefore not allocated to a treatment group by the chance of a randomization schedule.

Bias in minimization trials can be avoided when three conditions are met. First, those performing the clinical trial itself, that is, administering test medications and measuring endpoints, should be double-blind and unaware of which treatment the patient has received. Second, the independent coordinator need only allocate patients to anonymous groups A or B, and the study pharmacist need be the only person who knows which treatments these codes represent. Third, the criteria for which the treatment groups should be balanced must be prospectively identified and rigidly adhered to, using a recorded, quantitative system of scoring the factors.

In its simplest form, this class of minimization designs usually results in treatment groups of nearly equal size. By equitably assigning patients to three or more treatment groups, and yet having identical treatments for two or more of these, unbalanced sample sizes can be created. This is of use when, for example, it may be desirable to expose fewer patients to placebo than to active therapy, especially when conducting a trial of compounds whose properties are fairly well known or may be predicted with some confidence.

Note that minimization trials can only alter power calculations when assumptions of the size of worthwhile differences in effect are also prospectively defined. For example, from a clinical point of view, a small-sized improvement in outcome (perhaps a few percent of patients more than that observed for placebo treatment) may be viewed as very worthwhile in an extremely heterogenous patient population when subjected to multivariate analysis (this is common in large, simple studies; see the following section). On the other hand, when designing a minimization study, the assumption is that the treatment groups will be devoid of relevant differences in baseline characteristics and therefore clinical significance might only be assumed to follow from a large-sized difference in patient response. The size of the difference that is assumed to be of interest, as it increases, may compensate for the reduction in variability among study group samples, and thus have less than expected impact on the sample sizes needed to conduct the clinical trial.

Minimization designs are probably underused by the pharmaceutical industry. This approach is not well-designed for pivotal clinical trials, or for diseases with large numbers of prognostic factors, where in any case, large numbers of patients are especially needed for a tolerability database. If the controlled clinical trial is a gold standard, it would be wrong to assert that the independent treatment allocation design is the "platinum standard" (*pace* Treasure and MacRae, 1998). The interested reader is referred to a good published example (Kallis *et al.*, 1994), and to more detailed statistical treatments (Pocock and Simon, 1975; Freedman and White, 1976).

Stratification designs and the large simple study

These similar classes of study require large numbers of patients. The choice between them lies in being able to "hedge one's bets" with a partial indication approval versus "all or nothing" with huge logistical costs and potentially huge rewards.

Stratification studies

In pivotal studies, large numbers of patients are studied so that their diverse clinical characteristics can imitate better the ordinary patient population than in earlier, more selective, trials. When a variety of concomitant factors (e.g., other diagnoses, wider degree of disease severity, concomitant medications, etc.) are suspected, and may interact with drug tolerability or efficacy, patients may be stratified into randomization groups according to the presence or absence of such factors. For example, patients with Crohn's disease might be stratified according to whether or not they also have cutaneous manifestations, and each stratum then randomized to active or placebo for a total of four treatment groups, although only two test treatments. Separate statistical analyses for the strata can then be planned, and the study size adjusted accordingly. The efficacy of the new drug may be found to be restricted to a (some) particular patient subset(s). Regulatory authorities will often approve indications with caveats based on such subsets. For example, in the United States, one indication for aprotonin was ". . .to reduce perioperative blood loss . . . in selected cases of primary coronary artery bypass graft surgery where the risk of bleeding is especially high e.g. impaired hemostasis, presence of aspirin, or coagulopathy of other origin." The risk of stratification studies is that conservative regulatory authorities will want to see statistical significance in all patient subsets before allowing a short, broad indication in labeling.

Large, simple study

The large, simple study is a recognized alternative to stratification, pioneered by Peto. Large numbers of unselected patients are subjected to a single randomization. If enough patients are recruited, and if the randomization is truly unbiased, the large sample sizes will allow all the potentially interacting variables (concomitant drugs, concomitant diseases, demographic variables, etc.) to balance out between the treatment groups.

The "simple" part of this approach is that, in fundamental terms, the case report form can be very short. There is no need to collect lots of information about the patient's clinical condition because there is no use for these data. Trials of cardiovascular drugs, on an almost epidemiological scale, have been the most significant examples of this alternative approach. Literally tens of thousands of patients have been recruited under these protocols with case report forms having fewer than 10 pages for each patient. Dr Robert Temple (1997; Director of the Office of Drug Evaluation I, at the Food and Drug Administration (FDA)) has commented that it may even be possible to conduct large simple studies in Treatment IND situations, thus permitting the generation of efficacy data outside of orthodox "Phase III" clinical trial programs. However, in this case the endpoint would have to be just as simple, for example survival or death of the patient, during a documented period of observation; Kaplan-Meier analysis and other epidemiological approaches may also be applied to such databases.

Although the conditions under which large simple trials can provide efficacy data are fairly well worked out, it is important to consider whether (or which) tolerability issues can be precisely addressed in this way. If a tolerability factor (adverse event) relates to the efficacy variable of interest (e.g., a fatal adverse event in a patient survival study), a simple case report form may provide relevant information. However, if the adverse event type is rare or unanticipated (e.g., the test drug causes unanticipated, significant anemia in 0.1% of patients, and the protocol and case report form do not collect hemoglobin values before and after treatment), it is very likely that the adverse event will be missed. Large simple studies can thus create undue confidence in product tolerability ("thousands of patients were exposed to the agent during clinical trials").

Treatment withdrawal and other specialized designs

There are rare cases where established treatments are without strong evidence-based support. Two good examples exist for digoxin: the treatment of mild heart failure, and the treatment of cardiac asthenia, a diagnosis that is especially common in Europe, and for which relatively small doses are prescribed. When the effect of such treatments on the natural progression of disease is unknown, it can be ethical to recruit patients into a study with inclusion criteria that includes that they are *already* being treated with the drug of interest. Almost any of the designs discussed above may then be used, where patients are randomized either to remain on the treatment of interest or to be withdrawn from that treatment. All the usual needs for precisely defined prospective endpoints and sound statistical advice before starting the study apply.

Early-phase clinical trials in patients with cancer often use a two-stage design (Gehan, 1979; Ellenberg, 1989). With progressive, fatal diseases, the problem of preventing an untoward number of

patients from being treated with a useless therapy increases. These two-stage designs usually include a small number of open-label treated patients (usually $n \leq 14$) in the first stage. The proportion and degree of tumor responsiveness is then used to fix the number of patients in the second stage of the design, which may use an active comparator or no therapy as the alternative treatment, depending upon whether an active comparator therapy can be identified. Such studies cannot produce fundamental evidence of efficacy, but in the hands of experienced statisticians and development teams can predict whether wider trials are justified.

Stopping clinical trials

Safety issues

Stopping a clinical trial because of an emergent safety problem, either by a medical monitor or by a safety committee, is usually a unique situation and the specifics of the case are rarely generalizable. These are decisions that are always taken in consultation, and the safety of potential future trial recruits must be the paramount concern (including the abrupt cessation of therapy). Trial suspension is usually the best immediate option, allowing time for collective thought, notification of regulatory authorities, and wider consultations as appropriate.

Efficacy issues

Pocock (1992) has succinctly summarized most of the situations that pertain when considering whether to stop a clinical trial. Efficacy, like safety, can cause ethical concerns to the pharmaceutical physician when he or she suspects that patients will be exposed to alternative therapies that are suboptimal.

Interim efficacy analyses usually make a mess! These analyses require either that the overall size of the trial has to be greater than if no interim analysis was performed, or that a smaller α must be accepted as indicating statistical significance at the end of the whole study.

Clinicians will hear loud complaints about these drawbacks of interim analyses, especially from senior management with purely commercial backgrounds. Everyone will want to know as soon as possible whether "the drug is working," but lax scientific thinking is behind these complaints. Common statements are: "We don't want to stop the study at the halfway stage, we just want to see how it is going." When asked why, the answer is usually something like: "There would be no point in spending more money on the study if there is no chance of achieving a statistically significant result." This is a popular mis-rationalization: a decision not to stop a study is a decision to allow it to continue, and that introduces bias into the dataset that is eventually analyzed.

Spectacularly effective drugs may achieve a very small α at the time of the interim analysis. Stopping the trial by reason of the unethical basis for treating the patients with anything else is a rare and pleasant event for the clinical trialist. However, in that spectacular success, the clinician should ask whether a minimization design would have achieved the same thing with even fewer patients, and thus actually feel chastened.

It is not the purpose of this chapter to delve into the mechanics of statistics. However, a few comments about the relationships between values for α at the stage of an interim and complete statistical analysis of a clinical trial may be in order. There are several statistical points of view on this subject, and regulatory authorities have a habit of believing only the most conservative.

At the time of writing, the O'Brien and Fleming rule is becoming an acceptable standard. As a general rule, clinical trialists should expect statisticians to provide alternatives that obey a simple subtraction rule. For example, clinicians might agree that the study should stop due to great efficacy when $p \leq 0.01$ at an interim analysis of sufficient patients (power of 0.8) to detect such a difference. In that case, if the study continues after the interim analysis shows $p > 0.01$, the study as a whole will be required to achieve approximately $p \leq 0.04$ in the final statistical analysis for efficacy of the investigational drug to be assumed. Even so, Pocock and Geller (1986) have shown that trials stopped by reason of efficacy at an interim stage are likely to have exaggerated the size of the difference between treatment groups. Marketing departments should be aware of this error in their extrapolations to the commercial worth of the product.

Bayesian trial designs

A typical Bayesian design might be where, for example, there are several drugs with preclinical rationale for the treatment of cancer. Since none are clinically proven, one of the test treatments is placebo. Patients are then recruited sequentially into the study, and the results (e.g., tumor size reduction) are recorded. After a while, the proportions of patients responding to each treatment are compared using a sophisticated probabalistic method that takes into account the uncertainties associated with small and unequal treatment group sizes. The randomization code is then adjusted to favor more patients being allocated to the treatments that have started out looking better than the others, while very poor, placebo-equivalent, treatments might be dropped altogether. Eventually, the several test therapies are reduced to two and a definitive demonstration of superiority or nonsuperiority for that pair of treatments can be reported.

The difficulties with interim analyses do not arise when a Bayesian approach to the original design has been taken (Berry, 1985). The Bayesian methodology essentially revises the proportionate patient allocation among the test therapies according to the latest and best information available (e.g., Berry, 1995): in essence, after some minimum number of patients has entered the trial, an interim analysis is done every time another patient completes the trial. The important distinction between Bayesian and sequential designs (Dixon and Armitage, discussed earlier) is that although patient numbers required to complete a sequential design study are undefined at the beginning, the treatment allocations are nonetheless according to a fixed randomization schedule. Thus, the sequential designs are still, essentially, a frequentist methodology, and not Bayesian.

The potential benefits of Bayesian methods include the use of fewer patients to demonstrate efficacy, as well as potential seamlessness of Phase

II and III development. Bayesian approaches are therefore currently of interest to regulatory authorities, in their efforts to streamline clinical development. The US FDA has a draft guidance issued on the subject. Although, probably unduly, little used by generalists, there is every prospect that Bayesian methods will find increased uses in specialized areas, and this has already taken place for trials of cancer chemotherapy, medical devices, and studies of rare diseases.

General clinical trialists cannot be expected to be able to generate Bayesian statistical plans for themselves: These require an experienced statistician. Moreover, that statistician should not, him- or herself, be philosophically opposed to Bayesian or frequentist thinking. The decision to employ a Bayesian design for a clinical trial may well be viewed as courageous in most companies. There will also be many clinical trials for which an orthodox, frequentist approach will be selected for several good reasons. But, overall, when considering a new trial, one is well-advised to at least consider whether one of the adaptive designs described above might help. Even if that option is rejected, knowing the rationale why may still lead to a superior frequentist trial design.

Series of published cases

Some diseases are so rare that the prospects of ever conducting a clinical trial are remote because it is unlikely that enough patients could ever be collected at any reasonable number of study sites for any useful randomization. These diseases may be found in the literature as case reports. In these cases, probably the best that can be accomplished is to collect and retrospectively analyze as many such cases as possible. If the drug of interest has been used in a sufficient number of patients, retrospective risk ratios for benefit and harm can be calculated. This may be the strongest evidence that can ever be collected about a particular drug under these rare conditions, albeit never as strong as a controlled clinical trial. One example is the effectiveness of dantrolene in malignant hyperthermia (Strazis and Fox, 1993).

Objectives and pre-requisites of pivotal clinical trials

Licensing requirements typically are greater than reporting data by multi-center "Phase III" studies. Special populations may require small-scale studies to supplement a traditional two-study, large-scale registration development scheme. Similarly, if (in the United States) the proposed indication has an approved Orphan Drug designation, small-scale "Phase II-type" studies may be all that is possible due to disease rarity. Furthermore, even for conventional indications, the resource implications of pivotal studies are usually much greater than any earlier phase of development, and efficient resource utilization becomes exponentially more important than before. The incorporation of pharmacoeconomic and humanistic outcomes alongside the primary registration endpoints is becoming essential, and preparatory work is best done in conjunction with the smaller, earlier studies and must also factor treatment compliance.

Benefit–risk analysis

The cumulation of all the data from the clinical trials of a new drug product, assuming a fairly orthodox regulatory strategy for a typical dossier or NDA, will form the largest fraction of the application. However, these data are also needed for derivative documents within the application, one of which is a benefit–risk analysis, which forms the last part of an Integrated Safety Summary (Section 9 of the NDA). Benefit–risk analysis also underpins the Risk Management Plan that must accompany all Marketing Authorization Applications and their amendments in Europe. These benefit–risk assessments must be derived from the clinical study reports and summaries elsewhere in the applications.

All clinicians constantly weigh benefit–risk in their daily practice. Their assessment of this "ratio" in everyday practice, using approved drugs, is usually not as numerical as it sounds. In practice, clinicians make prescribing decisions based upon: a) a subset of the published information that might be available about the drug (labeling, drug representatives, comments from colleagues, etc.); b) their current and prior experience with this particular patient; and c) prior experience with other patients. This prior experience, even if personal, may or may not be recalled consciously. Furthermore, we all operate using algorithms taught to us by others whom we respect, and thus we use others' experience with drugs and patients, quite apart from the often hard-learned lessons from our own therapeutic adventures (*pace* "evidence-based medicine").

Clinical trialists also weigh benefit–risk, every time a protocol is written. Often, unlike for approved drugs, there is much less information to go on. In early clinical development, extrapolations are obligatory. However, unlike in general medical practice, these extrapolations are often not from clinical experience, but rather from pharmacokinetic models or animal data, or at best from patients who are clearly dissimilar from those proposed in the new trial. This is automatically the case: If the answers to the clinical trial questions were known, there would be little point in doing the trial.

There are some highly mathematical approaches to benefit–risk assessment, albeit of limited applicability. In the unusual case where a single (binary) efficacy endpoint can be balanced against a single adverse event type of concern, the number of patients required and the number of therapeutic events required to be observed can be defined. From there, making binomial, Normal, or other assumptions about event distribution, confidence intervals can be calculated (e.g., for GUSTO (Global Use of Strategies To Open occluded coronary arteries trial); Willan *et al.*, 1997). The numbers needed to treat and to harm (and their corresponding reciprocals) can then be used to compare drugs. However, this is a highly unusual, and artificial, situation, and the sophisticated statistical answers that result are unlikely to have more that a partial impact on the more *gestalt* approach that real-world clinicians must use.

In the end, clinical trialists usually have to stick out their necks to some extent. As in general medical practice, it is a rare clinical trial where

the benefit to the patient is measured by a single binary variable, and no drug possesses just one type of adverse event, whose probability may be prospectively estimated for any given patient. Even in the easiest case, with a great deal of information about a drug with substantial history and experience, the contrived mathematical approach described above has serious limitations. For example, Penicillin G has three adverse events of primary interest (anaphylaxis, bacterial drug resistance, and sodium load at high doses). Drug efficacy, when the infection recedes (if it is to recede), is only partly due to the action of the drug, and there is an additional source of extreme variability, namely by the concomitant condition of the patient. Whether or not to prescribe penicillin is a common decision for doctors and dentists: the mathematical analysis of the benefit–risk "ratio" is unlikely to affect most prescribing decisions.

If doctors cannot make precise benefit–risk assessments, neither can patients. The informed consent document is where we ask patients to make their own benefit–risk assessments, albeit with some guidance (Marsh, 1990). Certainly, the mathematical approach cannot be expected on the part of the patient, nor will it be useful in a balanced and fair communication with the patient about the nature of the clinical trial.

Benefit–risk, then, is a central part of the practice of pharmaceutical medicine and its regulation. It can almost never be reduced to a numerical exercise. Benefit–risk assessments of clinical trials data are an important part of all new drug applications. Good people will differ in their benefit–risk assessment even when using the same body of clinical trials data.

Summary

This chapter has attempted to provide a philosophy of clinical trials. The place of clinical trials in the overall development plan and what the clinical trialist must *know about*, rather than be able to implement him- or herself, has been emphasized. Almost all clinical trials are unique because of the infinite combinations of hypothesis to be addressed, pharmacological properties of the drug under investigation, the types of patients that are likely to be available, and likely users of the resulting data. The major categories of trial designs have been surveyed. It is hoped that, when challenged with testing any clinical hypothesis, the clinical trial team would consider all these broad categories, select the one most relevant to the clinical situation, and then refine the proposed trial design from that point. Some of the subtle interactions between statistical, financial, and psychological aspects of trial design have been hinted at. The clinical trialist will only really grow in this discipline through experience and good mentorship.

References

Amin HM, Sopchak AM, Esposito BF, Henson LG, Batenhorst RL, Fox AW, Camporesi EM. Naloxone-induced and spontaneous reversal of depressed ventilatory responses to hypoxia during and after continuous infusion of remifentanil or alfentanil. *J Pharmacol Exp Ther* 1995; **274**:34–39.

Bardolph EM, Taylor RH. Sailors, scurvy, science and authority. *J Roy Soc Med* 1997; **90**:238.

Berry DA. Interim analyses in clinical trials: classical vs. Bayesian approaches. *Stat Med* 1985; **4**:521–526.

Berry DA. Decision analysis and Bayesian methods in clinical trials. *Cancer Treat Res* 1995; **75**:125–154.

Chaput de Saintonge DM, Vere DW. Measurement in clinical trials. *Br J Clin Pharmacol* 1982; **13**:775–783.

Ebbutt AF. Three-period crossover designs for two treatments. *Biometrics* 1984; **40**:219–224.

Ellenberg SS. Determining sample sizes for clinical trials. *Oncology* 1989; **3**:39–42.

Freedman LS, White SJ. On the use of Pocock and Simon's method for balancing treatment numbers over prognostic factors in the controlled clinical trial. *Biometrics* 1976; **32**:691–694.

Freiman JA, Chalmers TC, Smith H, Kuebler RR. The importance of beta, the type II error and sample size in

the design and interpretation of the randomized control trial. *New Eng J Med* 1978; **299**:690–694.

Frey WG. British naval intelligence and scurvy. *New Eng J Med* 1969; **281**:1430–1433.

Gehan EA. Clinical trials in cancer research. *Environ Health Perspect* 1979; **32**:31–48.

Kallis P, Tooze JA, Talbot S, Cowans D, Bevan DH, Treasure T. Pre-operative aspirin decreases platelet aggregation and increases post-operative blood loss: a prospective, randomized, placebo-controlled double-blind, clinical trial in 100 patients with chronic stable angina. *Eur J Cardiothor Surg* 1994; **8**:404–409.

Laska E, Meisner M, Kushner HB. Optimal crossover designs in the presence of carryover effects. *Biometrics* 1983; **39**:1087–1091.

Lind J. *A treatise of the scurvy*. 8vo. Edinburgh, 1753.

Marsh BT. Informed Consent. *J Roy Soc Med* 1990; **83**:603–606.

Pocock SJ. When to stop a clinical trial. *Br Med J* 1992; **305**:235–240.

Pocock SJ, Geller NL. Interim analyses in randomized clinical trials. *Drug Information J* 1986; **20**:263–269.

Pocock SJ, Simon R. Sequential treatment assignment with balancing for prognostic factors in the controlled clinical trial. *Biometrics* 1975; **31**:103–115.

Spilker B. *Guide to Clinical Trials*. Raven Press: New York, USA, 1991. ISBN 0-881-67767-1, *passim*.

Strazis KP, Fox AW. Malignant hyperthermia: review of published cases. *Anesth Analg* 1993; **77**:297–304.

Taves DR. Minimization: a new method of assigning patients to treatment and control groups. *Clin Pharmacol Ther* 1974; **15**:443–453.

Temple R. Public hearings on "Myotrophin," Peripheral and Central Nervous System Drugs Advisory Committee, May 8, 1997. (Also in *Biocentury: The Bernstein Report* **5**(40): A2.)

Thomas DP. Sailors, scurvy and science. *J Roy Soc Med* 1997; **90**:50–54

Treasure T, MacRae KD. Minimisation: the platinum standard for trials? *Br Med J* 1998; **317**:362–363.

Whitehead J. A unified theory for sequential clinical trials. *Stat Med* 1999; **18**:2271–2286.

Willan AR, O'Brien BJ, Cook DJ. Benefit–risk ratios in the assessment of the clinical evidence of a new therapy. *Control Clin Trial* 1997; **18**:121–130.

CHAPTER 11

Phase IV Drug Development: Post-marketing Studies

Lisa R. Johnson-Pratt
Bryn Mawr, PA, USA

Objectives of the Phase IV clinical development program

Phase IV studies (in some companies sub-divided into Phases IV and V) are mostly conducted after initial product approval. A minority begin prior to product launch, at risk that product approval is delayed, but with the reward of a potential competitive advantage. The range of purposes of Phase IV studies is broader than for earlier phases of drug development, and there need not be constraints such as a need to provide pivotal evidence of efficacy. Table 11.1 summarizes the typical goals and tactics of Phase IV studies.

The conduct of Phase IV studies in some companies is carried out by the original development team that also did Phases II and III. This can be desirable because these are the people with a repository of information, for the entire history of the drug, who can spot or remember small events that might merit further study in Phases IV and V. Some of those people will enjoy following the drug through its entire life cycle, and will be glad for that opportunity. However, this opportunity brings with it a responsibility to evolve from a more regulation-oriented approach to clinical trials to a more market-oriented one; this challenge leads other companies to have separate Phase IV clinical trials departments (an essentially phase-oriented organizational structure).

Principles and Practice of Pharmaceutical Medicine, 3rd edition.
Edited by L.D. Edwards, A.W. Fox, P.D. Stonier.
© 2011 Blackwell Publishing Ltd.

Types of Phase IV studies

The typical characteristics of Phase IV studies, in comparison with Phases I, II, and III, are that they are larger, less technically complicated, have fewer inclusion/exclusion criteria, and are more likely to include subjective or qualitative endpoints (e.g., quality of life or patient satisfaction). Rigorous, placebo-controlled, parallel-group studies still find a place, however, when new indications are being investigated for drugs that are already approved. As a particular marketplace becomes more crowded, the competition for places in formularies, and for reimbursements increases, and some Phase IV studies are designed specifically to provide information for consumer and healthcare delivery "payer" organizations. Placebo-controlled studies are usually inadequate for this purpose (unless the product is unique). Table 11.2 summarizes some of the nuances and challenges of conducting Phase IV trials.

The type of investigator that one seeks during Phase IV development must clearly correspond to the nature of the study. Usually, larger numbers of investigators, each contributing fewer patients than the Phase II and III investigators, are sought. If such individuals are local or national thought-leaders, who will eventually advocate for the product, so much the better. But even at the local level, it is these investigators who might be found on hospital formulary committees, develop local treatment algorithms, see high volumes of patients, and are active in local medical societies.

Table 11.1 Typical goals and tactics of Phase IV clinical trials

Extension of tolerability information	Wider range of patients than in NDA/PLA database
	Larger numbers of patients
Competitive efficacy claims	Active comparator study designs
New indications	Supplemental efficacy studies
Ethnopharmacology	Additional approvals in non-ICH countries
Outcomes assessment	Pharmacoepidemiology and pharmacoeconomics in particular healthcare environments
Pharmacovigilance	Post-marketing commitments
Market expansion	All of the above

Comparative superiority trials

Well-designed, head-to-head, active comparator studies are always preferred over meta-analytical comparisons of placebo-controlled studies for competing drugs. The latter were conducted at different times and in different places. Generally, the active comparator will be a widely recognized "gold standard." This "gold standard" might be the prototypical drug in the same pharmacological class (e.g., a clinical trial comparing a new cephalosporin with an old one), or it could be a hitherto dominant therapy or procedure (e.g., comparing a proton pump inhibitor with an H_2 antagonist, or conservative management with a new drug versus surgery). Sometimes a change in pharmaceutical formulation may have occurred, and, even after approval, there may be questions over its superiority, patient preference, or economic advantage compared with the formulation that was initially approved (see Makuch and Johnson, 1986, 1989).

Table 11.2 Practical aspects of Phase IV clinical trials

Type of study	Challenges
Active comparators	Obtaining active comparator drug
	Blinding, reformulations, and bioequivalence
	Disclosure of trade secrets to competitors
	Placebo-control justifications
	Use of appropriate dose ranges
	Risks demonstrating superiority of competitor
Equivalence trials	Usually large patient populations needed
	Cannot demonstrate superiority
	Scientific demonstration of a negative
	"Standard of care" context challenged
Megatrials	Statistical complexity
	Few inclusion/exclusion criteria
	Representativeness to treated population known only towards the end of the trial
Open-label	Prescriber and patient biases
	Scientifically limited
New indication	Similarity to Phase III designs (q.v.)
Drug interactions	Almost unlimited alternatives
Special patient populations	See chapters in Section III
New formulations	Bioequivalence

Open-label studies

Conducting open-label studies can be a liberating and fascinating experience. When both the patient and the prescriber know the treatment being administered, many of the complexities of early-phase studies go away. Furthermore, when it is appreciated that double-blind clinical trials are always an abstraction from the ordinary clinical situation, to observe how one's new drug actually works in that latter environment is often eye-opening; one common and pleasant experience is to see with one's own eyes how conservative was the estimate of product efficacy prior to its approval.

This "real-world" environment can be studied at length and relatively cheaply, too. Longitudinal study designs (e.g., the Framingham Study, or the UK Physicians Cohort Study) can assess multiple effects of treatment: pathological, economical, quality of life, and even epidemiological impacts can be assessed. One can also find out what sort of patient one's drug will be prescribed to, which may or may not resemble the patient population pre-PLA/NDA (Product Licensing Agreement/New Drug Application), and which may suggest unknown benefits and hazards of the new therapy.

The open-label trial approach is, however, not without its critics. Friedman *et al.* (1985) drew attention to the need to observe whether

• The cohort being followed represents the larger population for whom the drug is being prescribed.
• The treatment groups are truly comparable, because patients are often matched on only one, or at most a small number of clinical characteristics.
• The need to check that randomization, or at least patient allocation, has not become unbalanced or biased as a result of some unspecified factor.

Another difficult aspect in the design of open-label studies is how one assesses those patients who withdraw from the study. The reasons for withdrawal can be at least as varied as in double-blind studies (intolerability, administrative difficulties, coincidental emergent disease, or concomitant therapies, etc.). However, in addition, in an open-label design patients may develop an opinion on the superiority of one or other treatment for reasons that may or may not be explicit. If completion

of a course of therapy is one endpoint of the study, all withdrawals can be accounted treatment failures, and the statistical handling is fairly straightforward. However, if there is another endpoint, and if withdrawals are imbalanced between the treatment groups and unrelated to product intolerability, the situation becomes a lot more clouded. Under these latter conditions, the entire trial may have to be abandoned when it becomes apparent that the trial design cannot answer the hypothesis under test one way or the other.

On the positive side, open-label trials are usually easy to administer and run quickly. Investigators have greater freedom in entering and allocating patients, and this is often more comfortable than a placebo-controlled situation in the ordinary clinical setting.

Equivalence trials

Sometimes the demonstration of equivalency (or "non-inferiority") is sufficient. Often the competing product cannot be expected to be inferior, and/or the successor product's only advantage is that it is marketed at a lower price than the innovator. In the special case of generic products, at the very end of a drug's life cycle when patent coverage has expired, equivalence need only be demonstrated pharmacokinetically (usually involving only a small number of normal volunteers, and the relevant, specific types of regulatory applications). However, when the new product is challenging the position of an older one, equivalence trials usually require very large numbers of patients (often hundreds per treatment group). The overall tactic is to show that with a well powered study (e.g., $\beta = 0.925$) that there is no *clinical* or statistical difference between the two treatments. The size of the clinical difference that is worth detecting is *sine qua non* defined prospectively, and forms the basis for the power calculations, and hence study size.

Mega-trials

When it is suspected that there may only be small differences between active treatments, and when placebo controls are unavailable for clinical or ethical reasons, it is often necessary to resort to large scale studies ("mega-trials"). A good, famous example was the clinical trial known by the acronym GUSTO (Global Use of Strategies To Open occluded coronary arteries), where streptokinase and recombinant tissue plasminogen activator (t-PA) were compared for acute coronary thrombosis (for a commentary, see Hampton, 1996).

Unlike more orthodox studies, mega-trials do not attempt to control for large numbers of confounding variables. Instead, huge numbers of patients (several thousands) are randomized, "the cards are allowed to fall where they may," and faith is placed in the notion that a large n will automatically lead to well-balanced treatment groups. This is not always the case, and imbalance can often be demonstrated between treatment groups of even several thousands when enough concomitant confounding factors are analyzed (Charlton, 1966).

Safety surveillance

The ICH Guidance (FDA, 2005) provides a framework for the pharmacovigilance of new drug products. Each new product should have a pharmacovigilance *specification*, which basically describes the clinical hazard landscape for the new product, as far as it can be known at the time of approval. The specification is essentially a problem statement. Each specification should then be accompanied by a pharmacovigilance *plan*; this may be part of the overarching Risk Management Plan. The plan might include routine adverse event reporting and periodic safety updates to be provided to regulators, and/or recommendations for clarifications to product labeling. In special cases, however, a post-marketing surveillance study might be recommended, and this forms another type of Phase IV study.

It is typical before conducting a post-marketing surveillance study to obtain the view of the regulatory authorities on its design. The study may have been a condition of product approval, and it is both reasonable and wise to ensure that the study design can be expected to provide the information that is needed both by the sponsor and the regulators. Unblinded designs that imitate the ordinary clinical situation are the norm.

New indications

As in the early phases of drug development, the identification of new indications for old drugs can be either rational or serendipitous. Rarely, even adverse events can be exploited as new indications, and the hair-growing properties of the antihypertensive drug minoxidil is a famous example.

Finding a new indication is an obvious opportunity to increase market size by enlarging the potential pool of patients that can benefit from the product. In this case, two pivotal, well-controlled Phase IV studies demonstrating efficacy will usually be required, at a minimum. If there is the potential for a new type of clinical hazard to be associated with the new disease being studied, a safety database of a size that regulators will find acceptable is also needed for the supplemental application. Clearly, whenever such a project is contemplated, a commercial assessment must precede the study, showing the positive balance between the cost of the program, the probability of success, and the size of the eventual revenue increment that may result.

The finding of a new, non-obvious use for an old drug can also be patented. This type of patent is known as a "Method of Use" patent, and its eventual enforcement is probably easier in the United States than in other jurisdictions. Nonetheless, the view of the corporate patent attorney on any proposed Phase IV exploration for a new indication should always be sought.

Stimulation of the process of finding new uses for old drugs is often done when companies offer investigator research grants. It is fairly common that individual prescribers will have bright ideas about the use of medical products, and indeed some specialties use most drugs "off-label" (e.g., intensive care physicians, anesthesiologists, and pediatricians). Small grants to such individuals, in order to observe such niche uses under organized circumstances, can lead to new indications. At the very least, such programs encourage disclosure of new ideas to the company, and allow for some review of the safety aspects of what these inventive individuals are getting up to!

New dosage forms

Initial dosage forms are usually those that are most easily developed, most stable, and at least reasonably acceptable to adult patients. Such formulations can often be improved upon, whether for matters of convenience (e.g., a bioequivalent melt-in-the-mouth wafer that, unlike a tablet, does not require access to water for its administration), or to enlarge the patient population that might use the product (e.g., a linctus instead of a tablet for use in children, or to permit smaller increments in dose adjustment). Again when there are serious physicochemical constraints on formulations, the discovery of a new one can itself be patentable.

A variety of regulatory approaches are needed when adding to the range of formulations, and each, in turn, dictates a different Phase IV clinical trial design. When the route of administration does not change (e.g., the wafer versus tablet example above), orthodox bioequivalence and absence of formulation-dependent intolerability might be all that is needed. A pseudo-Phase I approach during Phase IV might then be all that is required.

On the other hand, the new formulation might be deliberately designed *not* to be bioequivalent. Slow-release formulations are, by definition, not bioequivalent, but are often associated with therapeutic superiority due to reduced probability of C_{max}-related adverse events, C_{min}-related loss of efficacy, and better compliance because of reduced dosage frequency. In this case, efficacy data will normally be required of the scale and rigor of the earlier Phase III program.

It should be noted that the company might be wise to consider, when developing new formulations, that the minimum database acceptable to regulators might be insufficient for their own commercial purposes. The decision to launch a new formulation has to be based not only on its technical success, but also according to a financial analysis of the type referred to above for new indications. Crucial information on that question can usually only be obtained by studying the new formulation using one of the other authentic Phase IV approaches described in this chapter.

Special populations

Special populations have their own chapters in this book in Section III, to which the reader is referred. In the United States, many product approvals now come with the condition that future studies in children are mandatory. This is probably the most common special population with which Phase IV development units now routinely deal.

Other, newly identified special populations result from pharmacovigilance signals, unexpected use of the product in an unanticipated population, requirements for regulatory filings in non-ICH nations, or even the spread of disease into new geographical areas. Traditional pharmacokinetic approaches are usually the first step in assessing whether these events will alter product efficacy or safety.

Drug interactions

These are essentially another form of special population, and almost all drugs can exhibit at least some interactions. Many PLA/NDAs will contain studies of particular drug interactions that seemed relevant at the time, especially when combination therapy is the norm, or when there are biochemical predictions that a new drug will interact with older therapies (e.g., cytochrome P450 isoenzyme findings *in vitro*). Pharmacokinetic studies are typically done at small scale. But, in addition, the Phase IV team might be asked to do a retrospective case-controlled analysis of the existing clinical trials database, trawling for differences between patients who were and were not on a particular concomitant therapy.

The clinical–marketing interface

As mentioned, one purpose of a Phase IV clinical trial program is to gather new indications or information that can lead to a competitive advantage. Optimization of the clinical–marketing interface is critical to ensure success. It is the marketing team that is the keeper of the strategy, aware of the competitive environment (both current and future, within and outside the class of the drug under development), and closest to the commercial environment in which the drug will have to compete (e.g., formulary issues; pricing concerns). In order to ensure that the product is commercially successful, it is important for the clinical team to embrace this information when developing a Phase IV clinical trial program. It is especially important when entering a very competitive, highly developed marketplace (e.g., diabetes or hypertension) where there are multiple treatment options or a lack of perceived difference between members of a particular drug class. It is also important for new classes when there will be a within-class competitor launching within a short timeframe. In these cases, the label may be similar, especially in the US where there has been a trend in recent years to have drugs within the same class have similar labeling verbiage (i.e., "class labeling"). In the absence of "current" labeling differences between competitors, it is sometimes the robustness of the Phase IV clinical trial program that will differentiate competitors, as it is seen as a harbinger of future indications or positive data. These programs also highlight to the scientific community the "commitment" that the company has to the drug and the disease state.

For these reasons it is critical that the clinical and marketing teams collaborate extensively on the Phase IV development program, usually via a standing commercialization team with representatives from other functional areas that will provide sound input into the program to increase its chance of success (e.g., regulatory and legal). The marketing team should provide the commercialization team with a clear understanding of the market environment, including past promotional behavior of key competitors, so that a robust needs assessment can be formulated. Once the commercial case has been made, the clinical teams should provide a scientific risk assessment that includes the likelihood of success of achieving the desired outcome. If the ultimate goal of a given study is for promotional purposes, it is helpful for the marketing team to provide examples of how the data are intended to be promoted to ensure that the trial is designed to allow ultimately for those promotional messages.

With the financial stakes so high, it is no longer acceptable for clinical teams to view their roles as purely scientific. Success for a product is no longer dependent solely on approval of indications. Consumers of scientific information are always looking for new information to (dis)continue their support of a reimbursed product. Effective collaboration between clinical development and marketing teams

in the context of Phase IV trials can go a long way toward optimizing sales of an effective drug.

The clinical–legal interface

Concern about product liability can both decline and increase as Phase IV proceeds. If, on the one hand, the sudden exposure of large numbers of patients to a new drug (i.e., large in comparison to those in the Marketing Authorization Application and/or NDA) does not result in a flurry of serious adverse events, nor any signal of a qualitatively new type of adverse event, there is reassurance that the label is probably doing its job properly.

If, on the other hand, anything new is discovered about a drug in Phase IV, then, by definition, it will not be in the product label. Furthermore, sometimes, when such a signal is observed, a retrospective trawl through the preclinical and clinical databases can often uncover consistent information whose significance had not been earlier realized. In this case, a "gap" exists between what is known about a drug and what information has been provided to prescribers.

The gap may exist for a very short period of time because of a prompt change in product labeling, and the company will have done everything that is appropriate as fast as it possibly could. In some cases, the gap might exist due to a very rarely occurring adverse event of questionable direct association with the product, which does not warrant inclusion into the label.

However, on other occasions the gap will need to be urgently addressed. The range of actions that might be needed, in increasingly alarming order, are as follows:

- design/implement purpose-built Phase IV study;
- change in label at next routine printing;
- more urgent change in labeling;
- issuance of "Dear Prescriber/Doctor/healthcare professional" letter;
- institution of restrictive access program;
- product withdrawal.

The Phase IV development program will almost always generate information that is relevant in choosing from among these alternative actions. The corporate lawyers will always be depending upon the Phase IV clinicians to determine the appropriate course of action due to their knowledge of the post-marketing trial program, results, and how that information has been communicated to the medical community.

Conclusion

Phase IV clinical trials, in all their many forms, are the natural extension from the constrained environment of Phase II and III drug development, as well as a pivotal, interfacing position between the marketing, research, regulatory, and legal departments. Indeed, such distinctions can be seamless, especially when there is no change in development team post-approval, or when Phase IV is actually begun before approval. The variety of questions that Phase IV teams must answer are many and varied. This can be a liberating, stimulating, and educational assignment for those who have hitherto worked only in early-phase product development.

References

Charlton BG. Megatrials are based on a methodological mistake. *Br J Gen Pract* 1966;**46**:429–431.

FDA. Pharmacovigilance planning. *Federal Register* 2005;**70**(62):16827–16828.

Friedman LM, Furberg CD, DeMets DL. *Fundamentals of Clinical Trials.* Mosby-Year Books: St. Louis, Missouri, USA, 1985.

Hampton JR. Alternatives to mega-trials in cardiovascular disease. *Cardiovasc Drugs Ther* 1996;**10**:759–765.

Makuch RW, Johnson MF. Some issues in the design and interpretation of 'negative' clinical studies. *Arch Intern Med* 1986;**146**:986–989.

Makuch RW, Johnson MF. Issues in planning and interpreting active control equivalence studies. *J Clin Epidemiol* 1989;**42**:503–511.

Further reading

Hammer CE. *Drug Development.* CRC Press: Boca Raton, Florida, USA, 1990.

Spilker B. *Guide to Clinical Trials.* Raven: New York, USA, 1991.

CHAPTER 12

Site Management

Barry Miskin

Department of Surgery, Nova Southeastern University College of Osteopathic Medicine, Fort Lauderdale-Davie, FL, USA

Introduction

The investigative site serves a critical function in the clinical development process. As the physical location where clinical trials are conducted, its purpose is to produce clean, reproducible clinical data in a timely and safe manner. The site generates these data by performing the study protocol on human subjects that it recruits. By providing this valuable service, sites play a major role in moving investigational products through the clinical phases on their way to regulatory submission, and ultimately, to market.

This chapter describes different kinds of investigative sites around the globe and makes the case that operating a successful site requires an infrastructure that enables the generation of good quality data. The infrastructure must include critical business functions such as budgeting, patient recruitment, regulatory oversight, audit preparation, and the keeping of metrics on site performance. Investigators and clinical research coordinators well trained in Good Clinical Practice (GCP) are also key to site success.

Types of investigative sites

As the clinical trials industry becomes increasingly global, research is taking place in a variety of venues (see Figure 12.1), ranging from academic medical centers to Phase I units. To some degree,

Principles and Practice of Pharmaceutical Medicine, 3rd edition.
Edited by L.D. Edwards, A.W. Fox, P.D. Stonier.

the location of the study is dictated by the complexity of the protocol, the types of procedures required, and the availability of experienced staff. But there can be other factors at play that determine where a clinical trial occurs.

In many locales, clinical trials take place largely at academic medical centers, regardless of complexity, using investigators who are part of a national health service. In other regions, such as the United States, there are many public and private clinical trial options. Data suggest that in the US, approximately 35% of studies take place at academic medical centers (see Figure 12.2). The rest occur at a mix of public and private, dedicated and part-time, investigative sites.

The *dedicated site* functions with a staff and infrastructure in place to enable the conduct of clinical trials on a full-time basis. It is essentially a business. The elements needed to operate the dedicated site successfully are described in the Basic Infrastructure section below.

Some dedicated sites maintain loose affiliations with non-competing sites to share leads about upcoming studies. Others belong to a site management organization (SMO), which is a formal affiliation offering centralized management, contract negotiation, accounting, and patient recruitment services.

With more than one-third of US-based clinical trials taking place in *part-time sites*, they are a popular option. They are generally defined as trial locations in which the investigator(s) conducts a limited amount of clinical trials annually, usually less than four or five. They offer community-based, actual use settings, a feature that sponsors find attractive (Hart, 2007), and can be profitable

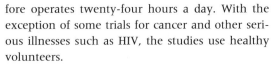

- Academic Medical Center

- Dedicated Clinical Trial Site

- Part-time Site

- Phase I Site

Figure 12.1 Clinical trial venues.

because they tend to require less infrastructure than their dedicated site counterparts.

Investigators may opt for part-time site status when they have commitments such as private practice and academic appointments that restrict their available time for clinical research. Also, they may simply prefer to conduct just a few studies each year to supplement income or to indulge a research interest.

There is a hot market for *Phase I* sites. Because pharmaceutical sponsors seek to limit costs and risk by weeding out weak drug candidates earlier, they are increasing their investments in Phase I studies. Data suggest that Phase I spending is rising more rapidly than other sectors of the clinical development market (Korieth, 2004).

Phase I is a collection of small safety studies using approximately 20 to 100 subjects to research the drug's pharmacokinetics and pharmacological effects. Substantial investment in staff and equipment is required to conduct these studies because the Phase I site often houses inpatients, and there-

fore operates twenty-four hours a day. With the exception of some trials for cancer and other serious illnesses such as HIV, the studies use healthy volunteers.

Phase I sites are found in many countries but have been prevalent in Europe, particularly the United Kingdom. Prior to the implementation of the European Directive on Clinical Trials on May 1, 2004, an investigational new drug (IND) application for studies on healthy volunteers was not required in Europe (UK), as it was and continues to be in the United States. Europe's then more lenient regulatory environment attracted business (Neuer, 2000), but with the advent of the European Directive, regulatory approval by ethics committee is now required to begin Phase I testing.

Basic infrastructure

Clinical trials cannot take place without an infrastructure designed to support the research function. With research studies becoming more complex and entailing more procedures per subject (see Figure 12.3), it is critical that the staff at the investigative site have an appreciation of what it takes to perform good quality clinical research in a timely, ethical, and fiscally responsible manner.

The basic infrastructure, particularly for dedicated sites, includes the following (Miskin and Neuer, 2002):

- clinical investigator;
- study coordinator;

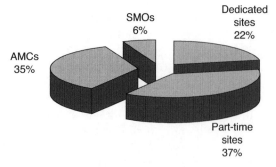

Figure 12.2 Clinical studies are conducted at various venues (source: Thomson CenterWatch, 2003).

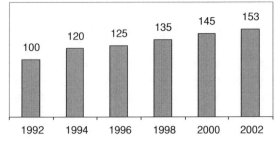

Figure 12.3 Mean number of procedures per patient (source: *Thomson CenterWatch Analysis*, 2004; *Parexel Sourcebook*, 2004–2005; *Fast Track Systems*, 2004).

- director of clinical operations;
- quality assurance;
- writing of standard operating procedures (SOPs);
- regulatory affairs;
- data management and increased use of electronic data capture (EDC);
- accommodation for record storage.

Clinical investigator

The clinical investigator is ultimately responsible for clinical research conducted at the site. According to FDA and GCP regulations (Sections 21 CFR 312.60 and 4 respectively), the investigator has broad-based responsibilities for protecting the rights and safety of study volunteers. This is accomplished through activities such as obtaining informed consent, administering study drug, maintaining and storing medical records, and reporting adverse and serious adverse events.

Physicians report that they participate in clinical research mostly because it is scientifically rewarding, but they are also attracted to the financial rewards and the opportunities to improve patient care (Lamberti, 2005). With clinical trials numbering in the tens of thousands, the current shortfall in the number of qualified US investigators is expected to grow unless more physicians start participating in clinical research (CenterWatch, 2006). There are several factors contributing to this dilemma.

First, the number of evaluable subjects per new drug application continues to rise and is now in the range of 5300, a dramatic increase from the 3200 needed for New Drug Applications (NDAs) submitted in the mid-1980s (Lamberti, 2005). To meet this demand, more investigators per study need to be recruited.

Second, the percentage of US investigators participating in clinical trials has always been low, in the range of 5% of physicians, and that number seems to be declining. A recent study from the Tufts Center for the Study of Drug Development indicates that only 3% of US board certified physicians are principal investigators (Tufts, 2005).

To complicate matters further, there is a high rate of drop out among investigators. Many conduct one or two trials and choose to never conduct another one leading to a dilemma in which 50% of US principal investigators have opted out of the clinical trials business. The reasons cited are that clinical research interferes too much with other responsibilities such as private practice medicine or academic obligations, or they lack the infrastructure to handle today's rigorous trials.

There is good news, however. The Tufts Center study (2005) reveals that the number of investigators in many regions of the world is actually rising. In addition, there are now certification programs for investigators, and so it is possible that those who invest in preparing for and receiving certification by examination may be less likely to drop out. Certification programs are offered by the Drug Information Association (DIA) and through the Association of Clinical Research Professionals (ACRP) affiliate, the Academy of Pharmaceutical Physicians and Investigators (APPI). Certification offered through DIA is the Certified Clinical Investigator (CII) (see www.diahome.org). The ACRP-APPI designation for physicians is Certified Physician Investigator (CPI). The ACRP offers the CTI (Clinical Trial Investigator) designation to non-physician investigators (see www.acrpnet.org).

Study coordinator

The study coordinator is generally considered the linchpin in the day-to-day activities of clinical research. Without this key individual, sites would be hard pressed to perform studies in a quality and timely fashion because the coordinator's responsibilities define clinical trial conduct.

The coordinator's job is detailed oriented and includes responsibilities such as the following (Miskin and Neuer, 2002):

- patient recruitment activities;
- completing case report forms;
- transmitting study data;
- scheduling patient visits;
- meeting with principal investigators;
- meeting with study monitors;
- shipping samples to laboratories;
- maintaining inventory and accountability of the investigational product;
- closing out the study;

- participating in preparing proposals for soliciting new studies;
- participating in budget preparation;
- attending investigator meetings;
- participating in ongoing training;
- collecting metrics.

Today's quality sites often encourage study coordinators to become certified either by the ACRP, an international organization with chapters in more than a dozen nations, or the Society of Clinical Research Associates (SoCRA), a organization with chapters in some half-dozen countries. The ACRP certification is known as "Certified Clinical Research Coordinator" (CCRC), and SoCRA's certification is the "Certified Clinical Research Professional" (CCRP).

To achieve either of these designations, the coordinator must sit for an examination following specified amounts of full-time or part-time experience by the date of the exam as defined by either organization (www.acrpnet.org and www.socra.org). The examinations test knowledge in study conduct, regulations, and ethical issues.

A major issue in clinical research today is that of the overwhelmed study coordinator. Because of the ever growing number of details that comprise clinical studies, coordinators can easily become bogged down and, ultimately, very frustrated. This situation can lead to a decline in work quality or a high level of employee turnover. According to a recent survey, 53% of study coordinators have been in their jobs for three years or less (Borfitz, 2004). This poses real challenges in terms of experience level, knowledge of GCP, and familiarity with site operations.

Sites interested in retaining their trained and certified coordinators are exploring ways to improve retention. This includes offering good compensation and benefits, offering ongoing training, and making decisions to hire more full or part-time coordinators if the workload expands beyond the capacity of the existing staff complement.

Director of clinical operations (DCO)

The DCO is the point person for daily clinical operations. This is the individual who interfaces with sponsors, investigators, study coordinators, and other professional staff on a regular basis to oversee clinical and budgetary status of ongoing and upcoming studies. Because of the intense, close attention to detail that the job demands, it makes sense to fill this position with a highly detailed-oriented individual with an understanding of the clinical trials process.

For small or part-time sites that cannot justify a full-time DCO, a well-trained coordinator can assume this function.

Quality assurance (QA)

Putting systems in place to ensure product quality is a standard business process. According to the International Standardization Organization (ISO 9000), quality assurance is defined as a set of activities whose purpose is to inspire the confidence of customers and managers that all quality requirements are being met for a product or service (ISO 9000 definitions).

The investigative site should have a keen interest in adopting quality assurance methods to assure its clients—sponsors and CROs—that it is achieving its goal of turning out a quality product: clean data. The way to accomplish this goal is by assigning an individual to review the site's adherence to GCP guidelines, its handling of clinical data, its attention to patient safety and protection, and its adherence to standard operating procedures. The QA professional should establish specific time intervals for routine review of case report forms (CRF), certainly at study start-up and once a month thereafter. Because mistakes in data collection and reporting are most likely to occur at study start-up, it is a good idea for the QA manager to review the first three to five charts.

Attention to detail will also serve to improve the outcomes of visits from study monitors. As a representative of the sponsor or CRO, the monitor's job is to ensure that the study protocol is being adhered to and that the clinical data are properly collected, recorded, and forwarded (Miskin and Neuer, 2002). A quality site treats the monitor with respect and provides a quiet space in which the person can work.

Writing of SOPs

The writing and implementation of SOPs forms the framework of a quality operation by defining expectations and providing a consistent approach to drug development at the sponsor, CRO, and site levels (Hamrell *et al.*, 2001). SOPs for the site are best developed with input from all levels of site management and should describe how each member of the clinical research team is to complete various tasks. The SOP should state its objective, mention to whom it applies, define terms or abbreviations, describe tasks in a step-by-step manner, include appropriate checklists or forms, and list any associated SOPs (Miskin and Neuer, 2002). Because the industry is not static but constantly changing, it is a good idea for the head of Quality Assurance to review the SOPs annually to evaluate the need for updates.

Standardizing procedures becomes particularly relevant as sites grow internally or eventually expand into more than one location. In addition, employee turnover is inevitable, and so the SOPs can serve as a basic element of the training program for new hires.

There is a whole host of SOP topics for the investigative site, ranging from study management to patient recruitment to handling of accounts receivable. Some study management SOPs appear in Figure 12.4 (Miskin and Neuer, 2002).

- Telephone Screening
- Sign-in Sheet
- Schedule Book
- Confirming Appointments
- Informed Consent Process
- Amended Consents
- Screen Failures
- Tracking Forms
- Serious Adverse Events
- Master Charts
- Source Documents
- Progress Notes
- Obtaining Medical Records and Notifying Primacy Care Physician
- Storage of Records
- Patient Stipend

Figure 12.4 Some study management SOPs (source: Miskin and Neuer, *How to Grow Your Investigative Site*, 2002).

Regulatory affairs

Clinical trials cannot operate without regulatory oversight. Regulatory agencies from each country or region promulgate guidelines and regulations for conduct of ethical clinical research by industry and government sponsors. As part of that chain, investigative sites share the responsibility for conforming to federal guidelines and regulations, and do so by receiving training that defines what their responsibilities entail. At the site level, there is a growing amount of regulatory responsibility, particularly in countries that have adopted ICH-GCP guidelines or similar regulations. Everything from submissions to institutional review boards (IRBs) or ethics committees, completion of the Statements of Investigator Form 1572 and financial disclosure forms (US), maintaining the regulatory binder and the credentials of investigators and sub-investigators, adverse event reporting, and participation in site inspections are some of the many responsibilities assumed by the regulatory affairs department.

Generally, small and part-time sites cannot justify creating a position for a full-time regulatory manager, but once the number of studies conducted annually approaches eight or more, a full or part-time regulatory affairs position needs to be created. Without this function firmly in place, it becomes increasingly difficult to maintain site quality. Signals that staffing in regulatory affairs needs to increase include the failure to submit important regulatory documents in accordance with established timelines, difficulty in keeping regulatory binders up-to-date, and failure to report adverse event (AE) and serious adverse events (SAE) to sponsors or ethics committees as required.

Data management and increased use of electronic solutions

As clinical trial protocols increase in complexity, there is an industry-wide shift toward adoption of electronic solutions to improve critical functions, most notably the collection, handling, analysis, and storing of clinical data, as well as the reporting of adverse and serious adverse events.

Traditionally, the collection of data at the investigative site has been, and to a large extent continues to be, accomplished using paper and pen, but in recent years there is growing emphasis on electronic methods. Estimates vary as to the percentage of electronic solutions used to collect and submit clinical data, but the figure is approaching 50% of clinical trials (Borfitz, 2007; Emam *et al.*, 2009). This number is expected to increase over time as more pharmaceutical sponsors commit to implementing electronic data capture (EDC) in virtually all their clinical trials (Bleicher, 2005).

For the investigative site, shifting away from paper in favor of electronic solutions means that staff must be trained in both types of data collection during this transition phase. The Quality Assurance department should create SOPs for both methods because the capturing and handling of clinical data are completely different for "paper-based" and "electronic" studies. In a paper-based study, clinical source data are handwritten onto paper case report forms that are mailed, faxed, or overnighted to the sponsor or CRO. In a study using EDC, data are entered electronically into a secured web-based case report form that is sent via the Internet to the sponsor or CRO. Data that are missing, placed in the wrong field, or out-of-range are immediately spotted, thereby reducing the number of queries. And to facilitate the more rapid sending of electronic data to sponsors or CROs, and allowing near real-time viewing of those data, the site should implement high speed Internet access.

Regulatory pressures are also driving increased use of electronic solutions (Beyster *et al.*, 2005).

Regulatory agencies around the globe are requiring that more trial-related information be submitted electronically. For example, on May 1, 2004, European Medicines Agency (EMA), the regulatory body for the EU Member States, started requiring suspected serious unexpected adverse reactions (SUSARs) to be reported electronically to EudraVigilance, the European data processing network. The Food and Drug Administration (FDA), the US regulatory agency, has established the Adverse Event Reporting System (AERS), a database that accepts electronic individual case safety reports. In addition, FDA is requiring electronic submission of NDAs in the format of the Common Technical Document (CTD), amended new drug applications (ANDAs), and biologics license applications (BLAs), using industry accepted standardized formats for data submission.

These trends have implications for the investigative site. First, GCP guidelines require investigators to report SAEs immediately to the sponsor unless otherwise indicated in the protocol or Investigator's Brochure (see Figure 12.5). AEs are to be reported to sponsors in accordance with the protocol. Complying with these reporting requirements can be greatly facilitated if they are done electronically. Second, to enable sponsors to conform to the growing number of electronic submission requirements,

---

4.11.1 All serious adverse events (SAEs) should be reported immediately to the sponsor except for those SAEs that the protocol or other document (i.e. Investigator's Brochure) identifies as not needing immediate reporting. The immediate reports should be followed promptly by detailed, written reports…

4.11.2 Adverse events and/or laboratory abnormalities identified in the protocol as critical to safety evaluations should be reported to the sponsor according to the reporting requirements and within the time periods specified by the sponsor in the protocol.

Figure 12.5 ICH-GCP Guidelines for SAE and AE reporting (source: *Safety Reporting Guideline for Good Clinical Practice*).

the clinical trial data they collect from dozens of sites across the globe are more easily compiled and analyzed if the sites use standardized electronic formats.

Accommodation for record storage

Clinical trials generate vast amounts of paperwork, all of which must be stored during and after the trials. With trials sometimes lasting for several years and generally requiring more patients per trial (Lamberti, 2005), storage requirements are important regulatory and cost considerations for the investigative site.

According to ICH-GCP Guideline 4.9.5, records are to be retained until at least two years after the last approval of a marketing application. Records may be retained for even longer periods if required by applicable regulatory requirements or if required by the sponsor.

Trial-related documents can be stored off-site once a trial is completed, but generally, while a study is ongoing, it is more convenient to keep them on-site. In particular, a visiting study monitor will expect to have direct access to trial documents, and so having them readily available is important.

It is a good idea for the investigative site to plan for excess document storage capacity in a location that is dry and can be locked. Storing documents in the basement of a building without special protection from water damage or rodent destruction is not a good idea and is actually a violation of GCP. ICH-GCP Guideline 4.9.4 states that the investigator is responsible for storing documents in a manner that will prevent their accidental or premature destruction.

Clinical site challenges

Once basic infrastructure is in place, the challenge of conducting successful clinical research begins. Basic infrastructure provides the necessary framework, but the essence of clinical research is defined by specific tasks such as the following:

- patient recruitment and retention;
- budgeting;
- FDA audits.

Patient recruitment and retention

The recruiting of study volunteers and retaining them throughout the study remains one of the industry's key bottlenecks. Data suggest that in North America, for example, 87% of clinical trials must extend the enrollment period beyond established timelines because of incomplete enrollment (Getz, 2008).

Patient recruitment and enrollment targets goals are set by the sponsor but become the responsibility of the selected investigative sites once they commit to conducting specific trials. If a site contracts to enroll 15 patients, for instance, it is committed to reaching that goal.

Often, a site expects to fill its enrollment quota from its own internal patient database, but statistics suggests that most of the time, this approach is less than successful. To improve their chances for recruitment success, site managers need to determine how to go about recruiting and enrolling patients if the database falls short.

Sites in some regions of the world, such as the United States, attempt to boost enrollment through active patient education and recruitment campaigns including advertising the study in electronic and print media as well as the Internet. Other locales have been more conservative, generally relying on practitioners to inform patients of appropriate clinical trial opportunities. That approach is starting to change, however, as more countries are allowing patient recruitment activities in their regulatory guidelines.

The EU, for example, permits patient recruitment activities for the Member States as described in a detailed guidance put forth by the European Commission in April 2004, revised February 2006 (European Commission, 2006). Section 7.5 of the guidance, entitled "Advertising for Trial Subjects," lists various aspects to be included in advertisements (see Figure 12.6) provided they are reviewed and approved by an ethics committee.

Once patients are recruited, retaining them becomes the next hurdle. Data suggest that only 70% of subjects enrolled in Phases I–III trials complete those trials (Lamberti, 2005). That retention figure is likely to increase if study volunteers are satisfied with the care and treatment they

All advertisements for trial subjects should be included in the submission for approval by the Ethics Committee. The review by the Ethics Committee might also include the procedures to take care of subjects responding to the advertisement.

The advertisement might contain information on the following points:

1. The research nature of the project
2. The scope of the trial
3. Which type/group of subjects might be included
4. The investigator clinically/scientifically responsible for the trial, if possible or if required by local regulations.
5. The person, name, address, organisation, to contact for information
6. That the subject responding will be registered
7. The procedure to contact the interested subjects
8. Any compensation for expenses
9. That a response on the part of a potential subject only signifies interest to obtain further information

Figure 12.6 Section 7.5—Advertising for trial subjects (source: *Detailed Guidance on the Application Format and Documentation to be Submitted in an Application for an Ethics Committee Opinion*, April 2004, revised February 2006).

are receiving (Miskin and Neuer, 2002). Proper treatment starts from the beginning, from the minute volunteers enter the site, extends to follow-up reminder telephone calls or postcards about upcoming visits, and continues by making them feel valued at every step of the process, essentially treating them like important customers (Neuer, 2003).

Budgeting

The clinical trials industry is a competitive business. Although thousands of clinical trials are ongoing at any given time, there are thousands of investigative sites competing for that business. Yet despite the strong competition, sites need to avoid rushing to accept studies before taking the time to determine if they make financial sense.

The clinical staff and financial manager need to evaluate the following (Gersch *et al.*, 2001):

- the study of study visits;
- the number and cost of procedures, i.e., physical examinations, chest X-rays, electrocardiograms, stress tests, and blood draws, including the cost of processing, packing, and shipping the samples to a central laboratory;
- supplies and equipment needed to conduct the trial;
- cost of recruiting subjects;
- the amount of screening or "pre-study" work involved to determine study eligibility and if the site will be paid for that work, even for prospects who ultimately fail to qualify for the study;
- personnel costs and time for performing procedures, and collecting and forwarding clinical data to the sponsor or CRO;
- records retention fee;
- administrative or overhead costs such as rent, utilities, and office supplies.

Many sites report cash flow problems because they accepted studies with insufficient budgets, the sponsor or CRO is very slow to pay for work already done, or the site failed to negotiate reimbursement for pre-study work. Regarding slow pay, a recent study of 111 investigative sites revealed that 71% of respondents reported that it is taking "somewhat longer" or "much longer" to receive payment from sponsors or CROs as compared to three years earlier (Lamberti, 2005). There is also research to suggest that pre-study work can quickly reach US$10,000 before successful enrollment of the first subject, and so during the budget negotiation process, sites should request compensation for screening costs whether they result in screen failures or subject enrollment.

If a budget is presented by the sponsor as "non-negotiable," it is the site's responsibility to determine the feasibility of accepting the budget as is, or attempt to negotiate a few favorable points such as receiving several thousand dollars in start-up expenses (see Figure 12.7) or adding a line item for patient recruitment costs.

FDA audits

Clinical sites should be in the habit of operating as if every day is inspection day. Operating in top form is not only in the best interest of the study volunteers, but also prepares the sites for FDA inspection,

- Time spent procuring the study, developing a proposal, and meeting with pre-study site selector
- Preparation of paperwork necessary for the study, i.e. tracking forms and screening forms
- Regulatory submissions
- Time spent for study initiation, typically an entire day
- Time spent training hospital staff, nursing and pharmacy personnel if study has an inpatient component

Figure 12.7 Start-up expenses (source: Miskin and Neuer, *How to Grow Your Investigative Site*, 2002).

- Who did what
- Degree of delegation of authority
- Where specific aspects of the study were performed
- How and where data were recorded
- How test article accountability was maintained
- How monitor communicated with clinical investigator
- How the monitor evaluated the study's progress

Figure 12.8 Facts surrounding the conduct of the study (source: IRB Information Sheets, 1998).

an inevitability if they are conducting studies for compounds or devices to be submitted to FDA. The purpose of inspections is to ensure the protection of research subjects and the integrity of data submitted to the agency in support of a marketing application.

Generally, inspections are done by appointment and begin with an opening interview with the investigator and study coordinator(s). The inspector will tour the facility, and review charts as well as the regulatory binder.

FDA conducts three types of inspections through its Bioresearch Monitoring Program (Information Sheets, 1998):
- study-oriented;
- investigator-oriented;
- bioequivalence study.

The *study-oriented* inspection is conducted almost exclusively to audit trials that are important to product evaluation such as NDAs and product license applications (PLAs) pending before FDA. The inspection consists of two parts: the facts surrounding the conduct of the study (see Figure 12.8), and the auditing of study data.

The *investigator-oriented* inspection is initiated for several reasons. Some include: the investigator conducted a study that is pivotal to product approval; representatives of the sponsor have reported to FDA that they are having difficulty getting case reports from the investigator or have some other concern with the investigator's work; a study volunteer complains about protocol or

subject rights violations; an investigator has participated in a large number of studies or has done work outside his or her specialty areas, or contributed many patients to a pivotal approval study.

Most inspections are of the study-oriented or investigator-oriented types. The *bioequivalence study* inspection is conducted when one study may be the sole basis for a drug's marketing approval.

At the end of the site inspection, the inspector(s) conducts an exit interview with the investigator and appropriate staff. If the inspector uncovered any significant issues, he or she may issue Form FDA-483, an "inspectional observations" form documenting deviation from GCP. The investigator will need to respond to the Form 483 and take corrective action.

Following the inspection, the clinical investigator will receive one of three types of letters:
- *NAI (No Action Indicated)*: A notice that no significant deviations from the regulations were observed. This letter does not require any response from the clinical investigator.
- *VAI (Voluntary Action Indicated)*: An informational letter that identifies deviations from regulations and good investigational practice. This letter may or may not require a response from the clinical investigator. If a response is requested, the letter will describe what is necessary and provide the name of a contact person.

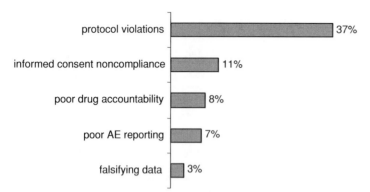

Figure 12.9 Top five deficiencies (source: Thomson CenterWatch, FDA CDER, 2004).

• *OAI (Official Action Indicated)*: Identifies serious deviations from regulations requiring prompt correction by the clinical investigator. The letter will provide the name of a contact person. In this case, the FDA may inform both the study sponsor and the reviewing IRB of the deficiencies. The agency may also inform the sponsor if the clinical investigator's procedural deficiencies indicate ineffective monitoring by the sponsor.

The vast majority of inspections, some 77%, result in "Voluntary Action Indicated." Of the other two categories, 16% result in "NAI" and 7% in "OAI" (Lamberti, 2005).

The number of annual inspections has been growing steadily, and in 2004 reached a total of 242 for US clinical investigators and 82 for foreign clinical investigators (Center for Drug Evaluation and Research, 2004). The top five deficiencies, led by protocol violations, appear in Figure 12.9.

Final thoughts

The purpose of the investigative site is to produce clean clinical data by performing a protocol on study volunteers. Sites that achieve this goal do so by building an infrastructure that supports the many functions involved in generating those data. The infrastructure includes standard business practices such as quality assurance, writing of SOPs, regulatory affairs, and data management. It must also include study coordinators and investigators who are well trained in GCP.

Because the conduct of clinical trials is a competitive business, sites should document their performance in terms of quality and timeliness. This entails keeping metrics of on-time completion of patient recruitment and enrollment, retention rates of study volunteers, success rates with different kinds of patient recruitment media, and numbers of studies completed in various therapeutic areas.

Sponsors looking to select sites for clinical trials can use these metrics to distinguish performing sites from nonperformers. In addition, sponsors are increasingly using metrics to identify sites with a higher probability of achieving trial objectives on time (Anderson, 2004).

By reaching objectives, sites begin to form relationships with sponsors who recognize and appreciate the contribution they make to the clinical development of investigational compounds and devices.

References

(Notes: all websites cited in the text were accessed April 24, 2010.)

Anderson D. *A Guide to Patient Recruitment and Retention*. Thomson CenterWatch: Boston, MA, USA, 2004, 10–11.

Beyster MA, Hardison DH, Lubin GM. *Improving Clinical Trials by Implementing Information Technology, Where Will You be in Three Years?* SAIC, April 2005; http://www.saic.com/life-sciences/pdfs/mcv.pdf.

Bleicher P. Tools are just the beginning. Pharmaceutical Executive Supplement 2005; **25**:16–19.

Borfitz, D. CRC loss tied to heavy workload. *CenterWatch* 2004; **11**(8).

Borfitz D. Connor: 2007 will be tipping point for EDC. *eCliniqua* 2007; May 21.

Center for Drug Evaluation and Research. *Report to the Nation Improving Public Health Through Human Drugs*. US Department of Health and Human Services, 2004; http://www.fda.gov/downloads/AboutFDA/ CentersOffices/CDER/WhatWeDo/UCM078941.pdf.

CenterWatch. Addressing the investigator shortfall, *CenterWatch Monthly*, 2006; **13**(9).

Emam KE, Jonker E, Sampson M, Krieža-Jerić K, Neisa, A, The use of electronic data capture tools in clinical trials: Web-survey of 259 Canadian trials. *J Med Internet Res* 2009; **11**(1).

European Commission. *Detailed Guidance on the Application Format and Documentation to be Submitted in an Application for an Ethics Committee Opinion on the Clinical Trial on Medicinal Products for Human Use*, February 2006, http://ec.europa.eu/enterprise/sectors/ pharmaceuticals/files/eudralex/vol-10/12_ec_guideline _20060216_en.pdf.

Gersch S, Cohen B, Hirshhorn B. The seven basic components of clinical trials budgets. *Clinical Trials Advisor* 2001; **6**(3):5.

Getz K. *Overview of the Investigative Site Landscape*, presentation at the DIA Annual Meeting, Boston, MA, June 25, 2008.

Hamrell MR, Wagman B. Standard operating procedures; a beginner's guide. *The Quality Assurance Journal* 2001; **5**(2):93–97.

Hart S. Planning late stage studies. *Evidence Matters*, 2007; **13**(3).

Information Sheets, Guidance for Institutional Review Boards and Clinical Investigators 1998 Update, FDA, http://www.fda.gov/oc/ohrt/irbs/operations.html# inspections.

ISO 9000 Definitions; http://www.praxiom.com/iso-definition.htm.

Korieth K. Phase I spending sizzles. *CenterWatch* August 2004; **11**(8).

Lamberti M (ed.). *State of the Clinical Trials Industry*. Thomson CenterWatch, 2005, 265, 291, 292, 261, 275.

Miskin BM, Neuer A. *How to Grow Your Investigative Site, A Guide to Operating and Expanding a Successful Clinical Research Center*. Thomson CenterWatch, 2002, 39–56, 27–38, **64**, 137–158.

Neuer A. Stirring up the Phase I market. *CenterWatch* October 2000; **7**(10).

Neuer A. Treating study volunteers as customers. *CenterWatch*, March 2003; **10**(3).

Tufts University. *Number of Principal Investigators in the U.S. is Declining, According to Tufts CSDD*, May 3, 2005; http://70.42.48.93/NewsEvents/NewsArticle.asp? newsid=54.

CHAPTER 13
Good Clinical Practices

*Lionel D. Edwards**

Pharma Pro Plus Inc., New Jersey, and Temple University, School of Pharmacy, Philadelphia, USA

*This chapter is based on the excellent chapter by Wendy Bohaychuk and Graham Ball in the 2nd edition.

The aim of this chapter is to describe the general framework for conducting good clinical practices (GCP)-compliant clinical research. As it is difficult to cover this broad topic in such a short chapter, the author will focus on those areas that are most discussed, most problematic, and most critical to achieving a GCP-compliant clinical study. Thus, there is particular emphasis on ethical issues, source data verification and data integrity, monitoring and safety review, and study medication/device management.

The current rules for conducting clinical research

Conducting GCP-compliant clinical research is a serious undertaking, and this has been recognized by numerous authorities internationally. It is difficult to achieve a fully GCP-compliant clinical study, but the expectation today is that the greatest effort will be made nevertheless and the documentation to provide evidence of this effort must be available.

The basic tenets of GCP

GCP is an international ethical and scientific quality standard for designing, conducting, recording, and reporting clinical trials that involve the participation of human subjects. Compliance with the 13 core principles of this standard provides public assurance that the rights, safety, and

Principles and Practice of Pharmaceutical Medicine, 3rd edition.
Edited by L.D. Edwards, A.W. Fox, P.D. Stonier.
© 2011 Blackwell Publishing Ltd.

wellbeing of trial subjects are protected—consistent with principles that have their origin in the Declaration of Helsinki—and that the clinical trial data are credible.

The primary reason for the presence of GCP is protection of the subjects and protection of the data. To safeguard human rights, structures must be set up because both the welfare of current study subjects and future patients are at stake. Therefore, systems must be in place (such as ethics committee review and informed consent) to protect study subjects. Collecting honest and accurate data is also a major objective of GCP to ensure that data have integrity and that valid conclusions may be drawn from those data. Further, data should be reproducible, that is if the study were to be conducted in a similar population using the same procedures, the results should be the same. In addition, if the study clinical case reports were destroyed, the original core source data must be available to reconstruct the study results. To ensure the integrity and reproducibility of research results, the whole process should be transparent, that is everything must be documented so that an external reviewer may verify that the research was actually conducted as reported by the researchers.

The general regulatory framework for GCP

The regulatory framework for compliance with research procedures has essentially developed on an international basis only in the last two decades, except for the United States where rules were first established in the 1930s. Today, countries in the European Union, other countries in Europe (e.g., Switzerland), and Japan have regulations on

GCP. Other countries have regulations controlling clinical studies, with guidelines on GCP, such as Australia and Canada. In the 1990s, an attempt was made to harmonize GCP requirements in the form of the ICH GCP document implemented in the three regions in 1997, which has since been adapted into their regulations by many countries.

Some countries have no guidelines or regulations, but guidance for researchers has been provided by organizations such as the Council for the International Organizations of Medical Sciences (CIOMS) and the World Health Organization (WHO). (A brief list of existing regulations and guidelines is presented at the end of this chapter.) Regulatory authority review and/or approval are usually necessary in all countries before, during, and after clinical studies. With the advent of the EU Clinical Trials Directive, compliance with the principles of GCP is now a legal obligation in Europe for all trials of investigational medicinal products. Further, it is now a legal requirement in Europe for these investigational medicinal products to be manufactured, handled, and stored to the standards of Good Manufacturing Practice (GMP) in order to prevent exposure of subjects to defective medicines.

In the past few years, there has been increasing interest in regulatory inspection of GCP compliance to ensure validity of the data and protection of study subjects and to compare the practices and procedures of the investigator and the sponsor/contract research organization (CRO) with the commitment made in the application to undertake a study. Although inspection has been a regulatory requirement in the United States for many years, inspectorates have only just started in countries such as Austria, Denmark, France, Finland, Germany, Japan, The Netherlands, Norway, and Sweden. There are problems in finding good inspectors, in deciding on the final standards for inspections and in imposing sanctions for noncompliance. An interesting recent development has been the initiation of inspections in Europe by the central regulatory authority, the European Medicines Agency (EMA). Regulation of compliance with requirements by ethics committees is also developing in some parts of the world (e.g., France

and Denmark). To date, the US Food and Drug Administration (FDA) is the only authority that is actively checking on the activities of institutional review boards (IRBs) by requiring registration with the Department of Health and Human Services, and by inspection of the IRBs.

For noncompliance with regulations, the three regions all imposed serious sanctions. The FDA "blacklist" (list of all investigators who have been found to be noncompliant and were placed on probation or barred from clinical research for FDA submissions) is publicly available through freedom of information rules. The United States has vast experience (thousands of inspections) in the US, compared to the couple of hundred of inspections it has undertaken in other countries. Nonetheless, comparison of FDA inspection findings is reassuring, and citations run at about the same rate internationally to the US.

Within a research organization, other independent review—auditing—is undertaken internally to check on compliance with standards and basically to pre-empt the inspectors. Auditing may be conducted at any time during a clinical study to ensure continued compliance with GCP. Almost all aspects under GCP could be audited. Auditing, by definition, must be undertaken by personnel who are independent of the research being audited.

Setting up clinical studies

To ensure that the standards for clinical research are established before studies begin and to check on compliance with those standards, many fundamental systems and processes must be pre-defined by study sponsors and CROs. These are outlined in Table 13.1.

The sponsor/CRO has a duty to place a study safely. That is, the sponsor (or the delegated CRO) must assess and choose a site where study subjects will not be harmed, and that adequate staff and facilities exist to treat emergency adverse events, whether study or disease related. This is not always easy due to the apparent lack of choice, in that there may be too few patients in a chosen demographic area or investigators in a particular

Table 13.1 General systems and procedures for implementation of GCP

The following systems and procedures must be established by clinical researchers to ensure compliance with GCP requirements:

Quality assurance: Systems for assuring quality and for checking quality must be established and followed at all stages.

Planning: Studies must be conducted for valid (ethical and scientific) reasons.

Standard operating procedures (SOPs): Research procedures must be declared in writing so that reviewers can determine the standards that are being applied and so that users have a reference point.

Well-designed study: All studies must have a valid study design, documented in a protocol, so that it can be fully reviewed by all interested parties. The data collection plans, as described in the CRF, are part of the protocol.

Qualified personnel: All personnel (sponsor/CRO and study site) must be experienced and qualified to undertake assigned tasks. Documentation of qualifications and training must be evident.

Ethics committee review and approval: All studies must be independently reviewed by ethics committees/IRBs, to assess the risk for study subjects, before clinical studies begin. Review must continue throughout the study.

Informed consent: All study subjects must be given the opportunity to assess personally the risk of study participation by being provided with certain information. Their assent to participate must be documented.

Monitoring: A primary means of quality control of clinical studies involves frequent and thorough monitoring by sponsor/CRO personnel.

Data processing for integrity of data: Data must be honest. Data must be reviewed by site personnel, monitors, and data processing personnel.

Control of study medications/devices: The product being studied must be managed so that study subjects ultimately receive a safe product and full accountability can be documented.

Archives: Documentation of research activities must be securely retained to provide evidence of activities.

therapeutic area (only 3% of practicing physicians have ever taken part in a research study and of those only 2% have participated in two or more studies). None of these reasons is as important as compliance with the basic GCP principle, which requires the sponsor/CRO to assess, select, and choose safe settings for research. This is done in a formal pre-study site inspection visit.

Setting up clinical studies is a lengthy process, because there are many documents to prepare (e.g., protocols and case report forms (CRFs)), study facilities to be assessed (e.g., study sites, CROs, clinical laboratories, Phase I units), regulatory review to be considered, and negotiations and agreements with study sites (e.g., contracts, finances, confidentiality, indemnity, insurance) to be undertaken. In addition, as will be dealt with in subsequent sections, ethical aspects of the study must be considered (e.g., ethics committee and IRB review and informed consent requirements), and study medications/devices must be organized.

Protocols and CRFs

The protocol, with the accompanying CRF, is the key document governing a clinical study. It formally describes how a clinical study will be conducted and how the data will be evaluated, and it must include all the information that an investigator should know in order properly to select subjects, collect safety and efficacy data, and prescribe the correct study medication/device. Protocols must be prepared in accordance with a specified and standardized format, which is described in guidelines and regulations (the reader is particularly advised to refer to the ICH GCP document, available at www.emea.europa.eu/pdf/human/ich/013595eu.pdf (accessed April 14, 2010)). Protocols are usually prepared, at least initially, by the sponsor or the delegated CRO, although investigator input is obviously necessary. It is also recommended that both sponsor field personnel and investigator study coordinators help in the review because this ensures the "do-ability" and later reduces the number of amendments. A recent change implemented in 2008, as a result of the Food and Drug Administration Amendment Act (FDAAA) of 2007, no longer requires a statement of compliance to the Helsinki agreement, but a statement of compliance with GCPs. The last rewrite of the Helsinki agreement in Edinburgh 2000 was very controversial and blurred the difference between good medical practice and good medical research; the two are not identical.

Any document used to collect research data on clinical study subjects may be generically classed as a data collection form. These completed forms provide evidence of the research conducted. The most common type of data collection form is the CRF. Other types of data collection forms include diary cards, dispensing records, quality-of-life forms, and so on. The CRF must allow for proper analysis of the data and proper reporting of the data in the final clinical study report, and it must reflect the protocol exactly: no more and no less data must be collected. Thus, a CRF must be created for each clinical study and must be prepared in parallel with the protocol. CRFs are usually also prepared by sponsors/CROs because of the demanding requirements for their design and contents.

Selection of investigators and study sites

The sponsor/CRO must go through a formal assessment procedure before placement of a study. Some of the most important areas requiring assessment are described in Table 13.2. All studies involving research of investigational medications and devices require qualified investigators, and the interna-

tionally accepted standard for "qualified" usually encompasses three main criteria: (i) medically qualified, that is legally licensed to practice medicine as a physician (or dentist if a dental product is being studied); (ii) experienced in the relevant therapeutic specialty; and (iii) experienced in clinical research.

Many contracts or agreements must be prepared, understood, and authorized before clinical studies begin. The most common contracts include the protocol and CRF; agreements for finances, confidentiality, insurance, and indemnity; and contracts between the sponsor and the CRO. A separate investigator agreement, specifying all responsibilities, is usually necessary in addition to the protocol to emphasize certain aspects of the protocol. Table 13.3 highlights some of the responsibilities of the main investigator GCP that might be included in contracts.

Ethical considerations

Part of the selection process for a study site involves confirming that ethics committee/IRB review will be safe and that all study subjects will be properly informed prior to consent to study participation. If the sponsor/CRO cannot obtain documented evidence of compliance with these two fundamental requirements, it is not safe to work with that site.

Ethics committee/IRB review

All clinical studies require review by an independent ethics committee/IRB before, during, and after the study. Before any study subject is treated,

Table 13.2 Selection of study sites

The following items should be assessed at study sites by sponsor/CRO monitors before studies begin:

Study site personnel, for example qualification, experience, training, availability; specific allocation of responsibilities.

Facilities, for example offices, wards, archives, pharmacy, clinical laboratory; study medication/device storage areas; clinical laboratories; access to source documents; ethics committee/IRB requirements.

Suitable study subject population, for example access to suitable subjects in sufficient numbers; method of subject recruitment; source, for example from investigator's subject population, or be referred by other physicians and, if referred, means by which investigator will obtain adequate evidence of medical history; use of advertisements; potential subject enrolment (recruitment) rate.

Table 13.3 Investigator GCP responsibilities

The following investigator responsibilities must be declared in agreements or contracts:

Adhere to the protocol exactly. No changes to the protocol may be undertaken without following a formal protocol amendment procedure and without agreement by the sponsor/CRO.

Be thoroughly familiar with the properties of the clinical study medications/devices as described in the investigator brochure. Have sufficient time to conduct and complete the study personally. If more than one investigator is involved at a specific study site, the specific responsibilities must be described for each investigator. The investigator must ensure that no other studies divert study subjects, facilities. or personnel from the study under consideration.

Maintain the confidentiality of all information received with regard to the study and the investigational study.

Medication/device

Submit the protocol, information sheet, and consent form, and other required documentation, to an ethics committee/IRB for review and approval before the study begins. During the study, the investigator is also responsible for submitting any new information, for example protocol amendments, safety information, which might be important for continuing risk assessment by the ethics committee/IRB.

Obtain informed consent from each study subject prior to enrolment into the study.

Inform the subjects primary care physician, e.g., general practitioner or family physician, of proposed study participation before enrollment into the study.

Maintain study subject clinical notes, that is source documents, separately from the CRFs. The source documents must support the data entered into CRFs and must clearly indicate participation in a clinical study. If the study subject is referred by another physician, the investigator must ensure that sufficient evidence is available in the clinical notes to support the eligibility of the study subject.

Maintain a confidential list identifying the number/code and names of all subjects entered into the study.

Allow authorized representatives of the sponsor/CRO and regulatory authorities direct access to study subject clinical notes (source documents) in order to verify the data recorded on CRFs.

Ensure CRFs are complete and accurate.

Allow monitoring visits by the sponsor/CRO at a predetermined frequency. During these monitoring visits, the monitor must be allowed to communicate with all site personnel involved in the conduct of the clinical study.

Report all AEs and SAEs to the sponsor/CRO and follow the special reporting requirements for SAEs.

Maintain the security and accountability of clinical study supplies; ensure that medications/devices are labeled properly; maintain records of clinical study medication/device dispensing, including dates, quantity, and use by study subjects; and return or disposition (as instructed by the sponsor/CRO) after completion or termination of the study.

Archive all CRFs and documents associated with the study for a minimum of 15 years. Notify the sponsor/CRO of any problems with archiving in potential unusual circumstances, for example investigator retires, relocates, dies; study subject dies, relocates and so on.

Provide reports of the study's progress whenever required.

Review the final clinical report, and sign and date the signature page after review.

Allow an independent audit and/or inspection of all study documents and facilities.

Agree to the publication policy.

Agree to the sponsor's/CRO's ownership of the data.

Agree to the stated time frames for the study, for example start and completion of recruitment, submission of completed CRFs.

Work to GCP as defined by the ICH, FDA, and local regulations.

review by the committee must be documented in compliance with international guidelines and the local regulations of the country in which the research is conducted. Clinical studies begin (for the study subjects) whenever the study subjects undertake any procedure that they would not normally undergo: ethics committee/IRB review must be sought before these events. Thus, if a study requires screening procedures, washout from normal treatment, and even completion of a questionnaire that poses personal questions, the study begins when those procedures are undertaken. It is a common misconception that studies begin only when study subjects are randomized to treatment.

Prior to selection of a clinical study site, the sponsor/CRO must confirm and document, in the pre-study assessment visit report, that the investigator has access to a local ethics committee/IRB. Local committees cannot be bypassed: the only official exception to this requirement is France, where by regulation, a central committee may rule for all sites in a multicenter study. However, in the United States, it appears to be common practice for a central IRB to rule for the widely geographically separated areas in the country, and occasionally researchers in error may not inform the local IRB.

Normally, the sponsor/CRO will prepare all necessary documentation for submission by the investigator to the ethics committee/IRB (it is not usual procedure for the sponsor/CRO to directly submit items to the committee, unless requested to do so by the committee). Whatever the local variations, the sponsor/CRO is usually responsible for ensuring the submission of the items shown in Table 13.4. Some committees require other additional items.

The membership of an ethics committee/IRB will vary nationally and regionally. However, the sponsor/CRO is only permitted to conduct studies that are approved by ethics committees/IRBs that have a sufficient number of qualified members to enable a medical and scientific review of the proposed study and a review of all other ethical aspects of the study. Ethics committees also have to be diverse in composition, and may vary by country: For example, in the US it is required that both genders

be represented, and in France that two lay people be present. Details of the membership of the ethics committee/IRB should be obtained and reviewed by the sponsor/CRO, prior to initiating the study, to ascertain the above and to determine that there is no serious conflict of interest (e.g., investigator voting on her or his study).

The sponsor/CRO should also request a written copy of the working procedures of the ethics committees/IRBs. These procedures should provide sufficient information to assure sponsors/CROs, investigators, auditors, and inspectors of the integrity and independence of the ethics committee/IRB. Unfortunately, today, it is still difficult to obtain working procedures from many committees.

Ethics committees/IRBs also have responsibility for review during and after clinical studies (see Table 13.5). In other words, committee review is an ongoing responsibility that extends beyond the initial submission and review of documents to proceed with the study.

Informed consent

Potential study subjects may enter a clinical study conducted by the sponsor/CRO only after being properly informed and consenting to participate. The researchers must consider who does what, when, what sort of information must be provided, and how this will all be documented. The general principles for the conduct of informed consent are noted in Table 13.6 (see also Chapter 8). All information sheets and consent forms should include the items listed in Table 13.7, and they must be provided before study participation. Obtaining informed consent is a complex issue, and it is not easy to comply with these requirements. Especially difficult is the "Readability," which the American Medical Association and the *New England Journal of Medicine* recommend to be at reading grades 6–8 or reading levels normally attained at 11–12 years of age in US and 10–11 years in Europe.

Monitoring and safety assessment

The conduct of clinical studies is a cooperative undertaking between the sponsor/CRO and the

Table 13.4 Review by ethics committees/IRBs before clinical studies begin

The following items should be reviewed by ethics committees/IRBs before clinical studies begin:

Protocol (including annexes, such as the CRF).

Consent procedures (described in the protocol and the appended information sheet and consent form), which specify who will provide information and who will obtain consent, how consent will be documented, and whether or not a witness will be present.

Consent form/information sheet. Most committees will be particularly interested in these documents to ensure that all necessary information is provided to study subjects.

Suitability of investigator and facilities, including support personnel. Some committees may request a copy of investigator and other site personnel CVs. The committee will be particularly interested in allocation of resources, whether the investigator has enough time and study subjects to conduct the study, and whether use of resources for clinical studies will detract from normal medical care requirements.

Delegation of responsibility by investigators.

Source of study subjects and means of recruitment. The committee will wish to know if study subjects are known to investigators, and if not (i.e., referred patients), how investigators will confirm eligibility and whether primary care practitioners will be informed. The committee will wish to determine that advertisements are not unduly coercive or misleading or too "inviting."

Appropriateness (eligibility) of study subjects (described in the protocol).

Primary care physician to be informed of study participation.

Number of subjects to be studied and justification for sample size (this information should be in the protocol). The committee will be interested in how many subjects will be exposed to the risk of treatment. In a multicenter study, the local ethics committee/IRB should be informed of the number of subjects to be enrolled at each site and the total number of subjects to be enrolled in the study.

Investigator brochure or other authorized summary of information (e.g., preclinical and clinical summaries) about the investigational products, including comparator products and placebo. If the study medication/device is a marketed product, the ethics committee/IRB must review the most current data sheet, product monograph, and so on. The brochure is particularly important for confirming the formal declared safety profile of the study treatment and therefore is of great assistance to committees in assessing the relevance of AEs. Also, the committee can verify, by reviewing the brochure or product labeling, that the information sheet for obtaining consent provides sufficient information with regard to safety.

Evidence of regulatory submission and review/approval (if applicable). Committees particularly wish to know whether the drug/device is on the market in their country or in other countries, and the details of the stage of the submission.

Adequacy of confidentiality safeguards, with regard to protection of identification of the study subject (described in the protocol and the appended information sheet and consent form).

Insurance provisions, if any, for injury to study subjects (described in the protocol or provided as a separate document). Committees must confirm that there is insurance for protection of the study subjects.

Indemnity/insurance provisions for the sponsor/CRO, investigator, institution, and so on (as relevant to the study and if required by local regulations).

Payments or rewards to be made to study subjects, if any. Committees must determine that the amount, and schedule of payments, is not unduly coercive.

Benefits, if any, to study subjects.

Payments or rewards to be made to investigators. Many committees are beginning to realize that the financial interests of the investigator might have a strong influence on some aspects of the study, particularly recruitment patterns.

Assurance of quality/stability of medication/device to be administered.

Review decision of other ethics committees/IRBs in multicenter studies.

Duration of study.

Plans to review data collected to ensure safety.

Table 13.5 Review by ethics committees/IRBs during and after clinical studies

The following items should be reviewed by ethics committees/IRBs during and after clinical studies:

Serious and/or unexpected AEs, if any occur during the study, including the follow-up period.

Protocol amendments, if any, and reasons for amendments.

Protocol violations that impact on subject safety, if any.

Discontinuation of study, if applicable, and any reasons for premature discontinuation.

Any new significant information, for example information arising from other studies, results of interim analyses, marketing approvals, changes in local procedures, updated investigator brochure, supply problems, during study, if any.

Amendments to consent forms/information sheets, if any.

Annual reports of the study. More frequent review may be necessary, depending on the working procedures of each individual ethics committee.

Final clinical report/summary of study. Some ethics committees/IRBs also review publications, if any.

investigator; each is responsible for ensuring that the study is in conformity with the protocol and in accordance with all applicable laws and regulations, and of course, that study subjects are protected at all times. This responsibility involves regular and conscientious review of the progress of the study by the sponsor/CRO and by the investigator and study site personnel.

Monitoring

One of the most important means of quality control of a clinical study is management by frequent and thorough monitoring. The monitors' aim is first to protect the agenda of the sponsor/CRO who employs them. Monitors (often referred to as CRAs or Clinical Research Associates or Assistants in the pharmaceutical industry) must ensure

Table 13.6 Principles for the conduct of informed consent

The following principles for conducting informed consent should be implemented for all clinical studies:

Informed consent must be obtained from each study subject. The person receiving the information and giving consent must sign the consent form. This is usually the study subject, but may be the study subject's legally acceptable representative (depending on national regulations) in the event that the study subject is incapable of providing informed consent, for example the subject is unable to write or understand the consent documents, or the study subject is in a "vulnerable" population, for example children, elderly. Informed consent must be obtained before the start of the study.

The person providing the information and obtaining consent must sign the consent form. This person should be an investigator who must be qualified to inform adequately the study subject, and her or his signature also indicates personal involvement in the consent process. If other personnel, for example study nurses assist in providing information or obtaining consent, they should also sign the consent form, clearly describing their role in the consent procedure.

A witness or patient advocate should be present during the consent procedure at the times of providing information and giving consent, and should sign the consent form. The witness will ensure that there was no coercion in the obtaining of informed consent and that the study subject was given adequate time to consider participation in the study. The witness must be able to confirm that the consent procedure was adequate and must have no vested interest in the clinical study, that is the witness should be impartial, independent, or neutral, as far as this can be achieved. The relationship of the witness to the study subject and to the investigator and the study should be documented.

All participants should personally date their signatures and all dates should precede the start of the study (for each subject).

Table 13.7 Information to be provided to study subjects before obtaining consent to participate in clinical studies

The information sheets and consent forms should contain the following items:

1. *Information about the consent procedure*:

Consent to be given by the study subject's free will

Adequate time (which should be defined in advance in the protocol) must be allowed for the study subject to decide on participation in study

Adequate time must be allowed to ask questions

Statement that participation is entirely voluntary

Statement that refusal to participate will involve no penalties or loss of usual benefits

Description of circumstances under which participation would be terminated

Right to withdraw at any time without prejudice or consequences

Study subject is allowed to keep the written explanation (information sheet and consent form) for future reference

2. *Information about the study and medications/devices*:

Instructions on use and storage of study medication/device, if relevant

Name of sponsor/CRO

Explanation that the study is a research procedure

Description of study type and research aims

Description of study medications/devices

Description of procedures to be followed

Description of experimental procedures to be followed, if any. Experimental procedures might include those that are not normally used for the presentation under consideration or procedures that are new or have never been used before

Comparator treatments (including placebo) described. It is important to explain "placebo" in simple terms

Randomization procedures. Randomization is not easily understood by many subjects and should also be explained in simple terms

Expected duration of participation

Required number of visits

Reason for selection of suitable subjects

Approximate number of other study subjects participating in the study

3. *Information about the risks/benefits*:

Foreseeable risks, discomforts, side effects, and inconveniences

Known therapeutic benefits, if any. The benefits must not be "oversold"

Availability of alternative therapies. If there are other treatments, this must be explained so that the subject does not feel the new treatment is the only option

Any new findings, which might affect the safety of the study subject, and that become available during participation in the study, will be disclosed to the study subject

Assurance of compensation for treatment-induced injury with specific reference to local guidelines (it must not be expected that the study subject is familiar with the guidelines, and therefore the guidelines must be explained and/or attached)

Terms of compensation

Measures to be taken in the event of an AE or therapeutic failure

(Continued)

Table 13.7 (*Continued*)

Financial remuneration, if any. Patients, whether receiving therapeutic benefit or not, are not usually paid for participation in clinical research, except for incidentals such as travel costs. Healthy volunteers are usually paid a fee for participation, but this payment should never be offered to induce the prospective subjects to take risks they would not normally consider

Explanation of additional costs that may result from participation, if any (this normally only occurs in the United States)

4. *Other items*:

Ethics committee/IRB approval obtained (some debate about this)

Name of ethics committee/IRB (if applicable by local and/or national requirements) and details of contact person on the ethics committee/IRB (if applicable by local and/or national requirements)

Explanation that participation is confidential, but records (which divulge study subject names) may be reviewed by authorized sponsor/CRO representatives and may be disclosed to a regulatory authority

Name, address, and telephone number (24-hour availability) of contact person at study site for information or in the event of an emergency (this information may be provided on a separate card)

Requirement to disclose details of medical history, any medicines (or alcohol) currently being taken, changes in any other medication/device use, and details of participation in other clinical studies

Medical records will clearly identify study participation

Conditions as they apply to women of child-bearing potential

Primary care physician (or general practitioner or family doctor) and/or referring physician will be informed of study participation and any significant problems arising during the study. Some subjects may not be comfortable with this requirement, for example in a study of sexually transmitted diseases, they may not wish the doctor, perhaps a family friend, to be aware of their situation. If this is the case, the subject is not eligible for the study as it is vital to confirm history with the primary care physician

The information sheet must be written in language that is understandable, for example technically simple and in the appropriate national language, to the study subject

maintenance of proper standards, compliance with the protocol, accurate and complete data capture, and standardization across sites in a multicenter study. Basically, monitors will undertake the review noted in Table 13.8.

In general, study sites should be visited by a monitor at least every four to eight weeks. At the beginning of a study, monitoring may be even more frequent. The frequency of monitoring visits will be defined for each individual study and will depend on details such as the study phase, treatment interval and overall duration, enrollment rate, complexity of the study methodology, occurrence of adverse events (AEs) or other significant events, and the nature of the study medication/device. Under US GCP, any open study site must be visited at least once a year. The most time-consuming task at the study site is the review of source documents to confirm entries in CRFs and compliance with the protocol.

The monitor will be ever-vigilant for protocol violations which can occur during a study and which can have a serious impact on eligibility and evaluability. Many researchers confuse the terms "protocol violations," "protocol deviations," and "protocol amendments." The FDA does not recognize "deviations," but only major or less serious violations. It is important to appreciate the differences between these terms and understand how to avoid protocol violations and how to manage protocol amendments. Perhaps the easiest way to explain the difference is to stress that violations are not planned changes (hopefully) to the protocol, whereas protocol amendments are planned changes and are enacted through a formal approval process (if violations are deliberate or

Table 13.8 Objectives of monitoring visits

The following tasks should be undertaken by the sponsor/CRO monitor at each study site visit:

Verify accuracy and completeness of recorded data in CRFs, including diary cards, quality of life forms, registration forms, consent forms, etc., by comparing with the original source documents (clinic or hospital records). Where discrepancies are found, arrangements must be made for corrections and resolution. Resolve any outstanding queries, ensuring completion of any issued data queries, since the last monitoring visit.

Verify compliance with entry criteria and procedures, for all study subjects, as specified in the protocol. If subjects are found to be ineligible or unevaluable, these events must be immediately brought to the attention of the investigator. There may also be implications for payment to the study site and requirements for reporting to ethics committees/IRBs. Finally, and most seriously, there could be implications for subject safety.

Review all AEs, including clinically significant laboratory abnormalities, that have occurred since the previous visit. If a serious or unexpected AE has occurred, which was not correctly reported by the investigator, the monitor must ensure that the correct reporting procedure is followed immediately.

Evaluate the subject recruitment and withdrawal/dropout rate. If recruitment is less than optimal, suggest ways in which it can be increased. In particular, query the reasons for withdrawals/dropouts, or unscheduled visits, in case these are related to AEs.

Confirm that all source documents will be retained in a secure location. Source documents must be legible and properly indexed for ease of retrieval. Check the study site file to ensure that all appropriate documents are suitably archived. Check that the investigator files are secure and stored in a separate area which is not accessible to individuals not involved in the study.

Conduct an inventory and account for study medications/devices and arrange for extra supplies, including other items, such as CRFs, blank forms, and so on, if necessary. Resolve discrepancies between inventory and accountability records, and medication/device use, as recorded in the CRFs. If a pharmacy is involved in the study, the pharmacy and pharmacist must be visited. Check that the medication/device is being dispensed in accordance with the protocol. Check that the medication/device is being stored under appropriate environmental conditions and that the expiry dates are still valid. Check that the medication/device is securely stored in a separate area that is not accessible to individuals not involved in the study. Check that any supplies shipped to the site since the last visit were received in good condition and are properly stored. If applicable, ensure that randomization procedures are being followed, blind is being maintained, randomization codebreak envelopes are intact (sealed and stored properly) and a chronological sequence of allocation to treatment is being followed.

Verify correct biological sample collection (especially number, type, and timing), correct procedures for assays (if applicable), and labeling, storage, and transportation of specimens or samples. All clinical laboratory reports should be checked for identification details, validity. and continued applicability of reference ranges, accuracy of transcription to CRFs (if any), comments on all out-of-range data, and investigator signatures and dates. The dates of sample collection, receipt, analysis and, reporting should be checked to ensure that samples are analyzed promptly, and that investigators are informed of results and review them promptly.

Ensure continued acceptability of facilities, staff, and equipment. Ensure that the reference range, documentation of certification and proficiency testing, licensing, and accreditation, for the clinical laboratory are still current. Document any changes in clinical site personnel and, if changes have occurred, collect evidence of suitability of new personnel. Ensure that new staff are fully briefed on the requirements of the protocol and study procedures and arrange any training of new personnel, if necessary. Document any changes in overall facilities and equipment and if changes have occurred, collect new evidence of suitability, maintenance, calibration, and reason for change of new equipment.

Advise the investigator and other site personnel of any new developments, for example protocol amendments, AEs, which may affect the conduct of the study.

planned and repeated, a case of fraud should be considered!).

Reporting and recording safety events

An issue over which site personnel and monitors will be particularly watchful is the observation and recording of safety information. In many studies, safety information is under-reported because of the tendency to make judgments that are often based on subjective and biased clinical opinion. It seems difficult to teach clinical researchers to operate as "scientists," that is, to observe and record all observations before making judgments. The monitor and all clinical research personnel must ensure that all safety information is documented. This means that all AEs occurring in clinical studies must be recorded in CRFs even if clearly not due to the medication or device, their significance must be assessed, and their possible attribution to the agent in the study: "definitely," "possibly," and "not related" are the usual terms used. Other information must also be provided for reporting AEs externally (e.g., to regulatory authorities and ethics committees/IRBs). This applies to any study treatment (including comparator agents, placebo, and nonmedical therapy) and any stage of the study (e.g., run-in, washout, active treatment, follow-up), from signing the informed consent to one month after the last patient completes the study.

All serious AEs must be reported in the annual Investigational New Drug (IND) or New Drug Application (NDA) updates; however, all unexpected serious AEs must be reported urgently to the three regional authorities, and to other regulatory authorities according to their applicable regulations wherever the product or investigational drug is under study or application. For investigational drugs, deaths and life threatening unexpected AEs must be reported in a written format within seven calendar days, and other unexpected serious AEs are required to be reported in a written format within fourteen days for marketed drugs. Unexpected also has a narrow definition, which is any serious AE not described in the Investigators' Brochure or Product Label (or unexpected increase in severity or incidence). For a fuller explanation of the different types of events to be reported the reader is referred to ICH's Clinical Safety Data Management for Expedited Reporting (1994). Not reporting attracts heavy fines, prison sentences, and even closing of research facilities. This applies to any responsible person, not just the sponsor and investigative staff, but also sales staff who hear of an event.

All research personnel must search for clues about safety events from many sources, such as information in clinical records at the study sites; information in data collection forms (e.g., CRFs, diary cards, quality-of-life forms, psychiatric rating scales, etc.), occurrence of missed and/or unscheduled visits, dropouts, and withdrawals; use of any concomitant medications/devices; and abnormal laboratory data. AEs may also occur simply as a result of study procedures and study participation. Information about definitions of AEs and requirements for reporting AEs must be clearly stated in the protocol and explained to the site staff, which must also be educated in the correct procedure and immediate requirement for reporting any AE suspected to be serious or unexpected as per the regulatory definitions.

All investigators and other study site personnel, ethics committees/IRBs, and possibly study subjects must be informed of all new significant safety information, including all events occurring with any treatment (e.g., washout, investigational product, comparator, placebo, etc.) in the study, even if these occurred in another study with the same treatment or in another country. Significant safety information includes all serious AEs and any other events (e.g., significant trends in laboratory data or new preclinical data) that might have an impact on the risk assessment of the study. Safety events may necessitate an update to the investigator brochure, the protocol and CRF, the information sheet and consent form.

Collecting data with integrity

Collecting accurate, honest, reliable, and credible data is one of the most important objectives of conducting clinical research. It is difficult to achieve.

However, in general, data in CRFs are not credible to the regulators unless they can be supported by the "real" documents (i.e., the source documents maintained at the study site for the clinical care of the study subject). This becomes very important when data are being entered electronically (Electronic Data Capture), and transferred, with strict protocols and audit trails for altered data (corrections). If the data are electronic, the generated electronic data are the original (e.g., electronic lab reports) and a paper copy is not.

Source data verification

Source data verification is the process of verifying CRF entries against data in the source documents. Source data verification is only carried out at the study site, usually by the sponsor/CRO monitor (auditors will also conduct source data verification on a sample of CRFs; inspectors may conduct source data verification on a sample or all CRFs).

Source documents (and the data contained therein) comprise the following types of documents: patient files (medical notes where summaries of physical examination findings, details of medical history, concurrent medications/devices and diseases are noted); and recordings from automated instruments, traces (e.g., ECGs, EEGs), X-ray films, laboratory notes, and computer databases (e.g., psychological tests requiring direct entry by patient onto computers or direct entry of patient information onto computers by physicians).

The primary purpose of source documents is for the care of the study subject from a clinical perspective: The primary purpose of CRFs is to collect research data. CRFs (and other data collection forms) generally cannot substitute as source documents. Data entered in CRFs should generally be supported by source data in source documents, except as specifically defined at the beginning of the study. Nevertheless, some data entered in CRFs may be source data (e.g., multiple blood pressure readings, psychiatric rating scales, etc.) and would not be found elsewhere. This may be acceptable, if these data would not normally be entered in medical records, and if knowledge of such data is not required by the investigator or other clinicians who concurrently or subsequently treat the study

subject (the protocol should specify which data will be source data in the CRF).

How much information is expected to be documented in source documents? This is a difficult issue, but one that must be discussed and resolved before the CRFs are completed. Some guidelines are provided in Table 13.9.

Direct access to source documents is required for all studies: Direct access means monitors, auditors, other authorized representatives of the sponsor/ CRO in country inspectors, even inspectors from foreign agencies must be permitted to view all relevant source documents needed to verify the CRF data entries. Other restricted methods of access to source documents (e.g., "across-the-table," "back-to-back," and "interview method") are not acceptable, because they do not allow proper verification of the data in CRFs. To ensure direct access, the study subject consent form must clearly indicate that permission for access has been granted by the study subject.

Other reviews to ensure data integrity

After retrieval from the study site, there are further means of assessing CRFs. First, there is the initial review at the sponsor/CRO premises: this process is sometimes referred to as "secondary monitoring." This is not just looking for missing data or incorrect entry but review of the still blinded safety and laboratory data by a physician looking for trends in the safety data that might warrant a protocol amendment or stopping of the study. Thereafter, review by the data management department is another extremely important means of quality control. Also, there may be another planned review by a data monitoring committee with or without an interim analysis. It is a lengthy and complex process and there are few guidelines and regulations for reference. These processes will inevitably result in queries about the data. It is critical that all data review procedures be prompt. As time goes by, it becomes more and more difficult to correct data. Slow processing usually means that data lose credibility.

To ensure that the integrity of clinical research data is maintained and that there is total

Table 13.9 Source data verification

For all study subjects, source data verification requires a review of the following items:

Existence of medical records/files at the study site. There must be a medical file, separate from the CRF, which forms a normal part of the clinical record for the study subjects. The medical file should clearly indicate the full name, birth date, and hospital/clinic/health service number of the study subject.

Eligibility of study subjects. The medical file must show compliance with the inclusion and exclusion criteria. At a minimum, demographic characteristics, for example sex, weight and height, diagnoses, for example major condition for which subject was being treated, and other "hard" data, for example laboratory results within a specified range or normal chest X-ray, should be clearly indicated. All required baseline assessments must be evident. If the medical file has little or no information concerning medical history, it would not support selection of the subject.

Indication of participation in the study. The medical file should clearly show that the subject was in a clinical study in case the information is necessary for future clinical care.

Consent procedures. The original signed consent form should be maintained with the subject's medical files or in the investigator files and an indication that consent was obtained (with the date specified) should be noted in the medical files. Signatures and dates must be checked carefully to ensure that the correct individuals were involved in the consent procedure and that consent was obtained prior to any study intervention.

Record of exposure to study medication/device. The medical file should clearly indicate when treatment began, when treatment finished, and all intervening treatment dates.

Record of concomitant medications/devices. All notations of previous and concomitant medication/device use must be examined. All entries in the CRF should be verifiable in the medical file by name, date(s) of administration, dose and reason (or indication). All entries in the medical file during the time period specified by the protocol must be noted in the CRF. Concomitant medication/device use must be explicable by an appropriate indication and must be consistent from visit to visit. The reasons (indications) for use of concomitant medications/devices, newly prescribed during the study period, must be noted as AEs.

The medical history should be reviewed to determine whether medical conditions arising during the study already existed at baseline. The dispensing records, which are normally separate from the medical file, must also be examined to determine consistency.

Visit dates. All visit dates should be recorded in the medical file. Interim visit dates recorded in the medical file, but not in the CRF, should be noted by the monitor in case they signify occurrence of AEs or protocol violations. The final visit date should be so indicated, for example "study finished" or "withdrew from study."

AEs. All AEs noted in the medical file during the time period specified by the protocol must be recorded in the CRF. The monitor must also carefully check other documents (e.g., diary cards, quality of life forms) for sources of information about AEs. Occurrence of out-of-range laboratory values, which are considered to be clinically significant by the investigator, must be reported and assessed as AEs.

Major safety and efficacy variables (to be decided and documented in advance). It is not necessary for all measured variables to be recorded in the medical file. Present and future clinical care of the study subject is the most important factor in determining whether or not measured variables should be recorded in the medical file. The investigator should record what he or she would normally record to care for the study subject, but also take into account any recording needed because of the special circumstances of a clinical study. The entire medical file should be reviewed to ensure that no additional information exists in the medical file that should have been recorded in the CRF.

agreement between the data recorded on CRFs, the data entered in the computer, the data recorded in data listings and cross-tabulations, the data entered into statistical and clinical study reports, and finally the data in the sponsor/CRO and investigator archives, it is essential that the data must only be changed by following a formal procedure. Thus, requests for data clarification and all resolution of queries must be documented. All data changes must be authorized by the investigator ultimately initialing and dating all data changes as well as the whole completed patient case report forms. Obviously, the sponsor/CRO cannot arbitrarily make changes of data.

Archiving

Systems must be in place to ensure that documents will be securely retained for a long period of time. The purpose of archiving is to safeguard all documentation that provides evidence that a clinical study has been conducted in accordance with the principles of GCP. Archives at both the sponsor/CRO and investigator sites must be reasonably secure with regard to indexing, controlled access, fire-resistance, flood-resistance, and so on.

The investigator must be held responsible for ensuring that all source documents, especially records acquired in the normal practice of care and treatment of a study subject, are safely archived and available for inspection by authorized company personnel or regulatory authorities. Further, the investigator must archive all necessary documents for a minimum of 15 years, the usual industry standard, although the ICH Topic E 6 regulations state that the documents must be retained for two years after registration in the last of the three regions, or after the product has been discontinued. All appropriate clinical study documents should be archived by the sponsor/CRO, essentially for the lifetime of the product. The specific documents to be retained are described in the ICH GCP document.

Managing study medications/devices

Management of clinical study medications and devices is a complicated activity, and many clinical researchers report that they are not particularly interested in this aspect of clinical studies: they assume that it is all handled by other personnel in the manufacturing facility. Meanwhile, personnel in the manufacturing facility usually report that they assume no further responsibility once the supplies are released!

Preparation of study medications/devices

The preparation of study medications or devices is often rate limiting in initiating the study, particularly with double-blind designs.

Requisition, labeling, and packaging are some of the important considerations. Requisition of study medication/device (including placebo and comparator products, if relevant) must be initiated at an early stage to allow sufficient time to procure the study medications/devices and to prepare the final labeling and packaging, taking into account any special circumstances for blind studies and for import requirements.

The principles of safe labeling and packaging require compliance with the following principles: the contents of a container can be identified; a contact name, address, and telephone number is available for emergencies and enquiries; and the study subject (or the person administering the medication/device) is knowledgeable about storing and administering the study medication/device, and that the packing process can be audited against a standard operating procedure. Study materials must bear an expiry date, and in Europe, individual containers or devices as well. In most cases this means only a short expiry time in early development, and often clinical supplies have to be relabeled during a study.

Shipment of study medications/devices

Clinical study medications/devices should not be dispatched to study sites until all pre-study activities have been completed and regulatory requirements have been satisfied. The receipt of each shipment of study medication/device should be confirmed in writing by the investigator or pharmacist (or other authorized personnel), who will be instructed to return a completed "acknowledgement of receipt form" immediately. The recipient at the study site will be instructed to contact the sponsor/CRO immediately if there are any problems (e.g., missing or broken items, defects in labeling, evidence of excursion from temperature ranges) with the shipment. The recipient must be particularly instructed to record the exact date of receipt of the clinical supplies at the study site. This information is necessary so that the monitor can determine that the supplies were secure and correctly stored environmentally during the entire period of shipment. This requires that a log be maintained.

After the clinical study supplies have been sent to the study site, the monitor must verify as soon as possible that the supplies have arrived satisfactorily. No subjects should receive medication until the monitor has checked the condition of the supplies. The monitor will verify that the amount shipped matches the amount acknowledged as received. If there is a lack of reconciliation, or if the shipment is not intact, recruitment may be delayed until the situation is resolved.

Control of study medications/devices at study sites

Evidence of careful control at the study site is imperative, and naturally it is difficult to standardize the situation across many study sites and many countries. Security, correct storage, and accurate documentation of dispensing and inventory are necessary. Systems to ensure and assess compliance with the required use of the product being studied must be established. Monitors must be trained to check on these features and ensure that all site personnel are fully briefed.

The expectations with regard to maintenance of study medications/devices at study sites focus on security and appropriate environmental conditions. Concerns for security require that supplies be maintained under locked conditions. All agreements between the sponsor/CRO and the study site must specify that supplies are only for clinical study subjects, and this information must also be clearly stated on the labeling. The main concern for appropriate environmental conditions is usually temperature requirements, especially with biologic supplies that are usually required to be kept refrigerated between 39–47° F (4–8° C) and so are recorded at all times, but other factors (e.g., light, humidity) might also be important. Terms such as "room temperature" and "ambient temperature," which have different meanings in different coun-

tries, should always be avoided and specific temperatures must be stated. At each monitoring visit, the monitor will ensure that the correct procedures are being followed.

Compliance with medication/device use (by the study subject) should be assessed in all studies. If supplies are dispensed to subjects for self administration, methods to ensure compliance (e.g., diary cards, instructions on labeling, supervised administration) and check compliance (e.g., tablet counts, plasma/urine assays, diary card review) must be in place. At each study visit, the study subjects should be asked to return all unused supplies and empty containers to the investigator, who will check the supplies for assessment of compliance and store them for return to the sponsor/CRO. The monitor will review all relevant documents (e.g., source documents, CRFs, medication/device inventory, dispensing forms) to ensure that the data in the CRFs reflect the subjects' compliance with the study medications/devices.

Overall accountability of study medications/devices

Overall accountability must be documented and reviewed. A reconciliation of the initial inventory and the final returns must be undertaken and all discrepancies must be explained. Final disposition and destruction must be carefully documented to also allow assessment of possible detrimental environmental impact. All unused and returned medications/devices, empty containers, devices, equipment, and so on, which are returned to the investigator by the study subjects, must be stored securely and under correct environmental conditions at the study site until retrieved by the monitor. The monitor will check the supplies returned and verify that they reconcile with the written specifications. All discrepancies and reasons for any non-returns must be documented and explained. Some supplies may be required for potency testing by the sponsor to reflect, for example, stability under field transport and storage conditions.

Generally, destruction of returned study medications/devices by the sponsor/CRO may not take place until the final report has been prepared and there is no further reason to question the accountability of the study medication/device. The actual destruction process must be documented in a manner that clearly details the final disposition of the unused medications/devices and the method of destruction. The information is particularly necessary in case of any query regarding environmental impact. In exceptional circumstances, unused study medications (e.g., cytotoxics, radio-labeled products) may be destroyed at the study site, with appropriate documentation.

Randomization and blinding

Randomization procedures are employed to ensure that study subjects entered into a comparative study are treated in an unbiased way. Blinding (or masking) procedures (e.g., single-blind or double-blind) further minimize bias by ensuring that outcome judgments are not based on knowledge of the treatment. If the study design is double-blind, it is essential that all personnel who may influence the subject or the investigator conduct of the study, are blinded to the identity of the study medication/device assigned to the subject, and therefore do not have access to randomization schedules.

Summary

The code of GCP was established to ensure subject safety and arose because of biases inherent in clinical research (e.g., pressures to recruit subjects for payment, publication, etc.), which needed some counterbalance, and frankly to try to avoid some the major patient subject abuse and fraud. GCP also helps to bring some standardization to the clinical process of research. It is hoped the reader will appreciate that GCP is not "bureaucratic nonsense" (as argued by some researchers) but a logical, ethical, and scientific approach to standardizing a complex discipline. This chapter has been but a brief overview of GCP, and the next section provides the serious student with material for fuller and more detailed understanding of the regulations and guidances in the US and other major regions. Many interweave with GCP and other guidances, and those on special populations are very specific in their application.

Sources of international guidelines/regulations for GCP

(Note: all the materials cited in this section are available on the Internet, although websites often change.)

Australia

National Statement on Ethical Conduct in Research Involving Humans, National Health and Medical Research Council Act, 1992. http://www.health. gov.au/nhmrc/publications/synopses/e35syn. htm.

Note for Guidance on Good Clinical Practice (CPMP/ICH/135/95). Annotated with TGA comments. Therapeutic Goods Administration (TGA) (Australia), Commonwealth Department of Health and Aged Care. The TGA has adopted CPMP/ICH/135/95 in principle but has recognized that some elements are, by necessity, overridden by the National Statement (and therefore not adopted) and that others require explanation in terms of "local regulatory requirements," July 2000. http://www. health.gov.au/tga/docs/html/ich13595.htm.

Note for Guidance on Clinical Safety Data Management (CPMP/ICH/377/95). Annotated with TGA comments. Therapeutic Goods Administration (Australia), Commonwealth Department of Health and Aged Care. The TGA has adopted the *Note for Guidance on Clinical Safety Data Management: Definitions and Standards for Expedited Reporting* in principle, particularly its definitions and reporting time frames. However, there are some elements of CPMP/ICH/377/95 that have not been adopted by the TGA and other elements which require explanation in terms of "local regulatory requirements," 2000. http://www. health.gov.au/tga/docs/html/ich37795.htm.

Canada

Code of Ethical Conduct for Research Involving Humans, Medical Research Council of Canada, Natural Sciences and Engineering Research Council of Canada, Social Sciences and Humanities Research Council of Canada, 1998. http://www. nserc.ca/programs/ethics/english/policy.htm.

Clinical Trial Review and Approval, Drugs Directorate, Policy Issues, Health and Welfare Canada, 1995. TPP (Therapeutic Products Program, Canada). http://www.hc-sc.gc.ca/hpb-dgps/therapeut/htmleng/whatsnew.html.

Clinical Trial Framework, Schedule 1024, Food and Drug Regulations. Therapeutic Products Directorate, Health Products and Food Branch, Health Canada, 2001. http://www.hc-sc.gc.ca/hpbdgps/therapeut/zfiles/english/schedule/gazette.ii/sch-1024_e.pdf.

European Union

Good Clinical Practice for Trials on Medicinal Products in the European Community, Committee for Proprietary Medicinal Products (CPMP) EEC 111/3976/88-EN, Brussels, 1990.

Commission Directive 91/507/EEC modifying the Annex to Council Directive 75/318/EEC on the approximation of the laws of Member States relating to the analytical, pharmacotoxicological and clinical standards and protocols in respect of the testing of medicinal products, Official Journal of the European Communities, 1991.

Commission Directive 2005/28/EC of 8 April 2005 laying down principles and detailed guidelines for good clinical practice as regards investigational medicinal products for human use, as well as the requirements for authorization of the manufacturing or importation of such products. Directive 2001/20/EC of the European Parliament and of the Council of 4 April 2001 on the approximation of the laws, regulations and administrative provisions of the Member States relating to the implementation of good clinical practice in the conduct of clinical trials on medicinal products for human use. http://europa.eu.int/eur-lex/en/lif/dat/2001/en_ 301L0020.html.

Good Manufacturing Practice (GMP) Directive 2003/94/EC. EU Directive on GMP. Guide to Good Manufacturing Practices, Annex 13, Manufacture of Investigational Medicinal Products, July 2003. The Rules Governing Medicinal Products in the European Community, Vol. 4, Biostatistical Methodology in Clinical Trials in Applications for Marketing Authorizations for Medicinal Products, Committee for Proprietary Medicinal Products (CPMP) EEC 111/3630/92- EN, 1994.

United Kingdom

Clinical Trial Compensation Guidelines, Association of the British Pharmaceutical Industry (ABPI), 1994.

Conduct of Investigator Site Audits, ABPI, 1993.

Good Clinical (Research) Practice, ABPI, 1996.

Good Clinical Trial Practice, ABPI, 1995.

Introduction to the Work of Ethics Committees, ABPI, 1997.

Patient Information and Consent for Clinical Trials, ABPI, 1997.

Phase IV Clinical Trials, ABPI, 1993.

Set of Clinical Guidelines, ABPI, 2000.

Structure of a Formal Agreement to Conduct Sponsored Clinical Research, ABPI, 1996. http://www.abpi.org.uk/.

Fraud and Misconduct in Clinical Research, Royal College of Physicians of London, 1991.

Guidelines for Clinicians Entering Research, Royal College of Physicians of London, 1997.

Guidelines on the Practice of Ethics Committees in Medical Research Involving Human Subjects, Royal College of Physicians of London, 1997.

Research Involving Patients, Royal College of Physicians of London, 1990.

Research on Healthy Volunteers, Royal College of Physicians of London, 1986. http://www.rcplondon.ac.uk/pubs/pub_print_bytitle.htm.

Governance Arrangements for NHS Research Ethics Committees: (Section A – General Standards and Principles), Department of Health (DOH), Central Office for Research Ethics Committees (OREC), 2001. http://doh.gov.uk/research/rec.

Guidelines for Good Pharmacy Practice in Support of Clinical Trials in Hospitals, Royal Pharmaceutical Society, 1994.

Guidance on Good Clinical Practice and Clinical Trials in the NHS, National Health Service, 1999. http://www.doh.gov.uk/research/documents/gcpguide.pdf.

Research Ethics Guidance for Nurses Involved in Research or Any Investigative Project Involving Human Subjects, Royal College of Nursing Research

Society, 1998. http://www.doh.gov.uk/research/rd3/nhsrandd/researchgovernance/govhome.htm.

The Medicines for Human Use (Clinical Trials) Regulations 2004, Statutory Instrument 2004, No. 1031, HMSO.

United States

Regulations

Code of Federal Regulations (CFR), 21 CFR Ch 1, Food and Drug Administration (FDA), Department of Health and Human Services (DHHS):

• Part 11—Electronic Records; Electronic Signatures. http://www.access.gpo.gov/nara/cfr/waisidx_01/21cfr11_01.html; accessed April 26, 2010.

• Part 50—Protection of Human Subjects. http://www.access.gpo.gov/nara/cfr/waisidx_01/21cfr50_01.html; accessed April 26, 2010.

• Part 54—Financial Disclosure by Clinical Investigators. http://www.access.gpo.gov/nara/cfr/waisidx_01/21cfr54_01.html; accessed April 26, 2010.

• Part 56—Institutional Review Boards. http://www.access.gpo.gov/nara/cfr/waisidx_01/21cfr56_01. html; accessed April 26, 2010.

• Part 312—Investigational New Drug Application. http://www.access.gpo.gov/nara/cfr/waisidx_01/21cfr312_01.html; accessed April 26, 2010.

• Part 314—Applications for FDA Approval to Market a New Drug. http://www.access.gpo.gov/nara/cfr/waisidx_01/21cfr314_01.html; accessed April 26, 2010.

Compliance Program Guidance Manuals for FDA Staff:

• Compliance Program 7151.02. FDA Access to Results of Quality Assurance Program Audits and Inspections, 1996. (Same as Compliance Policy guide 130.300.) http://www.fda.gov/ora/complianceref/cpg/cpggenl/cpg130-300.html.

• Compliance Program 7348.001. Bioresearch Monitoring—In Vivo Bioequivalence, 1999. http://www.fda.gov/ora/compliance_ref/bimo/7348_001/Default.htm, http://www.fda.gov/ora/compliance_ref/bimo/7348_001/foi48001.pdf.

• Compliance Program 7348.809. Institutional Review Boards, 1994. http://www.fda.gov/ora/compliance_ref/bimo/7348_809/irb-cp7348-809.pdf.

• Compliance Program 7348.810. Bioresearch Monitoring—Sponsors, Contract Research Organizations and Monitors, 2001. http://www.fda.gov/ora/ compliance_ref/bimo/ 7348_810/default. htm, http://www.fda.gov/ora/compliance_ref/bimo/7348_810/48-810.pdf.

• Compliance Program 7348.811. Bioresearch Monitoring—Clinical Investigators, FDA, 1997. http://www.fda.gov/ora/compliance_ref/bimo/7348_811/default.htm, http://www.fda.gov/ora/ftparea/compliance/48_811.pdf.

Information Sheets

Computerised Systems Used in Clinical Trials. FDA, 1999. http://www.fda.gov/ora/compliance_ref/bimo/ffinalcct.htm.

Enforcement Policy: Electronic Records; Electronic Signatures—Compliance Policy Guide; Guidance for FDA Personnel, FDA, 1999. http://www.fda.gov/ora/compliance_ref/part11/FRs/updates/cpg-esig-enf-noa.htm.

Guidance. Financial Disclosure by Clinical Investigators, FDA, 2001. http://www.fda.gov/oc/guidance/financialdis.html.

Guidance for Institutional Review Boards and Clinical Investigators, FDA, 1998. http://www.fda.gov/oc/ohrt/irbs/default.htm.

Guidance for Institutional Review Boards, Clinical Investigators, and Sponsors: Exceptions from Informed Consent Requirements for Emergency Research, FDA, 2000. http://www.fda.gov/ora/compliance_ref/bimo/err_ guide.htm.

Guideline for the Monitoring of Clinical Investigations, FDA, 1988. http://www.fda.gov/cder/guidance/old006fn.pdf.

Guideline on the Preparation of Investigational New Drug Products (Human and Animal), Department of Health & Human Services, FDA, April 1991. http://www.fda.gov/cder/guidance/old042fn.pdf.

Inspection and warning letters

Clinical Investigator Inspection List. http://www.fda.gov/cder/regulatory/investigators/default.htm.

Debarment List. http://www.fda.gov/ora/compliance_ref/debar/default.htm.

Disqualified/Restricted/Assurances List for Clinical Investigators. http://www.fda.gov/ora/compliance_ref/bimo/dis_res_assur.htm.

Notice of Initiation of Disqualification Proceedings and Opportunity to Explain (NIDPOE) Letters. http://www.fda.gov/foi/nidpoe/default. html.

Public Health Service (PHS) Administrative Actions Listings. http://silk.nih.gov/public/cbz1bje.@www.orilist.html.

Warning Letters. http://www.fda.gov/foi/warning.htm.

Forms

Form FDA 1571—Investigational New Drug Application (IND). http://forms.psc.gov/forms/FDA/FDA-1571.pdf.

Form FDA 1572—Statement of Investigator. http://forms.psc.gov/forms/FDA/FDA- 1572.pdf.

Form FDA 3454—Certification: Financial Interests and Arrangements of Clinical Investigators. http://forms.psc.gov/forms/fda3454.pdf.

Form FDA 3455—Disclosure: Financial Interests and Arrangements of Clinical Investigators. http://forms.psc.gov/forms/FDA/FDA- 3455.pdf.

International ICH

Clinical Safety Data Management: Definitions and Standards for Expedited Reporting, International Conference on Harmonization (ICH) of Technical Requirements for the Registration of Pharmaceuticals for Human Use, 1994. http://www.ifpma.org/pdfifpma/e2a.pdf.

Clinical Safety Data Management: Periodic Safety Update Reports for Marketed Drugs, International Conference on Harmonization (ICH) of Technical Requirements for the Registration of Pharmaceuticals for Human Use, 1996. http://www.ifpma.org/pdfifpma/e2c.pdf.

Note for Guidance on Structure and Content of Clinical Study Reports, International Conference on Harmonization (ICH) of Technical Requirements for the Registration of Pharmaceuticals for Human Use, 1995. http://www.ifpma.org/pdfifpma/e3.pdf.

Guideline for Good Clinical Practice. International Conference on Harmonization (ICH) of Technical Requirements for the Registration of Pharmaceuticals for Human Use, 1996. http://www.ifpma.org/pdfifpma/e6.pdf.

General Considerations for Clinical Trials. International Conference on Harmonization (ICH) of Technical Requirements for the Registration of Pharmaceuticals for Human Use, 1997. http://www.ifpma.org/pdfifpma/e8.pdf.

Statistical Principles for Clinical Trials. International Conference on Harmonization (ICH) of Technical Requirements for the Registration of Pharmaceuticals for Human Use, 1998. http://www.ifpma.org/pdfifpma/e9.pdf.

WHO

Good manufacturing practices for pharmaceutical products supplementary guidelines for the manufacture of investigational pharmaceutical products for studies in humans, 1994. http://saturn.who.ch/uhtbin/cgisirsi/ThuþSepþþ7þ13:17:28þMETþDSTþ2000/0/49.

International Ethical Guidelines for Biomedical Research Involving Human Subjects, Council for International Organizations of Medical Sciences (CIOMS) in collaboration with the World Health Organization (WHO), 1993; http://www.cioms.ch/frame_guidelines_nov_2002.htm; accessed April 26, 2010.

Guidelines for Good Clinical Practice (GCP) for Trials on Pharmaceutical Products, Division of Drug Management & Policies, World Health Organization, 1994. http://saturn.who.ch/uhtbin/cgisirsi/ThuþSepþþ7þ13:17:28þMETþDSTþ 2000/0/49.

Operational Guidelines for Ethics Committees that Review Biomedical Research, World Health Organization, 2000. http://saturn.who.ch/uhtbin/cgisirsi/ThuþSepþþ7þ13:17:28þMETþDSTþ2000/0/49.

World Medical Association

Declaration of Helsinki. Recommendations Guiding Physicians in Biomedical Research Involving Human Subjects, Adopted by the 18th World Medical Assembly, Helsinki, Finland, June 1964, amended by the 29th World Medical Assembly, Tokyo, Japan, October 1975, the 35th World Medical Assembly, Venice, Italy, October 1983, and the 41st

World Medical Assembly, Hong Kong, September 1989, the 48th General Assembly, Somerset West, Republic of South Africa, October 1996, and the 52nd General Assembly, Edinburgh, Scotland, October, 2000. http://www.wma.net/e/policy/17-c_e.html.

Other related publications

Bohaychuk W, Ball G. *Good Clinical Research Practices*. An indexed reference to international guidelines and regulations, with practical interpretation (available from authors), 1994.

Bohaychuk W, Ball G. GCP. A report on compliance (available from authors), 1996.

BohaychukW, Ball G. GCP audit findings—case study 1. *Qual Assur J* 1998; **3**(2).

Bohaychuk W, Ball G. 101 GCP SOPs for sponsors and CROs (available from authors: paper and diskette), 1998.

Bohaychuk W, Ball G. GCP audit findings—case study 2 *Qual Assur J* 1998; **3**(3).

Bohaychuk W, Ball G, Lawrence G, Sotirov K. A quantitative view of international GCP compliance. *Appl Clin Trials* 1998; **7**(2):24–29.

Bohaychuk W, Ball G. GCP compliance assessed by independent auditing: international similarities and differences. In *The Clinical Audit in Pharmaceutical Development*, Hamrell M (ed.). Marcel Dekker: New York, USA, 1999.

Bohaychuk W, Ball G. GCP compliance: national similarities and differences. *Eur. Pharm. Contract* 1999; September.

Bohaychuk W, Ball G. *Conducting GCP-compliant Clinical Research*. John Wiley & Sons, Ltd: Chichester, UK, 1999; http://www3.interscience.wiley.com/cgi-bin/book home/89013938?CRETRY=1&SRETRY=0; accessed April 14, 2010.

Bohaychuk W, Ball G. GCP compliance assessed by independent auditing. International similarities and differences. In *The Clinical Audit in Pharmaceutical Development*, Hamrell M (ed.). Marcel Dekker: New York, USA, 2000.

CHAPTER 14

Quality Assurance, Quality Control and Audit

Rita Hattemer-Apostel
Verdandi AG, Zurich, Switzerland

The aim of this chapter is to describe the general framework for Quality Management (QM) in clinical trials. Quality Assurance (QA), including audits, and Quality Control (QC) are components of quality management and their contribution to quality and integrity of clinical data is widely recognized, in particular in clinical research conducted according to Good Clinical Practice (GCP). Since it is difficult to cover all aspects of quality and auditing in one chapter, the particular emphasis here is on approaches to QM and general procedures for QA, QC, and audit. This should allow readers to develop QM systems for clinical trials that are tailored to their specific environment and organization.

Introduction

Quality management is not a new discipline in industry, but the concepts evolved and were refined over many decades and have been implemented in nearly all areas, in manufacturing industries, service providers, as well as non-profit organizations. It, therefore, comes as no surprise that QM found its way into pharmaceutical medicine, in particular in clinical research and GCP.

Research and development of pharmaceuticals is a time-consuming and complex process, demanding a good understanding of medical and regulatory requirements paired with the ability to man-

age sophisticated clinical trials, which are often to be conducted within an ambitious time schedule. Competition is fierce and time-to-market often dictates the "pulse" of drug development. Over the years, clinical studies have become increasing difficult because of heightened requirements stipulated be regulatory agencies, development and evolution of GCP guidelines and regulations, and technical advancements in data and document management.

The need for outsourcing parts or even all drug development activities to Contract Research Organizations (CROs) and specialized external providers contributes to the complexity of developing new pharmaceuticals.

Clinical research is a global business and multinational trials with globally dispersed investigator sites are one sign of it. Local, national, and international requirements for conducting clinical studies must be respected and, because of the variety of countries and languages involved, familiarization with those requirements is not always an easy undertaking, but essential. And, to add to the above, regulatory frameworks are subject to continuous refinement and revision. Monitoring of these changes is mandatory and requires regular review and update of internal processes and Standard Operating Procedures (SOPs).

An effective QM system for clinical research helps ensure that studies are planned, conducted, analyzed, reported, and managed in compliance with GCP guidelines and ethical principles as noted in the Declaration of Helsinki so that dependable trial results are achieved while ensuring that trial participants are protected.

Principles and Practice of Pharmaceutical Medicine, 3rd edition.
Edited by L.D. Edwards, A.W. Fox, P.D. Stonier.
© 2011 Blackwell Publishing Ltd.

Quality management

Surprisingly, "quality" or "quality management" are not included in the glossary of the International Conference on Harmonization (ICH) GCP (ICH, 1995a), although definitions for "quality assurance," "quality control," and "audit" are to be found in this guideline. Useful explanations related to quality are also included in ISO 9000:2005 (ISO, 2005), the "generic" standard that can be applied to any organization (large or small), whether its "product" is actually a service, in any sector of activity. Let us review some of the ISO definitions in the following sections.

Quality

In ISO 9000:2005, quality is defined as: "The degree to which a set of inherent characteristics fulfils needs or expectations that are stated, generally implied or obligatory."

Hence, the standards for conducting clinical trials must be known before they can be applied. Standards are (i) international (e.g., ICH GCP); (ii) European (e.g., European Union (EU), Clinical Trials Directive (EU, 2001), and GCP Directive (European Commission, 2005); (iii) national (i.e., national drug laws and GCP regulations); or (iv) even more local, such as state laws in the United States.[1] Apart from the regulations, the clinical trial protocol, SOPs, and other internal or external instructions document procedures how the trial should be carried out from start to finish. Compliance with these standards is expected.

Without clear standards prepared within an organization, or without adequate knowledge of existing standards, compliance with GCP requirements, ethical principles, and the trial procedures may be suffering, up and until the point that regulatory authorities reject the data because data validity and adherence to ethical standards cannot be demonstrated.

Quality management

ISO 9000:2005 defines quality management as "The coordinated activities to direct and control an organization with regard to quality." ICH GCP does not contain a definition for quality management.

Quality management is not a new concept; it is rooted in medieval Europe in the late 13th century where guilds were responsible for developing strict rules for product and service quality. Inspection committees enforced the rules by marking flawless goods with a special mark or symbol (Hattemer-Apostel, 2003).[2] This was the start of "quality control," a process to assess finished products to evaluate whether they fulfilled pre-established criteria. The statistical evaluation of data paved the way to focus on improving the manufacturing process rather than inspecting the final product by preventing errors instead of correcting them, that, "assuring quality" instead of "inspecting quality into a product or service." The benefits of QA soon led to the insight that quality is an attribute that can be managed. On one hand, quality can be influenced in that investments in process quality impact the outcome of the product or service. On the other hand, quality has increasingly become a task of management. ISO 9000:2005 describes the role of senior management and emphasizes the importance of leadership by top management in implementing quality management.

The absence of the term "quality management" in clinical research regulations and guidelines is surprising. Neither the US Code of Federal Regulations nor European documents, such as the (EU) Clinical Trials Directive 2001/20/EC (EU, 2001) and the EU GCP Directive 2005/28/EC (European Commission, 2005), describe the requirement for a comprehensive quality management system. "Quality assurance" is found in the US Food and Drug Administration's (FDA) inspection guide for sponsors, CROs, and monitors (FDA, 2001), stating: "Clinical trial quality assurance units (QAUs) are not required by regulation. However, many

---

[1] US State Laws; http://law.findlaw.com/state-laws/all-states.html; accessed November 20, 2009

[2] ASQ. Basic Concepts – The History of Quality; http://www.asq.org/learn-about-quality/history-of-quality/overview/overview.html; accessed November 20, 2009

sponsors have clinical QAUs that perform independent audits/data verifications to determine compliance with clinical trial SOPs and FDA regulations."

In Europe, the GCP inspectors expect that sponsors have implemented an audit system as part of their QA system.[3] Audits should cover key clinical trial processes, including monitoring, data management, safety reporting, clinical study report production, archiving, and computer system validation activities. Audits of contractors and subcontractors should also be performed.

Quality assurance

ICH GCP defines QA as "All those planned and systematic actions that are established to ensure that the trial is performed and the data are generated, documented (recorded) and reported in compliance with GCP and the applicable regulatory requirement(s)." In clinical development of pharmaceuticals, QA usually describes the audit function within a company; however, QA should not be limited to auditing.

According to ISO 9000:2005, QA activities are not confined to auditing, but comprise all activities suitable to ensure that company procedures are designed so that the product or service will comply with pre-established quality requirements: "The part of quality management focused on providing confidence that quality requirements will be fulfilled." This definition emphasizes that QA activities are future-oriented and should focus on improving systems and procedures to be followed to ensure that these are set-up in such a way that produces a quality result or service.

The conduct of audits is not a mandatory requirement in ICH GCP. ICH GCP does mention in section 5.19 "If and when sponsors perform audits, as part of implementing quality assurance," but this is not interpreted as an obligation to establish an audit program. Similarly, FDA does not mandate the conduct of audits (FDA, 2001). However, European

inspectors expect evidence of a comprehensive audit program.[3]

Quality control

The ICH GCP definition for QC is: "The operational techniques and activities undertaken within the QA system to verify that the requirements for quality of the trial-related activities have been fulfilled." ISO 9000:2005 uses a more precise definition, which nicely contrasts the above definition for QA: Quality control is "The part of quality management focused on fulfilling quality requirements."

Quality control activities in clinical research are manifold and comprise all activities undertaken by operational departments (such as clinical monitoring, project management, data management, etc.) to ensure that activities are performed in compliance with the trial protocol, SOPs, and other procedure guides. These in-process quality controls are vital to the quality of the documents prepared (e.g., trial protocols, study reports) and the integrity of the trial conduct.

Compliance

"Adherence to all the trial-related requirements, Good Clinical Practice (GCP) requirements and the applicable regulatory requirements," is how ICH GCP defines compliance.

A myriad of laws, regulations, and guidelines specify the requirements to be adhered to when conducting clinical trials. Responsibilities of clinical investigators, sponsors, CROs, Independent Ethics Committees (IECs), monitors, and auditors are described, including also activities such as pharmacovigilance/safety reporting, data management/statistics, notification of trials at regulatory authorities, and so on.

It is important to be aware of the enforceability of requirements laid down in documents (e.g., legal requirements versus industry best practice) and the geographic coverage of guidance documents (e.g., FDA regulations versus EU Directives).[3] Without dependable knowledge on the applicable regulatory requirements, it is unlikely that GCP compliance can be achieved. Key steps towards compliance are as follows:

---

[3] EMA Inspection Procedures and Guidance for GCP Inspections Conducted in the Context of the Centralised Procedure; http://www.emea.europa.eu/ Inspections/GCPproc.html; accessed November 20, 2009

1. Know the regulatory framework and keep abreast of changes.

2. Train employees and colleagues and implement the requirements in the standard processes.

3. Follow the rules and provide sufficient documentation so that compliance can be verified.

Implementing quality assurance

QA's task to identify non-compliance with regulatory requirements, the trial protocol, and internal procedures such as SOPs is not always an easy job. Communicating deficiencies and highlighting inadequate procedures is certainly a benefit for the company as a whole, but the individual may not appreciate being confronted with audit findings (Hattemer-Apostel, 2004). In order to be efficient and effective in QA, the items in the following sections should be observed.

Organization and independence of QA

According to ICH GCP, FDA (FDA, 2001) and European Medicines Agency (EMA),[4] the audit function must be independent of routine monitoring or quality control functions, so that auditors are able to provide an unbiased, objective assessment. Being involved in designing, conducting, monitoring, or analyzing a clinical study would undermine the requirement of independence.

QA's independence from operations should be identifiable in the organizational charts of a company or CRO. The reporting line of QA should go directly to senior management and in no case to any operational function. To preserve the independence of the audit function, audits are also often outsourced to external contractors; however, this is not a GCP requirement.

SOPs for QA

The requirement of having SOPs for all functions in clinical research also applies to QA and is emphasized in ICH GCP in section 5.19.3 ("The

sponsor should ensure that the auditing of clinical trials/systems is conducted in accordance with the sponsor's written procedures on what to audit, how to audit, the frequency of audits, and the form and content of audit reports"), by the FDA (FDA, 2001) ("Obtain a copy of any written procedures (SOPs and guidelines) for QA audits and operation of the QAU"), and by EMA[4] ("Procedures should be reviewed in order to verify their compliance with GCP standards and applicable regulations").

The number of SOPs and their topics depend on the scope of audits performed, the set-up and size of the QA department, and whether audits are outsourced to external contractors, which may decrease the scope of audits conducted by internal QA members. The QA department may also be tasked with activities such as SOP management and staff training; SOPs would also be needed for these areas.

Qualification of QA auditors

The need to use qualified and trained employees in all areas of clinical research also affects the QA department. QA auditors are verifying the work of their colleagues and are evaluating compliance with regulations, and so they must have a dependable knowledge of the clinical trials regulatory framework and practical work experience in clinical research to be credible in their role (Winchell, 2004).

There is no standard professional education for QA auditors and, therefore, practical experience is indispensable before embarking on the QA job. Before joining the QA department, the QA candidate may have worked in clinical monitoring, data management, pharmacovigilance, regulatory affairs, training, and other areas of clinical research.

ISO 19011:2002 (Hattemer-Apostel, 2000a) lists the following personal attributes for auditors (and includes further information on desired auditor qualifications):

- *Ethical*, i.e., fair, truthful, sincere, honest, and discreet.
- *Open-minded*, i.e., willing to consider alternative ideas or points of view.
- *Diplomatic*, i.e., tactful in dealing with people.
- *Observant*, i.e., actively aware of physical surroundings and activities.

---

[4] EMA Inspection Procedures and Guidance for GCP Inspections Conducted in the Context of the Centralised Procedure; http://www.emea.europa.eu/ Inspections/GCPproc.html; accessed November 20, 2009

- *Perceptive*, i.e., instinctively aware of and able to understand situations.
- *Versatile*, i.e., adjust readily to different situations.
- *Tenacious*, i.e., persistent, focused on achieving objectives.
- *Decisive*, i.e., reach timely conclusions based on logical reasoning and analysis.
- *Self-reliant*, i.e., act and function independently while interacting effectively with others.

The standard also outlines the areas in which QA auditors should be competent:

- *Audit principles, procedures, and techniques:* This includes knowledge on the ethical and professional conduct of audits, interaction with auditees and co-auditors, confidentiality, fair presentation of results and observations in an audit report, and the need to be objective throughout the audit process and base conclusions only on audit evidence.
- *Management system and reference documents:* This comprises the SOPs, working instructions, and other internal documents to demonstrate that the company's processes and procedures comply with GCP and regulatory requirements.
- *Organizational situations:* Organizational charts, internal reporting lines, and relationships with external service providers and partners fall into this category.
- *Applicable laws, regulations, and other requirements relevant to the discipline:* The QA auditor should be aware of international GCP regulations, regulatory requirements in the relevant countries where clinical trials are conducted, as well as any protocol requirements and trial-related procedures and contracts.
- *Quality-related methods and techniques:* Knowledge of methods applied in quality management, e.g., use of checklists and forms to record audit observations, sampling techniques, interview techniques, verification of information, and writing audit reports must be acquired by the auditor. Communication skills, both oral and written, are essential for QA auditors to ensure adequate communication with auditees and management.
- *Processes and products, including services:* QA auditors must possess a good understanding of all processes in clinical research and drug development and be familiar with the terminology and abbreviations used related to clinical trials.

Training of QA auditors

Induction training in QA may comprise the general audit procedures employed at the company, key audit SOPs, and documentation requirements in QA. A thorough review of the regulatory framework for GCP is recommended, because QA auditors are expected to be experts for clinical trial regulations and all GCP aspects. It would impair the QA auditors' credibility if they knew less than the auditees of the requirements that must be adhered to in drug development.

Auditing cannot be learned in a theoretical course and on-the-job training is mandatory. It is recommended that the QA auditor be accompanied during the first audits to learn from an experienced and competent auditor and to qualify for conducting audits alone (ISO, 2002).

With the changing regulatory environment and evolving internal company processes, continual training is also required in QA. Attending internal and external trainings and seminars, meeting QA peers to exchange experiences and discuss audit situations, and interpretation of regulations refines the QA auditor's knowledge (Hattemer-Apostel, 2000b). It goes without saying that QA auditors, like everyone in clinical research, should maintain a training file to document their qualification.

Scope of QA activities

Internal consulting

QA auditors are often consulted for advice in GCP because of their broad and profound expertise in the regulations. As they acquire knowledge in many areas and oversee a variety of different clinical trials, QA auditors are often requested for information and clarification. This aspect of interaction with employees and auditees is an opportunity for preventing errors and fostering communication between operational staff and QA. Auditors remain aware of day-to-day challenges in clinical research and learn early on about potential misinterpretations.

Auditing

QA auditors' core responsibility is to conduct audits in the various areas in clinical research. This requires the set-up of an audit program, which should be based on the clinical development plan for the substance(s), previous experience gained in audits, and the importance of the trials in the light of a marketing submission. Ideally, the audit program should cover all clinical trials.

ICH GCP defines an audit as "A systematic and independent examination of trial-related activities and documents to determine whether the evaluated trial-related activities were conducted, and the data were recorded, analyzed and accurately reported according to the protocol, sponsor's SOPs, GCP and the applicable regulatory requirement(s)."

The benefit of audits can be maximized if they are performed during the active phase of a clinical trial (e.g., when trial subjects are recruited and treated), so that deficiencies can still be corrected.

Training

QA auditors are often actively involved in providing training on GCP and regulatory topics related to clinical research. They gain first-hand experience regarding interpretations, shortcoming, and problem areas when conducting audits. This knowledge is a valuable resource to tap in trainings.

QA auditors should assess, for example, during audits, if adequate programs for induction training and continual education are established and followed. It has been observed that in some companies the QA department has been made responsible for maintaining the training files for all employees and for ensuring that training plans are available and training courses are attended.

SOP management

QA auditors are often tasked with responsibilities related to SOP management, such as maintaining originally signed versions, managing the dissemination (electronically and as hard copies), organizing SOP reviews (scheduled and ad hoc), and sometimes, even writing SOPs for departments other than QA.

SOP review by QA auditors is certainly recommended before issue to ensure that the SOPs are consistent with applicable international, country-specific, and regional regulations, ICH guidelines (not limited to ICH GCP), and company policies and procedures.

SOPs are considered to be controlled documents and as such require a system that controls the distribution of SOPs to ensure that only current versions are accessible for use. Outdated documents should be retrieved and identified as historical. It is QA's responsibility to verify that this system is being followed and is effective. Deficiencies in the SOP system are usually attributed to a lack of control and weaknesses of a company's quality management system.

Inspection readiness

The frequency of GCP inspections is increasing with many countries having established GCP inspectorates over the past years. Inspections can occur at sponsors, at investigator sites, laboratories, CROs, and other external providers. GCP inspectors may assess compliance with regulations, protocol requirements, and SOPs at various time points related to a clinical trial: before a trial starts (e.g., to evaluate the adequacy of the selected site), during an ongoing trial (i.e., surveillance inspection), or as part of a Marketing Authorization Application (MAA) (i.e., pre-approval inspection) (EU, 2001; European Commission, 2005).

The assistance of QA auditors in preparing, managing, and following up GCP inspections is vital. Auditors are familiar with audit and inspection situations and know how to interact with inspectors. The presence of QA auditors during regulatory inspections (in-house as well as at external facilities) is strongly encouraged. A wealth of information about approaches, needs, and expectations of GCP inspectors can be gained. This knowledge may be very helpful for preparing forthcoming inspections and for formulating responses to inspection reports.

Inspection readiness is another area in which the QA function can contribute considerably to establish systems and procedures that ensure that a company is always ready for an inspection. This includes a dependable SOP system in full compliance with guidelines and regulations, up-to-date training programs and documented training for all employees with complete training files, current résumés (CVs) for all persons involved in clinical research, current organizational charts and job descriptions, contracts in place with all external providers, and so on. QA auditors can help establish and maintain a state of inspection readiness at the company.

Suspected misconduct and fraud

Misconduct or fraud is a rare occurrence in clinical research, but when misconduct or fraud is confirmed the consequences can be disastrous (Eichenwald and Kolata, 1999; Hattemer-Apostel, 2001; Lock *et al.*, 2008). Fraudulent practices in clinical trials can lead to trial subjects being exposed to safety risks, to submitted or published clinical data being jeopardized, and if the product has been licensed based on false data, this may result in compromised patient safety. Therefore, any suspected case of misconduct or fraud needs to be taken serious and be assessed—this is when QA auditors should be involved.

Anyone who has access to or responsibility for collecting, transcribing, monitoring, or reporting data and who is motivated to deceive can commit fraud. Although misconduct and fraud is reported to occur at investigator sites rather than elsewhere, this should not preclude from finding obscure and questionable situations and documentation in other areas.

It is important to distinguish clearly between misconduct, fraud, and honest error. The FDA provides the following examples for fraud:

• *Altered data:* data that have been legitimately obtained, but that have been subsequently changed to bias the results.

• *Omitted data:* the non-reporting of data, which has an impact on study outcome, for example, the non-reporting of adverse events (AEs).

• *Fabricated data:* data that have been deliberately invented without performing the work, for example, making entries in case record forms when no data were obtained or patients not seen.

QA auditors should help investigate suspected fraud or misconduct by means of data and document review and audits at the concerned sites. Their independent and objective perspective of the situation will be important to provide an unbiased view and a valid assessment. Investigations of fraud should always be conducted by two auditors.

Training on how to detect and, even more important, prevent fraud is another area where QA should be involved.[5] QA auditors should play an active role in fraud prevention and awareness training measures so that all employees are adequately sensitized to reliably identify such occurrences.

Audits from A to Z

Audit program

Audits should be carefully planned and scheduled to maximize the potential and the use of QA resources. Ideally, the audit program should be aligned to the drug development program so that the audits are placed in accordance with the complexity and the importance of the clinical trials for a regulatory submission. Application of risk assessment and management methods may be helpful to identify high-risk areas in the company's clinical research environment.

For example, first-in-human studies and pivotal trials are more likely to be audited than Phase IV trials, and external providers selected for the first time who are responsible for key areas in clinical trials should be audited with a higher priority than CROs with a long history and reliable performance.

Audit plan

For each individual audit, it is useful to prepare an audit plan to provide the auditee with an overview on the audit components and the conduct of the audit. An audit plan may also be useful as a basis for agreement between the sponsor, the (external) QA auditor, and the audit team. It is common practice in clinical research to draw up an audit plan and distribute this information prior to the audit.

---

[5] EMA Inspection Procedures and Guidance for GCP Inspections Conducted in the Context of the Centralised Procedure; http://www.emea.europa.eu/ Inspections/GCPproc.html; accessed November 20, 2009

ISO 19011:2002 (Hattemer-Apostel, 2000a) suggests including the following information in the audit plan:

- type and scope of the audit; organizational and functional units and processes to be audited;
- audit objectives and reason for conducting the audit, if appropriate;
- audit criteria and reference documents;
- identification of the client/sponsor and trial protocol;
- date(s) and location(s) of audit activities at the site together with expected time and duration of activities, including any audit-related meetings;
- names, roles, and responsibilities of the audit team members and technical experts accompanying the audit team, if appropriate.

The following details may also be addressed in the audit plan, as required:

- language in which the audit will be conducted and the audit report will be written where this is different from the language of the auditor and/or the auditee;
- structure of the audit report;
- travel arrangement for auditors, where required, and logistic arrangements at facilities at the site (e.g., pharmacy, packaging area, laboratory. etc.);
- confidentiality agreements;
- follow-up activities to the audit.

Audit-related correspondence

For announced audits, it is good business practice to inform the auditee in writing of the planned audit and to agree on a mutually feasible audit date. Once the audit is scheduled, the audit plan should be sent with a cover letter to the auditee, audit team members, technical experts (if involved), and the client/sponsor (in case of third party audits).

After the audit, a letter to the auditee should confirm that an audit has taken place and the site staff should be thanked for their availability and assistance during the audit. The letter should not include deficiencies or observations made during the audit; however, general follow-up procedures can be outlined. For unannounced audits, only the audit confirmation letter is mandatory.

QA should keep records of all correspondence with the auditee and should check during the audit that the announcement letter and audit plan were received at the auditee's site.

Audit team

Prior to the audit, the audit team needs to be established if the audit is conducted by more than one auditor. The lead auditor must be nominated and responsibilities for the individual team members should be clearly assigned, considering competence and expertise. The same is true if technical experts (internal or external) are involved in the audit. Technical experts should be independent of the auditee and activities to be audited. In any case, the responsibility for the audit will rest with the lead auditor and the audit team.

Audit tools

Recording audit observations is an essential part of the audit to enable the auditor to prepare detailed, accurate, and complete audit reports that are based on factual observations. Checklists, audit questionnaires, and sampling plans are useful tools and should be prepared prior to the audit. Generic checklists may be a good start and can be refined as required for each audit to account for trial-specific issues. Source Data Verification (SDV) templates are always trial-specific because each clinical trial is unique. Although checklists and questionnaires are very useful to record audit observations, they should never restrict the extent and scope of audit activities, but allow for flexibility during the audit.

Opening meeting

An opening meeting should be held with the auditee and his/her management, if appropriate, and those responsible for the functions and processes to be audited, in order to confirm the audit plan and the sequence of reviews and topics and to present the audit procedures. The purpose of the meeting is also to confirm that documents to be audited and individuals to be interviewed are available.

Communication during the audit

Depending on the duration of the audit, interim meetings with the auditees may be necessary to discuss interim results, ideally at the closure of each audit day. For the audit team, it is very useful to confer periodically to exchange audit observations and information to assess the audit progress. The lead auditor is responsible for communication with the auditee.

The auditee and/or the sponsor should be informed without delay in case serious deficiencies are uncovered that may pose a high risk for either trial participants or the clinical data. Likewise, if the audit scope cannot be covered during the scheduled time for the audit, the auditee and/or the sponsor should be notified and appropriate action should be determined (e.g., extension of the audit time or modification of the audit plan, etc.).

Audit notes, audit evidence, audit findings, and audit conclusions

Audit *notes* are indispensable to allow QA auditors to write an accurate report after the audit. Detailed notes allow the auditor to prepare a meaningful audit report that is based on verified observations. All information collected during an audit is considered audit *evidence*. Information sources in an audit are, for example, document review, interviews, and observation of activities. If applicable, sampling techniques may be applied, for example, for SDV and verification of information in tables and listings. Audit observations are only considered audit *findings*, if it is determined after comparison with audit criteria that these are not or insufficiently fulfilled. And finally, audit *conclusions* can be drawn to assess whether the audit findings impact the validity of the clinical data and the safety of the trial subjects.

Closing meeting

It is good auditing practice at the termination of the audit to conduct a closing meeting with the auditee to present the audit findings and conclusions. This is also the last opportunity for the auditee to clarify potential misunderstandings by the audit team and to provide requested documentation. The lead auditor should chair this meeting and, if applicable, address follow-up activities.

Audit report

ICH GCP defines an audit report as "A written evaluation by the sponsor's auditor of the results of the audit." Format and layout of audit reports vary greatly between companies and can range from a simple list of audit findings to a detailed description of all audit areas, observations, and conclusions. The lead auditor is responsible for preparing the audit report and should be assisted by the entire audit team. Ideally, the audit report should be prepared as soon as possible after the audit. The report should be a complete and accurate representation of the audit conducted and not include opinions or assumptions.

Typically, the following details are included (Hattemer-Apostel, 2000a):
- type and scope of the audit;
- audit objectives and reason for conducting the audit, if appropriate;
- identification of the auditee and organizational and functional units and processes audited;
- identification of the client/sponsor and trial protocol;
- identification of the audit team leader and members and technical experts, if required;
- date(s) and location(s) of audit activities at the site; start and stop dates of the audit;
- audit criteria and reference documents;
- audit findings and conclusions.
  Further details may be useful, as follows:
- audit plan and any deviation to the audit plan;
- list of auditees and interview partners;
- recommendations for improvement and recommended follow-up activities;
- distribution list for the audit report;
- statement of the confidential nature of the contents.

The lead auditor should sign and date the final audit report, which should then be disseminated to the recipients as agreed with the sponsor.

It may be useful to remind the recipients of the confidential nature of audit reports, which means that they should not be made publicly available or distributed to persons outside the company. Regulatory authorities should not routinely be provided with audit reports. Audit reports should be securely filed (ideally with the QA department) and not included in the Trial Master File.

Audit certificate

According to ICH GCP, an audit certificate is "A declaration of confirmation by the auditor that an audit has taken place." It is kind of a "neutral" document and does not make reference to deficiencies or findings observed during the audit. It merely documents that an audit has taken place and is issued by the lead auditor at the termination of the audit.

Audit follow-up

The value of an audit would be considerably reduced if no corrective or preventive follow-up activities emerged from an audit report in case of identified deficiencies or recommendations for improvement. The auditee and/or recipient of the audit report are responsible for initiating follow-up activities. In the case of serious or critical observations made during the audit, QA auditors are often asked to review the corrections planned to resolve a problem.

Archiving

Like all documentation in clinical research, archiving is also required for QA documents, such as correspondence, audit notes, reports, and certificates.

Brief outline of audit types

Audits are conducted either for a specific trial or to evaluate an entire system in clinical research and development. Both approaches are value-adding and ensure that clinical trials are conducted according to accepted principles, that trial participants are treated ethically, and the trial data is valid.

Trial-related audits focus on a particular trial to assess compliance with the protocol, with related SOPs, and applicable GCP regulations. Of particular interest is how trial participants are informed of the trial, the study activities conducted at the investigator sites, and the procedures of clinical data handling, recording, processing, analysis, and reporting.

Systems audits are not specifically conducted for a particular trial, but may use a clinical trial as a guidance to assess the system. These audits evaluate whether a system (e.g., clinical monitoring) is capable of delivering the desired result (e.g., adequate oversight of investigator sites and appropriate documentation of monitoring activities). To this end, the adequacy and practicality of processes and procedures followed within a system are analyzed and SOPs, working instructions, and process descriptions are assessed for their suitability to lead to consistent services, documentation, and output. SOPs are checked for compliance with GCP regulations and guidelines and the education, training, and qualification of involved personnel is reviewed during systems audits. And finally, the interfaces to other internal departments and to external service providers and contractors are evaluated to identify potential process weaknesses or gaps, which may impair or even invalidate the clinical trial and its data.

Trial-related audits

Protocol audit

Protocol audits are best scheduled when the protocol is still in draft stage, immediately prior to finalization. The purpose of protocol audits is to assess if the protocol complies ICH GCP (ICH, 1995a), ICH E3 (ICH, 1995b), ICH E9 (ICH, 1998), the Declaration of Helsinki (World Medical Association, 2008), national regulations (e.g., FDA CFR requirements),[6-10] and company SOPs regarding format and contents of protocols. The audit also evaluates whether trial procedures are accurately, completely, clearly, and consistently described in

---

[6] FDA 21 CFR Part 50 Protection of Human Subjects; http://www.fda.gov/oc/gcp/regulations.html; accessed November 20, 2009

[7] FDA 21 CFR Part 54 Financial Disclosure by Clinical Investigators; http://www.fda.gov/oc/gcp/regulations.html; accessed November 20, 2009

[8] FDA 21 CFR Part 56 Institutional Review Boards; http://www.fda.gov/oc/gcp/regulations.html; accessed November 20, 2009

[9] FDA 21 CFR Part 312 Investigational New Drug Application; http://www.fda.gov/oc/gcp/regulations.html; accessed November 20, 2009

[10] FDA 21 CFR Part 314 Applications for FDA Approval to Market a New Drug; http://www.fda.gov/oc/gcp/regulations.html; accessed November 20, 2009

the protocol so that misinterpretations are prevented.

If a generic subject information sheet and informed consent form is attached to the protocol, these documents should also be reviewed for compliance with any requirements for informed consent, such as GCP, SOPs, and the Declaration of Helsinki, and for consistency with the trial protocol. The information sheet and informed consent forms must be written in a language understandable to the trial participant and should include information on data protection/privacy. Further information on protocol and informed consent audits is available in the literature (Bohaychuk and Ball, 1999; DGGF, 2007).

Case Report Form (CRF) audit

CRF audits should also be conducted on a draft version, just before finalization of the CRF. As the CRF is "the" data collection tool in a clinical trial, errors and inconsistencies in its contents and design and inconsistencies with the trial protocol may lead to serious problems if they are not identified prior to the CRF being used. This holds true for paper CRFs and electronic CRFs as well as the use of Remote Data Entry (RDE) or web-based data collection and transmission tools. The latter requires careful consideration of the related guidelines (FDA, 2007).[11]

The focus of the CRF audit is on consistency with the protocol, ease of completion (e.g., module-based style, chronology of events), and compliance with SOPs and any requirements outlined by data management (DGGF, 2007).

Trial Master File (TMF) audit

TMF audits can be conducted at any stage of a clinical trial, for example, before shipping investigational medicinal products to a clinical site, in preparation for an investigator site audit, or at trial termination and before archiving to ensure completeness of the essential documents as per ICH GCP.

Complete, consistent, and accurate trial documentation is the basis for any inspection by regulatory authorities or sponsor/client audit and is a proof that the study was conducted according to GCP regulations, the trial protocol, and SOPs. The TMF plays a vital role in providing confidence to auditors and inspectors that the clinical data is valid and the trial was conducted properly.

Although it may be possible in studies with only a few investigator sites to conduct a 100% review of the TMF contents, large trials require a sampling approach.

TMF audits may be conducted to review the filing system for trial documentation. Combining the TMF audit with an assessment of the archiving system allows evaluating the retrieval procedures of trial documents to ensure that the documents are accessible at any time within the agreed archival period.

Investigator site audit

Investigator site audits are probably the most frequent type of audits conducted by clinical QA departments and, therefore, deserve particular attention. The purpose of investigator site audits is to assess compliance with the GCP regulations (with a focus on the country-specific regulatory requirements) and the protocol. Further, the safety of the trial participants, the ethical conduct of the trial, and the validity, completeness, and accuracy of the data collected and recorded is verified during the audit.

Preparing for the site audit requires the *review of key trial documents* before visiting the site for the on-site part of the audit. The QA auditor should review at least the trial protocol (and amendments), the current investigator's brochure (to the extent necessary). Ideally, the following documents should be studied as well before the audit: any site-related documents, including the IEC submission and approval; approved informed consent form used at the site; monitoring reports for the site; Serious Adverse Event (SAE) reports and shipment forms of Investigational Medicinal Products (IMPs); and study materials, previous audit reports related to the site, and relevant SOPs followed for clinical monitoring.

---

[11] FDA 21 CFR Part 11 Electronic Records, Electronic Signatures; http://www.fda.gov/oc/gcp/regulations.html; accessed November 20, 2009

At the investigator site—after an *opening meeting* to introduce the audit team, the auditees, and the audit process—*interviews* with the site staff are conducted to determine procedures followed for recruiting and consenting trial subjects, method of recording source data and maintaining source documents, and communication and interaction between site personnel, sponsor, and any external providers. Also, delegation of responsibilities and tasks is discussed at this stage of the audit.

During the time on site, *facilities for storage and archival* of investigational medicinal products, biological samples, and trial-specific equipment are reviewed. These facilities should be secure and protect the items stored against loss or deterioration. Access should be restricted to authorized personnel and should be controlled. Storage and archival facilities for documents (e.g., investigator binder, trial records, CRFs, and source data) should be secure for the duration of the trial and the archiving period. Storage facilities for investigational medicinal products must be environmentally monitored (e.g., temperature, light, and humidity) and storage conditions must be recorded to allow for retrospective assessment of storage conditions. Biological samples must be kept at required temperatures, for example, in the refrigerator or in –20°C or –80°C (–4°F or –112°F) freezers. Regular maintenance, cleaning, and calibration is required and should be documented. If any specific equipment is required for the trial, records should be verified regarding maintenance, calibration, quality control, and SOPs.

Another important component of investigator site audit is to *review the investigator site file* for completeness to verify whether all trial-related documents are available at the site. Chapter 8 of ICH GCP lists the documents to be expected at the site. In addition, country-specific regulations may require additional documents to be included, such as the FDA form 1572 "Statement of Investigator" for investigators involved in Investigational New Drug (IND) trials. A particular focus of the document review is placed on ethics committee correspondence and approval; regulatory authority correspondence and notification/approval; documentation of IMP shipments, accountability, recon-

ciliation, and destruction; and randomization code break envelopes to determine that they are complete and intact. Any code breaking must be fully documented.

Verification of informed consent forms for all trial participants is a key task during audits. The auditor should check whether an informed consent form is present for all trial subjects and has been signed by the subject and the investigator prior to any trial-related activity.

A major component of investigator site audits is devoted to verify the validity of the clinical data generated and recorded at the investigator site. This step includes the *audit of a sample of CRFs* against source documents and original medical records. The purpose of the review is to determine whether the trial procedures followed at the site are complying with protocol requirements, the data gathered is complete and accurately transcribed onto the CRF or electronic forms, and the clinical monitoring and source data verification process is satisfactory (DGGF, 2007; FDA, 1988). If *computerized systems* are used at the site to capture data, these should also be reviewed to ensure security, retrievability, and validity (FDA, 2007).[12]

The investigator site audit concludes with a closing meeting with the investigator and key site personnel to review key audit findings and to suggest corrective and preventive action, if required.

Database audit

Following collection of the CRFs from the investigator sites, the clinical data are transcribed or transmitted on to an electronic database. Data entry and verification, data cleaning and consistency checks, and coding of medical terminology such as adverse events, concomitant medication, and medical history are procedures that are prone to error. Therefore, periodic checks, in-process quality control steps, should be implemented in the data management process. An audit of the database by QA helps ensure that data integrity and validity

---

[12] FDA 21 CFR Part 11 Electronic Records, Electronic Signatures; http://www.fda.gov/oc/gcp/regulations.html; accessed November 20, 2009

has not been impaired during data management procedures.

Clear procedures (SOPs) for conducting such audits must be established, detailing the sampling procedures for CRFs and acceptable error rates. Information is available in the literature on error levels and data verification procedures (Zhang, 2004; DGGF, 2007; Society of Clinical Data Management (SCDM), 2009).

For the database audit to be meaningful, the database should only be audited in a "frozen" or "defined" state and prior to database lock so that eventual changes are possible after the audit without requiring a database "unfreeze." When comparing CRFs and data queries against the database entries, data entry, data validation, and coding procedures should be taken into account. It is important to ensure that no changes were made to the clinical data without proper justification and complete documentation. Depending on the number and volume of CRFs to be verified, database audits can be quite time-consuming.

Clinical study report audit

The clinical study report is the essence of the clinical trial and summarizes trial data and their interpretation. Since trial reports are part of the package submitted to regulatory authorities for obtaining marketing authorization, the contents must be valid, complete, and accurate. Report audits verify that all necessary components and attachments are included in the report. Ideally, the last draft version is subject to audit, thus avoiding rework that may be necessary after audits of early drafts, which are substantially changed until they are considered final. In addition, all QC checks and activities should have been completed prior to the audit.

Apart from compliance with SOPs for biostatistics and report writing, the statistical analysis plan, the trial protocol, and regulatory requirements and guidelines (ICH, 1995a, 1995b, 1998), QA auditors check the internal consistency of the trial report and appendices and between data in tables, figures, and graphs and numbers cited in the text. All numbers and percentages must be substantiated by attached tables and listings. In summary, the

trial report should be an accurate representation of the clinical data. Allocation of trial subjects to the datasets analyzed and to treatment groups must be traceable and comply with the randomization scheme and the outcome of the data review meeting, if such a meeting occurred).

In contrast to Good Laboratory Practice (GLP) regulations, GCP does not require an audit for all trial reports. The number of report audits may depend on the audit plan, the importance of the trial for a regulatory submission, and the confidence in the procedures followed for evaluating clinical study data and writing reports, just to name a few.

Systems audits

The purpose of systems audits is to assess procedures and systems across clinical studies and departments to evaluate that adequate procedures are followed that are likely to produce a quality product or result.

Systems audits focus on the verification of quality control steps incorporated in the procedures, on interfaces between different functions and departments, and on the relationship to external providers. Although non-compliance may be detected in systems audits, such audits aim to assess the capability of a system to deliver a quality output.

Based on the above-described trial-related audits, systems audits can be composed of such "core audit elements" and "enriched" by additional elements to form a systems audit. In general, the scope of any study-related audit can be broadened into a systems audit. The following paragraphs describe selected systems audit; further information is available in literature (DGGF, 2007).

Phase I/clinical pharmacology unit

Early phase clinical trials, including first-in-human studies, are often conducted in dedicated Phase I CROs or clinical pharmacology units. Because of the very limited information on the drug's toxicological and pharmacological effects on the one hand and the importance of the trials to the entire drug development program on the other hand, audits of such trials are a valuable component of the audit program.

In addition to the components verified for investigator site audits, the QA auditor should check the quality management and SOP systems, compliance with particular requirements for early phase clinical trials (FDA, 1995, 2006, 2008; EMA, 2009; The Association of British Pharmaceutical Industry (ABPI), 2007), recruitment and informed consent procedures for volunteers (e.g., volunteer panels or database), medical oversight and organization of the trial (particularly on dosing days), and access to resuscitation equipment and proximity to emergency units and typical facilities for Phase I trials (e.g., sleeping and recreational rooms, standardized meals).

A detailed outline on the scope for Phase I unit audits is available in literature (Bohaychuk and Ball, 1999).

Clinical monitoring

Clinical monitoring is one of the core activities in clinical research and regular verification of the capability of the monitoring processes is recommended. A systems audit in clinical monitoring can be based on investigator site audits where clinical monitoring activities are assessed in detail. In addition, the systems audit should verify if adequate SOPs are available for clinical monitoring, which comply with GCP requirements (FDA, 1988). The SOPs should also address procedures for SDV and document and facility review. Training procedures and documentation for monitors should be reviewed to ensure that CRAs are adequately trained in GCP, SOPs, and protocol procedures. This includes the review of activities such as co-monitoring or supervised visits.

The systems audits should also evaluate procedures followed for investigator site selection and initiation, the scope and frequency of monitoring visits, and the SDV procedures applied as well as the timing of and process for conducting close-out visits. Handling of safety information (AEs, SAEs) by clinical monitors at the site and in-house is also an important area to review. Documentation of monitoring visits is essential and the audit should therefore evaluate the contents of monitoring reports and their timely preparation and also check whether contacts with the investigator sites between monitoring visits are adequate recorded.

Data management, statistics, and medical writing

This late phase in clinical trials "offers" many opportunities to introduce errors and inconsistencies in the clinical trial data as obtained on the CRFs by the investigator sites. No stage before included so many steps for data processing, coding, cleaning, programming, analysis, and reporting, and requires seamless interaction of many contributors.

Systems audits in this late phase in clinical trials aim at assessing related procedures to ensure that capable procedures exist for managing and cleaning clinical trial data, for conducting statistical analyses, and for preparing the final study report that represents properly the data collected and reported in the clinical trial. Such systems audits are performed across functional boundaries. Such systems audit can be combined with a database audit and/or an audit of the final study report.

Typical aspects of such audits are the capability of SOPs and project-specific instructions for data management, statistical analyses, and medical writing to provide an error-free report containing clinical trial data that is traceable to the original CRFs. This includes verification that software used in data management, for statistical analyses and report generation, is validated and validation is adequately documented. Audit of the reconciliation process between clinical and safety database is another key area of the audit. All programs written, including database set-up and statistical analyses programs, must be validated and approved prior to use. Adequate procedures for database freeze/lock and unfreeze/unlock should be established together with proper documentation so that post-final database updates are fully traceable and do not render the clinical trial data invalid. Conclusions drawn in the final study report must be valid and substantiated by clinical data included in the report. Documentation related to data management, statistics, and medical writing must be securely archived and, ideally, be part of the TMF.

All personnel involved in data handling, analyses, and reporting must be adequately trained.

Further details on and requirements to review during such systems audits are provided in the literature (Rondel *et al.*, 2000; DGGF, 2007; FDA, 2007; SCDM, 2009).[13]

Computerized systems

Systems audits in the area of computerized systems validation (CSV) are closely related to data collection and management, statistics, and pharmacovigilance, because these areas are fully dependent on validated and properly functioning systems.

The objective of QA is to provide assurance to management that computer systems are appropriately validated so that clinical trial data integrity is maintained. This includes verification of the system development life cycle (SDLC) documentation (or alternative documentation for systems that have been in place for a long time and are not validated according to current requirements) and adequate testing and user acceptance testing of specified requirements. System security (logical and physical) must be evaluated as part of the systems audit, including access to server rooms and back-up procedures. Handling and access to audit trails is a critical component of any CSV audit. System documentation, instruction manuals and appropriate training records for anybody involved in computer systems (either as developer or as user) must be available.

Revalidation and change control procedures for hardware and software should be checked during the audit.

Further details regarding CSV audits are available in the literature (Rondel *et al.*, 2000; Follett, 2003; Association for Clinical Data Management (ACDM), 2004; McDowall, 2005; DGGF, 2007; FDA, 2007; PIC/S, 2007a).[13]

---

[13] FDA 21 CFR Part 11 Electronic Records, Electronic Signatures; http://www.fda.gov/oc/gcp/regulations.html; accessed November 20, 2009

Investigational medicinal products

Procedures for manufacturing, packaging, labeling, shipping, accounting, reconciling, and disposing of IMPs must comply with relevant GCP and Good Manufacturing Practice (GMP) requirements (FDA, 1991, 2008; ICH, 1995a; EU Commission, 2003a, 2003b, 2006, 2007; PIC/S, 2007b, 2009).

The systems audit should follow the route of the IMPs and verify that all drug shipments between manufacturer, CRO, investigator sites, pharmacies (if applicable), and trial participants are fully documented, providing information on the nature of the drug, the amount, batch number(s), subject kit number(s), storage conditions, and expiry/retest date. Certificates of analysis should be available for all batches of IMPs (active and placebo) and comparators. Labeling should comply with GMP requirements as requested for the countries involved in the trial and release of the drug should be documented—if required by a "Qualified Person" (QP), for example in Europe.

According to Annex 13 GMP, a two-step release procedure is mandatory, consisting of a technical release by the QP and a "regulatory green light" to confirm that all GCP regulatory requirements have been fulfilled prior to shipment of IMPs to the investigator site.

All procedures related to IMPs should be adequately described in SOPs. Finally, accountability and reconciliation information for the study medication should be consistently performed during and after the clinical trial and be traceable. All involved persons must be trained in related GCP and GMP regulations and SOPs and training should be documented.

Safety reporting/pharmacovigilance

Safety reporting is a key area in clinical development and information on AEs experienced in clinical trials and after the drug has been launched must be reliably handled and reported within specified timeframes (DGGF, 2007). Companies must have a clearly defined pharmacovigilance system established even before they have a product on the market and when they are still in the drug development phase to be able to make proper assessments of the safety of a new drug and to meet regulatory obligations for safety reporting.

Systems audits in pharmacovigilance are useful to evaluate all processes and SOPs related to pharmacovigilance and to assess the interaction with investigator sites, CRAs, and related in-house personnel involved in handling safety information. QA auditors verify whether the pathways and timeframes for reporting AEs, SAEs, and Suspected Unexpected Serious Adverse Reactions (SUSARs) are followed and that all required recipients of such safety information are notified as needed. SOPs and if required protocol-specific instructions should be available to describe the management of AE information. Sufficient and transparent documentation is required to demonstrate the timely and satisfactory handling of AE reports, including expedited reporting, where required. The QA auditor should also assess the training of involved personnel and, where needed, review the validation documentation of computerized systems utilized in pharmacovigilance.

Training

As already mentioned in the descriptions above, training and education is a key component in systems audits. ICH GCP requires that "each individual involved in conducting a trial should be qualified by education, training and experience to perform his or her respective task(s)." Related requirements can be found in several paragraphs of ICH GCP.

Systems audits of the training department/function should assess whether procedures and SOPs are in place for all aspects of training. For each employee in clinical drug development, training records should be available to document the training and demonstrate the qualification and experience. Training files should be archived when employees leave the company. The training records should also include a current job description and previous versions should be retained. A résumé (CV) should be available and maintained. Attendance at internal and external training courses and conferences/meetings should be documented. Ideally, training programs are outlined for induction and continual training.

Closely related to training files are organizational charts, which should be available for all company departments/functions involved in clinical drug development. Organizational charts must be updated when necessary; previous versions should be maintained.

Archiving

At the termination of each clinical trial, the study-related documents should be archived so that they can be accessed in the future, if needed, for example, in case of regulatory inspections (ISO 9000:2005, 2005; GCP Directive, 2005). SOPs, AE reports/pharmacovigilance documentation, staff records, equipment and validation records, and audit files are also subject to archiving.

Systems audits in archiving should verify that SOPs and procedures are in place for timely archiving and adequate retrieval of clinical documents. This involves, for example, a dedicated facility/area for long-term storage with adequate access controls and environmental protection (e.g., against loss, flood, vermin, or fire). A dedicated person (and a back-up) must be responsible for the management and operation of the archive. Documents provided to the archive must be indexed to ensure retrievability. A reasonable timeframe should be specified for documentation to be moved into the archive after trial termination.

Retention times must also be specified because ICH GCP 5.5.1.1 does not provide a clear rule and only outlines that trial documents "should be retained until at least two years after the last approval of a marketing application in an ICH region and until there are no pending or contemplated marketing applications in an ICH region or at least two years have elapsed since the formal discontinuation of clinical development of the investigational product."

Retention times are typically laid down in country-specific laws and guidance documents.

Audits of external providers

CROs, SMOs, and AROs

A wide range of external providers is used to deliver services in clinical trials, for example, CROs, Site

Management Organizations (SMOs), and Academic Research Organizations (AROs). To ensure that they are capable of providing the services in a reliable manner and to the standards expected in compliance with current regulatory requirements, capability audits are conducted at service providers prior to contracting.

It is good business practice and a sign of due diligence to confirm (prior to outsourcing services) that the systems in place at, and procedures followed by, the external provider are compatible with the sponsor, that staff at the service provider are adequately trained and qualified, and that records exist to demonstrate this fact. A functioning quality management system including current SOPs and a QA audit program should exist; storage and archiving procedures and facilities should be available. To the extent applicable, required equipment and calibration/maintenance records should be assessed during vendor audits as well as computerized systems, validation records, and back-up procedures. The systems audit will also evaluate the training records and personnel qualifications.

The audit should also verify procedures in those functional areas that provide services to the sponsor.

Apart from systems audits conducted to assess the capability of an external provider, such audits can also be conducted to verify compliance throughout the clinical trial or retrospectively after trial termination.

Laboratory

In the majority of clinical trials, external (central) laboratories are contracted to analyze biological samples that are taken during the clinical trial. Laboratory results are often critical, for example, primary efficacy data, and therefore warrant systems audits in laboratories.

Based on the above items listed for CRO audits, the laboratory systems audit should assess whether the laboratory participates in routine external quality assessment schemes, sample handling is adequate and transparent, and the risk of mix-ups is minimized. Proper documentation should be available for all sample movements and adequate space at refrigerators/freezers/cold rooms is

mandatory. Refrigerators/freezers/cold rooms must be temperature-monitored, connected to an alarm system, be maintained, cleaned, and calibrated as required.

Analytical methods must be adequately validated following regulatory requirements and adequate validation documents should exist. Computerized systems must be validated and the reporting of laboratory results to investigator sites, CROs, monitors, and sponsors should be clearly described.

Conclusion

QA activities are manifold and require a broad set of skills and a dependable knowledge of GCP regulations and clinical development processes. Possible areas of occupation for QA auditors are diverse: some are focusing on auditing and specialize to become an expert in a specific area; others would like to be flexible and conduct a variety of audits. Moving into training and consulting is a valid opportunity and even moving out of QA into operational functions is possible. Most important, though, for QA auditors is the skill to work with a variety of functional areas and to work cross-functionally, to be detailed but also not to lose sight of the overall picture. Auditors should be able to deal with conflicts and critical situations that may emerge in auditing clinical trials and systems.

Regulatory authorities are expecting QA programs to be established at sponsors and external service providers. However, this should not be the only reason for implementing a proper QA program at a company. QA auditors can help ensure the integrity and validity of clinical trial data from the beginning to the end, from trial planning until the final study report, through trial-related and systems audits, training, and consulting. Although QA's contribution may not be easily measurable, its investment in error prevention, compliance assessments, and contribution to inspection readiness is a considerable benefit to companies and adds value to the processes and procedures. Management support and adequate resources, however, are mandatory to ensure that QA auditors and programs are effective.

Last but not least, one should remember that QA is not ultimately responsible for the quality of the services and products: that is the responsibility of the individual(s) involved in the clinical research process.

References

Association of the British Pharmaceutical Industry (ABPI). Guidelines for Phase I Clinical Trials, 2007; http://www.abpi.org.uk/publications/pdfs/phase1_guidelines.pdf; accessed November 20, 2009.

Association for Clinical Data Management (ACDM). Computer Systems Validation in Clinical Research – A Practical Guide, second edition. UK; February 2004; www.acdm.org.uk; accessed November 20, 2009.

Bohaychuk WP, Ball G. *Conducting GCP-Compliant Clinical Research – A Practical Guide*. John Wiley & Sons, Ltd: Chichester, UK, 1999.

DGGF (Expert Group of the German Society for Good Research Practice). GCP Auditing – Methods and Experiences, second edition. Editio Cantor Verlag: Aulendorf, Germany, 2007.

Eichenwald K, Kolata G. Research for Hire: A Doctor's Drug Studies Turn Into Fraud. *New York Times*, May 17, 1999; http://www.nytimes.com/library/national/science/health/051799drug-trials-industry. html; accessed November 20, 2009.

EMA. EMA Guideline on Strategies to Identify and Mitigate Risks for First-in-Human Clinical Trials with Investigational Medicinal Products (EMEA/CHMP/SWP/28367/07). July 19, 2007; http://www.emea.europa.eu/pdfs/human/swp/2836707enfin.pdf); accessed November 20, 2009.

European Commission. Commission Directive 2003/94/EC laying down the Principles and Guidelines of Good Manufacturing Practice in Respect of Medicinal Products for Human Use and Investigational Medicinal Products for Human Use, October 8, 2003a; http://ec.europa.eu/enterprise/pharmaceuticals/eudralex/vol-1/dir_2003_94/dir_2003_94_en.pdf; accessed November 20, 2009.

European Commission. European Commission, EudraLex Volume 4, Good Manufacturing Practices, Annex 13 Manufacture of Investigational Medicinal Products, July 2003b; http://ec.europa.eu/enterprise/pharmaceuticals/eudralex/vol-4/pdfs-en/an13final_24-02-05.pdf; accessed November 20, 2009.

European Commission. Commission Directive 2005/28/EC of 8 April 2005 laying down principles and detailed guidelines for good clinical practice as regards investigational medicinal products for human use, as well as the requirements for authorisation of the manufacturing or importation of such products. Official Journal L 91, April 9, 2005, 13–19; http://ec.europa.eu/enterprise/pharmaceuticals/eudralex/vol-1/dir_2005_28/dir_2005_28_en.pdf); accessed November 20, 2009.

European Commission. European Commission, EudraLex Volume 10, Guideline on the Requirements to the Chemical and Pharmaceutical Quality Documentation Concerning Investigational Medicinal Products in Clinical Trials, March 31, 2006; http://ec.europa.eu/enterprise/pharmaceuticals/eudralex/vol-10/18540104en.pdf; accessed November 20, 2009.

European Commission. European Commission, EudraLex Volume 10, Guidance on Investigational Medicinal Products (IMPs) and Other Medicinal Products Used in Clinical Trials, April 2007; http://ec.europa.eu/enterprise/pharmaceuticals/eudralex/vol-10/guidance-on-imp_nimp_04-2007.pdf; accessed November 20, 2009.

European Union (EU). Directive 2001/20/EC of the European Parliament and of the Council of 4 April 2001 on the approximation of the laws, regulations and administrative provisions of the Member States relating to the implementation of good clinical practice in the conduct of clinical trials on medicinal products for human use. *Official Journal L* **121**, May 1, 2001, pp. 34–44; http://ec.europa.eu/enterprise/pharmaceuticals/eudralex/vol-1/dir_2001_20/dir_2001_20_en.pdf; accessed November 20, 2009.

FDA. FDA Guidance for Industry: Guideline for the Monitoring of Clinical Investigations, January 1988; http://www.fda.gov/ICECI/EnforcementActions/BioresearchMonitoring/ucm135075.htm); accessed November 20, 2009.

FDA. FDA Guidance for Industry: Guideline for the Preparation of Investigational New Drug Products (Human and Animal), March 1991; http://www.fda.gov/cder/guidance/old042fn.pdf; accessed November 20, 2009.

FDA. FDA Guidance for Industry: Content and Format of Investigational New Drug Applications (INDs) for Phase I Studies of Drugs, Including Well-Characterized, Therapeutic, Biotechnology-derived Products, November 1995; http://www.fda.gov/downloads/Drugs/GuidanceComplianceRegulatoryInformation/Guidances/UCM074980.pdf; accessed November 20, 2009.

FDA. FDA Compliance Program Guidance Manual 7348.810 – Sponsors, Contract Research Organizations and Monitors, 21 February 2001; http://www.fda. gov/downloads/ICECI/EnforcementActions/Bioresearch Monitoring/UCM133770.pdf; accessed November 20, 2009.

FDA. FDA Guidance for Industry, Investigators, and Reviewers: Exploratory IND Studies, January 2006; http://www.fda.gov/downloads/Drugs/Guidance ComplianceRegulatoryInformation/Guidances/ UCM078933.pdf; accessed November 20, 2009.

FDA. FDA Guidance for Industry: Computerized Systems Used in Clinical Investigations, May 2007; http:// www.fda.gov/downloads/Drugs/GuidanceCompliance RegulatoryInformation/Guidances/UCM070266.pdf; accessed November 20, 2009.

FDA. FDA Guidance for Industry: CGMP for Phase 1 Investigational Drugs, July 2008; http://www.fda. gov/downloads/Drugs/GuidanceComplianceRegulatory Information/Guidances/UCM070273.pdf; accessed November 20, 2009.

Follett T. *Computer Validation: The 100 Worst Mistakes You Can Make*. CVSI Press: Richville, NY, USA, 2003.

Hattemer-Apostel R. GCP auditors: hard to find – hard to develop – hard to keep: part 1. criteria and methods for candidate selection. *Qual Assur J* 2000a; **4**(1):3–8.

Hattemer-Apostel R. GCP auditors: hard to find – hard to develop – hard to keep: part 2. initial training requirements for auditors. *Qual Assur J* 2000b; **4**(3):123–135.

Hattemer-Apostel R. GCP auditors: hard to find – hard to develop – hard to keep: part 3. continuous education and further development. *Qual Assur J* 2001; **5**(1):3–11.

Hattemer-Apostel R. A career in clinical quality assurance. In: *Careers with the Pharmaceutical Industry*, second edition, Stonier PD (ed.). John Wiley & Sons, Ltd: Chichester, UK, 2003, 188–202.

Hattemer-Apostel R. Quality assurance and clinical research. In: *Clinical Research Manual*, Luscombe D Stonier PD (eds). Euromed Communications Ltd: Haslemere, UK, 2004, **17**. 1–17.46.

ICH. ICH Note for Guidance on Good Clinical Practice (CPMP/ICH/135/95), 1995a; www.ich.org; accessed November 20, 2009.

ICH. ICH Note for Guidance on Structure and Content of Clinical Study Reports (CPMP/ICH/137/95), 1995b; www.ich.org; accessed November 20, 2009.

ICH. ICH Note for Guidance on Statistical Principles for Clinical Trials (CPMP/ICH/363/96), 1998; www.ich.org; accessed November 20, 2009.

ISO. ISO 19011:2002. Guidelines for Quality and/or Environmental Management Systems Auditing, October 3, 2002; http://www.iso.org; accessed November 20, 2009.

ISO. ISO 9000:2005. Quality Management Systems – Fundamentals and Vocabulary, September 20, 2005; www.iso.org; accessed November 20, 2009.

Lock S, Wells F, Farthing M (eds). *Fraud and misconduct in biomedical research*, fourth edition. Royal Society of Medicine Press: London, UK, 2008.

McDowall RD. Effective and practical risk management options for computerised systems validation. *Qual Assur J* 2005; **9**(3):196–227.

PIC/S. PIC/S Guidance Good Practices for Computerized Systems in Regulated "GXP" Environments (PI 011-3), September 25, 2007a; www.picscheme.org; accessed November 20, 2009.

PIC/S. PIC/S Aide-Mémoire GMP Particularities in the Manufacture of Medicinal Products to be Used in Clinical Trials on Human Subjects (PI 021-2), September 25, 2007b; www.picscheme.org; accessed November 20, 2009.

PIC/S. PIC/S Guide to Good Manufacturing Practice for Medicinal Products (PE 009-9), September 1, 2009; www.picscheme.org; accessed November 20, 2009.

Rondel RK, Varley SA, Webb CF (eds). *Clinical Data Management*, second edition. John Wiley & Sons Ltd: Chichester, England, 2000.

Society of Clinical Data Management (SCDM). Good Clinical Data Management Practices, 2009 edition. Milwaukee (USA); www.scdm.org; accessed November 20, 2009.

Winchell T. Start up: CQA. *Qual Assur J* 2004; **8**(1):13–20.

World Medical Association. Declaration of Helsinki – Ethical Principles for Medical Research Involving Human Subjects, last amended by the 59th WMA General Assembly, Seoul, October 2008; http:// www.wma.net/en/30publications/10policies/b3/index. html; accessed November 20, 2009.

Zhang P. Statistical issues in clinical trial data audit. *Drug Inf J* 2004; **38**(4):371–386.

CHAPTER 15

The Unique Role of Over-the-Counter Medicine

Paul W. Starkey
Merck Consumer Care, Whitehouse Station, NJ, USA

The expanding place of self-medication

In recent years, the role of over-the-counter (OTC) medication in the overall health system has increased dramatically. The increased interest in and availability of OTC medications is being driven by several factors:

• There is a growing recognition of the capability of patients to treat themselves in a rational and safe manner. The older authoritarian model of medicine is being gradually replaced by a more participative model.

• There is an increasing desire by patients to participate in their own medical care. This is not just a result of changes in philosophy but also of the dramatic increase in average educational level over the past half-century. The world increasingly possesses a well-informed and intellectually capable population that demands an active and inclusive role in its own healthcare.

• The democratization of information that has resulted from the advent of the Internet has revolutionized the availability of medical information for the average person. It is now easy and convenient to research both common and rare diseases. The Internet makes it possible for a lay person to develop quite a thorough understanding of almost any disease and its available treatment options quickly and easily. This level of readily-available information has resulted in a population that has at its disposal all the information needed to empower its members to take a very much more active role in their own healthcare. Indeed today it is not uncommon to find lay people whose knowledge of a disease that afflicts them approaches that of a medical professional.

• There is a growing need to contain medical costs. OTC drugs are not only cheaper than prescription drugs, due to their simpler and more efficient distribution channels, but they also eliminate the need for an expensive visit to the doctor for each episode of illness. The professional intervention required to prescribe pharmaceuticals represents the dominant cost in the handling of many common types of illness.

• There is a need to increase treatment effectiveness, which is not ordinarily considered an advantage of self-medication. Increase in effectiveness depends on the generally more rapid availability of OTC medications compared to prescription medications, so that treatment may begin sooner. This can significantly shorten the total length of suffering, especially when the natural course of a disease is brief or when severe discomfort makes prompt therapy especially helpful.

An example of this last phenomenon is in the treatment of vaginal candidiasis. Prior to the OTC availability of topical antifungals, it was often necessary for a woman who had already recognized the symptoms of the disease to call and arrange a clinician's appointment. This often took several days. Delaying treatment caused much unnecessary suffering and encouraged disease progression. Many

Principles and Practice of Pharmaceutical Medicine, 3rd edition.
Edited by L.D. Edwards, A.W. Fox, P.D. Stonier.
© 2011 Blackwell Publishing Ltd.

clinicians, recognizing these difficulties, would pre-scribe over the phone, based solely on the woman's description of symptoms. Research has shown that the accuracy of the clinician's diagnosis in this setting is no better than that of the woman herself. This constituted an ideal situation for the switching of an important class of drugs from prescription to OTC status. The patient obtains equally accurate diagnosis and far more rapid treatment for a disease that is very uncomfortable. Severe cases of vaginal candidiasis with heavy discharge are now much less common.

A second example is in the treatment of the common cold. Anticold medications have been available OTC for many years, because of the compelling need for rapid treatment. A cold evolves quickly, the entire illness lasting only a few days. A delay of only a day or two in seeing the clinician for a prescription may eliminate any possibility of obtaining effective treatment for half of the duration of the illness. The prompt availability of self-medication improves treatment efficacy while reducing costs and enhancing patient satisfaction with the medical system.

The above factors have combined to increase greatly public awareness of the importance of self-medication in the total healthcare scheme. The sponsor should recognize the opportunities for OTC use of medications and the advantages and pitfalls attendant upon such use. As self-medication becomes a central part of the healthcare system, the skillful and appropriate movement of pharmaceuticals from prescription to OTC availability will increasingly become a vital role of the sponsor in optimizing the nation's health.

Differing styles of over-the-counter distribution

What is meant by OTC availability differs substantially in different regions of the world. The United States has made a consistent effort to maintain a system of distribution with only two classes of availability. In America drugs are either prescription only or they are available for sale as ordinary merchandise, not only on open shelves in pharmacies but also in supermarkets and any other outlets that care to stock them. Thus, once a drug is designated as OTC in the United States, there is no intermediary of any kind. Patients simply self-select the drug based on its advertising and labeling and uses it as they chose. Recently the American FDA has found it necessary to create what amounts to a third class of drugs to be sold without a prescription but only behind the counter with pharmacist supervision. This new class is still considered to be a special exception for very few drugs and is not yet recognized as an official classification. The necessity for this *de facto* third class of drugs was not brought about by any safety consideration but rather it was due to the need to reduce greatly the availability of pseudoephedrine in order to prevent its use as a convenient starting material for the illicit manufacture of methamphetamine. The FDA was reluctant to completely remove this drug from OTC status since it is a highly effective and safe systemic nasal decongestant for which there is no equivalent substitute other than the relatively weak drug phenylephrine, which remains as the only fully OTC nasal decongestant in the USA.

The Continental European model for non-prescription distribution is quite different from that in the United States in that "OTC" drugs are in fact sold behind the counter in pharmacies only. In this style of distribution the pharmacist may provide advice and guidance to the patient over and above what is on the product's labeling. However, some patients may find that they are reluctant to discuss the need for a particular drug with the pharmacist and do not want to have to justify their request. This more restrictive form of OTC availability is well suited to the nature of Continental European pharmacies, which tend to be small independent specialty shops while American pharmacies tend to be part of large retail chain stores that operate in quite a different way.

The United Kingdom has yet another style of OTC distribution, which is intermediate between the highly customer-centered American system and the pharmacist-centered Continental European system.

Criteria for OTC use of medicines

The criteria by which a drug may be judged as suitable for self-medication are never absolute. The capability for OTC drug labeling is always a matter of careful judgment. The Food and Drug Administration (FDA) has been progressive in defining the requirements for OTC use in recent years. The old tendency to restrict OTC treatment to conditions of short duration and primarily to symptomatic therapy is rapidly disappearing.

The suitability of a medication for OTC use is not solely dependent upon its pharmacologic characteristics. Appropriate labeling and advertising of the medication can have a major impact on the extent to which patients understand its proper use. An OTC product should be envisioned not just as the drug itself but as the whole package of drug, labeling, and advertising, designed to encourage safe and effective self-medication. With this in mind, several vital considerations concern suitability of a drug for OTC marketing.

Self-diagnosis

The characteristics of the indication are just as important as the pharmacology of the drug itself in determining OTC suitability: Self-treatment implies self-diagnosis. Only diseases that are self-diagnosable with the assistance of appropriate labeling can be considered for OTC treatment.

Fortunately, there are many common conditions that are indeed self-diagnosable with the help of well-designed labeling. It should not be assumed that a diagnosis made by a patient is necessarily inferior to that made by a clinician. The patient can actually feel the symptoms as well as observe the signs of a disease—a real advantage in the diagnosis of diseases where symptoms predominate and signs are few. Of course, diseases where diagnosis depends on the interpretation of complicated laboratory tests or sophisticated imaging techniques are usually best diagnosed by the clinician and treated only by prescription.

An example of a self-diagnosable condition is headache, where the diagnosis rests largely on history and symptoms: The patient has lived the history and experienced the symptoms. The clinician has at best a description of these symptoms, which a particular patient may be able to communicate well or poorly. Even with the most skillful clinician eliciting the history, there is a degradation of information as it moves from patient to clinician. If patients can be educated about the criteria for diagnosis, they may be as capable of rendering the diagnosis as accurately as the clinician.

Even when a fully adequate description of symptoms and signs is not practicable for patient labeling, this barrier may be surmounted by limiting use to patients who have previously had the condition and had been diagnosed by a professional. Once some diseases have been experienced, they are unmistakable. This approach emphasizes the need for the sponsor to think creatively in evaluating whether or not a disease can be made self-diagnosable.

OTC products offer an opportunity for real and very meaningful creativity in devising wording and graphics that can explain a diagnosis in a way that lay persons can effectively understand and use. Usually, the best OTC labeling is obtained by an iterative process in which various labeling possibilities are tried out in label comprehension tests. These nonclinical trials do not actually use the drug but simply ask patients, preferably with the disease of interest, to read the proposed labeling and then take a test to find out what they understood. The results can be most illuminating and can guide the sponsor to far more effective ways of getting the right message across.

Differential diagnosis

Once a condition is established as self-diagnosable, a related consideration is the differential diagnosis—the potential consequence of confusing the disease with other similarly presenting ones, possibly resulting in a major delay in treatment. This consideration can often be a dominant factor in determining whether a condition is safely self-treatable. In conditions where minimal consequences are likely from a misdiagnosis, a modest level of diagnostic inaccuracy is tolerable to obtain the benefits of self-medication. If the major downside of misdiagnosis is simply the persistence or modest worsening of symptoms without serious health consequences, even more difficult self-diagnoses may be reasonable. However, it is usually wise to place a time limit on the length of self-treatment without a satisfactory response.

Drug safety

When evaluating the safety and tolerability of a drug for possible OTC use, one must first consider the quality of available information. Many drugs, particularly those used for a long time as prescription medications, have extensive safety databases. However, some do not, especially older drugs that predate modern research standards and newer drugs with insufficient usage. Also, with some drugs, the tolerability of one formulation may differ greatly from that of another. One example is benzyl peroxide, in which formulations may vary greatly, even at the same strength but with different excipients. Where such problems mean that there is an inadequate database for an intended OTC formulation, clinical testing will be needed before launch.

Safety is usually the controlling factor in determining suitability for OTC use, and involves several factors:

• The "therapeutic window" (or "therapeutic index", i.e., the size of the difference between therapeutic and toxic doses). This varies widely for both prescription and OTC drugs and is often less of a safety determinant than might be supposed. For example, the prescription drug sucralfate for the treatment of ulcers has extremely low toxicity, whereas OTC systemic decongestants typically have a narrower therapeutic window than most prescription drugs, as has recently been seen, leading to restrictions on ephedrine-containing products in the United States and Europe.

• The effects and consequences of toxicity and overdosage.

• The ease of recognition of early signs of toxicity to allow reduction in dosage or professional assistance.

Safety (negative propensity to cause genuine harm) can be distinguished from tolerability (negative propensity to cause limited adverse effects). Tolerability can limit OTC use even when safety is good. This is particularly true for topical agents such as anti-acne preparations, most of which are of little safety concern but can produce very substantial irritation.

However, the effect of a drug on the general population is only part of the story. The acceptability of a drug for market, particularly an OTC drug without a clinician intermediary, is often determined by its effect on special populations, including those patients who are particularly sensitive to its effects. Care should be taken to examine atypical patients in a study population, as well as individual adverse reaction reports. Precautions may be required in the labeling for populations at particular risk.

The conclusion that a drug is not acceptable for OTC use based on safety should be reached only after determining that satisfactory labeling cannot be developed. The sponsor must weigh safety and tolerability against efficacy, both in the general and special populations. Here the responsibility rests directly on the sponsor, because there will be no other medical professional between the drug and the patient using it.

Efficacy

Efficacy is a central issue with all pharmaceutical products. In the context of OTC products, it is traditional to accept a somewhat lesser degree of efficacy in order to improve the safety profile. Also, a lesser standard of efficacy is normally expected by the patient, because OTC medication tends to be a first step in therapy. Failure to obtain satisfactory efficacy typically results in the patient seeking professional advice, at which point more powerful treatments can be prescribed. This does not mean, however, that OTC drugs should not be effective for the conditions they treat.

Dosage selection

The extent of efficacy will depend considerably on dosage. In the past, there was an automatic tendency to reduce the dosage to half or less of prescription strength. Today, it is widely realized that dosage should not be reduced simply as a matter of course; rather, a considered judgment on optimum dosage should be made. It is being progressively appreciated by both the pharmaceutical industry and the regulatory agencies that inappropriate reduction of dosage can result in reduced efficacy with little or no safety and tolerability benefits, thus leading to needlessly ineffective treatment. The goal is to provide the lowest effective dose. It is vital to retain medically meaningful efficacy that will provide patients with satisfying results if self-treatment is to fulfill its proper role in the medical care system.

The unique characteristics of the OTC field from the sponsor's viewpoint

The role of the clinician working in the OTC division of a major pharmaceutical company is substantially different from that played in the research or medical affairs departments dealing with drugs intended for prescription. One might assume that OTC work is simpler and less involved than that related to prescription medications. In many ways, the opposite is true.

Clinicians overseeing OTC products must be generalists, requiring a broad expertise in medicine, toxicology, and regulatory affairs. The OTC clinician deals with a vast variety of drugs from many different areas of medicine, including some that are little taught in medical school and never encountered while working as a junior hospital doctor. This contrasts with research on new chemical entities, where clinicians generally focus on a single therapeutic area, enjoy a large support staff that provide them with in-depth assistance, and use a limited number of research protocols and techniques that can be thoroughly mastered. In contrast, the OTC clinician must be an expert on, for example, smoking-cessation one day, gastroenterology the next, and dermatology the next.

The regulations governing OTC medications are substantially different from those in the prescription field, and the OTC clinician is typically more involved in regulatory matters than non-OTC colleagues. The OTC clinician must also be concerned with detailed issues of formulation and manufacturing.

As staff are fewer and the hierarchy simpler, the OTC clinician has much more general authority, with broad responsibility for in-line, new, and forthcoming products. On the prescription side, this would not be true of any job short of the Vice President of Clinical Research.

Another difference concerns marketing. Typically in the prescription area, interaction with the marketing department is infrequent, although sometimes intense. In the OTC area, it is constant. The clinician educates the marketing department on medical issues surrounding a particular drug and on the opportunities and limitations that these present. In particular, the clinician must understand the needs of the brand managers and be able to offer guidance. For instance, when difficulties occur in the implementation of marketing plans, the clinician must be able to assist in developing alternative strategies. An OTC business is subject to intense market pressures. The clinician must help the marketers deal with them effectively by frequently playing the roles of educator and creative thinker, as well as medical expert.

One of the most surprising aspects of the clinician's role in OTC medication development is the very high degree of creativity that is required. With prescription medication, one must work with whatever compounds have been previously developed by chemistry and toxicology. These are brought to clinicians for clinical testing, and there is seldom any input by the clinicians into drugs they are required to work on. Sometimes the project on which the clinician will be spending years of his or her life is of considerable medical interest, in other cases it is not. Whatever the case, prescription clinicians will be able to exercise only minimal control over what compounds they are working on at any given time. Although it is possible for the clinical development of a new chemical entity to be poorly handled, it is not possible for the clinical researcher to add any characteristic that the particular chemical entity did not possess when it was synthesized.

In contrast, in the OTC area, clinicians are actually in a position to influence greatly the choice of compounds on which they and the company will do research. They can even creatively discover new indications suitable for OTC therapy. The OTC clinician typically enjoys major input into all decisions involved in the company's commitment to particular compounds and formulations. This is true for OTC switch and for new formulations of older products. The formulators in an OTC operation seek extensive input from their medical colleagues, and the corporation looks to the clinician for more than just straightforward opinions. Creativity is required and clinicians have an opportunity to devise concepts that are developed by the company.

Because the development cycle of OTC drugs is much shorter than that of prescription compounds, clinicians are often able to see their own ideas brought to fruition in the form of a tangible product. Typically, it requires only three years or less for the development of an OTC drug, as opposed to 7–10 years for a new chemical entity. The skillful use of medical knowledge and its creative application to new products can make all the difference in the medical and business success of an OTC company.

The extent to which the OTC clinician is a key decision-maker is especially clear in dealing with the release to market of new formulations of drugs that have monograph status. Here the sponsor makes direct judgments on the safety and marketability of products without the intervention of a regulatory agency. The US FDA has provided for the direct marketing of a wide variety of OTC drugs which it has pre-approved in the so-called "monograph" system. The underlying concept of this system is that there are many drugs that have long been on the OTC market and for which abundant information already exists. Therefore, it would be redundant and wasteful for a new New Drug Application (NDA) to be submitted each time a new formulation of one of these compounds is to be brought to market. The FDA has provided a series of numerous monographs, each one of which deals with a particular narrow therapeutic area, ranging from acne and antihelminthics to hormones and weight control. The therapeutic area is discussed in some detail and specific requirements for well-established drugs in that area are set forth. As long as a new formulation remains within the exact

requirements set forth in the monograph for type of drug, dosage, indication, and labeling statements, a compound may be formulated and marketed on the judgment of the sponsor alone. No further pre-approval or examination of any application to the FDA is necessary. However, if the requirements set forth in the monograph for a particular compound are to be changed in any way by a different dosage, a new indication, or by changes in labeling, the formulation no longer is covered by the monograph and it is necessary to submit a full NDA. As long as the monograph requirements are strictly met, the clinician in charge will make the final judgment on whether a new formulation is satisfactory for market. This system exists only in the United States and it provides for a striking amount of speed and flexibility in the OTC marketing of products.

However, the situation also places a very substantial amount of responsibility on the sponsor. You can never appreciate the value of having a regulatory agency review your work and make the final decision to allow marketing until you do not have them and must take the responsibility yourself. This is particularly true with regard to the tolerability of new formulations. It is unlikely that major safety problems will arise with well-known drugs dosed at well-known levels for indications that are thoroughly understood. With topical drugs, however, where irritation and allergenicity are a problem, the judgment of suitability for market can be difficult. These drugs tend to be very dependent on the contents of individual formulations, and so be sure of enough information before releasing them to market.

The need for specific clinical testing must be determined by the clinician in each individual instance. A wide variety of situations may arise, varying from those in which no particular testing is required to those in which an extensive series of tests is needed before full confidence can be felt in a formulation. In short, the American monograph system provides unparalleled speed and flexibility of drug development for those compounds that are covered by it, but special vigilance is also needed on the part of the OTC clinician. For all the delay and difficulty involved in obtaining approvals from FDA, it does have the major advantage that it provides a second source of learned judgment prior to the marketing of products. Even in the limited scope of monograph drugs, clinicians can often find it necessary to use all their abilities to ensure that adequate testing is done and that careful judgments are made before individual formulations are allowed to reach the marketplace.

Because of the monograph system, one of the more striking features of OTC drug development is the speed with which new formulations can be moved from the conceptual stage to actual product realization. This contributes in a major way to job satisfaction, but also creates the need to act with much more speed in advancing one's own portion of the development efforts. There is a need for the clinician to participate in every phase of early planning of a development program. This is the only way to ensure that it is properly handled and can be quickly executed. Frequently, several companies will be moving forward with similar projects. Both commercial and personal success rely upon being the first to market. Thus, the program must be planned for success on the first try. If major delays in research occur, the product will usually be so far behind the competition in reaching the market that it will have little commercial value.

Several factors can accelerate the entire process of research in the OTC area. As it is much quicker and simpler for a product to remain within the monograph requirements, every effort is made to do so if possible. For research with monograph drugs, it is perhaps surprising to learn that an Investigational New Drug (IND) exemption is not always required prior to undertaking research. This is only logical, however, because for a monograph drug there is pre-approval from the FDA to launch the product into the market. It would not be sensible to require special pre-approval to perform human research via the IND system. This considerably speeds and simplifies the course of the research effort but again results in greater responsibility for the OTC clinician. The clinician must ensure that the research undertaken will be complete and adequate for both safety and efficacy determination purposes and must make a solo judgment as to the safety of the research subjects involved, with no FDA oversight.

The details of the clinical research process are little different for OTC and prescription work. What changes most is the role of the sponsor. This role is greater in scope and responsibility in the OTC area and everything must be done with greater speed.

Prescription-to-OTC switch

One of the most dynamic areas in the pharmaceutical industry today is the prescription-to-OTC switch, commonly called the *Rx-to-OTC switch*. This is the process by which a drug that has previously been used only by prescription is converted to self-medication status. We have already considered the criteria for OTC use of medications and these criteria represent a sound guide in determining what drugs are suitable for switching. There are no hard and fast guidelines for determining which drugs may become suitable for OTC switch, but a consideration of self-diagnosability of the disease state to be treated, the general safety and tolerability of the drug, its ability to show efficacy in the hands of nonprofessionals, and a relative absence of problems with masking of symptoms, all contribute to making a drug more OTC-able.

The first question that arises when considering the possibility of an OTC switch is, why has the drug not been available OTC before and what can be done to remove the obstruction? It is possible that a drug may simply not have had adequate prescription experience in the past. It takes time to accumulate a substantial use database of real-world experience. This is essential to make it possible to form a judgment about safety in prescription use and, therefore, projected safety in OTC use. What constitutes substantial use is always a relative matter. Typically, at least three years of data accumulation with a widely marketed drug is required to be able to feel some security in making judgments from the adverse reaction database accumulated. For drugs with 1000 sales this can easily take 10 years or more. The fewer problems this database reveals, the better the drug will be as a switch candidate.

It is sometimes possible to accelerate the accumulation of data for a promising OTC candidate by specialized Phase IV studies. These studies accelerate the process of data collection by conducting what amounts to a survey among clinicians using the drug on a prescription basis. As the sole interest is the gathering of adverse reaction data, with special emphasis on rare and serious events, record forms are kept very minimal, often to a single page. The study design consists simply of a survey done without control groups. Hundreds of clinicians, or even thousands, must be contacted to participate in the survey by submitting brief record forms on patients they treat in their usual manner with the prescription drug. Such a survey can rapidly provide a much more reliable database than spontaneous reporting. With a survey, you get both a frequency of the various side effects and a reasonable estimate of the number of patients treated, which permits the calculation of accurate rates for the adverse effects observed. This is in marked contrast to the data obtained from an entirely spontaneous adverse reaction database, where it is impossible to determine the efficiency of reporting. Therefore, it is extremely difficult to estimate correct rates of occurrence of individual adverse effects. The spontaneous databases are more useful for the qualitative evaluation of what can happen with a drug than for the quantitative evaluation of its true frequency. This type of adverse reaction survey study can pave the way for a switch effort in much less time than needed if reliance is placed solely on spontaneous reports for collection of data.

If the principal barrier to switch has been a lack of clinical experience with a drug, this can be remedied by the collection of a large adverse reaction database. Once this is done, it is usually straightforward to establish that the drug is safe in prescription use. This is a major advance on the road to OTC approval, but it certainly does not yet prove that the drug will be safe and effective in the hands of consumers without the benefit of a learned intermediary. In order to establish this additional point, it is almost always necessary to supplement the analysis of adverse reaction databases with clinical studies in realistic conditions, using the labeling composed for the OTC product. We will discuss the peculiar aspects of the design of clinical studies suitable for such purposes

later, but for now, it is sufficient to note that they may usually proceed with the objectives of establishing efficacy and side effects *in a fully realistic OTC setting.*

When starting with a prescription-only medicine, it is extremely important to begin interactions with the regulatory agencies as soon as possible, if only to establish whether or not there are concerns that the company has not anticipated. Obstructions to an Rx-to-OTC switch might not be related to safety or efficacy, and can involve some other peripheral but still highly important considerations. Examples of such problems are indications that the FDA does not regard it as self-diagnosable, spread of antibiotic resistance, or inability to keep the OTC product out of the hands of children. It should be remembered that regulators' principal concern in considering an Rx-to-OTC switch is from a public health perspective. This is in contrast to the usual viewpoint of the pharmaceutical companies, which tends to be focused on the treatment of the individual patient. There is nothing that will facilitate the Rx-to-OTC switch of a drug more powerfully than convincing regulators that this will contribute toward the health of the public.

Other issues that may concern regulators are when a precedent is being set. It is possible that the precedent set by one particular Rx-to-OTC switch could be damaging in terms of the regulators' overall policy, even when they have relatively little concern about the switch itself; this may be the reason for hesitancy shown in approving "Plan B," a proposed OTC product for emergency contraception by the US FDA. Careful negotiation is called for. The corollary is that if your proposed Rx-to-OTC switch can be shown to follow some sort of precedent, your road with the regulators will be smoother.

Another broad-scale public health concern that may worry the FDA is the implied message given to the consumer by the OTC availability of a particular compound. This concern is illustrated by the situation with soluble fiber cholesterol-lowering agents of the psyllium-type. These agents have been shown to lower cholesterol but only to a very small degree. It was felt by the FDA that, if they become established with claims of cholesterol reduction, the population may be misled into feeling that they have made a major beneficial intervention in their lipid profile, when in fact, they have not. The message communicated to the consumer by making these compounds available constitutes a barrier to this Rx-to-OTC switch.

The timing of the Rx-to-OTC switch can be a major contribution to its success. The timing is influenced by both regulatory and commercial considerations. The completeness of the available database is critical, and the time this takes can dictate the timing of a switch. Often, however, it is a commercial factor that is the key to deciding when an Rx-to-OTC switch should take place. Before the end of patent expiration is one obvious opportunity for major benefits of a company obtaining OTC status, to offset the foreseen precipitous decline in unit price of the prescription product and reduction of the sponsor's share of that segment of the Rx market. Typically, once a drug has become an OTC product, it is sold at a lower unit price with smaller profit margins, but the total volume increases several-fold. On occasion, the rapid growth of an OTC market can be even larger than the original prescription sales.

Unfortunately, in many cases, an Rx-to-OTC switch at the time of patent expiration does not occur and there is a long hiatus before OTC status is secured; this is the consequence of failing to examine seriously the need for an OTC switch early enough. Unlike for monograph products, two years are quite insufficient for the necessary studies and regulatory applications in time for an Rx-to-OTC switch. Thus, realistic expectations of loss of patent coverage must be made to create the greatest opportunity. Organizations often exhibit an ebullience, exhibited in one form as the requirement of its staff to believe and promulgate that the weakest method of use patent will prevail against a generic challenge. This weak patent is inevitably the latest. Long-range revenue projections are created and published accordingly, and woe betide anyone suggesting planning for an Rx-to-OTC switch as a contingency.

Awareness of the OTC potential of the company's portfolio of drugs, and the time it will take to implement, should be constant.

There are two fundamentally different types of Rx-to-OTC switches from the standpoint of the scope of the research program required. Switch programs can vary from large NDA programs, as extensive and expensive as anything found in the new chemical entity development, to programs consisting of little more than a single study. What influences the basic size and expense for a proposed Rx-to-OTC switch is whether or not the indication or the dose of the drug will change.

New indication or dose size

If the indication or the dose is to be changed, you will be involved with an entirely new IND/NDA, which is needed to show the fundamental efficacy and safety of the drug, either at its new dose or in its new indication. Such a program obviously will require several years and involve extensive expenditure.

Same indication and dose size: actual use studies

In contrast to this are the programs of modest size often required for the switch of drugs that will be taken into the OTC market at their existing prescription dosage and for their existing prescription indications. Here, the regulatory agencies will generally accept the concept that there is no need to prove again the basic safety and efficacy of the drug, because this has already been done in the primary new chemical entity NDA. Such a repetition would not provide useful new data. What will be required is an actual use study, to show that the proposed labeling for OTC use is effective in enabling patients to use the drug properly. Also, it may be necessary to address whatever specific factor it is that has been obstructing the drug from OTC use hitherto.

For example, if there is a question as to whether the prescription indication that will now be taken OTC is self-diagnosable, then a study of self-diagnosis will be required. This occurred with the vaginal antifungal compounds, which were long kept on prescription status because of questions as to whether women could effectively diagnose vaginal candidiasis themselves. Only a single study was required to resolve this issue, and it was extremely unusual for the pharmaceutical industry in that it involved no drugs of any kind. It was simply a study of women's ability to self-diagnose, but it resolved the one outstanding issue that had blocked OTC approval. The time required to carry out studies on such special questions can vary considerably depending on the complexity of the question. However, it is typically a brief program and its budget is commonly small by the standards of the pharmaceutical industry. It is obvious that in the planning and preparation of a switch program, it is essential not to assume that a full safety and efficacy program will be required. Rather, early communication with the regulatory agencies is needed in order to establish what barriers actually exist.

Special study designs for the OTC area

The philosophy for OTC study design is significantly different from that of prescription medication studies. With the latter, you are typically striving to answer the basic scientific questions of "Can this drug work effectively?" and "Is it safe to administer to people?" Therefore, it is appropriate to study these new chemical entities primarily in highly controlled settings with extensive inclusion and exclusion criteria. This provides increased safety for the study participants, who will be using a drug of relatively unknown toxicity. Also, it allows a reduction in the inherent variability of the study population so as to obtain a clearer scientific answer to the questions of basic safety and efficacy. Every effort is made in studies of this type to control for all possible variables and to reduce random real-world circumstances to a minimum.

For drugs being prepared for the self-medication market, it is just the opposite. In this situation, a great deal of evidence is already available about the safety and efficacy of the drug. The key issue is whether the drug can work in the real-world context, with all the inherent happenstance and randomness in an environment that is relatively more chaotic than even outpatient IND/CTA (Clinical Trial Application) studies. Realism is the key to OTC research design.

Actual use studies are often called "slice-of-life" studies. In the real world, what will this OTC product do? It helps when inclusion and exclusion criteria are minimized, as they are in the supermarket or pharmacy. Every effort should be made to simulate the way in which patients will actually use the drug. Eliminating large segments of this population by strict admission criteria will simply give a result that is irrelevant. In some cases, it may even be necessary to even have patients pay for the drug, in order to assess the motivational factors associated with a purchase (they can be reimbursed post hoc and without their prior information).

In the same philosophical vein, it is important to design the study for minimum interaction with patients. They must be left free to act, guided only by the labeling. Intervention by the investigator will only distort the results.

These types of studies are not unscientific. Even if lacking well-matched placebo-controls among others, there is still a hypothesis under test, and these studies are addressing different sorts of questions. At the stage where a drug is being considered for a switch, the umbrella question is, "What impact will this drug have on the public health as it will really be used by the lay public?; this is the central question that the regulators and the sponsor need answered.

Real-world studies are tests of the labeling as much as they are tests of the drug itself. It is essential that the combination of the drug and its OTC labeling work closely together to enable patients to self-treat effectively. Not only is a great deal of creativity necessary in developing effective labelling, but also appropriate label comprehension studies are important in ensuring that the best labeling is obtained. The labeling may, in fact, make all the difference between approval of the Rx-to-OTC switch.

Research has shown that patients by and large do read labeling and they do heed it, particularly when they are using OTC products that are unfamiliar to them. Prior to any program being advanced to the stage of the definitive clinical studies, it is wise to develop a variety of different versions of the proposed labeling, so that these versions can be tested in label comprehension studies. These studies are sometimes organized by the medical department and sometimes carried out as market research, because they need not involve actual ingestion of drug. They consist of comparative studies in which patients in a realistic setting read the proposed labeling and then are quizzed on their comprehension of it. In this way, it is possible to see whether they understand how the drug ought to be used and whether they have understood key precautions. It is best to check both short-term and long-term comprehension to see how well the patients are able to remember what they have learned. This sort of pre-screening of labeling can be absolutely essential to success and it has saved many careers by avoiding disasters in large-scale definitive studies. Note that Institutional Review Board/ethics committee approval may still be required even when a drug is not being swallowed because, at the very least, there will still be issues of informed consent and confidentiality that must to be accorded to participants when documenting their experience of disease.

Market support studies

The market support study is the second major class of study that is used commonly to research OTC products. These often involve active comparator, head-to-head clinical comparisons between alternative formulations or against competitors. Only authentic differences will emerge as successful claims at the end of the study process.

Locating such possible advantages for quantification in market support studies can be done through usage and attitudes (U and A) studies, usually performed by marketing departments. Focus group sessions can be invaluable in discovering the possible existence of advantages for a particular formulation over its competitors, as well as individual interviews, and these are discussed elsewhere in this book.

Careful review and surveillance of the literature is another way in which differences can be identified. The term "literature" should be interpreted loosely; it should include the academic journals, newspapers, magazines, patients' newsletters, and any and all ephemera associated with the disease or drug of interest. Even small differences may be quite meaningful to patients, even though they may appear minor to the pharmacologist, who is not personally using the drug. For example, in the case of an antinausea drug, a difference in onset of action of 10–15 mins can be very important if you are the one who is nauseated, and yet completely insignificant to the medical reviewer of the original NDA at the regulatory authority. The other side of the coin is that differences that are not meaningful to patients will not generate sales: do not let the scientists run this part of the company! And do not allow expectations to grow out of hand; chasing after advantages that never existed in the first place leads to designing studies for bizarre purposes with a very high failure rate.

New claims

Once a probable new claim has been identified and the chances of its being scientifically valid have been assessed, two good-quality studies are usually necessary to support them (rarely, a single study may be enough).

A different regulatory milieu compared with prescription-only medicines drives what is needed to support a new claim for an OTC product. Typically, after a brief initial period, oversight of the OTC product passes to the government authorities that deal with consumer products and trading in general, rather than the European Medicines Agency or FDA (for example, in the United States, this is the Federal Trade Commission). In practice, advertising of OTC products must conform to the standards that might equally apply to, say, washing powder, fashion clothing, "herbal remedies," or shoes. The OTC pharmaceutical industry also tends to be self-enforcing; companies maintain eagle eyes on each other's advertising as part of the literature surveillance program described above, and often sue their competitors when unsupportable claims are suspected. The possession of scientifically sound studies is of great value in preventing, prosecuting, and defending such lawsuits.

Thus the medical director for OTC products often find him- or herself under oath, and there is less trepidation when you have carefully prepared a satisfactory scientific basis for the advertising claims that you have approved.

Summary

An OTC product has two components: the galleni-cal itself and its labeling. New OTC products are developed either by compliance with regulators' pre-approved monographs or by regulatory approval of Rx-to-OTC switches using the NDA/Marketing Authorization Application proce-dures. The former is often without direct govern-mental oversight and places a greater responsibility solely on the sponsor than the latter. Obstacles to Rx-to-OTC switches may or may not be related to product safety and efficacy, and the information needed to support such applications depends greatly on whether there will be any proposed change in indication or dose size; demonstrating a contribution to the public health and finding a rele-vant precedent make success more likely. The clini-cal data in support of a new OTC product should be obtained under conditions that are as close to the proposed ordinary use of the product as possible; in particular, investigator–patient interaction runs counter to obtaining real-world information about usefulness of labeling, capability for self-diagnosis, likelihood of product selection in the retail envi-ronment, and product effectiveness. Timing Rx-to-OTC switch applications well is key, and realistic anticipation of prescription product patent expira-tion usually offers one such opportunity. In spite of the generally lower unit price, the volume of sales of OTC products can on occasion mitigate the loss of, or even exceed revenues formerly realized by, the corresponding proprietary prescription-only drug.

SECTION III

Special Populations and Required Special Studies

Introduction

In 1993, the US Food and Drug Administration (FDA), Europe's Committee for Proprietary Medicinal Products (CPMP), and Japan's Ministries of Health and Welfare (MOHW) issued regulatory requirements for testing and labeling in a "special population," namely the elderly. These were not promulgated in isolation but after consultation with academia and industry. In the USA, initially this was done under the auspices of the American Society of Clinical Pharmacology and Therapeutics. Industry was allowed to participate and was largely credited with aiding the process. The First International Conference on Harmonization (ICH) held in Europe (November 5–7, 1991), again involved the regulators and the regulated and, for the first time, involved Japan as a major contributor. As a result of pre-, during-, and post- conference discussions, success was achieved. The "elderly" drug guidance was the forerunner of many future tripartite agreements in the clinical area.

Any subset of people or patients with disease may be labeled a "special population." However, gender differences and patients at the extremes of age, or with distinctive racial backgrounds, relative renal or hepatic failure, those using other concomitant drugs, and those with rare ("orphan") diseases have been included in this section because these are routine problems in pharmaceutical medicine.

Food and drug regulation has usually been stimulated by therapeutic disasters. Amongst special populations, perceived omissions of research and development have resulted in new regulatory requirements, if not after disaster, then due to political pressure from patient advocacy groups. Bluntly, these new regulations were necessary because the pharmaceutical industry formerly ignored these patient subsets because of the perceived costs of research, lack of direct revenues resulting from studying such special populations, and the ever-present fear of litigation resulting from the vulnerability of these patients.

For the pharmaceutical industry, it is ironic that attention to these special populations has actually proven to be "good business." In some cases, the mandated studies have led to extensions of patent lives or market segment expansion, plus the less tangible benefit of desperately needed positive public relations. Most of the chapters in this section therefore include a limited historical context; for example, the chapter on orphan populations not only describes what constitutes an orphan population and an "orphan drug," but also the history of legislation and the current inducements for industry.

Lastly, for those developing drugs, the study of special populations can often be a fascinating occupation. This fascination is not least because it often requires both lateral and integrative thinking.

The physiology, say, of hepatic function in the elderly must be reconciled against the inevitably incomplete information about a new drug; a plan of action must then be designed against that reconciliation, together with obtaining the regulatory input that such a plan is likely to be sufficient for product approval. This can become an integrated project on its own, which can pleasantly contrast with orthodox phase-oriented pharmaceutical company organizations.

CHAPTER 16

Drug Research in Older Patients

Lionel D. Edwards

Pharma Pro Plus Inc., New Jersey, and Temple University, School of Pharmacy, Philadelphia, USA

Demographics

The elderly (over 64 years old) comprise 12% of the US population and 17% of Sweden and Japan. This sector continues to grow. In the US, it is estimated that the elderly population would increase to 14% by 2010 and reach 17% by the year 2030 (US Bureau of the Census, 1996). This, together with their known sensitivity to medications (Everitt and Avorn, 1986), contributed to acceptance by the industry of additional requirements for testing in the elderly.

The US Bureau of the Census, International Database (1996) (National Center for Health Statistics, 1996) projected that, for the year 2020, developing countries would contain only 16.4% of the world population compared to 27.1% in 1996, and that by 2020 the mean age of the population in more developed countries would be 42 years, up from 36 years in 1996. In developed regions, the elderly would outnumber young children by 8:1, for example in Italy, based on current fertility and survival rates, only 2% of the population would be five years or younger, but 40% would be 65 years and older.

There were even more startling projections by the United Nations International Population Division (1996). They projected life expectancy in the developed countries to reach 81 years by 2050. For developing countries, this would still reach 76 years. However, this increase in the global elderly population would be proportionally offset by a decrease in birth rate, now under way, from 1.7 births per woman down to 1.4 in the Western world. This is below the replacement rate. For Second World regions, the rate of about 3.3 births per woman would decline to 1.6. Even in developing countries, five births per woman would fall to two by 2050. Thus, the whole world would actually start to "depopulate" in 40 years. In the US, the birth rate is 2.05 births per woman, mainly driven by new immigrants.

The social and healthcare impact of these demographics in the United States and across the globe will lead to an increased demand for better medicines directed at a healthy old age. This elderly population has more income than average per capita income. In the United States, 70 million "baby-boomers" are starting to retire to a total of 86.7 million retirees, 21% of the population (US Administration on Ageing, 2005). In addition, with more time on their hands to lobby, they are more likely to vote, and can be expected to use their political muscle to make demands on their governments. The governments will respond in the usual knee-jerk reaction—"more regulations and controls" on industry—while increasing funding for academic research aimed at improving the quality of life and the prolongation of active old age. It will be interesting to see whether a more extended life expectancy, over and above the current projections, will reverse the depopulation trend. A new census was taken in 2010.

Principles and Practice of Pharmaceutical Medicine, 3rd edition.
Edited by L.D. Edwards, A.W. Fox, P.D. Stonier.
© 2011 Blackwell Publishing Ltd.

Impact of an ageing population on the society

In developed countries, by 2017, the working population aged 15–65 years will fall from 59.7% in 2009 to 55.6%. Those aged 65 years and over will increase to 20 from 16% (US Bureau of Census, 1996); from five workers down to four workers to support each retiree. In the United States, 60 years ago, the retirement age for Social Security "pension" was designed for an expected average lifespan of 65 years. Already this has been pushed back to 67 years by year 2004, and additional legislation will probably push the age requirements back to 70 in 10 years' time, when the "baby-boomers" swell the retired population.

To encourage the healthy older person to continue working beyond 65 years, legislation was passed to remove the penalty (in workers 65–70 years) of the loss of US$1 for every US$2 earned from Social Security benefits in the United States. In December 2003, the Medicare Modernization Act (MMA) was signed into law by President G.W. Bush. Because the older people were the greatest users, they are now eligible for drug cost reimbursement under Medicaid. This would give the US Government reimbursement control on more than 58% of drugs prescribed and the power to "set price," as in other countries (e.g., Canada, the UK, France, Italy, Germany). This has sent a chill through the US pharmaceutical industry. The current situation is that the government will not use this volume to drive prices down. How long this legislation will remain un-amended is to be seen, because the Democratic Party is still in power (as of 2010) and pressing for changes.

Of great concern is the social and financial impact of Alzheimer's disease, whose incidence per capita increases to 32% of the surviving population at ages 80–85 (and declines rapidly after age 85). Many live with this disease for 5–10 years before succumbing. This causes enormous detriment to the surviving spouse and family and to family finances, and must eventually impact Medicaid and Medicare Federal and State budgets. The duration of financial burden of terminal care is 1–4 months in general (1–18 months for Alzheimer's patients) and, even with what would normally be an adequate pension, this burden can financially ruin the surviving spouse. In the United States alone, Alzheimer's disease will affect 16 million people by 2050 (Tauzin, 2008), and 91 medicines are being developed for Alzheimer's disease.

Immigration from the developing to the developed countries will increase as countries of ageing populations try to replace the loss of their labor pool. This is already happening in Europe and in the United States. This again will put further pressure on Medicare and Medicaid, because many of these immigrants will suffer from tuberculosis, hepatitis, and intestinal disease, endemic to many of their home countries. In 1997, 39% of tuberculosis cases in the United States were in foreign-born parents; in California, this rose to 67% (Satcher, 1999) and the annual cost of diagnosis and treatment of the one million immigrants was US$40 million (Muenning et al., 1999). This will cause further competition for available health dollars.

Prescribing and adverse events

Studies of drug utilization in the elderly show that older people receive disproportionate amounts of medication (Rochon and Gurwitz, 1995). A study in rural persons 65 years or older showed that, of 967 interviewed, 71% took at least one prescription drug and 10% took five or more prescription medications. Again, women took more medications than men, and in both groups, the number of drugs increased with age. The elderly comprised 18% of the population but received 45% of all prescription items (Lassila et al., 1996).

One in ten admissions to acute geriatric units was caused or partly caused by adverse drug reactions. The drugs involved most commonly were benzodiazepines, warfarin, digoxin, and non-steroidal anti-inflammatories (Denham and Barnet, 1998). Tamblyn (1996), in his review article, cites reports of adverse events causing 5–23% of hospitalizations, nearly 2% of ambulatory visits, and one in 1000 deaths in the general population. These rates increase in the elderly. Errors in prescribing accounted for 19–36% of hospital admissions due to drug-related adverse events.

In 2003, Gurwitz, *et al.* reported on an analysis of 27,617 Medicare enrollees aged 65 and older cared for by a multi-specialty group practice in a health screen finance organization over a 1-year period in 1999 and 2000. The report identified 1,523 adverse drug events, of which 27.6% were preventable. Of the events, 578 (38%) were considered serious, life threatening, or fatal, and of these, 42.2% were deemed preventable, either errors in monitoring (60.9%), and/or errors in prescribing (58.4%). In some instances of the preventable serious events, 21.1% were compounded by patient compliance problems.

In 2006, the US Center for Disease Control and Prevention (CDC) published a serious adverse drug event incidence of 6.7% as the mean of all US emergency departments leading to hospital admission (Budnitz *et al.*, 2006). This did not include suicide attempts or drug abuse. A similar earlier study in the UK (Pirmohamed *et al.*, 2004) gave a similar percentage of 6.5% of 18,820 admissions being for serious drug-related adverse events.

The CDC study also showed that the elderly were at greater risk: 8.8% of all events were due to serious adverse events due to medication (8.1% in women, 5.4% in men).

With one in 15 hospital admissions due to drug intoxication, greater concern to the unnecessary distress, damage, and the resulting human and dollar costs need to be addressed especially in the preventable areas and patient compliance.

To compound this worrying situation, there is the concomitant use of over-the-counter (OTC) non-prescription drugs. Only 50% of physicians or health workers ask about OTC drug use, and yet 40% of all drugs used by the elderly are non-prescription. In all, 69% of the elderly use OTC drugs, and 70% take at least one prescription, as described earlier. In addition, 31% take alcohol frequently (Conn, 1992).

Qato *et al.* (2008) reported from a survey undertaken in individuals 57 through 85 years of age: 81% used at least one prescription medication, 42% used at least one OTC medication, and 49% also used a dietary "supplement." Twenty-nine percent used at least five prescription medications, concurrently highest in men and woman 75 to 85 years old. Some individuals combined prescription, OTC, and dietary supplements. Overall, 4% of individuals were at risk of a major drug-drug interaction. More than half the drugs prescribed were anticoagulants or anti-platelet adhesion agents.

This new potential for adverse drug interaction is enormous. Interaction of NSAIDs and aspirin with anticoagulants, such as warfarin, can increase the bleeding tendency, and not just from the stomach. Antacids can decrease the excretion of antidepressant tricyclics as well as quinidine, pseudoephedrine, and indomethacin. They can also reduce the absorption of digoxin and β-blocker anti-hypertensive medication. These are only a few of the multitude of interactive drug effects. This is imposed on the reduced efficacy of hepatic metabolism and elimination, and renal excretion in the elderly (on average, about a 30% reduction). Thus, OTC drug use can add to the recipe for toxic drug accumulation and, in the latter case of antacids, cause further damage to the kidney by loss of blood pressure control and worsening cardiac failure.

Practical and ethical issues of drug research in older populations

Traditionally, elderly subjects were frequently excluded from clinical drug development (unless the disease being treated was more prevalent in that age group). The reasons given were that the elderly suffer from too many other concurrent diseases requiring concomitant medicines, are frailer, and are more vulnerable to adverse events. All these can cause "static" in the interpretation of the data, and give undue weight to adverse events in the labeling and product package insert.

In addition, the elderly can exhibit differences, both physiologic and pathologic compared with the younger population; the contrast in speed of disease progression of prostate cancer in the "younger elderly" compared to the slower rate in the "older old," is an example. The older elderly may be confused or demented, making informed consent and their continuation in a study questionable. Finally, the elderly indication may represent only a small use of a drug, for example, seasonal allergies that decrease with age; it is uneconomic to include the elderly in a drug's development program. These are some of the perceived concerns of both investigators and pharmaceutical firms.

What is "geriatric?" Strictly defined, it describes a person aged 65 years or over, but ageing is neither a homogeneous nor a linear process. There are very fit 80-year-olds who climb mountains, an 85-year-old former US President parachuting, and young children dying from genetic advanced ageing (progeria). The elderly therefore cover a spectrum of fitness. Therefore, many of the above concerns can be reduced by selecting "uncomplicated, healthy" older patients in Phase I studies, who are increasingly available due to the success of medicines and preventative medicine.

However, there is a need to know how medicines behave in the real world—not just their interactions with other medicines but also in other disease states suffered concurrently, which is often the case in a geriatric population and less so in younger age groups. For the elderly, of equal importance to life extension and cure is improvement or preservation of their activities. Thus, the results of quality of life, patient and disease outcomes, and pharmacoeconomic studies are of even greater relevance to this special population and to third-party payers.

Regulatory response

By the 1980s, most of the new medicines still had little or no information on elderly dosing or contained disclaimers. As a result, and the fact that 30% of prescription drugs by then were consumed by just 12% of the population (those over 65 years), a new guideline was issued. Thus, the Food and Drug Administration (FDA) *Guideline on Drug Development in the Elderly* (1990) recommended that, if a drug was likely to have significant use in the elderly, studies should be done in an elderly population. These studies should look at effective-

ness and adverse events by age. In addition, other studies should determine whether older people handle the new drug differently (a 30% decrease in renal excretion and liver metabolism is normal in a healthy elderly person). This Guideline also required studies of the pharmacokinetics (PK) and, where possible, pharmacodynamic (PD) studies of the new drug in the elderly. The FDA Guideline also urged the study of possible drug interactions with drugs commonly used concurrently in this age group. Digoxin was given as an example. Looking even further forward to the future, the Guideline encouraged the inclusion of patients over 75 years of age.

Medicines in the elderly had become a world issue and, in 1994, the FDA implemented the International Conference on Harmonization (ICH) tripartite guidance, *Studies in Support of Special Populations: Geriatrics* (Federal Register, August 1994). The agency followed up with specific requirements on content and format of labeling for human prescription drugs, the addition of a "Geriatric Use" subsection in labeling (Federal Register, August 1997). This set out priority implementation lists of drug categories for information in the geriatric population and gave the industry one year to comply. It also set out the specific content and format of wording to be used.

Overview of International Conference on Harmonization Guideline

This Guideline was very similar to the 1990 FDA *Guideline on Drug Development in the Elderly* in intent. It made the following requests:
• Studies should be done on new molecular entities (NMEs) or new chemical entities (NCEs) likely to be used in the elderly, either to treat a disease of ageing or because the disease is also common in the elderly.
• Studies should include patients 65 years and older, and preferably patients aged 75 years or older, and advised against arbitrary age cut-off (patients aged 60–65 are not considered elderly).

- Meaningful numbers, especially in Phase III: a minimum of 100 patients was suggested for a non-geriatric-specific disease (e.g., hypertension).
- Analysis of the database for age-related differences of efficacy, adverse events, dose and (gender) relationships. A geriatric database may contain data from the main Phase II and III studies or from a geriatric-specific study.
- PK studies, either formal PK studies or on a population basis, should be carried out. For the latter, a blood sample is taken from many patients on up to four occasions. The time of dosing is recorded, and the time of samples. The patients must be in "steady state." This way, an adequate population PK plot can be built.
- PK studies in renal-impaired patients if the drug or metabolites are renally excreted. If the NME/NCE is excreted and/or metabolized by the liver, a hepatic-impaired study should be undertaken. These studies do not have to be done in elderly patients (they are usually done on a new NME anyway).
- Although, usually, differences in the therapeutic response or adverse events are too small to detect at an equivalent plasma level between ordinary adult and elderly patients to make this a requirement, separate studies are requested of sedative hypnotic psychoactive drugs or drugs having a significant CNS effect, and similarly, if Phase II and III studies are suggestive of an age-related difference.
- Drug interaction studies should be done on digoxin and oral anticoagulants, because these drugs have a narrow therapeutic range and are commonly prescribed in the elderly, and these drugs frequently have their serum levels altered by other drugs. Where drugs are heavily metabolized by the liver, the effect of drug enzyme inducers and inhibitors should be explored. Similarly, drugs that will share the same cytochrome P450 enzyme pathways should be tested. Ketoconazole, macrolides, and quinidine are given as examples. Finally, other common drugs most likely to be used with the test drug are recommended to be explored for possible synergistic or antagonistic drug interactions.

Industry response

A survey conducted by the FDA in 1983 (Abrams, 1993) showed that, for 11 drugs recently approved or awaiting approval of New Drug Applications (NDAs), in seven applications 30–36% of patients were aged over 60. In one application, a study on a drug for prostate cancer, 76% of patients were, not surprisingly, over 60 years old (Everitt and Avorn, 1986). An additional survey by the FDA in 1988 of 20 NDAs showed similar results but, in addition, analysis by age and PK studies in the elderly were frequently included. A survey by the Pharmaceutical Research and Manufacturers of America (PhRMA) (Tauzin, 1995) showed that 917 medicines were being studied for potential use in the elderly. These included 373 drugs targeting indications of old age, 166 for heart disease and stroke.

A private survey of 19 pharmaceutical companies operating in the United States (Chaponis, 1998) ranked cardiovascular disease, depression, Alzheimer's disease, hypertension, rheumatoid arthritis, osteoarthritis, and oncology as the most important therapeutic areas in their company. All of these conditions are commonly found in the elderly. Why did companies target these therapeutic areas in the geriatric population? This drew the following responses: "It's a growing population," from 77% of respondents, and "increasing market size," from 58% of the 27 company respondents. Companies were asked which types of geriatric-based clinical trials they conducted. Safety, efficacy, PK, and drug interaction studies were quoted in that order of frequency, which because of the introduction of the guidelines, is to be expected. However, the next most frequent studies were quality-of-life, pharmacoeconomic, drug disease (outcomes), and patient satisfaction studies. The later studies reflect the elderly and third-party payers' influences (Chaponis, 1998). In its 2005 survey, PhRMA reported that more than 600 medicines were then being developed just for diseases of ageing. This reflects the increasing importance of medicines for the graying population of the United States.

Issues of diseases in the elderly

Hypertension affects about 50% of the elderly population. There is also a unique form called isolated systolic hypertension (ISH), which affects 9% of the geriatric population and is growing as the population ages. The challenges of doing studies in this area increase with the age of patients admitted, which correlates with increased concomitant medications and illness and compliance, but otherwise relates well to study designs in the younger age group. Hypertension is a major cause of three major events causing death in the elderly: *coronary heart disease*, *heart failure*, and *stroke*.

Coronary heart disease caused one in five deaths in 2002 at an average age of 65.8 for men and 70.4 for women (American Heart Association, 2005).

Heart failure is a leading cause of hospitalization of the elderly. About five million Americans suffer from this disease, which has a high mortality rate. Control of blood pressure, use of β-blockers, ACE inhibitors, and now spironolactone (Pitt *et al.*, 1999) will result in further improvement in mortality rates, which have started to fall from 117 per 110,000 in 1988 to 108 per 110,000 in 1995, according to the CDC.

Because of its severity, patients are on many concomitant medications apart from the aforementioned drugs, such as anticoagulants or "blood thinners": diuretics, digoxin, potassium supplements, medicines to improve pulmonary function, and antibiotics to control frequent infection in edematous and often emphysematous lungs. Measurements of heart function, and the long duration of these studies and large patient numbers required for mild to moderate heart failure (endpoint death), make these very challenging and expensive studies.

Stroke, thrombotic or hemorrhagic, is the third leading cause of death, killing 160,000 persons in the United States each year, 7 out of 10 victims being aged 65 or older. Of those that survive, one-third will be permanently disabled. Some improvements in these figures are hoped for, with earlier use of thrombolytics in the case of cerebral thrombosis. As of 2009, more than 22 (Tauzin, 2008) new drugs were in development to treat this condition.

Arthritis causing inflammatory and degenerative changes around joints affects 43 million people in the United States, and CDC projects that this will rise to 60 million by 2020. It can be caused by more than 100 different diseases, but the most common are osteoarthritis and rheumatoid arthritis. New medications, such as the anti-tumor necrotic factor antibody-blockers, raise fresh challenges to clinical study methodology because of limitations on nonclinical toxicity predictors and the application of biologic measurements to the traditional drug appraisal system.

The new non-steroidal anti-inflammatory drugs, including the Cox II inhibitors, because of the vast range of arthritic diseases, require careful selection of indications for initial product approval. Rarely do companies have the time or money to develop all the pain indications (acute, chronic use) or to study all the many arthritic diseases prior to product launch. As with hypertension, the numbers of patients required in the database will be large for product approval, especially for safety.

Depression is a frequently missed diagnosis in the elderly. The National Alliance on Mental Illness (2009) says that 18.5% of Americans aged 65 years and older experience clinically relevant depression. It can amplify the underlying disabilities in stroke, arthritis, or Parkinson's disease, slow or prevent recovery from hip fracture and surgery, and be mimicked or masked by an underactive thyroid. The latest receptor-specific medicines have a very much reduced potential for adverse events and drug interactions. Difficulties can arise from confusion, memory impairment, and disorientation, which are common in the depressed elderly. This brings challenges of ensuring both drug compliance and follow-up attendance in clinical studies. It also may require guardian or caretaker co-signature for informed witnessed consent.

Parkinson's disease affects more than one million Americans and about four in every 100 by 75 years of age. Ten new drugs are under development. The patients may become very physically disabled but still retain a clear sensorium until the very end stages of the disease, where plaques and neural tangles similar to those found Alzheimer's disease and older Down's syndrome patients are found.

Thus, drug compliance and follow-up visits are easier to achieve than with Alzheimer's or depressed patients.

Alzheimer's disease is the eighth leading cause of death in the elderly and already affects some four million Americans. The incidence rises from 2% at 65 years to 32% at age 85. The National Institute of Health (NIH) estimates that at least half of the people in nursing homes have this disease. A small study of donezil showed that this treatment avoided the need for home nursing care by half compared to those who did not receive the medicine (Small, 1998).The financial impact of this can be measured in billions of dollars.

The available drugs for the treatment of Alzheimer's disease at present only have a short-term effect, six months in most patients; estrogen is not brain-protective as hoped, nor are the statins (McGuinness *et al.*, 2009). Results in Alzheimer mice of the equivalent of caffeine, in three cups of espresso coffee/day, have yet to be replicated in humans (Arendash, 2009), although the discovery that APOE4 and TOMM40 genes are involved in 90% of all cases may help (Roses, 2009: announced at the July 2009 annual meeting in Vienna of the Alzheimer's Disease Association).

Clinical studies in this disease are very expensive, often requiring several collaborating disciplines at each investigative site. A gerontologist, a neurologist, a psychologist, and a psychiatrist may be required, in addition to the usual support staff. Multiple cognitive tests and behavioral ratings of the patient, often involving primary caregiver ratings, will be required—all this in addition to the basic Alzheimer's Disease Assessment Scale (ADAS–COG). More recently, positron emission tomography with the Radioactive Fluorine-18 test, along with the Fluorodeoxyglucose test, are bringing more accuracy to the diagnoses. Despite these tests the diagnosis is still regarded as presumptive until a post mortem or biopsy sample confirms the diagnosis. These studies, at present, require large numbers of patients to show the often small improvement, as well as months of observation to detect a slowing of progression. As well as large numbers, many of these studies are conducted at multinational sites, and so so it must be asked whether cognitive scales have been validated in different cultural backgrounds?

Issues in the conduct of clinical studies in the elderly

Informed consent

In general, the principles are no different with the elderly than with other adults (see Chapter 8); the elderly are just as subject to the relationship to the researcher if the clinician and researcher are one and the same. Not wishing to offend (by refusal) is very strong in the elderly, and also they are also subject to "therapeutic fallacy," that is, they find it hard to accept that, despite repeated descriptions of risks and possible benefits, the treating physician could be really offering them treatment of uncertain benefit or risk. The elderly are more likely to have cognitive impairment or mild dementia, and to be living alone, in poverty, or under institutional care. They are also vulnerable to caregiver abuse, often because of indifference, anger, or physical abuse triggered by the patients' behavior and difficulties derived from their disease.

Hearing or vision problems must be expected; bright light and large print, together with honest and simple language, are much used for eliciting the informed consent. Research subjects, whether elderly or not, should be able to understand the informed consent process, which regrettably is normally written at reading grade 12 or higher. They should understand that they may refuse to participate or to withdraw from the study without reprisal and understand the risks and uncertain outcomes of the new drug, the use of placebo, and the random allocation of treatment.

The most vulnerable elderly population is found in nursing homes or mental institutions and frequently comprises persons of diminished or fluctuating mental ability. Ironically, regulations governing research in these patients were proposed but never voted upon. The NIH established a policy that allowed a patient, when still in a good cognitive condition, to appoint a "Health Care Agent."

For industry, prior written agreement of a family member with the potential subject to act as "guardian" is preferred but not always attainable. It is best for the researcher to meet personally with relatives, nursing staff, and residents, and fully explain to them the study purpose, benefit, and risks, as well as to the patient. Not infrequently, any of these persons may feel protective of the patient and undermine the research objective. It is wise that all family members who are not involved be sent a letter explaining the research, including a form to be completed if they wish to prevent the patient being involved in research.

Compliance

Compliance in the elderly in general is similar to that of the general population. If more than six drugs are prescribed long-term, or more than three doses per day are required, compliance will suffer (Gately, 1968; Blackwell, 1979). These factors are more common in the elderly. Recommendations for improving compliance in older patients are similar to any other studies, except for one: The physician should set priorities for which medications are critical to patients' health in a polypharmacy setting. The medication regimens should be as simple as possible; the caregiver and patient should be educated about the name, dose, and reason for all medications. Patients should be given simple instructions on cards, together with suggestions on how to remind themselves: "tick-off cards on fridge," "diary notes" on bathroom mirror for morning dose, or on pantry door "with food" and so on. Patients and their caregivers should be given educational pamphlets about their diseases. They should be encouraged to ask questions or report possible adverse events or strange feelings. Patients should be asked to repeat back instructions. Finally, there are telephone call services that will call and remind patients to take the medicine, or help organize cabs or transport for follow-up visits, either to the laboratories for blood work and so on, or to the investigator appointments.

Screening and recruitment

The Chaponis (1998) survey of 19 US-based companies recorded also that 32% reported difficulty in finding suitable investigative sites for geriatric patients. In addition, those respondents involved in Phase IV outcome, quality-of-life and pharmacoeconomic studies, and so on, said that the lack of "in-company" geriatric expertise and resources was a barrier. Locating suitable investigative centers for geriatric studies is only part of the solution and works well for the smaller elderly experience studies. Nonetheless, in clinical studies undertaken for specific diseases in ageing, much larger numbers of patients must be enrolled.

Even the large resources of the NIH can be strained. The Systolic Hypertension in the Elderly Person (SHEP) investigation recruited 4736 patients aged 60–96 years (average 72). The patient screening and selection was organized from 16 sites but took 31 months to complete, which had initially been projected to be 24 months. Nearly 450,000 patients were screened (SHEP Cooperative Research Group, 1991). Hall (1993) reported on 15 cardiovascular studies funded by the National Heart and Lung Blood Institute (NHLBI) over 10 years. All overran their projected recruitment times by an average of 27%. Overoptimistic projections are the norm, and this norm has been called "Lasagna's Law" (Spilker and Cramer, 1972). For pharmaceutical clinical physicians and their staff, similar overruns are not excused by management, and raise the temptation to "move the target" by closing recruitment at a lower level. This solution compromises the statistical robustness of the study; both the problem and this solution are career busters. Better to project realistically and plan recruitment and fallback strategies.

Hall (1993) also varied the recruitment strategies used; the most successful was community screening. This can be done through appeals to senior centers, churches, shopping centers, and major industrial sites (Melish, 1982). Medical chart review is also productive if the condition has a International Classification of Disease (ICD) code and charts are available to the investigators.

For large studies, mass-mailing to registered voters, members of organized groups such as the American Association of Retired Persons (AARP) or members of a disease association can be helpful, with 7–12% response rate (McDermon and Bradford, 1982). Use of media campaigns can result in up to 11% of first protocol visits (Levenkrow and

Farquhar, 1982). These need at least 3–6 months of planning for resources to respond to the initial wave of inquiries. The approach can be a newspaper article and advertisements in regional papers, TV, and radio. Appeals to community physicians for referrals are usually disappointing, possibly caused by the physician believing that he or she will lose a paying patient to a research clinic.

Conclusion

The growth of the ageing population, regulatory overview, and increased business opportunities will ensure the growth of clinical research in the elderly. Recent reports of the high level of seniors' adverse events, many leading to deaths, both in and outside hospitals, will force more monitoring systems for medications. Soon, plastic medicine card chips with imprinted medication recorded by the pharmacist will be required by third-party insurers. This would ensure that all current concurrent medications are captured.

There is a shortage of geriatric specialists, which will take time to be corrected if the 600 drugs under development are to be adequately researched. The rapid growth of sheltered self-care communal housing for active seniors, which guarantee healthcare up to terminal status, illustrates that seniors wish to stay out of nursing homes. Their expectation of the pharmaceutical industry is that it should provide them with medications which allow for an active safe old age. The industry has heard.

References

Abrams WB. Food and Drug Administration Guideline for the study of drugs in elderly patients: an industry perspective. In *Inclusion of Elderly Individuals in Clinical Trials*, Wenger NK (ed.). Marion Merrel Dow: Kansas, USA, 1993, 213–217.

American Heart Association. 2005. www.americanheart.org; accessed March 29, 2010.

Arendash G. Caffeine reverses cognitive impairment and decreases beta-amyloid levels in aged Alzheimer disease mice, *Journal of Alzheimer's Disease*. 2009; **17**:661–680.

Blackwell B. The drug regimen and treatment complications. In *Compliance in Health Care*, Haynes RB, Taylor DN, Sackett DL (eds). John Hopkins University Press: Baltimore, Maryland, 1979, 144–156.

Budnitz DS, Pollock, DA; Weidenbach, KN *et al.* National surveillance of emergency department visits for out patient adverse events. *JAMA* 2006; **296**:1858–1866.

Chaponis R. Geriatic-based research in the pharmaceutical industry. Private survey (personal correspondence), 1998.

Conn VS. Self-management of over-the-counter medications by older adults. *Public Health Nurse* 1992; **9**(1): 22–28.

Denham MJ, Barnet NC. Drug therapy and the older person; the role of the pharmacist. *Drug Safety* 1998; **19**(4):243–250.

Everitt DE, Avorn J. Drug prescribing for the elderly. *Arch Inter Med* 1986; **146**:2393–2396.

Federal Register. Studies in support of special populations: geriatric. *Federal Register*, 2 August 1994, 59 FR; 390–398.

Federal Register. Specific requirements of content and format of labeling for human prescription drugs: addition of 'Geriatric Use' subsection (1997). *Federal Register*, **62**(166), August 1997; 45313–45326.

Federal Register. Guidelines for the study of drugs likely to be used in the elderly. *Federal Register*, March 1999, 55 FR; 7777.

Gately MS. To be taken as directed. *J R College Geriat Pract* 1968; **16**:39–44.

Gurwitz RH, Field JS, Avorn J. *et al.* Incidence and preventability of adverse drug reactions effects amongst older persons in the ambulatory settings, *JAMA* 2003; **289**:1107–16.

Hall WD. Screening and recruitment of elderly participants into large scale cardiovascular studies. In *Inclusion of Elderly Individuals into Clinical Trials*, Wenger NK (ed.). Marion Merrill Dow: Kansas, USA, 1993, 67–71.

Lassila HC, Stoehr GP, Ganguli M, *et al.* Use of prescription medications in an elderly rural population. *Ann Pharmacother* 1996; **30**(6):589–595.

Levenkrow JC, Farquhar JW. Recruitment using mass media strategies. *Circulation* 1982; **66**(Suppl IV):32–36.

McDermon M, Bradford RH. Recruitment by use of mass mailings. *Circulation* 1982; **66**(6, part 2):27–31.

McGuinness B, *et al.* Statins for the prevention of dementia. *BMJ* 2009; **338**:b158.

Melish JS. Recruitment by community screenings. *Circulation* 1982; **66**(Suppl IV):20–23.

Muenning P, Pallin D, Sel RC, Chan MS. The cost of effectiveness of strategies for the treatment of intestinal parasites in immigrants. *New Engl J Med* 1999; **340**(10): 773–779.

National Alliance on Mental Illness. 2009. http://www. nami.org/Content/NavigationMenu/Mental_Illnesses/ Depression/Depression_in_Seniors.htm.

National Center for Health Statistics. 1996. US Department of Health and Human Services (data from 1996).

Pirmohamed M., Meakin S, Green C. *et al.* Adverse drug reactions as a cause of admission to hospital: perspective analysis of 18,820 patients. *BMJ* 2006; **329**:15–19.

Pitt B, Zannad F, Remme WJ, *et al.* The effects of spironolactone on morbidity and mortality in patients with severe heart failure. *New Engl J Med* 1999; **2341**(10): 709–177.

Qato D, Alexander GC, Lindau ST, *et al.* Use of prescription over the counter medication and dietary supplements among older adults in the United States. *JAMA*; 2008: **300**(2):2867–2878.

Roses A. International Conference on Alzheimer's Disease, July 2009, proceedings in press.

Rochon P, Gurwitz JH. Optimizing drug treatment for elderly people: the prescribing cascade. *BMJ* 1997; **315**: 1096–1099.

Satcher D. Global health at the cross-roads: Surgeon General's report to the 50th World Assembly. *J Am Med Assoc* 1999; **281**:942–943.

SHEP Cooperative Research Group. Prevention of stroke by hypertensive drugs treatment in old persons with isolated systolic hypertension: final results of the Systolic Hypertension in the Elderly Program (SHEP). *J Am Med Assoc* 1991; **265**:3255–3264.

Small J. An economic evolution of donepezil in the treatment of Alzheimer's Disease. *Clin Ther* 1998; **20**(4): 838–850.

Spilker B, Cramer JA (eds). *Patient Recruitment in Clinical Trials.* Rowen: New York, 1972.

Tamblyn R. Medical use in seniors: challenges and solutions. *Therapy* 1996; **51**(3):269–282.

Tauzin W. *Survey of Medicines in Development for Older Americans* and survey on heart disease and stroke, 1995; details can be obtained on request from PhRMA: www.phrma.org; accessed March 29, 2010.

Tauzin W. *Survey of Medicines in Development for Older Americans* and survey on heart disease and stroke, 2008; http://www.phrma.org/publications; accessed March 29, 2010.

United Nations International Population Division. US Administration on Ageing, 1996. www.aoa.gov; accessed March 29, 2010.

US Bureau of the Census. *Current Population Report Series,* 1996.

CHAPTER 17

Drug Development Research in Women

Lionel D. Edwards

Pharma Pro Plus Inc., New Jersey, and Temple University, School of Pharmacy, Philadelphia, USA

Background

The pharmaceutical industry is in the business of developing, manufacturing, and selling drugs, vaccines, and devices. Although basic research has become more important in recent years, it is not the primary aim of industry. However, increasingly and usually dictated by opportunity, industry is investing in a highly targeted fashion in some aspects of basic research, but the development of a product is always to the fore. This thrust, however, need not exclude the gathering of basic data, which may prove invaluable to the research process. Regrettably, these data were frequently inaccessible, in some instances owing to the needs of confidentiality, product protection, or even legal concerns, but by far the greatest reason is that such data are regarded as a by-product, almost "waste data," because they are not part of the mainstream of product development. Such data are recorded but rarely utilized, frequently residing in notebooks, case records, mainframe databanks, statistical reports, or data tabulations in the back of appendices of regulatory submissions.

So it is with gender data: it is collected, analyzed, and tabulated by each study and by each drug, but data on drugs of the same class and between each government agency handling multiple applications are virtually inaccessible. Mining these data

requires more creative solutions than "regulations." This is now happening.

It has been estimated that the average cost of developing a new drug is now US$800 million–2 billion (Masia, 2008). This estimate mostly comprises costs in development, but includes the loss of other revenue if the development money had instead been invested cumulatively. These costs are passed directly on to the consumer.

Drug costs have risen slowly compared to other health costs, when adjusted for inflation. When compared to other health costs, in 1965, the drug/device cost was less than a dime (10 cents) per health dollar, in 2004 it was less than 12 cents (Health Care Financing Administration, 2009) and in 2008, again only a dime (Center for Medicare and Medicaid Services, 2008). Drug cost is, and must remain, one of the most affordable aspects of treatment. A large component of drug development cost is caused by regulatory needs to test for drug safety and efficacy, both for the USA and foreign agencies. Clearly, the cost of any additional regulation imposed on top of the current burden will also be directly reflected in the eventual cost to the consumer.

Women comprise 51% of the population of most nations. According to the United Nations, the global female population will increase by 48.4% from 2000 to 2050, compared to males (45.4%). The population of women over 65 years will increase by 24% over 2000–2010 in the United States and 12% in Europe, and even in 2000, women of 80 years outnumbered males by a 2:1 ratio (Source: United Nations Population Database). In Western

Principles and Practice of Pharmaceutical Medicine, 3rd edition.
Edited by L.D. Edwards, A.W. Fox, P.D. Stonier.
© 2011 Blackwell Publishing Ltd.

countries, 54% of women are of childbearing potential (15–49 years). Women account for 57% of physician visits (National Disease and Therapeutic Index, 1991) and 63.2% of drug products (Neutel and Walop, 2005). In the age group 20–39 years, women were found to be the biggest users of anti-infectives, especially ampicillin and amoxicillin; antidepressants are prescribed twice as often to women as to men (Stewart, 1998); and of some concern was that tetracycline, a known teratogen, was the eighth most prescribed drug in the 38% of women of childbearing age (FDA, 1986).

As major users, it might be postulated that women, including those of childbearing age, should be the group on which Phase I and II dosing (early efficacy and safety) should be based. Why is this not so? Critics of the industry, and indeed of the wider research process, claim that it is entrenched discrimination by males, which is disguised as "concern and gallantry." Critics also point out that both medicine and research are dominated by males, who place research into women's diseases on the back burner of their male priorities and only see data, even on women, from the male point of view. They point to a report by Coale (1991) on the "missing 100 million women" in Asia and the Indian subcontinent, who are speculated not to exist because of abortion and medical and nutritional neglect. They also point to the misuse of science (ultrasound or amniocentesis) for sex determination.

Although these are extreme examples of societal attitudes, it is true that women have been excluded from many large, well-published studies, such as the Physicians' Health Study of aspirin in cardiovascular disease (Henrekens *et al.*, 1989). It is also true that many early studies of drugs in Phases I and II were conducted in healthy white males 18–40 years old, and the results then extrapolated to women in Phase III studies, primarily aimed at expanded efficacy and safety. Paul Williams (1996) confirmed that exercise raised HDL cholesterol in women, many years later than when reported in men. It is, however, in most cases, grossly naive to attribute this to deliberate "male discrimination" to exclude research on women.

It is also frequently mentioned that fear of embryonic malformation, whether or not drug related, and subsequent litigation is the major determining factor for exclusion of females from therapeutic and basic research projects. This overly simple explanation covers up other difficulties, such as methodology, lack of relevant baseline information, and biochemical variables, both hormonal and gender-related. It also ignores the use of information derived from other groups of women, those of no childbearing potential, sterile, or postmenopausal, the elderly, or children just entering puberty, where the risk of fetal exposure is nonexistent or minimal.

The dilemmas

Do women respond to medications differently than men? If so, in what ways and how frequently are these changes clinically meaningful? Review of the literature shows some examples of differences between the sexes in drug handling, particularly with certain classes of drugs. These will be dealt with later, but it is important to bear in mind that, despite some detectable differences, usually no therapeutically significant differences are seen (Edwards, 1991). This is unlikely to be due to lack of compliance, because women are generally more reliable than men, although compliance does fall off to 67% over a few weeks for both genders (Cramer *et al.*, 1990). This does not exclude self adjustment of dose by female patients, a phenomenon seen in both sexes and probably much more common than reported.

It has also been claimed (because gender data are rarely mentioned in clinical studies, papers, or reports) that gender differences are not sought. This presupposes that data are neither collected nor examined. In fact, the opposite is much more likely: 94% of surveyed pharmaceutical firms were found to collect gender data in their studies (Edwards, 1991). The reality is that findings of no differences are rarely reported, but sometimes any findings may just be a function of small sample size for each individual study or the small degree of difference to be found. It must also be recognized that many drugs were introduced into medicine prior to the current modern-day comprehensive testing programs. Nonetheless, after many years and millions of prescriptions, it is of reassurance that few have shown significant clinically important gender-related differences.

Differences in disease presentations

A report from the National, Heart, Lung and Blood Institute (NHLBI, 2001) showed that there is a similar incidence in both genders of heart disease (slightly greater in women) but that the age of major incidents between gender is different: 24% of the 65–74 year-old males compared to about 18% of females in the same age group. This incidence rises in both genders at 75–84 years to about 28% males and 30% females, though stroke is 19% more common in males (Moscal, 1997).

Not only do women develop heart disease later but they also present differently. The signature symptom of a heart attack, severe chest pain, is often absent in women, and pain in the upper back or neck, or fatigue, breathlessness, and nausea, may present as a single symptom or as multiple symptoms. The American Heart Association (2008) states that 44% of women are likely to die in the first five years of their heart attack, compared to 33% of men.

It is not surprising that heart attack and angina are misdiagnosed more commonly in women than men during emergency room visits. The range between hospitals of misdiagnosis was 0–11%, with an average 2.3% for angina and 2.1% for heart attacks. The diagnosis was missed in 7% of women under 55 years (Pope *et al.*, 2000).

Finally a large NIH study (the Women's Health Study of 40,000 women), completed in 2005, showed that aspirin gave no cardiac protection to women as had previously been assumed, though it did reduce the incidence of ischemic strokes in women over 65 years. This compared to the reduction of heart attacks in men. A subsequent meta-analysis of six studies, including the Women's Health Study, confirmed this finding, and in addition, aspirin showed no benefit in reducing ischemic strokes in men (Berger *et al.*, 2006).

What is representative?

An additional dilemma is, what population is "representative" for female dose and efficacy determination? Women of childbearing potential (54%)?

These will have possible hormonal cycling changes and those on contraceptive hormones will have even greater changes, added to a possible basic gender difference, either amplifying or even suppressing effects.

The needs of women aged 66 years or more are already represented in regulatory drug testing guidelines in the elderly (Federal Register, 1990), but women 50–65 years old also can lay claim to specific consideration, given the special problems associated with combined hormonal loss and age changes (e.g., osteoporosis, loss of possible cardiac estrogen protection, and changes in body fat composition and its distribution). Pregnant women, already isolated from drug development by fear of legal tort laws and, indeed, by their physicians' reluctance to even prescribe in early pregnancy, can also stake a claim to require additional studies. Finally, when studying females of childbearing potential, should we include patients on oral contraceptives (OCs), with their large levels of regulated fluctuating but synthetic hormones, or rely on females not taking OCs? The latter option will increase the risk of potential fetal exposure.

It must now be apparent that the female population (51%) contains many potential subgroups, none truly "representative," for all have major physiological differences from each other. For industry to study all groups would be impractical, uneconomical, and would gravely slow the drug development process and compromise the number of agents placed into development. To include all groups within one all-encompassing study, unless extremely large, offends a basic research nostrum: that is, to "stabilize, reduce, or remove all the variables except the one to be measured," or the signals many be lost in the static. This is especially true in Phase II studies.

The phantom fetus

Teratogenic issues

The term "phantom fetus" has been used to describe the current apprehension regarding the use of drugs in women of childbearing potential. This apprehension has dominated industrial, institutional, and private research. The thalidomide tragedy of the 1960s—the 10,000 or so deformed children now grown to adults—continue to haunt us. It must be recognized that, despite careful animal testing, the full potential for teratogenic activity of any drugs in humans will only come to light once the drug is in the marketplace, and then only when sufficient multiple exposures have occurred in pregnant patients and their fetuses. It is extremely unlikely that deliberate drug testing in pregnant women will ever become routine. However, in special circumstances, such as HIV-infected pregnant women, it is justified to include them in appropriate clinical studies. Current predictive animal screening cannot give complete assurance that the potential for teratogenicity will be uncovered in all cases. It must be remembered that the then-current 1956 screens did not discover the teratogenicity of thalidomide, nor the 16-year delayed hyperplasia and neoplasia effects on the cervix and uterus of female adolescents exposed to stilbestrol (given to prevent miscarriages during their mothers' pregnancies).

Both historically and currently, the major determination of teratogenicity is made from findings from animal screening; many agents have been eliminated from further development, and only rarely does teratogenicity become uncovered in the marketplace. Nonetheless, it requires large numbers of exposures before the more subtle embryotoxic or teratogenic effects are found, as was demonstrated most recently by the ACE inhibitors, which had passed all the screens. Indeed, these events may never be exposed. How could this be? One must take into account the "background noise" level, the so-called "natural" incidence of congenital abnormalities. By far the most common is Down's syndrome, whose incidence is known to increase with the age of the mother, although nearly all other abnormalities appear not to increase with maternal age, according to a report (Wilson, 1973). Thus, a higher incidence of "typical" drug-induced teratogenic effects serve as an early alert. The commonest abnormalities most frequently associated with drug exposure in the first trimester are neural tube defects, cardiac and renal anomalies, shortening of limbs and digits,

and failure of closure of the palate and upper lip. More subtle changes associated with exposure to drugs occur in the third trimester, with hearing and eye abnormalities predominating (Wilson, 1973). Any such determinations require many, many thousands of exposures before they become apparent.

However, many millions of women become pregnant before being aware of their pregnancy and have been exposed to environmental chemicals (most of which have never been tested), as well as over-the-counter (OTC) and prescription drugs. Also, a number of embryos are spontaneously aborted and a delay to the menstrual period of perhaps two or three weeks passes unremarked or sometimes unnoticed in a background of a national miscarriage rate of one in three pregnancies (Yoder, 1984). Teratologists have concluded that there is a threshold dose for any drug before it shows potential teratogenicity (in other words, enough must be given), and the effect tends to increase with the duration of exposure, with higher concentrations in the plasma or tissues and with the timing of the developing fetal tissues and organs (Wilson, 1973). In the first seven to eight days, the embryo is refractory to any teratogenic effect but is most susceptible 20–55 days after conception. Of some reassurance is that most drugs prescribed to women of childbearing age are antibiotics and tend to be for relatively short durations. But the tetracyclines and anti-epileptic drugs are known to have effects on the developing fetus and are frequently prescribed to women (Stewart, 1998).

It is an irony that the normal tenet of US and UK law that an individual is "innocent until proven guilty" does not apply to prescribed pharmaceutical products or devices. They must be proven safe and efficacious before they are approved; in other words, they must be proven to be innocent. Thus, it comes as no surprise that industry and other research groups tend to avoid the potential exposure of women of childbearing age in the early clinical development of pharmaceuticals or devices, for many experimental drugs (perhaps nine out of ten tested in humans) will never achieve the marketplace.

The potential for pregnancy while on a trial drug

What is the risk of pregnancy occurring in a study participant while a new drug is being developed? The author is not aware of any published figures, but from the author's experience in industry and from questions to colleagues, pregnancy does occur during drug development, even in those patients apparently taking adequate contraceptive precautions. A typical New Drug Application (NDA) database for most drugs will involve between 2000 and 4000 patients, of which perhaps half are female and exposed to study medication. It is not surprising, therefore, that given an average failure rate of the contraceptive pill of 2%, or even with the most stringent compliance (double barrier), a failure fate of 0.5/100 women years will result in occasional pregnancy (Trussell *et al.*, 1990). Other methods, such as the diaphragm, condoms, and IUDs, can carry even higher failure rates, depending on whether "usual" or "perfect compliance" calculations of 18.6%, 12.2%, and 3.05%, respectively, are used (Trussell *et al.*, 1990). If we assume an average NDA database of 4000 patients, one-third or more being female, it is likely that half of these will be females of childbearing potential (the other half being post-menopausal or elderly). Thus, approximately 660 females of childbearing potential may be exposed to the drug, the comparator, or a placebo. In the best circumstances of perfect contraceptive compliance, in a one-year exposure and at a 0.5% failure rate, 3.3 fetuses are likely to be exposed. With a "typical compliance" of the contraceptive pill, a 3% failure rate would leave about 19 fetuses exposed to experimental entities, one-third of which would be lost due to spontaneous miscarriage.

Few patients would be exposed for a full year, but more typically only between two weeks and three months of study medication. Given all the above assumptions, between 0.8 and 5 early embryos will be exposed in a full drug development program. From the author's personal experience of over 36 years in industry, an average of two children are born exposed to a new chemical entity per NDA. This is most likely to occur in Phase III studies, which have many more patients and are often of longer duration. Currently, pharmaceutical firms, with the agreement of the Food and Drug Administration (FDA), follow up all possible exposures until any resultant child is 12–14 years of age, and a full medical examination (including a full neurological workup) is done at yearly intervals.

The potential for teratogenic damage during drug study programs

As previously mentioned, the best sources for the actual figures for the above calculations reside within the FDA but may, as alluded, be inaccessible. In recent years, figures given by the agency, for example in elderly drug-testing studies, appear to have been hand-tallied rather than garnered from composite computer access. However, the agency is now involved in a large effort to "mine" data across therapeutic classes, some of which, with meta-analysis, will provide data that individual drug programs never could, nor were designed to show.

The ability to access data across drugs and across drug classes will grow as firms put in computer-assisted NDAs (CANDAs) in appropriate and compatible programs and formats. What is the risk of a fetus being damaged during an "average" NDA drug development program? Obviously small. Clearly, toxic but "life-saving" treatment will carry a heavy embryotoxic risk; anticancer, anti-AIDS drugs, and fetal intrauterine surgical procedures are obvious examples, but the clear-cut risks involved are usually deemed acceptable. A more subtle judgment call involves the development of anti-epileptic drugs. Let us look at two examples. It has been estimated that exposure of pregnant women to normal therapeutic doses of valproic acid may give rise to 1% fetal abnormality rate involving the neural tube (Lindhaut and Schmidt, 1986); that is, 10 times the natural incidence. Many of these defects are correctable with modern surgical techniques. Exposure to phenobarbitone also has a reported higher incidence of cleft lip and palate defects (Frederick, 1973): most are surgically correctible. If used in combination, the incidences of anticonvulsant teratogenic effects are increased (Lindhaut *et al.*, 1984). Would either of these drugs be developed in today's litigious atmosphere? It's doubtful. But both drugs are valuable in many circumstances; they may be the only drugs suitable for some patients and, indeed, frequently can be life-saving. Certainly, maternal status epilepticus is very injurious to the fetus, often resulting in miscarriage or premature birth.

The incidence of neonatal abnormalities in mothers taking anticonvulsant treatment is 70/1000 live births (Frederick, 1973). This is 2.4 times the "spontaneous rate" in the general population (29 abnormalities/1000 live births). Thus, even using a known "low-incidence" teratogen could cause 40 additional cases/1000 live births, but to determine that accurately would require many thousands of female patient exposures to be detectable against the "spontaneous" background incidence.

So, back to the opening question. What is the likelihood of detecting low-incidence, drug induced congenital effects in a drug development program? With our presumed database of 4000 patients, only 0.8–5 fetuses would be exposed to a background "spontaneous" risk of 2.9%. Each program could carry a 1 in 33 to a 1 in 6 chance of a single "spontaneous" abnormality occurring. If the drug or procedure should have low teratogenic activity (at the level of an anticonvulsant), this risk rises from 1 in 14 to 1 in 2.5 that a child will be born with a congenital abnormality in any drug development program. Both "spontaneous" or drug-induced abnormalities may occur, for example, a neural tube defect. Thus, on a single-case basis, the abnormalities will be indistinguishable for drug causality. This, in turn, can lead to litigation, and certainly to a reference in the package label insert.

Wilson has estimated that both drugs and environmental chemical exposures only account for 2–3% of developmental defects in humans (Wilson, 1972). Thus, a product-label reference of such an occurrence will be undeserved at least 97% of the time, but also may be the first signal of a teratogenic risk. It may now be appreciated why this 2–3% risk is termed the "phantom fetus" and also why the difficulty in disproving liability dominates the mainstream concerns of research, regulatory authorities, and industry alike. This "ghost risk" creates "discrimination" against female patients of childbearing potential in drug research. This "ghost" must be exorcised and contained; possible solutions will be discussed later.

Industry practice: Factors in Phase I and early Phase II testing

Medical journalist Paul Cotton (1990) asked, in a thought-provoking article, whether there is still too much extrapolation from data on middle-aged white men. Inspection of the demographics of recent NDAs will give us numbers to debate; however, these data are not readily accessible. Some Phase I testing is still undertaken in only healthy young males, and even for Phase I testing of new hormonal contraceptives for women. The reason why this occurs is multifaceted.

Timing of mutagenicity fertility and teratogenicity testing

The complete battery of tests with full histology and the development of a final report can take as long as two years. In general, only some of the mutagenicity studies are completed, and perhaps one- to three-month reports of animal testing are available when male Phase I dosing volunteer studies commence. All animal studies do not commence at the same time but are usually sequential. Some, such as post-exposure weaning and subsequent second-generation drug effect studies, will be time-consuming and expensive. Often, if mutagenicity tests, for example Ames' test or mouse lymphoma test, are positive (Ames' test has 30% false-positive rate), women will be excluded until more data are collected. Thus, only limited data are available prior to the first human exposure (for further reference, see Federal Register, 1994, 1996).

Volunteer dose-ranging studies will, by design, include high enough doses to provoke unpleasant adverse effects; also, information on "target organs" (organs likely to be most affected or harmed) is usually predictable but unconfirmed at this point. Generally, as a result of animal studies, it is thought that the effect of drugs on reproductive function in males is less than that in females and only affects the sperm viability or, rarely, the size and function of the testicles, which is usually reversible.

This is unduly optimistic, because one report by Yazigi *et al.* (1991) suggests that spermatozoa may not be immobilized or destroyed by cocaine, but may interact, and the spermatozoa themselves have the potential to act as an active transport mechanism for drugs, pesticides, and even environmental chemicals to the unfertilized ovum. They may also alter the genetic makeup of either spermatozoa or ovum. In addition, spermatozoa can be made sluggish by calcium channel blockers, leading to male infertility while on medication. Hence, the European guidelines call for male animal fertility testing prior to the start of Phase II.

The blastocyst (early embryo) is relatively resistant to damage in the first seven days, because up to 75% of cells can be destroyed before tissue differentiation and the embryo can still survive. What might happen if garden pesticides, or house builders' hard board containing formaldehyde glue and chemicals, are combined into the genetic material? If it is ever confirmed, we may have an inkling of what makes up the 65% of the "unknown" causes of developmental defects mentioned by Wilson (1972). If it could be shown that the synthetic chemicals are incorporated into the blastocyst, the field of male Phase I testing would be transformed, as would that of genetic counselling.

Testing facilities

Largely because early testing of drugs occurred in males rather than females, for reasons discussed above, most commercial and hospital units devoted to human pharmacology testing were set up to deal with a unisex population. They ran one gender study at a time, usually male, in 1993. Sleeping and bathroom facilities in the units' dormitory accommodations did not provide for mixed gender groups. Minor, but not inexpensive, alterations were quickly adopted following the publication of the FDA *Guidelines for the Study and Evaluation of Gender Differences in the Clinical Evaluation of Drugs* (Federal Register, 1993).

Standardizing for the menstrual cycle (Phase I and early Phase II)

Of much greater concern is the issue of standardizing the drug administration to the menstrual cycle.

Women of childbearing age do not all have cycles for the same length of days; variations of 24–36-day cycles are not unusual between and within the same women. Thus, unless controlled by OCs, women volunteers could not start and finish in a study all together. Indeed, if OCs were used to standardize cycles, the issue of how really representative of all women of childbearing age this artificial hormone-boosted group might be would be debatable. Evidence suggests that even low-dose contraceptives can affect metabolism (Abernathy and Greenblatt, 1981). The logistics of running Phase I single-dose and multiple-dose ranging studies while controlling for a natural menstrual cycle are truly horrendous, both for the phase I testing units and for the volunteer. The duration of any study would be extended by at least one month (the time required for the last patient's cycle to start), and each patient volunteer would have to be measured separately because of the different days of her cycle. A small but frequently argued point is timing. Which is the preferred day in the cycle for single-dose studies? And for a multiple-dose study (usually only 10–14 days long), which segments of the cycle should be covered? This may seem academic, but in those clinically significant drug classes where women's responses to drug handling are different to those of men because of biochemical hormone effects (not just gender), the timing of drug dosing and measurement would be critical.

Too many young volunteer studies

Many volunteer studies, especially at commercial, academic, and university clinical units, frequently include young people of college age. Both males and females will volunteer for financial remuneration, a free medical check-up, and medical care, which all play their part in motivation. The young also have less career and family commitments interfering with their motivation. Time for studying, reading, and relaxation within an atmosphere of camaraderie also contributes to the availability of younger volunteers, who because of their age, also tend to be very healthy. It will readily be appreciated that most drugs or devices are not unique or life-saving, but it is hoped are an improvement on existing agents, and indeed this applies to most basic research experiments. Nearly all drug studies in Phase I are aimed at gathering data on a potentially safe and possibly efficacious dose range. As a result, it is often hard to recruit older, more mature women for these basic types of essential drug development phase.

What is a representative female population in Phase I?

It has been stated that large numbers of mature women are volunteering for the new lipid, heart-risk, osteoporosis, and arthritis Phase III studies, due to their concern that women have been represented so poorly as subjects in the past. Phase I studies are of short duration (one to two weeks), but usually require confinement of the volunteers. Because of this time commitment, far fewer mature women volunteer, due to career conflicts or because they are often additional burdened unequally with family management. Those that do volunteer are generally unattached young female students. Thus, most female volunteers may not be typical of a "representative," mature, childbearing population (if this can ever be defined).

One alternative, a study design of stratification by age and sex, would lead to inordinately long study recruitment times, because the last "cell" (group) always takes a disproportionately long time to fill. The most obvious way out of the quandary for Phase I testing would be to maintain a special cadre of "safe, standard" volunteers. How "representative" these much used "new-drug volunteers" would become is debatable. For example, studies in arthritic patients show that these "retread" volunteer patients will differ in their tolerance to pain and in their judgment of efficacy and severity of adverse events, when compared to drug-study "naive" patients (Coles *et al.*, 1988). This "training effect" increases with multiple drug exposure.

By far, the biggest issue of undertaking additional dosing Phase I studies on women is expense. Most of these studies cost US$100,000–250,000 each. Altogether, single, multiple, and multiple-dose ranging studies, with food effect studies and extra staff costs, could add US$5 million to development costs and very rarely show a difference

that would prove clinically relevant. Indeed, the difference may not show up at all in Phase I or II gender to gender studies due to other variables, for example, small numbers, estrogen-cycle levels, and OC levels and drug polymorphism.

Drug handling differences between males and females

Due to space limitations, this section cannot discuss the many reports of apparent gender differences of psychology, different anatomic brain location of functions, skeletal build, and muscle-to-fat mass ratios that might have marginal impact upon drug activity. But in an analysis of 300 FDA-reviewed NDAs between 1995 and 2000, of 163 that included a gender analysis, 11 drugs showed a greater than 40% difference in pharmacokinetics between male and female, which though while listed on the product label, were not accompanied by any variable dosing recommendations.

An analysis of 26 bioequivalence studies involving both sexes was undertaken by Chen *et al.* (2000). In 39% of cases, two datasets (area under the curve (AUC) or C_{max}) difference of 20% or greater was observed and was reduced to 15% after body weight correction, in men.

The US General Accounting Office (US GAO, 2001a) issued a report to the Congressional Oversight Committee on gender differences. They had reviewed 36 NDAs; 75% had some differences, less than one-fifth were statistically significant differences in drug safety, but none was judged clinical significant.

In general, the between-gender variations did not result in obvious pharmacodynamic dose–response differences, but care must be exercised with drugs having a steep dose–response curve and/or a low toxicity ceiling (e.g., digoxin) where titration and adjusted dosing is required.

The weight/dose problem
A casual appraisal of ideal weight-for-height tables for males and females (Metropolitan Life Insurance, 1999) shows clear differences between males and females. The mythical "average" 70 kg (154 lbs)

male would be five feet ten inches in height and his female counterpart five feet four inches, and weight 130 lbs. This is a 28% difference in weight. This mythical male is often used to calculate dose ranges for "optimal" dose determinations, around which Phase II and III efficacy and safety studies evolve. Even more striking is the range of normal heights and weights, remembering that the same dose is usually prescribed to individuals across the range. In males, this varies from 5 feet at 106 lbs to 6 feet eight inches at 226 lbs; in females, it varies from 85 lbs at 4 foot 9 inches to 185 lbs at 6 foot 5 inches; and yet all are ideal weights for their respective heights. For both sexes, this represents a 46% differential in healthy weight while taking the same dose of medication. Why should these great disparities be tolerated by the research community, industry, and agencies? Because most drugs work—even over these ranges. First, the majority of the population falls toward the middle of the height–weight levels, rather than the extremes. Second, most drugs have a wide range over which they exert therapeutic effect before efficacy levels off. Third, the level of unacceptable adverse events generally occurs at much higher doses than the therapeutic level for most drugs (there are some notable exceptions, e.g., lithium, digitalis, warfarin, etc.).

For lipophilic drugs, the composition of mass to fat/total body water is a further variable, increasing in women after puberty. The composition of "good fat and bad fat" changes with age, both in increased fat, increased bad fat, and its relocation to the fat around the heart and abdomen. The quantity and distribution differs between genders. This may have an effect on lipid-soluble drugs, regarding the level, the time to achieve steady state, and the time to eliminate the drug and its metabolites from such fat storage depots.

Different gastric emptying time

Some studies have shown that women demonstrate greater duration in the gastric residence time of medications, which is reflected in an increased lag time of absorption, compared to men. This effect is increased when medication is taken with food, even when adjusted for the timing of the menstrual cycle (Majaverian et al., 1987). This was consistent with other reports that men had faster emptying times for both liquid and digestible solids than women (Majaverian et al., 1988; Wright et al., 1983). The length of time and variability of gastric emptying in women was also reported by Notivol et al. (1984) to be altered in relation to the menstrual cycle and was shortest at mid-cycle (Booth et al., 1957; MacDonald, 1965).

These changes can affect the amount of drug in the blood. Miaskiewicz et al. (1982) showed that, after a single dose of sodium salicylate, absorption was slower and achieved a lower level in women. This has also been shown for ibuprofen. The T_{max} was observed to be more than 54 mins in females, compared to a T_{max} of 31.5 mins in males. One study even showed a delay of 9.5 hours before absorption occurred in one woman (Majaverian et al., 1987). Sex differences in plasma salicylate albumin binding capacity have been reported (Miaskiewicz et al., 1982) and, for other agents (Allen and Greenblatt, 1981), γ-globulin transport systems have been reported to be altered with the menstrual cycle.

Some effects on absorption can be subtle, such as the greater absorption of alcohol in women due to their reduced gastric mucosal and liver alcohol dehydrogenase activity compared to men. This results in higher circulating levels of alcohol, in spite of body weight corrections (Frezza et al., 1990), with obvious implications. Odansetron given for nausea from cancer treatments, on the other hand, is more slowly metabolized by women and thus may be more effective.

Metabolic gender differences

Propranolol is still one of the most frequently used β-blockers (National Prescription Audit, 1989), but Walle et al. (1985) reported that women had higher plasma levels of propranolol than men following single oral dosing and, in an additional study, showed that on multiple dosing, propranolol steady-state (trough) plasma levels were 80% higher than in men (Walle et al., 1985). This is probably because propranolol is metabolized through three pathways, but in women the P450 cytochrome oxidation pathways are less effective than in men (Walle *et al.*, 1989).

Methaqualone metabolism has been shown to be significantly increased at the time of ovulation (day 15), almost double than that of day 1, and this was reflected in an AUC reduced by half on day 15. It is of interest that men, used as a control, only sustained levels at the level of day 1 in women (Wilson *et al.*, 1982).

Both verapamil and erythromycin appear more effective in women than in men; this may be due to higher blood levels resulting from differences in liver metabolism and reduced glycoprotein transportation (Meibohm *et al.*, 2002).

Differences between males and females in the amount of free drug found in plasma, and of protein binding, have been reported for diazepam (Abel *et al.*, 1979; Greenblatt *et al.*, 1979) and for imipramine (Kristensen, 1983). In the latter instance, a direct correlation was found with differences in lipoprotein and orosomucoid protein (1-*a*-acid glycoprotein) fractions (Greenblatt *et al.*, 1980). In women, oxazepam has been found to be eliminated at a slower rate, about 10%, and for temazepam about 25% (Divoll *et al.*, 1981). Chlordiazepoxide was also found to be less bound to protein and this was even further reduced if women were also on estrogen OCs (Roberts *et al.*, 1979). Free lignocaine levels in women were 11% higher in estrogen OC users, and 85% of this effect was due to the reduction of the orosomucoid protein fraction (Routledge *et al.*, 1981).

Circulating hormones, such as aldosterone and renin, have long been known to fluctuate with the menstrual luteal phase. If an amenorrheic cycle occurs, these changes are not seen (Michelakis *et al.*, 1975). If OCs are given, an increase of these hormones is also seen in the first part of the cycle (M'Buyamba-Kabunga *et al.*, 1985). Androgens transported on the β-globulin and albumen fraction are influenced by estrogen, which increases their binding. This effect is enhanced by the use of OCs (Clark *et al.*, 1971).

In animals, estrogen has been shown to influence the effect of antidepressants on the brain. Wilson (1986a) showed that estradiol increased the binding of imipramine to the uptake of serotonin at membrane sites. Estrone had no effect, but the addition of progesterone to low doses of estrogen increased this effect. In all, the greatest effect seen was about a 20% enhancement of imipramine binding (Wilson *et al.*, 1986b).

For narrow ratio therapeutic/toxic drugs such as lithium carbonate, this might prove to be an explanation of the reduction in efficacy seen at the end of the menstrual cycle, when these hormone levels fall (Conrad and Hamilton, 1986). It might also explain the reduction in efficacy of other central nervous system drugs such as antiepileptics (Shavit *et al.*, 1984; Roscizeweska *et al.*, 1986) and anti-migraine medications, seen with the fluctuation of the menstrual cycle (Gengo *et al.*, 1984).

Young women appear to be the group most at risk of developing extrapyramidal reactions when taking the anti-nausea drug metoclopramide. This appears to be strongly age- and gender-related (Simpson *et al.*, 1987). Another age- or gender-related effect is seen in older women who have become newly postmenopausal and who are still taking antipsychotic medications, because the symptoms of tardative dyskinesia may appear or even worsen (Smith and Baldessarini, 1973). This is perhaps another example of the loss of estrogenic protection.

Many of the examples quoted involve central nervous system drugs. This is very important, because gender-related prescription usage is heavily weighted in this area toward women. The FDA 1985 drug utilization report showed that for benzodiazepines, the increased usage in women outnumbers men by 2:1 (339 versus 171 prescriptions/1000 women and men, respectively). Twice as many women are treated for depression and anxiety neurosis than men, first described by Raskin (1974), and confirmed by Weissman and Klerman (1977). It is by no means certain that this is solely due to biochemical differences, for women are more likely to seek help than men. Of importance from the prior discussion is that, if women are the greatest users of these medications, should not study recruitment members be biased in their favor? However, some of the psychotropic CNS drugs also have animal data—and a few, even some human data—suggesting an increased teratogenic potential (*Physician's Desk Reference*, 1991; Jefferson *et al.*, 1987). There is no consistent evidence of class teratogenicity (Elia *et al.*, 1987), but there is a high association of fractured hips with the use of psychotropic medicines, even when corrected for women's greater age-related hip fracture rate (Ray *et al.*, 1987). One of the most common causes of the elderly being admitted to institutional care is urinary incontinence. Women have been found to be more susceptible than men to medications that can cause incontinence to occur (Diokno *et al.*, 1986).

Adverse event differences

There is increasing evidence that gender is a risk factor in adverse reactions with female patients at 1.5–1.7-fold greater risk than men (Rademaker, 2002). Although it is true that women take more medicines than men, for eight out of ten prescription drugs removed from the market, women suffered more serious adverse reactions. At least four of these were taken in equal numbers by both genders (US GAO, 2001b).

One of the most striking differences between male and female responses to drugs is the finding reported by Martin *et al.* (1998) in 513,608 patients with serious adverse events, which occurred in 43.2% males and 55.7% females when adjusted for age. In women of all ages, Tran *et al.* (1998) also reported that, in findings from records of 2367 patients, female patients were at twice greater risk of adverse reactions than males. More than one agent was reported to be responsible in 50% of female patients versus 33.1% of all male patients. Drugs in both genders most likely to cause an adverse event were anti-infectives (60.4%) and nervous system agents (21.5%) (Martin *et al.*, 1998). The most common events were skin-related reactions (49%). It is possible that bare arms and exposed legs in women may cause more phototoxic reactions than in men; nonetheless, this cannot be said of nervous system agents. Clearly, these two classes of agents need special gender exploration in clinical development.

Women also have a higher risk of developing drug-induced cardiac arrhythmia (Ebert

et al., 1998) and life-threatening *torsades de pointes* arrhythmia may occur with drugs such as antihistamines, antibiotics, or antipsychotics, making it important that Cardiac QT interval studies be conducted in volunteers of both genders (Woolsey, 2005). This is now an FDA requirement.

Government agency and industry actions on gender-related research

The Public Health Service Task Force on Women's Health Issues (1985) and the National Institutes of Health (NIH) Guide (1989) both recommended that biomedical and behavioral research should be expanded to ensure emphasis on conditions unique to, or most prevalent in, women of all age groups: "in addition, studies are needed to study the metabolism and disposition of drugs and alcohol by age and gender." The National Institute for Drug and Alcohol Abuse (NIDAA) (1990) policy provides detailed, almost affirmative-action instructions for the inclusion of women and minorities into study designs, according to their prevalence in the diseases being studied.

Since 1988, the FDA has requested tabulations of gender, age, and racial distributions in NDA submissions. Many of their senior officials, for example Drs Peck and Temple, had forcefully stated that women should be included in drug development studies. Indeed, the 1977 guideline, *General Consideration for the Clinical Evaluation of Drugs*, included a policy for the inclusion of women of childbearing potential in clinical trials but excluded them, in general, from Phase I and early Phase II studies, with exceptions for lifesaving or life-prolonging treatments. Childbearing potential was strictly defined as "any woman capable of becoming pregnant," including women using reversible contraceptive precautions and those with vasectomized partners.

The FDA issued new guidelines in 1993 (Federal Register, 1993), perhaps spurred by its own findings in 1989, and confirmed by the GAO, that in only 50% of submissions were gender analysis discussed in NDA submissions. Temple (1992) reported that two FDA surveys demonstrated that women were included routinely and in proportion to the presence in the treatment population, and young women in large numbers (Bush *et al.*, 1993). Not recorded were his concluding remarks, in which he said that many NDAs did not adequately discuss gender difference, which would be addressed in the new amended guideline. The FDA, in its discourse in the 1993 guidelines, *Revised Policy on Inclusion of Women of Childbearing Potential in Clinical Trials*, mentions that it was swayed by a legal precedent. In 1991, the US Supreme Court found on behalf of the plaintiff workers union that their pregnant members had been unfairly excluded from jobs by the Johnson Control Company, because the working conditions exposed their fetuses to potential risk. The court wrote: "Welfare of future children should be left to the parents … rather than to employers who hire them." Although not quite the same circumstances, the FDA was of the mind that this opinion would also apply to pregnant (informed) women, giving them the right to enter drug trials irrespective of the phase of development.

The FDA revised guidelines on this and ethnic differences (Federal Register, July 1993) in essence abolished the prior informal ban on women of childbearing age from Phase I and II studies, and stipulated additional topics, including the embryotoxic and teratogenic risk potential, to be covered in the patients' informed consent.

Earlier, the NIH had issued its own guidelines to its staff, grant applicants, and the academic centers it supported. It called for all research on human subjects concerning drugs, devices, epidemiology, nondrug device studies, and treatment outcomes, to include both genders and minority representatives whenever possible. In Phase III studies, "women and minorities and their subpopulations in sufficient numbers should be included, such that valid analyses of differences can be accomplished." It stipulated that "cost was not an acceptable reason for exclusion, and that programs and support for outreach efforts to recruit these groups be undertaken" (NIH, 1986). Failure to ensure adequate effort to implement could be a reason for grant rejection or loss of financial support.

To amplify the female view, both the FDA and NIH during the last decade have appointed women to significant roles. Dr Bernadette Healy headed the NIH and created the Office of Research in Women's Health; Dr Jane Henney led the FDA until 2001; and within the FDA, Dr Janet Woodcock and Dr Kathy Zoon were appointed to head CDER (drugs) and CBER (biologics), respectively, two of the largest centers, perhaps partly in response to an article by LaRosa and Pinn (1993) that bemoaned the exclusion of women in decisions of research. In 2009, President Barack Obama appointed another woman to head up the FDA, Dr Margaret Hamburg.

The industry is now encouraged by the FDA to include women as subjects earlier in the clinical development program, but there are also still good reasons why the FDA might deny inclusion of women of childbearing potential: insufficient toxicology data; a disagreement over the interpretation of such data; agency knowledge of another company's confidential data indicating a potential risk with a drug class-related compound; and, finally, an FDA reviewer's individual comfort level with "high-risk population exposure." Such an event has now become more common after the Vioxx withdrawal from the market.

Pharmaceutical industry practice

In July 1991, a survey was completed by this author for the Pharmaceutical Manufacturers Association (PMA), Special Populations Committee on the current practice of the industry in handling gender and minority data (Edwards, 1991). Vice-Presidents of headquarters, clinical, and regulatory affairs were contacted at 46 companies; 33 companies responded (nearly all the major companies). All 33 responding companies collected gender related data on the participant patients in clinical studies. Over three-quarters of the companies reported that they deliberately recruit "representative" numbers of women. It should be noted that the term "representative" has not been defined by the FDA or by industry. However, only ten companies (30%) frequently or usually collected data on menstrual cycle; 56% replied that the FDA at some time or other had requested the inclusion of women in trials. When women of childbearing potential were included in protocol proposals, 21% of the respondents said that the FDA never disagreed, but 79% had experience of some FDA reviewers at one time or another excluding women of childbearing potential. When excluded, this was usually in the Phase I and II trials, 58% and 45%, respectively, correspondents reported.

Although this survey was qualitative rather than quantitative, the results should not be dismissed lightly; because the survey was confidential, no respondents or their firms were exposed to open criticism. Because of their experience and senior positions, respondents had reviewed many different drugs and NDA applications. The survey replies were, therefore, likely to be reliable and provide a good approximation of the then-current industry gender practices and the frequency of clinically meaningful differences.

When gender differences in safety or efficacy were found to be clinically significant, most respondent companies (94%) opted to put the data in the product label, the *Physicians' Desk Reference*, and the product literature (72%), and to publish in the medical journals (69%). Presumably, the two companies that did not amend their labels acted thus because the products were only intended for one-gender use. By 2009, there were 969 medicines in development for diseases only in women or where women are disproportionately affected; 163 of these are medicines for specific female cancers and 86 for obstetric or gynecological conditions (Tauzin, 2009). Not only has the industry stepped up its research efforts, but many large firms have units devoted to women's healthcare.

Finally, correspondents were asked how frequently gender differences were found; 73% said "occasionally," 3% said "frequently," and the rest said "never." Of those who saw differences, only one-third found these differences to be clinically significant 5% of the time, while 17% of respondents said that significant differences occurred 10% of the time. This was more than expected, and provides further justification for gender testing.

Possible solutions

The author must stress that the opinions and the suggestions that follow are personal, based on 36 years in industry, from Phase I–IV study experience, with five large international pharmaceutical firms and two small biotech firms.

Women's inclusion as drug research subjects

Women should be, and indeed are, included into new drug and device development programs when not specifically excluded due to male-only disease or existing pregnancy. If it is predictable that a drug or device will be used in women (though they may not be the majority users), a "reasonable number" should be included in Phase II and III studies. If the disease occurs more frequently in women, for example rheumatoid arthritis, women should be involved in Phase I studies. The reality is that of the many hundreds of drugs and devices approved for use today, very few show major gender-related differences in either side effects or efficacy. Clearly, in the drug classes that have been shown to demonstrate significant gender clinical differences, "specific" gender-related studies should be included for investigational drugs and devices. These could be similar to those now undertaken in the elderly. First, a single-dose study should be undertaken. If important differences are found compared to men, a multiple dose study ought to be undertaken, and then a shorter duration efficacy and safety study in women. Such studies can be conducted later, perhaps concurrently with Phase III of the development program.

What do we mean by "a reasonable number"? "Reasonable" is that number which would be expected to show a significant gender clinical difference if a real difference is present, and probably will only apply to efficacy and adverse events 5% or larger, because a difference in low-incidence adverse events will not show up until the drug is in the market. This would mean at least 300 women exposed to the new drug. The number of patients should be based on what is judged to be a clinically significant percentage loss or enhancement of efficacy, for example 30%, dependent on the disease or symptoms.

Representative population of women

This can be based on the incidence of disease proportional to gender distribution and can be studied when drug development and toxicity are well enough advanced, usually by Phase III. Women of childbearing age must be represented if the disease is prevalent in the age group of 15–50 years. Indeed, diseases such as endometriosis can only be studied in such a population, whereas drugs to treat urinary incontinence would be better undertaken in older patients of both genders.

In some diseases, such as hypertension, where both sexes are similarly affected, balanced numbers of male and female patients in phase III would not seem out of place, although many investigators are finding recruitment of sufficient numbers of female patients increasingly difficult.

In diseases such as osteoarthritis, where women patients outnumber males (80%), a legitimate case can be made for a "female-weighted database," and also when women are the majority users for medicines, such as psychotropic agents (although they are not necessarily the majority of sufferers). Provision and timing of adequate animal toxicology and fertility data are critical to avoid expensive delays and to allow adequate female recruitment, and so these animal data may be advanced on an "at-risk basis," depending on the drug's clinical significance and its market potential. A list of diseases more prevalent in women is provided in *Medicines in Development for Women* (Tauzin, 2009).

The potential childbearing population

The probability of potential early embryonic exposure occurring in a drug development program must be expected and confronted because, despite careful pregnancy testing and adequate contraceptive precautions being undertaken, it happens. Levine (1975) in his book suggested that, in the consent form, there should be "a statement that the particular treatment or procedure may involve risks to the subject (or to the embryo or fetus if the subject is or may become pregnant) which are currently unforeseeable." This is now mandated.

When a woman of childbearing age participates in a research procedure in which there is a risk to the fetus, the nature of the risk being either known or unknown, she should be advised that, if she wishes to be a subject, she should avoid becoming pregnant. Her plans for avoiding conception should be reviewed during consent negotiations. At times, if her plans seem inadequate and she does not consent to the investigator's suggestions, it will be necessary to exclude her from the research. She should be further advised that if she deviates from the plans discussed at the outset, she should advise the investigators immediately.

Halbreich and Carson (1989) made the point that not to include women of childbearing age could even increase liability.

The general policy of an academic institution should be to favor the conduct of research involving women and children in testing of new drugs with potential for major therapeutic value to those populations. Such research may expose the institution to risk of liability for damage to subjects; however, that is inherent in research involving human subjects anyway, and there are many ways of minimizing such risks. Not to do such research, although it may serve to protect the interests of the institution as narrowly conceived, would involve a failure to serve the public interest in a much more serious manner by exposing classes of persons to knowable but unknown risks, through the practice of clinical medicines using drugs not thoroughly tested and understood, and withholding drugs that may be of benefit.

It has been suggested that members of female religious orders, women who have had tubal ligation, or lesbians could provide a "no-risk pregnancy" pool of volunteers. Although possible, this is not generally a widely applicable solution, because geographic, environmental, and volunteer numbers now become added variables.

If women on OCs enter studies, could the high level of artificial hormones confound the results? Female OC users make up 28% of the potential childbearing population (Ortho, 1991), and these hormone concentrations (10–20 times higher than the natural hormone levels) may cause drug interactions that cannot occur during ordinary menstrual cycling. Intrauterine devices are currently regaining popularity, but subdermal implants have had little influence on contraceptive practice at the epidemiological level.

Liabilities for fetal damage

Given all the above reasons for including women of childbearing potential, the issue of the chilling effect of legal liability for fetal damage on firms and institutions is still present, and the necessary addition to the patient's informed consent does not help. The US Supreme Court in 1992 rejected an attempt to cap the amount juries could award in damages as "unconstitutional;" that is, it would require a constitutional amendment. This is highly unlikely to occur. The consequences of litigation, particularly in obstetrics, were dramatic increases in cesarean section to 31% of all live births (CDC, 2006), resignations from this specialty, and a broader rejection of "high-risk" or Medicaid patients (O'Reilly *et al.*, 1986; Bello, 1989). A possible solution might be to follow the example of the National Vaccine Injury Act of October 1988, where a trust fund was set up derived from an excise tax imposed on each vaccine. The funds, through an arbitration panel, are used to compensate persons injured by vaccination. It should be noted that a Drugs in Pregnancy Registry has been set up to follow up early embryonic exposure to the anticonvulsants and antiviral drugs acyclovir and retrovir. This is administered by the American Social Health Association (ASHA), Centers for Disease Control and Prevention (CDC), and GlaxoSmithKline. One wonders whether it could be expanded (with suitable support) to cover additional agents.

Current enrolment

The use of double barrier contraceptive requirements in many clinical studies in women of childbearing potential has resulted in better recruitment.

Analysis of regulatory applications by the health authorities in Europe, Japan, and United States reported (ICH, 2005) that near equal representation of both women and men were observed.

As a result of this, the ICH declined to issue a separate guideline on women as a special population (ICH, 2005). The Office of Research on Women Health (ORWH), National Institute of Health, in February 2005, reported in its monitoring that both NIH recruitment of women and minorities, in the

clinical studies, were now reaching substantial proportions. Even in industry-based studies, by 2000, 22% of subjects were female in early-stage studies.

Data gathering

Gender data are collected by major pharmaceutical companies; few, however, record the menstrual dates. Frequently, no drug-handling differences between the sexes are detected; much less commonly is the absence commented upon in reports or publications. It is suggested that LMP dates could be included in case report forms, and that publications and reports should contain statements on the presence or absence of gender differences, also giving the patient gender numbers and *p*-values. This would allow for later meta-analysis. Both of these suggestions would be inexpensive to implement, but still to date (2009) such data are rarely collected.

Gender-related data from the FDA are more readily available as the FDA continues to increase its computer ability, and pharmaceutical firms use computer-assisted NDAs and increase their efforts to power adequately the studies to find differences. Unified systems and formats would enhance this. The information is included in the Summary Basis for Approval or in the Medical Reviewer's Report. Either should be available through the Internet at www.fda.gov./cder under "New Approvals."

Conclusion

Gender-related differences do exist in drug handling, but in general are relatively clinically insignificant. Theoretically, because of weight differences, women may receive more medication than men for a standard dose when adjusted to mg/kg. Greater effects might be expected from the range of normal weights rather than from the effects of gender.

Clinically significant gender effects have been reported with CNS, anti-inflammatory, and cardiovascular drugs. It is suggested that women continue to be enrolled into most drug study programs, but that greater thought be given to obtaining "representative" numbers in the early program planning stage. For drugs intended mainly or entirely for women, even Phase I testing in women should be usually considered. Single-dose testing, even in women of childbearing potential, poses minimal risk if done early in the cycle, with adequate precautions and "consort" consent to short sexual abstinence. Alternatively, women with tubal ligation could be enrolled for these small studies.

"Representative" could be twofold: a reflection of the percentage of women suffering from the disease, or a "reasonable or sufficient" number to show clinically significant differences in efficacy or safety in the main efficacy and safety studies; alternatively, conducting at least one study just in women in Phase III. What constitutes a "clinically significant effect" would depend on the drug and disease, but effects with a less than 15% difference get harder to detect and generally will be less meaningful. Again, women of childbearing potential could be included, depending on the age/prevalence of the disease. Women using OCs may be compared not only with males but also with non-OC users. OC and drug interaction studies are currently required for most drugs.

Early embryo drug exposure and the potential liability for any damage continues to influence industry, agencies, and some research workers. It must be recognized that, if an agent has human teratogenic potential, it is better to detect this before it achieves the marketplace. Unfortunately, this is unlikely to be detected because the small numbers of women becoming pregnant in any NDA program make it impossible to detect drug-induced effects from spontaneous birth defects. Data in women are needed and the possibility is suggested of an expanded National Register along the lines of the International Clearing House for Birth Defects Monitoring to follow up the expected small number of embryos exposed and a Compensation Panel in the event of proven damage, funded by an excise tax, as with vaccines.

Finally, with all the great strides being made to unravel the human genome and determine the gene structures and their influence, we are much nearer to tailoring drugs to match male and female differences, and with enhanced computer power, this chapter may become moot.

Acknowledgment

The author wishes to acknowledge that much of this chapter was supported by a grant from the NIH branch, Office of Protection from Research Risks.

Recommended reading

DiMasi JA, Hansen RUS, Grabowski, HG. The price of innovation: new estimates of drug development costs. *J Health Econ* 2003; **22**:151–158.

Mastroianni AC, Faden R, Federman D (eds). *Women and Health Research: Ethical and Legal Issues of Including Women in Clinical Studies*. Academy Press: 1994.

References

Abel JG, Sellers EM, Naranjo CA, *et al.* Inter and intrasubject variation in diazepam free faction. *Clin Pharmacol Ther* 1979; **26**:247–255.

Abernathy DR, Greenblatt DJ. Impairment of antipyrine metabolism by low dose oral contraceptive steroids. *Clin Pharm Ther.* 1981; **29**:106–110.

Allen MD, Greenblatt DJ. Comparative protein binding of diazepam and desmethyldiazepam. *J. Clin. Pharmacol.* 1981; **21**:219–223.

American Heart Association. Heart disease and stroke statistics, 2008; www.americanheart.org/statistics; accessed July 9, 2010.

Bello M. Liability crisis disrupts, distorts maternity care. *Natl Res Counc New Rep* 1989; **39**:6–9.

Berger JS, Roncaglion MG, Avanzini F, *et al.* Aspirin for the primary prevention of cardiovascular events in woman and men: a sex specific meta analysis of randomized controlled trials. *JAMA* 2006; **294**:306–313.

Booth M, Hunt JN, Miles JM, Murray FA. Comparison of gastric emptying and secretion in men and women with reference to prevalence of duodenal ulcer in each sex. *Lancet* 1957; **1**:657–659.

Bush JK, Cook SF, Seigel E. Issues of special populations in drug developments. *Drug Inf J* 1993; **27**:1185–1193.

Centers for Disease Control and Prevention (CDC), 2006; www.cdc.gov/datastatistics/; accessed July 9, 2010.

Center for Medicare and Medicaid Services 2008 Drug Costs, National Health Expenditure Data.; www.cms.gov; accessed April 28, 2010.

Chen, ML, Lee, SC, Ng, MJ, *et al.* Pharmacokinetic analysis of bioequivalence trials for sex related issues in clinical pharmacology and biopharmaceuticals. *Clin Pharmacol Therapeut* 2000; **68**(5):510–521.

Clark AF, Calandra RS, Bird CE. Binding of testosterone and 5-dihydrotestosterone to plasma protein in humans. *Clin Biochem* 1971; 4189–4196.

Coale AJ. Population and development review. *J Popul Counc* 1991.

Coles SL, Fries JF, Kraines RG, Roth SH. Side effects of non-steroidal antiinflammatory drugs. *Am J Med* 1988; **74**:820–828.

Conrad CD, Hamilton JA. Recurrent premenstrual decline in lithium concentration: clinical correlates and treatment implications. *J Am Acad Child Psychiatr* 1990; **26**(6):852–853.

Cotton P. Medical news and perspective. *J Am Med Assoc* 1990; **263**(8):1049–1050.

Cramer JA, Scheyer RD, Mattson RH. Compliance declines between clinic visits. *Arch Intern Med* 1990; **150**: 1509–1510.

Diokno SC, Brock BM, Brown MB, Hertzog AR. Prevalence of urinary incontinence and other urological symptoms in non-institutionalized elderly. *J Urol* 1986; **B6**:1022–1025.

Divoll M, Greenblatt DJ, Harmatz JS, Shader RI. Effect of age and gender on disposition of temazepam. *Pharm Sci* 1981; **70**:1104–1107.

Ebert SN, Liu XK, Woolsley RL. Female gender as a risk factor for drug-induced cardiac arrythmias: evaluation of clinical and experimental evidence. *J Womens Health* 1998; **7**:547–557.

Edwards LD. Summary of survey results on including women in drug development. PMA. *In Development Series, New Medicines for Women*, December 1991; 22–28.

Elia J, Katz IR, Simpson GM. Teratogenicity of psychotherapeutic medications. *Psychopharmacol Bull* 1987; **23**:531–586.

FDA. Drug Utilization in the US 1986—Eighth Annual Review. Washington, DC: FDA, 1986.

Federal Register. Guideline for study of drugs likely to be used in the elderly. *Federal Register* 1990; 55:7777; Labeling: subsection, geriatric use. 1997; 21 CFR Pt 201.

Federal Register. Guideline for the study and evaluation of gender difference in the clinical evaluation of drugs. *Federal Register* 1993; **58**:39406–39416.

Federal Register. Detection of toxicity to reproduction for medicinal products. ICH Guideline SSA. *Federal Register* 1994; **59**:48746).

Federal Register. Detection of toxicity to reproduction for medicinal products. Addendum an toxicity to male

fertility. ICH Guideline 553. *Federal Register* 1996; **61**: 15360.

Frederick J. Epilepsy and pregnancy: a report from the Oxford Record Linkage Study. *Br Med J* 1973; **ii**:442–448.

Frezza M, DiPadova C, Pozzato G, *et al.* High blood alcohol levels in women. The rate of decreased gastric alcohol dehydrogenase activity and first-pass metabolism. *N Engl J Med* 1990; **322**:95–99.

Gengo FM, Fagin SC, Kinkel WR, McHugh WB. Serum concentrations of propranolol and migraine prophylaxis. *Arch Neurol* 1984; **41**:1306–1308.

Greenblatt DJ, Divoll M, Harmatz JS, Shader RI. Oxazepam kinetics: effects of age and sex. *J Pharmacol Exp Ther* 1980; **215**:86–91.

Greenblatt DJ, Harmatz JS, Shader RI. Sex differences in diazepam protein binding in patients with renal insufficiency. *Pharmacology* 1979; **16**:26–29.

Halbreich U, Carson SW. Drug studies in women of child-bearing age: ethical and methodological consideration. *J Clin Psychopharmacol* 1989; **9**:328–333.

Health Care Financing Administration US Health and Human Services, 2009; available on the Internet.

Henrekens CH, *et al.* Steering Committee of the Physicians Health Study Research Group Final report on the aspirin component of the ongoing Physicians Health Study. *N Engl J Med* 1989; **321**:129–135.

ICH (International Conference on Harmonization). Gender considerations in the conduct of clinical trials. Regional Experience, 2005; http://www.ema.europa.eu/pdfs/human/ich/391605en.pdf; accessed April 27, 2010.

Jefferson JW, Greist JH, Ackerman DL (eds). *Lithium Encyclopedia for Clinical Practice*. 2nd edition. American Psychiatric Press: Washington, DC, 1987, 640–645.

Kristensen CB. Imipramine serum protein binding in healthy subjects. *Clin Pharmacol Ther* 1983; **34**:689–694.

LaRosa GH, Pinn VW. Gender bias in biomedical research. *J Am Med Womens Assoc* 1993; **48**(5):145–151.

Levine RJ. *Ethics and Regulations of Clinical Research*, second edition. Urban and Schwarzenberg: Baltimore, 1975.

Lindhaut D, Happener RJ, Meinardi H. Teratogenicity of antiepileptic drug combinations with the special emphasis on epoxidation of carbamazepine. *Epilepsia* 1984; **25**:77–83.

Lindhaut D, Schmidt D. In utero exposure to valproate and neural tube defects. Lancet 1986; **i**:1392–1393.

MacDonald I. Gastric activity during the menstrual cycle. *Gastroenterology* 1965; **30**:602–607.

Majaverian P, Rocci MC, Connor DP, *et al.* Effect of food on the absorption of enteric coated aspirin correlation with gastric residence time. *Clin. Pharm. Ther* 1988; **41**(1):11–17.

Majaverian P, Vlasses PH, Kellner PE, Rocci ML. Effects of gender posture and age on gastric residence time of an indigestible solid: pharmaceutical considerations. *Pharmaceut Res* 1988; **5**(10):639–644.

Martin RM, Biswas PN, Freemantle SN, Pearce GL, Minow RD. Age and sex distribution of suspected adverse drug reactions to newly marketed drugs in general practice in England. *Br J Clin Pharmacol* 1998; **46**(5):505–511.

Masia N. The cost of developing a new drug, 2008; http://www.america.gov/st/econ-english/2008/April/20080429230904myleen0.5233981.html; accessed April 27, 2010.

M'Buyamba-Kabunga JR, Lijen P, Fagard R, et al. Erythrocyte concentrations and transmembrane fluxes of sodium and potassium and biochemical measurements during the menstrual cycle in normal women. *Am J Obstet Gynecol* 1985; **151**:687–693.

Meibohm B, Beierle I, Derendorf H. How important are gender difference in pharmacokinetics? *Clin Pharmacokinet* 2002; **41**(5):329–342.

Metropolitan Life Insurance. Height–weight trades. http://www.halls.md/ideal-weight/met.htm; accessed April 12, 2010.

Miaskiewicz SL, Shively CA, Vesell ES. 1982. Sex differences in absorption kinetics of sodium salicylates. *Clin Pharmacol Ther* 1999; **31**:30–37.

Michelakis AM, Yoshida H, Dormois JC. Plasma renin activity and plasma aldosterone during the normal menstrual cycle. *Am J Obstet Gynecol* 1975; **123**:724–726.

Moscal, Manson, J.E. et al., Cardiovascular disease in woman on statement for health care professionals from the American Heart Association, circular, 1997; **96**:2468–2482.

National Disease and Therapeutic Index. IMS Health: Plymouth Meeting, PA, USA, 1978–1989, 1991.

National Prescription Audit. IMS Health: Plymouth Meeting, PA USA, 1964–1989, 1989.

Neutel CI, Walop, W. Drug utilization by men and women: Why the difference? *Drug Inf Journal* 2005; **39**(3):299–310.

NIH/ADAMHA. 1990. Policy concerning inclusion of women in study populations PT 343, 11 : KW 1014002, 1014006. NIH Guide Grants Contracts 19: 18–19.

Notivol R, Carrio I, Cano LE, Estorch M, Vilardell F. Gastric emptying of solid and liquid meals in healthy young volunteers. *Scand J Gastroenterol* 1984; **18**:1107–1114.

O'Reilly WB, Eakins PS, Gilfix MG, Richwald GA. Childbirth and the malpractice insurance industry. In *The American Way of Birth*, Eakins JNP (ed.). Temple University Press: Philadelphia, PA, 1986, 195–212.

Office of Research and Women's Health, 2005; http://orwh.od.nih.gov; accessed April 27, 2010.

Ortho. 23rd Ortho Annual Birth Control Study. Survey by Ortho: Rariton, NJ, USA, 1991.

Physician's Desk Reference. Medical Economics: Montvale, NJ, USA, 56th edition, 1991.

Pope J, Aufderheide TP, Ruthazer R, Woodard RH, et al. Missed diagnoses of acute cardiac ischemia in the emergency department. *N Engl J Med* 2000; **342**(16): 1163–1171.

Public Health Service Task Force on Women's Health Issues. Report. *PHS Rep* 1985; **100**:73–105.

Rademaker M. Do women have more adverse drug reactions? *Am J Clin Dermatol* 2002; **2**(6):349–351.

Raskin A. Age–sex differences in response to antidepressant drugs. *J Nerv Ment Dis* 1974; **159**:120–130.

Ray WA, Griffin MR, Schaffner W, et al. Psychotropic drug use and the risk of hip fractures. *N Engl J Med* 1987; **316**:361–369.

Roberts RK, Desmond PV, Wilkinson GR, Schenker S. Disposition of chlordiazepoxide: sex differences and effects of oral contraceptives. *Clin Pharmacol Ther* 1979; **25**:826–850.

Roscizeweska D, Buniner B, Guz I, Sawisza H. Ovarian hormones anticonvulsant group and seizures during the menstrual cycle in women with epilepsy. *J Neurol Neurosurg Psychiatr* 1986; **49**:47–51.

Routledge PA, Stargel NW, Kitchell BB, Barchowski A, Shand DG. Sex-related differences in plasma protein binding of lignocaine and diazepam. *Br J Clin Pharmacol* 1981; **11**:245–250.

Shavit G, Lerman P, Konczyn AD, et al. Phenytoin pharmacokinetics in catamenial epilepsy. *Neurology* 1984; **34**:959–961.

Simpson JM, Bateman DN, Rawlins MD. Using the adverse reactions register to study the effects of age and sex on adverse drug reactions. *Statist Med* 1987; **6**:863–867.

Smith JM, Baldessarini RJ. Changes in prevalence, severity and recovery in tardise dyskinesia with age. *Arch Gen Psychiatr* 1973; **29**:177–189.

Stewart DE. Are there special considerations in the prescription of serotonin reuptake inhibitors for women. *Can J Psychiatr* 1998; **43**(9):900–904.

Tauzin B. Medicines in Development for Women, Pharmaceutical Research and Manufacturers Association, 2009; http://www.phrma.org/files/attachments/09-110%20PhRMA%20Women09%200921.pdf; accessed April 27, 2010.

Tran C, Knowles SR, Liu BA, Shear NH. Gender differences in adverse drug reactions. *J Clin Pharmacol* 1998; **38**(1):1003–1009.

Trussell J, Hatcher RA, Cates W, Stewart FH, Kost K. Contraceptive failures in the United States—an update. *Stud Fam Plan* 1990; **21**(1):51–54.

US GAO. Women's Health: Women sufficiently represented in new drug testing, but FDA oversight needs improvement, GHO 01-754. Washington, DC, USA, 2001a; http://www.gao.gov/new.items/d01754.pdf.; accessed April 26, 2010.

US GAO. Most drugs withdrawn in recent years had greater health risks for women. Drug Safety, GAO 01-286R. Washington, DC, USA, 2001b; http://www.gao.gov/new.items/d01286r.pdf; accessed April 26, 2010.

US Public Health Services Office of Women's Health. *Heart disease and stroke in women*. Report on data collected by the National Heart, Lung, and Blood Institute. Chart Book: Bethesda, Maryland, USA, 1996.

Walle T, Byington RP, Furberg CT, *et al.* Biologic determinants of propranolol disposition. Results from 1308 patients in the β-blocker heart attack trial. *Clin Pharmacol Ther* 1985; **38**:509–518.

Walle T, Walle U, Cowart TD, Conradi EC. Pathway selective sex differences in metabolic clearance of propranolol in human subjects. *Clin Pharm Ther* 1989; **46**(3):257–263.

Weissman MM, Klerman GL. Sex differences and the epidemiology of depression. *Arch Gen Psychiatr* 1977; **34**:98–111.

Williams PT. High density lipoprotein cholesterol and other risk factors for coronary heart disease in female runners. *N Engl J Med* 1996; **334**(20):1298–1303.

Wilson JF. *Environment and Birth Defects*. Academic Press: New York, USA, 1973.

Wilson JG. Environmental effects on development—teratology. In *Pathophysiology of Gestation, Vol 2*, Assali NS (ed.). Academic Press: New York, USA, 1972, 269–320.

Wilson K, Oram M, Horth CE, Burnett D. The influence of the menstrual cycle on the metabolism and clearance of methaqualone. *Br J Clin Pharmacother* 1982; **14**:333–339.

Wilson MA, Dwyer KD, Roy EJ. Direct effects of ovarian hormones on antidepressant binding sites. *Brain Res Bull* 1986a; **22**:181–185.

Wilson MA, Roy EJ. Pharmacokinetics of imipramine are affected by age and sex in rats. *Life Sci* 1986b; **38**:711–718.

Women's Health Study, Ridker PM, Cook NR, Lee IM, *et al.* A randomized trial of low dose aspirin in the primary prevention of cardiovascular disease in women. *N Engl J Med* 2005; **352**:1293–1304.

Woolsey R. Center for Drug Evaluation and Research Semina and Arizona Center for Education. *New Approaches to Safety Surveillance*, June 22, 2005. http://www.arizonacert.org; accessed April 12, 2010.

Wright RA, Krinsky S, Fleeman C, *et al.* Gastric emptying and obesity. Gastroenterology 1983; **84**:747–751.

Yazigi Odem RR, Polakoski KL. Demonstration of specific binding of cocain to human spermatozoa. *J Am Med Assoc* 1991; **266**(14):1950–1960.

Yoder MC, Belik J, Lannon R, Pereita GR. Infants of mothers treated with lithium (Li) during pregnancy have an increased incidence of prematurity. *Pediatr Res* 1984; **18**:163A.

CHAPTER 18
Clinical Research in Children

Lionel D. Edwards

Pharma Pro Plus Inc., New Jersey, and Temple University, School of Pharmacy, Philadelphia, USA

Background

The world's population reached six billion in June 2009, with half (three billion) being less than 15 years old. Sadly, the mortality rate of children in the developing world is ten times higher than in the developed world. Before 1850, half of the children born in the United States died from infections before five years of age. The introduction of sanitation, antiseptics, vaccines, and medicines have made such early deaths in the United States now very uncommon. Infant mortality at birth is 6.4 deaths per 1000 live births.

Today, accident is the largest killer of children in the US, accounting for 2500 deaths in children less than five years old, comprising in order, motor vehicle, drowning, and fire. This compares to 700 deaths from congenital abnormalities, 518 from cancer, and 473 from murder. AIDS is the leading infectious cause of death in under-five-year-olds (200). The major causes of death in 5–14-year-olds are accidents (3500), cancer (1053), and murder (570). Again, in this age group, AIDS is the leading infectious cause of death (National Center for Health Statistics, 2000).

Many of the childhood cancers are hematologic, and great improvements in survival have been achieved. For example, the acute leukemia survival rate in children has risen from 53% in 1970 to 80% (American Cancer Society, 2009); and new surgical techniques and new devices are improving and sometimes correcting (even by intrauterine surgery) many previously fatal congenital abnormalities, for example hypoplastic heart.

This chapter focuses on the current regulatory requirements, their background, the clinical study challenges, and the clinical issues of drug research in the pediatric population.

It was estimated in 2000 that over 2500 studies in the US Food and Drug Administration's (FDA) defined pediatric subgroups needed to be conducted over the next three years (Still, 2000). This includes completion of pediatric studies on the FDA priority list of marketed products. Estimates of the annual cost to the industry of these studies vary. The FDA estimated in 1994 that US$13.5–20.9 million per year would be spent by industry (Federal Register, 1998). At a press conference, Christopher Jennings, President Clinton's principal healthcare advisor, said that pediatric label studies would only be about 1% of the development cost of a drug. Henry Miller (1997), a former FDA Director of the Office of Biotechnology, said that applying Jennings' figure will mean an industry cost of US$200 million (1% of the US$20 billion spent on R&D). Still, presenting at the 36th Drug Information Association (DIA) Annual Meeting (1999), estimated the cost at US$892 million if all five pediatric subgroups were to be studied (based on 1999 study costs).

These additional costs for pediatric studies may be justified if these studies satisfy all global markets. MacLeod (1991) estimated that "developing countries" by the year 2000 will comprise 36% of the total pharmaceutical market and that half of their populations are children (accounting for 18% of the market). In the developed countries, children under 18 years of age account for 20% of

Principles and Practice of Pharmaceutical Medicine, 3rd edition.
Edited by L.D. Edwards, A.W. Fox, P.D. Stonier.

the market. It would seem that the 38% pediatric share of the global market is worth an extra effort because the current 2009 pediatric market is worth US$56.9 billion and estimated to reach US$80 billion by 2013 (BCC, 2009).

Children, the therapeutic orphans

The Food, Drug and Cosmetic Act, first passed in 1906, was dramatically altered by the 1962 Kefauver–Harris amendments as a direct result of the thalidomide tragedy. This amendment required that drugs must be both safe and effective before marketing approval could be given. In addition, adequate animal, toxicology, and fertility testing had to be concluded prior to the first dose in humans. Substantial additional testing in animals and in humans was required prior to marketing approval. This led to the era of the Science of Clinical Trial Design. Regrettably, the testing of drugs in children did not advance at a similar pace, and most drugs (unless specifically intended for children) were never tested in children by the sponsors of new medicines.

Physicians were thus forced to use most drugs "off-label" and extrapolate the child dose on a comparative weight basis from those in adults. This often involved parents splitting or crushing tablets, hiding medication in spoonfuls of honey, or sprinkling a crushed tablet onto a meal. Each time this happened, a little more confidence in and knowledge of the drug was gained, but each child was a "one-off experiment" and only provided a learning curve for the individual physician. Eventually, academia published a series of cases, so giving guidance on dosing and likely toxic effects. Even so, the average pediatrician and family practitioner felt uneasy and legally vulnerable about off-label use.

A few drugs were developed for children in such categories as antibiotics, antihistamines, and anti-epileptics. Otherwise, few firms undertook studies to develop full pediatric label instructions or even pediatric formulations. Liquid formulations did exist for some drugs, but mainly for use in the elderly. In 1975, Wilson surveyed the 1973 *Physician's Desk Reference* for labeling instructions

for pediatric patients and pregnant or breastfeeding women. He found that 78% of listed drugs either had no information for pediatric dosing or contained a disclaimer. A subsequent survey by Gilman and Gal (1992) showed that this situation had not improved qualitatively and that the percentage had also risen to 81%. Eventually, the FDA issued the 1994 rule, which sought to strengthen the 1979 guideline on pediatric labeling requirements (Federal Register, 1994).

The Pediatric Use Working Group, chaired by Miriam Pina (1995) (FDA Division of Pulmonary Drugs) examined the data that the FDA had acquired on 1994 pediatric prescriptions from IMS. From these they identified the top ten drugs used "off-label" in children: Albuterol, Phenergan, Ampicillin i.m. or i.v., Auralgan otic solution, Lotison, Prozac, Intal, Zoloft, Methyl Phenidate (under six years), and Alupent syrup (under six years). A combined total of over five million of these ten products were prescribed in 1994.

Clearly, firms needed further encouragement to submit additional pediatric data, so in 1997 Congress passed the FDA Modernization Act (FDAMA), part of which called for firms to submit data on children to support labeling for a new pediatric subsection before the drug could be approved. This applied to drugs that could be projected to provide therapeutic benefit to substantial numbers of children. In exchange, Congress felt that an inducement was required and wrote into the Act provision for an extension of a drug's patent life by six months if pediatric studies were done. For a US$4 billion drug such as Loratadine, six months' extra exclusivity is not "chump change." The FDA was requested to provide guidance and, in December 1998, it issued the Final Rule Amendments to the Pediatric Subsection S to be implemented April 1999, governing the need for pediatric studies, and extending the requirements to biological drugs and already-marketed drugs. The FDA identified drugs for which supplemental data were still needed for pediatric labeling. The FDA has issued an annual list of "priority drugs" for which additional pediatric information may be "beneficial."

The FDA chose to interpret the patent life extension as applying to all indications, not just to pediatric use. As might be expected, the Association of Physicians and Surgeons appealed this interpretation of the pediatric rule, and it was overturned by a Washington DC judge. Subsequently the pediatric incentive program was enacted and the prior act intent contained within the Food and Drug Administration Amendment Act (FDAAA) of 2007.

1994 and 1998 final rules on pediatric studies (Federal Register, 1994, 1998)

Products subject to the rule

For drugs that are new molecular entities (NMEs), a determination should be made by the sponsor of the potential usefulness of the new drug in a pediatric population. If it is likely to generate over 100,000 prescriptions per year, this would indicate the need to develop a pediatric formulation and suitable pediatric studies. If it is likely to generate less than 50,000 prescriptions per year, the sponsor may be granted a waiver by the FDA for pediatric data, and a disclaimer statement allowed. Either way, in a children's disease, if less than 200,000 patients per year may benefit, then orphan-drug status with seven per year exclusivity may be applicable. This would then apply only to that pediatric indication.

The requirements of the Pediatric Final Rule now include marketed drugs and biologics. The FDA has already listed products affected and sent pediatric data requests to firms. The firms had until April 2001 to provide the extra data.

Data to be provided

If considerable data exist, or are planned, for the same indications in adults, it may be appropriate to extrapolate safety and efficacy from adults to children. But pharmacokinetic (PK) studies to determine dosing and, if possible, pharmacodynamic data will usually be required for children. Discussion with the FDA is recommended early on, to establish whether pediatric data will be required and which of the five groups should be covered: preterm, 37 weeks gestation; neonate, 0–1 month; infants, 1–2 years; children, 2–12 years; and

adolescents, 12–16 years. One or more adequately-sized efficacy and safety studies may be required, especially if the drug or disease behaves differently in children, or the drug uses different metabolic pathways. This may occur if the particular adult enzyme is not present in children, or is only present in low quantities. If a different indication to that in adults is being sought, one or two sizable safety and efficacy studies, in one or more age groups, are likely to be required. This is in addition to pediatric PK data. Sponsors should also plan for the major ethnic groups to be represented in these studies. Recent requests for hypertensive agents have indicated that 50% African-American patients be enrolled, costing over US$1.3 million.

Frequently, the FDA may allow a waiver or approval of a drug with incomplete pediatric data and defer the completion to a Phase IV commitment, especially when the product is life-saving and the only treatment available.

Major physiologic variations in pediatrics

In the past, the statement that "children are little people" dominated research thinking. Recently warnings have been required on package labeling for antidepressants that use in adolescence leads to higher rates of attempted or completed suicide in 20-year-olds, increasing in frequency the younger the patient (Hammad and Laughren, 2006). This brings home that children may have different responses than adults to drugs. But in general, both in children and in the elderly, drugs and biological products behave similarly to that in the 18–65-year old population, although this expectation must be adjusted for size and age-related differences in PK variables, such as immature or ageing enzyme metabolism systems as well as elimination rates affected by immature or ageing organs of excretion.

The National Health and Nutrition Examination Survey (NHANES, 2007) reported that 31.9% of children were overweight (BMI above 85 percentile) and 16% were frankly obese (at or above 95 percentile), and Ogden *et al.* (2008) found that in 20 years the number of obese children has doubled. Both these finding have short-term and serious long-term disease consequences, let alone practical body mass dosing issues.

In neonates, the gastric pH is biphasic, being high in the first few days after birth and decreasing by day 30, but it takes 5–12 years for the adult pattern and value to emerge (Signer and Fridrich, 1975). On the other hand, the methylation pathway, unimportant in adults, is well developed in children. Furthermore, acetaminophen is less toxic to children than to adults, probably because it uses the sulfate metabolic pathway (Rane, 1992).

Most infants are slow acetylators and may accumulate toxic levels of those drugs that are metabolized by this second phase of metabolism route. Renal perfusion and glomerular filtration rates (GFR) vary: for the premature, 2–4 ml min^{-1}; for neonates, 25 ml min^{-1}; and by 1–1.5 years old, 125 ml min^{-1}, which is equivalent to adult clearance rates (Arant, 1978). The potential toxic implication of renal metabolites and elimination of unchanged drug in the very young are obvious (Stewart and Hampton, 1987).

Dosing

Without pediatric PK data, dosing in children has depended on extrapolations from the adult data, either by weight or by body surface area. Using weight may result in overdosing neonates but underdosing infants and children. Using body surface area may be better because of its linear increase with age and its good correlation with cardiac output, renal flow and GFR—more so than weight. Neither method compensates for the varying metabolism aforementioned, or for differences in drug disposition between children and adults.

Concerns in formulations for pediatrics

If a drug is to be given by injection, i.m. or i.v., this may require only volume variations. But most drugs developed for adults are given by the oral route, as tablets, capsules, or caplets. The adult formulation is usually determined by marketing considerations. Invariably, for children, especially under age seven years, liquid or syrup must be formulated. Most drugs taste bitter or unpleasant (which is why most tablets are sugar-coated). Sometimes, it may be impossible to mask the taste completely. A commitment to a pediatric formulation requires a whole gamut of testing and the development of specific product specifications. If the liquid formulation changes the bioavailability (faster or slower absorption), further efficacy and safety studies may be required. A further concern is that liquid formulations usually have a shorter shelf life than tablets. Finally, stability characteristics or other factors may make it impossible to make a liquid or syrup or glycolated elixir, and so sprinkle beads or powder sachets, and split or crushed tablets in apple sauce, may be a last resort. In the latter two cases, an even distribution of active compound and other inactive excipients must be demonstrated. In addition, a lack of effect of apple sauce on bioavailability must be proved if such advice is to appear in the dosing instructions.

Toxicology

The plastic nature of immature organs such as kidney, liver, brain, and lung may indicate the need for more animal toxicology. Frequently, neonatal acute and subacute toxicology studies are undertaken in two animal species. Because of the small size of mouse and rat pups, this may prove a challenge to administer the active drug. The common "mixing with chow" is inappropriate in neonates. Dog pups usually provide one of the two species, and so a special liquid formulation for animals may be required (if the product is intended for oral delivery), and given by dropper or gavage.

Clinical studies

Pharmacokinetics (PK)

The traditional PK volunteer study in healthy children has proved very hard to set up, because of the attitude of many parents and over-viewing independent review boards (IRBs). Even in pediatric patients, the frequency and total volume requirements for samples for conventional PK studies can cause the same refusals. However, there are pediatric research units that specialize in these studies, with minimum needle sticks, minute blood volumes, and IRBs sympathetic to the needs of the pediatric community. The National Institute of Child Health and Human Development has set up a "network of pediatric pharmacology units," usually in academic regional centers, now numbering 13 units. There are other nongovernmental specialized units also available for pediatric PK work.

An alternative method of getting PK data is to take a small extra sample of blood (and urine) at a child's regular scheduled visit when blood is drawn for routine blood work. The time of day of this sample is predetermined by the time of the administration of the medicine. If samples are obtained from many children, a weight–age corrected, scatter-plot graph can be constructed and a PK profile be calculated. This is the "pharmacokinetic screen" method. A version of this method is also used to gather ethnic data for labeling in adults as well as children, and is called "population pharmacokinetics" (Sheiner, 1985).

Recruitment

One of the major problems in running pediatric clinical trials is the availability of pediatric patients, who tend to be scattered, because they are numerically less likely to have diseases (other than asthma and the usual childhood illnesses). This affects the logistics of screening and subsequent clinic visits. Another hurdle is finding trained pediatric investigators or pediatric pharmacologists, and outside the US they are even harder to find. In Europe, there is collaboration between the US-based Pediatric Pharmacology Research Units (PPRU), the European Society of Developmental Pharmacology, and the European Network for Drug Investigation in Children (ENDIC). For diseases of children, there are often self-help organizations that can prove invaluable in recruiting children and in reassuring their parents.

A large package of data and two well-controlled pivotal studies of safety and efficacy are rarely required, with the exception of diseases specific to childhood, such as surfactant studies in respiratory distress syndrome. This is especially the case if the drug has similar effects in both adult and pediatric populations, for example antihistamines.

However, if a disease or drug behaves in different ways in children compared with adults but a large body of safety data exists in adults, usually only a single efficacy and safety study is required.

Ethical concerns

The American Academy of Pediatrics formed a Committee on Drugs to examine ethical issues of pediatric studies for its members and for the guidance of IRBs dealing with pediatric studies. The Committee released its report in 1995. This report (Committee on Drugs, American Academy of Pediatrics) is very comprehensive, but the following three sections highlight some areas of its many recommendations.

Vulnerability

In this special population, there is a special duty to avoid (unintended) coercion of the patient, parent, or guardian. This coercion may arise because the investigator is usually also the treating physician. It would be better to have a colleague explain and obtain the informed consent. There are varying degrees of vulnerability. Patients handicapped mentally, emotionally, or physically are frequently institutionalized and may be supervised as Wards of Court or by a social welfare agency. These patients should be rarely used, unless the treatment is for serious diseases specific to institutional settings and no other treatment is available.

Emergency situations can arise where it may be impossible to obtain written informed consent from a parent or guardian. Medications for this type of problem will require intense IRB review and overview; only in special circumstances will informed consent be waived, and then it must "not adversely affect the rights and welfare of the subject" (Abramson et al., 1986). The last category is the use of a research medicine in a child close to dying who has either no response to standard therapy or where no alternative therapy exists. The agent to be considered must have some evidence of efficacy (animal proof of concept or clinical data and a good chance of a beneficial result). The risk of unintended coercion of desperate parents is especially to be guarded against.

IRBs' special emphasis

IRBs have a duty to make sure that the study is of value to children in general and in most cases to the patient personally, is robust enough to give answers, and attempts to minimize risk and maximize benefit. In reviewing the protocol, the IRBs should involve healthcare specialists who are aware of the special medical, psychological, and social needs of the child, and the disease as might be impacted by the study.

In studies conducted on diseases mainly affecting pediatric patients, the development will be entirely in pediatric patients. However, in addition to the appropriate usual toxicology and neonate animal toxicology, the first-in-humans studies for toxicity and safety are usually done in healthy adult volunteers. Clearly, drugs such as the surfactants would yield no useful data from adult testing. For these unique pediatric situations, new measurements and endpoints may need to be developed and validated. Frequently, the FDA will involve an advisory panel to help determine what these might be.

The use of a placebo control

Placebo control is desired whenever possible if using a placebo does not place the pediatric patients at increased risk. The AAP Committee on Drugs (1995) outlined some other circumstances:
• When no other therapy exists or is of questionable efficacy, and the new agent might modify the disease.
• When the commonly used therapy has a high profile of adverse events and risk greater than benefits.
• When the disease fluctuates frequently from exacerbations to remissions and thus the efficacy of the (new) treatment cannot be evaluated.

Conclusion

The ICH draft guidance on pediatric issues has been published in the Federal Register (2000). This guidance covers pediatric formulation, development, ethics, regional and cultural issues, regulatory expectations, duration and type of studies, and age ranges to be studied. The guidance is similar to the FDA Final Rules (Federal Register, 1994, 1998) with the addition of a fifth group, preterm newborn infants. It also seems better organized and informative, but then hindsight is always helpful.

The face of pediatric pharmacologic medicine has been changed. In the future, for pediatricians there will be less uncertainty and better predictive information available; for children, safer and more effective dosages will result. For the industry, the added cost of research will be more than recouped in a new global market to which previously they could not promote their products. This is supported by the 1998 survey by PhRMA (Tauzin, 1998), which showed that medicines and vaccines in development for children were up 28% from the previous year. More recently they reported 219 medicines were being tested to meet the special health needs of children of which 39 were for childhood cancers, 29 for infectious diseases such as AIDS, hepatitis, and ear infections, and 26 for genetic disorders.

The FDA Modernization Act of 1997, the Best Pharmaceutical for Children Act of 2002, and the Pediatric Research Act of 2003 have brought about improvements (see Chapter 34 on US Regulations).

Meanwhile in Europe similar efforts are undertaken with the EU issuing the European Draft Document for Pediatric Regulation, *Medicines for Children* (2006). It gives ten-year exclusivity for "off" patent drugs if required pediatric studies are done, two years for an orphan drug in pediatric indication, and six months for patented medicines. This was entered into law January 2007 and implemented in July of 2008. It requires studies in children to be conducted in compliance with a Pediatric Investigational Plan (PIP), agreed by the European Medicines Agency (EMEA) Pediatric Committee.

In addition, the ICH issued the E11 Pediatric Guideline on Federal Register 2000. This outlines conduct of studies in children and is used by many countries. This Guideline also addresses availability of formulations and labeling for children.

In addition, as of 2007, the Office of Pediatric Therapeutics has been formed in the FDA to monitor and enforce pediatric requests.

So, finally, the inclusion of the needs of children in clinical trials, as envisioned by the then FDA

Commissioner, Dr Charles Edwards, in 1972 to the American Academy of Pediatrics is almost fulfilled, albeit after 38 years.

References

Abramson VS, Meisal A, Sufar P. Deferred consent – a new approach for resuscitation research on comatized patients. *J Am Med Assoc* 1986; **225**:2466–2471.

Arant BS. Developmental patterns of renal function maturation compared to the neonate. *J Pediatr* 1978; **92**:705–712.

American Academy of Pediatrics (AAP), Committee on Drugs. Guidelines for the ethical conduct to evaluate drugs in pediatric populations. *Pediatrics* 1995; **95**:286–294.

American Cancer Society, 2009; www.cancer.org/cancer/cancerinchildren/index; accessed July 9, 2010.

BCC Research Report, March 2009. www.bccresearch.com/report/hlc059a; accessed March 29, 2010.

FDA Food and Drug Administration Modernization Act (Pub. Law 105–115), November 21, 1997, USDC 355a, 111 Stat. 2296.

Federal Register. Specific requirements on content and format of labeling for human prescription drugs revision of 'pediatric use' subsection in the labeling. *Federal Register* 1994; **59**(238):64240–64250.

Federal Register. Final rule regulations requiring manufacturers to assess the safety and effectiveness of new drugs and biological products in pediatric patients. *Federal Register* 1998; **63**:66632.

Federal Register. International Conference on Harmonization: clinical investigation of medicinal products in the pediatric population. *Federal Register* 2000; **65**(71).

Gilman JT, Gal P. Pharmacokinetic and pharmacodynamic data collection in children and neonates. *Clin Pharmacokinet* 1992; **23**:1–9.

Hammad T, Laughren T. Suicidality in pediatric patients treated with antidepressant drugs. *Arch Gen Psychiatry* 2006; **63**:332–339.

MacLeod SM. Clinical pharmacology and optimal therapeutics in developing countries: aspirations and hopes of the pediatric clinical pharmacology subcommittee. *J Clin Epidemiol* 1991; **44**(Suppl. II):89–93.

European Union. European Draft Document for Pediatric Regulation: *Medicines for Children*, 2006, http://www.ema.europa.eu/htms/human/paediatrics/regulation.htm; accessed March 29, 2010.

Miller telephone interview. 1997. Script No. 2260, 22 August 1997.

National Health and Nutrition Examination Survey (NHANES). National Center for Health Statistics. 1996. Based on data from US Department of Health and Human Services.

Ogden C, Carroll M, Flegal C. High body mass for age amongst US children and adolescents 2003–2006. *JAMA* 2008; **299**(20):2401–2405.

Pina LM. Drugs widely used off-label in pediatrics. *Report of the Pediatric Use Survey Working Group of the Pediatric Subcommittee*, 1995.

Rane A. Drug disposition and action in infants and children. *Pediatric Pharmacology, Therapeutic Principles in Practice*, Yaffe SJ, Arand AJV (eds). Sanders: New York, USA, 1992, 10–12.

Sheiner LB and Benet LZ. Premarketing observational studies of population pharmacokinetics of new drugs. *Clin Pharm and Therap* 1985; **38**, 481–487.

Signer E, Fridrich R. Gastric emptying in newborns and young infants. *Acta Paediatr Scand* 1975; **64**:525–530.

Stewart GF, Hampton EM. Effect of maturation on drug deposition in pediatric patients. *Clin Pharm* 1987; **6**:548–564.

Still JG. The pediatric research initiative in the United Statesa: implications for global pediatric research. *Drug Inf J* 2000; **35**:207–212.

Tauzin B. More than 200 medicines in testing for children. 1998, http://www.phrma.org/node/644; accessed March 30, 2010).

Wilson JT. Pragmatic assessment of medicines available for your children and pregnant or breastfeeding women. In *Basic Therapeutic Aspects of Perinatal Pharmacology*, Morsell PL, Garattini S, Serini F (eds). Raven: New York, 1975.

CHAPTER 19

Racial and Ethnic Issues in Drug Regulation

Lionel D. Edwards[1], J-M. Husson[2], E. Labbé[3], C. Naito[4], M. Papaluca Amati[5], S. Walker[6], R.L. Williams[7], & H. Yasurhara[8]

[1]Pharma Pro Plus Inc., New Jersey, and Temple University, School of Pharmacy, Philadelphia, USA
[2]Paris, France
[3]UCB S.A., Brussels, Belgium
[4]Teikyo University, Tokyo, Japan
[5]European Agency for the Evaluation of Medicinal Products, London, UK
[6]Centre for Medicines Research, International Institute for Regulatory Science, London, UK
[7]US Pharmacopia, Rockville, MD, USA
[8]Teikyo University, Tokyo, Japan

Background

The international need for quicker national approval of significant drugs offering improved therapy, less toxic effects, and even cure had been delayed and restricted by differing mandatory regulatory requirements between nations. Thus, by 1980, the need for an international cohesive policy was apparent. Discussions between the regulatory authorities of Europe (European Medicines Agency (EMEA)) and the United States (Food and Drug Administration (FDA)) were aimed at the harmonization of regulations governing the approval process of drugs and devices and have been going on since the first International Conference of drug regulatory authorities, which met in October 1980 (Annapolis, USA), and latterly under the auspices of the International Conference on Harmonization (ICH). In their first meeting in Brussels (November 1991), the Japanese regulatory authorities (Ministry of Health and Welfare (MHLW)) participated as a full member; these three major regional members were joined by representatives from the pharmaceutical industry of Japan (JPMA), Europe (EFPIA), and United States (PhRMA) and observers from the World Health Organization (WHO), Nordic countries, and Canada's HPB, thus covering about 92% of the current regulatory activity and global spending on pharmaceuticals.

The ICH continuing series of meetings has resulted in success in the areas of quality control, toxicology, pharmacology, and clinical development, including good clinical practice (GCP) and the recent issue of guidance on the acceptability of foreign clinical data, the Common Technical Document (CTD), adoption of MedDRA, and electronic submissions.

The clinical area had proved much harder to harmonize because of the lack of clear-cut regional or national concordance on many clinical issues. The very existence of some diseases is in dispute, for example, temporo-mandibular joint dysfunction (TMJS) and premenstrual syndromes in the United States, and hypotension syndrome (Pemberton, 1989) in Europe. The emphasis on treatment over prevention and the real physical and genetic differences between national populations with a variety of healthcare systems can cause disparity of results, observations, and conclusions. Again,

Principles and Practice of Pharmaceutical Medicine, 3rd edition.
Edited by L.D. Edwards, A.W. Fox, P.D. Stonier.
© 2011 Blackwell Publishing Ltd.

diversity within a national population, geographic influences, diet, varied measurement standards, religious and cultural effects, and patient–doctor relationships also play a part in making interpretation and agreement difficult.

To date, it is by no means clear that harmonization has reduced the overall burden of regulations for either the regulators or the regulated, but it has eliminated some inconsistencies. To those ends, "Ethnic Factors Influence on the Acceptability of Foreign Data" was proposed by Japan and Europe and accepted as an ICH 2 topic by the ICH Steering Committee, Washington (March 24, 1992). This chapter will give an account of the ethnic issues faced by the working party, ending in the tripartite implementation of the "Guidance" of 1998. A working party made up of representatives from each of three major regions was set up and met many times for two-day working sessions. A major study of approved drug dosage and pharmacokinetics (PK) between the three regions was undertaken by Japan's MHLW and JPMA. A further study, commissioned by EFPIA, was undertaken by the Centre of Medicines Research (CMR, UK). In addition, the type and incidence of spontaneous adverse events reports occurring with eight drugs marketed in the European Community were examined for consistency by the EC representative, and concurrently, the data files of one pharmaceutical company of four drugs in different therapeutic areas was examined for any variations of PK, dosage, and adverse events between regions by the EFPIA member. Only their major findings are included in this chapter, more information can be found in the individual reports (Naito and Yasuhara, Harvey and Walker; Papaluca; Labbé; Edwards; and Williams (ICH Orlando, 1993)).

Terminology

The terms "race" and "ethnicity" are often used interchangeably, but the Office of Management and Budget (OMB) issued in 1997 revised recommendations for the collection of race and ethnicity data by Federal Agencies. This led to the issue of Guidance for Industry (2005) by the FDA adopting the OMB categorization.

The non-binding recommendations were for the US database if collected separately.

Race would include American Indian/Alaska Native, Asian, Black or African-American, Caucasian Native Hawaiian, or Other Pacific Islanders. *Ethnicity* would be Hispanic or not Hispanic.

If a combined format is used, six categories are recommended by adding Hispanic or Latino as a group. Subsequently, Hispanic is now divided into Non Black Hispanic and Black Hispanic; the term Latino has been discontinued.

The agency admits that these are arbitrary groupings and not based on anthromorphic, genealogic, or genetic grouping. Indeed if the evolutionary human tree was used as a guide, African, the later evolving Caucasian, and the last major group Mongoloid/Asian Caucasians might be a better way to define race. The word ethnicity could be used to describe subgroups, either genetic sub-variations or culturally different—for example, Asian Indians and Japanese—thus affecting ethnic ancestral origins.

For the purpose of this chapter, the words race and ethnicity will be used interchangeably.

Regulatory practice

Initially in the United States, non-US studies, not under the investigational new drug applications (INDs), were considered primarily as a source of supportive safety data. By the early 1970s, it was appreciated that well-controlled non-US clinical data could be utilized to support US new drug applications. US regulations have allowed for the use of non-US data as the sole basis for approval, so long as certain conditions were met, including the stipulation that "foreign data are applicable to US populations and US medical practice" (FDA, 1975, 1985). No specifics were given regarding the definition of "applicable." Thus, clinical data from Phases I–III were allowed; but in practice, such data could not be the sole source of safety and efficacy for new drug approvals. The reasons given for not using Japanese data more widely in the US and Europe involved differences in medical practice, such as the use of different endpoints, lower dosages, and differences in research methodology, such as the emphasis on a large number of physicians and their experience in Phase III, resulting in a large number of investigators with a low ratio of patients enrolled. In Europe, although there may be preference by individual countries to have local clinical data developed, it did not appear that actual regulations precluded the use of "foreign" (usually US) data in most European countries (Safety Workshop ICH 1, 1992), although some nations (France, Italy, and Germany) required some clinical experience in their countries prior to approval.

In Japan, there has been harmonization with the other regions in the area of toxicology (animal studies); the Japanese Ministry of Health, Labor and Welfare (MHLW) accepts appropriate foreign animal data and animal safety studies performed according to ICH guidelines. Indeed, Japan has played a major role, and its then current fertility and reproductive animal studies requirements have been adopted by the other two regions.

However, the acceptance of "foreign" clinical data has been a major issue for all the health authorities for a long time. Previously, all Phase II and III clinical studies needed to be performed. Mandatory clinical studies were required in many European countries and in Japan on Japanese people. Phase I studies could be done outside Japan, but only if the drug was in wide use in that country (which had to be a developed country) and if the drug's performance was unaffected by racial differences in physiology. The Japanese position has been that diet, and perhaps genetics, can play a significant role in PK/PD, and that a drug's safety or efficacy may be different in the Japanese than in other races (MHW Notification 660 and Notification, June 1987) because of subsequent metabolic differences. Clearly, there are a few drugs where this rationale is justified, but there are many others where metabolism may be largely irrelevant (e.g., ophthalmological and topical medicines). However, these differences appear to constitute a major reason why (without exception) Phase II and III trials had to be carried out on Japanese patients (Uchida, 1988; Fairburn, 1989; Homma, 1991; for further discussion, see Apple and Weintraub, 1993).

Objective differences

Now to first examine those differences that can be quantified more readily.

Population demographics between tripartite areas

The United States is a nation of many racial, ethnic, and national origins and is the most heterogeneous population of the three areas. Given the successive waves of European, African, and Asian immigrants, themselves imposed upon even earlier waves of Bering Straits immigrants (Native North and South American Indians, and Eskimo), makes the US population the most diverse in the world. Although inter-marriage has occurred, many major racial groups remain regionally or locally clustered and still adhere to cultural aspects of their area of origin. However, many of the smaller distinct racial and ethnic groups may not be represented in the US pharmaceutical databases, either due to the realities of setting up clinical studies or because only small numbers are present in that population. In general, only Caucasians, Blacks, Asians, and Hispanics may have measurable populations in a database (Edwards, 1992). As of 1990, American Indians comprise 0.8% of the population, with the other minorities comprising larger or smaller percentages of the population: Hispanic (any race) 9.8%; Pacific Asian 2.9%; Black 12.1% (US Bureau of the Census, 1991). Europe has a Caucasian "heterogeneous" population made up of Anglo-Saxon/Celtic, Germanic, Gaelic, mid- European, and "Latin" races. There are sizeable populations of migrant foreign workers, as much as 10% in Germany, and many resident Asian and African citizens of Britain and in France (5%). In contrast, Japan is populated almost entirely by ethnic Japanese, truly homogeneous, although a sizable non-national immigrant population of other guest Asian workers exists, mainly Korean.

The definitions of racial groups are not totally satisfactory (e.g., what is "Black?"), and ethnicity and geography can wreak havoc on the meaning of "representative," for example, Pacific Islanders and Asians make up 9.8% of the Pacific states population and 61.8% of the US State of Hawaii (US Bureau of the Census, 1991). What is Hispanic, other than a language group that contains a combination of genetic groups from Europe, Africa, and Native America? Diseases such as stroke are associated with high levels of VonWillebrand factor (Folsom *et al.*, 1999), found commonly in the Black population. Sickle cell anemia, thalassemia, and glucose dehydrogenase deficiency are ethnically linked, but how do they affect drug metabolism?

The small genetic variation (DNA)—only 0.5 of the 11% total variations between individuals of these groups among the three major divisions of humans (Caucasian, Negroid, and Mongoloid)—makes up the total variation between individuals of these groups (Vessell, 1989). Thus, it would not be a surprise if race gives rise to fewer differences than does individual variation of drug metabolism and dynamics. That is, genes of race have less influence than an individual's total genetic make-up.

PK/PD and ethnic differences

One of the earliest reports of differences was described by Chen and Poth (1929). They noted that the mydriatic response to cocaine was greatest in Caucasians, less in Chinese, and least in Blacks. When PK differences were first reported in the literature, they usually involved the genetic polymorphisms of acetylation, the debrisoquine–sparteine and mephenytoin pathways, the second phase of metabolism, or selective protein transport systems. Drugs such as clonazepam, hydralazine, sulphonamides, isoniazide, nitrazepam, and procainamide undergo acetylation in the liver. Most Asians, especially Japanese (88–93%), are fast acetylators compared to 50% of Caucasians and Blacks (Wood and Zhou, 1991). Fast acetylators may be at greater risk of isoniazide hepatitis from toxic metabolites (Drayer and Reidenberg, 1977), whereas slow acetylators may respond better to treatment (sustained levels) but be at greater risk of toxic reactions. Those drugs that extensively use acetylation as to second phase of metabolism, and also use either of two cytochomes enzymes in the first phase, are more likely to induce Lupus (Hess, 1982) and/or hypersensitivity reactions (Reider, 1999). The two cytochromes were identified as

CYP2D6 and CYP2C19, part of the extensive P450 cytochrome enzyme systems not only found mainly in the liver but also present in other tissues such as gut, lung, and brain. Ethnic differences in these two pathways have also been found: CYP2D6 enzymes are lacking in 8% of Caucasians and 1% of Asians, but is hyperactive in East Africans, Ethiopians, and Saudi Arabians. This enzyme can be affected by the presence or absence of up to 21 alleles. But in 99% of the population, only 4–5 alleles are involved: Star 10 in Asians, Star 17 in Africans, and Star 29 in African-Americans (Zanger *et al.*, 2004). Frankiewicz (1999) reported that Hispanics had a faster response to Respiridone but more adverse events, suggesting that they had slower metabolism than the Caucasian group in the study. Even with Hispanics, there are differences: Mexicans have a faster metabolism by CYP2D6 than Dominicans or Puerto Ricans. CYP2C19 is lacking in 20% of Asian, 4–8% of Blacks, and 3% of Caucasians. These are two of the three most common first phases, metabolic pathways. The most common CYP3A4 has also demonstrated ethnic sensitivity. One of the most popular antihypertensives, nifedipine, (Mendoza *et al.*, 2001) has been shown to have three times the plasma levels in steady state in Mexicans than Caucasians; this reflects that 60% of Mexicans are slow CYP3A4 metabolizers.

Perphenazine and over-the-counter (OTC) ingredients codeine and dextromethorphan are made active by the debrisoquine–sparteine oxidative pathway. The percentage of an ethnic or racial population poorly metabolizing by this pathway varies greatly; for example Switzerland 9–10%, Hungary 10%, United States 7%, Nigeria 3–8%, and Japan 0.5% (Wood and Zhou, 1991), but if not will gain no pain relief.

Clinically, this has been shown to make a difference in a small study in males, involving ten Chinese and nine Caucasian subjects; the Chinese metabolized propranolol more rapidly, clearance was 76% higher, with a lower area under the curve (AUC) and plasma levels lower than that in the Caucasians at all time points. In this study, when dosage was adjusted upwards to equilibrate to Caucasian therapeutic blood levels, a greater response was noted in the Chinese subjects (lower blood pressure and pulse rate) (Zhou *et al.*, 1990). Conversely, the presence of very fast metabolizers in a population may also vary.

The mephenytoin metabolic pathway is utilized by commonly used drugs, such as mephobarbital, hexobarbital, diazepam, imipramine, and omeprazol, but only 3–5% of Caucasians and 8% of Blacks are poor metabolizers of mephenytoin, compared to 15–20% of Chinese and Japanese populations (Kupfer *et al.*, 1988). This enzyme's activity is inhibited by fluconazole and fluoxetine and induced by drugs such as barbiturates and nicotine (smoking).

The lack of digestive enzyme lactase in many Hispanics, especially Mexican-Americans and African-Americans, causes lactose intolerance, with nausea, diarrhea, and occasionally vomiting. It is understandable that lactose is no longer preferred as a filler (non-active excipient) in tablets and capsules.

Some drugs, such as phenothiazines and tricyclic antidepressants, show greater preference for binding and transport on α–1 acid glycoprotein rather than on albumin. Thus, 44% of Swiss and US Caucasian and Black populations have higher levels of this protein, compared to 15–27% of the Japanese population (Eap and Bauman, 1989; Lin *et al.*, 1991). This might explain the higher fraction of free drug found in Asians (with a greater volume of distribution and clearance), as well as the fact that the metabolism of some benzodiazepines appears to be slower in Asians than in Caucasians (Kumana *et al.*, 1987). One study (Zhang *et al.*, 1990) showed that Chinese subjects who were either poor or extensive mephenytoin metabolizers when taking diazepam (mephenytoin pathway) still metabolized diazepam at the same rate as Caucasian poor metabolizers. The higher proportion of slow metabolizers of mephenytoin pathways is thus not the only difference. However, ethnic differences in the percentage of body fat between the two groups could also account for this. The "p" protein transport system is also being explored for ethnic drug variations, especially in the maintenance of the blood–brain barrier.

As previously noted, drugs such as propranolol and imipramine each have two major pathways, and even poor metabolizers of any significant pathways usually have alternative pathways, which might be expected to show some increased handling ability over time. Thus, in many cases, plasma levels and clinical differences between poor and good polymorphic metabolizers may be insignificant. In others, especially where the therapeutic index is small, it may be critical—usually these drugs are titrated for efficacy and safety and so the effect is avoided. In other cases, such as antihypertensive agents, the clinical effect of genetic differences may not be seen, because the patient's dosage is titrated to blood pressure response (Eichelbaum and Gross, 1990) and only a large meta-analysis may show ethnic optimal dosage.

Prescribing differences

Of great concern are findings that ethnicity may affect prescribing habits. Sleath *et al.* (1998) looked at the patient's ethnicity and the likelihood of a psychotropic being prescribed: they found that Caucasians received medication 20% of the time and non-Whites only 13.5%. A similar finding was made by Khandker and Simoni-Wastilia (1998) concerning any prescription drug. Differences were found at all ages, with Black children receiving 2.7 fewer prescriptions than their Caucasian counterparts. This rose to 4.9 prescriptions in adult Blacks and 6.3 in elderly Blacks. All the patients were on Medicaid, and so ability to pay was not a factor. Dinsdale *et al.* (1995) confirmed a similar pattern in prescriptions issued for analgesics for postoperative pain to be self-administered by the patient, with Caucasians receiving prescriptions significantly more frequently than minorities ($p < 0.01$).

Genetic and ethnic susceptibility

Therapeutic effects may vary between ethnic populations, due either to a sizeable representation of poor metabolizers present or to a genetic or ethnic related "susceptibility." Clozapine is associated with the development of agranulocytosis in 20% of Ashkenazi Jews, compared to 1% of the general population treated for schizophrenia. This was found to be highly associated with specific linked genes for agranulocytosis and especially those of Ashkenazi Jewish origin (100%) (Leiberman *et al.*,

1990). Yet again, the best known example was the sensitivity to quinine and its derivatives in Blacks given to prevent malaria, resulting in many deaths in World War II.

Another example of PD differences is that of reports on lithium in the manic phase of bipolar depression. Asian patients, including Japanese, are reported to have therapeutic blood levels at 0.5–0.8 mEq/L compared to required levels in US Caucasian patients of 0.8–1.2 mEq/L (Takahashi, 1979; Jefferson et al., 1987; Yang, 1987); these findings, however, are disputed by Chang et al. (1985). African-Americans require less drug dose, but this is because of higher blood levels due to a slower clearance rate than Caucasians (Lin et al., 1986; Jefferson et al., 1987).

Asians have been reported to require smaller doses of neuroleptic drugs and to suffer adverse events at lower doses than Caucasians, even after body weight was accounted for (Lin et al., 1986, 1991; Wood and Zhou, 1991). With tricyclic agents, the picture is more confusing between Asians and Caucasians, but Asians appear to show more variability overall and African-Americans tend to have higher plasma levels, faster therapeutic effect, but more side effects than the other groups (Strickland et al., 1991).

Essential hypertension is a symptom of modern society, and its treatment accounts for a sizeable portion of global prescriptions. As a result, there is a great interest in reported ethnic and racial differences reported in the literature. The use of appropriate therapy in Black patients has been best studied. As monotherapy, calcium channel blockers and diuretics appear to be most effective in Blacks, whereas β-blockers and ACE inhibitors produce smaller reductions in blood pressure (Kiowiski et al., 1985; Freis, 1986; Hall, 1990). However, this may more reflect the lower plasma renin, salt and water retention, and intercellular sodium and calcium in Blacks, compared to other groups (Kiowiski et al., 1985). There are individual exceptions among patients and among drugs, even within these classes; for example, labetalol, a combined α-blocker and β-blocker, can be equally effective in both African-Americans and Caucasians and, as mentioned previously, the Chinese appear twice as sensitive to propranolol as Caucasians (Oster et al., 1987; Zhou et al., 1990).

Receptor sensitivity

Salzman (1982) described a down regulation of benzodiazepine and β-blocker receptors linked to ageing. It has been postulated that Asians have fewer benzodiazepine and β-blocker receptors than Caucasians. Down regulation of these receptors with age has been described and postulated by Zhou et al. (1990), but hard evidence of racial or ethnic differences is still awaited. If the Chinese are more sensitive to propranolol in spite of their high catabolic rate, it might be linked to adrenergic receptor sensitivity.

Looking at the broader picture, part of today's discovery process is the incorporation of isoenzyme detector screens and computer predictor modeling, to eliminate potential drugs posing major metabolic problems or interference patterns. This is being done as part of the screening process for lead candidates prior to preclinical screening. Drugs such as terfenidine and mibefradil would not pass these screens today.

In-depth drug case studies

The European Federation of Pharmaceutical Industries and Associations (EFPIA) commissioned a third party, the Centre for Medicines Research (CMR, UK), to collect data on a small number of targeted drugs. By direct appeal to manufacturers through an independent third party, compliance information between regions was made available, as well as PK data. In addition, data on efficacy and safety were also requested from firms operating in the three major areas.

The CMR conducted this study among European and American companies to assess the significance of inter-ethnic differences in clinical responsiveness and to determine the implications of such differences for international clinical development. Information was collected for all three phases of clinical development. Data from 21 compounds developed since 1985 in the West and Japan, and covering a wide range of therapeutic categories, were analyzed. Overall, there was no indication that the metabolism of any of these drugs was affected by genetic polymorphism. One compound is known to be eliminated by an enzyme that is polymorphic, but there was no evidence of altered phenotype or subset population within any ethnic group. Although three compounds displayed some regional variability in PK, further analysis of the data provided rational explanations for all such perceived differences. All the regional variations were attributable to different pharmaceutical formulations, reduction of initial doses, and alteration in sampling times and techniques, and none of these differences had any significant impact on clinical development.

There was considerable regional variation in dosing or frequency of dosing, with a tendency toward lower Japanese doses, because of cultural differences in medical practice. The type and frequency of adverse reactions observed during clinical trials was generally lower in Japanese subjects, although there was no correlation between reduced adverse reactions and lower doses. Cultural attitudes relating to the use of preferred terms, different assessment methods, and reporting differences were provided as explanations for the lower incidence of Japanese adverse reactions. More Western subjects were included in trials for a given indication than Japanese subjects, and Japanese dose-ranging trials were frequently of an open design. Phase III trials were controlled, although regional differences in the numbers of subjects and the use of placebos and reference drugs were observed, placebo controls being more frequent in the United States.

The only apparent difference in clinical effectiveness between the West and Japan was not considered to be significant, because all 21 compounds displayed no geographic differences in risk–benefit assessment (for further details, see Harvey and Walker, 1993).

Other ethnic factors with pharmacologic implications

Differences seen across regions and nations, both in reports of efficacy and incidence of adverse reactions, are much greater than can be accounted for by ethnic variations of PK and PD. Other objective differences are now discussed.

Alcohol

Even modest amounts of alcohol may induce enzyme activity of many hepatic-metabolized drugs; thus, it is conceivable that data derived from a French, Italian, or Spanish European population, who regard wine or beer as a "digestive" and part of the daily diet, might enhance, albeit slightly, a higher metabolism of some drugs, thus requiring higher dosages to achieve efficacy. Contrast this with the same drug developed in a Moslem or Mormon society, or in populations who have less tolerance of alcohol, because of poor metabolism due to a reduction or absence of either aldehyde dehydrogese or gastric alcoholic dehydrogenase (Agarwal, 1990). This reduction or absence of enzyme occurs in Japanese (44%), Eskimos (43%), or South American Indians (41–43%) and to a much lesser degree in other ethnic groups (Mendoza *et al.*, 1991). Initially, this reduced enzyme might exaggerate possible adverse events with drugs competing for the same metabolic pathway.

Other influences on drug differences

Some curiosities, such as delay of ductus arteriosus closure in the neonate at high altitudes and its resistance to indomethacin closure, are interesting but hardly relevant to most populations. Of greater impact is the effect of ultraviolet light on skin. Black pigment gives about 30% extra protection from sunburn, but Caucasian populations living in tropical areas not only suffer exaggerated sunburn and photosensitivity when ingesting some classes of drugs, for example, tetracyclines and quinolones, but also develop a higher incidence of skin cancers, basal cell carcinomas, and malignant melanomas.

Concurrent presence of diseases dominating in a region, for example, chronic hepatitis B, which is endemic in Asia and may affect up to 30% of the population, might distort laboratory normal ranges of liver enzyme to drugs and population baseline measurements. Heterozygous sickle cell anemia gene confers immunity against falciparum malaria to Africans (Medawar, 1961), but this benefit is unneeded in African-Americans in the malaria-free US, and homozygous genes (two sets) confer illness and sickle cell anemia episodes may confuse drug assessment. Indeed, drugs such as chloroquine give rise to occasional fulmanent hepatitis in these patients and diltiazam has been shown to produce greater sensitization of the PR interval in sickle cell type C and S patients (Weintraub and Rubio, 1992).

Although nutritional status is good in Japan, much of Asia lives on less than optimal nutrition, and it might be argued that the US and Europe suffer from nutritional excess, with about 30% of their populations overweight. Either status has implications regarding lipophilic drug storage, metabolism, and tissue distribution.

Ethnic variations in diet, additives, or salt content may alter metabolism rates. Lin *et al.* (1986) and Henry *et al.* (1987) report that antipyrine metabolism was different in rural Asian Indians than in Asian Indian immigrants resident in England for some years. Dietary environmental differences may also account for the findings of Gould *et al.* (1972) and Kato *et al.* (1973) of a gradation of heart and stroke incidence, lower in residents of rural Japan, higher in Japanese in Hawaii, and highest in Japanese in California.

High- or low-fat diets can affect ingestion of drugs, as a high intake of salt can affect diuretic efficacy. Findings that some spices may influence metabolism have been reported. Baily *et al.* (1991) showed the enhanced bioavailability of calcium channel blockers (felodipine can be more than doubled; nifedipine to a lesser extent) with concurrent consumption of grapefruit juice compared with water (an effect not seen with orange juice) (Rau, 1997).

Age, height and, weight differences

Currently, there is an obvious difference in average height–weight of US/European citizens versus Japanese. This reflects in a difference in blood/tissue volume, which alone probably accounts for more real drug differences than pharmacogenetics and other factors previously discussed. In the US and Europe, from the largest normal to the smallest normal males in terms of height and weight, there is a 70% difference (Metropolitan Life Insurance Tables, 1999). Add to this a 30% lower height–weight for the smallest normal-sized female.

To compound this, the Japanese small normal female is 20% smaller than her European counterpart. Despite this, in general, blood level differences are not as great as might be supposed. However, these regional size differences appear to be decreasing as the average increase of height in the US is slowing, whereas in other nations, such as Japan, it is increasing.

A final physiologic population difference to be considered is the relative ages of the three populations: United States 32.9 years, Europe 34–38 years, and Japan 38.2 years (World Almanac, 1992; World Population Prospects (by WHO), 1990). The differences between the average age of the three populations may cause a slight "age effect" change in the average function of organs such as kidney and liver and the metabolism and excretion of drugs. Japan and Sweden have a greater proportion of their population over 80 years compared to the other regions and this segment, whereas generally increasing worldwide, is increasing faster in Japan.

Subjective factors

The previous objective factors can produce, on occasion, a real although usually small/difference in drug levels and effect. The next group of factors to be discussed are largely subjective but still have an even more profound effect on protocol design, execution, measurement, outcome, recording, and interpretation of the data collected. The subjective biases of doctors, patients, study monitors, experts, investigators, and regulatory assessors are affected in different ways by variations of the three regional medical cultures and practices, and their population's cultural values. It is also an area that is poorly researched by comparative studies. Many of the observations reported in this next section come from the experiences of the authors or from the literature of anthropology and social biology.

Medical practice

Physicians in Japan try to achieve effectiveness with no adverse effects with what, by US standards, appear to be almost homeopathic doses at times. In Europe, the aim is to achieve effectiveness with some minimal side effects, often by titrating the dose upwards. In the US, the aim is to achieve optimal effectiveness with acceptable adverse effects and then titrate downwards. Thus, the highest total daily dosage tends to be greater in the US than in the other two regions.

The pressure to prescribe is greater in the US than in Europe; for example, antibiotic usage per capita is twice as great in the US compared to the UK, and four times more than in Germany. Cesarean section is 31% of all births in the US (CDC, 2006), but only 21% (NICE, 2004) in Britain. Defensive medicine is only part of the story; the need for an aggressive approach, with the need to cure as opposed to treat, is a major factor in the US. Less litigation may reduce this pressure, but this is unlikely to occur. Conversely, fear of litigation also increases drug attribution and reporting of adverse events.

In Japan, concurrent prescribing of different drugs of the same class in small doses is not unusual. Disclosure of cancer diagnosis to the patient is frowned upon in Japan, and reporting of GI side effects by the patient may be discouraged by the culture.

Differences in preferred dose form—availability of suppositories in France, injections in Italy, pills in the United Kingdom, and poly-pharmacy in Japan—reflect medical practice, education, and practice conditions. There is great emphasis and concern in Germany over the heart and diet; in France over the liver; in the United Kingdom over viruses; and in the US over hypertension and obesity. Only in 1999 were oral contraceptives approved in Japan, a brave action, for it may increase the falling rate of Japanese population replacement, shared with Italy and Western nations (excluding the United States). All these can reflect a different emphasis on a drug's development.

In the different regions, the physicians and investigators are held in varying degrees of esteem by their patients. In Japan, the ability to depend on others, to lean and to be leaned on, is considered healthy (Doi, 1973). The doctor is held in great respect by the patient, and both the doctor and patient regard the chief investigator with even greater respect. This can interfere with adverse event reporting (avoidance of offense) by the patient, and perhaps lack of critical observation by their sub-investigators. These factors can influence the use of placebo, and "informed consent format" in clinical studies. However, great strides are being made in Japan to share the responsibility with the patient for mutual benefit.

Physicians in the three regions deal differently with failure to achieve the desired clinical effect. In the US, the tendency is to change medications. In other countries, dose titrations of the same medication may be used more frequently. The different approaches reflect both medical school teaching and expectation of the results of therapy. In many areas of Europe, the physicians and investigators are free, to a certain extent, from suspicion of monetary influence because of extensive socialized or government-backed health schemes. This has its pitfalls, but allows a degree of benevolent, autocratic meritocracy to emerge, which resulted in the evolution of the "expert system" for regulation in Europe and the "doctor knows best" for the patient in Japan, which works quite well in those cultures. Again, the reporting, anticipation, or recognition of adverse effects may be diminished. This contrasts with the US, where frequently almost twice the number of adverse events is reported compared to European studies (except Sweden) and, not infrequently, placebo response rates are also increased. It has been postulated that these increased effects spring from both the aggression of American medical practice in search of cure and from the higher doses used. In addition, US physicians often focus on extensive data gathering in an attempt to achieve diagnostic certainty. This leads to an increased search for, and investigation of, adverse reactions and their causality. This may also be due to the litigious nature of the US system. The diagnostic approach "blitz" has been heavily impacted by the inroads of managed care to reduce costs.

Ethnic effects on European adverse drug reactions

As part of an ongoing effort by the EC's General Directorate for Scientific Research, the European "concertation" procedure's impact on the ability to monitor and detect changes in clinical safety was studied. Some of the information gathered on spontaneous adverse drug reactions (ADRs) was made available to the ICH EC Working Party by Dr M. Papaluca Amati.

The nature and incidence of serious spontaneous ADRs on three different new agents approved by, at the time, 11 EEC member states (1989–1991) were examined. As expected, the reporting rate varied between regions, according to the reporting framework and regulatory requirements, but qualitatively, the same serious adverse events were reported appropriately per capita in all member states where the drug was available. It thus appears, for serious ADRs, that ethnic variation in Europe does not influence the pattern of adverse events or its reporting. Other preliminary findings also showed a similarity of serious ADRs in multinational, multicenter European studies, provided that similar methodology and reporting formats are used. These observations did not apply to nonserious ADRs, where marked national differences were seen.

For further discussion, see sections on Evolution of ICH Topics and Ethnic Factors and Clinical Responsiveness (Papaluca Amati, 1993).

National socioeconomic influences

National reimbursement policies, therapeutic policies on patients, and third-party reimbursement differences between nations and national or private insurers can all have an impact on how drugs are used. One obvious example is the 1999 refusal of the UK government on the advice of the National Institute of Clinical Excellence (NICE) to reimburse the Glaxo Wellcome antiflu drug Relenza™ and Tamiflu™. Since the advent of the Swine Flu H1N1 pandemic in Britain (2009), this policy has been reversed. In another example, Germany, France, and Italy's policy on pricing grants only improved drugs a higher price than the advertised therapy, even to the denial of some "me-too" drugs. The pricing policy in Japan, with the compulsory dropping of a company's drug price after a few years, irrespective of patent life, is a further example. Lastly, the lately rescinded Canadian legislation, which basically denied research costs against developers' taxes and also shortened patent life, nearly crippled research in Canada and slowed the applications until a price structure had emerged for drugs in the US and Europe.

Finally, the US population and US third-party insurance, government, and private industry, all pay 30–50% higher prices for the same medicines than Canada, Mexico, or Europe. Pressures on the US manufacturers to reduce US prices will have a chilling effect on the development of new medicines and, hence, on the availability of new medicines globally (the US is the origin of about 60% of the world's new chemical entities).

Terminology, diagnosis, and other subjective factors

As previously mentioned, some diseases and syndromes are not universally recognized in the three regions. Until recently, neither AIDS nor depression was diagnosed in Japan. Conditions such as "cardiac fatigue" and "postural hypotension" in Germany; "liver crisis" in France; "heavy leg syndrome" (pre-varicose-vein development) in Switzerland; and "anxiety neurosis" in the US are unique to these regions. The endpoints for medicines to treat may also be different, for example, that for blood pressure in Japan is >160/95, in Europe >140/90, and in the United States >129/90. Indeed, even in the same language, the (British) phrase "I am in the pink" and the (American) phrase "I feel blue" have opposite meanings, and when used in self-rating scales they have no or different meanings for the other country.

The end result of these differences, although apparent rather than real, may be why the recommended dose of captopril (an ACE inhibitor, antihypertensive drug) is 75–450 mg per day in the US and 37.5–122.5 mg per day in Japan (with overall adverse events of 39% and 3.8% respectively). With a non-steroidal anti-inflammatory agent, overall adverse events were 45–51% in the United States and 24% in Japan at the same dosage; however, efficacy was the same (Dziewanowska, July 1992). In general, the British, Dutch, and Scandinavian data are closer to those observed in the United States, with the German and Swiss data "least reactive" and French, Italian, and Spanish in between. As mentioned previously, severe ADRs in clinical studies tend to be the same; the major difference was in "minor" adverse events, such as nausea, headache, and so on. Thus, national temperament also may play a part in the expectation of efficacy and ADR. This finding was reflected in a study of attitudes of 4000 nurses from 13 countries to ethnic tolerance of pain (Davitz and Davits, 1981), in which Jews, Hispanics, and Italians appear to suffer more than Germans, Anglo-Saxons, and Asians, but such differences may simply appear to be the socially acceptable level of expression of pain versus the actual pain severity itself.

In many African Animist cultures, Western medicine may cure the disease but not the patient, who continues to languish. Western medicine is regarded in Africa in the same way that the Western world regards naturopathy: as ineffective, and this can cause the reverse placebo effect. This can be seen to the extreme in the severe mental function and physiologic systemic shutdown produced by a witch doctor's curses, which seem totally unresponsive to antidepressant medication (Cannon, 1957), and the first author of this chapter has witnessed and successfully treated such an episode but had to use unconventional methods.

In addition, Third World patients who report seeing spirits and ghosts may not be equated to "hallucinating patients," as in a Western culture, for they may be experiencing the prevailing expectations of their culture (Hartog and Hartog, 1983). Even within the US, 70–90% of self recognized episodes of sickness are managed outside the formal healthcare system (Zola, 1972). Thus, the incorporation of clinical social sciences is essential if physicians are to understand, respond to, and help patients (Eisenberg, 1973); this is also applicable to the interpretation of clinical results.

The evolution of ICH topic E5

Background
In November 1991, in Brussels, the International Conference on Harmonization (ICH) of Technical Requirements for Registration of Pharmaceuticals for Human Use was held. A new topic was proposed to, and accepted by, the ICH Steering Committee. This was the thorny issue of tripartite mutual acceptance of "foreign" data. It was assigned the prefix E5 (efficacy, fifth topic approved) but was to be one of the slowest to be resolved: As the reader by now will appreciate, slowly resolved because of its complexity, not because of ill-will. It is true that initially, mutual suspicion reigned, with regional rights and pride. This was quickly replaced by mutual respect, first among the regulators and then between the regulators and the pharmaceutical industry representatives.

At a meeting in Washington in 1992, Professor Chikayuki Naito from Teikyo University, Japan, was handed perhaps the toughest job of the ICH. He was appointed chairman of the E5 working party. He selected his working party members from the three regions, including this chapter's first author. He then immediately set to work. One of the most interesting discussions was the topic's title; should it be "ethnic" or "racial?," so interwoven were these descriptors with cultural, religious, and language differences. Eventually, "ethnic" was selected, because it allowed more regional incursion than "racial," which was too restrictive. Then tasks were assigned on a regional basis; the United States representative (the first author) to a literature search, review, and compilation; Japanese members were to research the dosing differences between the three regions on the 80 common drugs, backed up where available by matching PK data; Europe was assigned two tasks, first to review of the European adverse event database (national variations) and second, through an independent third party (Center for Medicines Research, CMR), to review of dosage, efficacy, and safety differences. The reports were issued in October 1993 at the ICH 2 Orlando meeting. Professor Naito reported for the Japanese delegation that, among 42 drugs examined, daily doses of β-blockers and ACE inhibitors in the US and Europe were twice as high as in Japan. Hypolipidemic drugs were similar in all the regions but, surprisingly, the highest doses were in the EC. Similarly with antibiotics: higher maximum doses were prescribed in EC and also in the US, than in Japan.

H_2-blockers, a protein pump inhibitor, and NSAIDs showed no difference in daily doses in the three regions, but again, maximum and lowest doses allowed were all lower in Japan. They had also reviewed the PK factors in 80 drugs approved in the three regions but largely concluded that intra-ethnic variation in drug metabolism was as large as or larger than inter-ethnic differences; however, this variability was greater in the Japanese population. Professor Naito concluded that, if the metabolism of a new drug was influenced by genetic polymorphism, then additional regional PK and dose-ranging studies might be required.

Dr S. Walker of CMR approached European and US companies for information on 21 drugs available in the three regions. Within this narrow sample, only one drug had genetic polymorphism, but even this did not translate to ethnic variations. Three other drugs showed regional variability in PK, but these were attributable to different formulations, different sample times, and reduction of the initial dose. The CMR survey confirmed that the reported levels of adverse events were lower in Japanese patients, even when adjusted for dose—a cultural variation.

The US reports on findings in the literature were given by the first author of this chapter and Dr R. Williams of the FDA. Much of the earlier part of this chapter was drawn from these reports.

Deciding what to do about this complex issue took another four years! Two more conferences were needed to resolve the issue, but finally in July 1997, Step 3 was concluded, Europe and Japan referred it to their governmental bodies, and the United States published the draft guidelines in the Federal Register. Phase IV acceptance by the ICH Steering Committee occurred in February 1998, and the final guidance document was implemented in the US in June 1998 (Step 5) (Federal Register, 1998).

Outline of the "Guidance" ICH topic E5

Overall, it will not be necessary to repeat the entire clinical drug program in each of the other two regions. Each regional authority will judge whether the clinical data fulfill its regulatory regional requirements (i.e., a complete package). If so, can the data be extrapolated to the region's population? If the authority is concerned that a drug could be subject to ethnic factors impacting on efficacy or safety, limited clinical data gathered in people of that region may be required to "bridge" the clinical data between the data generated in one region to those of the area in which the data were generated. If new data are required by the new region anyway (found inadequate for regional requirements), the study could become a full Phase III clinical study.

What is a complete package?

Studies should have adequately well-controlled endpoints and medical and diagnostic definitions appropriate to the region. The specific needs are mostly covered in other ICH guidance: GCPs (E6), dose response (E4), and adequacy of safety data (E1 and E2), studies in elderly (E7), reports (E3), clinical trials (E8), and statistics (E9). Occasionally, a region may feel that other studies are needed in areas that other regions are less concerned with; a different "golden" standard as comparator or at a dosage as approved in that region, as well as patients with renal or hepatic insufficiency, are given as examples.

Ethnic factors and population extrapolation of a drug

Some properties of a drug or its class may make it insensitive to ethnic factors. This will make it easier for extrapolation to different regions and reduce the need for "bridging" clinical data. Properties that make it susceptible to ethnic influences (see Table 19.1) will require bridging studies, sometimes of PK/dynamics studies or safety and efficacy, or both.

Assessing the potential sensitivity of a drug to ethnic factors

If a drug is of a known class, the sensitivity may already be determined, but by the end of Phase I most of the PK and PD of a drug will be known. The properties of the compound that may indicate

Table 19.1 Classification of intrinsic and extrinsic ethnic factors (ICH Guidance, 1997)

Intrinsic	Extrinsic
Physiological and	
Genetic pathological conditions	Environmental
Gender Age (children–elderly)	Climate
Height	Sunlight
Bodyweight	Pollution
Race Liver	Culture
ADME Kidney	Socioeconomic factors
Receptor sensitivity Cardiovascular functions	Educational status
Genetic polymorphism Diseases	Language of the drug metabolism
Genetic diseases	Medical practice
	Disease definition/diagnostic
	Therapeutic approach
	Drug compliance
	Smoking/alcohol
	Food habits
	Stress
	Regulatory practice/GCP
	Methodology/end points

potential ethnic variation (ethnically sensitive) are as follows:

- nonlinear PK;
- a steep efficacy and safety PK dose curve;
- narrow therapeutic dose range;
- highly metabolized, especially if through just one pathway (potential for drug–drug interaction);
- metabolism by enzymes known to show genetic variation;
- a pro-drug relying on enzyme conversion subject to ethnic variation;
- low bioavailability (ethnic dietary effects);
- projected common use in multiple co-medication;
- potential for inappropriate use.

Properties that reduce a drug's potential for ethnic variation (ethnically insensitive) are the converse of the above, with the addition of low potential for protein binding and nonsystemic use.

Bridging data package

This consists of information from the complete clinical data package selected for its relevance to the new region. PK, PD, and early dose–response data should all be included. If a bridging clinical study between the foreign data and the new region's population is needed, this may be a PK study, or PD demonstration of efficiency, or a center running a PK study additionally on volunteer patients. A bridging clinical study may not be needed (a regional regulatory decision). This is most likely (i) where the medicine is ethnically insensitive and medical practice and conduct of trials are similar, (ii) if ethnically sensitive but the two regions have similar clinical make-up of populations, and (c) when extrapolation from drugs of a similar class can be made. If the drug is ethnically insensitive and clinical data are derived from dissimilar ethnic populations, provided that other nonphysiological factors are similar, a simple PD dose–response study may suffice. This could utilize an endpoint predictive of clinical value (surrogate), for example, blood pressure. If PK were also undertaken in the same study, dynamic effects may be directly reflected by the blood levels.

If the bridging study shows similarity to the dose–response study in safety and efficacy, this is usually sufficient, even if this study shows that a different dose is indicated. That is especially so if at that new dose (range) a similar safety and efficacy profile has been demonstrated.

Where the differences are greater (medical practice, a new drug class to the region, different comparator from that of the region standard), a controlled, randomized clinical study for efficacy will be required. This might utilize shorter duration surrogate endpoints, rather than the clinical endpoints common to Phase III studies.

The ICH issued further Questions and Answers Guidance (FDA, 2004) to provide further explanations of when bridging studies may be required following six years of experience.

Bridging safety studies

The new region may also have concerns regarding the relevance of the safety data of common serious adverse events and their incidence to its ethnic population. The guidance recommends that the clinical efficacy study should be powered to capture a 1% incidence of an event, namely 300 patients for six months on the new medicine. Additional patients will be needed for the control group in a controlled trial, given an expected dropout rate of 15–30%, dependent on disease and severity of efficacy depends on the balance of the groups (1:1, 1:2, 1:3). A small safety study might be done initially to assure the sponsor and the region that a high incidence of serious events is unlikely to be seen in the larger study.

Practical implications to sponsors of new medicines

Most major clinical pharmaceutical manufacturers recognize that it is not profitable to develop a drug just for one region. In the past, most drugs were introduced first in Europe, even by US-based firms for pricing reasons, often country by country, and then in Japan even later. This has dramatically changed since the introduction of the "centralized procedure" of Application for Europe. Frequently, firms will conduct multicenter studies in both the US and Europe and submit them almost simultaneously to the FDA and EMEA. This was not possible to do for Japan; now it is! Indeed, Japan now can conduct studies in other regions on its drugs and combine them with confidence into its own more extensive clinical data package for foreign submission. Differences of Japan's chemical, manufacturing, and quality control section (CMC) still have to be resolved before full interchangeability (mutual recognition) of its Common Technical Documents occurs. Many firms now do PK and PD dose–response studies on Japanese patients in Japan. In addition, even if not needed, they conduct a controlled local comparison clinical study to expand the database and for sound marketing reasons.

In the United States, because of legislation previously discussed, data on major ethnic groups are collected and analyzed and may in general provide reassurance that the most obvious ethnic differences are observed. This is of less concern to the other regions.

For many years, the FDA has encouraged a wide geographic distribution of Phase III multicenter studies. This can be used to enroll minority and cultural ethnic groups, because they tend to congregate in regional clusters, for example Hispanics in Miami, New Mexico, and New York. Placement with a physician investigator of similar ethnic origin can enhance the enrollment, because frequently they will attract patients of that group.

In 2005, the FDA approved a drug for heart failure only for use in African-Americans. Originally, it had turned down the drug in 1997. When the combination isosorbide and hydralazine was tested in only African-American patients, it was shown to work (Taylor, 2004). As of 2007, there are 691 medicines under development for diseases that are disproportionately present in the Black community. Similarly, as of 2006, there are 258 medicines for Hispanic common diseases (Tauzin, 2007).

The current regulatory position of the three regions has been outlined in the notes for *The Guidance for the Mutual Use of Foreign Data in the EC, Japan, and US, Part 1*. The ADME concern has been well-defined and quantified in separate reports.

Does it matter? The reality

Despite this huge list of possible factors influencing the drug development and assessment process, the following realities are emerging.

For most drugs the therapeutic range is broad, and rarely is an optimal dose so critical for effective treatment. Exceptions, such as cardiac glycosides, anticonvulsants, and anticoagulants, have a narrow therapeutic/risk window (therapeutic index) and must be individualized by titration. Such drugs, if not useful, are soon discarded (Benet, 1992). Despite the presence of multiple conflicting factors, the global dosage trend is toward a global "mean." Over time, the same dosage range emerges in many countries, adjusting to the "real world" as opposed to the narrow demographics of research or cultural expectations.

Generally, where dosages are the same, the incidence of serious adverse events tends to be the same in the three regions (Edwards, 1993; Papaluca Amati, 1993).

Objective differences, when found, are largely due to physiologic influences (blood/body volume and metabolic intra population differences) and less commonly due to ethnic variation. In the US, an estimate of less than 5% of drugs subject to significant clinical ethnic variation was reported by participating companies in a USA/PMA Survey (Edwards, 1991) and confirmed by the retrospective surveys undertaken for ICH 2 (Harvey and Walker, 1993; Natio and Yasuhova, 1993).

Data are more interchangeable between the US and Europe than between Japan and the US, or between Japan and Europe, but this is less often due to PK differences, body size, and diet but more often to the even larger differences in medical and cultural attitudes of Japan, Europe, and the US that influence dose selection and data compatibility.

The future

Technology, television, transcontinental travel, and international scientific and medical conferences continue to narrow the subjective variations. Differences in diagnosis, data measurement, and interpretation will diminish with such exchanges. It is possible that methodology, study design, and case report forms can be constructed that correct for culture, diet, and at least some subjective factors, which will allow comparability of efficacy and adverse events on dose/mg/kg body weight measured between European, US, and Japanese data. The days of personalized medicines are upon us where the genome and alleles will be more discriminatory than ethnicity, even while recognizing some will be more or less dominant in the major racial divisions.

In conclusion, most but not all differences will disappear and indeed, from such diversity, there may spring new understanding of both clinical and therapeutic mechanisms for the development and applicability of more specific and better medications.

References

Agarwal DP, Goedde HW. *Alcohol Metabolism, Alcohol Intolerance and Alcoholism*. Springer-Verlag: Berlin, Germany, 1990.

Apple P, Weintraub M. Notes for Guidance: The Use of Foreign Clinical Data in the EEC, Japan and USA. ICH: Orlando, FL, 1993

Baily DG, Arnold JM, Munoz C, Spence JD. Interaction of citrus juices with felodipine and nifedipine. *Lancet* 1991; **337**(8736):268–269.

Benet L. IOM Workshop, 1992.

Cannon W. Voodoo death. *Psychosom Med* 1957; **19**: 182–190.

Centers for Disease Control and Prevention (CDC), 2006; www.cdc.gov/datastatistics/; accessed July 9, 2010.

Chang SS, Davis JM, Ku NF, Pandey GN, Zhang MY. Racial differences in plasma and RBC lithium levels. Presented at the Annual Meeting of the American Psychiatric Association. Continuing Medical Education Syllabus and Scientific Proceedings, 1985; 239–240.

Chen KK, Poth EJ. *J Pharmacol Exp Ther* 1929; **36**.

Davitz JR, Davits LL. *Interferences of Patients' Pain and Psychological Distress: Studies of Nursing Behaviors*. Springer: New York, USA, 1981.

Dinsdale JE, Rollnik JD, Shapiro H. The effect of ethnicity on prescriptions for patient-controlled analgesia for postoperative pain. *Pain* 1995; **66**(1):9–12.

Doi T. *The Anatomy of Dependence*. Tokyo Kadansha International: Tokyo, 1973.

Drayer DE, Reidenberg MM. Clinical consequences of polymorphic acetylation. *Clin Pharmacol Ther* 1977; **22**: 251–258.

Dziewanowska ZE. International harmonization of clinical trials. In Fifth World Conference on Clinical Pharmacology and Therapeutics, Yokahara, Japan, July 1992.

Eap CB, Bauman P. The generic polymorphism of human a-1-acid glycoprotein: genetics, biochemistry, physiological functions and pharmacology. *Prog Clin Biol Res* 1989; **300**:111–125.

Edwards LD. Most major companies test medicines in women, monitor data for gender differences. In *Development: New Medicines for Women* (1991 Survey). Pharmaceutical Manufacturers' Association: Washington DC, USA, 1991, 27–28.

Edwards LD. *Gender and Ethnic Monitoring Survey*. Reported PERI Workshop. Pharmaceutical Manufacturers Association, 1992.

Edwards LD. Paper delivered at The International Conference on Harmonization (ICH), Orlando, FL, November 1993.

Eichelbaum M, Gross AS. The genetic polymorphism of debrisoquine/sparteine clinical aspects. *Pharmacol Ther* 1990; **46**:377–394.

Eisenberg L. The future of psychiatry. *Lancet* 1973; **2**: 1371–1373.

Fairburn WD. Japan drug regulations – a United States industrial perspective. *Regulat Affairs* 1989; **1**:25–33.

FDA. New drugs for investigational use: adoption of informational clinical research standards: acceptance of foreign data. *Federal Register* 1975; **40**(69):16052–16057.

FDA. New drug and metabolic regulations; final rule. *Federal Register* 1985; **50**(36):7452, 7483–7485, 7505.

FDA. E5 – Ethnic Factors in the Acceptability of Foreign Clinical Data – Questions and Answers, 2004; http://www.fda.gov/RegulatoryInformation/Guidances/ucm129314.htm; accessed April 12, 2010.

Federal Register. Ethnic factors in the acceptability of foreign clinical data (E5). *Federal Register* 1998; **63**(111): 31790–31796.

Folsom AR, Rosamond WD, Shahar E, Cooper LS, *et al.* Prospectual study of markers of hemostatic function with risk of ischemic stroke. The Athero Sclerosis Risk in communities (ARIC) study investigators. *Circulation* 1999; **100**(7):736–742.

Freis ED. Antihypertensive agents. In *Ethnic Differences in Reactions to Drugs and Xenobiotics*, Kalow W, Goedde HW, Agarwal DP (eds). Alan R. Liss: New York; 313–322, 1986.

Frankiewicz EJ, Sramek JJ *et al. Rispiridone in the Treatment of Hispanic Schizophrenics, Cross Cultural Psychiatry,* Herrera JM, Lawson WB (eds). John Wiley & Sons Inc.: New York, USA, 1999, 1360–1369.

Gould SE, Hayashi T, Nakashima T, Shohoji T, *et al.* Coronary heart disease and stroke. Atherosclerosis in Japanese men in Hiroshima, Japan and Honolulu, Hawaii. *Arch Pathol* 1972; **93**(2):98–102.

Hall DH. Pathophysiology of hypertension in Blacks. *Am J Hypertens* 1990; **3**:366S–371S.

Hartog J, Hartog EA. Cultural aspects of health and illness behavior in hospitals. *West J Med* 1983; **139**(6):910–926.

Harvey C, Walker S. Review of European CMR database for 21 drugs common to the West and Japan. In E5 Workshop Report ICH-2, Orlando, FL, USA, 1993.

Henry CJ, Emery B, Piggot S. Basal metabolic rate and diet-induced thermogenesis in Asians living in Britain. *Hum Nutr Clin Nutr* 1987; **41**(5):397–402.

Hess EV. Drug-related lupus. *Arthritis Rheum* 1982; **25**(7).

Homma M. Ministry of Health and Welfare Report. In *Proceedings of First International Conference on Harmonization,* ICH-I: Brussels, 1991.

Jefferson JW, Ackerman DL, Carol JA, Greisi JH. *Lithium Encyclopedia for Clinical Practice.* American Psychiatric Press: Washington, DC, USA, 1987.

Kato H, Tillotson J, Hamilton HB, Nichaman MZ, *et al.* Epidemiologic studies of coronary heart disease and stroke in Japanese men living in Japan, Hawaii and California. *Am J Epidemiol* 1973; **97**(6):372–385.

Khandker R, Simoni-Wastilia LJ. Differences in prescription drug utilization and expenditures between Blacks and Whites in the Georgia Medicaid population. *Inquiry* 1998; **35**(1):78–87.

Kiowiski N, Bolli P, Buhler FR, Ernep P, *et al.* Age, race, blood pressure, and renin predictions for hypertensive treatment with calcium antagonist. *Am J Cardiol* 1985; **16**:81H–85H.

Kumana CR, Chan M, Ko W, Lauder J, Lin HJ. Differences in diazepam pharmacokinetics in Chinese and White caucasians: relationship to body lipid stores. *Eur J Clin Pharmacol* 1987; **32**:211–215.

Kupfer A, Preisig R, Zeugin T. Pharmacogenetic aspects of biological variability. *J Gastroenterol Hepatol* 1988; **3**:623–633.

Leiberman JA, Canoso RT, Egea E, Kane JM, Yunis J. HLA-B38,DR4, DQW3 and clozapine-induced agranulocytosis in Jewish patients with schizophrenia. *Arch Gen Psychiatry* 1990; **47**:945–948.

Lin KM, Lesser JM, Poland RE. Ethnicity and psychopharmacology culture. *Med Psychiatry* 1986; **10**:151–165.

Medawar PB. Immunological tolerance. *Nature* 1961; **189**:14–17.

Lin KM, Poland RE, Smith MW, Strickland TL, Mendoza R. Pharmacokinetic and other related factors affecting psychotropic responses in Asians. *Psychopharmacol Bull* 1991; **27**(4):427–439.

Mendoza RP, *et al.* CYP2D6 polymorphism in Mexican American population. *J Clin Phararmacol Ther* 2001: **70**(6):552–560.

Ministry of Health and Welfare Notification 660 (June 1985); and Notification of PAB Director General: Acceptance of Data on Clinical Trials Conducted in Foreign Countries, Japan (29 June 1987).

Metropolitan Life Insurance. Male, Female, Height and Weight Tables, 1999; http://www.halls.md/ideal-weight/met.htm; accessed April 12, 2010.

Natio C, Yasuhova H. Retrospective survey of pharmacokinetics: dosage of 80 drugs approved in the EC, Japan, and US. E5 Workshop Reports, ICH- 2, Orlando, 1993.

Office of Management and Budget: Directive 15, 1997; http://ameasite.org/classification/omb15v97.asp; accessed April 12, 2010.

Oster G, Huse DM, Deles TE, *et al.* Cost effectiveness of labetalol and propranolol in the treatment of hypertension among Blacks. *J Natl Med Assoc* 1987; **79**:1049–1055.

Papaluca Amati M. Ethnic factors and clinical responsiveness: basic concepts of the retrospective survey. ES Workshop Report, ICH-2, Orlando, 1993.

Pemberton J. Does constitutional hypotension exist? *Br Med J* 1989; **298**:660–662.

Salzman C. Increased receptor sensitivity, psychoactive drugs, and analgesics. A prime of geriatric psychopharmacology. *Am J Psychiatry* 1982; **139**:67–74.

Sleath B, Svarstad B, Rotes D. Patient race and psychotropic prescribing during medical encounters. *Patient Educ Counsel* 1998; **34**(3):227–258.

Strickland TL, Lin KM, Mendoza R, *et al.* Psychopharmacologic considerations in the treatment of Black American populations. *Psychopharmacol Bull* 1991; **27**(4): 441–448.

Takahashi R. Lithium treatment in affective disorders: therapeutic plasma level. *Psychopharmacol Bull* 1979; **15**:32–35.

Tauzin W. Medicines in development, 2007; reports www phrma.org; accessed April 12, 2010.

Taylor AL, *et al.* Combination of isosorbide dinitrate and Hydrazine in blacks with heart failure. *N Engl J Medicine* 2004; **351**:2049–2057.

US Bureau of the Census. Press release C891–100, 1991.

Uchida K. Acceptability of foreign clinical trial data in Japan. *Drug Inf J* 1988; **22**:103–108.

Vessell E. Ethnic differences in reactions to drugs and xenobiotics. *Prog Clin Biol Res* 1989; **214**:21–37.

Weintraub M, Rubio A. Scoring system in a pilot effectiveness study of patients with sickle cell anemia. *J Clin Res Pharmacoepidemiol* 1992; **6**:47–54.

Wood AJJ, Zhou HH. Ethnic differences in drug disposition and responsiveness. *Clin Pharmacokinet* 1991; **20**:350–373.

World Health Organization. *World Population Prospects.* United Nations Publications: New York, 1990.

Yang YY. Prophylactic efficacy of lithium and its effective plasma levels in Chinese bipolar patients. *Acta Psychiatr Scand* 1987; **71**:171–175.

Zanger U, Raimundo S, Eichelbaum M, *et al.* Cytochrome P450 2D6, overview and update of pharmacology genetics and biochemistry. *Arch Pharmacol* 2004; **369**:23–37.

Zhang Y, Bertilsson L, Lou T, *et al.* Diazepam metabolism in native Chinese, poor and extensive hydroxylators of S-mephenytoin: inter-ethnic differences in comparison with White subjects. *Clin Pharmacol Ther* 1990; **48**:496–502.

Zhou HH, Adeloyin A, Wilkinson GR. Differences in plasma-binding of drugs between caucasians and Chinese subjects. *Clin Pharmacol Ther* 1990; **489**:10–17.

Zola IK. Studying the decision to see a doctor. In *Advances in Psychosomatic Medicine, Vol 8*, Lipowski Z (ed.). Karger: Basel, Switzerland, 1972, 216–236.

Recommended further reading

Federal Register (1999) Ethnic factors in the acceptability of foreign clinical data. *Federal Register* 1999; **63**(111):31790–31794.

Payer L. *Medicine and Culture*, H. Holt: New York, USA, 1988.

Walker S, Lumley C, McAuslane N. *The Relevance of Ethnic Factors in the Clinical Evaluation of Medicines*. Kluwer Academic: Hingham, MA, USA, 1994.

Suggested further reading

Reyes C. *et al. Genes, Culture, and Medicines: Bridging gaps in treatment for Hispanic Americans*. National Alliance for Hispanic Health and the National Pharmaceutical Council, 2004.

CHAPTER 20

Special Populations: Hepatic and Renal Failure

Anthony W. Fox

EBD Group Inc., Carlsbad, CA, USA and Munich, Germany, and Skaggs SPPS, University of California, San Diego, USA

Drug development programs are obligated to consider whether specific dose adjustments, warnings, or contraindications should be recommended in patients with varying degrees of hepatic or renal failure. In some regards the issues are analogous for patients with disease in one or other of these organs, and indeed, renal failure can be secondary to hepatic disease (even if the reverse is more controversial). The objective here is to review the issues surrounding these special populations. In doing so, readers should also review the two excellent US Food and Drug Administration (FDA) guidances on these subjects (1998, 2003).

General principles

(a) The issues surrounding hepatic or renal insufficiency are obviously greater for drugs (or their active or toxic) metabolites that are eliminated by the liver, kidney, or both.

(b) From a safety perspective, drugs whose effective doses are close to the harmful dose (a narrow "therapeutic ratio") are more likely to have critical limits on exposure, and thus in general, more likely to need careful study in patients with disease in these organs. A general useful rule is: "If there is (going to be) a clinical assay for drug concentration, then watch out for renal and hepatic disease associated adverse effects."

Principles and Practice of Pharmaceutical Medicine, 3rd edition.
Edited by L.D. Edwards, A.W. Fox, P.D. Stonier.
© 2011 Blackwell Publishing Ltd.

(c) Both renal and hepatic function can decline with age and differ with gender, pregnancy, and so on. When studies are needed (see below) the appropriate controls are not the typical young, fit, normal volunteers in Phase I studies, but rather patients or volunteers with relative renal or hepatic failure who are age and sex-matched as closely as possible to the patients with the disease state that will form the indication for the drug.

(d) Population kinetics can often provide much useful information. This is especially true when the intended patient population is elderly and may well have naturally reduced degrees of hepatic or renal reserve. This requires documentation of each patient's hepatic and renal status in ordinary clinical trials of unrelated diseases, within the ordinary Phase II/III database.

(e) For drugs administered chronically, consider carefully whether single-dose pharmacokinetics are truly predictive of the multiple-dose situation. Normal volunteers may not be predictive of patients with hepatic or renal disease. In case of doubt, conduct the studies described below in patients with liver or kidney disease at steady-state, or at least under conditions where the effects of the organ insufficiency can be assessed at both peak and trough drug concentrations.

(f) Be aware that pharmacokinetics and patterns of metabolism can change in patients with hepatic and renal insufficiency. With serious liver disease, many drugs' eliminations convert from first-order to zero-order. With serious renal disease, new metabolites may appear in the circulation because the urinary excretion of unchanged drug or the fastest generated metabolites is diverted to the liver. Dialysis often causes the opposite phenomena.

(g) There is a need to study the effect of *varying degrees* of hepatic or renal sufficiency on new drugs, according to the relevance of every degree to the promulgated indications. Almost all new drugs that will be administered to persons over 65 years of age will therefore need information about the effects of *mild* renal or hepatic insufficiency. Additionally, some drugs may need to be studied in patients with *moderate or severe* insufficiency(ies). In general, degree or severity of failure is easier to measure in the kidney than the liver.

(h) For drugs that are excreted entirely and unchanged by the lung (e.g., inhaled anesthetic gases), it is possible to provide a rationale to regulators that hepatic and renal insufficiency studies are unnecessary. Similar arguments can often be made for single dose drugs with wide margins between dose-response curves for wanted and unwanted effects, even if they are eliminated by either the kidney or the liver. However, note that this will not apply if the inhaled drug has intrinsic hepato- or nephro-toxic properties (e.g., halogenated gases).

(i) Drug interaction studies should not be overlooked as clues to drug behavior in hepatic and renal failure. As described in Chapter 21, these studies can mimic relative degrees of failure of the kidney and liver and thus guide the necessity for studies in these special populations.

Renal insufficiency

The central question is whether the degree of renal insufficiency that exists in patients that are likely to be exposed to the drug of interest could be sufficient to warrant an alteration in dosing. Note that the kidney is also an organ of metabolism, and therefore renal disease (especially when severe) can affect clearance in multiple ways, not just in urinary clearance.

Are studies needed?

The resolution of this central question, and thus the perceived need for special studies, hinges on multiple factors:

(a) Is the reduced excretion likely to cause a pharmacokinetic effect that is likely to be associated with a deleterious pharmacodynamic effect (reduction in efficacy or increase in intolerability)?

(b) Is the drug and its indication likely ever to be administered to people with renal insufficiency, and if so, to what degree of the latter?

(c) Is there an active metabolite for which these considerations are more important than the parent drug?

(d) Can fluid overload or other factors that change plasma protein concentration, and hence binding, interact with the anticipated effects on renal excretion?

(e) Are there some rare, special factors that can even theoretically be imagined (e.g., drug-induced diabetes insipidus and lithium)?

(f) Does the drug have intrinsic nephrotoxic properties?

Excluding an effect of renal failure

It is usually straightforward to conduct brief studies confirming the absence of any effect of renal failure that would impact pharmacodynamics. This is usually done when the circulating concentration response relationship for the wanted effects of the investigational drug is well-understood, of orthodox sigmoid form, when there is no active metabolite(s), and when the dose- or concentration-response relationship for unwanted effects is also well understood and some distance to the right of the concentration-response curve for efficacy. Small studies with dense sampling, or population kinetics with sparse sampling during the Phase III program, can accomplish this. Note that the latter cannot be accomplished when renal failure has been a routine exclusion criterion during the clinical development program. When study sponsors are confident, a small study (say $n = 4$–6 subjects with severe renal insufficiency) may serve to exclude an effect on pharmacokinetics of the investigational drug.

Quantifying the effect of renal failure

Assuming that studies are needed, patients with mild or moderate renal failure (estimated creatinine clearances 50–80 and 30–50 ml min^{-1}, respectively) must be studied. Age-, sex-, diet-, and smoking-matched controls for the disease state being treated should be used. Young, fit, volunteers will bias towards false-negative conclusions.

A single-dose study will usually be acceptable to regulatory authorities, provided that there is clear evidence elsewhere in the dossier/New Drug Application (NDA) that single-dose data can predict multiple-dose pharmacokinetics. If multiple-dose studies are needed, these should include an observation period at steady-state. The study size (i.e., number of patients per group) will be determined by a power calculation using the known variability of the pharmacokinetic parameters of the drug in question; in practice there is seldom the need for more than 15 subjects per renal function stratum, unless a population kinetics approach has been preferred. The nonlinear and non-compartmental modeling procedures for use in a population kinetics scheme are beyond the scope of this chapter, and should certainly be discussed in advance with the relevant regulatory authorities.

When possible, pharmacodynamic assessments should be made in conjunction with the pharmacokinetic estimates. The reason for this is that it can check that there has not been some supersensitivity state induced in the biophase by the disease causing the renal insufficiency. This will exclude a false-negative conclusion when purely pharmacokinetic data are analyzed.

Assays will usually be on plasma and urine. Plasma protein binding should be estimated simultaneously because renal disease can alter plasma protein binding of some drugs.

Note on estimation of creatinine clearance

Formal measures of creatinine clearance (CrCL), using intravenous inulin or radio-iodinated sodium iothalamate, will not have been performed on most patients with relative renal failure in ordinary clinical practice. Of several alternatives in adults, the Cockroft-Gault estimate of CrCL, from a point measure of serum creatinine, currently enjoys widest acceptance by regulatory authorities.

For men, the Cockroft-Gault estimate is

$$\text{CrCL (ml min}^{-1}) = [140 \times \text{age (y)} \times \text{weight (kg)}]/[72 \times \text{serum creatinine (mg dl}^{-1})]$$

For women, the Cockroft-Gault estimate is the same as for men, except that the result is multiplied by 0.85.

In infants, the Cockroft-Gault estimate is inaccurate. Currently, the US FDA guidance for children is

Under 1 year: $\text{CrCL (ml min}^{-1}) = [0.45 \times \text{length (cm)}]/\text{serum creatinine (mg dl}^{-1})$

1 – 12 years: $\text{CrCL (ml min}^{-1}) = [0.55 \times \text{length (cm)}]/\text{serum creatinine (mg dl}^{-1})$

Dialysis

End-stage renal disease is characterized by the need for routine dialysis. These are the patients with renal failure *for whom an increase in dosing* may be necessary to compensate for drug/active metabolites being lost into the dialysate. Understanding the pharmacokinetics of the drug during dialysis is essential unless it is anticipated that exposed patients will not be treated with it. Even then, knowing whether a drug can or cannot be dialyzed is helpful in providing advice to clinicians dealing with overdoses or poisonings after the drug has been marketed.

Labeling

The US FDA guidance provides several specimen pieces of wording for use by those drafting product labeling: They are highly recommended. Generally speaking, if renal insufficiency causes a change in pharmacokinetics that exceeds the latitude granted to generic copies of previously approved drugs, there should be careful consideration to adding specific dosing recommendations for patients with renal insufficiency. Currently this latitude is for the mean C_{max} to lie outside a range of 70–143% of the control mean, with the simultaneous mean AUC to lie outside 80–125 % of the control mean.

Hepatic insufficiency

Many of the guiding principles offered above for renal insufficiency find their corollaries in hepatic insufficiency. However, there are two fundamental differences. First, hepatic disease causes secondary renal failure more often than the other way round. Second, it is more difficult to quantify severity of insufficiency of the liver than for the kidney. This section of the chapter is again based upon the excellent US FDA guidance (see Further Reading section at the end of the chapter).

The literature contains hundreds of reports on the influence of liver disease on drug elimination. Most commonly the patients in these studies have various degrees of fatty degeneration or cirrhosis (the former often associated with alcohol or diabetes, and the latter most commonly due to hepatitis viruses, alcohol, but sometimes obliterative biliary disease, or auto-immune disease). These diseases are often associated with intrinsic alterations in pharmacodynamic responses. For example, liability to seizure is common in patients suddenly withdrawn from chronic alcohol abuse (e.g., bupropion for smoking cessation).

Assessing severity of hepatic dysfunction

Most widely accepted by regulatory authorities (i.e., you have to have a good reason not to use it) is the Child-Pugh scoring system. This was originally developed as a method for assessing anesthesia/surgical hazard in patients with varying degrees of hepatic disease.

It is a point-scoring system, according to Table 20.1.

The only other commonly used alternative is the Maddrey Discriminant Function (MDF), which was developed to assess acute alcoholic hepatitis. This is more easily calculated than the Child-Pugh score, as

$$MDF = [4.6 \times \text{prothrombin time (sec)}] + \text{serum total bilirubin (mg dl}^{-1})$$

Table 20.1 Child-Pugh point scoring system.

	Points scored		
	1	2	3
Encephalopathy grade*	0	1 or 2	3 or 4
Ascites	None	Slight	Moderate
Serum bilirubin mg dl^{-1}	<2	2–3	>3
Serum albumin mg dl^{-1}	>3.5	2.8–3.5	<2.8
Prothrombin time prolongation (sec)	<4	4–6	>6

Total points: good operative risk ≤6; moderate risk 7–9; poor risk >9 points.

*0 = normal; 1 = restlessness 5 Hz waves on EEG; 2 = lethargic, disoriented, asterixis; 3 = somnolent/stuperous rigidity; 4 = unrousable coma (each grade >0 can have other symptoms).

Disease was labeled not severe when MDF <54, severe at 55–92, and probably lethal at ≥93. In practice, most modern clinical trials will document both the Child-Pugh score and the MDF at all relevant time points.

Methods that involve studying the disposition of some exogenously administered agent (e.g., indocyanine green, antipyrine, galactose, or dextromethorphan) have now been superceded by functional (often multi-component) tests. Monoethylglycinexylidide formation has not found wide acceptance. More complicated Cox proportional hazards models may exist for other liver diseases, but are only used specifically for them (e.g., the Mayo Clinic Survival Model for primary biliary cirrhosis; see the US FDA guidance).

When studies are needed

In general, studies are needed for all drugs to which the liver is exposed, unless

- drug excretion is entirely non-hepatic;
- hepatic metabolism accounts for <20% of clearance *and* the drug has a clearly demonstrated, wide therapeutic window; or
- the drug is volatile and it (and its metabolites) are readily excreted by the lung *and* the drug has no intrinsic hepatotoxic properties.

Most regulatory authorities allow some relaxation of the requirement for studies when the drug is for single dose only, and when adverse events are C_{max} rather than AUC-related (because C_{max} usually varies little with reduced rate of clearance under these conditions).

Study design

Generally, there should be a clear understanding of the pharmacokinetics of the drug of interest in all three Child-Pugh classes of liver disease, unless the sponsor is willing to accept strong labeling against administration in severe liver failure (and then has to study only the other two grades of severity). The size of each treatment group depends upon the variability in the pharmacokinetics of the agent, although the US FDA guidance recommends that this should be at least six patients, regardless. As before, single-dose studies may suffice when there is reason to believe that for all the stages of liver disease that are being studied, the pharmacokinetics of a single dose are indeed predictive of the multiple-dose/steady-state situation. When drugs are being developed for more than one route of administration, usually one can be chosen that provides the maximum information, and the need to study the second route is obviated. Population kinetics approaches are also sometimes feasible if incorporated into Phase III development schemes, and when appropriate nonlinear and non-compartmental models can be defined.

Conclusions of no effect are based upon the pharmacokinetic tolerances accorded to generic versus innovative products. However, small numbers of patients usually make this quite difficult.

In general, regulatory authorities are keen to provide advice on particular study designs that are appropriate on a case-by-case basis, and this should always be an agenda item at end-of-Phase II meetings in the USA, or during scientific advice procedures in the European Union.

Labeling

The US FDA guidance provides specimens for labeling. In practical terms, another useful approach is to review some recent product labels in commonly used compendia (such as *Physician's Desk Reference*, *Drugs Sheet Compendium*, *Rote List*, and so on) to find the sorts of wordings that national regulatory authorities have recently found to be acceptable.

Further reading

Figg WD, Dukes GE, *et al.* Comparison of quantitative methods to assess hepatic function: Pugh's classification, indocyanine green, antipyrine, and dextromethorphan. *Pharmacotherapy* 1995; **165**:693–700.

Food and Drug Administration. *Guidance for industry: Pharmacokinetics in patients with impaired renal function: study design, data analysis and impact on dosing and labeling.* US Dept Health and Human Services: Washington DC, USA, 1998; http://www.fda.gov/downloads/Drugs/GuidanceComplianceRegulatoryInformation/Guidances/ucm072127.pdf; accessed April 24, 2010.

Food and Drug Administration. *Guidance for industry: Pharmacokinetics in patients with impaired hepatic function: study design, data analysis and impact on dosing and labeling.* US Dept Health and Human Services: Washington DC, USA, 2003; http://www.fda.gov/downloads/Drugs/GuidanceComplianceRegulatoryInformation/Guidances/ucm072123.pdf; accessed April 24, 2010.

Maddrey WC, Boitnott JK *et al.* Corticosteroid therapy of alcoholic hepatitis. *Gastroenterology* 1978; **75**:93–199.

Pugh RNH, Murray-Lyon IM, *et al.* Transection of the oesopgahus for bleeding oesophageal varices. *Br J Surg* 1973; **60**:646–649.

CHAPTER 21

Drug Interactions

Anthony W. Fox[1] & Anne-Ruth van Troostenburg[2]

[1]EBD Group Inc., Carlsbad, CA, USA and Munich, Germany, and Skaggs SPPS, University of California, San Diego, USA
[2]Takeda Group R&D, London, UK

Definition

A drug interaction is an effect observed with two or more drugs that is not seen with one drug alone. The effect can be qualitative or quantitative, and can create clinical hazard or therapeutic benefit.

Patients often receive multiple drugs. Every physician will be aware of the benefits of pharmacodynamic interactions of medications—such as additional effects on blood pressure when combining ACE inhibitors, calcium antagonists, beta blockers, or diuretics to treat hypertension. The interactions of these drugs result in additional blood pressure lowering effect, which can be both wanted or unwanted in its magnitude. Equally, all physicians will be aware of the potential for adverse effects of commonly used drugs such as warfarin when another drug, such as non-steroidal anti-inflammatory drugs (NSAIDs) are introduced. Interactions matter when one drug alters the pharmacokinetics of the other, or the therapeutic target is the same for both drugs.

It is impossible to remember all drug interactions. The purpose of this chapter is to offer a description of drug interactions in a systematic manner. In ordinary clinical practice, information technology (IT) and ready-reference manuals should always be used, and the physician and pharmacist should collaborate. Currently, a recommendation for IT-based systems would be to use at least two of the

proprietary programs because they widely overlap but are not comprehensive.

Within the realm of pharmaceutical research, additional aspects must be borne in mind. First, interactions must be described and quantified on paper, whether in product labeling, regulatory submissions, or scientific reports. Second, interactions must be considered when designing clinical protocols. Third, for investigative products, there may not yet be sufficient information to predict where interactions may lie.

Description and quantitation of drug interactions

Drug interactions may be described as *additive*, *synergistic* (or *potentiating*), or more commonly, *antagonistic*. These three categories are regardless of whether the underlying mechanism is pharmacodynamic or pharmacokinetic in nature.

Drug interactions may be quantitated and illustrated using *isobolograms*. An isolobolgram is simply a method of illustrating data with three variables in two dimensions, that is, on the surface of a piece of paper. This form of plotting should not be unfamiliar. Analogous examples of such plots are found (three dimensions) on topographical maps (latitude, longitude, and elevation above sea level using contour lines) and meteorological charts (latitude, longitude, and barometric pressure using isobars); in both cases the third variable is shown by the contours. In the simple case of an interaction between two drugs, the three variables that are

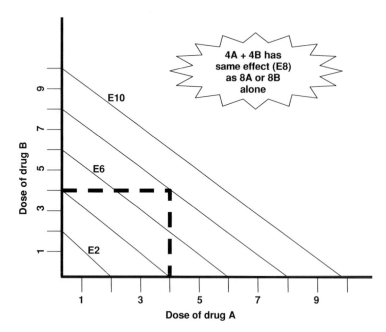

Figure 21.1 Isobologram illustrating simple additivity. The lines connect equal amounts of drug effect (E), with each having the general equation $ay + bx = kE_c$, where a, b, and k are constants and c is the percentage of maximal effect on the dose-response curve (in this case $a = b = k = 1$).

plotted are the dose (or plasma concentration) of drugs A and B, and the size of effect shown by the contours.

Additivity is where two drugs have the same effect, and neither potentiates or antagonizes the other. The contours of the isobologram are parallel line segments (see Figure 21.1). Antibiotic combinations frequently are additive. Nonetheless, the results of this efficacy analysis still need to be reconciled against clinical hazard, which is measured in different ways.

Antagonism is an interaction where one or other drug reduces the activity of the other. The contours of the isobologram are convex away from the origin of the plot (see Figure 21.2). Several examples of antagonistic interactions are discussed below in connexion of the locus where such interactions take place.

Synergy or potentiation is where the combination of two drugs have an effect that is greater than simply additive. The contours of the isobologram are concave towards the origin of the plot (see Figure 21.3). In most cases, an effect with this type of drug combination can exceed the effect that is achievable with even maximal doses of either

alone. Combination antihypertensive therapy or chemotherapy are good examples.

More complicated isobolograms also exist. The *N*-acetyl cysteamine dosage algorithm is an isobologram with time and acetaminophen (paracetamol)

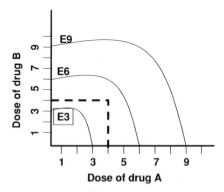

Figure 21.2 A classical isobologram illustrating antagonism. Uses the same notation as in Figure 21.1. The broken lines show how a combination of 4 units of drug A plus four units of drug B have an effect that is much less than E8 (as would be the case if the interaction were additive). The formulae for the contours are $ay + bx < kE_c$.

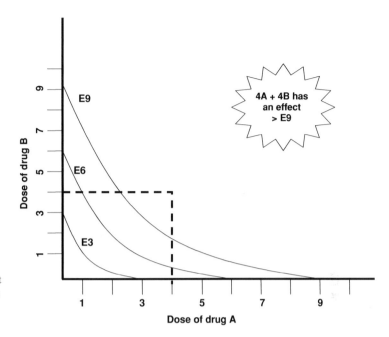

Figure 21.3 Classical isolbologram for a synergistic or potentiating drug interaction. The dotted lines show how 4 dose units of drug A plus four dose units of drug B result in an effect that exceeds E8. The formulae for the contours are $ay + bx > kE_c$ using the same notation as in Figure 21.1.

plasma concentration on the axes in the plane of the paper and a two-step measure in the third dimension (probability of toxicity that requires treatment). Somewhat as famous is Professor Herxheimer's depiction of the interaction between coffee and wine: Two glasses of each provides the maximum possible beneficial effect (the effect being "happiness"). The contours are thus of a hill on a plane.

Systematic consideration of drug interactions

The key to considering the potential for drug interactions lies in considering all the places that drug molecules may occupy. In this section we shall present a *repertoire* of drug interactions sorted by locus, which the reader may like to consider, and those sitting the Diploma in Pharmaceutical Medicine might like to be able to deliver to the examiners. The full set of drug loci are the sites of drug storage, absorption, distribution, action, metabolism, and excretion, plus, in some cases, the presence of the drug in blood and urine samples that reach the clinical laboratory; clearly there are

exceptions. For example, some drugs act at the site of absorption, and others are excreted unchanged.

Prior to administration: Drug storage
These interactions are always unwanted. A good example is the inappropriate mixing of insulins. Slower release insulins are complexed with protamine zinc in excess, while the conjugation of insulin with such adjuvant takes place slowly, especially in the relatively low temperature of a refrigerator. Drawing up the *lente* insulin first, and then sticking the needle into the soluble insulin, gradually transfers the excess protamine zinc into the soluble insulin, thus converting it into *lente* insulin. Chelation is usually a chemical reaction: heparin is the most acidic drug in common usage, and it chelates almost everything (for some reason, penicillins are reported as the most chelated combination in the infusion bag). Other examples include almost any drug in blood or elemental foodstuffs.

Site of absorption
There are common examples of both wanted and unwanted drug interactions at the site of absorption. Examples include activated charcoal/any

overdose (wanted), metoclopramide–naproxen (the absorption of the latter being hastened by the former for improved efficacy when treating migraine acutely), lipid or olefin fecal emulsifiers and fat-soluble vitamins (the latter being unabsorbed, an unwanted interaction), and tetracyclines–calcium containing drugs (e.g., milk, an unwanted interaction because of the calcium chelating properties of tetracyclines). Note that the epinephrine–lidocaine (adrenaline–lignocaine) interaction can be both wanted or unwanted. At most injection sites, localized vasoconstriction reduces the rate of systemic absorption, reduces the lignocaine (lidocaiane) dose needed, prolongs local anesthesia, and reduces the potential for central nervous system adverse effects (i.e., a wanted interaction). However, in tissues that form a salient (fingers, toes, nose, ear pinna, penis) the vasoconstrictor can cause necrosis because of the absence of collateral circulation.

Drug distribution

Most of these drug interactions involve displacement of drug from plasma proteins, thus increasing the free/bound ratio for drug concentration. When the free moieties are those that are pharmacologically active, unexpectedly exaggerated responses result from standard doses. Most (but not all) such interactions are unwanted. Almost any non-steroidal anti-inflammatory drug (NSAID) displaces warfarin, elevating the prothrombin time and rendering the patient liable to unexpected ecchymosis or more serious hemorrhagic adverse events. Similarly unwanted are the interactions between phenytoin and thyroxine (sedation and thyrotoxicosis), and salicylates with tolbutamide (hypoglycemia). Oral contraceptives compete for albumin binding sites, and phenytoin doses may need to be adjusted when the former are introduced. A rare example of a beneficial drug interaction at this locus are the use of NSAIDs with some glucocorticoids, where enhanced anti-inflammatory effects of the latter can result, even though a relatively low dose of the steroid has been administered.

Drug interactions at the site of action are manyfold and familiar. All receptor antagonists, when used in the face of an agonist challenge are clini-

cally desirable. Obvious examples include naloxone for opioid overdose and physostigmine for reversal of tubocurarine in anesthesia. Note that succinylcholine paralysis during anesthesia is only made worse with anticholinesterase administration (an adverse drug interaction at the receptor, beloved by multiple-choice question setting examiners!).

Sequential biochemistry interactions also fall within this category. Sulfamethoxazole and trimethoprim inhibit different stages of the folate metabolism pathway. Concomitant administration reduces the probability that a bacterial strain can mutate in any single step to evade the antibiotic effects of both drugs.

Physiological interactions are a subset of site-of-action interactions. Adding spironoloactone to furosemide (frusemide) provides no extra diuresis, but does antagonize the potassium loss that occurs when the latter drug is used alone. Both progestagens and estragens (progesterones and estragens) such as ethinyl(o)estradiol and levonorgestrol inhibit ovulation and uterine deciduation, thus being positive or wanted interactions, albeit acting at different receptors.

Unwanted interactions at the site of action classically include the highly undesirable concomitant use of tetracyclines and penicillins. The latter are bacteriocidal when the organism is dividing because it obstructs cell wall manufacture, and thus exposes the new bacterial membrane to osmotic destruction. Bacteriostatic compounds, such as tetracyclines, reduce the rate of bacterial division and thus reduce the effectiveness of penicillins.

Other nonreceptor site-of-action interactions include MAOIs–pethidine (acute dystonias and hyperthermia), ethanol–benzodiazepines (synergisitic sedation and respiratory depression), cocaine–amphetamines (hypertensive crisis), and dihydrocodeine–morphine (the former is a partial agonist and reduces the efficacy of the full agonist).

As far as drug metabolism is concerned, it is essential to understand some of the basic biochemistry before being able to anticipate the interactions that can occur at this locus. Mobile omnivore mammals are constantly exposed to xenobiotics, many of which can be toxic. An efficient defense against these toxins resides in the gut and the liver, with the general aim of metabolizing such toxic molecules into smaller and less toxic metabolites; these are generally more water soluble and thus more capable of urinary excretion. Reduction of exposure of the rest of the body to high concentrations of the parent toxin is the result. Drugs fall foul of the same defense mechanisms.

Cytochromes are a diverse class of enzymes, and are so-named because they are brightly colored when in solution. This color is because these enzymes contain heme groups and transition metal ions (e.g., Fe^{++}, Cu^{++}, etc.). Since they are colored, these enzymes may be classified by the wavelength of light that they absorb maximally. Although a comprehensive discussion of cytochrome classification is beyond the scope of this chapter, suffice it to say that cytochrome class P enzymes, with a maximal absorption of 450 nm (CYP450) are the most important for drug metabolism. These CYP450 enzymes themselves exist as several hundred isoenzymes, denoted by code letters and digits, e.g., CYP450 2D6. Each isoenzyme has a preferential substrate. Different species (including *H. sapiens*) exhibit different patterns of isoenzymes in their phenotype, and there may be further variation in the activity of particular isoenzymes between individuals, whether or not this is predictable on the basis of membership of particular ethnic groups.

CYP450 isoenzymes reside on the smooth endoplasmic reticulum. They are stereotypical mixed-function oxidases (or oxygenases). These enzymes oxidize and reduce two substrates simultaneously, and atoms from molecular oxygen usually are incorporated into one of the substrates. Alternatives include the loss of hydrogen atoms or alkyl groups, with the corresponding formation of water or formate. The loss of hydrogen atoms (i.e., the substrate becomes less reduced) is another form of molecular oxidation within the Lowry-Brønstein formulation. Thus, drug metabolism by CYP450 can involve hydroxylation, dealkylation, aromatic oxidation, sulfation, ring opening with hydroxylation, and so on. Sometimes, the isoenzyme itself is oxidized, and in this case it is usually regenerated by reduced nicotinamide adenine phosphate (NADP-H).

When thinking about interactions at the site of metabolism, one must therefore think about classical enzymology, and *from the enzyme's point of view*. Drugs can be substrates, inhibitors, or enzyme activators (i.e., inducers or promoters). Competition by two drugs for saturated enzyme is mutual competitive antagonism and elimination times for both will increase (when the enzyme is saturated, zero-order metabolism will supervene). Drugs that are enzyme inhibitors will prolong the elimination time for another substrate, but the pharmacokinetics of the inhibitor itself will not change (unless the drug is itself both a substrate and an inhibitor for the enzyme). Some drugs, for example, rifampicin, barbiturates (barbitals), and cigarette smoke are enzyme inducers. In molar terms per gram protein, the concentration of enzyme increases during exposure to the inducing drug a period of several days and there is secondarily hastening of the metabolism of some other drug substrate. Barbiturates (barbitals) are classic enzyme inducers; by enhancing the elimination of warfarin, anticoagulant effect can be lost. Some drugs (e.g., opiates) auto-induce their own isoenzyme, and this is one reason why doses tend to escalate in palliative care (note that there is no adaptive reduction in the gut, and oral opiate-induced constipation under these conditions gets only worse because this is a local effect at the site of absorption which is unprotected by hepatic metabolism of absorbed drug).

For a census of commonly prescribed drugs, the predominant CYP450 isoenzyme for drug metabolism is 3A4 (about 55 % of all prescribed drugs). Next comes 2D6 (25%). About 15% of drugs are metabolized by isoenzyme 2C9 (although this number probably includes small contributions by 2C10, 2C18, and 2C19, as well). A few percent of all drugs are metabolized by either CYP450 1A2 or 2E1 isoenzymes in humans.

Genetic polymorphisms in CYP450 isoenzymes are common. Among so-called "caucasians," 5–10% of the population carries a mutation of CYP450 2D6, causing them to be "slow metabolizers" of debrisoquine, mephenytoin, quinidine, metoprolol, and dextromethorphan. Standard doses are more likely to be associated with adverse events as a consequence, especially when a second substrate drug is interacting.

The elderly have livers that are functionally less effective than younger adults and CYP450 enzyme activity reduces correspondingly. The newborn has relatively reduced CYP450 capability, although this is uneven, and glucuronidation of bilirubin at birth is especially poor. The human fetus uniquely expresses CYP450 3A7; this disappears soon after birth, for reasons that are unknown.

Wanted interactions at the site of metabolism include acetaminophen (paracetamol)–N-acetyl cysteamine; note above the comments that this is an atypical isobologram. "Methylated spirits"—a mixture of methanol and ethanol—is used as a fuel for lamps or heating in some places. The methanol component is supposed to deter ethanol abusers, but nonetheless methylated spirits are still drunk in pursuit of intoxication, especially by the indigent. Both alcohols are substrates for the same dehydrogenases. Formaldehyde is more toxic than acetaldehyde, and formate is more toxic than acetate, with the optic nerve being an especially vulnerable tissue to these toxins. Thus, treating methylated spirits toxicity with *pure* ethanol can save the patient's eyesight because, at the expense of greater acetaldehyde exposure, enzyme competition will lead to increased excretion of unchanged methanol.

Site of excretion

The principal site of excretion that is liable to drug interactions is in the kidney. The classic example is forced alkaline diuresis using intravenous sodium bicarbonate solution to hasten the excretion of aspirin. Aspirin is freely filtered by the glomerulus into the nephron, and is then reabsorbed across the lipid membrane into the renal parenchyma, and thence the renal vein. When not ionized, resorption across the lipid membrane is more than when salicylate is ionized. Salicylate (like sulfate, nitrate, etc.) is the ion resulting from dissolving an acid. Making the urine alkaline increases the proportion of salicylate that is ionized, reduces its resorption, and hence increases its urinary excretion. Note also that this all works *vice versa*. Metamphetamine (like other compounds ending -amine) is a base: its excretion can be hastened by acidifying the urine

by using oral ammonium sulfate. These interactions are also beloved by multiple-choice question composers.

The techniques of forced diuresis must be contrasted with the tactics that can be employed to alter the excretion of drugs that are actively secreted into the post-glomerular nephron. Acidic drugs (e.g., penicillin) are good candidates for these transporters. The co-administration of another organic acid (classically an otherwise redundant analgesic called probenecid), by competing for the acid transport mechanism, can reduce the urinary excretion of penicillin, and hence enhance its residence in the body. Historically, this was used for economy of penicillin supplies when this drug was very precious during the Second World War; today, the same tactic can be used for single-dose treatment of gonorrhoea.

There are rare alternative examples for drug interactions at other sites of excretion. For example, volatile general anesthetics are exhaled, and drugs that reduce minute ventilation (e.g., benzodiazepines peri-operatively) consequently reduce the rate of excretion of isoflurane. Arguably, because one might also consider these as site-of-absorption interactions, drug excretion rates in the stool can be increased using oral polyethyleneglycol to reduce the absorption of oral poisons (wanted), and oral paraffins (used for constipation) can increase fat-soluble vitamin excretion (unwanted).

The clinical laboratory is the final place where drug interactions can occur. In the developed world it is likely that only a small proportion of false positive, false negative, and inaccurately quantitated clinical laboratory results are the result of interference by concomitant drugs. One somewhat historical example is that for some of the older, less-specific antibodies, spironolactone, vitamin D, and carbamazepine can all interfere with digoxin radioimmunoassays; this remains a problem in less wealthy countries.

Preclinical investigations and clinical trials to investigate interactions

Development plans for new drugs should include screening for potential drug interactions at an early stage. Structural chemistry and other chemical properties will give a broad idea of how the drug may be absorbed, transported, metabolized, and excreted. Mechanistic studies to elucidate the mechanism of action will give indications for possible interactions with other drugs acting at the same site. *In vitro* and *in vivo* investigations on hepatic enzyme systems can be carried out to investigate the substrate potential and/or capability for inhibition or induction of liver enzyme systems; this information can then be used to guide investigations of metabolic interactions that may be of eventual clinical significance. The animal toxicokinetics may also provide information about what can be expected in humans.

These batteries of preclinical tests will often generate questions that can only be answered by studying potential interactions in humans. Understanding whether a new drug will interact with other drugs that are likely to be co-prescribed for the disease of interest is essential for good product labeling. Oral contraceptives are used by about 50% of women in their reproductive years in the developed world, and must always be considered as a concomitant medication.

Clinical trial design for drug interactions

Drugs in development usually have to undergo a number of human interaction studies, before they can be administered to patients (often on stable co-medications) whether in Phase III clinical trials or after marketing authorization is obtained. It is hard to generalize about the number and type of interaction studies that are needed for new drugs because these depend on so many aspects of the preclinical profile and target disease (see above).

The design of individual studies that address possible interactions through the CYP450 metabolic pathway are, although often somewhat stereotypical, never completely standard. Usually these are Phase I healthy volunteer studies that have primary endpoints of a pharmacokinetic nature. The studies can usually be done in an open-label fashion and without the use of placebo because the endpoint is objective: Drug concentrations reported in the laboratory cannot be influenced by investigator bias.

Prior to study design, the available data need to be examined to understand whether the study drug is expected to be an inhibitor or inducer of any important CYP450 isoenzyme, or is a substrate competing for one of them. If there is a priori understanding of the putative metabolic pathway(s), it can be possible to design a single study that screens broadly across all those isoenzymes that are commonly involved in drug metabolism in humans.

Enzyme competition or inhibition occurs quickly and can often be demonstrated with a single-dose design. Inhibition tends to be very specific for a given isoenzyme. Offset of inhibition can be fast or slow. Straightforward substrate competition wears off as quickly as the fastest of the interacting drugs is eliminated. However, covalent binding of drug to the receptor or enzyme of interest is irreversible. A good example is proton-pump blockade, in which recovery requires regeneration of the proton transporter, and takes several days. Many inhibitory effects are dose-dependent and only reach clinically significant levels of inhibition at greatly supratherapeutic doses. It is therefore important in first interaction studies to plan for more than one dose level.

Enzyme induction is usually dose-dependent and typically needs 10–14 days of repeat dosing to develop to its full extent. Enzyme induction is generally less specific than enzyme inhibition and can be observed across a broad range of isoenzymes simultaneously. Barbiturates (barbitals), rifampicin, and cigarette smoking are all well-known enzyme inducers, and can affect the metabolism of a wide variety of drugs. A redundant non-steroidal agent (known as antipyrine) was the classical probe drug for enzyme induction, and its metabolism is increased compared to baseline when a 14-day challenge by an enzyme inducing drug is administered. Modern "cocktail" studies have now superseded antipyrine.

Substrate "cocktails" are now used so as to study efficiently the effect of the test drug on several CYP450 isoenzymes at once. The cocktail comprises a mixture of drugs where each is metabolized wholly by a sole and different isoenzyme. Several established "cocktails" have been published. For example, the "Indiana Cocktail" contains (isoenzyme) caffeine (1A2), tolbutamide (2C9), dextromethorphan (2D6), and midazolam (3A4). All such studies need to have adequate monitoring for safe administration of drugs in place—such as oxygen saturation monitoring when midazolam is given. Acute attention to detail and timing is vital in order to obtain reliable, interpretable results. In particular the timing of blood sampling for drug concentrations must be carefully designed in accordance with the known pharmacokinetic profiles of each drug administered and executed with the greatest precision.

For studies of CYP450 isoforms involving large phenotypical differences in humans, pre-screened volunteers, with known isoenzyme activity and capacity, are needed. In this way, experimentally-induced extreme plasma concentrations and the consequent clinical hazard can be avoided (e.g., due to pre-existing slow metabolism).

Two typical, Phase I, drug interaction clinical trial designs are shown in Figure 21.4. Pharmacokinetic profiles are found within each subject for each substrate with and without concomitant exposure to the study drug. These designs are applicable to both enzyme induction and inhibition effects (Fig-ure 21.4, upper half). The same study schematic can be used to study the effects of inhibitors or inducers on the study drug as a substrate for CYP450 systems (as illustrated in the lower half of Figure 21.4).

Some drug interaction studies must be done in patients and use longer durations of exposure, and these are usually conducted in small groups of patients (rarely more than 12). These investigate not only pharmacokinetic interaction considerations, but also the potential for interference with the efficacy of a proven agent. For example, drugs in development for rheumatoid arthritis must undergo an interaction study with methotrexate prior to the execution even of Phase II clinical trials because it is essential to ensure that the new agent neither interferes with the therapeutic effect of methotrexate nor potentiates its adverse effects. These studies are more complex and need to be designed carefully on a case-by-case basis.

Regulatory considerations of drug interactions

This chapter has concentrated on drug interaction studies during the development of new drugs. Just as important is that the development of a drug does not stop after marketing authorization has been obtained, because new information on a marketed drug can emerge at any stage of its lifespan. Marketing Authorization (MA) or New Drug Application (NDA) holders are obligated to monitor this emerging information for its relevance to prescribers and patients. This includes any new information on the potential for drug interactions.

When drug interaction information emerges late in the product life cycle it is almost always a matter of clinical importance. This information must be made available to prescribers and patients, and can be communicated by inclusion into the product labeling, or more quickly for issues of serious hazard, as a "Dear Healthcare Professional" letter. All such new information to be included in the label is subject to regulatory scrutiny and approval, and the initiating entity can be the MA or NDA holder or regulatory authorities themselves. However, the

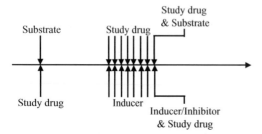

Figure 21.4 Two typical designs for a Phase I drug interaction clinical trial. The horizontal arrow represents time, at a scale of several days. Above the horizontal line is a typical screening study, where the test medication (Study drug) is being screened for any sort of interaction (inhibitory or inducing) with a known isoenzyme substrate; note that a cocktail of several substrates can also be used with this design. Below the horizontal arrow is a study design testing whether elimination of the test medication is itself susceptible to enzyme induction or inhibition by some other drug (Inducer/inhibitor); note that the roles of the known and unknown drugs have essentially been reversed.

pharmaceutical physician should be aware of the important differences between regional regulatory systems.

In the USA, pharmaceutical companies have the option of including important new safety information (such as a relevant drug interaction) in the label and sending a notification with the new label text to the FDA. The changed label will come into effect at the time of sending the notification to the agency. This "changes being effected" notification is justified on the grounds of an immediate improvement in notifying product hazards. Usually, the relevant FDA medical reviewer will communicate with the NDA holder and state whether the label change was accepted or whether he/she considers the change subject to prior approval. The latter allows the FDA reviewer more time and the option to adapt the proposed label text. In any case, this is a quick and effective way to ensure communication to all relevant parties in a minimum of time.

In the European Union matters are slightly more complex. Whether products have been approved using the central or mutual recognition procedures, the MA will have harmonized the product labeling across all EU Member States. European regulations require that all changes to product labeling must have prior approval. Thus, important new drug interaction findings will require the submission of a type II variation to the MA and an (albeit abbreviated) Common Technical Document. The Summary of Product Characteristics and Patient Information Leaflet must all be changed accordingly, and approval by the regulatory authority(ies) will inevitably take several months. For very significant clinical hazards, a more rapid and direct communication of such important new information from the MA holder to prescribers and patients will be needed.

Prospectus

As in many areas of drug development, the amount of information about drug metabolism in children is limited. More work on the ontogeny of drug metabolism systems will be needed in the future. Regulatory authorities are actively encouraging this with certain incentives both in Europe and the USA, which generally find support not only from academic societies of pediatric medicine, but also from MA and NDA holders themselves. Studies of drug interactions will form a part of this pediatric metabolic research, and should be able to exploit these regulatory initiatives.

Furthermore, as more information is wrung from the human genome, it is likely that many drug interactions that we currently view as idiosyncratic will acquire mechanistic explanations. This form of personalized medicine, with the capability to predict a pharmacokinetic or pharmacodynamic interaction by knowing the patient's phenotype in advance, will be a powerful therapeutic tactic in the interests of patient safety and optimization of therapy.

CHAPTER 22

Orphan Drugs

Bert Spilker[1]
Bert Spilker Associates, Bethesda, MD, USA

Introduction

"Rare disease" is defined by US law as a disease with a prevalence of fewer than 200,000 patients. Other countries have defined a rare disease based on a prevalence of 0.1–0.5% of the population. A rare disease is sometimes also referred to as an orphan disease, and an orphan drug is a drug to treat a rare disease. The term "orphan drug" originated from the belief that there were drugs that no pharmaceutical sponsor wanted to develop and market, and thus they were like homeless orphans.

The US National Institutes of Health estimates that there are 7000 rare diseases, but no one has a comprehensive count. Many of these diseases involve genetic problems and often are related to birth defects that are poorly characterized or involve permanent defects of nerve, muscle, or bone that cannot be corrected with drugs.

Almost all marketed drugs are used to treat some rare diseases. A few examples among the largest selling drugs in the world include: propranolol, which is used to treat idiopathic hypertrophic subaortic stenosis (in addition to the better known cardiovascular diseases); cimetidine, which is used to treat Zollinger–Ellison Syndrome (in addition to duodenal ulcers); and all antibiotics, which are used to treat rare bacterial infections as well as common ones.

Principles

One of the most important principles about orphan drugs is that they are a very heterogeneous group of drugs. In fact, they are as heterogeneous as any other group of drugs and, in most cases, should not be considered as a separate group. Orphan drugs are heterogeneous for the reasons given in Table 22.1.

Pharmaceutical companies have always developed orphan drugs. This did not change suddenly when the Orphan Drug Act was passed in 1983 in the United States, but the Act significantly stimulated the development of more such drugs.

If one compares the desirability of having orphan drug status with having a patent, generally it is more advantageous for a company to have a compound or use patent. However, there are some exceptions depending on the degree of patent coverage and the number of years left on the patent at the time of initial marketing. There are also various states of a patent to consider. For example, patent status may be characterized as nonpatentable, applied for, in interference, under final rejection, approved but not issued, approved and issued, or another scenario may apply.

Drugs are either investigational or marketed, and orphan drugs are no different. They may be used to treat only rare diseases, or both rare and common diseases. Under the law, they are deemed orphan only for the rare disease indication.

The clinical value of drugs being developed for rare diseases varies along the same spectra that

[1] The author acknowledges the help of NORD (National Organization of Rare Disorders) with the revisions in this chapter

Table 22.1 Reasons why orphan drugs are a heterogeneous group

Orphan drugs differ according to:
1. medical value
2. patent status
3. investigational or marketed status
4. availability in a generic equivalent form
5. use for a common disease too
6. costs of development
7. commercial (and profitability) potential
8. disease prevalence (stable, increasing or decreasing)
9. availability of alternate therapies
10. manufacture by conventional or biotechnology methods

exist for all drugs. This runs from having no clinical efficacy or medical value (for any of many reasons) to extremely high medical value that will revolutionize medical practice. One of the arguments used to support greater US federal funding for orphan drug research is that the research can identify mechanisms that may lead to the development of drugs for common diseases.

Development costs, time to market, and commercial potential vary enormously among orphan drugs, as with all drugs. It is usually meaningless to develop an orphan drug if a generic is available on the market or will be shortly, because any exclusivity would in effect be meaningless. Even if the generic version is not officially approved for treating the rare disease, it is likely that it would also be used to treat that disease.

Classification of orphan drugs

No single classification of orphan drugs has been accepted universally. In fact, several classifications have been proposed (Spilker, 1991). This section briefly mentions the criteria on which a classification scheme could be based and describes a simple classification based on economic value combined with medical value.

The major criteria that may be used to create a classification of orphan drugs include the following:
• Therapeutic or disease target of the drug.

• Marketing status of the drug (i.e., marketed or investigational).
• Patent status of the drug (e.g., patent issued and in force, patent expired, nonpatentable, patent pending).
• Generic drug availability (yes or no). Availability in the same dosage form, strength, with same excipients, and any other factor that is relevant to consider.
• Size of patient population. This refers not only to those in the parent country, but in other countries as well. Considerations of closely related subsets of patients must be considered because it is not possible to obtain orphan drug designation in the US if the drug can be used by a closely related subgroup of patients (e.g., one type of epileptics versus another; or a large number of moderately ill who can readily benefit from a drug as well as a small number (under 200,000) of severely ill patients with a particular disease).
• Can drug development costs be recovered through sales? This is a critical factor for pharmaceutical companies that are considering developing orphan drugs.
• Are alternative treatments available? The competitive position of the disease area must be considered. There are several categories in which alternative treatments may be used to treat the rare disease (e.g., none exist, all alternatives are highly toxic, alternatives are very expensive, alternatives are limited in availability, alternatives only work in a small number of patients).
• Medical value of the drug. In the author's opinion, this is the single most important criterion to judge (or classify) orphan drugs. If the drug does not have, or is not expected to have, high medical value, there are very few instances where its development would make sense. A classification of medical value may be as simple as high, medium, and low.
• Potential use in a more common disease, as well as in other rare diseases. This is often difficult to predict at the outset of development, but most drugs that reach the market are tested by the medical community in other diseases.
• Type of drug. This category considers whether the drug is a biotechnology-derived and produced

drug or a conventional pharmaceutical synthesized in a laboratory.

• Patient support group. If a patient support group exists, it may facilitate the development of the drug by notifying its members about participation in clinical trials. The group could also have its members write letters on behalf of the product to increase awareness in the medical community and to expedite the regulatory review process.

Economic classification of orphan drugs

An economic classification is one of the most relevant alternative classifications to consider, particularly for companies considering the development of orphan drugs. Five categories of drugs are as follows:

• *Drugs with little commercial potential, but with high medical value.* The commercial value may be subdivided as to whether the product will lose money and never pay back its development costs or whether the sales are expected to be below an arbitrary hurdle rate (e.g., internal rate of return) and achieve less profit than desired for new products added to the company's portfolio. In the former case, only wealthy companies that wish to perform a community service, or have reasons other than profits for developing the drug, could undertake the development of a money-losing drug. If the drug has high medical value and will not lose money, some companies would at least consider developing it if it met other criteria (e.g., a therapeutic area of interest).

• *Drugs of moderate or high commercial value and high medical value.* This category of orphan drugs should never have a problem finding a sponsor to develop the drug, as long as certain caveats are met. For example, no generic version of the drug should be on the market, or else pharmacies would fill prescriptions with the generic. This category is meant to imply that the commercial potential would be real if the product was to reach the market.

• *Variable commercial potential and low medical value.* This category is a very realistic description for many, if not most, drugs at an early stage of their development, before the clinical efficacy and safety profile are well understood. The wisest and best educated person or group of experts can only guess the value of a drug before it is tested and its profile is known. One exception is drugs that are developed in a new dosage form, but whose activity and safety are well known. Nonetheless, a drug of low medical value will rarely be developed unless a company knows that the commercial value is significant. A "me-too" drug is an example of a drug in this category.

• *Unprofitable drug for a common disease.* This category of drug is described in the orphan drug legislation and could refer to tropical diseases that are not prevalent in the US or to a drug that may be medically important for a subset of patients with a common disease but would not be expected to recoup the company's investment. Few drugs in this category have been developed.

• *Variable commercial potential for both a rare and common diseases.* Virtually every pharmaceutical company that develops an orphan drug hopes that the drug will be found useful in treating a more common disease, but this seldom occurs, though the knowledge gained during product development can prove valuable in identifying other development opportunities.

The interested parties

There is considerable interest in orphan products. The following sections describe eight groups involved in orphan drug development and use. These parties have a variety of motives for their interest in this area.

Government legislative bodies
Government legislative bodies can become involved in orphan drug development, primarily through passing legislation. For example, governments can provide incentives such as tax benefits or grants, or marketing exclusivity, or otherwise incentivize pharmaceutical companies to develop and market such drugs.

Regulatory authorities

The motivation of regulatory authorities is usually to improve and protect the public health of the community they serve. This is most obviously apparent through the approval of orphan drugs for marketing. These authorities are primarily motivated by their perception of the drug's medical value and less by whether the drug is considered to have commercial value.

Patient organizations

These groups focus primarily on one specific disease or one type of disease process (e.g., inborn errors of metabolism, muscle disease, glycogen storage diseases, autoimmune diseases). Since these organizations often are small, they need the support of umbrella organizations representing the interests of the rare disease community. Two such organizations, which work together on an international basis, are the National Organization of Rare Disorders (NORD), which is the umbrella group in the US representing the rare disease community, and Eurordis, which operates in Europe. The goal of the disease-specific organizations is to stimulate the discovery and development of new treatments for their diseases. Another important function of many of these groups is to provide information to their members, and often to the public and medical community as well. As the national umbrella organization in the US, NORD runs medical assistance programs for people with rare diseases and also advocates for policies in the interests of its members.

Pharmaceutical companies

The motivation of pharmaceutical companies is not solely profit oriented, because many orphan drugs that have been developed and marketed are of little commercial value. In most cases, pharmaceutical companies accept social responsibilities for the patients they serve with their more profitable drugs. In addition to the small amount of profit they may make on orphan drugs, there is an enhancement of the company's image, which is becoming more and more important in our critical society.

Trade associations

Professional trade associations representing pharmaceutical companies or other groups are concerned with the image of the industry, as well as providing social benefits through publicizing the products of their members. The Pharmaceutical Research and Manufacturers of America (PhRMA), which represents the large drug manufacturers in the US, had a "Commission on Drugs for Rare Diseases" that focused on issues relating to orphan drugs for many years.

Patients and families

The motivation of those with the disease or those with relatives with the disease is clear: They want better treatments that are affordable and will improve the quality of life for the patient. Those patients interested in clinical trials or who wish to join a trial should contact www.clinicaltrials.gov for information.

Physicians and other healthcare providers

The motivation of these people is also clear: They seek to find better treatments for their patients and are often willing to test new drugs in clinical trials.

Academicians

Orphan drugs offer research opportunities for scientists and clinicians. Another important motivating factor is the opportunities presented for career enhancement.

Peter Saltonstall, the President and CEO of NORD, says that bringing together all the various groups with an interest in rare diseases and orphan products is a challenge because many have competing interests, but that banding together leads to the enhancement of information in the marketplace and the implementation of better programs and more advanced therapies for patients.

Sources of information on orphan drugs

The Food and Drug Administration (FDA) publishes an annual list of orphan drugs that have been approved for marketing since the signing of the Orphan Drug Act in 1983. The FDA also publishes a monthly list of drugs that have received orphan drug designation within the last month and an annual cumulative summary of the current designations. There is also a home page on the Internet and an annual publication of grants to evaluate orphan drugs in clinical trials (see www.fda.gov).

Most specific disease organizations, as well as umbrella disease organizations, provide information of relevant diseases for members and sometimes for researchers, and for the public. These groups may also provide current scientific information. For example, the NORD database is a valuable source of information for many groups of people interested in a particular disease (see www.rarediseases.org).

Discovery, development, marketing, and distribution of orphan drugs

The process of discovering new orphan drugs is not different from that used to discover drugs for more common diseases (Spilker, 2009). (This is a broad topic and will not be discussed further in this chapter.)

Similarly, the methods used to develop drugs for rare diseases do not differ from those used for more common diseases in terms of strategies, methodologies, and criteria for success (see Chapter 4). However, there could be differences in the amount of clinical data needed to demonstrate safety and effectiveness. If there are only 500 patients with a particular disease, it is probably impossible to have two randomized, well-controlled placebo trials. At the same time, the quality and amount of manufacturing data required for regulatory submissions do not differ for orphan drugs than for more common drugs.

The same marketing tools are used to market orphan drugs and non-orphan drugs. Probably the greatest difference between orphan and non-orphan drugs from a marketing perspective is that the amount of money spent to market orphan drugs will be significantly less. Although the same

mix of marketing tools can be and are often used, the number of symposia and the number of advertisements will usually be fewer. Another difference is that a company marketing an orphan drug may not use sales representatives. There can be instances when a large company may in fact be developing the orphan drug so that the sales representatives can discuss the orphan drug (and non-orphans too), whereas a small company may have decided to develop an orphan because sales representatives are not necessary to promote the product.

Distribution methods differ more between orphans and non-orphans than the other categories discussed in this section. Conventional drugs are generally sold through wholesalers, as well as directly to institutions. Orphan drugs more often use what are referred to as alternative distribution systems such as mail order pharmacy and direct distribution to patients, physicians, and institutions.

Marketing benefits to selling orphan drugs

Most pharmaceutical companies that market their own products can benefit from marketing orphan drugs. These benefits include the following:
• It is useful for sales representatives to use orphan drugs as an entree to see physicians. In this busy world, physicians want new and important medical information and are not as willing to see sales representatives as they used to be. Thus, a sales representative who can discuss an important new treatment, even for a rare disease, is likely to have better access to physicians.
• It is useful to develop orphan drugs to keep competitors out of a therapeutic or disease area of importance to a company. A company may choose to develop a drug to prevent competitors from doing so and not because they want to develop an important orphan drug.

It is possible to bundle products more easily with a whole portfolio of products in a given therapeutic area. Several companies that have merged in recent years initially felt that some of the smaller products would be divested or dropped from the portfolio because of their small size. However, they soon realized that there was value in even the smallest products, and that the sum of their value was much greater than the sum of their sales, particularly when the company approaches managed care or other groups (with formularies) with a wide selection of products.

• Image enhancement of the company is likely to occur through development of drugs for rare diseases. Reporters are more likely to write heart-warming stories of patients with rare diseases who are helped by orphan drugs. Word of mouth and other public relations methods also help enhance a company's image.

• It may be possible to have a patient support group promote a drug by telling their members, writing articles in their newsletter or in the popular press, or informing the regulatory agency about the need to have the product available for patients to use.

Common issues for a company to consider when developing an orphan drug

When developing orphan drugs, companies need to consider the following aspects:

• If a company has approval for a drug indicated for a common disease and the drug may also be useful for a rare disease, the issue arises as to whether the company should seek to obtain approval for the rare disease, or allow off-label use of the drug to provide whatever commercial value it obtains. This problem is often viewed as an exercise in cost accounting, where the company totals all the costs and resources needed to obtain the rare disease indication and compares the total with the potential sales and profits that would accrue. It is important to consider the opportunity cost of working toward a new indication (i.e., if one spends x dollars and uses y staff months to obtain the indication, those staff cannot be working on other projects and the money cannot be applied elsewhere).

• If a company can develop a drug for either a common disease or a rare disease, the question arises as to which to pursue first. Assume that the orphan indication can be obtained in a much shorter time than the more common one and that the time to submit the New Drug Application (NDA) is less for the orphan indication. In this situation, there is a "trade-off" between the smaller amount of sales that will come sooner with the orphan indication along with the possibility of off-label use for the more common indication. The trade-off is with waiting longer for the larger indication that will be much more important commercially. Initially, many people think that the orphan drug development route is preferable, but a regulatory authority will have much less pressure to approve the more common indication when the NDA is submitted and approved for the orphan indication because of the availability of another form of the product. This means that during this period, the company will not be able to promote the drug for the common indication. Thus, it is usually preferable to try to obtain regulatory approval for the more commercially important indication first. There are some important exceptions to this rule. For example, start-up companies have limited funds and may seek approval for the rare indication first out of necessity.

Another consideration regarding this issue is that a company seeking an orphan approval and hoping for off-label use for a more common disease may find a strong regulatory backlash when the company's strategy becomes apparent. There are real cases where a company submitted an NDA for a rare disease and then shortly thereafter submitted an investigational new drug (IND) application for a more common disease. In these cases, the FDA realized the company's ploy and significantly raised the standards for approving the rare disease indication.

Benefits of orphan drugs from a development perspective

The most obvious benefit for a company is that the number of clinical trials and the quantity of clinical data required for marketing approval often will be less for an orphan drug. This is primarily because of the limited number of patients with certain rare diseases available for clinical trials. Even though the numbers are fewer, however, FDA insists that the data be convincing, and the standards of trial design are generally unchanged. In some situations, where a disease is extremely rare, the clinical trial standards may be altered if a company realistically can only obtain a small number of individual case studies.

A possible benefit in some drug development programs is that less toxicology data may be required. A regulatory requirement for less toxicology data is based both on the difficulty of obtaining the data as well as the benefit-risk ratio for getting the product to market rapidly.

A more rapid regulatory review may be anticipated for products of high medical value. This is due to the medical need of society for the drug, the smaller application (dossier) compared to other drugs with substantially more data, and the high priority of the application. In most circumstances, there will be a waiver of administrative fees charged (e.g., user fees) for orphan drugs to be reviewed.

Standards of manufacturing and quality control for orphan drugs are identical to those of drugs for common diseases. In some situations, fewer validation batches may be required and the duration of stability tests may be addressed while the drug is being evaluated by the regulatory authority, or in exceptional cases, after the product is on the market. Thus, the time to develop the chemistry and the technical package of data for the regulatory submission of an orphan drug may or may not differ from that needed if the drug were for a common disease.

The opportunity costs of developing an orphan drug must always be considered. In considering whether or not to develop orphan products, many large companies have taken the view that they will not do so because they have implemented financial hurdles (x million dollars in sales per year) that few orphans could meet. As a result, companies usually have specific reasons for developing orphan drugs.

An approved indication is not always necessary for a marketed drug to capture a rare disease market. In some countries, physicians may prescribe a marketed drug to treat a disease before it is approved by the regulatory authorities for that use: so called "off-label" use. This is often understood and accepted by the regulatory authority and the reimbursement officials. For example, the FDA did not approve acyclovir for the rare disease Herpes encephalitis for more than five years after the NDA was submitted because it was already the drug of choice for that disease and the FDA knew that it was widely used and that it could be viewed as malpractice not to use it. Nonetheless, when a particular indication is not approved despite its widespread use, companies could not promote the drug for the off-label use or educate physicians and patients about the data supporting this use.

One factor that influences the willingness of a regulatory authority to approve a new drug for a rare disease is the pressure from outside sources such as patient groups or the legislature. For example, the US Congress pressured the FDA to approve valproic acid for seizures in children many years ago, even before the company was ready to make its submission.

The medical value of a drug may be independent of the efficacy and rarity of the disease. For example, for Wilson's disease there are several products on the market that are effective, yet additional ones are still being developed. Penicillamine is often effective, but often causes serious adverse reactions. Zinc acetate and trientine are newer products and molybdenum was evaluated for the same indication.

Disincentives and obstacles for orphan drug development

There is no limit to the number of disincentives and obstacles that potentially stand in the way of developing orphan drugs, including the following:
• The tax credit offered in the US for developing orphan drugs is not much more than the tax credit for research and development of any new pharmaceutical.
• Resources of the company could be applied to developing more profitable drugs.
• Development may not be required if the drug is already marketed for a more common use. This

implies off-label use, which is acceptable in some countries but very difficult or impossible in others.

- Because the safety and quality standards of manufacturing are the same, orphan drug development may create challenging and costly technical problems.
- The medical need for the drug may not be great and/or the medical effectiveness of the drug may not be strong.
- The regulatory authority may require more data than the company thinks are warranted.
- The liability risks may be unacceptably high: A drug to treat patients with a rare disease that causes a serious adverse event could increase the exposure of the company to a major court suit.
- Difficulty in finding a small number of patients widely dispersed through the US (or other countries) for conducting clinical trials or for marketing products.

Additional obstacles may include lack of a patent or other proprietary position, availability of a generic equivalent, large amount of competition, technical difficulties in any area of formulation, analytical, stability, scale-up, or other related issues. Manufacturing issues or costs of any aspect of the manufacturing, from obtaining the raw products to final manufacturing and packaging to distribution, are other possible disincentives.

The United States Orphan Drug Act of 1983

The US Orphan Drug Act was signed by President Reagan in 1983. In its original form, the Act provided for the following:

- A seven-year period of exclusivity for designated drugs.
- Establishment of an Orphan Products Board within the US government.
- Tax credits for certain expenses in clinical trials.
- A grant program that included medical foods and medical devices, although they cannot obtain orphan designation.
- Assistance to corporations and academic investigators by the FDA.

It is important to note that medical foods and medical devices were not eligible for orphan drug designation or for the marketing exclusivity provisions of the Act. The Act was originally designed for unprofitable and unpatentable medicines only.

Amendments to the Orphan Drug Act

In 1984, an amendment to the Act changed the standard for orphan drug designation from profitability to prevalence of the target disease, which was set at less than 200,000 patients in the US. The requirement of unprofitability was dropped from the Act.

In 1985, another amendment to the Act made it possible for patented and patentable medicines to receive orphan drug designation (a pre-marketing classification) and orphan drug status (a post-NDA approval classification).

In 1988, a further amendment established the time period for filing for orphan drug designation. This clarified that the designation must be prior to filing the NDA.

In 1990, the US Congress passed an amendment that would have allowed shared exclusivity for companies that developed an orphan drug virtually simultaneously and to lose exclusivity under certain conditions. However, this amendment was vetoed by President George H.W. Bush, in whose judgment it was anticompetitive.

In 1991, an amendment was proposed that would have established a sales cap after which an orphan drug would lose its exclusivity. This and other amendments to the Act, proposed in 1992 and 1994, did not pass the Congress.

The benefits of the Act as it now exists actually emanate both directly from the Act itself, as well as from outside the Act.

Within the Act itself, the four major benefits are: (i) the period of marketing exclusivity, which may be considered as a type of patent; (ii) the tax benefits on clinical trials between the date of orphan drug designation and NDA approval; (iii) the FDA's Office of Orphan Products Development grants to support clinical trials on orphan drugs; and (iv) protocol assistance from the FDA, which was always available for important new drugs (as well as others) and is important, but not necessarily new.

The benefits from outside the Act (i.e., unofficial benefits) are as follows:

• Potential for more rapid regulatory review of NDAs. This is considered extremely important by many companies, but the author believes that it is the medical value of the treatment, rather than the number of patients treated, that influences the speed of regulatory review.

• Enhancement of the company's image by developing important orphan medicines. This often can be parlayed into valuable publicity.

• Build a portfolio of products. Orphan drug benefits may enable a company to develop and market a new drug and help build a portfolio of products in a therapeutic area of importance.

• Hope for a larger market. It is always possible that a new use for an orphan drug may be found that may give the medicine greater commercial potential than originally believed.

• Help fill important gaps in the company's development. There are often gaps in a company's portfolio that orphan drugs could fill. This would provide a wide variety of benefits to a company, including the stimulation of staff that recognizes the medical importance of the product.

• Have a new message and product for sales representatives to give to physicians.

Unintended consequences of the Orphan Drug Act

When the US Congress passed the Act, there were several factions with different views. All sides had to make compromises, but everyone knew that some incentives had to be given to pharmaceutical companies in order for the Act to have any impact or to influence their behavior. Nonetheless, the incentives worked too well in some people's opinion, in that there was concern that some of the Act's loopholes were exploited or were found to benefit companies in unintended ways.

For example, companies with orphan drug protection sometimes charge very high prices, which raised questions of appropriateness. In situations where the medicine had a reasonably strong patent, such as with Retrovir (zidovudine, azidothymidine), the orphan drug designation and exclusivity was not of consequence to the company, at least not for market protection. For drugs such as growth hormone, erythropoietin, pentamidine, and Ceredase, orphan drug designation and resultant exclusivity on FDA approval were essential. To some people, the high price of the drugs represented an abuse of the Act.

An important issue for US politicians was that the Medicare and Medicaid programs had to pay large sums of money for protected medicines. One final issue to some people outside the pharmaceutical industry, and also a few companies, was the inability of a second company to market a drug with an approved NDA. Of course, this was always a clearly known and obvious consequence of marketing exclusivity.

A current trend is that more biotechnology products (see Chapter 24) are applying for orphan drug designation. The main reason for this phenomenon is that biotechnology patents are so difficult to obtain and orphan drug protection is valuable, while the inventors wait to see if a strong patent will issue.

Establishing prevalence or incidence of a disease

The FDA recognizes any authoritative evidence to support the prevalence of less than 200,000 patients in the US. The major sources of evidence include the following:

• Peer-reviewed literature.
• Textbooks.
• Surveys by patient support groups.
• Data from the National Disease and Therapeutic Index.
• Hospital discharge data based on ICD codes or other clear classifications.
• Data from the Centers for Disease Control.
• Data from the National Center for Health Statistics.
• Data from IMS or other reliable market data organizations.

- Sales data of companies.
- Testimony of experts, based on evidence from their (or other) hospitals or practices.
- Testimony of experts, based on personal experience unsupported by hard evidence, although this is regarded as the weakest evidence.

Establishing differences among medicines

It is often important to establish that a company's medicine for which it desires an orphan drug designation differs from another medicine. There are a number of principles that will help a company establish such a difference:

- *Different chemical structures.* If it is unequivocally shown that two structures differ and it makes a biological or clinical difference, both will be given orphan drug designation. However, if the chemical difference is minor (e.g., one amino acid difference in a protein or the terminal carbohydrate portion of a large molecule) and no clinical differences can be shown, they will usually be viewed as the same product.
- *Differences in clinical effects.* This is often a very difficult criterion to demonstrate, but if it can be shown, a difference would be established.
- *Contribution to patient care.* If a marketed dosage form of a medicine cannot help certain patients with a problem, or not help them adequately compared to a different dosage form (e.g., parenteral), then the parenteral form would be eligible for orphan drug designation.
- *New production methods to purify a drug.* If such methods lead to a difference in safety or efficacy, this would qualify for orphan drug designation. A real example is a new Factor IX.
- *New excipients.* Differences in excipients that lead to a difference in clinical safety or efficacy would qualify for orphan drug designation.

Rear-Admiral Marlene Haffner MD MPH FRCP, former Director of the FDA's Office of Orphan Products Development, has summarized this issue best by saying, "For a difference to be a difference it must make a difference" (personal communication). A lower cost of a second form of a medicine, or of the same dosage form, is not a criterion to establish a difference between two drugs, even if the original is considered extremely expensive and a new breakthrough allows the new product to be sold at a markedly reduced price.

What is an orphan drug indication?

It is obvious that arthritis, epilepsy, depression, asthma, and other similar diseases are not rare and drugs to treat them do not qualify for orphan drug designation. But would a medically plausible subset of each disease qualify as an orphan indication if there were fewer than 200,000 patients with, for example, a severe form of the disease? The FDA's principle in addressing this common question is to ask the question: "Could (and would) patients with less severe forms of the disease use the new treatment?" If so, the FDA says that the indication is not a true orphan and usually denies the application for orphan designation.

A rare variant of depression, asthma, or other common disease might qualify as an orphan indication if it is deemed to be a medically plausible separate indication. In this situation, it is possible that the company may receive the designation, but the reviewing division of the FDA may impose much higher standards for regulatory approval of an orphan drug for marketing if it believes that the product will be widely used in medical practice. For example, a drug to treat a rare rheumatologic disorder that could also be useful in rheumatoid arthritis would likely have to provide much more data to obtain approval than if the drug were limited to treating a very small patient population. On the other hand, a toxic medicine that could only be used to treat severe cases of patients with a common disease (because of benefit to risk considerations) could receive orphan designation and regulatory approval for marketing as an orphan drug with relatively little data. This assumes that there was a significant medical benefit to using the medicine in patients with severe forms of the disease.

Rating the effects of the Orphan Drug Act in the United States

With more than 340 orphan drugs approved and more than 2000 designated as orphan drugs since enactment, plus numerous grants awarded since 1983, it is clear that the Act has been very successful and a major stimulus for certain pharmaceutical companies. The fact that some blockbuster drugs have been approved under this legislation is a controversial topic for reasons relating to drug cost. The tax credit for clinical trial costs has been very modest and does not represent a significant sum of money to most companies.

The number of designations have increased in recent years not only because of the incentives of the Act, but also due to advances in science and medicine, increased investments made in research and development by companies and academic institutions, increased competition within the pharmaceutical industry, and an increased interest in this legislation by the biotechnology industry.

Lessons of the Orphan Drug Act for Europe

By 1996, a number of European countries and organizations started to pay much more attention to orphan products. The US experience offered a number of lessons for the Europeans to consider as they discussed and considered numerous issues:

• True incentives for the pharmaceutical industry are required in order for any orphan drug legislation to be successful. Without true incentives, the legislation will have little, if any, effect. The major incentive required is a period of exclusivity for marketing. Without this incentive, the industry is not likely to modify its activities in this area. Europe established a ten-year period of marketing exclusivity as compared to seven years in the US.

Other incentives are secondary and are not really necessary for legislation to be successful.
• Abuses of the law by the pharmaceutical industry must be prevented. The simplest way of avoiding abuses is to have a sales cap. This means that the market exclusivity disappears when the cumulative sales of a drug reach a predetermined level. This amount of money should be set at a fair value to incentivize the companies and to protect the government or other groups that pay the bill for excessive charges.
• All potential medicines for indications or diseases meeting prevalence numbers should qualify for designation and a drug's potential profitability should not be a barrier to receiving orphan drug designation.
• A specific regulatory group must be in place to decide on "gray" issues. There will always be issues to resolve, such as determining whether or not an indication is real or represents salami (wurst) slicing of a larger one. Another commonly encountered "gray" issue is to decide whether or not a new dosage form qualifies for designation. The Committee on Orphan Medicinal Products within the European Medicines Agency (EMA) is now well established.
• Regulatory review of orphan drugs should be based on the drug's medical value and medical need and not on whether or not an official orphan drug status is present.

References

(Note: all websites cited in the text were accessed April 24, 2010.)

Spilker B. *Guide to Clinical Trials*. Raven Press: New York, USA, 1991.

Spilker B. *Guide to Drug Development: A Comprehensive Review and Assessment*. Lippincott, Williams and Wilkins: Philadelphia, USA, 2009.

CHAPTER 23

QT Interval Prolongation and Drug Development

Bruce H. Morimoto[1] & Anthony W. Fox[2]

[1]Allon Therapeutics Inc., Redwood City, CA, USA

[2]EBD Group Inc., Carlsbad, CA, USA and Munich, Germany and Skaggs SPPS, University of California, San Diego, USA

Introduction

Drug-induced cardiac QT interval prolongation has been the focus of considerable investigation and regulatory oversight for the past 15 years. The risk to human health is not QT prolongation *per se*, but drug-related sudden cardiac death. The drug-induced ventricular arrhythmias that lead to sudden death are rare events and not typically associated with the initial onset of drug treatment. Therefore, in the course of drug development, clinical documentation of arrhythmogenic risk potential is difficult, if not impossible.

To deconstruct the core danger, namely sudden cardiac death or cardiac arrest, it is important to appreciate the complexity of factors that can ultimately result in the final outcome (see Figure 23.1). The proximate cause of cardiac arrest is ventricular fibrillation (VF), a sustained failure of the coordinated electrical currents that are needed to empty the right and left ventricles. Uncoordinated contraction of cardiac muscle fibers leads to circulatory stasis.

Ventricular tachyarrhythmias generally precede VF. *Torsades de pointes* (TdP) is a sustained, polymorphic ventricular tachyarrhythmia and was first described in 1966 by Francois Dessertenne (see Figure 23.2). Commonly, TdP resolves sponta-

neously to normal sinus rhythm spontaneously (see Figure 23.2A). These self-limiting episodes are not fatal and may present as syncope, palpitations, or (more rarely) hypoxic seizures. Short periods of TdP may even be an incidental finding on Holter monitoring and without any clinical sequelae at all. But when TdP is sustained, VF and cardiac arrest surely follow (see Figure 23.2B).

TdP is also closely associated with prior, marked QT prolongation. The surface ECG represents a composite of the electrical activity of the heart as measured by electrodes placed on the skin, and corresponds to the electrical activity of the cardiac action potential (see Figure 23.3). The resting membrane potential is typically –70 mV, and the beginning of the action potential involves the opening of sodium channels giving rise to a rapid influx of sodium ions producing sodium current (I_{Na}) or the upstroke velocity (see Figure 23.3A). The movement of sodium ions into the cell results in membrane depolarization, and as the sodium channels inactivate, the membrane potential becomes slightly positive. Membrane depolarization in turn activates calcium channels, which open and allow calcium influx; this gives rise to the slight increase in membrane potential as seen in the cardiac action potential. Membrane depolarization also opens potassium channels and the efflux of potassium ions from the cell results in repolarization or resetting the membrane potential to –70 mV. The beginning of the action potential corresponds to the start of the QRS complex and

Principles and Practice of Pharmaceutical Medicine, 3rd edition.
Edited by L.D. Edwards, A.W. Fox, P.D. Stonier.
© 2011 Blackwell Publishing Ltd.

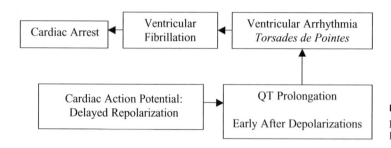

Figure 23.1 Relationship of QT prolongation to cardiac arrest and human risk.

the end of the T-wave corresponds to complete repolarization. Therefore, inhibiting potassium efflux by blocking the potassium channels will result in a time-lag or delay in repolarization. This in turn results in a lengthening of the QT interval.

Heterogeneity of electrical conduction occurs within the various layers of the myocardium. For the left ventricle, action potentials are longest in the subendocardial Purkinje fibers as well as in the mid-myocardium (M-cell layer). Shorter action potentials are recorded in the outer epicardial and endocardial layers. Abnormal spatial difference or

transmural dispersion may be an important factor in development of unstable (so-called "reentrant") arrhythmias such as TdP.

The factor(s) that allow an arrhythmia to self-limit or be sustained are mostly unknown. A complex series of factors appear to contribute to an increase in risk, and "repolarization reserve" has been proposed to provide a unifying framework for integrated risk assessment (Roden, 2004). Some factors that affect reploarization reserve include ion channel polymorphism (congenital long QT syndromes), differences in ion channel

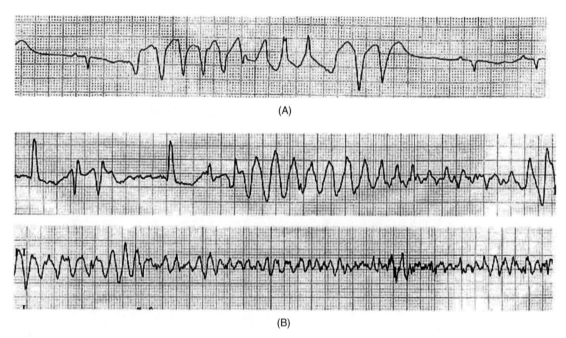

(A)

(B)

Figure 23.2 (A) ECG of self-limiting *Torsade de Pointes* in which ventricular arrhythmia resolves back to sinus rhythm. (B, middle) ECG of TdP resulting in ventricular fibrillation; (B, lowest). Reproduced from Yap & Camm (2003), with permission from BMJ Publishing Group Ltd.

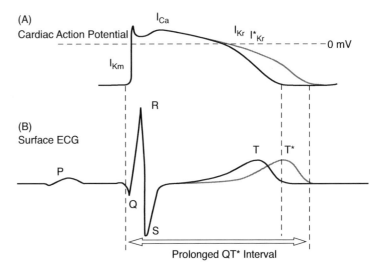

Figure 23.3 Schematic representation and temporal relation between ECG and cardiac action potential. An increase in the action potential duration (APD) results in an increase the QT interval. Source: Charles River Laboratories. *Drug Disc Dev* 2009; **6**:26–28 (http://www.dddmag.com/Article-Guarding-the-Heart-060109.aspx). Reproduced with permission

density (gender-related), metabolic disturbances, electrolyte imbalances (hypokalemia), and general cardiac health (congestive heart failure, left ventricular hypertrophy).

QT prolongation is a key precursor of TdP. The QT interval is the time from the start of the QRS-complex to the end of the T-wave as measured by surface ECG (see Figure 23.3B). Often Lead II is used for QT interval measurement because that is where the end of the T-wave is most pronounced; however, other leads should not be ignored.

QT prolongation is a risk factor for the development of a ventricular arrhythmia (leading to cardiac arrest) because when the interval becomes long enough, and if heart rate is fast enough, cardiac depolarization occurs before repolarization from the previous beat is complete ("R on T" phenomenon). The effect occurs not only due to drugs but also from a spontaneous disease state.

Prolongation of the surface ECG QT interval reflects an increase in the action potential duration (see Figure 23.3). The molecular entities involved in time-dependent repolarization include inward potassium ion flux predominantly mediated by two channels: the rapid delayed rectifier, I_{kr}, and the slow delayed rectifier, I_{ks}. Inhibition of the inward potassium current results in an increase in the action potential duration (APD). Mechanistically, an increase in APD can also result from enhance-

ment of inward current mediated by sodium or calcium channels, and their contribution to QT prolongation should not be overlooked.

The QT interval is therefore used as a marker for potential of R on T phenomenon. There is a correlation among drugs between observed clinical hazard for arrhythmia and QT interval prolongation. But within this correlation, QT prolongation lacks predictive specificity, and its sensitivity is also limited because the QT interval is just one of several factors predisposing to arrythmia (e.g., concomitant heart rate, structural heart or coronary disease, ambient potassium concentration, etc.). Thus, it is impossible to quantitatively state the risk factor based solely on the degree or magnitude by which a drug is observed to prolong the QT interval. However, as imperfect as QT measurements may be, the length of the QT interval is currently our best surrogate for a lethal adverse event type that cannot be studied proactively.

The length of the QT interval can be influenced by many factors including parasympathetic/vagal activity, cardiac disease, genetic abnormalities, or electrolyte imbalances. Diurnal variation can be as much as 75–100 msec during the course of a day. Therefore appropriate comparisons and controls need to be made, because a drug effect on QT interval may be a secondary consequence of changes in these other parameters.

A major factor influencing the QT interval is heart rate. As the heart rate slows, and while the QT interval becomes longer, the succeeding R wave moves farther away from the previous T wave. For the former, the relationship between heart rate and QT interval is not simple; it takes a period of one to two minutes for the QT interval to reach a steady state after a period of heart rate change. Thus, it is prudent to ensure that the complexes used in the analysis of QT interval be preceded by a period of stable heart rate.

For drugs with the potential to alter heart rate, the QT interval needs to be mathematically corrected. On an ECG, heart rate (HR) is inversely proportional to the time interval between two R-waves (RR interval; i.e., the time between two consecutive QRS complexes. Thus, HR (per minute) = 60/RR (sec). Two common formulas for adjusting QT for heart rate are both based on population measurements:

Bazett's formula: $QT_{cb} = QT/RR^{1/2}$

and

Fredericia's formula: $QT_{cf} = QT/RR^{1/3}$

Bazett's formula has a tendency to overcorrect at higher heart rates, whereas Fredericia's undercorrects at lower heart rates.

QTc is considered prolonged if it is greater than 460 msec for males and 480 msec for females. An analysis correlating QTc with cardiac events in patients with long-QT syndrome (see below) found that the probability of cardiac risk was significant when the QTc interval was greater than 500 msec (Priori *et al.*, 2003). When comparing drugs, there appears to be no correlation between the magnitude of observed, corrected QT prolongation and clinical risk of TdP.

Cisapride is a stereotypical example of a drug that increases the QT interval and the APD (see Figure 23.4). Cisapride has an IC_{50} at what is known as the *in vitro* potassium-conducting hERG channel of 20–30 nM (Hanson *et al.*, 2006), to which we shall return below. The mechanism for increasing APD is delayed repolarization because of inhibited potassium influx to the cardiac myocyte at the end of the action potential. Increases in APD can also

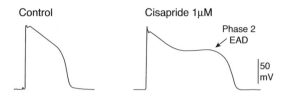

Figure 23.4 Effect of cisapride on rabbit cardiac action potential. Cisapride results in an increase in the action potential duration and results in an early after-depolarization (EAD). Reproduced from Joshi *et al.* (2004). Copyright 2004, with permission from Elsevier

be caused by morphologic changes in the trajectory of the repolarization wave, referred to as an early after-depolarization (EAD). EADs can trigger spontaneous depolarization (see Figures 23.4 and 23.5), and when they propagate through the heart, a ventricular ectopic beat results. EADs are also thought to be candidates for TdP initiation. Slow depolarization rates, low potassium levels, and treatment with QT prolonging drugs are thus all known risk factors for TdP, can experimentally produce EADs and triggered beats, and doubtlessly interact synergistically.

Historical context and regulatory reactions

In the late-1990s, several high profile drug withdrawals in the US focused attention on drug-induced QT prolongation, including the antihistamines terfenadine in 1997, astemizole in 1999, the antibiotic grepafloxacin in 1999, and cisapride

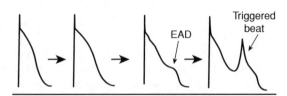

Figure 23.5 Development of after depolarization (EAD) at the level of the myocyte. Reproduced with permission from D. Roden, *New Engl J Med* 2004;350:1013–22. Copyright © 2004 *Massachusetts Medical Society. All rights reserved*

in 2000. Prior to this, many anti-arrhythmic drugs were also known to result in QT prolongation, such as dofetilide, ibutilide, quinidine, and sotalol; however, the appearance of ventricular arrhythmia from drugs without obvious cardiovascular properties was unexpected.

In Europe, the Committee for Proprietary Medicinal Products (CPMP) issued the first formal regulatory guidance on how to address the potential of drugs to cause QT prolongation. This was a "Points to Consider" document in 1997, which focused on the assessment of QT prolongation specifically by non-cardiovascular drugs.

In 2001, the International Conference on Harmonization (ICH) published the first draft of an industry guidance document, ICH S7B, titled "The Non-Clinical Evaluation of the Potential for Delayed Ventricular Repolarization (QT Interval Prolongation) by Human Pharmaceuticals." The initial draft document outlined a nonclinical approach to identify signals of QT risk. The guidance was adopted by the Committee for Medicinal Products for Human Use (CHMP) in May 2005.

Concurrent to the discussion of the draft ICH S7B guidance, the Therapeutic Products Directorate of Health Canada published a preliminary concept paper on the clinical assessment of QT prolongation. Extensive discussion between academia, industry, and regulators resulted in the ICH E14 guidance document titled, "Clinical Evaluation of QT/QTc Interval Prolongation and Proarrhythmic Potential for Non-Antiarrhythmic Drugs," which was adopted by the CPMP in 2005.

Approach to risk assessment

As a result of these regulatory developments, QT prolongation risk potential is now a standard part of nonclinical assessment. These include: (i) *a priori* chemical or pharmacological class; (ii) observed molecular interactions with ion channels *in vitro*; (iii) effects on the cardiac action potential; and (iv) effects on the ECG. The prevailing regulatory guidance for these studies is the current ICH S7B document.

Chemical or pharmacological class

Certain classes of compounds are known to be associated with QT prolongation. Although class membership is an imperfect predictor, new molecular entities with a similar chemical structure or pharmacological mechanism to drugs in these suspicious classes attract especially careful nonclinical evaluations. In many instances, a competitive advantage can be assessed to a new molecular entity without QT risk. An up-to-date list of potential drugs with QT risk can be found on the Arizona Center for Education and Research on Therapeutics website (www.azcert.org).

Anti-arrhythmic drugs

Many anti-arrhythmics prolong the QT interval and an early indication of this association was the report of syncope and ventricular fibrillation or flutter with quinidine use. Class Ia anti-arrhythmics such as quinidine, procainamide, and diisopyramide can promote QT prolongation and TdP; however, the incidence appears to be lower than expected possibly because of the concurrent inhibition of sodium channels, which can suppress QT prolongation. Class III anti-arrhymic drugs such as sotalol, which do not have activity at sodium channels, appear to have a higher incidence of TdP. This generalization does not hold true for all class III drugs since the incidence of TdP is low for amiodarone despite prolonging the QT interval as much as sotalol. Possessing risk for TdP is accepted for some anti-arrhythmic drugs because QT prolongation is an intrinsic part of their mechanism for effect. Paradoxically, these anti-arrhythmics then need little preclinical evaluation for QT prolongation because the hazard is assumed to be present and product approval then depends upon potential benefit being balanced against that definite hazard.

Antihistamines

Non-sedating antihistamines such as terfenadine and astemizole were found to cause QT prolongation and TdP, fortunately at low incidence, was also observed clinically. These adverse effects were predominantly observed when plasma concentrations of drug were supra-therapeutic, resulting from exceeding the recommended dosing or due to a metabolic drug–drug interaction. Terfenadine and astemizole are predominantly metabolized by the cytochrome P450 (CYP) 3A4 isoenzyme, and the antifungal agent ketoconazole and even grapefruit juice can inhibit CYP3A4 activity. Renal and hepatic impaired patients can also be at a higher risk for QT prolongation and TdP because of the reduced ability to eliminate these drugs from the circulation.

Anti-infectives

Several classes of anti-infectives have QT prolongation liability. Macrolides such as erythromycin and clarithromycin can prolong the QT interval and induce TdP. Erythromycin is also a potent inhibitor of CYP3A4, which can result in supratherapeutic levels of other QT-prolonging drugs (see above). Quinolones such as ciprofloxacin, levofloxacin, gatifloxacin, and moxifloxacin, used for respiratory and urinary tract infections, inhibit the inward potassium current (I_{kr}) and thus prolong the action potential, predisposing the patient to TdP. Grepafloxacin was voluntarily withdrawn for this reason. Sparfloxacin, another quinolone, increases the action potential duration, but may not be capable of inducing TdP. Newer fluoroquinolones are selected with a limit on QT prolongation, and with a delimited incidence of TdP at less than one per million prescriptions. Antifungal drugs such as ketoconazole and itraconazole can also inhibit I_{kr} and result in QT prolongation. As with erythromycin, these antifungal agents are also inhibitors of CYP3A4 and changes in drug metabolism must be considered.

Anti-psychotics

Phenothiazine, thioridazine, haloperidol, chlorpromazine, trifluoperazine, pericycline, prochlorperazine, and fluphenazine have all been associated with QT prolongation and TdP hazard. The precise mechanism is unknown but appears to include inhibition of the I_{kr} potassium current, again leading to an increase in the action potential duration (delayed repolarization), which is plasma concentration dependent. Therefore, metabolic drug–drug interactions can increase the risk of these drugs; however, whereas many drugs that prolong QT are metabolized by CYP 3A4, anti-psychotics are often metabolized by CYP 2D6.

Nonclinical evaluation techniques

In vitro evaluation of I_{kr} (hERG) inhibition

Delayed repolarization can be mediated by multiple mechanisms involving potassium, sodium, and calcium currents. The predominant ion channel responsible for the I_{kr} current is the hERG (human *Ether-à-go-go* related gene) channel, also known as KCNH2 or Kv11.1. The unusual name for this potassium ion channel is because it is the human homolog of the *Ether-à-go-go* gene in the fruit fly *Drosophila*. Discovered in the 1960s, when anesthetized with ether, fruit flies with a mutation in this gene shake their legs, thus imitating the then popular go-go dancers.

The structure of the hERG channel is unusual in that it includes predominantly aromatic amino acids lining the central pore, and these provide the common target for inhibition by many classes of small molecule drugs, and screening for drug-induced inhibitory activity toward the hERG channel has now become routine. The cloned hERG channel can be expressed in various heterologous systems, allowing for quantitative assessment of the acute inhibition of hERG-mediated potassium current by drugs *in vitro*. Single cell electrical recordings are made with voltage-clamp techniques. The concentration-effect of various drugs on current through this channel can be measured accurately. The ability of a compound to block or inhibit the current is expressed as the concentration required for 50% inhibition or IC_{50}.

Like the QT interval, the hERG channel assay is not perfectly sensitive or specific for clinical arrythmogenic risk. Some drugs are potent hERG channel inhibitors ($IC_{50} < 10$ nM) and, correspondingly, are known to be associated with TdP risk, for example, dofetilide (3.9 nM), cisapride (6.5 nM), and astemizole (0.9 nM). However, there are examples of other drugs associated with TdP risk in which the hERG IC_{50} is at the very high concentration (e.g., 0.1–0.6 mM for d-sotalol).

A reasonable approach to interpret hERG data is to compare the hERG IC_{50} to the potency for the intended target and the projected therapeutic plasma concentration. These ratios provide a margin for off-target interaction with hERG: the larger the ratio, the lower the risk. A retrospective study of 100 drugs to assess the value of hERG data in predicting TdP risk, found that a 30-fold margin is sufficient for early drug development, with the caveat that integrated risk assessment (including other assays) should also be considered in assessing human TdP risk (Redfern *et al.*, 2003).

Cardiac action potential: *in situ* evaluation

The *in situ* cardiac action potential provides an integrated evaluation of the potential drug effect on multiple ion channels and currents. The most common experimental preparations include isolated Purkinje fibers (rabbit or dog), ventricular myocytes, or intact papillary muscles. The preparation is electrically stimulated and the resulting action potential recorded. Several concentrations of drug are typically tested in the same preparation by means of perfusion or superfusion. The time required for the action potential to reach 50% repolarization (APD_{50}) or 90% (APD_{90}) is generally correlated with the surface ECG QT interval (see earlier Figure 23.3). Inhibition of the I_{kr} or I_{ks} currents would increase both the APD_{50} and APD_{90}. The drug effect on *in vitro* action potential duration measurements is known to be influenced by the frequency of electrical stimulation; most drugs that delay repolarization have greater effect at slower stimulation rates.

Delayed repolarization is only one potential cardiovascular liability assessed by *in vitro* or *in situ* action potential preparations, and additional information can be also obtained from the cardiac action potential in these tissues. For instance, drugs that block sodium channels reduce the initial depolarization or upstroke velocity (V_{max}), and calcium channel blockers shorten the APD_{50}. Moreover, effects on the resting membrane potential as well as changes in the upstroke velocity and amplitude can slow ventricular conduction and also have the potential to promote arrhythmia.

Action potential heterogeneity and electrical dispersion within the myocardium may be important contributors to ventricular arrhythmia and TdP. Action potentials in the endocardium, M-cell layer, and epicardium can all be measured in a "wedge" preparation, which is a perfused, cross-section of the left ventricular wall. A quasi-ECG can be recorded simultaneously from the endocardial and epicardial surfaces.

Nonclinical *in vivo* assessments

A variety of animal models are used to evaluate the potential of new drugs to prolong the cardiac QT interval. In addition to a variety of species (rat, guinea pig, dog, pig, monkey), both conscious and anesthetized can be compared, while telemetry with surface or implanted electrodes in mobile animals can also be studied.

The context of human risk based on data from various model systems requires an understanding of the limitations of such models. For example, the rat lacks I_{kr} completely and is thus unusable. The dog has a large heart (~1% of body weight) with a Purkinje architecture that is similar to humans; however, it has a short QT interval, and the dog is prone to respiratory sinus arrhythmia. The architecture of the porcine Purkinje system is unlike that of humans because it has evolved from larger animals (in this respect, pigs resemble whales, hippopotami, etc.). Unsurprisingly, among laboratory species, the primates resemble humans mostly closely. Species differences need to be considered when interpreting results from these model systems.

Since many physiological factors can affect the QT interval, including stress and activity, all these factors need to be well-controlled in order to adequately interpret data from conscious animal studies, in particular, the comparison of QT intervals between dose periods. Prior training to accustom the animal to dosing and/or restraint is important. For conscious animal studies, often 3–4 animals per group are evaluated. Telemetry transmitters can be surgically implanted, which measure blood pressure, heart rate, and the Lead II ECG. Surface electrodes are also be used in restrained (sling) animals or more recently with a jacket that allows the animal greater mobility. The vagal tone of a relaxed dog in a sling restraint dramatically changes the QT interval.

Anesthetized animals have advantages in that heart pacing can easily be done. This is useful when drug-induced heart rate change *per se* confounds QT measurement. Invasive catheter measurements are also facilitated, such as cardiac contractility, and systemic vascular resistance while the electrophysiological properties of the test drugs are studied.

Predictability of nonclinical studies

To better understand the validity and predictability of nonclinical QT evaluation, two major initiatives were undertaken by ILSI-HESI (International Life Sciences Institute Health and Environmental Sciences Institute) and the JPMA (Japan Pharmaceutical Manufacturer Association). The assays outlined in the ICH S7B guidance document were conducted in multiple laboratories using drugs that are known to prolong QT and others as negative controls.

The JPMA initiative, QT-PRODACT (QT Interval Prolongation: Project for Database Construction) studied 21 compounds, 11 of which were known to prolong the QT interval and 10 QT negative compounds. All 21 compounds were studied in an Action Potential Duration (APD) assay as well as in conscious and anaesthetized dogs and the *Cynomolgus* monkey (Omata *et al.*, 2005).

The QT-PRODACT study assessed action potential duration in guinea pig papillary muscle. Seven of the 11 positive control compounds tested resulted in an increase in APD_{90} of more than 10%; whereas, 9 of the 11 compounds increased the APD_{30-90}, an index of I_k or "triangulation." Therefore, the APD_{30-90} had better predictability for inhibition of potassium-mediated repolarization. This basic observation was confirmed by the ILSI-HESI initiative in dog Purkinje fiber, in which the APD_{90} was an imperfect predictor of delayed repolarization; triangulation (APD_{90-40} in this case) was more reliable.

In the QT-PRODACT study, there was very good correlation ($R^2 = 0.947$) between the results obtained in conscious dog and conscious monkey. Monkey appears to be more sensitive than dog to

ventricular arrhythmias with astemizole, cisapride, and sotalol at equivalent plasma exposures. A good correlation ($R^2 = 0.816$) was observed between conscious and anesthetized dog with the anesthetized dog expressing haloperidol-induced ventricular arrhythmia but not in conscious animals.

Meanwhile, the ILSI-HESI initiative looked at three nonclinical assays: hERG current inhibition, Purkinje fiber repolarization, and *in vivo* QT evaluation in conscious dog (Hanson *et al.*, 2006). For *in vivo* evaluation of QT prolongation, all positive control compounds in the ILSI-HESI conscious dog study increased QTc by approximately 20 ms during periods of high drug plasma concentrations. However, QTc did not necessarily correlate directly with plasma concentrations, possibly the result of delayed drug distribution or interaction of active metabolites. The conclusion of this observation is that timepoints for QTc analysis may not be coincident with plasma drug profiles. Equally important to validating positive controls is the observation that none of the negative control compounds produced a signal of QT prolongation when QT was corrected for heart rate using Fredericia or individual formulas. QT correction by Bazett's misidentified some negative control compounds as QT prolonging, possibly because Bazett's formula overcorrects QT at higher heart rates. The conclusion of the ILSI-HESI study is that QT evaluation in dog is a good predictor of potential risk.

The results of the ILSI-HESI and PRODACT projects confirm that the nonclinical safety pharmacology studies outlined in ICH S7B are sufficient to evaluate potential human risk. But there must also be a caveat, which is that single tests are always imperfect and an integrated risk assessment, using multiple assay systems, is prudent.

Clinical testing: Human thorough QT study

The thorough QT study (TQT) arose from the ICH E14 guidance with the goal of testing for QT prolongation in healthy volunteers. ICH E14 recommends that all drugs be evaluated in a TQT study (except when redundant, e.g., certain classes of anti-arrythmic drug). Measurement of drug-induced QT changes in TQT studies is often conducted in healthy volunteers at peak blood concentrations of the drug or its major metabolites. In order to conclude that a drug does not prolong the QT interval, appropriate controls are needed to establish the sensitivity of the study to detect changes in QTc. For TQT studies as specified in ICH E14, a positive or active control is included to be able accurately to measure a 5 millisecond change in QTc. Moxifloxacin is mostly used. Biologics are neither specifically mentioned nor explicitly excluded in ICH E14, but the overall risk of QT prolongation by antibodies and other biological therapeutics is generally low.

Sufficient understanding of drug exposure and metabolism is needed to properly design a TQT study. In addition, the anticipated range of therapeutic doses must be tested. ECGs need to be captured at the time of maximal plasma concentrations and also for supra-therapeutic exposures that imitate likely clinical drug–drug interactions and patients with impaired renal or hepatic clearance. When selecting doses for a TQT study, variability as well as drug exposure needs to be considered. Both the drug and its active metabolite concentrations, often modeled from the known pharmacokinetics, will dictate whether a single dose study is sufficient, or perhaps that dosing to steady state is warranted.

TQT studies should be double-blinded not only during treatment but also during the subsequent ECG analyses. Both crossover or parallel group designs have been used. A smaller number of subjects are needed in crossover studies because intra-individual variability of QTc is lower than inter-individual variability. Parallel group designs may be necessary if drug carryover between periods is problematic or if the washout period is impractically long (long elimination half-life or irreversible interaction with the target substrate).

Correction of the QT interval for heart rate is again important in TQT studies. A powerful standardizing technique is to correct for heart rate, using the individual's observed QT versus RR relationship ("within-subject QT correction"); this can reduce variability compared to using population-based corrections (e.g., Bazett or Fredericia). Despite general agreement regarding QT correction, QT_{cb} and QT_{cf} are still reported in TQT studies, if only to allow for comparison with historical data.

Data reported from a TQT study are often expressed as the mean effect or central tendency. The mean effect is determined by comparing the change-from-baseline values of placebo and drug at corresponding time points. The conclusion of a negative TQT study (no drug effect on QT interval) requires that the study be valid and that the upper bound of the 95% one-sided confidence interval for the largest time matched mean placebo-corrected drug effect is less than 10 ms. A valid study is when the point estimate for the positive control is greater than 5 ms and the lower bound of the 95% confidence interval is greater than zero.

TQT studies typically use positive control arms. This is to demonstrate that if a small QT prolongation had occurred with the test drug, it could have in fact been detected. TQT studies are designed and powered to detect a 5 msec change in QTc. Moxifloxacin is the most common active control drug in use at present.

Although TQT study sensitivity is high, its specificity to detect arrhythmogenic potential is often lacking. Verapamil, amiodarone, and ranolazine all prolong the QT interval but their clinical proarrhythmic hazard is very low. A negative TQT study does not guarantee drug safety, and a positive TQT study likewise does not necessarily mean that a drug will cause cardiac arrhythmia.

The results of a TQT study have a major impact on subsequent drug development. In particular, a positive signal would increase the extent of patient ECG monitoring in late-stage clinical trials. A positive TQT study also has implications on drug labeling and the possible contraindication for certain patient populations.

Other clinical assessments

Careful ECG monitoring in Phase 1 studies can be helpful in the assessment of QT prolongation. These early clinical pharmacology studies often explore a range of doses including the maximum tolerated dose and therefore provide an understanding of the effect-size for QTc prolongation—crucial information for the later TQT study power calculations. The safety and tolerability of certain classes of drugs, such as chemotherapeutics and neuroleptics, preclude the TQT testing in healthy volunteers; alternative strategies such as expanding ECG collection in Phase 2 and 3 clinical studies then need to be considered and discussed with regulatory agencies.

Spontaneous long QT syndrome

Spontaneous long QT syndrome is not obviously related to new drug development. However, it often goes undiagnosed, and it is occasionally encountered in normal volunteer studies. Moreover, unexpected adverse events involving long QT syndromes also arise in Phase 3 studies or in the post-marketing environment. Some understanding of the spontaneous syndrome can therefore help in the differential diagnosis of serious adverse events.

From first principles, the defective ionic currents that can prolong the action potential in the cardiomyocyte, and therefore lengthen the QT interval, are as follows:

- increased potassium efflux;
- increased sodium influx;
- increased calcium influx.

All these have human genetic equivalents. Although some 15 human mutations causing long QT syndrome are known at present, there are numerous patients with the phenotype without any of the 15, and it is likely that more will be found in the future.

There are two inward potassium channels (Ks and Kr) both of which have multiple mutations causing the same electrophysiological result. Mutations on the alpha subunit of the inward potassium channel IK_s are by far the most common, and, clinically, those patients do not shorten their QT interval with exercise. Notched T waves are supposed to be the defining characteristic for the IK_r mutation. Interestingly, the human hERG (or KCNH2) gene has two known mutations, one of which prolongs

the QT interval by inhibiting potassium influx, whereas the other shortens the QT interval with an effect on exactly the same part (alpha subunit) of the same channel, thereby accelerating potassium influx.

The inward sodium channel is known to have two mutations on the same gene (Brugada mutations SCN5A and LQT3). In contrast to the potassium channel mutations, these sodium channel mutations increase action potential duration by slowing the rate of initial depolarization (they increase the APD at its front end).

The inward calcium channel interference is known for only a single mutation at present (gene CACNA1C). These patients also often present with hemiplegic (or "basilar") migraine. However, a non-ion channel, ryanodine complex, mutation is a second known cause for long QT syndrome due to reduced calcium influx.

Etiologically, if TdP is automatically lethal in the natural environment, the multiplicity of these ion-channel mutations, and their reasonably wide distribution and persistence in modern populations, suggests that they are not actually as lethal as other causes of tachyarrythmias (e.g., myocardial infarction), at least until the age of fertility has passed. Moreover, most men with spontaneous long QT syndrome have had an initial clinical episode before the age of 20 years. But when TdP does appear, it is surely as dangerous, if not more so, than other sustained ventricular tachycardias. But, nonetheless, the underlying predisposition (congenital long QT) itself cannot be so, and the persistence of these traits in modern populations is something of a conundrum.

The conventional boundaries for risk are Bazette's corrected QT interval (QTcB) > 460 msec for men and > 480 msec for women. The traditional gender difference is unexplained, and possibly lacking in solid evidence. Except under circumstances of extreme sinus bradycardia (vasovagal collapse, cholinesterase inhibitor poisoning), possibly with escape ventricular systoles, any observed QT interval > 500 msec in the drug-free state must always suggest spontaneous long QT syndrome (the relative merits of Bazette and Fredericia corrections for various heart rates are discussed above).

Without the genetics, unexplained syncope remains a clinical challenge for the patient and the prescriber. Many of the phenotypes deriving from these 15 mutations present intermittently. R on T phenomenon, reckoned on both theoretical and observational grounds to provoke TDP, is logically more likely at fast heart rates. Thus, the treatment of spontaneous prolonged QT is based on limiting heart rate with either adrenergic beta receptor antagonists ("beta-blockers") or, now rarely, effective doses of digoxin (risking complete AV node blockade). Obviously, d-sotalol would not be the beta-blocker of choice!

Brugada syndrome is found most commonly in south-eastern Asian, young males. The mutation is with the inward sodium channel. Beta-blockers do not help these patients, and drugs such as procainamide and flecainide make it worse. These are the extremely rare patients, for whom beta-1 agonists (*sic*) or implanted defibrillators might be the only solution.

It is unknown how drugs and spontaneous long- and short-QT syndromes interact, and whether the effects are additive, synergistic, or independent. A concern, however, is that a potentially lethal cocktail is being mixed: (i) the current penchant for relatively large-scale normal volunteer thorough QT studies; (ii) the lack of genotyping of the participants; (iii) the natural prevalence of spontaneous long QT syndrome; and (iv) its often intermittent observation and diagnosis that will be missed in ordinary normal volunteer, phase one-unit screening.

Future considerations

Accurate risk assessment in drug development requires confidence in the tools and assays used. The Cardiac Safety Research Consortium and the Health and Environmental Sciences Institute organized a public forum in 2008 to discuss the strengths and limitations of the current paradigm for cardiac safety assessment. The panel con-

cluded that cardiotoxicity and non-QT proarrhythmia evaluation are not adequately addressed in drug development, and that assays need to be developed to assess non-I_{kr} mediated proarrhythmogenic risk.

References

(Note: all websites cited in the text were accessed April 24, 2010.)

Hanson LA, Bass AS, Gintant G, Mittelstadt S, Rampe D, Thomase K. ILSI-HESI cardiovascular safety subcommittee initiative: Evaluation of three non-clinical models of QT prolongation. *J Pharmacol Toxicol Methods* 2006; **54**:116–129.

Omata T, Kasai C, Hashimoto M, Hombo T, Yamamoto K. QT PRODACT: Comparison of non-clinical studies for drug-induced delay in ventricular repolarization and their role in safety evaluation in humans. *J Pharmacol Sci* 2005; **99**:531–541.

Priori SG, Schwartz PJ, Napolitano C, *et al.* Risk stratification in the long-QT syndrome. *N Engl J Med* 2003; **348**:1866–1874.

Redfren WS, Carlsson L, Davis AS, *et al.* Relationships between preclinical cardiac electrophysiology, clinical QT interval prolongation and Torsade de Pointes for a broad range of drugs: evidence for a provisional safety margin in drug development. *Cardiovascular Res* 2003; **58**:32–45.

Roden DM. Drug-induced prolongation of the QT interval. *N Engl J Med* 2004; **350**:1013.

Further reading

Darpo B, Nebout T, Sager PT. Clinical evaluation of QT/QTc prolongation and proarrhythmic potential for nonantiarrhythmic drugs: the International Conference on Harmonization of Technical Requirements for Registration of Pharmaceuticals for Human Use E14 Guideline. *J Clin Pharmacol* 2006; **46**:498–507.

Fenichel RR, Malik M, Antzelevitch C, *et al.* Drug-induced Torsades de Pointes and implications for drug development. *J Cardiovasc Electrophysiol* 2004; **15**:475–495.

Joshi A, Dimino T, Vohra Y, Cui C, Yan G-X. Preclinical strategies to assess AT liability and torsadogenic potential of new drugs: the role of experimental models. *J Electrophys* 2004; **37**(suppl):7–14.

Marchlinski F. The tachyarrythmias. In *Harrison's Principles of Internal Medicine*, seventeenth edition. Fauci AS, Braunwald E, Kasper DL, Hauser SL, Longo DL, Jameson JL (eds). McGraw Hill: New York, USA, 2008, 1441–1442. ISBN 978-0-07-159991-7.

Piccini JP, Whellan DJ, Berridge BR, *et al.* Current challenges in the evaluation of cardiac safety during drug development: Translational medicine meets the Critical Path Initiative. *Am Heart J* 2009; **158**:317–326.

Roden DM. Cellular basis of drug-induced Torsades de Pointes. *Br J Pharmacol* 2008; **154**:1502–1507.

Shryock JC, Song Y, Wu L, Fraser H, Belardinellin L. A mechanistic approach to assess the proarrhythmic risk of QT-prolonging drugs in preclinical pharmacologic studies. *J Electrophys* 2004; **37**:34–39.

Yap YG, Camm AJ. Drug induced QT prolongation and Torsades de Pointes. *Heart* 2003; **89**:1363–1372.

SECTION IV
Applied Aspects

Introduction

With this section we begin to move from the ortho-dox, center of traditional pharmaceutical medicine to more applied aspects. In many cases, these chapters tackle relatively modern sophistications, either in the drug development process or in their corresponding regulatory processes. These developments may require special approaches, say, beyond tradi-tional clinical trial designs (e.g., pharmacoepidemi-ology, patient compliance, plasma level sampling times), standard ethical considerations (e.g., some biotechnology products), or regulatory processes that assess product efficacy (e.g., homeopathy). The quantitative sciences are also included here, because they are fundamental to the entire discipline of pharmaceutical medicine, including its applied aspects.

CHAPTER 24

Biotechnology Products and Their Development

David A. Shapiro[1] & Anthony W. Fox[2]

[1]Intercept Pharmaceuticals, San Diego, CA, USA
[2]EBD Group Inc., Carlsbad, CA, USA and Munich, Germany, and Skaggs SPPS, University of California, San Diego, USA

Introduction

The objectives of this chapter are to describe what biotechnology products are, and where their regulation is similar or different from chemically-synthesized, small molecule drugs. It is a common assumption that biotechnology has sprung from nothing, *de novo*, within a small number of recent years. This is not the case, and we shall show how the growth of this field actually has a basis that is, in many ways, common and interconnected with development of all other types of drugs. But, in general, the chemical properties and synthesis of biological products are less important than their pharmacological properties.

Ethical aspects of this area of therapeutics are dealt with at the end of this chapter, after the various technologies have been discussed. In practice, ethics comes first. But the ethical issues can best be considered after the scope and complexities of this field have been considered.

Definitions

Biotechnology products are those that are prepared using biological organisms, rather than the usual types of industrial chemical synthesis. Biological organisms may be used *in vivo*, *ex vivo*, or *in vitro*

Principles and Practice of Pharmaceutical Medicine, 3rd edition.
Edited by L.D. Edwards, A.W. Fox, P.D. Stonier.
© 2011 Blackwell Publishing Ltd.

to make these products. Yeast, fungi, bacteria, viral vectors, and mammalian cells may all serve this synthetic purpose.

Meanwhile, the compositions of biological products are diverse. They include poly-peptides, biological organisms themselves (living, dead, or attenuated), genes, any type of fermented product (even when these may be alternatively synthesized chemically), synthetic inhibitory RNAs, and antisense compounds. To date, polypeptides have formed the largest group among these, themselves being functionally very diverse: hormones, antibodies, cytokines (including interferons), and immune adjuvants, including non-mammalian examples, such as Key-hole Limpet (*Megathura crenulata*) hemocyanin.

Biological products have a longer history than is generally assumed. At one time smallpox accounted for 10% of deaths in some countries. The development of the cowpox vaccination in 1796, and later the *Variocella* vaccine, led to smallpox being the only infectious disease ever to have been eradicated from the planet; the final outbreak was a small number of cases after a laboratory accident in 1979.

It is beyond the scope of this chapter to discuss all potential applications and all present technologies associated with biological drugs. This chapter concentrates on the newer technologies that are actually used on either an investigational or approved basis in human beings, and given the current breadth of the field, we can only provide an overview. Thus, vaccines, fermented antibiotics, blood products, diagnostic products (e.g., antibody-based assay systems), and devices using biotechnology products will not be covered, although these could be classed as biological products. Similarly, pluripotent stem cells are currently being investigated for the manufacture of tissues for grafting, but these are not biotechnology therapeutics themselves.

There are approximately 1250 biotechnology companies in the US and Canada, about half that number in Europe, and smaller but growing numbers throughout the rest of the world (especially Israel, Korea, Australasia, and in the recent past, India and China). These companies are usually much smaller than the large, fully integrated "pharmaceutical" companies ("large pharma") headquartered on the US east coast and in Switzerland. Small companies' research activities may be restricted to the preclinical discovery and early-stage clinical investigation of compounds; therefore, their business environment and practices differ from large pharma. Somewhat arbitrarily, we shall use the term "biotechnology company" rather loosely in this chapter to mean this type of small organization. An irreverent wit offered an alternative definition: a biotechnology company is a pharmaceutical company without revenues! Note, however, that the term "biotechnology products" refers to the compounds themselves, regardless of the size of the organization developing them, and in fact, most of large pharma are themselves engaged in biotechnology, one way or another.

Before we turn to the products themselves, we would like to draw attention to when biotechnology brings special ethical aspects to clinical trials. As we shall see below, some of these therapies require extraordinary procedures, such as the deliberate immunization of normal volunteers to foreign blood groups, or the introduction of exogenous genes into patients. Ensuring that consent is truly informed is *sine qua non*, even though, sadly, this was not the case in an infamous disaster when a patient in an early-phase gene therapy study died at an eminent US teaching hospital (Couzin and Kaiser, 2005). We return to ethical issues at the end of the chapter because they must be considered in relation to the technical aspects of investigational

biological products; nonetheless, these should be foremost and not an afterthought.

Regulatory considerations

In most countries, regulation of drug and biological compound development and marketing has usually derived from governmental response to crisis.

US perspective

The initial legislation affecting biologics was the Safe Vaccines and Sera Act of 1904. The focus of the Act was the development of safe, pure, and potent vaccination preparations, which at that time, were the responsibility of the Department of Agriculture. This legislation was updated by the Public Health Service Act (1944), written principally with blood products and prevention of the transmission of disease by intravenous infusion in mind.

It was not until 1972 that biological products were brought under the same regulatory framework as chemically-synthesized, small molecule drugs. The Food and Drug Administration (FDA), a branch of the US Department of Health and Human Services, accepted the responsibility for biologics, upon their transfer from the Department of Agriculture. Within the FDA, a designated Center for Biologicals Evaluation and Research (CBER) was created. This unified approach progressed further in 2005, when most (but not all) biological products were transferred within FDA from CBER to the Center for Drug Evaluation and Research (CDER), the latter comprising the "ordinary" Investigational New Drug (IND) and New Drug Administration (NDA) reviewing divisions with which readers will be familiar. Similar historical events stimulated other models in other countries.

In the US and elsewhere, evidence of this convergence of biological and nonbiological products is evidenced by the following:
• IND regulations (there are no unique regulations for biologics undergoing experimental study);
• similar good clinical practices guidelines;
• various International Conference on Harmonization initiatives;

- good manufacturing practices;
- "fast track" designations for accelerating review and approval.

In the USA, however, illogicalities still persist. For example, the Waxman-Hatch legislation gave authority for generics and provided patent term exclusivity for drugs, but not for biological products licensed prior to 1972. This has led to controversy over quasi-generic ("follow-on") biological products, which are considered below. Similarly, the pediatric "exclusivity" that the Act initiated currently does not extend to Biological License Applications (BLAs). Finally, the Centers for Disease Control remains involved with compensation issues for pediatric vaccines, a unique administrative arrangement.

Biotechnology versus conventional drug products

There is a widespread, but largely unreasonable, perception that biotechnology products differ in their properties to conventional small molecules drugs. For example, it is widely believed that simple pharmacokinetic models cannot adequately describe the behavior of biological agents *in vivo*. Although quantitative data relating to the intracellular distribution of these agents may not be known (largely due to inadequate assay methods), the underlying principals of Absorption, Distribution, Metabolism, and Excretion (ADME) are the same, even though new paradigms and different quantitative models may be required to describe the properties of biological compounds. Table 24.1 lists the factors that need to be considered when modeling pharmacokinetic–pharmacodynamic relationships for the extreme case of gene therapy products, most having correlates with features of orthodox drugs.

Although biotechnology products can have complicated PK–PD relationships, this can also be the case for orthodox drugs; for example, for antidepressant therapies, three weeks or more is usually needed before any therapeutic response is seen, and angiotensin converting enzyme (ACE) inhibitors remain antihypertensive after several

Table 24.1 Pharmacokinetic considerations for gene therapy agents (adapted from Ledley & Ledley, 1994)

Pharmacokinetic property	Gene therapy property
Absorption	DNA vector distribution
Distribution	Vector fraction target cell uptake
Distribution	Genetic material traffic in organelles
Metabolism	DNA degradation
Metabolism	mRNA production
Metabolism	Protein production: quantity
Excretion	Protein production: stability
Metabolism, Excretion	Protein production: compartmentalization
Excretion	Protein production: secretory fate

months of therapy, and yet serum ACE activity will have returned to normal. Likewise, both corticosteroid therapy and gene therapies require access to the cell nucleus; the intercompartmental transfer coefficients (serum/cytosol/nucleus) are complex and unmeasurable in human beings in both cases. In contrast, complexity among biotechnology products include antibody complement fixation, cellular attack may be an all-or-none phenomenon, DNA lysis in sputum may not require drug absorption at all, and clot lysis may depend on a wide range of endogenous plasma proteins, each with its own concentration–response relationships. An example of the all-or-none phenomenon was tragically demonstrated in six cases of cytokine storm during a biological product first-in-human study in London in 2006 (Suntharalingam *et al.*, 2006). The problems and analysis of tachyphylaxis are common to both orthodox and biotechnology products.

Manufacturing issues

Arguably, manufacturing changes are more likely to affect the clinical profile of biological compounds than small chemical entities. Small changes in the three-dimensional folding, post-translational modification, or glycosylation of proteins can significantly alter biological activity. The potential for the replication of viruses or bacteria in fermenters, and their persistence in finished drug product, raise additional safety concerns arising from the manufacturing process for such compounds. For the clinical trialist, this leads to a generality: when studying biologicals there is usually a greater need for early-stage test medications to be as similar as possible to the eventual marketed product than for "orthodox" small chemicals. The same reasoning is the current concern of regulators when trying to understand and approve quasi-generic (or "follow-on") biological products that have not been subjected to large-scale clinical trials demonstrating bioequivalence. An interlocking factor is that if small production differences or uncertainties of identity are to be allowed for "follow-on" products, can the same latitude be given between small scale, early clinical-phase investigational products and late-stage, large-scale, commercial production for innovative products?

Product classes and resultant clinical trial issues

Many of the principles outlined in other chapters in this book for Phase 1 and 2 studies of small molecules are equally applicable to the testing of most biotechnology products. Other chapters also discuss some specific toxicology and drug discovery aspects of biotechnology products.

The general design of a development program for a biological product also must obey the same principles as for ordinary drugs, and these should be familiar to the competent clinical trialist. Equally useful in the case of biologics, is to begin development with an agreed, desirable package insert or product label, which can then be used to define the development strategy. Those tactics (i.e., clinical trial designs, milestones, and product-killing findings) that are justified or validated by that strategy should be implemented. The development program should be tailored to the nature and needs of the disease; often the pharmacological activity of a biological product is likely to be very precise. For example, an antibody will bind to a previously identified, narrow range of antigens, and the pathogenesis or source of antigen presentation will

have a fixed relationship to a well-described disease or set of diseases. The nature and seriousness of the disease being treated is just as important as in more orthodox clinical trials. The degree of lethality or morbidity associated with the disease treated with existing therapies is correlated positively with the degree of intolerability of the test agent that may be accepted (e.g., oncologic products whether "biologic" or not).

The trialist's first concerns, of course, are for safety and tolerability. Compared with small molecules, most biological products carry a higher probability of antigenic immune response, because of their large size. However, the range of target-organ toxicities is usually narrower for a biological product, and more likely to be directly related to the specific receptors (using that term in a loose sense), which govern the product's pharmacodynamics. Clinical trialists should also be careful not to ignore the toxicological potential of the often large amounts of vehicle, often with unusual ionic strengths, buffering materials, or nonphysiological pH. Unusual preservatives that may be required to maintain complex peptides in a stable form may also present themselves (e.g., cresols for insulin). These "inactive" product ingredients often have their own nephrotoxic, hepatotoxic, and allergenic properties.

The clinical trialist who switches from small molecules to a biological product will nonetheless use familiar tactics to prove efficacy. The central ethical consideration will usually be about whether standard treatment (if any) can be withheld, and the debate is not about the use of placebo in an absolute sense. With "breakthrough" agents that offer the potential for a new type of therapy, clinical trials can still be conducted comparing the trial agent to a placebo.

Dose–response relationships need to be evaluated for biological agents prior to approval even when the biological response is of the "all or nothing" type (e.g., serological conversion, when the proportion of responding patients may be the endpoint of interest), because dose–response relationships must be understood for populations, as well as within individuals. Therapies such as vaccines must also be evaluated in different racial populations, and in other types of special populations, such as the elderly.

Peptides

For a long time, interest in biotechnology centered on the production and properties of administered hormones ranging from tri-peptides (e.g., corticotrophin releasing factor; CRF), through cyclic nonapeptides such as vasopressin analogues, to longer polypeptide chains, for example, insulins, growth hormones, and monoclonal antibodies. As the length of the poly-peptide increases the three-dimensional structure becomes an important determinant of *in vivo* activity and properties.

However, there are also important freedoms that an increase in protein size can bring. Single peptide mutations usually become less important as protein size increases. The scope for post-translational modification is also greater in large polypeptides than in small ones. Good biological examples of this are the large qualitative changes in pharmacology of a single amino acid that distinguishes arginine-vasopressin (the human anti-diuretic hormone) from human oxytocin (both nonapeptides) compared with the many minor and clinically irrelevant variants of human hemoglobin (Harrison *et al.*, 1998; Viprakasit *et al.*, 2006). The marked differences in pharmacodynamics between calcitonin and calcitonin gene-related peptide, which are both encoded by the same gene, require a major post-translational structural change (Andreotti *et al.* 2008; Brain *et al.*, 1985).

Immunologic adverse events can be viewed as either active or passive, i.e., first what the drug does to the patient (histamine release, B lymphocyte proliferation, etc.) and second what the patient does to the drug (enhanced clearance, peptide cleavage, hapten formation, etc.). The clinical correlates of these cellular processes range from tachyphylaxis (need for ever-increasing doses to maintain biological effect) to the acute emergencies of anaphylaxis. For example, around 13% of patients given aglucerase (indicated for Type 1 Gaucher's disease) develop IgG antibodies to the enzyme, and of those so immunized, approximately 25% have clinical symptoms of hypersensitivity.

Hormones

Insulin is an early and classic example of a biotechnology product. It illustrates some of the general problems that are associated with peptide drugs and how modern technology leads to improved therapy. Prior to the production of human insulin by cell-based fermentation processes, treatment was with pancreatic extracts of porcine or bovine origin. Many patients developed insulin resistance, and this correlated with specific antibody responses directed against the insulin of the species of origin. Patients then had a "career" of increasing insulin dose, punctuated by hypoglycemia when changing from one animal source to another without changing dose size. Some patients became so competent at clearing bovine or porcine insulin that they needed extracts from exotic species such as whales. The modification of recombinant chimeric or pure cell lines to secrete human insulin, the development of large-scale fermenters to multiply such cultures, and the ability to purify cell-free insulin from other materials in the culture medium led to a sufficient supply of exogenous, but nonetheless human, insulin. Now in use by almost all patients with diabetes in the western world, immune responses to this molecule are much rarer than before, and dose sizes tend to remain stable.

In addition to insulin, various other hormones made by recombinant methods have been approved or are under development. The most commonly prescribed examples at present include growth hormone (somatrem, Protropin™; Genentech, Inc.) or erythropoietin (epoeitin alfa, Epogen™; Amgen Inc.).

Enzymes

Several peptide drugs are enzymes. Dornase alpha (Pulmozyme®; Genentech Inc.) is an example, which is used to improve the management of chest infections and pulmonary function in patients with cystic fibrosis. It works because the rate of DNA release from dead and dying leucocytes is sufficient significantly to increase sputum viscosity. The enzyme (inhaled through a specific type of nebulizer) digests this released DNA, thus liquifying the sputum, and enhancing expectoration.

The clinical trials of this product were of generally orthodox design, using dose–response analysis and placebo-controlled designs. The fact that the product is made by fermentation of genetically-engineered Chinese hamster ovary cells containing DNA encoding for the native human protein, deoxyribonuclease I (DNAase) was essentially irrelevant to the design of the clinical development program.

Other enzymes in clinical use, manufactured using similar processes, include tissue plasminogen activator, other thrombolytic agents, and aglucerase (Ceredase™; Genzyme Corp.) for Type 1 Gaucher's disease. These illustrate the diverse clinical applications that enzymes may find.

Antibodies

Since antibodies bind to antigens, their function is often to augment intrinsic clearance mechanisms as well as potentially exerting definitive therapeutic effects. It is not surprising therefore that the range of therapeutic applications for antibody therapy is broad, ranging from anti-tumor therapy to specific immunological diseases, for example, rheumatoid arthritis, even though the use of each product is, contrastingly, narrow.

At least one biotechnology company (COVx Inc., now subsumed into Pfizer Inc.) has been able to create a range of peptides that are attached to the crystalline fragment (Fc) of an antibody whose binding fragment (Fab) can be independently selected. This prolongs the half-time of elimination of many peptide "pay-loads," and can target their delivery to tissues containing the corresponding antigen. Theoretically, this technology also allows for the admixture of different peptides, all attached to the same crystalline fragment of the same monoclonal antibody.

Antibodies can be targeted more or less specifically, either against a single or a variety of antigens. An example of a "broad-spectrum" antibody therapy is anti-Rhesus antigen antibody (WinRho®), which has been used *post partum* for many years to prevent rhesus immunization of an Rh- mother by an Rh+ neonate. The product is made from pooled plasma of Rh- male volunteers who have been deliberately challenged with small Rh+, ABO compatible blood transfusions. There are at least 60 known epitopes of the rhesus D antigen. The resulting product binds to red cells from 99.7% of all Rh+ blood donors.

Specific targeting of single, infrequently expressed antigens forms the basis of the large number of monoclonal antibody therapies. These are generally manufactured by mammalian cell fermentation process, as described above (see Chapter 7 for issues relating to the manufacturing process and viral contamination of these products). Rituximab (Rituxan®; IDEC Pharmaceuticals) is a highly targeted antibody that binds principally with CD-20 positive B lymphocytes that characterize one form of non-Hodgkin's lymphoma. More recently, clinical trials on this agent have been conducted evaluating its effects on other putatively B-lymphocyte mediated diseases such as rheumatoid arthritis. Another example of a specific therapeutic is anMuromonab-CD3 (Orthoclone OKT3, Ortho Pharmaceuticals), which is used to reverse acute rejection of transplanted kidneys.

The presence of single antigen targets in or on tumor cells can be further exploited by conjugating the antibody to a radioactive or cytotoxic molecule. For example, human milk fat globule I monoclonal antibody complexed with ^{90}Yttrium (Theragyn™) is under development for the treatment of ovarian carcinoma by Antisoma, PLC.

Antibody development tactics can be learned by reviewing the product labeling for some of agents mentioned. Anti-tumor necrosis factor alpha (infliximab, Enbrel®; Amgen Inc., Wyeth Inc.) has revolutionized the treatment of rheumatoid arthritis, even if its labeling, in small font, occupies both sides of a small poster.

Cytokines

On phyllogenetic grounds, cytokine responses to infection or tumors are thought to be the most ancient form of immune response. Cytokines are generated in response to antigen challenge and have a large part in innate response and impact on the clinical management of many diseases. However, their properties are considerably different to antibodies. Cytokine responses are nonspecific, and, mostly, their principal biological effect is to enhance general, lymphocyte-mediated attack on the antigen-bearing cell. Since cytokines have non-specific effects, existing biological products often find additional indications. Similarly, their adverse effects also reflect their nonspecificity with symptoms such as fever, myalgias, flu-like symptoms, and rhabdomyolysis.

Cytokines include the large and ever-increasing set of therapeutically-useful interleukins, various interferons, trophic factors such as tumor necrosis factor, and the many growth factors. Granulocyte macrophage colony stimulating factor (GMCSF, sargramostim, Leukine™; Immunex Corp.) is used for myeloid reconstitution after bone marrow ablation, exploiting its eponymous property (which was initially identified *in vitro*). Interleukin-2 (aldesleukin, Proleukin™; Chiron Corp.) is approved in the US for the treatment of renal carcinoma and metastatic melanoma. Platelet-derived growth factor can be used to heal diabetic foot ulcers, presumably by imitating normal physiology that is blunted in patients with diabetes (gel becaplermin, Regranex®; Ortho-McNeil/Chiron Inc.). Pegylated interferon alpha has revolutionized the treatment of hepatitis due to virus type C.

The Te Genero disaster in London illustrates many of the hazards of biologics research (Suntharalingam *et al.*, 2006). The test material had been given to chimpanzees, which (evidently) have the same target receptors. However, it was a vigorous all-or-none response in the normal human volunteers that led to such severe adverse events even at an appropriately small, properly allometrically scaled dose.

Immune adjuvants

Immune adjuvants can be classed as
- nonspecific, e.g., BCG vaccine for bladder cancer;
- specific, e.g., Salk vaccine for polio prevention;
- genetic, to elicit cytokine responses (see below).

Traditionally, vaccines have been directed against the prevention of specific infectious diseases. *Vacca* is a latin female nominative meaning a cow, and vaccines have been used widely in medicine since Jenner's pioneering work. Live, live-attenuated, and killed microrganisms may all be used as antigens to elicit cellular and humoral responses. They may be viewed as adjuvants because it is the enhancement of endogenous physiology that protects against the pathogen, and not the vaccine itself.

The great scope for preventing infectious disease remains, and there is a continuing need for worthwhile research programs. Current challenges include malaria, sleeping sickness, HIV, and prion-mediated disease. The last of these may (controversially) also be regarded as an "autoimmune" or "congenital" disease, if it turns out to be truly due to the de-repression of prion genomes, lurking dormant in many normal mammals, including human beings. Drug resistance is a huge problem that has limited the utility of so many anti-infective agents, attempting to treat almost any class of microorganism ranging from viruses (e.g., HIV and Hepatitis B), bacteria (e.g., *Staphylococcus aureus*) to protozoa, such as malaria.

Not surprisingly, there is considerable interest in using adjuvant tactics for the prevention or treatment of noninfectious disease. Spontaneous tumor regression (although observed clinically only very rarely) and the development of rare tumors in immunocompromised patients (such as Kaposi's Sarcoma in patients with AIDS) are both consistent with the usefulness of endogenous host mechanisms to either prevent or retard cancer. Tumor specific antigens may be used as therapeutic targets for exogenous therapy.

Anti-sense drugs

Anti-sense drugs are exogenous oligo-nucleotides that bind to specific endogenous nucleic acid sequences. Binding to mRNA prevents translation to proteins by ribosomes, and similarly, binding to specific gene sequences on DNA can prevent transcription (i.e., inhibit mRNA synthesis). The application of antisense technology is broad because this approach can be used to inhibit the production of a wide range of proteins including stimulatory and inhibitory molecules.

Although the synthesis of antisense molecules using modern combinatorial chemical approaches is easily automated, the delivery of these molecules to the appropriate intracellular and intranuclear targets is more difficult. The first antisense drug to be approved is for the treatment of cytomegalovirus retinitis in patients with AIDS (fomivirsen, Vitravene®; ISIS Pharmaceuticals, Inc.). This must be administered by direct intraocular injection, illustrating well how ADME complexities can severely limit biological product utility.

To date, most regulatory authorities have treated antisense drugs in the much same way as any other biological product, and without the additional constraints that apply to gene therapies. Since these oligonucleotides have specific binding activities, safety considerations are usually dependent on the potential for nonspecific effects of protein synthesis inhibition. At present, with the current limited experience, there would appear to be sound *in vitro* methods for the testing of the specificity of antisense drugs to be predictive for their tolerability in humans. Furthermore, when the properties of the protein that is inhibited are discrete and consistent both across species for preclinical efficacy evaluations, and in humans, it is likely that the potential adverse effects will be predictable. Generally, if an antisense compound is specific to only one 18-mer or 19-mer, specificity of its action can be assumed.

Gene therapy

Gene therapy may be defined as the administration of exogenous DNA, in the form of intact gene(s) for therapeutic purposes. There are some *a priori* characteristics for diseases that are likely to be attractive targets for gene therapy, and a fundamental contrast between the gene therapy of protein replacement in comparison with protein synthesis regulation.

The absolute or relative deficiency of a particular protein needed for health may be correctable, for example, the enzyme needed to reverse Gaucher's disease. If the gene product can be manufactured and administered effectively and tolerably, the need for a gene therapy is reduced.

However, there are also congenital disorders involving relative deficiencies of a particular protein, and where, importantly, therapeutic-induced overexpression can be as harmful as underexpres-

sion. Attempting to down-regulate gene expression can be more difficult than inducing it. The thalassemias are *a priori* a good example of this problem. Overproduction of the missing hemoglobin chain is unlikely to be helpful to the patient. Similarly, when the principal desired target for gene therapy is a specific target organ, overexpression of genes in other tissues may create tolerability problems.

Gene therapies usually have two major components: the DNA molecule itself (the "construct"), and an administration adjuvant (the "vector"). Initially, constructs were injected directly (i.e., without a vector, "naked DNA"); however, this has proved not to be an efficient method of transfection. Vectors may be viral or nonviral (e.g., "zinc-finger" proteins, and various types of liposomes), and are designed to carry genes (which are large, hydrophilic molecules) across lipid membranes. Liposomal envelopes may be constructed that are either anionic or cationic. Complex liposomes, coated with antibodies that will target specific antigen presenting cells, can also be designed. Gold-coated DNA may also be inserted into cells by a "gene gun," where electrostatic or gas pressure powered displacement from a plastic matrix occurs.

Viral vectors include the following:
- *Potentially pathogenic DNA viruses:* These include adenoviruses and pox or vaccinia viruses. Both virus types can replicate in mammalian cytoplasm, whether or not the host cell is in mitosis or quiescent; both can elicit a host immune response.
- *Herpes simplex virus I (HSV1):* This also contains double-stranded DNA, but it replicates in the nucleus of cells that are successfully infected, again without need for mitosis.
- *Nonpathogenic adeno-associated viruses:* These parvoviruses carry single stranded DNA and are able to integrate into a broad range of nondividing cells.
- *Retroviruses:* These RNA-containing viruses exist in an envelope derived from host cell membrane, and thus do not usually elicit vigorous immune responses. Retroviruses also tend to replicate only in dividing cells.

Human gene transfer experiments in lymphocyte marking studies began in 1989. These early studies showed that gene transfer was feasible and could be well-tolerated although there was no demonstrable therapeutic benefit. The first human gene therapy clinical trial was in 1990, in a patient with adenosine deaminase (ADA) deficiency; initial responsiveness proved not to be uniform when the series of cases was extended, possibly due to the fact that the disease phenotype could be elicited by a variety of genotypes.

Two-stage delivery systems for gene therapies are also under development. This usually requires initial manipulation of somatic tissue *ex vivo*. A good example is following the transformation of bone marrow biopsies. The gene therapy can be introduced into the biopsy material *ex vivo* using either a viral or a nonviral vector. Successful expression can then be definitely demonstrated *in vitro*, following which the transformed marrow biopsy can be infused as an autologous transplant, with the intention of its proliferation and generation of the desired protein product *in vivo* (Wasserfall and Herzog, 2009).

The pharmacokinetics of gene therapy and its relationship to dynamic effects are very different from the orthodox pharmaceutical situation (see earlier Table 24.1). Ledley and Ledley (1994) have proposed a corollary of traditional PK/PD modeling, predicated upon the specific events in the cellular response to gene uptake and activation. These authors have developed a six-compartment model, which appears to have general applicability, to evaluate the apparent kinetic properties of a therapeutic gene product. This leads to the possibility of designing dosing regimens and relating them to measurements of expression and efficacy responses.

There are two major concerns about specific tolerability of gene therapies. These relate separately to the expressed gene product and the vector. Both are immunological in nature, and may lead to therapeutic ineffectiveness.

If the gene therapy causes the production of a protein that was previously absent in the body, an immune response to the novel protein may occur and should be anticipated. It cannot be predicted which sort of immune response may (or may not) then follow.

Resistance to gene therapy can also result from immunization against either the construct or the vector. The former is analogous to the patients who used to become resistant to xenobiotic insulins (see above), and is also seen in the case of human factor VIII in some patients with hemophilia. Escalating doses may be needed to maintain efficacy, or efficacy may be eventually lost. On the other hand, viral vectors are liable to replicate and also to elicit immune responses, as in any vaccination.

One approach has been to develop strains of many of the viruses listed above as "replication defective" or "replication incompetent." These viruses are mutations that are cultured initially in conditions that provide some crucial nutrient or element of the replicating machinery that neither the virus nor, importantly, the patient can synthesize. These strains of virus are therefore replication-incompetent after human administration. There is nonetheless always the concern that after injection the virus will find some way to overcome its incompetency, for example by recruitment of the host cell machinery for this purpose.

Safety issues in gene product development

Although issues surrounding sterility, mutagenicity, stability, and carcinogenicity, and the attendant good laboratory and manufacturing practice issues are much the same for gene and other biotechnology therapies in principle, there is often greater complexity associated with the former. These complexities include uncertainties with preclinical toxicology and the potential for germ cell line incorporation.

First, the toxicology of any gene therapy needs to be considered as a combination of three products: the construct; nongenetic elements in the construct (e.g., pharmaceutical adjuvant stabilizing materials); and the vector.

Second, there is a need to test in animals the possibility of incorporation of the therapeutic gene into the germ cell line. Many constructs contain multiple genes: not only is the therapeutic gene present, but also genes that assist in manufacturing, for example those conferring antibiotic resistance to the microorganism that is being used for production, or a gene for a marker enzyme. All these genes require toxicological assurance that they do not incorporate into the germ cell line, and thus will not be replicated in the offspring of the treated patient. This special field of toxicology is still in its infancy; in some cases clinical trials have to be restricted to surgically-sterile patients in the absence of this information. Understanding the relevance of the animal species used in germ cell safety evaluations and the test product effects to their human correlates is paramount.

Regulatory issues specific to gene therapies

In the US, gene therapy protocols attract an additional degree of regulatory review. Not only must an IND be approved by the FDA, but also the protocol must be approved by the Recombinant DNA Advisory Committee of the National Institutes of Health (the "RAC"). To date, many dozens of such protocols have been approved, with the largest group for therapies that are designed to increase production of a specific cytokine in a specific tissue location. In Europe there is no equivalent to the RAC, and regulatory requirements are handled within the national regulatory authorities reviewing research protocols for investigational agents and the European Medicines Agency (EMA) and Committee for Medicinal Products for Human Use (CPMP) reviewing the final product license applications. Gene therapies are exempt from the time limits that usually apply to the review of clinical trial protocols by national competent authorities in Europe.

In 2009, a milestone was reached, however, with the first US approval of a human pharmaceutical made in a genetically-engineered animal. Human anti-thrombin is now made in goats containing the human DNA construct and is indicated for the treatment of patients with congenital anti-thrombin deficiency who suffer repetitive thromboembolic episodes (Human Recombinant Antithrombin, ATryn®; GTC Biotherapeutics, Massachusetts and Lundbeck Inc., Illinois).

"Follow-on" biologicals

Hitherto, regulatory authorities have taken the position that the manufacturing process for any given biological process defines the product. This has been a consequence of the hypothesis that a quaternary change in structure is unlikely to be detectable by conventional means for assessing product purity. For product innovators, this has meant (compared to small molecules) relatively early and expensive scale-up, so as not to be accused of trying to conduct Phase 3 studies with a product that differs from that used in Phase 1. The biopharmaceutical industry has correspondingly benefited by not having the same (quasi-) generic challenges at the end of patent lives.

However, there is a competing pressure to this conservative regulatory approach: product cost. Just as small molecule generics reduce costs for third-party payer systems, the same is being demanded for patent-expired biological products. The EMA is probably ahead of the US FDA in this process, predicated by the predominantly socialized healthcare systems in Europe. But it is likely that during the currency of this edition of this book the US FDA will be pressured into finding a way to approve "follow-on" biologicals, as part of the comprehensive legislation to change healthcare in 2010.

Cell and tissue products

There are various clinical conditions where administration of cultured whole cells or tissue may be desirable. The sources of these tissues are as diverse as the disease targets. For example, cultured fibroblasts from human prepuces have been manufactured as "artificial skin" for the treatment of leg ulcers and burns (Advanced Tissue Sciences, La Jolla, California). Other companies are developing implantable pancreas generated from isolated pancreatic islet cells. Unlike matched transplantations, such therapies may involve treatment of large numbers of patients from a limited or sole initial human source or may be autologous albeit after some *ex vivo* manipulation and culturing of the cell mass before reimplantation.

Ex vivo therapeutic strategies may take different forms. Chronic lymphocytic leukemia has been treated for long periods of time by using cell separators to reduce the burden of lymphocytosis, and to permit red cell transfusion. Laser-directed cell sorters may be used to select appropriate subpopulations of lymphocytes, which are then transfected with an appropriate gene product *ex vivo* and returned to the patient, where these cells will hopefully target some diseased tissue such as widespread melanoma. Expense, availability of therapy, and the duration and specificity of effect currently limit the widespread application of these approaches.

General ethical issues

Modern biotechnology creates numerous ethical issues. Care should be taken in relating directly the therapy type and the ethical issue. Moreover, ethical standards vary among highly-respected "experts." Indeed, it can be said that, to some extent, everyone is an ethicist. But those involved in biological product development certainly should be.

It is easy for those without technical training to extrapolate that *all* biological products have the same range of ethical issues that *actually* only affect *some* of these therapies. For example, the cloning of mammals (sheep at Roslin Therapeutics, Scotland; mice at the University of Hawaii) forces the consideration of cloning of humans. On one hand, much of this technology can be used for genetic screening of fetuses to exclude an inherited disease. On the other hand, the same techniques could be used to provide parents with a deliberate choice of the sex of their next baby. Science is likely always to be ahead of the lay public and politicians in creating these dilemmas in the absence of agreed guidelines or consensus. The biggest problem for the lay public to grasp is there is always an ethical continuum, without bright lines of demarcation or absolute limitations.

Another current ethical problem is that diseases that plague tropical countries and the developing world are in great need for drug development and research, but offer little financial incentive to a for-profit pharmaceutical industry. This is well-recognized (for example) by the Wellcome and Gates' Foundations. Biological products that evade microorganism resistance remain a huge therapeutic need and opportunity.

If it is the ethical continuum that is the central difficulty, there are nonetheless analogies in the "pre-genetic engineering" era of medicine. Consider, for example, the parents of a child who needs a kidney transplant, and who find themselves without any suitable living donor. Without any modern technology at all, they may choose to have another baby with the hope or intent that the new child can serve as a suitable donor for their existing child. In this case, tissue proliferation *ex vivo* and implantation seems to be a simpler ethical situation than parents having offspring by entirely ordinary means. Consensus guidelines are needed: but in our opinion they must remain flexible in order to deal with ever-faster technological innovation that is not going to stop, and they must also be consistent with guidelines that have wide acceptance in other areas of medicine.

Informed consent

More prosaically, the difficulties of explaining the nuances of biotechnology products to potential clinical trials subjects may be more difficult than for orthodox small molecule drugs. Often, candidate clinical trial patients will be experiencing life-threatening disease, and the apparent novelty of, say, a gene therapy, could under the wrong conditions create undue hope and bias in deciding to provide what should be truly informed consent. It is crucial that the same principles apply for biotechnology as for conventional drugs; the protocol and therapy must still be clearly explained in a noncoercive manner that does not raise false hopes in the patient. It should not be forgotten that a major ethical lapse (largely due to excessive optimism and expectations of benefit) led to the death of Jessie Gelsinger at a famous university during a clinical trial of a biotechnology product in the United States, in 1999 (Couzin and Kaiser, 2005).

Finally, progress in computational science and informatics has been one of the enablers of biological products, but they are beyond the scope of this chapter. Similarly, the underlying science of the human genome and human proteomics could not possibly be dealt with comprehensively in this sort of chapter. Some further reading is nonetheless recommended below.

References

Andreotti G, Mendéz BL, Amodeo P, Morelli MA, Nakamuta H, Motta A. Structural determinants of salmon calcitonin bioactivity: the role of leu-amphipathic alpha-helix. *J Biol Chem* 2006; **281**:24193–24203.

Brain SD, Williams TJ, Tippins JR, Morris HR, MacIntyre I. Calcitonin gene-related peptide is a potent vasodilator. *Nature* 1985; **313**:54–56.

Couzin J, Kaiser J. Gene therapy. As Gelsinger case ends, gene therapy suffers another blow. *Science* 2005; **307**:1028.

Harrison R, Chui DHK, Roemer C, *et al.* Access to "A Syllabus of Human Hemoglobin Variants (1996)" via the World Wide Web. *Hemoglobin* 1998; **22**:113–127.

Ledley TS, Ledley FD. Multicompartment numerical model of cellular events in the pharmacokinetics of gene therapies. *Hum Gene Ther* 1994; **5**:679–691.

Suntharalingam G, Perry MR, Ward S, Brett SJ, Castello-Cortes A, Brunner MD, Panoskaltsis N. Cytokine storm in a phase 1 trial of the anti-CD28 monoclonal antibody TGN1412. *New Eng J Med* 2006; **355**:1018–1028.

Viprakasit V, Chinchang W, Chotimarat P. Hb Woodville, a rare alpha-globin variant, caused by codon 6 mutation of the alpha1 gene. *Eur J Haematol* 2006; **76**:79–82.

Wasserfall CH, Herzog RW. Gene therapy approaches to induce tolerance in autoimmunity by reshaping the immune system. *Curr Opin Investig Drugs* 2009; **10**:1143–1150.

Further reading

Auaje F, Dopazo J (eds). *Data Analysis and Visualization in Genomics and Proteomics.* John Wiley & Sons Ltd: Chichester, UK, 2005. ISBN 0-470-09439-7.

Holm L, Sander C. Mapping the protein universe. *Science* 1996; **273**:595–603.

International Human Genome Sequencing Consortium. Initial sequencing and analysis of the human genome. *Nature* 2001; **409**:860–921.

International Human Genome Sequencing Consortium. Finishing the euchromatic sequence of the human genome. *Nature* 2004; **431**:931–945.

CHAPTER 25

Health Economics

Daniel C. Malone[1], Edward P. Armstrong[1], & Mirza I. Rahman[2]

[1]Pharmacy Practice and Science, College of Pharmacy, University of Arizona, Phoenix, AZ, USA

[2]Health Economics & Reimbursement, Evidence Based Medicine, Ortho-Clinical Diagnostics, Inc., Rochester, NY, USA

Health economics has been defined as a branch of scientific inquiry that tries to establish value by understanding the outcomes of specific healthcare practices and the cost of achieving those health outcomes. It includes studying clinical, economic, and humanistic consequences of these healthcare interventions in real-world settings.

Introduction

As new healthcare technologies emerge, a significant amount of effort is expended to assess their value. These new technologies include medications, medical devices, and *in vitro* diagnostics (IVDs), and their emergence has had a profound positive impact on the health of patients. However, they have also had a significant financial impact on healthcare organizations and payers, such as hospitals, managed care organizations, pharmacy benefit managers, and governments.

The use of health economic evaluations has also impacted the development of these new technologies, because they place certain financial constraints on the manufacturers of these medications, medical devices, and IVDs. Both creators and users of new technologies are expanding their utilization of methods simultaneously to assess health outcomes and costs, while instituting policies that incorporate the results of these analyses into their decision-making.

Principles and Practice of Pharmaceutical Medicine, 3rd edition.
Edited by L.D. Edwards, A.W. Fox, P.D. Stonier.
© 2011 Blackwell Publishing Ltd.

Several terms are used to describe these analytical methods that are used, including health economics, outcomes research, and pharmacoeconomics (often used when assessing medications). When a new medication becomes available in the marketplace, a health economic analysis may be designed to quantify the impact of any improvements in clinical outcomes (e.g., more successfully treated patients) and any change in health system costs. Such an analysis may estimate the incremental improvement in successfully treated patients, along with the incremental increase in health system costs for a new technology, and compare this to an existing treatment.

Health economic analyses are used to identify, quantify, and contrast the outcomes and costs among various healthcare interventions. The term "outcomes" is used to describe both clinical and humanistic outcomes. Clinical outcomes include long-term outcomes such as mortality, measures of morbidity, or measures of disease control (e.g., blood pressure control in hypertensive or A1C control in diabetic patients). Humanistic outcomes typically include measures of health-related quality of life (e.g., results from questionnaire assessing the impact of asthma) and patient satisfaction.

Within health economics, costs are often stratified by different categories and are impacted by the perspective of an analysis. The broadest perspective is the societal perspective, where direct medical costs are included, as well as the impact of a disease or treatment, on the ability to work (defined as indirect costs). Commonly, many health economic analyses are conducted from the perspective of a hospital (for inpatient treatments) or from the perspective of a managed care organization (to include both ambulatory and inpatient costs). Analyses from hospital or managed care perspectives often emphasize direct medical costs. Direct medical costs include the cost of medications, physician clinic visits, laboratory tests, emergency department visits, and hospitalizations.

Health policy and the pharmaceutical industry

Healthcare costs are growing significantly and this has caused significant concerns on the part of patients, physicians, hospitals, managed care organizations, government entities, and politicians. The growth of healthcare costs is an important driver for reforms to health systems. This dramatic rise in healthcare costs has focused attention on the need to be sure that healthcare dollars are being spent wisely. Payers, patients, and healthcare organizations need and want to know how limited financial resources can be spent most effectively and efficiently, to attain important improvements in healthcare. This has resulted in greater scrutiny of new technologies.

Currently, hospital pharmacy and therapeutics committees often closely scrutinize new medications to determine whether newer, more expensive products truly provide greater clinical or humanistic outcomes. These tougher questions by payers have placed a greater burden on the pharmaceutical industry to provide additional information about new products. Formerly, placement on a medication formulary was based largely on product efficacy and safety. Now, a new hurdle is being created. Not only does a pharmaceutical company need to have strong data demonstrating clinical efficacy and safety, but also there is a greater need for these companies to demonstrate the "value" of its new products.

Value involves demonstrating the incremental improvement in clinical or humanistic outcomes for a reasonable increase in cost. If the incremental cost is too great, a payer may judge the product as not being cost-effective, and discourage its use.

On the other hand, if a new product provides significant improvement in clinical outcomes for a reasonable increase in cost, a payer may judge the product to be quite cost-effective, and encourage its use.

Although price controls do not exist for pharmaceuticals in the US, this is not true for the rest of the world. In most western countries, the prices of pharmaceutical products are regulated by the national payer. However, price controls do exist in the IVD market in the US, where the Medicare Clinical Laboratory Fee Schedule has set the prices that the government pays for IVD tests.

Additionally, in an attempt to utilize healthcare resources most efficiently, many nations have made the decision to allocate the delivery of healthcare services in a rational manner, as opposed to chance, inconvenience, or a person's individual ability to pay. They have proposed the use of comparative effectiveness research (CER) as a method to try and get the most value possible for the amount of money that they will spend. This type of study, though likely to be expensive, will entail direct head-to-head comparisons of similar drugs, devices, or diagnostics, in an attempt to determine which has the greatest clinical utility and the highest health economic value.

Specifically, in the US, President Obama's "stimulus package" allocated significant money for CER. The American Recovery and Reinvestment Act (2009), contains US$1.1 billion for CER in the US. CER compares treatments and strategies to improve health, and provides this essential information to clinicians, payers, and patients to help them decide on the best treatment. The CER agenda is to help.

• Conduct, support, or synthesize research that compares the clinical outcomes, effectiveness, and appropriateness of items, services, and procedures that are used to prevent, diagnose, or treat diseases, disorders, and other health conditions.

• Encourage the development and use of clinical registries, clinical data networks, and other forms of electronic health data that can be used to generate or obtain outcomes data.

Guidelines and regulatory guidance

Many countries have significant financial concerns about how tax revenues are spent on healthcare. Also, many governments are involved in negotiating and setting prices, making formulary and reimbursement decisions, and rigorously evaluating what value new health technologies provide to their citizens. Given this increased focus on documenting the value of new technologies in many countries, several of them have implemented guidelines to assess these new technologies. Typically, these guidelines outline what information needs to be provided by a manufacturer to have a new technology evaluated for approval and reimbursement.

The International Society for Pharmacoeconomics and Outcomes Research's (ISPOR) website (www.ispor.org/peguidelines/index.asp) provides pharmacoeconomic guidelines from over 30 different countries. Within the US, the best known pharmacoeconomic guideline is the Academy of Managed Care Pharmacy Format for Formulary Submissions (which can be found at www.fmcpnet. org). In addition, several ISPOR Task Forces have produced principles of good practice for budget impact analysis and for decision analytic modeling to help standardize the methodology of various types of health economic research (Weinstein, 2003; Mauskopf, 2007).

Outside the US, there is little need for regulatory guidance with respect to the use and dissemination of the results of health economic studies. This is because the various national payers routinely decide on how this will be done based on their review of the new technologies. However, in the US, the use of health economic studies is governed by the 1997 Food and Drug Administration Modernization Act, Section 114, which set a new, less stringent standard for promotional dissemination of healthcare economic information to managed care organizations formulary committees (Radensky, 2000). Section 114 states that health economic studies must provide "competent and reliable scientific evidence" versus the more stringent "adequate and well-controlled studies" required for general promotion on efficacy and safety.

Health technology assessment organizations

There are numerous health technology assessment (HTA) organizations globally (see Table 25.1), and these can include governmental, quasi-governmental, and private organizations, set-up along local (state/provincial), national, or international auspices.

The role of various HTA organizations is to conduct or support studies evaluating the effectiveness, outcomes, and cost-effectiveness of new drugs, devices, and diagnostics. They try to gather the best available evidence and synthesize that information so that it can be converted into appropriate coverage policies and help to inform good public policy.

Principles of health economic assessments

While the field of pharmacoeconomics and technology assessment is relatively new, there have been rapid advances in methodological approaches over the past 15 years. However, the basic methods have been utilized for non-health technology assessment for decades.

Many refer to the health economic assessment of pharmaceuticals as pharmacoeconomics. The field of pharmacoeconomic assessment is a subset of the broader field of health economic technology assessment. For purposes of this chapter, those terms will be used interchangeably. Most technology reports currently published involve pharmaceuticals, but evaluations of other technologies such as devices, diagnostics, and even screening programs, such as cancer screening, are becoming more common.

One of the initial steps in conducting a health economic evaluation is discerning what resources to include and how to value them. Costs in health economic evaluations are different from accounting costs. The overriding principle in health economics is the efficient allocation of resources. Therefore,

Table 25.1 A select group of health technology assessment organizations

Country	Organization name	Scope
Australia	Pharmaceutical Benefits Advisory Committee (PBAC)	To use evidence-based assessment of health benefits and costs associated with new drugs, to recommend which medicines should be subsidized (http://www.health.gov.au/internet/main/publishing.nsf/Content/health-pbs-general-listing-committee3.htm#pbac).
Canada	The Canadian Agency for Drugs and Technologies in Health (CADTH)	This national body provides Canada's federal, provincial, and territorial healthcare decision-makers with credible, impartial advice and evidence-based information about the effectiveness and efficiency of drugs and other health technologies (http://www.cadth.ca/index.php/en/home).
France	The Haute Autorité de santé (HAS) (French National Authority for Health)	To provide health authorities with the information needed to make decisions on the reimbursement of medical products and services. To encourage good practices and the proper use of health services by professionals and users; To improve quality of care in healthcare organizations and in general medical practice. To provide information for the public and generally improve the quality of medical information (http://www.has-sante.fr/portail/jcms/c_5443/english?cid=c_5443).
Germany	Institute for Quality and Efficiency in Health Care (IQWiG)	IQWiG is an independent scientific institute that investigates the benefits and harms of medical interventions for patients. It regularly provides information about the potential advantages and disadvantages of different diagnostic and therapeutic interventions (http://www.iqwig.de/institute-for-quality-and-efficiency-in-health.2.en.html).
Spain	Healthcare Technology Evaluation Agency (AETS)	Offers objective assessments of the healthcare, social, ethical, organizational, and economic impact of medical-healthcare techniques and procedures to bolster the decisions taken by authorities and other healthcare agents (http://www.isciii.es/htdocs/en/investigacion/Agencia_quees.jsp).
UK	National Institute for Health and Clinical Excellence (NICE)	NICE is the independent organization responsible for providing national guidance on the promotion of good health and the prevention and treatment of ill health (www.nice.org.uk).
	National Institute for Health Research (NIHR) Health Technology Assessment program	The HTA program produces independent research about the effectiveness of different healthcare treatments and tests for those who use, manage, and provide care in the National Health Service. (www.ncchta.org).
	The Cochrane Collaboration	The Cochrane Collaboration is an international not-for-profit and independent organization, dedicated to making up-to-date, accurate information about the effects of healthcare readily available worldwide. It produces and disseminates systematic reviews of healthcare interventions and promotes the search for evidence in the form of clinical trials and other studies of interventions. (www.cochrane.org).
USA	Agency for Healthcare Research and Quality (AHRQ)	AHRQ's mission is to conduct and support studies of the outcomes and effectiveness of diagnostic, therapeutic, and preventive healthcare services and procedures. (www.ahrq.gov).
	Blue Cross Blue Shield Association Technology Evaluation Center (TEC)	The TEC provides scientifically rigorous assessments that synthesize the evidence on the diagnosis, treatment, management and prevention of disease (http://www.bcbs.com/blueresources/tec/).
	Drug Effectiveness Review Project (DERP) Oregon Health & Science University	To obtain the best available evidence on effectiveness and safety comparisons between drugs in the same class, and to apply the information to public policy (http://www.ohsu.edu/ohsuedu/research/policycenter/DERP/).

Table 25.1 (*Continued*)

Country	Organization name	Scope
EU	European Network for Health Technology Assessment (EUnetHTA)	The overall aim of EUnetHTA is to establish an effective and sustainable European network for health technology assessment that informs policy decisions. The EUnetHTA Collaboration is implementing a proposal for a sustainable, permanent collaboration for HTA in Europe. Partners come from 28 EU countries, in addition to the US, Canada, Australia, and Israel. (www.eunethta.net).
Global	Health Technology Assessment International (HTAi)	The mission of HTAi is to support and promote the development, communication, understanding, and use of health technology assessment (HTA) around the world, as a scientifically based and multidisciplinary means of informing decision-making regarding the introduction of effective innovations and the efficient use of resources in healthcare (http://www.htai.org/index.php?id=121).

use of resources is an opportunity cost. Given that resources are scarce, health technology assessment analyses seek to inform a decision-maker on the anticipated value for selecting one health technology over another.

Costs in health economics can be classified as direct, indirect, and intangible (Berger *et al.*, 2003). *Direct costs* represent products and services that are consumed in the treatment or management of a disease or condition. Direct costs include such items as drugs, physician services, hospitalization, home health services, concomitant therapy, durable medical equipment, medical supplies, and adverse drug events. Nonmedical direct costs include such items as child-care, exercise programs, transportation to and from medical facilities, and nutrition and diets.

In health economic evaluations, *indirect cost* refers to lost or reduced productivity or premature mortality. Indirect costs represent the notion that individuals have human capital and that reduction in productivity or removal from the workforce due to a disease or condition is a lost opportunity. That said, some national guidelines, such as in Australia, do not allow the inclusion of indirect cost when presenting economic models to the Pharmaceutical Benefit Advisory Committee (Pharmaceutical Benefits Advisory Committee, 2008).

Intangible costs are represented by the notion of pain and suffering. These costs are real costs to the patient, but are difficult or impossible to value. Some analysts have used willingness-to-pay methodologies to attempt to capture pain and suffering, as well as other costs. In general, intangible costs are recognized, but they are often not included in the analysis.

The decision of which costs to include in a specific analysis is driven entirely by the perspective of the study. That perspective can of the patient, a healthcare purchaser, such as a managed care organization or government, or a provider. Most analyses are conducted from the perspective of a healthcare purchaser. In the US, where commercial insurance firms are common, the inclusion of costs is limited to direct medical costs. In countries where the government is a major or sole payer, analyses may include both direct and indirect costs, when the government also bears the responsibility for disability payments. The patient perspective would include both direct and indirect costs.

Health economic methods

There are four fundamental approaches to evaluating a healthcare technology using a health economic framework:

- cost minimization;
- cost effectiveness;
- cost benefit;
- cost utility.

All these approaches combine information concerning costs and benefits, but primarily differ with respect to how the benefits are valued. We describe these four approaches below along with decision analysis methods and quality of life concepts, because they are intimately intertwined with some of these health economic methods.

Cost-minimization analysis

Cost minimization is the most straightforward of the four methods because this approach assumes that there are no differences in benefits gained from one technology relative to another. For example, if an analysis was comparing two different medications used to treat hypertension, the change in blood pressure for the two agents would be assumed to be identical. In this case, one would then only be concerned with the cost of each respective agent. This is an oversimplification to some degree, because we know that medications often differ with respect to effectiveness, side effect profiles, route of administration, frequency taken, and other factors. Many times these attributes have not been well-studied, but a cost-minimization analysis permits the analyst to ignore these obvious differences and focus solely on the costs that accompany each product.

In practice, true cost-minimization analyses should be relatively rare because there are almost no situations where the efficacy of medications is identical. The most common situation where cost minimization might be appropriate is when one is comparing a brand-name product to a generic equivalent. Thus, one can focus almost exclusively on the acquisition cost of the two entities.

Cost-effectiveness analysis

Cost-effectiveness analysis (CEA) is the cornerstone of pharmacoeconomics and economic evaluations of health technologies. Unlike cost-minimization analysis, cost-effectiveness analysis does not assume that the value derived from each product is identical. Cost-effectiveness analysis compares the difference in costs between the technologies divided by differences in effectiveness in the denominator. The key distinguishing feature of CEA is that the health benefits are measured in "natural" units; clinically meaningful

outcomes. For example, antihypertensive medications might be evaluated using added years of life (Edelson *et al.*, 1990). Adding misoprostol to non-steroidal anti-inflammatory drugs has been evaluated using the number of gastrointestinal events avoided (Gabriel *et al.*, 1993), and macrolide antibiotics for the treatment of community-acquired pneumonia has been evaluated using events avoided as the measure of effect (Tasch *et al.*, 1997). Therapies used to treat asthma may be evaluated using symptom-free days (Weiss *et al.*, 2006). Cost-effectiveness analysis is appealing because clinically-orientated decision-makers are more likely to be familiar with the measure of effect.

In many situations, cost-effectiveness analysis is really cost-efficacy, with the denominator representing differences in effect that is measured from randomized controlled trials. The substitution of the word effectiveness, with efficacy, is not a trivial issue, because there are a multitude of reasons why a clinical trial may be different to the "population" of actual recipients, once the products reach the market.

In CEA, the ratio of the difference in costs to the difference in effect is called the incremental cost-effectiveness ratio (ICER), as shown in Figure 25.1. One should note that an ICER is a comparative value, requiring the analyst to make a decision as to which therapy is the current standard. The resulting value from an ICER is the additional gain/loss in benefits relative to the additional gain/loss in terms of costs.

$$ICER = \frac{Cost_{New} - Cost_{Current}}{Effect_{New} - Effect_{Current}}$$

Figure 25.1 The basic formula for the incremental cost-effectiveness ratio.

The interpretation of the ICER is not straightforward. ICERs can have both positive and negative values. Each can represent different situations for the healthcare decision-maker. In order to interpret an ICER, the original values must be known, or the result must be plotted on a cost-effectiveness (CE) plane. The CE plane contains four quadrants, each representing a different scenario. Figure 25.2

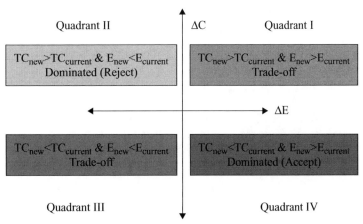

Figure 25.2 A cost-effectiveness plane.

TC_{new} = Total cost of new technology; $TC_{current}$ = Total cost of current technology; E_{new} = Effectiveness of new technology; $E_{current}$ = Effectiveness of current technology

shows a cost-effectiveness plane, where the quadrants are labeled I to IV in a counter-clockwise direction. The origin on the CE plane represents the value and cost of a "baseline" or comparator therapy. The vertical axis is the change in cost, relative to the baseline therapy. The horizontal axis represents the change in effectiveness, relative to the comparator therapy.

Quadrant I of the CE plane is a trade-off situation because the "new" agent is more effective but more expensive than the baseline treatment. This is a common situation for the development and marketing of new therapeutic agents. For example, selective serotonin reuptake inhibitors are "more effective" than traditional tricyclic antidepressants (TCAs) from the standpoint that patients tolerate the SSRI medications much better than the older TCAs (Canadian Coordinating Office for Health Technology Assessment, 1997). However, when first marketed, brand-name SSRIs were considerably more expensive than TCAs. Thus, the healthcare decision-maker had to balance the difference in "effect," relative to the increase in cost.

Quadrant II represents the situation where the new agent is more costly but less effective. When this occurs, the new technology is considered to be "dominated" by the older agent. Quadrant III is another trade-off situation, where the new agent is less effective and also less costly. This may occur with a second, third, or fourth product in

a therapeutic class that may be less potent and hence, priced accordingly. Quadrant IV represents situations where a technology is more effective and also less costly. This new technology is said to dominate the older agent.

It is important to note that the ICER value alone cannot determine in which quadrant the new technology is located. A negative ICER value will indicate the new technology is either in quadrant II or IV. Conversely, a positive value results in the ICER being in quadrant I or III.

There are several issues with ICER values that should be recognized (Coyle, 1996; Polsky *et al.*, 1997). First, it is possible to obtain an undefined value when the difference is zero. Second, the threshold for determining cost-effectiveness is largely unknown. Due to these issues, many analysts prefer the use of cost-effectiveness acceptability curves (CEACs). These diagrams use the notion of net monetary benefit, whereby the incremental change in effect is multiplied by a "willingness to pay" (WTP) for each additional unit of benefit.

The difference in cost is then subtracted from the product of WTP multiplied by the incremental gain in effect. The advantage of this approach is that the analyst can run the calculations using a variety of WTP values and then generate a diagram like the one shown in Figure 25.3. On the y-axis is the probability that a given technology is cost-effective. The x-axis is a range of WTP values.

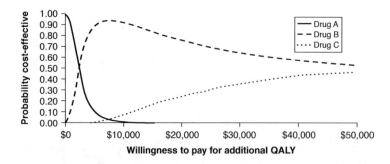

Figure 25.3 Cost-effectiveness acceptability curve (QALY = quality-adjusted life years).

The decision-maker then selects the WTP value that represents the organization's value for that outcome and then draws a horizontal line from zero to 1. The technology with the highest probability of being cost-effective is the preferred technology. When a decision-maker has a low willingness to pay, say US$10,000, Drug B has the highest probability of being cost-effective. However, as the WTP increases, the difference between Drugs B and C narrow.

Cost-benefit analysis

The third approach to health economic technology assessment is cost-benefit analysis (CBA). This approach values health benefits in monetary units, but is used less often because it requires one to transform the value, into monetary units. The lack of a standard approach for this transformation has limited the usefulness of CBA in the healthcare arena.

Unlike CEA, interpreting the results from CBA is more straightforward. When the net benefits exceed the net costs, the technology should be adopted. An alternative approach is to divide the benefits by the costs. If the resulting value is greater than zero, the technology should be adopted.

Economic evaluations of vaccination programs are typically evaluated using the cost-benefit framework. For example, a CBA of a varicella vaccination program for children was conducted in the US (Lieu *et al.*, 1994). In this study, the benefits of the vaccine were measured as the cost offsets in terms of additional healthcare utilization, fewer hospitalizations, and a reduction in long-term disability. In this analysis, indirect costs asso-

ciated with work-loss were included. The results were expressed as cost per life saved as well as a benefit to cost ratio. The value of the program was estimated to be US$5.40 for every dollar invested in the program.

Cost-utility analysis

With a cost-utility analysis (CUA), the main differentiating feature from CEA and CBA is how the units of effectiveness are measured. In a CUA, the denominator is quality-adjusted life years (QALYs). This approach assumes that one can value the quality of life when a person has a given disease.

Quality values are then multiplied by the number of years of life spent living in that particular disease state. Often various health states, reflecting the severity of the disease, exist. Therefore, the degree to which a new technology will keep a disease process under control, the more QALYs will be assigned to that technology. The difference in QALYs between competing technologies becomes the denominator in the CEA formula. Many analysts view CUA as a subset of CEA. Due to the need to calculate utilities over time, most CUA are conducted using Markov models. These models require "time" to be explicit in the analysis.

Assessing utility is done by the use of a simple rating scale, time trade-off board, or the standard gamble technique. Each method has its own set of advantages and disadvantages (Torrance, 1987). The *rating scale* is a visual analog line with two anchor points: best and worst possible health. A health state description is read to a participant and they are then instructed to place a mark that indicates where the health state falls in the continuum of health. The distance between the anchor points is divided into equal units, like a measuring stick, and the health state is rated as a proportion of the total length. This is called a "utility" value.

The *time trade-off board* calculates utility by first determining the number of years of life remaining for a participant (Smith and Dobson, 1993); the person is then read a health state description. The participant is asked to choose between living "X" years with the condition or living fewer life years without the condition. Typically the instrument is administered in an iterative fashion, going from few life years remaining to almost all life years remaining. When the participant exhibits no preference for living in the health state the remainder of his or her life or living fewer years in perfect health, the amount of life in perfect health is expressed as a percentage of life expectancy. The resulting value is the utility of that health state.

The *standard gamble* approach uses an iterative approach as well, except that the options given to the participant are: (i) living in a reduced health state; or (ii) a probability of perfect health or immediate death. In this approach, the probabilities between perfect health and immediate death are changed until the participant has no preference between the two options. Given the standard

gamble's inherent uncertainty, it is the preferred method of assessing utility (Gafni and Birch, 1995). However, patients often have difficulty in understanding the scenario and can make irrational choices.

Utility values have also been mapped to other quality of life instruments, such as the EQ-5D or the SF-36. More information on these instruments is provided below in the section on Quality of Life Assessment.

Decision analysis

As data for economic models often come from a variety of sources, the use of decision analysis models is common in pharmacoeconomic evaluations. This permits the analyst to combine data across treatments that may not have been studied in a head-to-head fashion. In addition, costs will vary by locale and institution, and so the ability to change input prices is required. Decision analysis provides a framework for explicitly valuing and evaluating the cost-effectiveness of a technology.

An example of a decision model is shown in Figure 25.4. Decision models are constructed using three types of nodes: decision, chance, and terminal. Decision nodes are represented by squares and tend to occur on the left side of the model,

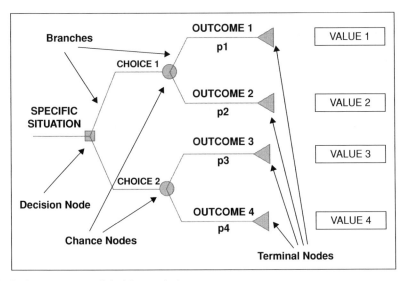

Figure 25.4 The basic components of decision analysis.

whereas chance nodes are represented by a circle and terminal nodes are triangular in shape.

The steps in decision analysis are as follows:
1. Frame the question.
2. Structure the clinical problem.
3. Estimate the probabilities.
4. Determine the values for cost and effect inputs.
5. Analyze the tree.
6. Test the assumptions.
7. Interpret the results.

Framing the question is obviously the most important aspect of a decision or cost-effectiveness analysis. A poorly framed question will not be answerable and generate a lot of "trash-can" models. Once the question has been clearly defined, the next step is to structure the model to reflect clinical reality and also be able to answer the question.

There is often a trade-off in the simplicity of the model versus the accuracy (Detsky *et al.*, 1997). The model must reflect clinical reality but every nuance of clinical decision-making is impossible to include. Rather, the model must capture the most relevant aspects of the decision. Incorporating the key elements that reflect the clinical reality is often a process that involves clinicians, epidemiologists, and health-service researchers to give the model face validity.

Step 3 of the model construction process relates to providing probabilities to the model. Probabilities occur at chance nodes. For any given chance node, the sum of the probabilities for the branches must sum to one. Probabilities come from epidemiological studies, clinical trials, or meta-analyses. In many situations, there are numerous studies that provide estimates that could be used for chance probability. Probabilities can be combined using a weighting scheme, providing more weight to those studies that have larger sample sizes or reflect high-quality evidence. Data from meta-analyses or Bayesian models can also be used to estimate probabilities.

Step 4 in constructing a decision model is to value the input and outcomes associated with each pathway. Two components are assigned: (i) costs; and (ii) effect, such as utilities. For costs, the resources associated with each pathway are likely to be different, reflecting the clinical approaches to treatment. Treatment costs that are not different between the branches are not included because they cancel out. In CEA, the outcomes for each branch will be valued using utilities. At other times, the outcome will reflect success or failure, or another measure of effectiveness.

Once the model has been populated with probabilities, costs, and outcomes, the analyst "rolls back" the tree. In this step the path probabilities are calculated by multiplying the chance probabilities for each path. Figure 25.5 shows the calculation of the path probabilities for a model comparing the use of misoprostol with non-steroidal anti-inflammatory drugs for the prevention of gastric bleeding. The path probability is simply the multiplication of each of the chance node probabilities. For this model,

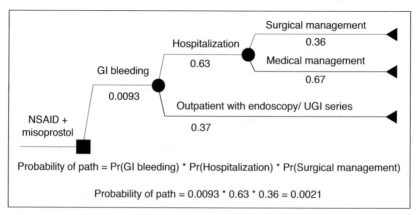

Figure 25.5 An example of decision analysis.

the path probability associated with the surgical management of a bleeding ulcer for persons treated with NSAIDs and misoprotol is 0.0021, or 0.21%. The path cost is the cost of the treatments and other services multiplied by the path probability. In this situation, the cost was US$9,013, and so the path cost is US$18.92.

After the primary analysis has been conducted, a series of sensitivity analyses are often conducted to test the robustness of the results. The key questions for the sensitivity analyses include: (i) which variables to evaluate; and (ii) what range of values to test. Variables that should be evaluated include those that are likely to influence the results, such as the chance node probabilities. In addition, costs are also frequently varied.

A more objective method of determining which variables to include in a sensitivity analysis is to use a tornado diagram. These diagrams rank-order the variables from those that have the most influence on the results, to those that have a minimal or no effect. In an analysis examining multiple treatments for depression, a decision was constructed evaluating five hypothetical therapies. In the tornado diagram shown in Figure 25.6, the cost of treatment failure was the variable that had the greatest influence on the results, while the cost of Drug C had a negligible effect.

Another approach to conducting sensitivity analyses is to construct the model using stochastic values for probabilities and input parameters. Once the parameters have been estimated, a Monte Carlo simulation can be used to sample values for each the parameters (Briggs, 2005). This approach

assumes that the analyst has the mean and variance or other similar metrics on the parameters of interest. This is more likely to be the case for measures of effect, but is often unknown for costs.

Quality of life assessment

Health-related quality of life (HR-QOL) is another common outcome that is measured in health technology assessments. The term "quality of life" is a multi-dimensional construct. Although HR-QOL is narrower, with a focus on health, it is still a broad theoretical construct that attempts to measure and explain the interrelations between health status, values, satisfaction, and general well-being (Berger *et al.* 2003).

Measurement scales can focus on health or life as a whole. Quality of life is considered to be a final health outcome (MacKeigan and Pathek, 1992). Two basic instrument types are used to measure HR-QOL: disease specific or generic instruments. Generic HR-QOL scales are designed to measure the continuum of function, disability, and disease. The main advantage of generic instruments is that differences across disease states can be compared.

Generic instruments can be further classified into health profiles and utility measures. Health profiles consist of a series of questions that measure varies aspects of quality of life, such as physical function, social function, mental health, pain, and emotional well-being. Profile scales include instruments such as the Sickness Impact Profile (SIP) and the SF-36. Some profile scales can be collapsed into a single measure, like the SIP. Other scales, such as the SF-36, were designed to be reported as a profile only.

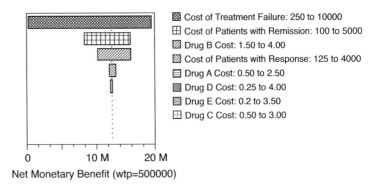

Figure 25.6 A tornado diagram sensitivity analysis.

Case Study: NICE, Bortezomib, and Cost-Effectiveness (2006–2007)

20 October 2006: Final NICE Appraisal Determination–bortezomib monotherapy for relapsed multiple myeloma.

The Committee concluded that bortezomib monotherapy for the treatment of relapsed multiple myeloma is clinically effective compared with high-dose dexamethasone, but that it has not been shown to be cost effective. Therefore, bortezomib monotherapy is not recommended for the treatment of patients with relapsed multiple myeloma.

4 June 2007: Draft NICE Guidance–bortezomib monotherapy for relapsed multiple myeloma.

This draft guidance followed the evaluation of a refund scheme proposed by the manufacturer after NICE initially rejected bortezomib in October 2006 on the grounds of cost:

- Bortezomib monotherapy is recommended as an option for the treatment of progressive multiple myeloma in people who have received at least one prior therapy and who have undergone, or are unsuitable for, bone marrow transplantation under both of the following circumstances:

  - The response to bortezomib is measured using serum M-protein after a maximum of four cycles of treatment, and treatment is continued only in people who have a reduction in serum M-protein of 50% or more (that is, a complete or partial response).

  - The manufacturer rebates the full cost of bortezomib for people who, after a maximum of four cycles of

treatment, have less than a 50% reduction in serum M-protein (that is, less than a partial response).

24 October 2007: Final NICE Guidance–bortezomib monotherapy for relapsed multiple myeloma.

- Bortezomib monotherapy is recommended as an option for the treatment of progressive multiple myeloma in people who are at first relapse having received one prior therapy and who have undergone, or are unsuitable for, bone marrow transplantation, under the following circumstances:

  - the response to bortezomib is measured using serum M protein after a maximum of four cycles of treatment, and treatment is continued only in people who have a complete or partial response (that is, reduction in serum M protein of 50% or more or, where serum M protein is not measurable, an appropriate alternative biochemical measure of response) and

  - the manufacturer rebates the full cost of bortezomib for people who, after a maximum of four cycles of treatment, have less than a partial response (as defined above).

October 2010: Scheduled to be reviewed: Final NICE Guidance–bortezomib monotherapy for relapsed multiple myeloma.

Utility measures are designed to reflect the preferences of patients for a given treatment or disease. The most common and widely accepted utility instrument is the EQ-5D. Another instrument is the Quality of Well-Being Scale. The EQ-5D includes a rating scale as well as questions for the five dimensions of mobility, self-care, usual activities, pain/discomfort, and anxiety/depression. Each of these dimensions is divided into three levels of perceived problems, resulting in 243 health states. These values have been mapped to utility values for specific populations, such as the United Kingdom (Dolan, 1997) and the United States (Shaw *et al.*, 2005).

Disease-specific instruments for HR-QOL are designed to be responsive or measure specific aspects of health status. Instruments can be developed for a disease or condition (e.g., asthma, chronic lung disease, rheumatoid arthritis, etc.)

or related to specific function (e.g., sexual functioning, emotional well-being, etc.). Attributes included in disease-specific instruments are more closely related to signs and symptoms assessed by clinicians. Hundreds of disease-specific quality of life instruments exist and new instruments are constantly being developed. The development of instruments over the past 20 years has been staggering. In fact, the US FDA developed a guidance document for the development of patient-reported outcome measures, which encompasses HR-QOL.

The process for developing and validating a HR-QOL instrument is not a trivial one. An instrument must show evidence of validity, reliability, and responsiveness to change. In general, a single study is insufficient to accomplish these tasks. For many instruments, the validity and reliability is established over many studies that span several years.

The advantage of including HR-QOL and other patient-reported outcomes in the drug development process is that the data are allowed in certain countries for promotional claims. For example, GlaxoSmithKline (formerly GlaxoWellcome) was able to include a claim of improved HR-QOL in the US product label for its asthma combination product of salmeterol and fluticasone. This labeling claim was based on an asthma specific quality of life questionnaire, the Asthma Quality of Life Questionnaire (Juniper *et al.*, 1993).

Caveats for health economic studies

Although the health economic determination of the value of a new drug, device, or diagnostic test is important, it must be recognized that its clinical utility is of even greater importance. If a new technology is unable to demonstrate that it is clinically useful, it is irrelevant how cheap that new technology is.

Additionally, since there are few clinical trials that directly compare new technologies, health economic methods and models are used to try and make such surrogate comparisons. These health economic models can be useful in terms of the direction they provide, however, they are built on assumptions that must be tested by conducting sensitivity analyses. Moreover, the data used in such models should be real-world data, to get to clinical effectiveness, as opposed to randomized controlled trial data that is gathered under ideal conditions and reflects the efficacy of the product. If models are to be truly valuable to clinicians and payers, they should try as best as possible, to simulate real-world clinical practice.

References

(Note: all websites cited in the text were accessed April 24, 2010.)

American Recovery and Reinvestment Act of 2009 and Comparative Effectiveness Research, 2009; http://www.hhs.gov/recovery/programs/cer/index.html.

Berger ML, Bingefore K, Hedblom E, Pashos CL, Torrence G, Smith MD. *Healthcare Cost, Quality, and Outcomes: ISPOR Book of Terms*. International Society for Pharmacoeconomics and Outcomes Research: Lawrenceville, NJ, USA, 2003.

Briggs A. Probabilistic analysis of cost-effectiveness models: statistical representation of parameter uncertainty. *Value in Health* 2005; **8**(1):1–2.

Canadian Coordinating Office for Health Technology Assessment. A Clinical and Economic Evaluations of Selective Serotonin Reuptake Inhibitors in Major Depression. Canadian Coordinating Office for Health Technology Assessment (CCOHTA): Ottawa, 1997.

Coyle D. Statistical analysis in pharmacoeconomic studies: a review of current issues and standards. *Pharmacoeconomics* 1996; **9**(6):506–516.

Detsky AS, Naglie G, Krahn MD, *et al.* Primer on medical decision analysis: part 1 – getting started. *Medical Decision Making* 1997; **17**:123–125.

Dolan P. Modeling valuations for EuroQol health states. *Medical Care* 1997; **35**(11):1095–1108.

Edelson JT, Weinstein MC, Tosteson ANA, Williams L, Lee TH, Goldman L. Long-term cost-effectiveness of various initial monotherapies for mild to moderate hypertension. *JAMA* 1990; **263**:408–413.

Gabriel SE, Jaakkimainen L, Bombardier C. The cost-effectiveness of misoprostol for nonsteroidal antinflammatory drug-associated adverse gastrointestinal events. *Arthritis and Rheumatism* 1990; **36**(4):447–459.

Gafni A, Birch S. Preference for outcomes in economic evaluation: an economic approach to addressing economic problems. *Social Science and Medicine* 1995; **40**(6):767–776.

Juniper EF, Guyatt GH, Ferrie PJ, Griffith LE. Measuring quality of life in asthma. *American Review of Respiratory Diseases* 1993; **147**:832–838.

Lieu TA, Cochi S, Black SB, *et al.* Cost-effectiveness of a routine varicella vaccination program for US children. *JAMA* 1994; **271**(5):375–381.

MacKeigan LD, Pathak DS. Overview of health-related quality of life measures. *American Journal of Health-System Pharmacy* 1992; **49**:2236–2245.

Mauskopf JA, Sullivan SD, Annemans L, *et al.* Principles of good practice for budget impact analysis: Report of the ISPOR Task Force on Good Research Practices: Budget Impact Analysis. *Value Health* 2007; **10**(5):336–47.

NICE (National Institute for Health and Clinical Excellence). Guidance Documents for Bortezomib Monotherapy for Relapsed Multiple Myeloma: http://www.nice.org.uk/nicemedia/pdf/MultipleMyelomaBortezomibFAD.pdf; October 2006; http://www.nice.org.

uk/niceMedia/pdf/207018BortezomibACD2.pdf; June 2007; http://www.nice.org.uk/nicemedia/pdf/TA129 Guidance.pdf; October 2007.

Pharmaceutical Benefits Advisory Committee. Guidelines for preparing submissions to the Pharmaceutical Benefits Advisory Committee (Version 4.3), Commonwealth of Australia, 2008.

Polsky D, Glick HA, Willke R, Schulman K. Confidence intervals for cost-effectiveness ratios: a comparison of four methods. *Health Economics* 1997; **6**:243–252.

Radensky P. Outcomes research: When can the results be communicated? 2000; http://www.medscape.com/viewarticle/409968_3.

Shaw JW. Johnson JA. Coons SJ. US valuation of the EQ-5D health states: development and testing of the D1 valuation model. *Medical Care* 2005; **43**(3):203–220.

Smith R, Dobson M. Measuring utility values for QALYs: two methodological issues. *Health Economics* 1993; **2**:349–355.

Tasch RF, Kunz KC, Marentette MA, Redelmeier DA. Macrolides in community-acquired pneumonia and otitis media. Canadian Coordinating Office for Health Technology Assessment (CCOHTA): Ottawa, 1997.

Torrance GW. Utility approach to measuring health-related quality of life. *Journal of Chronic Disease* 1987; **40**(6):593–600.

Weinstein MC, O'Brien B, Hornberger J, *et al.* Principles of good practice of decision analytic modeling in healthcare evaluation: Report of the ISPOR Task Force on Good Research Practices: Modeling Studies. *Value Health* 2003; **6**(1):9–17.

Weiss K, Buxton M, Anderson FL, Lamm CJ, Lijas B, Sullivan SD. Cost-effectiveness of early intervention with once-daily budesonide in children with mild persistent asthma: results from the START study. *Pediatric Allergy & Immunology* 2006; **17**(Suppl):21–27.

CHAPTER 26

Pharmacoeconomics: Economic and Humanistic Outcomes

Raymond J. Townsend[1], Jane T. Osterhaus[2], & J. Gregory Boyer[3]

[1]Elan Pharmaceuticals, San Diego, CA, USA
[2]Wasatch Health Outcomes, Park City, UT and Carlsbad, USA
[3]Accreditation Council for Pharmacy Education, Chicago, ILL, USA

Increased competition makes it imperative to hold down healthcare costs while maintaining or increasing quality. This has dictated changes in the traditional drug development path. For most of the past 40 years, the development of most pharmaceutical products has followed a stereotypical path from discovery to preclinical and clinical development, approval, and marketing. To maximize the commercialization and clinical use of a product, successful drug development today must now focus on measuring other outcomes of a pharmaceutical intervention. It is no longer adequate to capture data that only documents some clinical trial endpoints during drug development programs.

Economic and humanistic outcome evaluations have also become part of healthcare governance. The information gained from validated outcome measures can be used on a national level to allocate expenditures for treating various sectors of the population (e.g., the elderly, neonates, etc.) or to determine which programs will receive financial resources (e.g., vaccine programs versus acute influenza treatments). Outcome information can be used to help make decisions regarding the inclusion or exclusion of drugs on formularies. Complete information about the economic, humanistic and clinical impacts that medications have on specific patients can help healthcare providers make better prescribing and expenditure decisions.

Decision-makers, including prescribers, providers, payers, and patients, all want to maximize the value received for the money spent. Value to a prescriber might mean achieving a desired clinical effect for the cost of drug; value to a payer could mean spending more for a drug that reduces the number of days in a hospital, thus reducing the total economic impact of a condition. Value to a patient or employer might also be making sure that the drug prescribed maintains quality of life or worker productivity. To be successful, the pharmaceutical developer must address the needs of all these decision-makers. To do this, it is imperative that drug development programs today include quantitative measures of economic, clinical and humanistic value of the drugs they develop. It is never too early to begin to think about how the value of a product will be demonstrated.

The intent of this chapter is to help pharmaceutical developers and researchers understand how to document the economic and humanistic value of pharmaceuticals through appropriate pharmacoeconomic development programs.

Outcomes, health economics, and pharmacoeconomics

Outcomes research is the study of the end-results of medical interventions: Does the healthcare intervention improve the health and well-being of patients and populations?

Principles and Practice of Pharmaceutical Medicine, 3rd edition.
Edited by L.D. Edwards, A.W. Fox, P.D. Stonier.
© 2011 Blackwell Publishing Ltd.

The field of outcomes research emerged from a growing concern about which medical treatments work best and for whom. Outcomes span a broad range of types of intervention, from evaluating the effectiveness of a particular medical or surgical procedure to measuring the impact of insurance status or reimbursement policies on the outcomes of care. Outcomes research touches all aspects of healthcare delivery, from the clinical encounter itself to questions of the organization, financing, and regulation of the healthcare system. Each of these factors plays a role in the outcomes of care or the ultimate health status of the patient. Understanding how these factors interact requires collaboration among a broad range of health service researchers, such as economists, sociologists, physicians, nurses, political scientists, operations researchers, biostatisticians, and epidemiologists (Foundation for Health Sciences Research, 1993).

Health economics offer basic tools and criteria with which to analyze these issues of efficiency and the distribution of healthcare. These tools include techniques of optimization and the perturbation of equilibrium situations (e.g., predicting change in demand for services). A set of criteria is used to determine whether the patient or the population is better or worse off as a result of a particular action. Health economics tools are often used to evaluate how much money should be allocated to a healthcare program services or priorities. Health economic analyses can clarify the costs of alternative medical treatments and make the values underlying those alternatives explicit; it is therefore a useful approach to the study of medical care (Feldstein, 1983). Health economics focuses on all aspects of healthcare and as such can be very useful for generating data to make policy decisions involving multiple, interacting healthcare programs and systems. While some health economists take a big-picture or macro-view and focus on issues involving healthcare policy, others may focus specifically on pharmaceutical industry issues such as drug pricing, the cost of drug development, and whether it is justified.

Pharmacoeconomics is the science that identifies, measures, and compares the costs and consequences of pharmaceutical products and services (Bootman *et al.*, 1996). As such, pharmacoeco-nomics focuses primarily on pharmaceuticals, and attempts to evaluate the economic and humanistic impact of drug therapy. Pharmacoeconomic tools are derived from a variety of sources, including the fields of economics and outcomes research. The pharmacoeconomist can offer skills and experience in assessing quality of life, patient satisfaction, and other patient-centered measures to a clinical development team. Although the terms are sometimes used interchangeably, health economists and pharmacoeconomists differ, in having stronger backgrounds in the theoretical and applied aspects of health economics, respectively.

A researcher with solid pharmacoeconomic skills may not be a very good health economist, and *vice versa*. When hiring pharmacoeconomists or health economists, first determine what they will do, and then evaluate their skills and experiences to make sure that they will be able to deliver what is needed for your specific drug development program.

New paradigm: three-dimensional outcome assessment

Healthcare used to be constrained mainly by the technologies available to assist in delivering care. As technology becomes increasingly sophisticated, its cost is potentially outpacing the resources available to pay for such care. Which patients should get which treatment? How should healthcare be allocated, or in some cases rationed?

Health outcomes are the measured, end-result of a medical intervention. They represent what happened to patients. Being cured of an illness is an outcome, as is succumbing to it. However, this primitive, epidemiological distinction tells us very little about the current functional status of the patient. Being alive but relying on a respirator to breathe is very different from being alive and fully functional. Additionally, intermediate outcomes (e.g., alleviation of pain or other symptoms of arthritis) are sometimes as important an outcome as the final outcome.

The measurement of outcomes is critical to the conduct of pharmaceutical research. Clinical outcomes (efficacy and safety) are the hallmarks of US Food and Drug Administration (FDA) approval of a product for marketing. Clinical outcomes are necessary but no longer sufficient as a sole consideration in making development and prescribing decisions, as well as for reimbursement in socialized healthcare systems (where reimbursement essentially governs marketability).

During the last three decades, patients have become involved in healthcare decisions that affect them, and economic considerations at this level have also increased in importance. Hence the need today to measure outcomes beyond the traditional clinical endpoints associated with pharmaceutical research. Healthcare decision-makers must now know more than simply the safety and efficacy parameters of an intervention. It is important for them to know how a specific intervention will impact budgets and the use of other resources (including those of the patient). How will this therapy impact the patient from the patient's perspective?

Pharmacoeconomic information demands are often not anticipated early enough in the clinical development program. For example, several million people in the USA are taking antihypertensive medications to lower their blood pressure, something we would generally think of as good, since the medications can possibly extend life by reducing the risk of stroke and coronary artery disease. However, in some cases the potential benefits of antihypertensives may not outweigh the negative effects of the drugs on quality of life; one study reported that the health of a person treated with antihypertensive medication is comparable to that of an otherwise similar person 5–15 years older. Clearly trade-offs between the side effects and benefits of the medications should be presented to patients so that they can make informed decisions about treatment (Lawrence *et al.*, 1996).

It may seem obvious, but if a pharmaceutical company is developing a new antihypertensive medication targeted for chronic use, preparing a submission with a goal of having the drug prescribed should be the objective. Part of this objective is enabling the prescriber to persuade the patient to take the drug on a regular basis, as well as to ensure that patients understand the pros and cons of taking the medication from their own perception of quality of life. An astute pharmacoeconomic researcher will therefore incorporate a quality of life component into appropriate comparative studies, so that patient-derived and patient-reported aspects of treatment are considered in addition to the management of physiological symptoms such as blood pressure reduction.

Although clinical outcomes remain critical, they are no longer the sole factor reviewed in making a decision to use a therapeutic intervention. Just as the information requirements increased from safety, to safety and efficacy in the 1960s, the bar has been raised once again, and these requirements now include not only clinical safety and efficacy, but also economic and humanistic outcomes. This paradigm shift has been represented in a model termed the economic, clinical, and humanistic outcomes (ECHO) model, described by Kozma *et al.* (1993). Economic outcomes include direct medical resources used to provide a service or achieve an outcome, such as preliminary diagnostic procedures, healthcare providers' time pursuing risk management tactics, and laboratory services (such as adverse event or plasma concentration monitoring, if needed).

In contrast, humanistic outcomes include health-related quality of life, patient satisfaction with interventions, and patient preferences. Patient productivity is another economic outcome; time spent at repetitive clinic visits detracts from it.

Under the new paradigm for decision-making, all decision-makers will increasingly be forced to take into account the perspectives of the other players affected by their decisions. Prescribers must no longer consider just the clinical impact of the prescribing choice. The economic impact their decision will have on the payer, and the quality of life impact the decision will have from the patient's perspective, must also be factored. The payers and the patients must also consider the impact of their decisions on the rest of the system. Successful drug developers now evaluate these three-dimensional outcome data (prescriber, payer, patient) as early as possible in the product development life cycle. This information will also be useful to investors who are making decisions regarding the ultimate potential for success or failure of a newly discovered therapeutic product.

Table 26.1 Examples of outcomes

Type of outcome	Examples
Clinical	Symptoms, diagnosis
	Adverse events
	Drug interactions
Economic	Hospitalizations
	Physician visits
	Prescription drugs
	Productivity
Humanistic	Quality of life
	Satisfaction with treatment
	Preference for one treatment versus
	another

Table 26.1 provides examples of clinical, economic, and humanistic outcomes. Each outcome type is not mutually exclusive, for example, pain could be a clinical or a humanistic outcome, but only needs to be measured once in a study.

Pharmacoeconomics in development programs: advantages, disadvantages, and challenges

Pharmacoeconomic tools will not *make* a decision, but are useful as an aid to decision- makers regarding the appropriate use of a product. Although typically considered to aid the end-user, pharmacoeconomic data also have great applicability at the drug development level. This is not an entirely altruistic concern for the pharmaceutical company: if incorporated early into the development of a drug, a strategic advantage due to a more complete package of outcomes information is available at the time of product approval.

Pharmacoeconomic tools can even assist in selecting an area of preclinical exploration, choosing which drugs should move forward into Phase I, and whether to progress a drug from Phase II to Phase III. An understanding of the current burden of the illness or condition, in terms of its natural history, resource use, and quality of life profile, can help a research team put the estimated development costs and the desired return on invest-

ment in proper perspective. A drug that "cures" an illness that is common but not very debilitating is not likely to be seen as worthy of a premium price by many formulary committees. But this does not necessarily mean that the drug should not be developed. The expected return on the drug must be put in the appropriate context. Early research may also identify targets for comparative studies; a *sine qua non* under the new paradigm. If research is conducted in the most severe patients with a particular condition, but they constitute only 5% of the diseased population, the perspective of those patients needs to be compared with that of patients with less severe forms of the same disease. This will help to demonstrate how patients with less severe forms of the disease might respond to treatment and to determine what the impact of the condition is on their quality of life.

Does pharmacoeconomic research slow down development programs?

A perception exists that disadvantages of incorporating pharmacoeconomic parameters into the development program necessarily delay the filing of the New Drug Application/Product License Application (NDA/PLA), while gathering data that will not be "useful." First of all, the same statements could apply to any secondary clinical endpoint; every efficacy endpoint, including pharmacoeconomic ones, must be carefully considered before incorporating it into a study or program. Similarly, not every program requires all conceivable pharmacoeconomic components. Acute treatments (e.g., antibiotics for otitis media) may not require quality of life components; "me-toos" (e.g., a new NSAID) may only require a simple cost-comparison study.

Drugs for chronic use should be considered as a prime target for pharmacoeconomic study especially. If a disease is not going to be cured, and the patients are expected to take a product for the rest of their lives, there should be some message that can be provided to the patients that will support their use of the product in a compliant fashion for that long period of time.

It must be remembered that the ultimate objective of the pharmaceutical company is the successful launch of a worthy, profitable, new product. If Phase III studies are already completed by the time pharmacoeconomic components are considered, the likelihood of having any outcomes data beyond traditional safety and efficacy at product launch is small. Delay to gather such data may then become obligatory, and a strategic advantage for the product will have been lost. One of the most frequently requested pieces of information by formulary committees and reimbursement agencies is "what is the impact on my budget?". From the patients, it is "What will be the impact on me? Will I feel better?" It is tempting to ignore pharmacoeconomic and humanistic outcomes under the guise of "it is not required by the agency" or "it will slow things down." But ultimately, neglecting these issues will cost the company.

The challenges associated with successfully incorporating pharmacoeconomic components into a clinical development program include making sure that the right people are involved early enough. Adding pharmacoeconomic components to clinical development programs need not be rate-limiting, but *will automatically be so when the project team fails to bring the pharmacoeconomist into the project at an early stage*, that is, Phase I. Early involvement will enable the pharmacoeconomist to understand the characteristics of the investigational drug and the targeted conditions, and as the trials program is laid out, pharmacoeconomic components can be selected that are the most appropriate for the studies in the program. A thoughtful and documented pharmacoeconomic development plan should be available at the same time as the clinical and marketing development plans. Then the three plans can be synchronized and mutually supportive.

Value-added versus traditional clinical development programs

The magnitude of the challenge of incorporating pharmacoeconomics into a traditional clinical development program will depend on the type of program being studied, the willingness of the research team to be open to new types of outcome measures, and the capability of the pharma-

coeconomist. As research-orientated companies avoid "me-too" products, and forge new areas of unmet medical needs, the need for value-added development programs with scientifically valid pharmacoeconomic outcome data will increase. When the need to demonstrate value has been discussed long enough, the real debate should be why to *exclude* pharmacoeconomic measures, not whether to *include* them. Including pharmacoeconomic measures should be the default.

The training and experience of the pharmacoeconomist will impact the conduct of how well value is added to a drug development program. Does the pharmacoeconomist understand the clinical trial process? Is the goal to have a pharmacoeconomic message that will be useful to marketing? Does the pharmacoeconomist understand what messages a sales representative can communicate and what materials can be disseminated as promotion? Has the pharmacoeconomic scientist experience in interacting with the FDA and other regulatory agencies? Will he or she be able develop a pharmacoeconomic strategic plan that will complement the clinical and marketing plans and fulfill the goals of the company? All these questions should be asked before selecting a staff or consultant pharmacoeconomist and embarking on a value-added development program.

Pharmacoeconomic baseline

The important first step in developing a pharmacoeconomic strategic plan is to start by finding out what is currently known about the disease and the economic and humanistic burden that it has on patients, payers, and providers. This may entail a review of the epidemiology and clinical aspects of the condition to verify that pharmacoeconomic components would be a worthwhile addition to a clinical program. After this review the pharmacoeconomist should then formulate the plan for measuring economic and humanistic outcome, and this will ultimately become a component of the full development plan.

If adequate baseline measures do not exist, an important part of the strategic plan will be to research and document the baseline burden of illness as it is currently being treated (or not treated, as may be the case). This can be done separately from the clinical trials that are taking place, although placebo-treated patient measures may also be important in finding this baseline. The goal is to identify a benchmark, documenting the *status quo*. This baseline is critical to being able to show the impact (improvement) that the new drug will have.

Table 26.2 lists some of the important questions to consider when documenting the baseline burden of illness. Full answers will never be available for every question, and neither will perfect data always be available for those answers that can be provided. The risk–benefit assessment of taking the time to answer each question thoroughly versus applying some "quick and dirty" estimates to the questions should be considered. Not every program requires a large-scale major prospective study to answer each question, for many of the reasons discussed above. However, in the long run it is usually less costly in terms of time and money to research the unknown issues before committing to the pharmacoeconomic development plan. The *post hoc* piecemeal approach almost always fails.

Table 26.2 Considerations when documenting baseline burden of illness

---

- Who has the condition (men, women, children, elderly, Blacks, Asians, Caucasians, etc.)?
- How long does the condition last?
- What is the impact of the condition and current treatment on the patient's functional status or quality of life?
- How satisfied are patients with current treatment options?
- Does the disease impact productivity?
- What healthcare and other resources are currently used to manage the condition?
- What percentage of patients with the disease are seeking treatment?
- What is the economic and humanistic impact if treatment is not received?
- What treatments or interventions are currently used to manage the condition?

Case study: data sources

Hirsch and Van Den Eeden (1997) studied antiepileptic drug outcomes, and have demonstrated some of the challenges associated with collecting burden of illness data. The traditional clinical measure of seizure frequency is no longer considered appropriate as the sole measure of outcome of treatment or surgical intervention. The additional variables to document the burden of illness that were found illustrate the gap between the type of data desired and what is available. Hitherto, quality of life had been assessed in epilepsy patients using no fewer than 12 different instruments (both disease-specific and general). The economic impact of epilepsy had previously been assessed at a national level and in a few small studies. Using a retrospective cross-sectional design in a managed care organization these authors sought to define the overall disease impact for patients with chronic epilepsy. Multiple data sources were required, and no existing, single database held the various types of data required; these included administrative databases, medical charts, pharmacy databases, outpatient databases, hospitals, laboratories, outside services, memberships, etc. All the identified sociodemographic variables were available in at least one automated database, as were two of the clinical variables, and 26 of the economic variables. None of the humanistic variables were available in any database.

In this case, about half of the data desired were available electronically, most of which were related to health as heavily weighted toward economic information. To gather the remaining desired data the investigators needed to collect prospectively humanistic as well as some additional clinical variables (Hirsch and Van Den Eeden, 1997). It is quite typical that clinical data available electronically often are not complete and therefore not very useful, and that humanistic data are missing completely from the databases held by Health Maintenance Organizations.

When setting out to document the burden of illness, it is critical to ensure that the patients in the databases really are truly patients with the disease of interest. In come cases, the ICD-9 codes are known to be inaccurate regarding patient capture, and means other than electronic data bases must be used. One advantage of using clinical trial patients is the certainty of having patients with the condition of interest—the trade-off being a concern for the generalizability of information to the general population.

Pharmacoeconomic baseline data should not be considered in isolation, but as one aspect of data that must be considered as a part of the whole. Once the burden of illness information is collected and analyzed, the development team must plan for ways to measure and document the clinical, economic, and humanistic impact of the new pharmaceutical entity or other intervention.

Studies within clinical trials: techniques

wThe information generated from the burden of illness component of a pharmacoeconomic strategy can then serve as a guide for the design of pharmacoeconomic endpoints within clinical trials. Obviously, this must be factored against the prior judgment of whether or not disease-specific quality of life instruments are required at all. Healthcare resource use, measures of lost productivity, and indirect financial cost measures may be all that is required. The process of incorporating pharmacoeconomic measures into clinical trials should begin before a draft protocol is ever created.

Both the quantity and the types of data able to be collected will be affected by the nature of the clinical study: patients may be inpatients or outpatients, and this in turn will govern the nature of pharmacoeconomic data that can be recorded. It is also important whether a clinical trial is intended as a pivotal trial for registration or not: if a study is pivotal, a clinical efficacy measure will have to be the primary endpoint. Pharmacoeconomic parameters can still be incorporated into such a study as secondary endpoints, and still provide valuable information. If, on the other hand, the clinical research addresses a health system delivery issue, the pharmacoeconomic endpoints may well be primary, and the study design need not be constrained by FDA-mandated requirements for the double-blind, placebo-controlled aspects of proof of efficacy.

As the development moves from early Phase II through to Phase IV, the rationale for incorporating pharmacoeconomic parameters into studies should evolve. Initially, measures may be used in studies with small sample sizes to gain experience with certain instruments, or to determine which instrument is preferred for use in larger studies. Early on, the project team may think that everything conceivable ("all but the kitchen sink") is being included in a study. In some cases, the instrument feasibility study could be done as a separate study, but the costs in terms of additional patients needed, and other resources required, need to be carefully considered before a decision to reject the inclusion of several pharmacoeconomic instruments in one early clinical study.

As the product moves from Phase II into Phase III, the number of seemingly redundant instruments should decline as the obvious choice, or best guess, rises to the top. If the goal of Phase III studies is to file an NDA or gain regulatory approval, the studies may not be appropriately designed to capture the additional information deemed necessary for the product's success. In some cases, separate pharmacoeconomic studies may be needed prior to marketing.

Good advice is to prioritize at this stage of development: Which pharmacoeconomic components are and are not critical for product launch or shortly thereafter? Thus, there is usually a need to strike a balance between getting information in a timely fashion, meeting regulatory demands, and meeting the demands of the marketplace. That balance is often struck pragmatically.

Confidence and validity of data

As in any other scientific endeavor, the validation of the database is as important as its interpretation. Pharmacoeconomic variables require two degrees of confidence: in the accuracy and validity of what has been measured.

Consider two opposite examples of pharmacoeconomic measurement. In one case, patients could describe their impression of the impact of an intervention on their quality of life (QOL) following completion of a two-week, open-label course of treatment. At the other extreme, a randomized controlled trial (RCT), using a double-blind, placebo-controlled protocol and a 12-month follow-up in several hundred patients, could use a statistically validated QOL instrument. The results of the latter would probably inspire more confidence than the "informal" scenario, all other things being equal. However, it does not mean that the answers given using the informal method are wrong, it simply requires an appreciation of the trade-offs involved in how data are collected. Furthermore, the former method might be of more use than the latter in exploratory pharmacoeconomic research conducted in the earliest stages of drug development.

The RCT, although regarded as a gold standard in much of drug development, offers real challenges to the pharmacoeconomist. The RCT is costly, time-consuming, and may have ethical constraints (12 months of placebo?). Some types of outcomes, such as compliance, do not lend themselves to double-blind designs because such designs mask one of the effects being measured. RCTs generally strive to maintain high levels of internal validity at the risk of reducing external validity. Biases to internal validity affect the accuracy of the results of the study, because they apply to those who participated in the study (e.g., patient selection bias, cross-over bias, and errors in measurement of outcomes). Biases to external validity affect how well the results may be generalized to the public at large. Obviously, the choice of study design must take potential biases into account. These factors are somewhat analogous for pharmacoeconomic and traditional clinical research.

Selecting a QOL instrument

It is always important to select an instrument that has adequate reliability and validity. Although many instruments have been published, many of these have little supporting validation. Another source of information is the Medical Outcomes Trust (2001; www.outcomes-trust.org). Some instruments, such as the MOS-SF-36, a generic QOL instrument, currently have popularity, and it is tempting to incorporate these routinely into clinical studies. Many experts in the field

recommend that both a disease-specific and a generic instrument should be used in each study, in order to capture the broadest QOL information. Yet, excess burden on patients can defeat the accuracy and completeness of what is collected. Generally, if resources or patient burden threatens, most experts would argue for retention of a disease-specific instrument when it is only possible to use a single measure.

Standard operating procedures and quality analysis should be a part of every study in which the company invests money to collect endpoints, be they traditional or pharmacoeconomic endpoints. The handling and analysis of pharmacoeconomic data should follow Good Clinical Practices (GCP) guidelines. Data collection instruments need to be selected, or created and incorporated into case report forms, just as for any other endpoints. Data collection and statistical analysis plans should be created prospectively (see Table 26.3). The type

Table 26.3 Points to consider: incorporating pharmacoeconomic measures in clinical trials

---

- Document the pharmacoeconomic objectives, methodology, and analysis plan within the study protocol.
- Measure outcomes in the most appropriate and most disaggregate units. Categories can always be collapsed at a future time, but it is impossible to split out variables beyond their original units. The sources of process and outcomes data may vary.
- Clinical data may be captured from providers, patients, and medical records.
- Resource use data may be obtained from patient, administrative databases, providers, or charts.
- Quality of life data should come from the patient. In some cases (very young, very old, mentally unstable) patient proxies are used, but the patient should be considered the optimal choice.
- The study design can affect the *types* of outcomes that can be reliably collected, and the *manner* in which the outcomes can be collected.
- Study design affects several parts of the evaluation process:
  - cost of evaluation;
  - time required to conduct the evaluation;
  - accuracy of the information gained;
  - complexity of administering the evaluation;
  - ease of defending subsequent decisions made, based upon the evaluation.

---

of data collected should drive the level of analysis (continuous versus categorical data). If there is an investigators' meeting for the study, the pharmacoeconomic components should be presented at the meeting so the investigators and/or the study coordinators fully understand their role in data collection. As the study is ongoing, appropriate levels of monitoring should be conducted. Queries that arise during the study and reconciliation of the data afterwards should be handled in the same manner in which clinical queries and data reconciliation are handled.

Reporting and publications

The principles outlined in Chapter 46 on study publications apply just as well to pharmacoeconomic outcomes reporting. Most companies have some form of standard operating procedure by which they generate clinical study reports. Pharmacoeconomic data should be handled and reported in the same way. In some cases it may be appropriate to issue the pharmacoeconomic component of a study as an appendix to a larger clinical report. This will depend on the level of pharmacoeconomic involvement in the study and how closely related the endpoints may be to the pathological measures. If just a few pharmacoeconomic measures were being tested, an appendix to a clinical report might be appropriate. In contrast, for example, where recovery from anesthesia is measured by "street fitness" (the humanistic outcome) and neurological measures of balance and coordination (the physiological endpoint), it could be cogent to report these two types of data together, and to examine how well they correlate; this would not be suited for an appendix for the humanistic data.

External reports are most likely going to be manuscripts submitted to peer-reviewed journals. Placement of pharmacoeconomic articles in non-specialty journals is important but difficult. Some editors do not understand the intrinsic properties of pharmacoeconomic data, and some reviewers will blindly apply statistical constraints that are inappropriate or not valid to humanistic outcomes (e.g., power calculations to measures of the adverse effects of drugs on quality of life measures).

The basic principles of scientific writing and reporting apply to pharmacoeconomic research, and little need be said here. The structure of the paper is the same (Introduction, Methods, Results, Discussion, etc.). It is important to be consistent and appropriate in the use of terminology (e.g., "costs" is not synonymous with "charges," and cost-effectiveness is not a cost–benefit analysis; Sanchez and Lee, 1994). Obviously, the Internet also offers possibilities for publication, dissemination, and debate (see: Medical Outcomes Trust, 2001; www.outcomes-trust.org; American College of Clinical Pharmacy, 1996).

It must be said that how such information gets disseminated is controversial in the USA. A good recent example is an investigation of atovaquone versus intravenous pentamidine in the treatment of mild to moderate *Pneumocystis carinii* pneumonia. This report included a decision tree to estimate the costs and cost-effectiveness of atovaquone versus pentamidine for cotrimoxazole-intolerant patients (Zarkin *et al.*, 1996). Clinical outcomes were based on data from a previous Phase III RCT, which compared the two medications. Economic outcomes were based on treatment algorithms derived from discharge data, published reports, and clinical judgments by the co-authors. The clinical data were from a randomized, double-blind study. A sensitivity analysis was conducted. The major conclusion of the study was that there were significant cost savings to be had from treating *Pneumocystis carinii* pneumonia on an outpatient basis. An FDA representative, during a platform presentation of this paper, even indicated that these data could be used in promotion.

Current and future uses of pharmacoeconomic outcomes

Pharmacoeconomics now has a well-established place in the current healthcare environment. However, like any discipline, pharmacoeconomics has its limitations (Jennings and Staggers, 1997):

• *Competing perspectives create tension:* for example, pharmacoeconomics versus clinical importance. Differences in perspective may be irreconcilable because they relate to a perceived encroachment:

"turf wars" can erupt between clinical, marketing, and pharmacoeconomics departments within the same company, in spite of all three professing the same goal, that is, to market successfully a worthwhile drug in a proper fashion.

• *Need for rapid response.* Protocol in two weeks versus six weeks? Sometimes it takes longer to develop the pharmacoeconomic portion of a protocol. There may be fewer people to do it, there are likely to be more unknowns than for purely clinical endpoints, and there may be a need to decide which instrument to use; worse yet, there may be no baseline data to validate any chosen instrument. Studies that examine efficiency are especially likely to require more planning.

• *Lack of prototype.* Some groups want these studies to be pragmatic and relevant to everyday practice, and yet there is no prototype to delineate the basic tenets of such studies, meaning that the data may be riddled with inaccuracies and misrepresentations. Additionally, the regulatory agencies may be more concerned with internal validity than the pragmatic approach would allow.

• *Performance measure pitfalls.* What gets measured reflects system values. If clinical groups are measured on the ability to meet target filing dates, peak sales potential will be ignored. Relevant clinical indicators of performance may not be known, neither is it the best mix of data.

• *Dearth of patient-centered outcomes measures in traditional drug development.* Physicians are usually relied upon for clinical data. Data from the patient is sometimes perceived to be "soft." Patient perspectives can also be missed when the traditional clinical focus is disease- or organ-dominated.

• *Discrepancies in terminology.* A new lexicon is emerging. The lexicon must be carefully and precisely translated in its application to healthcare to avoid miscommunication.

• *When to measure.* A major challenge for clinical studies is when to measure. At what point in the process is the endpoint reached? The decision can significantly affect the cost and time of conducting a study. Unfortunately, there are no obvious guides, but there should be sufficient proximity between process and outcome measures to believe the linkage.

• *Value.* To what extent is value related to quality? If there is no standard definition of quality, it may be overridden by cost. It is difficult to quantify nonmonetary value into a neat formula. The challenge is to propose quality indicators that allow calculating a balance of quality and cost.

• *Absence of clearly delineated perspective(s).* Outcomes can be categorized in a variety of ways, including disease, patient, provider, and organizational. There will likely be multiple perspectives, but it still needs to be orderly.

• *Outcomes are not processes.* Patient care and quality dimensions of outcomes must be considered.

The applied discipline of pharmacoeconomics is slowly evolving. Despite its lack of maturity, many people and systems are embracing it as a savior. Although pharmacoeconomics is an important addition to decision-making, it does need to be put in appropriate context. It is a new and essential part of older and previously less sophisticated processes of drug development and product selection. Used appropriately, pharmacoeconomic research can assist in rational decision-making at every level of drug development and drug therapy.

References

(Note: all websites cited in this chapter were accessed April 24, 2010.)

American College of Clinical Pharmacy. *Pharmacoeconomics and Outcomes: Applications for Patient Care.* A series of three modules created to develop in-depth working knowledge of pharmacoeconomic and outcomes assessment. ACCP Kansas City, MO, USA, 1996; http://www.accp.com.

Bootman JL, Townsend RJ, McGhan WF (eds). *Principles of Pharmacoeconomics*, third edition. Harvey Whitney: Cincinnati, OH, USA, 2005.

Feldstein PJ. *Health Care Economics*, second edition. John Wiley & Sons Inc: New York, USA, 1983.

Foundation for Health Sciences Research (1993) *Health Outcomes Research: A Primer.* Foundation for Health Services Research: Washington, DC.

Hirsch JD, Van Den Eeden SK. Epilepsy: searching for outcomes data beyond seizure frequency in a managed care organization. *J Outcomes Managem* 1997; **4**(1):9–11, 14–17, 23.

Jennings BM, Staggers N. The hazards in outcomes management. *J Outcomes Managem* 1997; **4**(1):18–23.

Kozma CM, Reeder CE, Schulz RM. Economic, clinical and humanistic outcomes: a planning model for pharmacoeconomic research. *Clin Ther* 1993; **15**:1121–1132.

Lawrence WF, Fryback DG, Martin PA, *et al*. Health status and hypertension: a population-based study. *J Clin Epidemiol* 1996; **49**(11):1239–1245.

Medical Outcomes Trust. 2001; www.outcomes-trust.org.

Sanchez LA, Lee JT. Use and misuse of pharmacoeconomic terms: a definitions primer. *Top Hosp Pharm Managem* 1994; **13**:11–22.

Zarkin GA, Bala MV, Wood LL *et al*. Estimating the cost effectiveness of atovaquone versus intravenous pentamidine in the treatment of mild to moderate pneumocystis pneumonia. *Pharmacoeconomics* 1996; **6**:525–534.

Further reading

Bowling A. *Measuring Health: A Review of Disease-specific Quality of Life Measurement Scales*. Open University Press: Buckingham, UK, and Bristol, PA, 1995.

Bowling A. *Measuring Health: A Review of Quality of Life Measurement Scales*, second edition. Open University Press: Buckingham, UK, and Bristol, PA, 1997.

Drummond MF, Stoddart GL, Torrance GW. *Methods for the Economic Evaluation of Health Care Programmes*. Oxford University Press: Oxford, UK, 1986.

Drummond MF, O'Brien B. Clinical importance, statistical significance and the assessment of economic and quality of life outcomes. *Health Econ* 1993; **2**:205.

Eddy DM. Should we change the rules for evaluating medical technologies? *In Modern Methods of Clinical Investigation*, Gelijns AC (ed.). National Academy Press: Washington, DC, USA, 1990.

Freund DA, Dittus RS. Principles of pharmacoeconomics analysis of drug therapy. *PharmacoEconomics* 1992; **1**:20–32.

Jolicoeur LM, Jones-Grizzle AJ, Boyer JG. Guidelines for performing a pharmacoeconomic analysis. *Am J Hosp Pharm* 1992; **49**:1741–1747.

Lee JT, Sanchez LA. Interpretation of "cost-effective" and soundness of economic evaluations in pharmacy literature. *Am J Hosp Pharm* 1992; **48**:2622–2627.

McDowell I, Newell C. *Measuring Health: A Guide to Rating Scales and Questionnaires*, second edition. Oxford University Press: New York, USA, 1996.

Patrick DL, Deyo RA. Generic and disease-specific measures in assessing health status and quality of life. *Med Care* 1989; **27**(suppl):S217–S232.

Sederer L, Dickey B (eds). *Outcomes Assessment in Clinical Practice*. Williams and Wilkins: Baltimore, MD, USA, 1996.

Spilker B (ed.) *Quality of Life Assessments in Clinical Trials*. Raven: New York, USA, 1990.

Ware JE Jr. The status of health assessment 1994. *Ann Rev Public Health* 1995; **16**:327–354.

CHAPTER 27

Pharmacoepidemiology and the Pharmaceutical Physician

Hugh H. Tilson

School of Public Health, University of North Carolina, Chapel Hill, NC, USA

The specialty practice of preventive medicine extends into the realm of pharmaceutical medicine just as deeply as better-recognized disciplines such as clinical pharmacology or toxicology. Preventive medicine physicians may often be found practicing pharmaceutical medicine under the guise of clinical research or regulatory affairs, or in separate departments of pharmacoepidemiology, health economics, or outcomes research, as well as the perhaps more predictable aegis of drug safety and pharmacovigilance.

Preventive Medicine/Public Health physicians, alias pharmacoeconomists and pharmacoepidemiologists, are trained in the core sciences of public health—epidemiology and statistics—along with their nonphysician pharmacoepidemiology colleagues. But, being physicians, they are also steeped in pathophysiology, diagnostics, therapeutics, and behavioral sciences. Additionally, specialization in preventive medicine requires detailed education in environmental health, general management, and health policy. Many of these areas of expertise are shared with other types of pharmaceutical physicians, for example clinical trialists. It is not uncommon to find professionals moving (or oscillating) between pharmacoepidemiology and other departments within the same company or regulatory agency.

Public health physicians use all these tools to identify, and control, public health hazards. In the pharmaceutical sector, these skills extend to such hazards associated with pharmacotherapy. Pharmacoepidemiologists have an additional dimension to their work, in that they may use their unique observational methods to study drugs not only as a potential hazard to the public health (perhaps through drug surveillance programs), but also as a potential benefit to the public health (e.g., in large-scale interventional or observational, clinical outcomes, or economics studies). Identifying the types of patients who are most likely to benefit (or be harmed) by a therapeutic intervention is merely an extension of the orthodox world in which the public health physician practices. Thus, preventive medicine physicians may be found in pharmaceutical companies, contract research organizations (CROs), and academic, governmental, and international political environments.

Epidemiology

The word has three components, from the Greek *epi*, upon; *demos*, the people; and *logos*, the study. These elements describe the fundamentals of what epidemiology is all about: The application of scientific principles to the understanding of health issues that are "upon the people." All pharmaceutical physicians need an understanding of the fundamentals of this field, in order to understand and harness the value that epidemiology, and epidemiologists, can bring to drug development and product surveillance programs. Epidemiology is taught in all schools of public health and, in

---

Principles and Practice of Pharmaceutical Medicine, 3rd edition.
Edited by L.D. Edwards, A.W. Fox, P.D. Stonier.
© 2011 Blackwell Publishing Ltd.

varying depth and quality, in schools of medicine. Epidemiologic techniques are used by many people who would not describe themselves as epidemiologists. Board certification in preventive medicine requires a Master's degree (or its equivalent) with a large epidemiology component, and further tough examinations.

Such epidemiology training emphasizes observational research methodology as the core approach of the field. However, emphasis is also given on building expertise in clinical trials design and biostatistics. These disciplines require expertise and experience in the management of huge quantities of data and the attendant expertise in scientific computing/informatics. These are skills that find natural places in Phase III and Phase IV clinical study design and conduct within industry, and evaluation within the regulatory environment. However, it is in the understanding of the applications (and often more importantly the limitations) of the nonexperimental/observational method that the epidemiologist adds special value to the pharmaceutical sector.

It is important to remember that epidemiology represents another set of tactics to address the same underlying challenges as others working in and with the development enterprise. Just as much as a molecular biologist or clinical pharmacologist, the epidemiologist is trying to find out which set of conditions causes a particular disease or benefit or adverse event (AE). The additional perspective of the impact on actual populations (the actual effectiveness) complements the emphasis on the experimental subject (the efficacy) of much of clinical research. The epidemiologist is faced with the substantial challenge of observational approaches. Without the benefits (comforts) of randomization and blinding afforded by the experimental method, only rarely can the epidemiologist imitate the pharmacologist, who can premeditate an intervention in a confined population, and then prospectively observe its effect. However, even when constrained by the observational approach, the epidemiologist is like other scientists in that findings are in the context of comparison among various structured observational groups, differing in their known exposures or out-

comes (Strom and Kimmel, 2006; Hartzema *et al.*, 2008).

Epidemiologic methodologies

Prospective cohort studies

A prospective cohort epidemiologic study approximates to a parallel-group clinical trial in its scientific basis, and epidemiologists will be as aware as clinical trialists of the bias that can be introduced if the study groups do not contain comparable, well-balanced and homogeneous groups of people. Although the experimentalist uses exclusions, randomization, and blinding as tools to control for unseen biases, the epidemiologist is, rather, required to measure and document attributes and control for those that may lead to skewed results, by selection in ascertainment and stratification in analysis. Furthermore, like others calling themselves drug surveillance specialists, the epidemiologist will be well aware that the size of the groups that must be studied increases with the rarity of the phenomenon that is sought. The latency of the effect (e.g., the duration between exposure to an unsuspected atheromatous stimulus and coronary artery disease) can define the desirable duration of follow-up, in a manner analogous to the study of the probability of AEs arising only after prolonged multiple-dose drug exposure. Often, rather, the size of the available population and the duration for which it has already been followed (e.g., for other, administrative or clinical purposes) will dictate the extent to which an observational study is able to state the level of certainty of its observations.

Case–control study designs

These were developed to provide information more rapidly than when cohorts are followed for prolonged periods of time, using traditional hands-on methods. Case-based research is, however, necessarily retrospective. Analysis begins with the characterization of a group of people that already have the disease of interest, the "cases." Control subjects are then drawn from a population with attributes as closely parallel as possible to those of the population from which cases are selected (often a very difficult task!). The antecedent demographic, therapeutic, and environmental factors of both groups are documented, often by a combination of record abstraction and interview. If differences are found in the proportion (rate) for some factor between the two groups, this becomes suspected as an etiological agent for the disease of interest. This suspicion is strengthened when either the discovered factor corresponds with a predictive hypothesis at the start of the study, or when there is consistent evidence that would support its identification (perhaps a biochemical link between the factor and the disease).

Drug risk as an epidemiologic problem

Drug-related epidemics have occurred, mercifully relatively infrequently. However, with each unfortunate episode, there is inevitably a variety of regulatory and clinical fallout. Indeed, the illnesses associated with ingestion of glycol-tainted linctus led to the Food, Drugs and Cosmetics Act in the United States, and the disastrous association of phocomelia with thalidomide propelled reforms of drug regulations worldwide. Other famous examples include, of course, practolol-induced oculomucocutaneous syndrome, and more recently, fenfluramine-induced myocardial fibrosis, isotretinoin-associated birth defects, and unexpected heart complications with long-term use of Cox-2 inhibitors.

The major driver for the field of pharmacoepidemiology is the nature of the drug development process itself. Relatively small and often quite carefully selected clinical trials populations are followed for only limited periods, during and after exposure to the agent under study, in the populations that comprise typical product license applications and New Drug Application (NDA) safety summaries. This leaves, for the post-approval scientific environment, the challenge to apply methods that can detect AEs with relatively low frequency or relatively specific risk situations. Those who call for transfer of these burdens to the pre-approval environment would benefit from training in epidemiology, with the associated understanding that

the only way to understand the real world is to study the real world!

Pharmacoepidemiology and pharmacovigilance do not pretend to be able to eliminate the occurrence of drug-associated epidemics. The challenge is to detect and quantitate problems as rapidly and accurately as possible, so that changes in the benefit–risk balance, as understood at the time of approval, can be quickly recognized and possible public health actions considered. Thus, pharmacovigilance may be understood as "epidemiologic intelligence." And thus, in turn, the physician pharmacoepidemiologist is a strong contributor to drug surveillance departments in industry and drug safety groups in regulatory agencies. Typically, these epidemiologists will be supervising and/or providing expert counsel to groups of less specialized or highly trained health scientists who implement the day-to-day running of these programs. Teamwork becomes an indispensable skill.

Consideration about the need for and technical considerations regarding one or more structured observational studies is a frequently recognized contribution of the epidemiologist in this enterprise. Less frequently extolled are the great contributions that epidemiologists make to consideration of approaches, which seductive because of their apparent simplicity, will not be likely to contribute, as options for reducing uncertainty around estimates of possible risk are considered. Observational science is very complicated, and the opportunities of failure of study are considerable! When epidemiologic studies are undertaken, and results are known, it falls to the physician epidemiologist to put on the public health hat and recommend whether an intervention in the interests of public health might be needed, and if so, to suggest what its parameters might be.

The "wired" epidemiologist

It probably goes without saying in the cybernetic environment of the twenty-first century that effective epidemiology of all types, including pharmacoepidemiology, can only be seriously conducted with the addition to the epidemiologist's armamentarium of the skillful use of large, automated, multipurpose, population-based systems (the LAMPS): known by shorthand as "the databases."

Often these databases have been developed wholly outside the research context, with a primary intent of submitting or paying the bills, creating economic efficiency, quality assurance, or management controls within organized systems of healthcare. Hence, in the United States, the organizations that construct these databases include insurance companies, hospitals, health maintenance organizations, and other companies in the healthcare business. In Canada, and increasingly in Europe, such databases are emerging from provincial/regional or national reimbursement programs. If the database is equipped with patient identifiers (e.g., a unique membership number), hospitalizations, prescriptions, and combinations of healthcare transactions can be linked to a single individual across components of the system and over time: a so-called "record-linkage" system. More recently, the evolution of a powerful clinical management tool, the electronic medical record, further powers the availability of linked data for entire populations under care. Note that *not* all databases are created equal, For most effective use in epidemiology, the databases must provide information about all important medical encounters for an entire defined population. Such databases render it feasible to assemble cohorts of drug-exposed individuals and computer-matched comparator populations from historical (extant) data and observe them (using cohort analyses) forward over the time in the database (often decades) for evidence of excesses of events under study. Similarly, case–control methods may assemble cases and comparators, and use the powerful databases as the source of the antecedent information, so elusive in hands-on methods.

Recent regulatory efforts on behalf of the needs to protect patient privacy have established a long and successful record of systems that protect patient privacy while ensuring access to necessary population-level, individual-linked data. The excellent and durable policy positions on data privacy protections of many professional organizations (notably the American College of Epidemiology (ACE) and the International Society for Pharmacoepidemiology (ISPE)) stand as evidence of this competence. The reader is referred to the websites of these organizations.

A recent pioneering effort has been the emergence of "sentinel surveillance" using LAMPS. In this application, frequent powerful automated scans are applied to multiple databases operating in parallel to ascertain any events that are occurring with an unexpected/unpredicted frequency in association with a specified (drug, biologic, device) exposure. Such "signals" are then subjected to further, rigorous investigation. With the projected numbers exceeding one hundred million "covered lives" in such data resources in the US by the year 2012, sentinel surveillance should have the power for early detection of relatively common AEs and the size to detect even relatively rare, important drug-associated morbidity and mortality.

It is to be emphasized that such database work is often complicated, and requires a team of professionals comprising physician and nonphysician pharmacoepidemiologists, statisticians, and specialists in information technology. Perhaps one of the greatest contributions that a clinician can make to such a team is to provide relevance to the hypotheses that are tested and as a reality check on the results that the computers generate, and which those less close to the field tend to regard automatically as "fact."

Despite the deserved enthusiasm for the contribution of the LAMPS to epidemiology, more traditional hands-on, structured observational studies, and registries, with enrollment of cohorts of persons exposed to an agent under study and proper comparator populations, and selection of cases (e.g., from medical records) and appropriate controls, still have specific applications in pharmaceutical medicine, thus characterizing part of the activity of pharmacoepidemiologists.

Definitions

The pharmaceutical physician, epidemiologist or not, must understand the concepts of prevalence and incidence *sine qua non*. Prevalence is the frequency of disease in a defined population, at any one moment. Incidence is the frequency of new cases of a disease in a defined population during a defined time interval.

Thus, influenza may have an incidence of 15% for the months December–April 1999 in the United Kingdom, whereas the prevalence of influenza in the United Kingdom probably ranges between 0 and 10% on any given day. Perinatal (and maternal) mortality rates are usually stated annually and for specified country or region.

These are thus measures of incidence. The proportion of a population that will experience at least one seizure or one migraine attack in their lives is a measure of incidence and would likely be expressed as a number per thousand (or per hundred thousand) person-years, whereas the proportion of a population suffering from epilepsy or migraine during the year 2010 is an expression of prevalence.

In pharmacovigilance terms, the "true frequency" in a treated population in a specified period, if it was known, of an AE observed in a marketed product, would be considered an incidence. All too often, the frequency of reported AEs (definitely not the complete or even estimated numerator), perhaps weighed against known sales (scarcely a true denominator), is mistakenly used to calculate a rate and called an "incidence." At best, such spontaneous reports data should be termed "reports rates."

Other, more complex terms are defined and described in standard textbooks of epidemiology and statistics (*q.v.*) and included in two excellent lexicons, the *Dictionary of Epidemiology* (Last, 2001; Porta 2008) and a very useful Lexicon from the International Society for Pharmacoeconomics and Outcomes Research (ISPOR).

Epidemiology in drug development

The complexities of drug development include a decision web that is inevitably informed by incomplete information. Although past, focused research may comprise some of the information for the next step, epidemiologic information can be of valuable assistance. The capturing and extension of population-based studies, often concerning the natural history of disease rather than the pharmacological properties of the test agent itself, can guide the choice of indication, market strategy, and even the viability of an entire project. Furthermore, the place of existing therapies, in the context of the natural history of disease, can also be investigated epidemiologically. "If they don't need it, we can't sell it; then let's not pursue it" is an aphorism: but whether they need it is, of course, an epidemiologic challenge.

Population-based measures of burden of disease involve a formal quantitation of the opportunity for a new drug. These measures vary among organ systems, but typically involve the interaction of lifestyle interference, duration of disease, prevalence, incidence, effectiveness and adverse effects associated with existing therapies, and reduction in lifespan. Such objective measures can be ascertained from population-based studies and existing national databases, for example from major ongoing population health surveys, and can often allow the pharmacoepidemiologist to contribute a substantial and useful evidence base to inform the difficult and emotion-laden decisions that must be made by senior executives in drug development.

During Phases II and III, an additional capability can be offered to the development team that might hitherto be comprised purely of clinical department staff. Are infrequently observed but highly dangerous AEs being seen in a clinical trials program within the expected range for that study population? If so, then entire development programs in jeopardy could be saved; if not, appropriate actions may be undertaken more rapidly and decisively. Under some circumstances, in the United States, widespread distribution of an investigational agent prior to NDA approval, involving large-scale populations, is permitted. Under these conditions it is, of course, necessary to monitor safety in such broader use, and usually with greater scrutiny that might ordinarily apply after product approval. Thus, the best practice is to structure such programs as observational studies. AEs are bound to occur, thus providing an ideal opportunity for early detection of infrequent but important adverse reactions; conversely, trouble-shooting these—in the context of a sound epidemiologic and clinical understanding of AEs associated with the disease itself, and with alternative therapies—is also often needed to protect against false conclusions. Such interpretations also eventually are translated into labeling, either by exclusion or inclusion. The landmark report of the Institute of Medicine, *The Future of Drug Safety* (2006) calls for a lifetime approach to drug safety and the creation of a "cultures of drug safety," particularly within regulatory authorities.

Epidemiology in drug registration and licensing

During the registration process, there is typically repeated interaction between an NDA/PLA sponsor and the regulatory authority. Often these interactions revolve around whether the tolerability of the new drug is sufficiently well characterized, and the criteria for the inclusion and exclusion of particular observed intolerabilities in labeling, as well as the weight that should be applied to each (e.g., AE list, warning, contraindication, or rarely, precluding drug approval). Often the question "What level of risk is acceptable?" becomes quickly answered with "Acceptable, compared to what?" These considerations are clearly based on an insight into public health decision-making and are often well served by the inclusion of epidemiologists working with and/or consulting with regulators and sponsors, assuring the culture of drug safety.

Furthermore, the scientific proof of a negative is virtually impossible when fewer than an infinite number of patients have been studied. The more elusive problem, then, is to define acceptable uncertainty. Some of these decisions are based on precedent rather than observation. Pharmacoepidemiology is often a useful source of precedents, as well as available for further, future study in the post-approval period to clarify residual questions and/or reduce the remaining uncertainty.

The emerging world of risk management

Although many of the activities described can then be orientated toward support of registration with fair and balanced labeling or education that is useful to the prescriber, recently regulators have requested and sponsors have proposed programs of "risk management". These would apply under circumstances in which an unacceptably serious risk has been identified or can reasonably be anticipated and risk factors or situations can be specified, which if addressed, can reduce that risk to a level that, balanced against anticipated benefits, could be accepted for clinical use. To manage such situations, sponsors are asked to develop, test, and field interventions with the provider, distributor, or consumer to accompany the marketplace activities with a drug with a residual safety concern. The FDA has issued official guidance regarding action programs to minimize such risks (RiskMaps) (FDA, 2005) and the European Medicines Agency (EMA; the European drug regulatory authority) followed suit (EMA, 2005). Expectations regarding these programs likewise include documentation of the effectiveness of the intervention, once again a challenge for the public health researcher, that is, the pharmacoepidemiologist (FDA, 2009).

Post-marketing surveillance studies

Approval (especially in the United States) to introduce a drug into the market is now often contingent on the agreement of the sponsor to conduct one or more post-marketing surveillance studies. Typically conducted on a scale of 5000 or more patients, the design of such studies poses classic epidemiologic challenges: the choice of control cohorts (if any), appropriateness of historical controls, power calculations, and the nature and range of confounding variables among others. Many of these may be addressed using the databases described above. It should be noted that post-marketing surveillance studies are often implemented by companies without any imposed regulatory requirement, simply due to the value that they bring in understanding a new product that may formerly only have been tested in several hundred patients. The strategic or forward thinking company will initiate such studies well in advance of the appearance of a signal of a potential problem, recognizing that large-scale and long-term studies need to be in place before a problem emerges if they are to be of use in clarifying the extent and nature of that problem in time to be of use, particularly in a closely regulated and often adversary environment.

General pharmacovigilance

Whether or not a post-marketing surveillance study is used, all drugs undergo pharmacovigilance when in the marketplace. This can be especially challenging but vital during the early period after launch, and will become yet more complex with emergence of sentinel surveillance systems. The assessment of pharmacovigilance findings, particularly the initial few reports of AEs with low incidence and/or unexpected disproportionality, has obligatorily to include an epidemiologic component. The epidemiologic interpretation of a finding of excess prevalence requires the sophisticated epidemiologic understanding of baseline, or population-expected risks, and application of this understanding to the vagaries of uncertain ascertainment that characterize spontaneous reports. The usual disposition of a "signal of a potential problem" from pharmacovigilance is introduction into the product's core safety information ("product label").

However, further, recent product withdrawals provide a litany of more extreme examples that need not be repeated here, but average one or two major products and several minor ones each year. Product withdrawals are often misunderstood, particularly by the lay press hungry for a scandal. It is neither feasible nor desirable to "know everything about a product" at the time of approval. But judicious product withdrawal, based on substantial evidence properly collected and analyzed in the post-marketing environment, is a classic example of a robust and balanced system, with each component functioning as it should. Pharmacoepidemiology contributes to the pursuit of the best-informed decision making, with the shared goal of optimization of the balance between patient benefit and the inevitable patient adversity.

Prescription-event monitoring (PEM)

This is essentially an extension of traditional, hands-on epidemiology, which assembles all patients who are prescribed a drug into a cohort that is then followed. In the UK, for example, through the Drug Safety Research Trust, all or a sample of this cohort is assembled from the records of the prescription pricing authority, generally within the first year or two of initial marketing of the product. Each patient can be followed up with a confidential enquiry for serious AEs using a form that, in the UK is popularly called by its appearance: the "Green card" (this term has an entirely different meaning in the US, and, curiously, describes a pink document!). It is a classic example of an observational as opposed to an experimental method, in which all uses and all outcomes (events) are observed, generally without a simultaneously collected comparison population. Thus, data stemming from these sorts of activities are fraught with analytical and methodological traps. However, PEM is a good method for generating hypotheses for further testing, usually after reconciliation with the known pharmacology of the drug of interest, other drugs in the same class, and the natural history of the disease and kindred disorders. These, of course, shed further light on these data, and may be gathered, for example, from the spontaneous reports system. Indeed, sometimes this is also the first evidence of an unsuspected drug intolerability, perhaps in a previously unsuspected subset of the treated patient population. The ability in certain European areas and New Zealand to aggregate prescriptions from entire countries or regions, often as part of the reimbursement system, is obviously strategic to this approach.

Pregnancy registries

Pregnancy registries (or, more properly, pregnancy follow-up studies) are being recommended with increasing frequency for products that are likely to be used in women with child-bearing potential. Inevitably, all new drugs have not been studied in women who are, or become, pregnant, and equally inevitably, labeled warnings to that effect do not prevent exposures of embryos and fetuses to new drugs. The anticipated, spontaneous incidence of anomalies detectable post partum is in the range 3–7%. This wide range is cited because of the wide variations in criteria such as severity (e.g., is a minor birthmark a "birth anomaly?"), degree of scrutiny (follow-up until the age of four years or beyond is needed to detect some anomalies; some types of inguinal hernia presenting in adulthood are even thought to be congenital; changes in the use of ultrasound can "cause" false alarms by early detection of clinically unapparent heart defects), geography, concomitant disease or toxin exposures (including tobacco, illicit drugs, and alcohol), and socioeconomic status (including differences in rates of access to early intervention). The key to a successful pregnancy registry is that pregnancies should be registered before their outcome is known: the diagnosed birth anomaly can cause bias in reporting frequency, and converts a prospective approach into a retrospective one. The choice of comparison population is highly complex. In general, the assumption of such registry studies is that the appropriate comparison is the general population, effectively a prospective controlled cohort approach. Thus, the objective of such studies is to detect increases of specific defects over the expected rates in the general population. However, the detected occurrence of defects is a function of follow-up method and definition, and may be influenced by many (undocumented or even unknown) factors. Therefore, the conduct of registries and development of such comparisons must be done with great caution. Guidance on these matters has been supplied by the FDA (2002).

Balancing benefits against risks

Critical to understanding the evolving picture of risk with a marketed product is to recognize that such risks emerge with progressively greater experience in increasingly broad and diverse populations over time, experiences that include patients who differ in age, underlying disease state and stage, or even indication from those who were studied in the development process. These uses will have varying impacts, and may materially change the benefits profile from that in the approved product information. Often these issues become particularly important when a newly identified risk may appear to change the balance of benefits against risks to an unacceptable extent, precipitating consideration of possible regulatory withdrawal.

Thus, a program of ongoing research may well be needed which calls upon the skills of the pharmacoepidemiologist, observational studies of drug utilization patterns, often tied to medical outcomes. The professional epidemiologist is the first to caution against cavalier approaches to such effectiveness research. Without the protections of randomization and blinding, many of the biases that have plagued clinical research since its inception can creep in to such studies and render them uninterpretable, or perhaps worse, lead to wrong interpretations. Thus, the research team contemplating the use of observational follow-up studies to understand effectiveness, particularly as part of a revised benefit to risk assessment, needs a pharmacoepidemiologist onboard.

Training to be a pharmacoepidemiologist

No parent has ever heard the statement: "Mummy (or Daddy), I want to be a pharmacoepidemiologist when I grow up"! Very few physicians and pharmaceutical physicians choose this route. But what is along that route? The "high road," in the US at least, is graduation from medical school, obtaining at least one year of intense clinical postgraduate training (often leading to internal medicine or other primary care boards, the equivalent of MRCP in the UK), and then to undertake a further formal residency training program that leads to certification by the American Board of Preventive Medicine. Residencies are inspected and approved by the Board, and may be in one of four areas: public health, general preventive medicine, occupational medicine, or aerospace medicine. Various concentrations in medical management are also becoming recognized. In the UK, registrar positions in most of these specialties are advertised, and the Diplomas in Occupational or Public Health, membership of the Faculties of Occupational or Public Health, and the Diploma in Aviation Medicine would provide equivalent experience and certification.

In the US, the academic equivalent of these, which can often be pursued in parallel, is to obtain the additional degree of Master of Public Health (MPH). Board certification through a preventive medicine residency requires such formal academic training and an MPH degree as well as at least one additional year of structured training or "practicum" entirely within preventive medicine. Again, European equivalents exist. A four to five-year program following graduation in medicine can accomplish all of these. Additionally, those interested in pharmaceutical matters that involve epidemiology, but who do not aspire to board certification, can often attend specialized courses, and use case studies in this area to fulfill their academic requirements, or of course, at least enroll in a MPH degree program. Many of these now exist as "off-campus" (so-called executive) degree programs, particularly for physicians.

Complicating the training challenge for the pharmacoepidemiologist has been the relative paucity of academic centers of excellence specializing in this field. Thus, as part of the FDA Modernization Act of 1997 in the US, Congress created, and the agencies working together have jointly developed, a network of Centers for Education and Research on Therapeutics (CERTs), with particular emphasis on outcomes research and the capacity in pharmacoepidemiology. For further details, the reader should consult the CERTs website (www.ahrq.gov). The International Society for Pharmacoepidemiology maintains a registry of academic centers currently training and conducting research in pharmacoepidemiolgy (www.pharmacoepi.org).

More commonly, if not the "high road," a pharmaceutical physician will stumble into this area by lateral transfer within a company, or due to the chance happening of being assigned a development project that requires extensive pharmacoepidemiologic support. Such physicians can supplement their training with *ad hoc* programs in statistics and epidemiology that are commonly offered on a short-term or part-time nondegree basis by many universities and training groups, or an executive MPH. All physicians seeking to be "credentialed" in Pharmaceutical Medicine will have, as part of the required core competencies for the field, extensive and substantial orientation to the broad field and approaches of pharmacoepidemiology, so that they may be effective demanders and intelligent users of the fruits of pharmacoepidemiology and partners with their physician pharmacoepidemiologist colleagues.

The future

Pharmacoepidemiology has proved itself over the last 20 years since the creation of the International Society for Pharmacoepidemiology in 1989, and will only grow in numbers and in the strength and value of its contributions during the next 20 years. It is unlikely that society as a whole will understand the subtle but vital nuances of the concepts of risk and uncertainty or the complex concept of the balance of harms against benefits any better in 20 years time than it does now. Governments and the general public will require the pharmacoepidemiologist to protect their interests, and to assess accurately the hazards and benefits that today's powerful drugs will also bring. And tomorrow's drugs, driven by the genomics revolution, will only further underscore the need for epidemiology, to help us map the genome to the "phenome," that is, the population manifestations of our genomic makeup, and closely monitor the revolution of personalized therapeutics.

Although it is by no means clear where our earliest experiences with genetic alteration will lead, it is clear that any efforts in this arena will require long-term population-based follow-up. Cost containment will become increasingly a constraint on pharmaceutical medicine, and we must ensure that it does not bring its own hazard. Risk management, with its accompanying accountability, is emerging as a classic epidemiologic challenge. And sentinel surveillance, with the enormous power of large population automated databases, will require the vigilant epidemiologist-physician to ensure medical meaning for statistical findings. The future for the pharmacoepidemiologist trained in both epidemiology and medicine is bright indeed. The lucky men and women who choose pharmacoepidemiology will be highly fulfilled in this subspecialty of pharmaceutical medicine.

References

(Note: all the websites cited in this chapter were accessed April 24, 2010.)

American College of Epidemiology (ACE). *Data Privacy Protections*, 2000; www.acepidemiology.org.

EMA. *Guideline on Risk Management Systems for Medicinal Products for Human Use*. CHMP, December, 2005; www.ema.europa.eu.

FDA. Guidance for Industry: Establishing Pregnancy Exposure Registries, August 2002; http://www.fda.gov/Drugs/GuidanceComplianceRegulatoryInformation/default.htm.

FDA. Guidance for Industry: Risk Minimization, March 2005; http://www.fda.gov/Drugs/GuidanceComplianceRegulatoryInformation/default.htm.

FDA. Proposed Guidance: Format and Content of Proposed Risk Evaluation and Mitigation Strategies, REMS, 30 Sept 2009.

Hartzema AG, Tilson HH, Chan KA (eds). *Pharmacoepidemiology and Therapeutic Risk Management*. Harvey Whitney Books: Cincinnati, USA, 2008.

Institute of Medicine. The future of drug safety. National Academies Press: Washington DC, USA, 2006.

International Society for Pharmacoepidemiology (ISPE). *Data Privacy Protections*, 2003; www.pharmacoepi.org.

Last JM. *Dictionary of Epidemiology*, fourth edition. Oxford University Press: New York, USA, 2001.

Porta M. *Dictionary of Epidemiology*, fifth edition. Oxford University Press: New York, USA, 2008.

Strom BL, Kimmel SW (eds). *Textbook of Pharmacoepidemiology*. John Wiley & Sons Ltd: Chichester, UK, 2006.

CHAPTER 28

Statistical Principles and Application in Biopharmaceutical Research

Dan Anbar
DANA Pharmaceutical Consulting, Inc., NJ, USA

The scientific method and the role of the scientific experiment

The purpose of science is to explain natural phenomena by uncovering the natural laws that give rise to them.

The scientific method is a three-step process:
1. Formulating theories as explanations of phenomena.
2. Making predictions based on these theories.
3. Testing the theories through experimentation.

Most people engage daily in the first two activities. Explaining the environment in which we live is an innate human urge. However, people rarely subject their theories to testing by experimentation.

What characterizes the scientific method is that it does not accept an explanation as valid until it has been validated through testing. However, a scientific experiment can never *prove* a theory. At best, it can provide evidence for the usefulness of the theory in predicting the consequences of given experimental conditions and help to define more precisely the relationship between these conditions and their consequences. The greatest value of a scientific experiment is in its ability to *disprove* a theory or identify limits of its applicability, either of which is key to scientific advances. An experimental finding inconsistent with a theory suggests that the theory should be revised or rejected. Popper (1959) states that a necessary condition for a valid

Principles and Practice of Pharmaceutical Medicine, 3rd edition.
Edited by L.D. Edwards, A.W. Fox, P.D. Stonier.

theory is the condition of *falsifiability*. That is, it must be capable to generate predictions that can be tested experimentally. Experimental outcomes contradicting the theoretical predictions necessitate a reassessment of the theory and lead to a revision or rejection. In other words, a scientific theory is always tentative and entirely dependent on experimental verification. Theories that are not falsifiable may be the subject of religious or philosophical discourse but not of scientific investigation, according to Popper.

Experiments designed to confirm a theory (or to falsify it) are called *confirmatory*, and those designed to merely accumulate information and generate hypotheses are termed *exploratory*. Exploratory experiments are a useful first step in the process of formulating scientific theories. Either type must follow strict methodological procedures and adhere to a detailed experimental protocol describing the conditions of experimentation, the methods of measurement, and all other aspects that might affect the results. The experimenter must record the raw data prior to any analysis and document any protocol deviations, documenting all aspects of the experiment such that another scientist can precisely repeat it.

The statistical method: Making decisions under conditions of uncertainty

The scientific method runs into difficulties when applied to the study of *random phenomena*. A random phenomenon is one where the outcome cannot be predicted with certainty from the experimental conditions. One cannot guarantee the repeat of a coin toss, no matter how hard one tries to keep the conditions constant. Neither can one expect a drug to produce an identical effect in the same patient under identical conditions on separate occasions. Such phenomena can be described probabilistically. That is, one can assign numerical values describing the likelihood, or *probability*, of the possible outcomes. Because of the uncertainty, an isolated failure of a drug to produce an expected therapeutic effect does not prove that the drug is non-efficacious. Similarly, an isolated successful drug treatment outcome does not prove that the drug is efficacious.

Unfortunately, it is impossible to design an experiment that will totally disprove a theory based on random phenomena. Various outcomes may occur, some of which may be unlikely but not impossible. Thus Popper's falsifiability condition does not apply. The statistical method advocated by Fisher (1956) attempts to overcome this problem by substituting "unlikely" for "impossible," but otherwise follows the principles of the scientific method. With this substitution, Fisher and others proposed conceptual structures for testing theories and scientific hypotheses under conditions of uncertainty that are analogous to the scientific method. However, these approaches, although being very useful in practice, have raised a host of conceptual issues that are the subject of ongoing debates.

Let us illustrate the statistical method with an example.

A pharmaceutical company has developed an antihypertensive drug that is theorized to lower diastolic blood pressure when given to subjects with moderate to severe hypertension. If the diastolic blood pressure were constant under given conditions, failure to lower diastolic pressure by any amount in any human subject treated with this drug under a constant set of conditions would disprove the theory. In reality, the subject's blood pressure is a random phenomenon: It varies with or without treatment. Thus, administering the drug to one subject and measuring the resulting change

in blood pressure cannot be used to prove or disprove the hypothesis that the drug has no efficacy. How can one tell whether the difference in blood pressure before and after treatment is due to the effect of the drug or due to the inherent randomness of blood pressure? To answer this question, one must (i) have knowledge of degree of the natural variability of diastolic blood pressure and (ii) determine the likelihood that the observed change in blood pressure is the result of the inherent variability. Measuring variability requires the study of more than one subject. Thus, a statistical experiment always consists of the study of groups of subjects rather than individual ones.

A typical experiment might look like this: Subjects are selected from a target population to participate in the study. They are assigned to one of two groups, A and B. Group A receives no treatment or a placebo. Group B receives the test drug. A quantitative variable that is hypothesized to be affected by the drug (e.g., the measured diastolic blood pressure), the *efficacy variable*, is measured in all subjects before treatment (baseline) and at some time point when the drug effect should be measurable if the drug is efficacious. Mean change from baseline in the efficacy variable is compared between the groups. If the magnitude of the difference appears to be consistent with what would be expected due to the randomness of the measurements, the drug is probably ineffective. If the magnitude is substantially larger, and nothing else has changed in the experimental conditions between the two time points, it is probably due to the effect of the drug. The starting point for the experimenter is the hypothesis that the drug is ineffective. Thus, the smaller the probability that the observed difference is due to randomness, the more confidence the experimenter has that the hypothesis of no efficacy is incorrect.

This example illustrates the basic steps in statistical research methodology:

1. A scientific question is posed ("the drug effect is to reduce blood pressure").

2. An experiment is designed so that in the absence of randomness it would yield distinctly different outcomes ("treat one group of subject with the presumed active drug and another with inert

Table 28.1 Type I and type II errors in statistical decision-making

Real state	Decision	
	Accept hypothesis	Reject hypothesis
Hypothesis is true		Type I error
Hypothesis is false	Type II error	

substance, or placebo") and a test variable is defined ("the mean change from baseline to post-treatment blood pressure").

3. A statistical hypothesis is formulated, that is, the scientific hypothesis is formulated in terms of the test variable ("the mean reduction in blood pressure in the group treated with the new drug is greater than that of the placebo-treated group").

4. A decision criterion is formulated, that is, which outcomes of the experiment would lead to the rejection and which to the acceptance of the hypothesis.

5. The experiment is conducted, the data are collected, and the test variable observed in the experiment is calculated ("the mean change from baseline to post-treatment blood pressure is calculated for the two groups of subjects").

6. A decision is made using the decision criterion.

The key difference between the statistical method and the scientific method is that statistically the result, no matter how unlikely, is not impossible. Therefore, any decision to confirm or reject a hypothesis is liable to error. Depending on whether the hypothesis is in fact true or false, two types of error are possible: *type I error* and *type II error*. As can be seen from Table 28.1, type I error is committed when a true hypothesis is rejected wrongly and type II error is committed when a false hypothesis is declared as true.

The statistical test: The null hypothesis, error probabilities, statistical power

Seemingly, the decision whether a drug is efficacious or not, is a dichotomy. In reality, however, it is a continuum. If we consider the measurable

effect (E) of our drug in lowering diastolic blood pressure, then lack of efficacy corresponds to $E = 0$. Positive efficacy corresponds to $E > 0$, which consists of a continuum of possibilities depending on the magnitude of the effect. Thus, the hypothesis of no efficacy is very specific in terms of the size of the effect and is called a *simple hypothesis*, whereas a hypothesis corresponding to a range of values is called a *composite hypothesis*.

As we have seen, both the scientific method and the statistical method are designed to prove a claim false rather than true. In drug testing, the statistical experiment is designed to reject the *null hypothesis*: the hypothesis of lack of efficacy, or that there is no difference between the treatments being tested. Applying the definitions of type I and type II errors to the null hypothesis we obtain the following;

• *Type I error:* Rejection of the null hypothesis when it is true (an ineffective drug is judged effective).

• *Type II error:* Acceptance of the null hypothesis when it is false (an effective drug is judged ineffective).

Type I error is often also called "False Positive" and type II error "False Negative." Because rejection of the null hypothesis enables one to make the scientific claim that the study was performed to prove, statisticians label such a rejection as *significant*. When the result of a statistical test is declared significant, the only error that could have occurred is type I error. Clearly, the smaller the probability of type I error, the more secure one is in rejecting the null hypothesis. The probability of a type I error is called the *significance level* of the test and is denoted by α. The probability of a type II error is denoted by β and 1 − β is called the *power* of the test, often expressed as percent. Thus, the power of the test is the probability of rejecting the null hypothesis when it is false. When the null hypothesis is that the drug is not efficacious, the power is the probability that the test would declare the drug as efficacious when indeed it is so. The null hypothesis is usually a simple hypothesis. Therefore, α is usually a single number. The alternative to the null hypothesis, however, is typically a composite hypothesis.

In our antihypertensive drug testing example, this alternative was the whole region $E > 0$. In this case, the value of β and the power $1 - \beta$ depend on the specific value of E. Thus, it is meaningless to talk about the power of a statistical test without specifying the alternative for which it applies. In our example, the power of the test at $E = 10$ is the probability that the statistical test would be significant if the effect of the drug is to reduce the diastolic blood pressure by 10 mmHg on average.

It is desirable that a statistical test should have as small α and β (i.e., a small type I error and high power) as possible with regard to alternatives of interest. The perfect test would have $\alpha = \beta = 0$. However, as we will see, this is not possible in practice due to the fact that all experimental measurements involve errors. If, in our example, the clinician estimates that the drug should lower diastolic blood pressure by an average of about 10 mmHg, the statistician would want α to be small, say ≤ 0.05, and $1 - \beta$ to be large, say ≥ 0.95, for the alternative $E = 10$. Can the statistician design a study such that the test would have any desirable α and β? The answer is generally, yes, by selecting an appropriate sample size; that is, by including a sufficient number of subjects in the study. Once the sample size is fixed, the relationship between α and β is determined. Any further reduction in α must be compensated by a corresponding increase in β, and vice versa. For a given study design, the only way to decrease α and β simultaneously is by increasing the sample size. We will discuss this topic in greater detail in the later section, "Study design: determining the sample size."

Causality

The ultimate goal of clinical research is to establish causality: to determine efficacy outcomes that are caused by the drug, to measure their magnitude, and to identify adverse effects associated with the drug.

How does one know whether an effect A (e.g., giving a particular drug at a particular dose) causes an event B (e.g., diastolic blood pressure is reduced)? Two conditions must be satisfied. First, A must precede B. Second, whenever A occurs, B must occur too. These, of course, are not suf-

ficient, because both A and B could be caused by an effect C. In addition, therefore, a theory is required that links A to B. This requirement is the Achilles Heel of "causality," because all theories are necessarily tentative. In an experimental science such as pharmaceutical research, the second condition can be established by conducting an experiment both when effect A is absent and when effect A is present, whereas all other conditions remain unchanged. If B requires the presence of A, one can conclude that A causes B. However, if B is present regardless of A, no causality is proven.

In studying drug effects in humans, the controlled clinical trial is the preferred method to establish causality. In its simplest form, a controlled clinical trial is an experiment in human subjects in which some subjects are treated with an investigational drug and some are not, whereas all other conditions remain the same for the two treatment groups. In this way, differences in clinical outcomes can be attributed to the investigational drug (Controlled Clinical Trials (CCT) will be discussed in greater detail in the later section "The Controlled Clinical Trial: basic design elements."

Variability: The source of uncertainty

Virtually no drug has an identical response in all patients. For example, an effective antibiotic will almost certainly be ineffective in some patients, possibly because such patients are infected with a resistant strain or have a deficient immune response. Variability in response introduces uncertainty in establishing cause and effect. The fact that administering a drug to a given subject has not resulted with the desired therapeutic effect does not necessarily imply that the drug is ineffective. Causality in the strict sense discussed in the previous section can no longer be established when outcome of an experiment is subject to variability. However, one can still talk about causality in a *probabilistic* sense by modifying the requirement that "whenever A is present B *must* be present too" necessary for the establishment of causality, to "the *probability* that B will occur is *greater* in the presence of A than when A is not present."

Another issue is that when the measurement of efficacy is variable, it is impossible to determine what part of the measured outcome is due to the effect of the drug and what part is due to variability unrelated to the drug effect. The size of a drug effect is called the "signal," whereas the variability associated with it is referred to as the "noise." Clearly, the larger the "signal-to-noise ratio," the easier it is to establish a causal relationship. Thus, in a clinical drug trial, it is equally important to measure both noise and signal. How are these measured? The nature of variability is that the effect of interest is random. When we measure the blood pressure of an individual subject repeatedly, the measurements will be dispersed around some central value in a random fashion; some will be larger and some smaller. The effect, however, is systematic. If, for example, we measure the blood pressure of an individual repeatedly before and just after administering an antihypertensive drug, the pre-treatment and post-treatment measurements will be dispersed around different central values, the post-treatment value being lower than the pre-treatment value. The magnitude of the effect (signal) is usually calculated as the mean of the individual effects in a population of subjects. The variability (noise) is usually calculated as the standard deviation.

Example: Suppose ten hypertensive subjects are treated with a novel antihypertensive drug. The subjects' blood pressure is measured at 8 a.m., just prior to the administration of the drug, and then again 1 hour later. Data are as shown in Table 28.2.

The first and the second rows of Table 28.2 give the diastolic blood pressure of subjects before and after treatment, respectively. The third row gives the change (*D*) in diastolic pressure (value in row 1 minus the value in row 2). The mean, given in the last column, is 12.8 mmHg. On the face of it, 12.8 looks like an impressive effect. However, as we have discussed earlier, we cannot assess its significance without considering the inherent variability, the noise. Indeed, the values of *D* range from −4 to 33, a substantial range.

To assess *D*'s variability, we calculated the deviations of the values of *D* about their mean 12.8. These values are given in the next row. Naturally, as the mean is a value somewhere in the middle, some deviations are positive and others are negative. One property of the mean is that the sum of these deviations is always zero. Thus, the average (mean) of the deviations around the mean is always zero, and therefore is not useful as a measure of the variability. Instead, we calculate the mean of the squares of the deviations about the mean as a measure of variability. This measure is called the *variance*. The variance is an average of nonnegative numbers and it is, therefore, always a nonnegative number. It is equal to 0 if and only if all the deviates are equal to zero, meaning that all the measurements are the same and thus equal to their mean, that is, there is no variability at all. The *standard deviation* (S.D.), the most commonly used measure of variability, is the square root of the variance. In our case

$$S.D. = \sqrt{110.16} = 10.50$$

The advantage of using the standard deviation over the variance is that it is measured with the same units as the mean. The mean does not

Table 28.2 Diastolic blood pressure before and after treatment (mmHg) (hypothetical data)

	Subject										
	1	2	3	4	5	6	7	8	9	10	Mean
Before treatment	102	78	95	86	109	107	100	86	96	92	95.1
After treatment	75	82	80	81	76	93	92	80	90	74	82.3
Difference (*D*)	27	−4	15	5	33	14	8	6	6	18	12.8
(*D* − mean *D*)	14.2	−16.8	2.2	−7.8	20.2	1.2	−4.8	−6.8	−6.8	5.2	0
(*D* − mean *D*)^2	201.64	282.24	4.84	60.84	408.04	1.44	23.04	46.24	46.24	27.04	110.16

represent the response to treatment of any particular individual. It does, though, give us an idea of the magnitude of the response to treatment produced by the drug. Can we conclude, then, that the drug is efficacious? If the drug is ineffective, there should be no systematic change in blood pressure measurements taken 1 hour after treatment as compared to pre-treatment measurements and thus the mean change should equal approximately to zero. The observed mean change of 12.8 mmHg is then due entirely to chance. Statistical theory shows that the likelihood that a sample of ten numbers drawn at random from a set of numbers with mean zero (in our example, the set of all possible post-treatment minus pre-treatment blood pressure measurements) with standard deviation of 10.5 would have a mean of 12.8 or larger is less than 0.15% (or 15 in 10,000). Although this outcome is not impossible, it is highly unlikely. Thus, it is more prudent to conclude that the drug is efficacious and that the observed mean of 12.8 is due to a systematic effect caused by the drug rather than to chance.

The above example encapsulates many of the ideas and concepts behind the theory of statistical inference. The standard deviation quantifies how widely a measurement is expected to deviate from a theoretical typical value of the variable being measured. In our example, the variable being measured is the change between pre-treatment and post-treatment in a patient's diastolic blood pressure. So, if the drug is ineffective, any change is due entirely to chance and therefore one would expect the change to be zero. This expected typical value is theoretical. In reality, blood pressure is affected by a variety of factors independent of the treatment and therefore actual measurements will not necessarily be zero. The standard deviation enables us to calculate the probability that the measurements will fall close to or far away from zero. For example, the probability is 95% that a measurement will fall within ± 2 S.D. That is, assuming the drug is ineffective and the standard deviation is 10.5, 95% of patients treated with the drug should have a change in their pre-treatment and post-treatment diastolic blood pressure between -21 and 21.

This is a fairly large range and indeed all but two of the measurements in our example are within this range. This observation does not contradict our previous conclusion that the drug is effective. This is because our conclusion that the drug is effective was based on the mean of ten measurements rather than on a single measurement. The mean change is also associated with experimental error. If we calculate the mean change for another set of ten measurements obtained from different patients, it is unlikely that the result will be exactly 12.8. However, the variability associated with a mean is smaller than that of a single measurement. The standard deviation associated with the mean is called the *standard error of the mean* (SEM) and is smaller than the S.D. by a factor equal to the square root of the number of measurements used to calculate the mean. In our example, SEM $= (10.5/\sqrt{10})$ $= (10.5/3.16) = 3.32$. Thus, in our experiment, the probability is 95% that the mean change will fall between -6.64 and $+6.64$. The mean of 12.8 is well outside that range. In fact, $(12.8/\text{SEM}) = 3.85$. The probability of observed sample mean to be a distance of 3.85 SEMs or more from the actual population mean is approximately 0.15 %.

To summarize, statistical methods are not intended to establish a cause and effect relationship between treatment and the response of any *individual* subject; rather, they establish a cause and effect relationship in the aggregate response (e.g., the mean) of a *population* of subjects. The key to this is the fact that by considering aggregates, one can control the variability of a measured quantity. By increasing the sample size, one can reduce the standard error of the mean to a level that would make it possible to determine whether a signal is likely or unlikely to be due to chance and thus decide whether a causal relationship is likely or unlikely to exist.

The Controlled Clinical Trial: Basic design elements

Randomization

The CCT is the scientific tool for demonstrating causality. Two essential elements characterize the CCT: (i) it contains a control group and an experimental group; and (ii) with the exception of treatment, all other conditions and procedures to which the subjects are exposed during the trial are constant. These two characteristics of the CCT enable the researcher to establish a causal relationship between treatment and the outcome of the trial. The tool for standardizing the trial is the study protocol, which is the document defining the subjects eligible for inclusion in the study and the study procedures, schedules, and methods.

A key element is the method of allocating subjects to the treatment groups. Subjects may possess a variety of characteristics that could influence their response to treatment. These could be related to the subject's demographic background, such as age, sex, ethnic origin, genetic disposition, or other prognostic variables: factors that could influence the response to treatment. The method of allocating subjects to treatment must be such that the resulting treatment groups are balanced with respect to such factors. The most effective way to achieve this is by randomization. That is, each subject is assigned to a treatment group using a chance mechanism. Of course, one could achieve the desired balance by using a systematic, nonrandom allocation scheme that will force the balance. Randomization, however, has some important advantages. Any nonrandom method inevitably involves a decision by the individual making the allocation. This potentially could result with the preference of a certain type of subjects for one of the treatments that may not be reflected as an imbalance in any of the identified prognostic variables. Furthermore, there might be some other variables that affect the response to treatment and which are either unrecognized as such at the time the study is planned, or are impossible to balance for logistical reasons. A random allocation, at least in large trials, will typically protect the investigator against such problems.

To achieve a completely random allocation, one could use a mechanism such as a simple toss of a balanced coin or anything equivalent to it and assign a subject to receive treatment A if the coin lands on Heads ("H"), say, and treatment B if the outcome is Tails ("T"). Although the result of a coin toss is a perfect random sequence of Hs and Ts, the number of Hs and Ts in any random sequence of coin tosses is rarely the same. The result of using a coin toss mechanism for treatment allocation would typically result in an unequal number of subjects allocated to the different treatment groups, an undesirable statistical design property.

The most common method of randomization that will guarantee that approximately equal number of subjects is allocated to the different treatment groups is the *randomized blocks* method. Let us illustrate this for a trial with three treatment groups: A, B, and C. Blocks containing the letters A, B. and C in a random order, with each letter repeated the same number of times, are generated. Such a block of length 6 might look like (B, B, A, C, C, A). The requirement that each letter appears in the block as frequently as any of the other two letters implies that the length of the block must be a multiple of 3. Thus, for the case of three treatment groups, the block size must be 3, 6, 9, and so on. The number of such random blocks generated must be such that the number of letters in the resulting string equals or exceeds the number of subjects to be enrolled in the trial. Subjects are then assigned sequentially to the treatment group corresponding to the next unassigned letter in the randomization string. Because each individual block contains the same number of each of the letters, the treatment assignment sequence obtained from the randomized blocks method is not exactly a sequence of random numbers. However, it is approximately so and has the advantage that it guarantees a maximum balance in the resulting sizes of the treatment groups. In fact, the number of subjects allocated to two treatment groups cannot differ by more than the number of times each treatment is repeated within the block.

Bias and blinding

Statisticians routinely use data obtained from a sample to estimate unknown characteristics of the population from which the sample was drawn. The estimate is subject to variability inherited from the data. Thus, different samples would result in different values of the estimate that are distributed around a mean value. *Bias* is the difference between that mean value and the quantity it intends to estimate. The bias, then, is a measure of the magnitude by which a statistical estimation method is systematically overestimating or underestimating the parameter it is designed to estimate. We refer to this type of bias as *statistical bias*. Clinical researchers often use the term "bias" in a broader, though less precise, fashion. They refer to bias as t*he effect of any factor, or combination of factors, resulting in inferences, which lead systematically to incorrect decisions about the treatment effect*. Although this usage has the appeal that it corresponds to our intuitive understanding of the word "bias," it cannot be quantified because of its imprecision. It is, nevertheless, useful in discussing problems that could result from a faulty design or inadequate conduct of a trial.

The most common source of bias is one resulting from subjects being selected to the different treatment groups in a way that creates an imbalance in one or more prognostic factors. This type of bias, known as *selection bias*, is usually the result of unconscious action on the part of the investigator or other people involved in the enrolment of subjects into the trial, or of a faulty treatment allocation method. Randomization is designed to take the treatment assignment decision away from the enrolling investigator and place it in the hands of chance. Unfortunately, it is not foolproof. An investigator who has a personal preference for one treatment over another for a particular type of subject may decide to postpone enrolling a subject until the "right" treatment comes up on the randomization schedule. Also, there are many other ways that are not affected by randomization, in which the investigator can influence the trial outcome. A simple talk with a subject reinforcing the subject's confidence in the efficacy of treatment can often have a real or transient effect on the subject's response to treatment.

Another potential source of bias is the subject him- or herself. Often, the mere expectation that the drug will have a therapeutic effect produces an effect. This effect is known as the *placebo effect*, and in some cases, it could be considerable.

To counteract these types of bias, subjects are assigned to treatment in a *blinded* fashion. That is, the identity of the assigned treatment is concealed from everybody who can influence the treatment assignments and any procedure that could impact the trial outcome. When the treatments are masked from both the investigator and the subject, the trial is called *double blind*. In drug trials, blinding is accomplished by using placebo, an inert substance, as a nonactive control along with identically looking packaging, for the different treatments, with coded labels that do not reveal the identity of the drug.

The use of double-blind randomized clinical trials has become the gold standard for good clinical research. However, it is not always possible to mask the treatments. A trial designed to compare the effectiveness of two surgical procedures, for example, or a trial comparing an intravenous drug to an oral drug, cannot be blinded. In principle, one could blind such a trial by delivering an inert substance (e.g., saline) intravenously to the oral drug group and an oral placebo to the intravenous group. However, this procedure might be controversial for ethical reasons because subjects are exposed to additional risk, albeit small, without direct potential benefit to them. When the comparators have distinct characteristics that would identify them such as smell or taste, route of administration, etc., blinding can be achieved by encapsulation of the drug substance or by using the so-called "double-dummy" method unless it is ethically unacceptable. The "double-dummy" method means that all subjects receive identically looking treatments only one of which is active and the others are placebos. For example, in a comparison of two oral drugs, one of which is a tablet and the other a capsule, each subject receives a tablet and a capsule, one of which contains the treatment assigned to that subject and the other is placebo. Sometimes even the "double-dummy" method is not helpful. The drug might have a characteristic profile, such as characteristic adverse event or other biological effect that would reveal the identity of the treatment either to the investigator or to the subject or both, no matter how the drug is packaged or labeled. When blinding is not possible, special efforts must be made to minimize the possibility of introducing bias by incorporating appropriate bias prevention methods in the study design. Once bias

Table 28.3 Heartbeat measurements of 20 students

Student	Heartbeat
1	60
2	53
3	56
4	56
5	56
6	57
7	56
8	52
9	63
10	51
11	59
12	63
13	55
14	58
15	56
16	53
17	64
18	56
18	58
20	55
Mean	56.8
S.D.	3.57

Table 28.4 Heartbeat measurements of 20 students by exercise status

	Subject	Heartbeat
Group A	2	53
	8	52
	7	56
	13	55
	20	55
	5	56
	4	55
	18	56
	10	51
	16	53
Mean		54.2
S.D.		1.81
Group B	12	63
	15	56
	14	58
	1	60
	11	59
	6	57
	9	63
	3	56
	17	64
	19	58
Mean		59.4
S.D.		2.99

is introduced, it is very difficult and sometimes impossible to adjust for it at the analysis stage.

Stratification

An efficient study design is one that maximizes the "signal-to-noise ratio." Therefore, controlling the "noise," or variability, is an important aspect of a good design. Consider the following example.

A graduate student in Public Health is conducting a research project on the health-related habits of the students at her university. As part of the project, she measured the resting heartbeat of 20 student subjects. The results are listed in Table 28.3.

The mean and standard deviation are 56.8 and 3.57, respectively. The student further divided the subjects into two groups: Group A consists of subjects who do aerobic exercises regularly and Group B of those who do not. The results are presented in Table 28.4.

We notice that the two groups of subjects have different means and different standard deviations. Both standard deviations are smaller than the one obtained before separating the subjects into sub-

groups. That is, the two groups are more homogeneous than the original group. When one combines the standard deviations into so-called pooled standard deviation, the result is $S.D._{pooled} = 2.47$, which is substantially lower than the standard deviation of the original group. The reason for this is that when we calculated the mean of the combined group, we ignored the fact that the group consisted of two subgroups with different means. Thus, the calculated mean was in fact, a mean of the two subgroups' means. Indeed, the overall mean 56.8 equals the average of the means of the two subgroups, that is, $56.8 = (54.2 + 59.4)/2$. Similarly, the standard deviation represents the sum of two sources of variation: the intra-group variability represented by the two subgroups' standard deviations, and the intergroup variability represented by the difference between the two subgroups' means.

In general, if one combines two groups of measurements with the same number of measurements in each group and if the standard deviations of the two groups and the combined group are denoted by S_1, S_2 and S, respectively, and if the means of the two groups and the combined group are denoted by M_1, M_2 and M, respectively, then the following relationship holds:

$$S^2 = \frac{1}{2}\left(S_1^2 + S_2^2\right) + \frac{1}{2}\left((M_1 - M)^2 + (M_2 - M)^2\right)$$
$$= \frac{1}{2}(S_1^2 + S_2^2) + \left(\frac{M_1 - M_2}{2}\right)^2$$

The variance of the combined group is the sum of the two parts: The first is the average of the variances of the two individual groups, and the second is the square of one half of the difference between the means of the two groups. The first part represents the intra-group variation and the second the intergroup variation.

This example illustrates well the idea behind stratification. The study population is usually quite heterogeneous. If one measures the effect of treatment by calculating the overall mean effect in the population, although this mean represents an estimate of the treatment effect in this population, it might be associated with a large error that could make it difficult to distinguish the signal from the background noise. In other words, the overall mean may be an estimate of the treatment effect, but an inefficient one. If one can identify *a priori* certain subgroups, or *strata*, in the study population that are more homogeneous with respect to the efficacy variable of interest in the trial, then by estimating the effect within each of these strata and combining these estimates one may increase substantially the power of the analysis because the noise masking the effect of interest is reduced.

It is well known, for example, that in multicenter trials, the measured effect often varies from one investigator to another. This could be due to many reasons such as the physician's procedures, his or her instruments, the method of evaluating the subject's response, the hospital care protocol, diet, etc. This is particularly the case when the measurements have a great degree of subjectivity. Sometimes the difference is due to the characteristics of subject populations from which the different investigators draw their subjects. Whatever the reason, it is common practice to stratify the subjects by investigators. It is also wise to identify important prognostic variables and design the trial so as to stratify according to them. Examples of some common stratification variables are sex, race, age, disease severity, Karnofsky status score in cancer studies, disease staging, and so forth. When strata are identified the randomization process performed within the strata. This helps to equalize the number of subjects in the various treatment groups within each of the strata and balance them with respect to the stratification variables. The drawback is that as the number of important prognostic variables increases, the number of strata increases by multiples, thus complicating the trial's logistics. For example, if one wants to stratify by sex and race, then sex has two categories (male and female) and race has four (White, Black, Hispanic, other), and the number of strata is eight. Adding another variable with three categories, such as disease severity at baseline (mild, moderate, severe), will bring the number of strata to 24. If, in addition, investigator is a stratification variable, this would mean that each data center performing the randomization will have to manage 24 randomization tables for each investigator, one for each stratum, which is utterly impractical. For a study of moderate size of 100–500 subjects, a large number of strata may mean that some strata may contain very small number of subjects, which complicates the statistical analysis and its interpretation.

In summary, stratification is a very useful tool for noise reduction, but it has its limitations. Usually, the one stratification variable used in multicenter trials is the investigational site. More than one additional variable can introduce serious logistical and methodological difficulties. If one is not concerned about the investigator's effect, central randomization procedures can be very useful in situations of complex stratification requirements. Computerized central randomization procedures are now available that make complex stratification schemes possible.

Blocking

Another common method employed to decrease the background variability is *blocking*. Like stratification, blocking involves the subdivision of the subject population into homogeneous subgroups. The experimenter defines block of subjects and randomizes the subjects within each block to the study treatments such that the same number of subjects are assigned to each treatment within each block. The blocks are defined so that the intra-block variability is minimal. For example, to determine whether a drug is carcinogenic, rats of the same litter are randomized to receive several doses of the drug or placebo. This way, effects due to genetic variation are minimized.

To take advantage of the block design, the treatments are compared within each block and then the information is pooled across blocks. When the "within-block" or "intra-block" variability is substantially smaller than the "between-block" or "inter-block" variability, blocked designs could be very efficient in the use of subject resources. One disadvantage of blocked designs is that they do not allow for missing data. If data from one subject in the block are missing, the entire block may be disqualified.

A variation on the idea of blocking is the *crossover* design. Here, each block consists of one subject who receives the study treatments in a random order. Crossover experiments are frequently used in bioavailability and pharmacokinetic studies. The reason is that the pharmacokinetic parameters that determine the absorption, distribution, and metabolism of the drug in the body and its elimination from the body depend on the biological makeup of the subject and vary, often considerably, from subject to subject. Thus, the inter-subject variability is typically much higher than the intra-subject variability.

In crossover studies, the treatments are compared within each subject and then summarized across subjects. The crossover design is different from the blocked design described above in that each block consists of a single subject, which means that measurements within each block are not independent of each other. Furthermore, it is possible that a residual effect of one drug carries over to impact the effect of another drug administered subsequently. Statistical analytical methods are limited in their ability to adjust and correct for such effects.

This is why the use of crossover designs in clinical research is limited.

In summary, the design of a clinical trial incorporates methods of minimizing noise and the prevention of bias. This is done through the use of appropriate subject allocation procedures, such as randomization and blinding or through the use of stratification and blocking.

The study population: Inclusion and exclusion criteria

Generalizability

The study of the pharmaceutical effect of a drug is always done in reference to a population of prospective patients. For example, the clinical dose to be recommended for an older patient is often different than for a younger patient. Thus, the target population for the study must be well defined in advance. Obviously, it is impractical to study the entire patient population of interest. Fortunately, this is also not necessary. Statistical sampling methodology enables us to draw conclusions from a sample to the population from which the sample had been drawn, to any desirable degree of accuracy and confidence. But there is one important caveat to this ability: The sample must be "representative" of the population of interest, meaning that the sample must preserve all the relevant characteristics of the population. That is, samples should have the similar proportions of men and women, similar racial composition, similar numbers of hypertensive patients, and so on. Clearly, the creation of an exact replica of the population on a small scale is an impossible task. However, statistical sampling methods can produce very close to representative samples with very high probability. These are the methods utilized by pollsters to make highly reliable predictions and inferences on the population from relatively small samples.

In clinical research, the random selection of subjects to be included in the trial from the target population is not practical. Subjects are usually selected from the patient pools available to the investigators participating in the trial. This, in and of itself, is problematic. The subject pool available to a particular center usually reflects the population in the geographical area where the center is located,which may not represent the general potential patient population. To complicate things even further, some of the subjects available at a given center may not be suitable for enrollment in a trial with an experimental drug. The investigator may wish to exclude certain subjects because of certain known or unknown risks. The possible effects of drugs on the unborn fetus and infants are often unknown, and thus pregnant or lactating women are usually excluded. Potential subjects may be excluded if they are taking another medication, which can potentially interact with the study drug. Also, some potential subjects may refuse to participate in the trial for one reason or other. Finally, for the purpose of studying the efficacy of a drug, it is desirable to enroll only subjects who are most likely to have a measurable response to treatment. Thus, every trial protocol contains a list of inclusion and exclusion criteria defining the subject population to be studied. Obviously, such a population is hardly ever fully representative of the target population. This raises a question regarding the generalizability of the trial's conclusions.

When defining a set of inclusion and exclusion criteria for a trial, the issue of generalizability must be kept in mind. The rule is that the more restrictive the criteria, the less generalizable the results. On the other hand, setting criteria for eligibility to participate in the trial provides the investigator with an important tool for controlling the variability. Thus, the choice of eligibility criteria must be guided so as to balance the statistical efficiency of the trial design against the need to ensure that the results are generalizable. Some of the guiding principles for defining subjects' eligibility are described in the following sections.

Homogeneity

Homogeneity of the subject population is an important factor in controlling variability. The more homogeneous the subject population generating the data, the more informative it is. Thus, fewer subjects are required to achieve the desired control of the statistical errors when a study is conducted in a homogeneous subject population as compared to

when the subjects are drawn from a heterogeneous population. The problem is that the more homogenous the group of subjects, the less representative of the general potential patient population it is. In the early stages of drug development, where the goal is to establish the general perimeters for the drug safety and efficacy, and provide information for the design of future studies, studies are usually carried out on a limited number of subjects. In these early trials, it is the subjects' safety that is of primary concern, and the question of efficacy is secondary. The scope of the efficacy-related questions is limited to the "proof of principle," that is, a demonstration of clinical activity, the identification of a safe dose range, and information leading to the choice of dose and regimen for further studies. Subjects are selected who are most likely to respond to treatment, present no obvious potential safety risks and are as similar as possible. Later stage studies such as confirmative Phase III trials, those providing pivotal information for the proof of the drug's efficacy and safety, are generally less restrictive.

Safety

The safety of the subjects enrolled in the trial is always the primary concern of the researcher. Individuals at high or unknown risk to treatment with the drug are excluded from the study. For example, women of childbearing potential are usually excluded or required to use an acceptable method of birth control. Similarly, patients who are taking medications that might interact with the experimental drug, or who have medical conditions that place them at increased risk, are also excluded from participation.

Selection of subjects: maximizing the signal-to-noise ratio

Clinical trials are very expensive undertakings. Also, because they involve human subjects, there is always an ethical imperative to use the subject resources judiciously. Often, the researcher has only one chance to conduct a trial designed to answer a given question. Thus, the efficiency of the trial design is critical. In other words, the design must be such that the signal-to-noise ratio is maximized. The selection of subjects by specifying certain inclusion and exclusion criteria may go a long way in this direction. The exclusion of patients with poor prognosis who are unlikely to respond to treatment, the inclusion of only patients with more than minimal severity of their condition, and similar measures are often used to achieve this goal. Again, one must be careful not to narrow the subject population to the extent that the results could not be generalized to a broader patient population.

The placebo effect

Placebo is the preferred control in the double-blind Randomized Controlled Clinical Trial (RCCT). Although placebo is not supposed to have any relevant biological activity, it is well known that it often produces remarkable therapeutic responses. This phenomenon occurs across the therapeutic board. It seems that mere knowledge that the subject is being treated for a condition often produces a measurable favorable response (Bok, 1974; Gribbin, 1981). A high placebo response will tend to mask the response of the experimental drug. Since placebo is rarely used outside the clinical research setting, some people argue that the comparison with placebo tends to show lower response rates for the drug than would later be observed in general use. Thus, goes the argument, the placebo-controlled trial puts the test drug at a disadvantage. The counter argument is that what one sees in the clinic is perhaps the combination of the placebo effect plus the drug's biological effect, and therefore, establishing the residual effect of the drug over its inherent placebo effect should be the true objective of the trial.

Whatever the case might be, the placebo effect invariably results in a decrease in the signal-to noise ratio. Therefore, measures are often taken to select subjects whose placebo response is low or nil. One way of accomplishing this is by treating prospective subjects with placebo for some time prior to randomization. Patients whose response during this screening phase is high or very variable are then disqualified from participating in the trial.

In summary, the selection of subjects to be enrolled in the trial using a list of entrance criteria is an important tool that helps to sharpen the signal-to-noise ratio, thus making the study more powerful. It also helps in understanding the extent to which the study conclusions can be generalized to a broader population of patients than those studied under the artificial conditions of a clinical trial.

The statistical model

The statistical model is the mathematical framework in which the statistician operates. It provides the statistician with the tools to quantify the information obtained during the trial and defines relationships among the various measurements. It provides a framework for evaluating the properties of the statistical methods used to analyze the data and answer the questions the study is designed to address.

What is a statistical model?

A statistical model consists of a set of assumptions about the nature of the data to be collected in the trial and about the interrelationships among various variables. These assumptions must be specific enough that they could be expressed by a set of mathematical expressions and equations.

For example: In a placebo-controlled clinical trial for testing a new analgesic for treatment of migraine headaches, the key efficacy variable is the number of subjects whose headache is eliminated within 1 hour of treatment. A statistical model appropriate for this situation is as follows.

Let p denote the probability that a subject treated with a drug will have their headache disappear 1 hour after treatment, following an episode of migraine headache. If the responses of different subjects are independent of each other, this probability can be expressed as

$$\text{Prob. (no. of responses} = k) = cp^k(1 - p)^{N-k},$$
$$\text{for } 0 \le k \le N$$

where N is the number of subjects treated and c is a constant representing the number of possible combinations of k elements out of N. This model is known as the Binomial Model.

The trial objective is to determine if the new drug is more efficacious than placebo. Within the context of this model, one could declare the drug as "more efficacious" if $p_d > p_p$, where p_d is the probability of response for a subject treated with the new drug and p_p the probability of response of a placebo-treated subject.

The data collected during the trial will provide information about p_d and p_p, enabling the statistician to test the null hypothesis H_0: $\Delta = p_d - p_p = 0$ against the alternative hypothesis H_1: $\Delta = p_d - p_p > 0$.

This very simple model provides sufficient structure for the statistician to design a statistical test to test these hypotheses. As was discussed in earlier in the section "The statistical test: the null hypothesis, error probabilities, statistical power," the statistical test is a device providing a rule for decision-making associated with possible errors. The study design must be such that the error probabilities are properly controlled. In other words, the researcher must decide on acceptable levels of α and β, the probabilities of type I and type II errors. Typically, α is chosen to be 0.05, or 5%, and β between 0.05 and 0.20, depending on how serious the consequences are of committing a type II error ("False Negative"). As the type II error probability is calculated under the assumption that the alternative hypothesis is true, it depends on the value of Δ. The investigator must specify a value of Δ for which the type II error should be calculated. This value is *the smallest clinically important* Δ. In our example, the clinician might consider an increase in the probability of response, of less than 50% to be not clinically meaningful. So, if it is known that 15% of patients treated with placebo report the disappearance of their headache, $\Delta = 0.075$, or 7.5%. Using the model and this information, the statistician can calculate the number of subjects required in the trial to guarantee that the statistical test will have the desired power, say 90%, to detect this increase if it is true, while maintaining the type I error below a desired low level, say 5%.

Another commonly used statistical model is the Linear Model, which represents a family of models of a similar structure. The most commonly employed linear model is the analysis of variance model (ANOVA). We shall illustrate this model using the simplest case, the one-way ANOVA model. The model is used to describe continuous data such as blood pressure.

The model assumes that the observed variable of interest Y (e.g., diastolic blood pressure) can be expressed as a sum of a number of factors:

$$Y = \mu + t + \varepsilon \tag{28.1}$$

Here μ represents the overall mean diastolic blood pressure in the population under study, t represents the increase (or decrease) of the blood pressure due to treatment, and ε represents a random error. The model makes two additional assumptions:

(a) ε behaves like a Normal (Gaussian) variable with mean zero and some (unknown) standard deviation.

(b) The measurements obtained from different subjects are independent of each other.

The quantities μ and t are called the *model parameters*, sometimes referred to as the *independent variables*. There is one additional parameter in this model, which is the standard deviation of the random error ε. It is not explicitly evident from Equation (28.1) but is implicit in assumption (a). The model parameters are unknown quantities that must be estimated from the data. The data here are represented by the symbol Y, sometimes referred to as the *dependent variable*. The relationship between the data and the model parameters is expressed by the linear equation (28.1), hence the name Linear Model.

Linear models can be quite complicated when additional structure, parameters, and assumptions are introduced. For example, one may include another term c in the model to account for the effect of the investigator (center) on the measurements, or another parameter $t*c$ to account for the interaction between the treatment and the investigator effect. We will discuss this important parameter in some detail in the later section, "Issues in data analysis."

There are two common features to all linear models: The relationship between the data and the model parameters is always assumed to be linear, and the errors are assumed to be Normal.

It is important to remember that all the statistician's quantitative work and calculations are model-dependent. That is, their application to real life depends on the extent to which the model assumptions are satisfied in reality. Much of the work the statistician does in planning the trial, in discussing the nature of the efficacy and safety variables, randomizing, blinding, and so forth, is expressed in the model. Obviously, the more complex the model and the more specific the model assumptions, the more the final results of the analysis will depend on it.

Statisticians are advised to always start the statistical analysis by performing certain diagnostic procedures on the data to check to what extent the model assumptions are supported by the data. This process involves a certain level of subjective judgment, and different statisticians may reach different conclusions looking at the same data. Statisticians have at their disposal certain tools by which they can manipulate the data so as to conform better to the model assumption. For example, the distributions of measured pharmacokinetic (PK) parameters is typically skewed. The assumption of Normality of the distribution implies that the distribution is symmetric. It turns out that if one calculates the PK parameters using the natural logarithms of the blood concentrations rather than the raw measured concentrations, the distributions of the estimated parameters are less skewed. The choice of model is part of the study design. It is, therefore, done before any data are available.

It is not uncommon that at the analysis stage, it becomes evident that the model assumptions are grossly violated. It may become necessary to use different methods that are not as dependent on the model assumptions to analyze the data. This should be done with great care so that spurious patterns in the data would not lead the researcher to reach wrong conclusions. Additionally, changing the analysis methods after an inspection of the data could result in an introduction of bias if the statistician is aware of the treatment assignments. For this reason, it is prudent to perform these diagnostic examinations of the data without revealing the treatment assignments. In blinded studies, this means that these procedures are executed prior to

the breaking of the blind. The statistical guidelines issued by the International Conference on Harmonization (ICH), which were adopted by the Food and Drug Administration (FDA) and the European regulatory authorities, address this issue as follows:

> The [statistical] plan should be reviewed and possibly updated as a result of the blind review of the data ... and should be finalized before breaking the blind. Formal records should be kept of when the statistical analysis plan was finalized as well as when the blind was subsequently broken. If the blind review suggests changes to the principal features stated in the protocol, these should be documented in a protocol amendment.
>
> (ICH, 1998, E9, 4.1)

It is important to remember that the question is not whether the statistical model is true or false. The statistical model is a theoretical construct, and thus it is always false. The question is how well it approximates the situation under study. Or, in the words of a famous statistician, "All models are wrong, but some are useful."

Statistical inference

Hypothesis testing revisited: the *p*-value; power

In the earlier section "The statistical test: the null hypothesis, error probabilities, statistical power," we discussed the concept of the statistical test and defined some basic terms. In this section, we take a closer look at this idea and see, through an example, how this is actually done. Let us revisit the data presented in Table 28.4. The graduate student who generated the data did not, in fact, study 20 randomly selected students. The purpose of her study was to demonstrate that engaging in aerobic workout on a regular basis has a beneficial effect on the cardiovascular system, including the slowing down the heart rate. To do this, the researcher set out to test the null hypothesis (H$_0$) that the mean heart rate of exercising students, μ_A, is the same as the mean of the nonexercising students, μ_B. The alternative hypothesis (H$_1$) is that $\mu_A < \mu_B$. In order to test H$_0$ against H$_1$, one would need to identify a variable (or a *statistic*), the distribution of which is sensitive to the difference between the heart rates of the different groups. Such a statistic is the signal-to noise ratio,

$$T = \frac{\bar{X}_B - \bar{X}_A}{S.E.(\bar{X}_B - \bar{X}_A)} \qquad (28.2)$$

where the signal is the difference between the sample mean of Group B, $\bar{X}_B$, and the sample mean of Group A, $\bar{X}_A$, and the noise is the standard error of the difference $\bar{X}_B - \bar{X}_A$.

We saw in the earlier section "Variability: the source of uncertainty" that the standard error of the mean is $1 = 1/\sqrt{N}$ times the sample standard deviation. The variance of the difference $\bar{X}_B - \bar{X}_A$ is the sum of the variances of $\bar{X}_B$ and of $\bar{X}_A$. Therefore, from Table 28.4 we obtain:

$$\bar{X}_B - \bar{X}_A = 59.4 - 54.2 = 5.2$$
$$\text{VAR}\,(\bar{X}_B - \bar{X}_A) = 1.8^2/10 + 2.99^2/10$$

and thus,

$$\text{S.E.}(\bar{X}_B - \bar{X}_A) = \sqrt{(1.8^2 + 2.99^2)/10} = 1.104$$

Therefore, $T = 5.2/1.104 = 4.7$.

Statistical theory teaches that under the assumption that the population means of the two groups are the same (i.e., if H_0 is true), the distribution of variable T depends only on the sample size but not on the value of the common mean or on the measurements population variance and thus can be tabulated independently of the particulars of any given experiment. This is the so-called Student's t-distribution. Using tables of the t-distribution, we can calculate the probability that a variable T calculated as above assumes a value greater or equal to 4.7, the value obtained in our example, *given that H_0 is true*. This probability is <0.0001. Thus, if H_0 is true, the result obtained in our experiment is extremely unlikely, although not impossible. We are forced to choose between two possible explanations to this. One is that a very unlikely event had occurred. The second is that the result of our experiment is not a fluke; rather, the difference $\mu_B - \mu_A$ is a positive number, sufficiently large to make the probability of this outcome a likely event. We elect the latter explanation and reject H_0 in favor of the alternative hypothesis H_1.

The steps we have taken in the above example are quite generic. They can be summarized as follows:

1. Describe a statistical model and identify the variable measuring the effect of interest.
2. Define the statistical hypothesis to be tested.
3. Define the test statistic to be used for testing H_0. This test statistics is always the signal-to-noise ratio.
4. Perform the experiment and collect the data.
5. Calculate the value of the test statistic based on the data.
6. Calculate the probability under the assumption that H_0 is true, that the test statistic will assume a value equal or greater than the value obtained in the experiment. If this probability is sufficiently small for you to decide that the value obtained in the experiment is highly unlikely, declare the test as statistically significant and reject H_0.

Step 6 reflects the logic driving statistical inference. It is based on the expectation that if an event occurs in an experiment it is not an unlikely event.

The probability that the test statistics will assume a value as large, or larger, than the value obtained in the experiment is called the *significance probability* of the test, or the *p-value*. In our example, the *p*-value was less than 0.0001. Most people would consider such a value extremely unlikely and declare the test statistically significant. The question of what values should be considered small enough to declare statistical significance is a matter of judgment. Over the years of statistical practice, the number 0.05 became the standard cutoff point. Any *p*-value smaller than 0.05 is considered significant, and any *p*-value greater than 0.05 is considered not significant.

It should be emphasized, though, that 0.05 is an arbitrary value and that there is no real difference between a *p*-value of 0.049 and a *p*-value of 0.051; although, if one follows the cutoff rule of 0.05 to the letter, one will declare statistical significance in the former but not in the latter case. This is, of course, absurd. These two *p*-values should not lead the researcher to conclusions with such diametrically opposed consequences. A choice of any other cutoff value will lead to a similar situation if followed strictly. A good measure of common sense is always useful. There is, of course, no reason why anyone should not use a cutoff point other than the customary 0.05 if he or she feels it is more appropriate. But as in any other situation when one deviates from a standard, one must provide an acceptable explanation for the reasons for doing so *before* the experiment is performed and before the data are known.

The statistical testing setup, as we have already seen, is geared toward the declaration of statistical significance. When a test is significant, we draw a conclusion about the cause of the effect of interest. If we decide to reject the null hypothesis, the *p*-value is the type I error associated with this decision. Therefore, the level of confidence in the correctness of the decision depends on the *p*-value; the smaller the *p*-value, the more confident one is that the decision is correct.

What if the statistical test is not statistically significant? If one accepts the null hypothesis in this case, the error to be concerned about is the type II error (see the earlier Table 28.1). At the design stage of the trial, the statistician usually ascertains that the test to be employed at the end has desired power at clinically important alternatives. As the power is 1 minus the probability of type II error, a well designed study has built-in protection against making a type II error when one of these alternatives is true but generally does not have this protection at other alternatives. In fact, for most statistical models used in practice, for alternatives close to the null hypothesis, the probability of type II error is near $1 - \alpha$, where α is the significance level of the test. As the alternative hypothesis is usually composite, not all alternatives can be protected uniformly. Thus, accepting the null hypothesis when the test fails to achieve statistical significance is a decision associated with uncontrolled probability of type II error. For this reason, statisticians prefer to declare the test as inconclusive when it fails to achieve statistical significance.

Confidence intervals: precision and confidence

Testing statistical hypotheses is a decision-making tool. The outcome of the test is a dichotomy; either the test is declared "statistically significant" or it is not. The test provides directly very little information on the magnitude of the effect of interest. In the example of the heart rate data of Table 28.4, we declared the test statistically significant and rejected the null hypothesis that the effect is zero. But we did not identify how large the effect is. It is often important to take the next step and estimate the magnitude of the effect.

The obvious starting point is the "signal" $\bar{X}_B - \bar{X}_A = 5.2$. This value is an estimate of the difference between the two population means, $\Delta = \mu_B - \mu_A$, and as we have already seen, it is associated with a certain amount of variability measured by its standard error. This means that if the experiment was to be repeated under exactly the same conditions, it is most likely that a value different than 5.2 is obtained; but how different? How much should one expect the values obtained from repetitions of the experiment to spread about the true Δ? This information is provided by the standard error.

A method of simultaneously providing information on the magnitude of the estimated parameter and the range of likely values of the estimate is the *confidence interval*. The key idea rests on a fundamental mathematical fact that if $\bar{X}_n$ is a sample mean of a variable calculated from n independent samples of a variable, whose population mean and standard error are μ and σ, respectively, then the quantity

$$Z = \frac{\bar{X}_n - \mu}{\sigma/\sqrt{n}} \tag{28.3}$$

has approximately Standard Normal distribution (Gaussian distribution). The Normal distribution has the familiar bell-shaped curve and is tabulated in almost any elementary statistics textbook. The word "approximately" here means that the actual distribution of Z may be different from the Normal distribution, but it becomes closer and closer to it as the sample size n increases. For all practical purposes, when the sample size is greater than 30, performing probability calculations on Z using the Standard Normal Distribution tables, will result in only minor errors.

Using the Standard Normal Distribution tables, one can find for every number $0 < \gamma < 1$, a pair of numbers $Z_1(\gamma)$ and $Z_2(\gamma)$, such that

$$\text{Prob}\{Z_1(\gamma) < Z < Z_2(\gamma)\} = 1 - \gamma \qquad (28.4)$$

For example, for $\gamma = 0.05$, the pair $Z_1(0.05) = -1.96$ and $Z_2(0.05) = 1.96$ satisfy this equation. Since the Normal distribution curve is symmetric about zero with area under the bell-shaped curve equals one, we can always find a value $Z(\gamma) > 0$ such that $Z_1(\gamma) = -Z(\gamma)$ and $Z_2(\gamma) = Z(\gamma)$ so that Equation (28.4) holds. Now, by substituting the definition of Z in expression (28.3) with $Z(\gamma) = Z_2(\gamma) = -Z_1(\gamma)$ and rearranging terms, the inequality $Z_1(\gamma) < Z < Z_2(\gamma)$ can be re-written as

$$L_\gamma = \bar{X}_n - Z(\gamma)\sigma/\sqrt{n} < \mu < \bar{X}_n + Z(\gamma)\sigma/\sqrt{n} = U_\gamma \qquad (28.5)$$

Now, let us take a closer look at expression (28.5). The value at the center, μ, is the population mean, which is the unknown quantity we are estimating. The population standard deviation, σ, is also usually unknown. However, as we have seen earlier, we can estimate σ by S, the sample standard deviation. With the estimate of the standard deviation substituted for σ the two expressions on the right-hand and the left-hand sides of (28.5) are variables calculated from the data. Thus, expression (28.5) represents an event that the random interval with endpoints (L_γ, U_γ) contains the population mean μ. Expression (28.4) assigns a probability $1 - \gamma$ to this event. The interpretation of this is that if we conduct an experiment and calculate the lower and upper limits of the interval, L_γ and U_γ, respectively, then the interval (L_γ, U_γ) will contain the true (and unknown!) population mean with probability $1 - \gamma$. The interval (28.5) is called a *confidence interval* for the population mean, and $1 - \gamma$ is called the *confidence level* of the interval, often expressed as a percent.

Let us illustrate these concepts using the data from Table 28.4. Suppose we wish to estimate the difference Δ between the population means of the nonexercising and the exercising students by constructing a confidence interval with confidence level 95%. Then substituting D for $\bar{X}_n$ and SE_D for

$\sigma/\sqrt{n}$ in Equation (28.5), and recalling that $Z(0.05) = 1.96$, we obtain the confidence limits

$$L_{0.05} = D - Z(0.05) \times SE_D$$
$$= 5.2 - 1.105 \times 1.96 = 3.03$$

and

$$U_{0.05} = D - Z(0.05) \times SE_D$$
$$= 5.2 + 1.105 \times 1.96 = 7.26$$

Thus, the interval (3.03, 7.26) is a 95% confidence interval for the effect Δ. It should be emphasized that the probability statement about the confidence level of 0.95 does not relate to the specific interval (3.03, 7.26), because this specific interval is an outcome of the specific sample used for the calculation and either contains the parameter Δ or does not. It is a theoretical probability pertaining to a generic interval calculated from a sample following the steps we described above. Thus, if we could repeat the experiment many times, each time calculating a confidence interval in the way we have just done, we should expect approximately 95% of these intervals to contain the true mean effect Δ. Of course, when calculating a confidence interval from a sample, there is no way to tell whether or not the interval contains the parameter it is estimating. The confidence level provides us with a certain level of assurance that it is so, in the sense we just described.

One might ask, why not choose γ to be a very small number, say, 0.01 or 0.001 and thus obtain a higher confidence level? The answer is that one can see from the way $Z(\gamma)$ is defined that it increases as γ decreases. For example, $Z(0.01) = 2.58$ and $Z(0.001) = 3.25$, which would correspond to the confidence intervals (2.35, 8.05) and (1.54, 8.86), respectively. So the answer becomes self-evident: Yes, one can choose an arbitrarily high confidence level but this will come at the price that the resulting confidence interval will be so wide that it becomes meaningless. In other words, there is a trade-off between confidence and accuracy. It seems that 95% confidence achieves a satisfactory balance between the two in most cases.

Confidence intervals are often calculated after performing a statistical test. When the test is statistically significant, we have reason to believe that the effect is real. The confidence interval gives us additional information as to the size of the effect. Confidence intervals are also calculated during exploratory analyses. The purpose of such analyses is to explore the data, identify possible effects, and generate hypotheses for future studies rather than make specific inferences. Confidence intervals are extremely useful tools toward this goal.

Another common use of confidence intervals is in the establishment of equivalence between two treatments. Here "equivalence" is not synonymous with "equality." It means that the difference, if any, between the effects of the two treatments is not considered to be of material importance. Let us illustrate this with the following example: Suppose one is interested in determining whether two antihypertensive drugs are equivalent in their effect on diastolic blood pressure after four weeks of treatment. Let μ_A and μ_B denote the mean change from the pre-treatment baseline for patients treated with drug A and drug B, respectively. Let $\Delta = \mu_A - \mu_B$. Blood pressure varies from measurement to measurement, even when the measurements are taken within minutes from each other so that measurements within ± 3 mmHg are not considered to be clinically different. Therefore, as long as the two means are within ± 3 mmHg, the two drugs are considered as having equivalent effectiveness. A trial to establish whether the two drugs are equivalent must be then designed so that a confidence interval for Δ with confidence level of 0.90 or higher (or another level considered by the researcher to be adequate) will have width not exceeding 6 mmHg. When the trial is concluded, the confidence interval is constructed. If it is entirely contained within the interval $(-3, +3)$, the two drugs are considered equivalent. Otherwise, they are not.

It is possible to design a trial so that a desired confidence interval of a given confidence level will have a desired width. The width of a confidence interval for a parameter is the estimate's *precision*. It depends on (i) the confidence level, (ii) the inherent variability of the data, and (iii) the sample size. The inherent variability of the data can be controlled only to a limited degree. For a fixed sample size, the width of the confidence interval is determined by the confidence level. As we have seen in the previous example, the researcher can increase the precision of the estimate only by lowering the confidence level associated with the confidence interval and *vice versa*. The only way to guarantee an acceptable level of confidence and precision is to include sufficiently large number of subjects in the trial. In our example, if the interval's width is larger than 6 mmHg, the trial could never establish equivalence because the criterion for this cannot be met. However, it could establish the lack of equivalence if the entire confidence interval is either lager than 3 or smaller than -3.

To summarize, when estimating the magnitude of a parameter is an important objective of a trial, thought must be given at the design stage to what levels of confidence and precision are considered acceptable and to make sure that the trial is designed to enroll sufficient number of subjects to accommodate these requirements. There are no hard and fast rules about what levels of confidence are considered acceptable. However, rarely do researchers go below 80%, and more typically, they require a confidence level of 90% or higher. The desired level of precision depends entirely on the particular situation.

Study design: Determining the sample size

We have already seen through a number of examples the interplay between sample size, variability, and the performance of the statistical procedures employed to analyze the data. The sample size determines the amount of information that will be available at the end of the trial. Therefore, the determination of an adequate sample size is one of the most important aspects of the trial design. A trial accumulating an inadequate amount of information is hopelessly flawed, because it will not enable the researcher to answer the questions the trial is intended to answer.

The determination of the sample size is intimately related to the trial objectives, the inferences the researcher wants to be able to make, and the error probabilities in the case of hypotheses testing, or the confidence and precision in the case of estimation that the researcher is willing to tolerate. We revisit our previous example to illustrate the process of determining the required sample size for a clinical trial.

Suppose one wishes to conduct a trial to test the efficacy of a new antihypertensive drug. The clinical research physician plans to enroll a certain number of subjects with mild to moderate hypertension and randomize them to receive either the experimental drug or placebo. The primary efficacy variable is the decrease in the diastolic blood pressure as compared to a pre-treatment baseline. The subject's diastolic blood pressure is measured twice: once prior to treatment when the subject is free of any antihypertensive medication, and once following the administration of treatment (experimental drug or placebo). The change in diastolic blood pressure between the two measurements is the primary efficacy variable. The researcher knows that to justify further development, the treatment must reduce the subject's diastolic blood pressure by at least 10 points. So, if we denote the mean decrease in diastolic blood pressure for the drug group by μ_D and the corresponding decrease for the placebo group by μ_P, the null hypothesis the researcher is set to test is

$H_0 : \mu_D = \mu_P$; or $H_0 : \mu_D - \mu_P = 0$

versus the alternative hypothesis

$H_A : \mu_D > \mu_P$; or $H_A : \mu_D - \mu_P > 0$

One particular alternative of interest is $H_{10} : \mu_D = \mu_P + 10$; or $H_{10} : \mu_D - \mu_P = 10$.

In order to guarantee that the statistical test of H_0 will have a significance level α and power not less than $1 - \beta$ at the alternative $H_\Delta : \mu_D = \mu_P + \Delta$, each of the two treatment groups must have at least N subjects, where N is given by the formula

$$N = 2(Z_{1-\alpha/2} + Z_{1-\beta})^2 (\sigma/\Delta)^2 \qquad (28.6)$$

σ is the standard deviation of the raw measurements (i.e., the decrease in diastolic blood pressure). For simplicity, we assume that it is the same for both treatment groups. $Z_{1-\alpha/2}$ and $Z_{1-\beta}$ are two constants depending on α and β, that can be obtained from tables of the standard normal

distribution. If in our case, we assume that $\sigma = 12$, $\Delta = 10$, $\alpha = 0.05$ and $\beta = 0.10$, then $Z_{1-\alpha/2} = 1.96$, $Z_{1-\beta} = 1.28$, and Equation (28.6) yields $N = 30.23$. That is, a sample size of at least 31 subjects per group is required. Expression (28.6) is specific to situations similar to our example. In general, the sample size required is calculated by a formula that looks like expression (28.7) below:

$$N = C_{\alpha,\beta}(\sigma/\Delta)^2 \qquad (28.7)$$

where $C_{\alpha,\beta}$ is some constant depending on α and β.

There are a number of important observations on Equation (28.7):
- The sample size is proportional to σ^2, the measurements variance. That is, the more variable the measurements, the larger must be the sample size to enable one to distinguish the effect of interest from the noise.
- The sample size is inversely proportional to Δ^2. That is, the smaller the effect of interest, the larger must the sample size be to enable one to separate it from the background noise.
- The sample size depends on the squares of the parameters σ and Δ; meaning that if we are able to reduce the noise in the experiment by half, the payoff is that the clinical trial will require one-fourth of the number of subjects. Similarly, if we wish to ensure sufficient power to detect half of the effect, the clinical trial would have to enroll four times as many subjects.

During the design phase of the trial, the statistician will typically ask the clinical researcher questions leading to the determination of σ and Δ. The anticipated standard deviation is often very difficult to estimate, and the best way of arriving at a useful number is to look for such an estimate either in the published scientific literature or estimate it from data obtained in similar studies performed by the pharmaceutical company. Underestimating σ can result in an underpowered study resulting with unacceptable errors rates leading to ambiguities and an inability to make reliable inferences. For this reason, it is always preferable to overestimate σ rather than underestimate it when information on σ is scanty. The value of Δ, the minimal clinically important effect, is usually arrived at by the clinician based on past clinical experience.

The abuse of power: pitfalls of overdesign

Equation (28.7) is expressing N in terms of σ and Δ. It is very easy to rewrite this equation and express any of the three parameters N, σ, and Δ in terms of the other two. If we express Δ in terms of N and σ, we could see that by increasing N, the statistical test could have high power to detect very small differences. Thus, it is sometimes tempting to "overdesign" the study; that is, to enroll more subjects than required so that if the drug is not quite as efficacious as one hopes, the statistical test would still be significant at the end; sort of buying an "insurance policy." By enrolling a large number of subjects, one can ensure that the statistical test is so powerful that it would declare very small and possibly meaningless differences as statistically significant.

This approach is not only wasteful but may also lead to false inferences, and is outright unethical in the drug development arena. Clinical trials are very expensive enterprises, and it is typically not feasible to repeat a trial to demonstrate that the results are reproducible. Furthermore, in studying therapies for life-threatening diseases, a trial resulting with a significant outcome often precludes the possibility of conducting a second confirmatory trial. The variables studied in clinical trials are random, thus there will always be differences between the treatment groups that are due to chance. An overpowered study could find such differences statistically significant and lead the researcher to a false conclusion that a drug is efficacious when it is not, or that it is harmful when it is not. In the absence of a second chance, these findings may never be repudiated.

An underpowered trial is wasteful and unethical for a different reason. Such a trial may not have enough power to detect clinically meaningful differences resulting in missing clinically important medical advances. The subjects enrolled into such a trial are exposed to the risks involved in all clinical trials using experimental drugs, without the anticipated benefit to them or society.

For these reasons, it is important that the size of the trial is just right: not too small and not too large. The discussions taking place among the project research team leading to the appropriate choice of the sample size are therefore very important, and although in the end, it is the statistician who performs the calculations, the input from the other team members is critical.

Issues in statistical trial design

Multicenter trials

Most Phase III clinical trials are multicenter trials; that is, they are conducted in more than one clinical center. The number of centers participating in a clinical trial can vary greatly.

There are a number of good reasons to conduct phase III trials as multicenter trials. The most obvious is an administrative and logistical reason. Spreading the burden of subject recruitment among many centers will reduce the duration of the subject enrollment phase of the trial. This is an important reason considering that often the key to commercial success or failure of a new drug is the timing of its introduction to the market. There are also important scientific reasons to conduct the trial as a multicenter trial, as described in the following sections.

Noise reduction

Different centers often draw subjects from different types of patient populations. Also, different centers may utilize different procedures and medical practices that are not controlled by the study protocol. It is, therefore, reasonable to expect that the within-center variability is smaller than the overall variability. In a multicenter trial, the center often serves as a stratification variable, thereby reducing the variability and increasing the efficiency of the trial design. In order to take advantage of this aspect of the multicenter trial, the number of subjects per center cannot be too small so that the estimate of the intra-center variability is stable. A general rule is that the number of subjects per treatment group within each center will be at least five.

Generalizability

A multicenter trial may be viewed as a number of identically designed small trials each conducted at

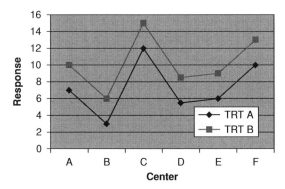

Figure 28.1 Center effect

a single center. From this perspective, each center can be viewed as repeating the study conducted in other centers. In addition, different centers draw their subjects from different geographic areas and thus a multicenter trial is more likely to enroll subjects who are representative of a cross-section of the general population. Consistency of the results among the different centers adds to the level of confidence that the results could be replicated anywhere. It is possible that the results across centers are inconsistent. There are two types of inconsistencies.

Center effect

When the magnitude of the response to treatment is different across centers but the relative effect between the two treatments is approximately constant, this is referred to by statisticians as "center effect." The existence of a center effect means that the different centers contribute differently to the measured effect of both treatments, but this contribution is the same for both the experimental treatment and the comparator. This situation is illustrated in Figure 28.1.

Figure 28.1 shows schematically the effects of two treatments across six centers. The magnitude of the treatment differs from center to center, but the difference between the effect of treatment A and treatment B is the same. Such a situation does not present a problem in comparing the treatments because what one is interested is the response to the experimental treatment relative to the response to the control. It makes it impossible, though, to

talk about the absolute magnitude of the treatment effect, because it is not constant. Observing a center effect is not unusual in clinical trials. The reasons for this may be many. It could be the result of a difference in the type of patients seen at the different centers, the center procedures and general nursing care, subjects compliance in taking their medication, the equipment used in the different centers, and so on.

Treatment-by-center interaction

We say that there is a treatment-by-center interaction when the relative response to the different study treatments is different across centers. This is the type of inconsistency that may cause an invalidation of the entire study. There are two situations that present qualitatively different levels of difficulties:

• *Quantitative interaction.* We say that the interaction is quantitative if the relative effect of the different treatments is in the same direction across centers, although the magnitude may be different. Figure 28.2 illustrates this type of interaction. This type of interaction means that the relative efficacy of the treatments is different in different centers, but the direction is always the same. That is, treatment A is more efficacious than treatment B at all centers, but the magnitude of the difference between the treatment effects is different in different centers. When this type of interaction exists, one can say that one treatment is more efficacious than the other, but cannot say by how much because the relative efficacy of the two treatments is not constant.

• *Qualitative interaction.* This occurs when the relative efficacy of the two treatments is different across the different centers both in magnitude and direction. This type of interaction is the one that could invalidate the entire study. This is illustrated in Figure 28.3. Here, treatment A produces a larger effect than treatment B in some centers and a smaller effect in other centers. If the researcher cannot find the cause of this interaction and correct for it, the study will be inconclusive. This type of interaction would occur if, for example, the data center mislabeled the treatments for some centers. This would be easy to rectify. However, often there is no

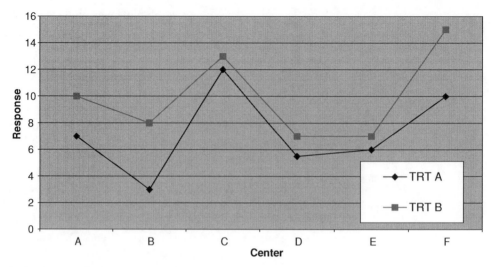

Figure 28.2 Treatment by center interaction: quantitative interaction

obvious explanation for this, and the entire study has to be invalidated.

The ICH guidelines address this issue as follows:

If heterogeneity of treatment effects is found, this should be interpreted with care, and vigorous attempts should be made to find an explanation in terms of other features of trial management or sub-ject characteristics. Such an explanation will usually suggest appropriate further analysis and interpreta-tion. In the absence of an explanation, heterogeneity of treatment effect, as evidenced, for example, by marked quantitative interactions implies that alterna-tive estimates of the treatment effect, giving different weights to the centers, may be needed to substantiate

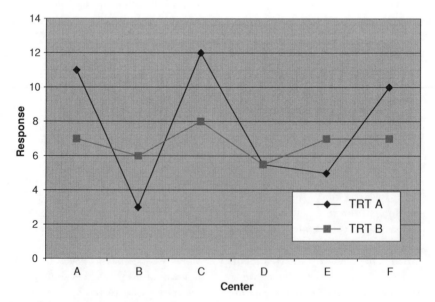

Figure 28.3 Center by treatment interaction: qualitative interaction

the robustness of the estimates of treatment effect. It is even more important to understand the basis of any heterogeneity characterized by marked qualitative interactions, and failure to find an explanation may necessitate further clinical trials before the treatment effect can be reliably predicted.

(ICH, 1998, E9, 3.2)

Multiplicity

Clinical trials always include multiple endpoints and/or multiple comparisons between treatments. For example, in a clinical trial of a new drug for asthma, one may want to analyze the change in the Forced Expiratory Volume in 1 second (FEV1) as well as the change in the total asthma symptoms score, the subject's morning and evening symptoms severity scores, the investigator's global improvement score, and perhaps other endpoints. In a dose–response trial with placebo, low dose, intermediate dose, and high dose, the investigator may want to compare the three dose groups to the control and perhaps the different dose groups with each other.

The issue of multiplicity is that when performing multiple statistical tests, the error probability associated with the inferences made is inflated. To see this, let us consider a simple situation where one is interested in performing two statistical tests on independent sets of data, each at a significance level of 0.05. Thus, the probability that each of the two tests will be declared significant erroneously (type I error) is 0.05. However, the probability that at least one of the two tests will be declared significant erroneously is 0.0975. The probability that at least one of the tests of interest will be declared significant erroneously is called the *experiment-wise error rate*. If we perform three 0.05 level tests, the experiment-wise error rate increases to 0.143. In practical terms, this means that if we perform multiple tests and make multiple inferences, each one at a reasonably low error probability, the likelihood that some of these inferences will be erroneous could be appreciable. To correct for this, one must conduct each individual test at a decreased significance level with the result that either the power of the tests will be reduced as well, or the sample size must be increased to accommodate

the desired power. This could make the trial prohibitively expensive. Statisticians sometimes refer to the need to adjust the significance level so that the experiment-wise error rate is controlled, as the statistical penalty for multiplicity.

The need to control the experiment-wise error rate may not apply to exploratory analyses. Statisticians often perform formal statistical tests for exploratory purposes; that is, to explore the data for promising signals that could be pursued further in future studies, or for signals consistent with the primary analysis thereby enforcing the confidence in the study outcomes. So, no formal hypotheses are stated and no inferences are made based on them. Even though the act of formally performing an exploratory test involves the same steps as testing, it is conceptually different because of the absence of a null hypothesis. The *p*-value obtained in such a test should be viewed as a measure of the level of inconsistency of the data with the underlying assumptions of the test rather than error probabilities involved in making causal inferences.

In summary, one should limit the number of inferential tests to be performed to the minimum necessary for making the desired causal inferences. They must be specified in the study protocol and the appropriate adjustments to the error probabilities must be made. Similarly, one should remember that when multiple tests are performed without adjustment, as the case would be in exploratory testing situation, one should expect to see spurious statistically significant results that may or may not be meaningful. This last comment applies particularly to statistical tests performed on adverse events and laboratory data. Adverse events reported in a study are often summarized by reporting their incidences summarized by body system. Often, dozens of categories are listed. When formal statistical tests are applied to these data, some of these tests will result with *p*-values less than the customary 0.05. The researcher should be cognizant of this issue and not jump to conclusions. It is strongly advisable to specify in advance the particular safety tests to be performed inferentially if there is a recognized or suspected safety concern with the drug or the class of drugs tested.

Interim analysis

For long-term clinical trials in life-threatening disease areas or in diseases involving serious morbidities, or in the study of drugs with possible serious toxicities, it is imperative to monitor the data on an ongoing basis and perform periodic interim analyses.

Interim analyses are performed for a variety of reasons. Some of the main reasons are as follows:
• Stop the development of an ineffective treatment.
• Stop the development of a toxic treatment.
• Terminate a trial in a life-threatening disease as soon as enough evidence accumulates to conclude that one treatment is significantly more efficacious than the other.
• Interim design adjustment (e.g., verification of assumptions on variability, power recalculation, and sample-size adjustment; verification of assumptions on expected drug or control group response rate).
• Plan additional trials.
• Plan for capital expenditures and product launch.
• Make a regulatory submission for a short-term portion of a long-term trial.
• Other regulatory reasons (e.g., opening the trial to previously excluded high-risk subjects).

The first three reasons in the list include the possibility of terminating the trial based on an interim inferential analysis. The fourth reason can potentially alter the trial's conduct. The other reasons should not, in principle, impact the trial.

Essentially, there are two separate issues involved in performing an interim analysis: a statistical issue and an administrative or trial management issue. The statistical issue is similar to the multiplicity issue discussed in the previous paragraph and applies to the first three items in the above list. If we perform an interim inferential test, the overall error probability is inflated. Therefore, if one contemplates to perform an interim analysis with the option of making inferences early and possibly terminating the trial before its planned end, the procedure used for making this determination must be planned in advance and documented in the study protocol just as any other inferential procedure. As we

discussed above, there will be a statistical penalty in the sense that each of the interim analyses and the final analysis will have to be performed at a lower level of significance than the overall type I error rate. The statistical penalty depends on the decision-making procedure to be used. It must be emphasized that the penalty must be paid for the option of changing the course of the trial before the planned end whether this option was exercised or not. Some non-statisticians are often puzzled when they are told that a p-value of 0.04 will not be significant at the end of the trial even though no changes were made in the conduct of the trial subsequent to the interim analysis. A decision was made at the interim analysis that was to continue the trial unchanged. The decision process that led to this decision included the option of terminating the trial early, a decision that by design had a built-in protection against a type I error. Similarly, the terminal decision at the end of the trial had a protection against type I error. If the protection at the terminal decision is at the level 0.05, any protection at the interim stage would necessarily make the overall type I error probability larger than 0.05. The allowance for the terminal type one error must necessarily be at some level less than 0.05.

Interim analysis for the purpose of reassessment of the design assumptions and sample size recalculation has become rather commonplace, especially in large, long-term Phase III trials. The assumptions driving the design of these trials are typically based on published or unpublished previous exploratory research or on extrapolations from preclinical work. These assumptions often involve a great deal of uncertainty. To reduce this uncertainty, an interim analysis at some time point early in the trial is planned, the sole purpose of which is to use the data accumulated thus far and estimate the parameters used to perform the power calculations and make appropriate adjustments to the trial design. Recalculation of the sample size is the most typical purpose of such analysis.

A number of procedures for an interim sample-size adjustment have been proposed in the statistical literature in recent years. One such approach is to calculate the probability that the trial, when continued as planned, will result in a significant outcome conditioned on the accumulated data. When this probability is calculated under the alternative hypothesis, this (conditional) probability is called the *conditional power*. If the conditional power is equal or higher than the power used in the original design of the trial, the trial will continue as planned. If the conditional power is smaller, the sample size will be increased. The increase of the sample size may not depend solely on statistical considerations but also on budgetary or other considerations.

Although there is no reason in principle why one would not allow reducing the sample size if it turns out that the trial is overpowered, all the methods for sample-size adjustment allow only for increasing the size of the trial. The reason is a practical one. As the trial sponsor has already committed the resources to conduct the trial as designed, they would rather use them all and have a more powerful trial rather than saving and risking that the trial may be underpowered. Clearly, if one incorporates the option of an interim sample size adjustment, at the outset, the expected sample size of such a trial will be larger than a trial designed without such an option using the same design assumptions. Therefore, if the criterion for statistical significance at the end of the trial is the same, such a design will result in a more powerful trial than if this option was not available. This gain comes, of course, with a price tag: the type I error probability is increased as well. Therefore, the inclusion of an interim redesign must be planned as an integral part of the trial design and proper adjustments must be made to ensure that the resulting decision procedure has the desired power while still properly controlling the type I error rate.

The timing of an interim analysis for reassessment of the sample size is very important. One would want to conduct this analysis after sufficient amount of data have accumulated so that the estimated design parameters are stable and reliable. However, one would also not want to wait too long either. For a typical large trial, when a sample-size adjustment procedure is planned after 30–50% of the data are available, the estimates are reasonably stable and the statistical penalty involved in the *p*-value adjustment is relatively small. In addition, some procedures leading to an early decision to stop the trial for lack of efficacy, or a *futility analysis*, also involve the calculation of conditional power. The same calculations involved in sample-size adjustment can be used to assess futility. If the conditional power is very low (which would lead to a substantial increase in the sample size, should the trial continue), the sponsor may want to consider terminating the trial and reallocating the unused resources to more promising investigations.

The idea of allowing the clinical researcher to make interim decisions during the trial based on accumulated data has been investigated extensively in recent years leading to the development of methods allowing a great deal of flexibility in changing the trial conduct as data are accumulated. Such designs are known as *adaptive designs*. Adaptive designs are used to make decisions not only on extending the enrollment of patients, but also to drop one or more of the trial's arms, increase or decrease the dose, or even to change the endpoint of interest. Designs that allow this level of flexibility yet maintain the type I and type II error probabilities under control are necessarily complicated and require very complex computations for the calculation of the decision rules. Although a number of computer programs are available for calculating the decision rules for some flexible designs, many appealing methods have been developed by statisticians and are available in the statistical literature, although no software is readily available at this time that is accessible to pharmaceutical clinical trialists.

The administrative issue involves the potential for the introduction of bias. Any interim analysis, regardless of whether or not it is done with the intention to affect the ongoing trial, involves the possibility of introducing bias if the analysis requires the breaking of the blind. The FDA is particularly wary about these types of analyses, because even if every step and decision is well documented it is impossible to anticipate the impact on the trial that a partial, even preliminary, knowledge of the efficacy results might have. For this reason, it is imperative that such analyses, regardless of their declared purpose, are performed with strict guidelines as to who will be unblinded, and how the results will be disseminated. It is important to make sure that individuals directly involved in the trial conduct and management, such as investigators, monitors, and other project personnel, should remain blinded to the data and the results of the interim analysis. It has become standard practice in the pharmaceutical industry to appoint a Data Monitoring Board consisting entirely of people uninvolved in the trial conduct to review the interim data and analyses and make recommendations. The Pharmaceutical Manufacturers Association published a position paper discussing in detail the various aspects of this issue as it relate to the specific circumstances of new drug development (PMA Biostatistics and Medical Ad-Hoc Committee on Interim Analysis, 1993). The ICH guidelines address this issue as well:

> The execution of an interim analysis should be a completely confidential process because unblinded data and results are potentially involved. All staff involved in the conduct of the trial should remain blind to the results of such analyses, because of the possibility that their attitudes to the trial will be modified and cause changes in the characteristics of patients to be recruited or biases in treatment comparisons. This principle may be applied to all investigator staff and to staff employed by the sponsor except for those who are directly involved in the execution of the interim analysis. Investigators should be informed only about the decision to continue or to discontinue the trial, or to implement modifications to trial procedures. [...] Any interim analysis that is not planned appropriately (with or without the consequences of stopping the trial early) may flaw the results of a trial and possibly weaken confidence in the conclusions drawn. Therefore, such analyses should be avoided. If unplanned interim analysis is conducted, the clinical study report should explain why it was necessary and the degree to which blindness had to be broken, and provide an assessment of the potential magnitude of bias introduced and the impact on the interpretation of the results. (ICH, 1998, E9, 4.5)

Issues in data analysis

Clinical trials present unique problems during the analysis phase that other experiments do not. The inherent complexity of the clinical trial is compounded by the fact that it uses human subjects, and therefore it is governed by a set of ethical rules, paramount of which is the voluntary and informed participation of the subjects in the study. Subjects must be mentally competent to understand the risks as well as the potential benefits they would be subject to should they participate in the trial. They are required to sign an informed consent form prior to their enrollment in the study in which they confirm their understanding of the trial procedures, the potential risks and benefits, and state their voluntary agreement to participate. Notwithstanding the informed consent form, subjects can at all times exercise their free will and choose to terminate their participation, refuse to undergo a procedure, skip a visit, or violate any of the study protocol procedures without penalty.

Similarly, the clinical investigator's foremost commitment is the patient's safety. Thus, although participating clinical investigators are committed to follow the study protocol, they could at any time decide to treat a patient in violation of the protocol if in their clinical judgement it is in the patient's best interest. The result is that clinical trials rarely are conducted exactly as planned. Some of the issues resulting from this reality are discussed below.

Noncompliance, dropouts, and missing data

Noncompliance

In testing the efficacy of a new drug, or studying a dose–response relationship, it is of critical importance that subjects take their medication as prescribed in the protocol. Most drugs exhibit a direct dose–response relationship in terms of the drug's efficacy and safety. Noncompliance with respect to the schedule and dose of the study medication may have serious impact on the researcher's ability to determine the recommended dose or even to show efficacy. When subjects underdose themselves, the drug efficacy may be missed and the true adverse event pattern of the drug may be underestimated. Clinical researchers always try to build in mechanisms into the trial's procedures designed to maximize compliance. However, it is not uncommon that despite such efforts, some subjects will miss some doses.

It is impossible to adjust for noncompliance at the analysis phase without making assumptions about the dose–response relationship, which is often not well understood and might vary greatly from one subject to another. It is always important to assess the level of compliance at the end of the trial so that one might gain some appreciation, qualitative and incomplete as it may be, of what one should expect when the drug is taken as prescribed.

Another type of noncompliance is the subjects' (lack of) adherence to the protocol procedures and schedules. It is the role of the investigator to make sure that the protocol is adhered to. Lack of adherence to the protocol complicates the analysis and may make the result difficult to interpret.

Dropouts

Subjects may drop out of the trial for a variety of reasons. Some could be unrelated to the trial such as relocation, but others, such as experiencing adverse events, the perception of no efficacy, or perception of well-being, could be strongly correlated with the study drug effect. The result is that some subjects will have no data to evaluate from some time point onwards. When the reasons for dropping out are treatment related, the patterns of dropouts will be typically different between the different treatments, and ignoring the missing data will introduce bias into the analysis.

There are a number of methods for handling dropouts, none of which is entirely satisfactory. One common way is to use the Last-Observation-Carried-Forward (LOCF) method. In this method, the last available value is substituted for all missed measurements. The problem with this approach is that it assumes that had the subject not dropped out, he or she would continue to respond exactly the same way as on their last visit before dropping out. This assumption is never verifiable and often unreasonable. Another approach is to substitute

the worse possible value for the missing data. The rationale for this approach is that the results of the analysis will show "worst case scenario" and if the drug passes this test and can be labeled safe and effective, it would still be so had subjects not dropped out. This rationale is certainly plausible. The trouble is that efficacy of important and moderately efficacious drugs may be missed, or mildly toxic drugs may end up with unnecessarily serious safety warnings on their labels. There are other methods of statistical "imputation" where a value is calculated using some algorithm and is substituted for the missing value. The reasonableness of these procedures must be judged on a case-by-case basis by examining the underlying assumptions and judging their appropriateness in the given situation.

Missing data

Dropouts present one type of missing data; namely, data are not available from a certain time point onward. Data could also be missing in many other ways. A subject may miss a visit, a sample could be invalid, or a subject may fail to fill out a form or a questionnaire. When data are missing at random, the effect is generally some loss in the power of the statistical analysis. When data are missing according to some pattern, bias can be introduced in addition.

Some statistical study designs are particularly sensitive to missing data. Crossover designs are such designs. In crossover designs, each subject is randomly assigned to a sequence of treatments administered at certain time interval apart. The reason for using these designs is that each subject serves as his or her own control, and the comparisons between treatments are done within subjects. When the within-subject variability is substantially smaller than the between or inter-subject variability, the crossover design may be quite powerful and offer great savings in the utilization of subject resources. The loss of one value in a crossover study may result in a loss of the entire sequence. Some designs require certain balances among the treatments and schedules of treatment. Missing data can destroy such balances, seriously handicapping the statistician's ability to analyze the data. Here too, imputation, with all the caveats going along with it, is the method of "correcting" for the missing data. When much data are missing, say 20% or more, one should seriously question the validity of the conclusions drawn from the study, because they might be over-influenced by the assumptions made on how to handle the missing data rather than by the data themselves.

Intent-to-treat analysis

One possible way of handling protocol violations, noncompliance, missing data, dropouts, and so on is to remove all subjects whose violations are considered to be serious from the analysis and analyze only the data obtained from the subjects who reasonably complied with all the requirements stated in the protocol. Such analysis is sometimes referred to as *per-protocol analysis* (PP). The problem with this approach is that the effectiveness of the randomization process as a mechanism to bestow balances among latent and known prognostic factors, and set the stage for making causal relationship inferences, is disturbed. Also, if the reasons for these violations are not independent of treatment or the subject's condition, the removal of these subjects for the analysis may introduce a bias in the analysis.

Therefore, it is an accepted rule to always perform an *intent-to-treat-analysis* (ITT) in which all subjects randomized, or all subjects randomized who received at least one dose of study medication, are included. The proponents of this approach argue that in addition to the preservation of the randomization process, the ITT reflects "real life" results. They argue that in "real life," as opposed to the artificial setup of the clinical study, neither patients not their physicians follow a specific rigorous protocol. So, if the outcome of noncompliance, for example, is reduced efficacy, this is what one should expect to see when the drug is used in clinical practice. Although, the arguments for the ITT analysis are valid, the inclusion of patients with incomplete or missing data, poor complying patients, and/or patients with major protocol violations, complicates the analysis and if the number of such patients is large it may either obscure or distort the actual drug effects.

Statisticians have developed data imputation methods for handling missing data by reconstructing the missing information on the basis of avail-

able data. However, these methods are all based on assumptions about the relationship between the available data and missing data that are hard or impossible to verify. Therefore, any conclusion derived from imputed data must be viewed with caution and different imputations should be applied to see the extent that the conclusions depend on the imputation method.

The use of ITT is required by the FDA as the primary analyses that must always be presented to them. The problems we highlighted earlier in this section present challenges to the data analyst that can be addressed at the analysis phase only to a limited extent. It is impossible to design a trial so that these problems will be prevented entirely. However, a careful design and diligent execution and monitoring of the trial can minimize them.

The dissemination of clinical trials results

Clinical trials are complex and expensive scientific endeavors. For this reason, most clinical trials are supported by either pharmaceutical companies or government. Pharmaceutical companies conduct clinical trials not only as part of their clinical development of new therapies, but also to discover new indications or special features of their approved drugs as part of their marketing activities. The results of trials conducted as part of the drug approval process are summarized and submitted to the FDA. In addition, the FDA requires sponsors to summarize and submit the results of all other studies of the drug conducted by the sponsor or that were published in the scientific literature. This information becomes part of the public knowledge after the drug is approved. Studies conducted outside of the New Drug Application (NDA) process are treated quite differently. As these studies are conducted for the purpose of promoting the sales of the drug or in exploration of additional indications, there is no requirement to submit the results to any governmental agency unless the company decides to submit a supplementary NDA. Many such trials result with negative outcomes and the sponsors as well as the clinical investigators have little or no incentive to expend the resources of analyzing data from trials and publish the results. Contributing to this is the fact that scientific publications must make editorial decisions as to what they will and will not accept for publication. Negative studies are often found uninteresting scientifically and are refused publication. The result of this is that the information available to the medical community is selective and incomplete. This might have serious public health consequences, because it could influence medical practice. Medical practitioners may not be aware of certain adverse effects of a drug they prescribe, the usefulness of drugs in the treatment of certain conditions may not be known, or worse, treatments proven ineffective may continue to be employed.

This problem was recognized, and a Federal law was passed in 1997 requiring the sponsors of clinical trials to register trials to the FDA to be included in a trial registry and available to the public. The law has been largely ignored by the pharmaceutical industry, and the FDA did little to enforce it. A registry was established in 1998 but only a small percentage of industry-sponsored trials were posted in it. This issue came to the attention of the American public recently after it became known that one of the nation's major pharmaceutical manufacturers has been withholding information of serious adverse events of one of their antidepressants in children and adolescents (*Bloomberg Business News*, 2004; *The Washington Post*, 2004a, 2004b). In 2007, a law was enacted requiring all but Phase I studies of drugs and devices that are subject to FDA regulation to be registered. Furthermore, the new law required that the results of these studies be reported as well. The new law also established penalties for noncompliance with it. The trials and the reports are posted on a special website (http://clinicaltrials.gov; accessed April 24, 2010) and are available to all.

The statistician's role

Information derived from data collected in a clinical trial is the ultimate product of the trial. Every aspect of the trial from its conception to its execution impacts the quality of the data and the information they contain. The final step in the process, the analysis, is nothing but the application of statistical methods for organizing the data, summarizing them, and extracting relevant information; that is, separating the signal from the noise. The statistician's ability to make up for design deficiencies and for noisy data is limited, and the same rule defining good practice of medicine applies here as well: the best treatment of a disease is to prevent it. The statistician's greatest impact could, therefore, be at the front-end, during the trial planning, rather than the back-end, at the analysis phase.

The study protocol and case report forms (CRF)

A clinical trial is a complex scientific undertaking that requires the collaboration of many people: clinical investigators, subjects, study coordinators, data managers, statisticians, programmers, and many more. It is, therefore, of critical importance that a study plan, procedures, and conventions will be laid out clearly in advance in a document so that all the participants in this journey will follow the same road map. The study protocol is this road map. Like any good road map, the study protocol must be very clear about the ultimate goal and direction of the journey: that is, the study objectives. Often, the clarity of the study objectives in the protocol determines the coherence of the rest of the protocol. Clearly and specifically stated objectives will help identify when the primary measures of efficacy, for example, are inadequate, or when the design is flawed, or when superfluous data, which will not contribute anything to answer the questions posed in the objectives, are going to be collected.

The creation of the study protocol is a multidisciplinary and collaborative effort. Every aspect of the protocol impacts all other aspects. A medical procedure may impact the response of subjects to treatment, their compliance, or other important aspect that ultimately will impact the data and the conclusions that can be drawn from them. For this reason, every member of the study design team must assume responsibility for the entire protocol. The statistician may be responsible directly for writing the statistical design considerations and the analysis plan, but his or her involvement in all other aspects of the design that feed into it are equally important.

The CRF is the data collection tool for the clinical trial. Often, the design of the CRF is viewed as a technical task auxiliary to the trial, and the statistician may not see it until the trial is ongoing and the data start coming in for processing. The CRF design is an important activity that can make a difference in the quality of the data obtained in the trial. It should be viewed as an integral part of the protocol development process, and input from the clinician, the clinical monitor, and the statistician must be obtained. The CRF is a multipurpose instrument. It serves the investigator as the tool for recording the data obtained in the trial, must facilitate the review of the data by the clinical monitor, and is the document used by the data manager to build the database for statistical analysis. The organization and structure of the CRF, the way the questions are phrased, and the use of codes, all impact the data quality.

Since the early 1980s, technology has been available for electronic transfer of the data from the investigational sites to the data center. However, this technology had very limited used until recently. Electronic data collection (EDC) systems have become very powerful and attractive in the last few years due to the maturity and growing power and speed of the Internet. The use of EDC systems can speed up the data processing and thus ultimately reduce the entire new drug development process. The procedures involved in the use ECD systems are still evolving, but one can predict with certainty that these methods will become the dominant mode of data acquisition in the not too distant future.

Analysis and reporting

The analysis of the data at the end of the trial is, of course, the statistician's domain. A successful analysis is one that reaches unambiguous conclusions, not necessarily the ones the clinical researcher is hoping for. As we emphasized earlier, the success of the analysis depends entirely on the way the trial was conducted and monitored, and the way the data were generated and collected. The statistician's

role is to utilize the appropriate tools designed to most effectively extract the information from the data. The analysis tools do not create information. We emphasized the need to prepare for the analysis at the design stage. It is also important to think one step ahead and consider the need to analyze the data obtained from a number of different studies. A new drug application usually consists of many different studies. The approval of the application is not based on any single study but rather on the synthesis of the information obtained from all the studies. Data from some studies will have to be combined and analyzed. Such an analysis, called *meta-analysis*, must be planned for in advance, too.

Two examples of meta-analysis are the integrated summary of safety (ISS) and the integrated summary of efficacy (ISE). These analyses must be planned for just as if the combined database represented data from a new study. Ideally, plans for meta-analyses should be made at the time the individual studies are planned. This is not always possible, but this is the best way to ensure that the meta-analysis database used for the analysis is coherent. For example, if the adverse events information is collected in two studies using different data collection forms, the combination of the individual databases may be difficult and some information may be lost.

Epilogue

An anonymous cynic once said that there are three types of liars: liars, damned liars, and statisticians. This statement reflects the discomfort many researchers feel when working with statisticians. The image of the statistician taking the data to his or her dark room, performing incomprehensible manipulations behind closed doors, and coming back with results, charts, and magic numbers, and throwing around vaguely understood terms, is unfortunate. It is my hope that this chapter helps to disperse the haze and clarify the statistician's role and mode of thinking. The statistician is neither a liar nor a magician; rather, the statistician is a professional trained in scientific methods devised to establish causal relationships under conditions of uncertainty. My goal in writing this chapter was not to turn the reader into a statistician. Instead, it was to bring the statistician out of the dark room into the open, and by reviewing the issues he or she is concerned about and clarifying basic terminology, to facilitate communication between the statistician and the rest of the study team.

References

Bloomberg Business News. U.S. doctors may seek rules for drug makers to disclose studies. *Bloomberg Business News*, June 15, 2004.

Bok S. The ethics of giving placebos. *Sci Am* 1974; **231**:17.

Fisher RA. *Statistical Methods and Scientific Inference*. Hafner: New York, USA, 1956.

Gribbin M. Placebos: cheapest medicine in the world. *New Sci* 1981; **89**:64–65.

ICH (International Conference on Harmonization). E9: Statistical Principles for Clinical Trials. No. 1, *Federal Register*, 1998; **63**(179):49583–49598.

PMA Biostatistics and Medical Ad Hoc Committee on Interim Analysis. Interim analysis in the pharmaceutical industry. *Control Clin Trials* 1993; **14**:160–173.

Popper K. *The Logic of Scientific Discovery*. Basic Books: New York, 1959.

The Washington Post. Drugmakers prefer silence on test data. Firms violate U.S. law by not registering trials. *The Washington Post*, July 6, 2004a.

The Washington Post. Drug firms flout law by failing to report test data, FDA says. *The Washington Post*, July 7, 2004b.

Further reading

Armitage P. *Statistical Methods in Medical Research*. John Wiley & Sons Inc.: New York, USA, 1971.

Freedman D, Pisani R, Purves R. Statistics.W.W. Norton & Co.: New York, USA, 1978.

Friedman LM, Furberg CD, DeMets DL. *Fundamentals of Clinical Trials*. John Wright: Boston, MA, USA, 1981.

Pocock SJ. *Clinical Trials: A Practical Approach*. John Wiley & Sons Ltd: Chichester, UK, 1983.

CHAPTER 29

Data Management

T.Y. Lee[1], Michael Minor[1], & Lionel D. Edwards[2]

[1]Clinical Development and Asian Ventures, Kendle International Inc., Cincinnati, OH, USA
[2]Pharma Pro Plus Inc., New Jersey, and Temple University, School of Pharmacy, Philadelphia, USA

Pharmaceutical research and development is a lengthy (8–12 years) and costly process (approximately US$1.3 billion in 2007). It starts from discovery of the compound and moves through biological screening, animal toxicological studies, formulation, assay development/validation, clinical pharmacology, stability testing, clinical trials, data management, statistical and clinical evaluation, new drug application, and promotional marketing. At each stage of the research and development, data are generated, processed, and validated before being subject to statistical analysis. Data management plays a significant role in assuring the government agency and consumers that the database represents a pool of information that was accurately collected and processed and logically presented. With the advancement of pharmaceutical technology in identifying new compounds, and improved efficiency in software support and information processing, the duration of exclusivity enjoyed by a new drug has been drastically reduced before a competitive drug of the same or a similar class reaches the market. For example, the duration of exclusivity (PhRMA, 1997) of several major drugs is summarized in Table 29.1, and in 2009–2012 a record number of blockbuster medicines will lose their patent protection.

Because of the accelerated shortening of the duration of the exclusivity, pharmaceutical companies tend to initiate clinical trials in several countries simultaneously to obtain worldwide clinical data. This strategy will give them a chance to market the drug in many countries within a relatively short time and recover as much cost as possible before the competitors join in. To collect worldwide data and pool them together presents a special challenge to data management professionals. It is necessary to consider differences in culture, medical practice, laboratory standards/units, classifications of disease and medication, drug reactions, religion, self-medication, drug interactions, and so on. Therefore, a detailed and coordinated data management plan, standard operation procedures, quality control (QC), and quality assurance (QA) are essential to produce a reliable database.

Obtaining the project material

To develop a data management plan pertinent to the project, a checklist of the project material is necessary to enhance the planning. The items to be collected include the protocol, annotated case report forms (CRFs), literature, log-in and tracking forms, file structures, coding rules, CRF review conventions, query handling procedure, required edit checklist, central laboratory address/file format, laboratory normal ranges, clinically significant ranges, timelines, QC rules, QA sampling, error analysis, criteria to release the database, disaster recovery plan, and so on. Most of these rules and conventions are preliminary and collected from earlier studies. These rules and conventions will be discussed by the project team from time to time to make them pertinent to the current studies.

Principles and Practice of Pharmaceutical Medicine, 3rd edition.
Edited by L.D. Edwards, A.W. Fox, P.D. Stonier.

Table 29.1 Duration of exclusivity for some major drugs

Drug name	Year approved	Exclusivity (years)
Inderal	1968	10
Tagmet	1977	7
Capoten	1980	5
Prozac	1988	4
Diflucan	1990	2
Recombinate	1992	1
Invirase	1995	0.25

Formation of the project team

Pharmaceutical companies usually assign a project manager to coordinate the formation of the project team (see Table 29.2). The project manager works closely with the functional department heads to select the team members. The team usually includes representatives from the departments of regulatory affairs, clinical research, medical writing, biostatistics, data management, programming, and document support. The project manager should coordinate the activities to make sure that the team has adequate resources; the project information is distributed in a timely fashion; the status is issued; milestones are reached at each stage; and the team members have a clear and detailed instruction of the priorities of the various protocols. For multinational projects, the quality of CRFs varies from

Table 29.2 Project team personnel list

Protocol No.	Project team coordinator:
Name of drug:	Directory location:
1. Regulatory associate:	
2. Clinician and medical writer:	
3. Primary statistician:	
4. Secondary statistician:	
5. Scanner:	
6. Primary CDC:	
7. Secondary CDC:	
8. Data entry screen designer:	
9. Edit check programmer:	
10. Quality assurance:	
11. Data entry:	
12. Data verifier:	

country to country. It requires a great deal of management skill on the part of the project manager to balance national pride and quality requirements without sacrificing the quality of the final database.

Project setup

From the data management perspective, the clinical data coordinator (CDC) is the central team member receiving and distributing data-related information to the project team members. The CDC meets with the project team members to review the project material collected and to elicit the rules and special requirements from the statistician, clinician, safety officer, medical writer, and regulatory associates. These project materials, rules, and special requirements will be considered in conjunction with data management requirements to develop the data management plan. The CDC should prepare the following documents before the clinical trials are initiated:
- data creation flow chart (see Figure 29.1);
- project team personnel list (see Table 29.2);
- CRFs log-in sheet (see Table 29.3);
- CRFs cover sheet (see Table 29.4);
- preliminary edit check document (see Table 29.5);
- data query sheet (see Table 29.6);
- data processing status (see Table 29.7);
- audit sheet (see Table 29.8);
- audit document (see Table 29.9);
- summary of audit results (see Table 29.10);
- sample memo of notifying formal closure of database (see Table 29.11).

Data processing

Log-in and scan process
To prepare the CRFs to be scanned into the computer, carry out the following tasks:

1. Verify the shipment of CRFs from clinical research department to the inventory of data management department (see Table 29.3).

2. Check the CRFs to ensure that the header information is accurate and complete.

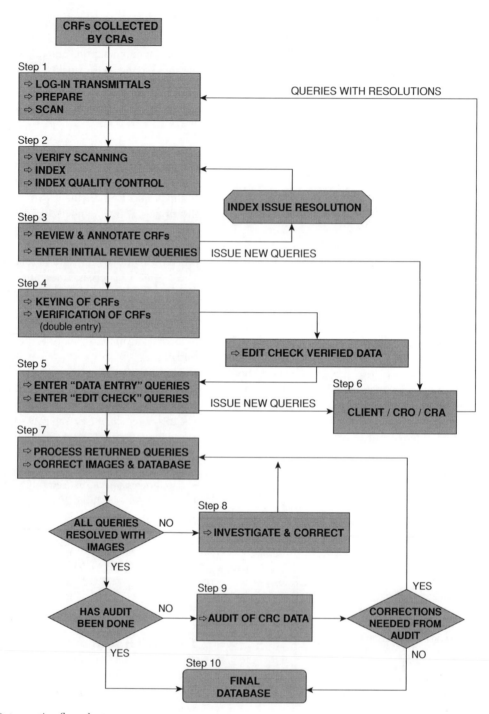

Figure 29.1 Data creation flow chart.

Table 29.3 CRFs log-in sheet

Protocol No.:
Name of drug:
Data clerk name:
1. Log-in date:
2. Investigator number and name:
3. Patient number/initial:
4. Book/visit number:
5. Batch name:
6. Comments:

---

3. Prepare the CRF file folder with the cover page (see Table 29.4), which carries the following information: batch number, site, patient ID, visit number, log-in date, and the initials of the person who logged the CRFs. This will ensure that the scanner assigns the patient information to the correct fields of the electronic image files.
4. Scan CRFs into the computer image files.

CRFs image review process

This process is to ensure that unexpected data problems or unusual inter-data relations in various data fields are identified. It is a very important step in the data process: many companies have encountered data quality problems because of the lack of this step, which is not included to replace the computer edit check but rather to enhance it. The basic principles for the image review are checking the "accuracy," "completeness," and "consistency" of the data within a subject and across subjects.

This review and timely computer edit checks will provide feedback to the monitoring staff concerning a problematic investigator or CRF page,

Table 29.4 CRFs cover sheet

Protocol No:		Site/investigator:
Name of drug:		Patient No/Visit No:
Data clerk name:		Batch No:
Process	Date	Initial
Log-in		
Review		
Key		
Verify		
Query		
Audit		

so that corrective action of monitoring practice or enhancement of the computer edit checks can be implemented promptly. The review should include the following steps:
1. Are there missing header information, missing pages, and visits?
2. Are randomization numbers allocated sequentially?
3. Are blanks are properly answered?
4. Check adverse events and prematurely discontinued subjects, with special attention to the comments for hidden information.
5. Has clinically significant laboratory abnormality been followed by the investigator?
6. Does the drug inventory match the number consumed?
7. Clarify all text items, for example adverse events, concomitant medications, physical examinations, ECG, progress notes, and so on.

Data entry and double entry using CRF images

Carry out the following tasks:
• Autocode the data using structured glossaries, including drug class, body system, preferred term, and verbatim term.
• Manual code the "no-hit" terms and update the glossary.
• Run computer edit checks (see Table 29.5) and generate queries. Reconcile the discrepancies between the queries generated by manual review and computer edit check. Issue the queries (see Table 29.6) to the investigators.

Query resolution and database update

When the answers to the queries are returned, the CDC updates the database and CRF images. This is a continuous process during the course of the clinical trials.

Create test datasets for various analysis population

To make the adequate inferences of the efficacy and safety of the study drug, Federal Register should be followed (ICH, 1996): in Section 11.1, "Data Sets

Table 29.5 Preliminary edit check document

Protocol No: Edit check programmer:
Name of drug: Version date:
CDC name: Revision date:

General checks:
(D-1) Subject initials should be consistent throughout casebook
(D-2) All dates should be within valid ranges

Inclusion criteria:
(D-1) Inclusion #1 should be yes or no
(D-2) Inclusion #2 should be yes or no
(D-3) Inclusion #3 should be yes or no
(D-4) Consent date should be equal to visit date

Exclusion criteria:
(D-1) Exclusion #1 should be yes or no
(D-2) Exclusion #2 should be yes or no
(D-3) Exclusion #3 should be yes or no
(D-4) Exclusion #4 should be yes or no
(D-5) Exclusion #5 should be yes or no or n/a
(D-4) Exclusion #6 should be yes or no or n/a
Demographics:
Efficacy:
Safety:
(etc.)

Analyzed," it states:

> Exactly which patients were included in each efficacy analysis should be precisely defined, e.g., all patients receiving any test drugs/investigational products; all patients with any efficacy observations or with a certain minimum number of observations; only patients completing the trial; all patients with an observation during a particular time window; or only patients with a specified degree of compliance. It should be clear, if not defined in the study protocol, when (relative to unblinding of the study) and how inclusion/exclusion criteria for the datasets

analyzed were developed. Generally, even if the applicant's proposed primary analysis is based on a reduced subset of the patients with data, there should also be, for any trial intended to establish the efficacy, an additional analysis using all randomized (or otherwise entered) patients with any on-treatment data ... A diagram showing the relationship between the entire sample and any other analysis groups should be provided.

Therefore, an algorithm has to be developed to define precisely how each analysis population of the dataset is defined. There are at least four analysis population datasets, for example, the intent-to-treat (ITT) population, the per-protocol (PP) population, the safety population, and the microbiological population, as indicated in Figure 29.2. During the derivation of various analysis populations, it may be necessary to issue new queries and update the database, based on the resolution of the queries.

Status reporting (Table 29.7)

Carry out the following tasks:
1. From the image files and the database, generate a weekly production report.
2. A cross-check of milestones and progress achieved should be made and the status reported to the department heads for review and action.
3. The department heads may adjust the resources, depending on the progress report.

Create audit sheet for audit

The computer-generated audit sheet (see Table 29.8) should be formatted in the same sequence as the fields in the CRFs. This will enhance the speed of the audit task. The QA auditor will check the audit sheet against the CRF images.

Table 29.6 Data query sheet

Protocol No: Data submitted:
Name of drug: Date returned:
CDC name:

Site/pat. no	Page	Visit	Problem	Resolution	
Investigator signature:					Date:

| CRA signature: | | | | | Date: |

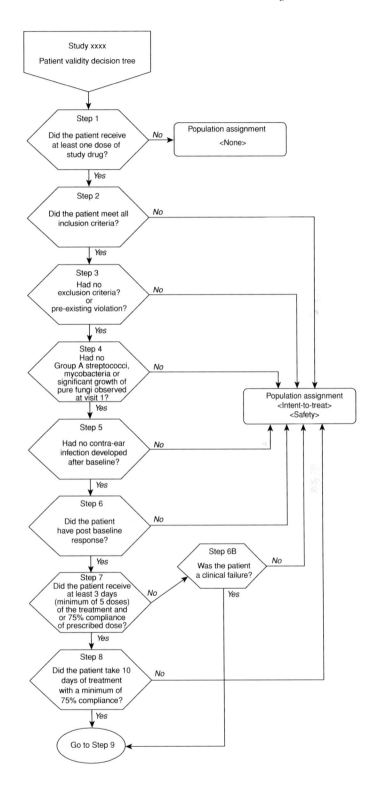

Figure 29.2 Derivation of study population.

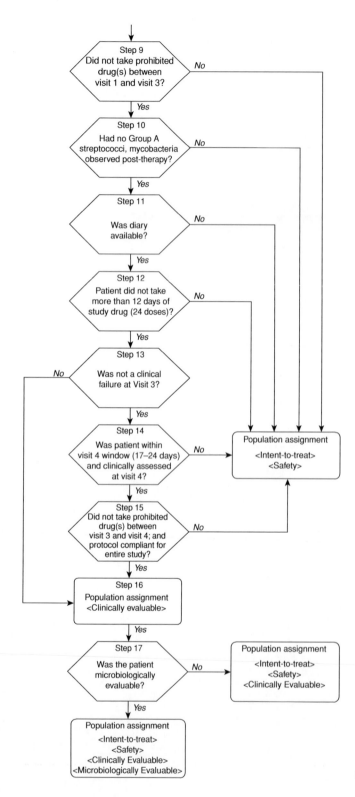

Figure 29.2 (*Continued*)

Table 29.7 Data process status

Protocol No:					
Name of drug:					
CDC name:					
Site/inv.	Logged (no.) (%)	Reviewed (no.) (%)	Keyed (no.) (%)	Verified (no.) (%)	Audited (no.) (%)
Total:					

Issue interim audit document and audit summary

When 10% of the CRFs have been scanned and entered into the computer, the interim audit should be conducted in order to tune up the CDC review manual and edit-check programs. Findings regarding the quality of the database should be given to the head of the data management group for possible action. The audit document (see Table 29.9) should include patient ID, the initials of the keyer and verifier, CDC, editing programmer, type of audit, number of errors, and description of errors. It is a tool to find out which records tend to produce more errors and who tends to make most of the mistakes. Is CDC review ade-quate? Are the programs written for the computer edit checks sufficient? Did the data entry verifier find the problems of the keyer and fix them? Once the CDC review manual and computer edit checks have been improved, a second interim audit should be repeated when 50–60% of the CRFs have been scanned and entered. Final audit should be performed when all the CRFs are scanned and entered. In addition to the audit memo issued during the interim audits, an audit summary report (see Table 29.10) should be issued to summarize the quality of the final database. This will also give management an index of the error rate, which measures the confidence level of releasing the database.

Table 29.8 Audit sheet

Protocol No:										Audit sheet programmer
Name of drug:										Version date:
Name of CDC:										Revision date:
CRF Page 1:										
Eligibility criteria:										
Initial: RLD										Visit date:
Inclusion criteria										
1	2	3	4	5	6	7				
1	1	1	1	1	1	1				
Exclusion Criteria										
1	2	3	4	5	6	7	8	9	10	11
2	2	2	2	2	2	2	2	2	2	2
CRF Page 2:										
Infection history:										
Initial: RLD										Visit date:
Number of infections in past year: 3										
Therapy for infection in past year: 2										
Medication: Drug aaa				Effective: 1						Complete med: 1
(etc.)										

Table 29.9 Audit document

Protocol No: Date audit start:
Name of drug: Date audit stop:
Auditor name:

Pat. no.	Keyer	Verifier	CDC	Auditor	Type of audit	No of errors	Description of errors
½	ka	jp	sr	et	Full	0	
01/005	ka	jp	sr	et	Full	0	
01/009	ka	jp	sr	et	Full	1	Med. His—"Pnemonia" should be "Pneumonia"
01/014	ka	jp	sr	et	Full	0	
01/018	ev	cc	jf	wa	Full	0	
02/005	js	cc	jf	wa	Full	1	Diary—3/24/98 bedtime 11:10 pm should be at 11:00 pm
(etc.)							

Database release memo

Once all the queries have been resolved and updated to the image files and database, the database is officially locked. A database release memo (see Table 29.11) should be issued to the project statistician, all other team members, and management. The project statistician will then merge the file of the randomization codes to the database to generate the analysis datasets.

Disaster recovery plan

The data files and the completed CRFs generated from the clinical trials are more precious than the hardware. In addition to daily and monthly back-up, pharmaceutical companies should have a detailed recovery plan in case of unexpected disaster. The disaster recovery plan should include the following items:

Table 29.10 Format of summary of audit result

Protocol No: Date audit start:
Name of drug: Date audit stop:
Auditor names:

Page description	Data set No	Variables/ patient No	Patient audited No	Records checked No	Values checked No	Errors found	Error rate (%)
Adv. Exper	Adverse	26	497	558	14 508	0	0.0000
Study Complete	Complete	7	497	497	3 479	2	0.0575
Conc. Med.	Conmed	18	497	602	10 836	4	0.0369
Eligibility Criteria	Criteria	29	497	497	14 413	1	0.0069
Diary	Diary	160	497	497	79 520	17	0.0214
Drug Accountab.	Drugacct	6	497	497	2 982	1	0.0335
Overall					27 0771	51	0.0188

Table 29.11 Database release memorandum

Date:
To: Project statistician
From: CDC
Subject: Database Release
The master files of the following study have been audited
by the QA department and passed. The database is
therefore signed off and released by Data Management.
Drug:
Protocol number:
Investigator number and name:
Date master files signed off:
Time master files signed off:
Please verify that you have received the master files.
Via this memo, QA department is requested to release the
randomization codes to the project statistician. Thanks.
Clinical Data coordinator
cc: Project team members

• *Key personnel contact list*, with home telephone
and pager numbers listed.
• *List of critical applications and operations.* It should
be a company's policy to set up an off-site processing center with the same hardware–software
setup. This should be able to be made operational
within 2 hours should it become necessary if a
disaster strikes the data center. Critical applications
and operations include upcoming New Drug Application (NDA) studies, safety database, and NDA
summaries.
• *Off-site storage.* In order to be operational at the
off-site process center for critical applications, the
files that need to be updated to the off-site center
are master files for all completed projects, daily
back-ups for ongoing studies, monthly system files,
monthly glossary updates, monthly safety monitoring, NDA files, and production job streams. The
protocols, CRFs, regulatory documents, rules, and
manuals should also be stored off-site. A drill of the
disaster recovery plan should be put to the test at
least every six months to reveal any unanticipated
problems.

Interactive voice response system (IVRS) and electronic data capture (EDC)

IVRSs have been used in clinical studies since
around 1989, and are increasingly being utilized

in a variety of ways: patient recruitment, screening
and randomization, medication management, electronic patient reported outcomes, real time patient
compliance data, and data quality and data management. The systems are commercially available
but many will need some custom work. They
feature secure telephone-based access, which can
be site-based, sponsor-based, patient-home-access-
based, or a combination of all three. IVRSs are useful in randomization especially where various doses
of drugs are being used such as combination drugs
and adaptive design Phase 1–2 studies as well as
studies requiring stratification of different cohorts,
because they provide a centralized randomization
and the random code can be accessed only centrally
by the sponsor.

An IVRS provides a useful tool for monitoring
study recruitment and drug management (Byron,
2002), especially where a drug is in short supply, as
well as location of expiring batch dates, a frequent
occurrence in the early Phase 1–2 studies. Its value
to data management is in the provision of a safe
electronic memory storage and ease of appropriate
access and retrieval. Initially these systems were
not welcome at many sites because early versions
were poor at speech recognition, Today's versions
are much more user-friendly and often requested
by the sites to speed up the randomization
process without tedious waiting to contact a live
person, especially when patients cannot take time
off work and are seen in evening clinics. The best
use is when an IVRS is used in conjunction and
integrated with electronic data capture (EDC).

The early versions of electronic case report forms
appeared in the mid-1980s, and were designed
with data management in mind (that is, ease of
data collection), rather than being inclusive of the
investigators' needs and the sponsor's data review;
thus, they were not very user-friendly (Edwards,
1990). It took years to align all the needs into a reliable bundle that also complied with good clinical
practice (GCP) and emerging electronic regulatory
requirements. An early report (Edwards, 1990)
compared the time to close out four sites using
EDC and two sites using paper CRFs once the last
patient, last visit occurred. The four EDC sites were
all closed out in 24 hours and the two paper sites
took ten weeks until the last was closed.

The uptake of EDC has been slow; many systems were disappointingly unfriendly and slow—the first modem of 18 and 22 bauds could take 20–30 minutes for transmission for a single page over telephone landlines. Of course, Moore's law of data processors (every two years processing speed will double) proved very accurate, but now it is slowing, and superconductor and nana silicate methodologies together with lateral processing are functioning or being explored in order to increase speed and computer ability. We have quite enough computing power, storage, speed, and software to run the current programs of fully integrated IVRSs and EDC, so much so that many firms are utilizing integrated systems. As these still tend to be custom built, this is a drawback.

Even the integrated system is less efficient than it could be, unless it is combined into a "life cycle" Clinical Trial Management System (CTMS) with SOPs and Best Practices built in.

The FDA requires the NDA be submitted in its entirety as an electronic Common Technical Document (CTD), and so it is easier and more efficient to record, transfer, and store for submission, data in electronic format. This not only reduces paperwork but also time-consuming double data entry, transcribing errors, and missing data queries. To define electronic data standards, the FDA has assigned the Clinical Data Interchange Consortium (CDISC) the task of producing the best standards and format for FDA submissions. Getting agreement among the many "stake holders" is a large effort and very time-consuming. In addition, as technology has increased ability, so has the complexity increased, making the task of validating systems, processes, and data even harder to do.

Much better software and technology have converted many firms into making the necessary technology investment and training to nearly all their studies. Of course, there is still some latter-day Luddites. But the shortening of the time to NDA submission and the reductions of labor and time spent in data retrieval, data transfer, double entry, and data queries have persuaded most people to adopt the integrated systems.

Aiding in this are newly launch-based systems such as i3cube (an application developed by i3global.com). This runs on Adobe and provides both sponsor and site staff with real-time "dash boards" to access for reports accrual and many other functions.

The American Recovery and Reinvestment Act (February 2009), among other stimulus grants, directed US$19 billion in funds to physician offices and hospitals to upgrade their clinical patients' records electronically, and although the primary reason was to reduce errors of treatment and prescribing, this could also be a powerful tool in pharmocovigilance, patient outcomes monitoring and analysis. How this may be aligned with Phase 4 vigilance and efficiency studies under the Health and Insurance Portability and Accountability Act (HIPAA) confidentiality regulations is yet to be worked out.

References

American Recovery and Reinvestment Act. February 2009; http://www.recovery.gov/About/Pages/The_Act .aspx; accessed April 12, 2010.

Byron B. Using IVRS in clinical management. *Applied Clinical Trials* 2002; Oct: 36–38.

Edwards LD. Multinational Experience Using Remote Data Entry in Clinical Studies. *Drug Info Journal* 1991; **24**:629–633

ICH. International Conference on Harmonization: Guideline on Structure, Content and Clinical Study Reports; availability; notice. *Federal Register* 1991; **61**(138):37326.

PhRMA. *Facts and Figures*, 1997.

Further Reading

Katz HI, Edwards LD, Survey results of Remote Data Entry by Clinical Investigator Site. *Drug Info Journal* 1990; **3**.

CHAPTER 30

Patient Compliance: Pharmionics, A New Discipline

*Dr. Jean-Michel Métry**

*This chapter has been updated by Anthony Fox and is a tribute to the late Jean-Michel Métry who died in August 2009.

Summary

The term *pharmionics* refers to a new area of study, namely the investigation of what the patient actually does with the drug after it has been prescribed. Pharmionics-guided measurements have, as one aim, to accelerate and improve clinical development of new drugs for ambulatory patients. Another aim is to improve clinical outcomes of ambulatory pharmacotherapy. The fundamental data for achieving both aims are full and reliable measurement of the time and amount of drug exposure.

A major aspect of this area is patient noncompliance. It has long been recognized that patients often do not take the drugs that they have been prescribed. But it is only during the last 25 years, relatively recently, that this has become an analyzed aspect of ambulatory healthcare, as objective, satisfactory methods became available for compiling drug dosing histories in ambulatory patients; this is now the cornerstone for measuring compliance. Since then, much new information has been gained.

Pharmionic terminology and definitions

It is important to understand the terminology of pharmionics. The term *persistence* is the length of

Principles and Practice of Pharmaceutical Medicine, 3rd edition.
Edited by L.D. Edwards, A.W. Fox, P.D. Stonier.
© 2011 Blackwell Publishing Ltd.

time between the first-taken dose and the last-taken dose in a course of ambulatory pharmacotherapy. *Adherence* is a blanket term for the three phases of ambulatory pharmacotherapy, which are as follows:

- *Acceptance:* The first phase is whether the patient accepts the principle and regimen of the prescribed treatment. If acceptance is forthcoming, the patient commences to engage with the drug dosing regimen.
- *Execution:* The second phase, measured by *compliance*, is the extent to which the patient engages with the therapy: that is, how well the dosing history corresponds to the prescribed dosing regimen.
- *Discontinuation:* The third phase is when the treatment ceases; this may be because the prescriber called for it to cease, or the patient may have partially or wholly stopped engaging with the dosing regimen; discontinuation is when, for whatever reason, drug intake levels have fallen so low as to be therapeutically inconsequential.

The three phases are separated because the first and third are binary, or dichotomous, phenomena, in that they either happen or they do not. The second phase, however, is continuous, and capable of varying from day to day, sometimes quite widely. One cannot have a single parameter that describes both dichotomous and continuous phenomena, and for that reason, the term *adherence*, which has a certain convenience, is inherently nonquantitative. Someone can be accurately termed a "poor adherer," because of nonacceptance, acceptance but poor execution, or short persistence, with either good or poor compliance during the period of time that the patient was engaged with the drug dosing regimen.

From a methodological point of view, the most challenging of the three phases of ambulatory pharmacotherapy to measure has been execution and compliance, which is the subject of this chapter. Subjective methods to assess patient compliance in drug trials or medical practice grossly overestimate patient execution. To measure drug exposure in ambulatory patients reliably, methods are needed that make it difficult for patients to censor evidence for delayed or omitted doses. Electronic monitoring has emerged as the gold standard for measuring drug exposure in ambulatory patients.

Introduction

A major reason for poor compliance is simple negligence. Neither good intention nor a professional level of understanding of medicine and pharmacology competes well for priority in busy lives: 35–40% of well-informed, cooperative patients frequently delay or omit scheduled doses. This range and pattern of imperfect drug intake are irrespective of drug, disease, prognosis, or even symptoms. The medical and economic consequences, however, vary widely, and do depend on drug, disease severity, and comorbidity. This need for intervention thus varies, and requires proper prioritization to those patients who will incur the most clinical trouble or other high cost.

Two fundamental factors in the intervention, therefore, are (i) reliable detection of poor compliance and (ii) reliable measurement of the effect of steps taken to improve it. Given that we typically grossly underestimate poor compliance without any special tools, real-time electronic monitoring becomes the gold standard.

From the patients' points of view, feedback about dosing history data probably has a future role. Well-timed, audible, or visual alerts can help, and modem- or pager-mediated alerts for professionals who assume responsibility for pharmaceutical care are another approach. Obviously, given the required labor, the latter must be focused on well-defined, high-risk situations.

What does "compliance" really mean?

With the advent of electronic monitoring methods, described below, it has become practical to use a definition of compliance that has a pharmacologic meaning, in terms of drug exposure. A recorded history of dosing measures drug exposure in respect to the timing of individual doses. In order to get full therapeutic benefit from the drug, with least toxicity, certain standards can be created for the quantity of drug taken and the timing of doses during each therapeutic course.

Methods of evaluating compliance

Direct evaluation of compliance

The most basic, direct method is to sample blood for drug concentration. But unfortunately, this method reflects only the recent prior dosing history, and perhaps only the taking of the most recent dose (see Chapter 31, which covers plasma concentration). Moreover, patients' dosing behavior usually improves during the day or two known to be prior to a scheduled visit with the clinician (so-called "white-coat compliance"; see below). Thus, for most drugs, the measurement of drug concentration in plasma at the time of a scheduled examination only reflects atypical good compliance. One could, of course, contrive to do unannounced sampling of blood, but that is costly and intrusive. Finally, although true negatives are easy to interpret (zero plasma concentration of drug usually means that the drug was not taken within five half-lives in the past), interpretation of positives is more difficult.

Plasma concentration monitoring can also be adapted. A useful, but rather cumbersome direct method is based on adding a slow turnover chemical marker with the therapeutic drug. Low doses of phenobarbital can serve as such a marker because its elimination and its assay is sufficiently sensitive; it can estimate exposure during the previous week for a daily drug. Similarly, fluoroscein will appear in the urine for about 24 hours after dosing, and can easily be checked by holding a dipstick in front of a fluorimeter. However, marker methods do not indicate the actual timing of doses, and are generally only poorly quantitative.

Indirect evaluation of compliance

Prior to 1987, the indirect methods in use were methods that made it easy for patients to censor evidence for delayed or omitted doses. These included paper dosing diaries and counts of returned dosage forms. These have repeatedly been shown to be unreliable, giving results that "grossly overestimate compliance" in both trials and practice (Pullar *et al.*, 1989).

But in 1987 there came the first electronic monitor for solid dosage forms (Norell, 1984; Pullar and Feely, 1990; Cramer, 1995; Urquhart, 1997). These recorded every opening of the drug package, by means of time-keeping micro circuitry. The only disadvantage is that the actual intake of the drug cannot be confirmed, except with complicated, simultaneous pharmacokinetic sampling (Urquhart, 1997). Experience has shown that patients not wishing to take their medicine rarely go to the length of opening the drug package at scheduled times, especially over long time periods.

Compliance during clinical trials

Early-phase studies

A growing consensus supports the measurement, by reliable means, of compliance with the protocol-specified regimen during clinical trials (Efron, 1991; Meier, 1991; Rubin, 1991, Cox, 1998; Efron, 1998; Rubin, 1998). The gold-standard method for evaluating patient compliance is now accepted to be electronic monitoring (Cramer, 1995; Kastrissios and Blaschke, 1997; Urquhart, 1997; Urquhart and de Klerk, 1998). The difficulties of trying to interpret data from unreliable alternative methods (e.g., counting returned, unused tablets, which are confounded by the high incidence tablet-dumping by poorly/partially compliant patients), are now well-documented (Rudd *et al.*, 1989; Waterhouse *et al.*, 1993; Pocock and Abdalla, 1998), or by drug diversion if something really effective is being tested (this was the case for sumatriptan in early

trials among migraineurs). Research with electronic methods for compiling dosing histories in ambulatory patients can now be incorporated economically and with little risk in all phases of research (Sheiner, 1997; Urquhart, 2002). Novel statistical methods (Loeys and Goetghebeur, 2003) have also been developed for this sort of data.

Population pharmacokinetic studies in outpatients are the most obvious situation in which an accurate dosing history is important. This can allow for estimates of variation, not only between-but also within-patient, when an ordinary clinical situation prevails (Vrijens *et al.*, 2003). Avoidance of erroneous dose-PK relationships can also lead to better dose-ranging information and fewer adverse events post-marketing; after all, perfect compliance is frequently presumed in such decision-making. Typically, when relying on the assumption of steady state, more than 20% of observed concentrations have to be queried in a typical study. With electronic compilation of dosing histories these queries could fall to <2%. The economic and time-saving advantages of this are obvious.

Later-phase studies

With larger patient samples, questions about treatment adherence usually arise for a wider range of reasons than during early-phase studies. In a confirmatory trial it is crucial to guarantee that patients get the optimal exposure to the test drug. Testing for similar adherence between placebo and active therapy (or low dose versus high dose) is crucial when comparison of treatment groups as a whole makes or breaks the trial. Supportive pharmionic analysis is in addition to conventional intent-to-treat (ITT) analysis.

Beyond the ITT analysis, a pharmionic program can also provide robust estimates of the treatment response in the subpopulation of patients who dose essentially correctly, which types of dosing errors have the greatest potential to undermine effectiveness, and which errors cause the greatest hazard (e.g., rebound effects after sudden cessation of dosing, recurrent first-dose effects, emergence of resistance to anti-infective agents, and the like). Products can be inherently weak simply because of poor compliance, and this is another factor that should guide development decisions (Urquhart and Chevalley, 1988; Urquhart, 2001; Delmas *et al.*, 2003; Eastell *et al.*, 2003; Vrijens *et al.*, 2003).

Standards for analyzing real-time compliance

Most electronic monitors are designed to transfer their data to a computer. The compliance report is then automatically generated and can be compared with pro- or retrospectively designed criteria. Calendar plots show the number of daily dose units taken by the patient; this checks for assignments of drug intake to certain days, and can control for white-coat and weekend compliances. Actual consumption can also be reconciled against the timing of adverse events and chronopharmacological benefit.

The chronology diagram is the next level of resolution. It shows how dose units were used by the hour. Regularity of dosing can be assessed, and treatment effects (or resistance) can again be reconciled.

Therapeutic coverage is defined as the percentage of time during which the patient had a therapeutically adequate effect of medication during the observation period. It depends on the pharmacokinetic properties of the drug and the patient's dosing history (Urquhart, 2000).

The term "forgiveness" has been adopted from engineering slang, and means how well a pharmaceutical product continues to provide therapeutic drug action in spite of the most common errors in dosing. In quantitative terms, forgiveness is the size of the gap between post-dose duration of therapeutically effective drug action, the recommended interval between doses, and the intervals between when it is actually taken by the patient. "Uncovered hours," during which drug action is inadequate, cumulate and can be measured as the percentage of the entire observation period. Deliberate supratherapeutic dose sizes of some drugs are used to increase their forgiveness (e.g., some oral contraceptives).

For the patient, knowledge of therapeutic coverage heightens the understanding of the impact of a particular level of compliance. For the doctor and the pharmacist, these data can guide counseling.

How is compliance classified: typical pattern

Full compliance

This is when the patient executes the prescribed dosing regimen to a high degree of punctuality. Limits for deviation will vary from study to study mostly depending on the forgiveness of the drug of interest (Urquhart, 1998).

Partial compliance

Partial compliance is a dosing history that is sufficient only to elicit a partial therapeutic response. With exceptionally unforgiving drugs, a patient can take 100% of prescribed doses, but nevertheless have an inadequate therapeutic response simply because of erratic timing of doses taken. It is a product-specific matter, dependent on the forgiveness of the product in question.

Noncompliance

This is a level of drug exposure that is too little to matter. Although again product-specific, and in the absence of reliable data on forgiveness, an intake that is less than 50% of what was prescribed could be called "noncompliance."

Overcompliance

This term is used when there is evidence that the patient has taken more than the prescribed amount of medication. The outcomes of overcompliance are product-specific, but can be expected to include increased numbers and severity of adverse effects, with or without increased levels of therapeutic action.

Which forms of partial compliance and noncompliance are particularly relevant?

Skewed dosing

The statistical distribution of drug exposure among ambulatory patients is strongly skewed downwards, with relatively little overdosing, but a great deal of underdosing, relative to the prescribed dosing regimen. The consequences of this prevalent pattern of drug exposure for treatment outcomes are product-specific.

White coat compliance

A few days prior to the consultation with his doctor, many patients improve their compliance and, hence, present with optimized clinical parameters. This leads to the doctor wrongly assuming that the patient's long-term treatment with the prescribed medication is adequate. This is particularly well documented for antihypertensive drugs.

Drug holidays

This term implies that the patient discontinues the intake of his or her medication for three or more consecutive days. These so-called "drug holidays" tend to occur on days when the patient changes usual daily activities, for example, weekends and holidays (Kruse *et al.*, 1990). If a "drug holiday" occurs shortly before a medical consultation, the doctor may have the impression that the patient is not under satisfactory control with the medication so far prescribed. The consequence may be an increase in dosage or an unnecessary change of medication.

Skipped dosing

This pattern is when the daily intake of the medication is not at regular, set times. There may be long deviations or the pattern may be completely unstructured. This type of noncompliance fails to ensure adequate therapeutic coverage, depending on the product's forgiveness.

Actions to enhance compliance and persistence

The prevalence of suboptimal compliance in all fields of chronic, ambulatory pharmacotherapy is well established (Jones *et al.*, 1995; Caro *et al.*, 1999; Catalan and LeLorier, 2000; Benner *et al.*, 2002). What can be done about it?

In this effort, the patient holds a key position, since his or her ability to cope with the prescribed regimen is crucial for good compliance, and through good compliance with rationally prescribed medicines, good outcomes. Health professionals have an important role to play in helping patients comply properly and thus get the fullest possible benefit from their prescribed medicines. When compliance is insufficient, the outcome of the treatment is put in jeopardy and the costs of care rise, due to the needless addition of second or third agents, dose escalations, or diagnostic tests to ascertain the nature of a clinical problem that has been created by persistent, clinically unrecognized poor compliance.

The crucial step is to use the objective record of the patient (prior dosing) as a management tool. This allows the patient to see what errors were made, and can open discussions about how to avoid repeating them in the future. This step is wholly new, because prior efforts to improve compliance have relied on patients' self-reported compliance, which is subject to errors due to imperfect memory, mixed feelings about the treatment program, and a desire to please the physician.

There must also be recognition that compliance is not a static quantity but a dynamic process. Many studies have clearly shown that the compliance of most patients deteriorates as treatment progresses, particularly in diseases with few or no symptoms. The differential diagnosis, when in ignorance of compliance, is between a progressive disease course, drug tachyphylaxis, or inadequate compliance (Kass *et al.*, 1986; Cramer *et al.*, 1989; Cramer *et al.*, 1990). Compliance-monitoring with feedback of the results to the patient has been clearly demonstrated to enhance compliance (Psaty *et al.*, 1990; Waterhouse *et al.*, 1993).

What is the relevance of compliance in daily practice?

About one third of patients appear to underdose to an extent that is likely, for most drugs, to be clinically relevant. About 50% of the patients comply well enough, if not perfectly, to get full benefits of the prescribed treatment. Only one patient in about six is strictly punctual. "How much compliance is enough?" is a key question in order to secure full therapeutic benefit. Diagnostic confusion and hospital admission are the direct consequences of poor or partial compliance with medically crucial prescribed drug regimens (Didlake *et al.*, 1988; Rovelli *et al.*, 1989; De Geest *et al.*, 1998; Nevins *et al.*, 2001). The associated economic problems have, for the most part, not yet been quantified, although some initial efforts have been made (Urquhart *et al.*, 1999).

Here it is important to re-emphasize that the clinical signs of overdosing are often recognizable, but the clinical signs of underdosing–which is far more common–are usually misinterpreted as worsened disease, with ensuing lack of responsiveness to the pharmaceutical in question.

What should interactive packaging offer to improve patient compliance?

It is clear that patients have individual preferences and needs, and so will decide what fits them best: audible, visible alerts, and integrated or not with the phone system. Technology is available to meet foreseeable preferences. It seems highly unlikely that a single type of electronically monitored packaging will accommodate the whole range of patient needs. Instead, one can expect a variety of electronically-monitored packages to emerge as the recognized need for such information grows.

Consider the following scenario: a 60 year-old patient is diagnosed as having high cholesterol levels, and is prescribed a once-daily cholesterol synthesis inhibitor, essentially life-long therapy. The patient has a certain tendency to forget doses, which can be minimized by use of a simple reminder device. Perhaps, with practice, the patient develops a strong routine of drug intake, linked to some regular routine in his life. If that occurs, the reminder device becomes superfluous, although it has served its purpose during the start-up phase of treatment, to make the patient aware of the frequency of missed doses. Meanwhile, the consequences of missing an occasional dose of cholesterol-lowering drug are, as far as anyone knows, negligible. After a decade of treatment, however, the patient develops coronary heart disease with congestive heart failure, and now is in a situation where the punctual maintenance of a strict regimen is essential to prevent hazardous retention of fluid. In this setting, the types of errors that had little or no consequence for cholesterol regulation can create major problems: omission of the daily diuretic dose for as few as three days in sequence can trigger acute pulmonary congestion, requiring hospitalization that costs on the order of US$7,000 per day.

In this common scenario, the changing nature of drugs, diseases, severity of diseases, and comorbidity can radically change the medical and economic implications of compliance errors.

The type of devices needed for this particular patient might be as follows:
• A device with an acoustic or visual reminder for the patient and a memory capability so the treating physician will get that patient's actual history of dosing. When a strong routine exists, this device may be used then only sporadically to check if the patient is continuing to dose satisfactorily.
• For elderly patients with multiple diseases and multiple medications, an electronic dose organizer may help them cope with the more complex regimens.
• An effective program of medication management may prevent the patient having to abandon home-based care: an obvious issue in both the economics of care and the quality of life.

Of course, some patients will not agree to any kind of monitoring, but the hazards and costs of suboptimal care have become well-understood.

Nonetheless, in this world of technology, the patient should come before, not after, the technology. Technology by itself will not solve all the problems created by erratic compliance. Technology is a tool that can help healthcare professionals identify, track, and potentially solve many of the issues created by partial and poor compliance. The patient may or may not respond, and external attempts to force the patient into an unnatural behavior that he or she will simply not internalize are sure to fail. When all is said and done, the patient will have to perceive the value of available services, him or herself, adopt one of them, and adapt to it (Métry and Meyer, 1999).

What will be the reaction of third-party payers?

If proven cost-effective, third-party payers will support improvements in compliance. Certain diseases appear to be good candidates for this cost-effectiveness, for example, patients with congestive heart failure, epilepsy and xenografts, where the benefits of avoiding hospitalization as a result of improving compliance have ample evidence. There are probably many other areas.

The field of therapeutics is vast and complex. Doubtless, many other areas will benefit from investigation as to whether compliance is causing inadequate response, and why the drug is not as effective in the market place as it was in the clinical trials.

Conclusion

Almost two decades ago the problem was how to measure drug intake in ambulatory patients (Averbuch et al., 1990; Kruse and Weber, 1990). That problem has been solved by a variety of approaches, which integrate time-recording microcircuitry into a variety of drug packaging. Electronic monitoring is now well-established as an indirect method of measuring drug intake by ambulatory patients, even though it does not document actual ingestion of the dose and requires no special effort on the part of the patient (Wagner, 2002). Naturally, it must be used with common sense, for it does have certain "blind spots" that can occur if, for example, the patient removes doses at times

remote from actual ingestion, uses a second, non-monitored package, or diverts the drug for one reason or another. However, these are errors made mainly by patients who are striving for full compliance, not the errors of the negligent, who often seek to minimize the errors they make.

Today's key question is how best to target the methods we have (World Health Organization, 2004). Can we use them to improve care and reduce costs?

References

Averbuch M, Weintraub M, Pollack DJ. Compliance assessment in clinical trials: the MEMS device. *J Clin Res Pharmacoepidemiol* 1990; **4**: 199–204.

Benner JS, Glynn RJ, Mogun H, Neumann PJ, Weinstein MC. Long-term persistence in use of statin therapy in elderly patients. *JAMA* 2002; **288**: 455–461.

Caro JJ, Salas M, Speckman JL, Raggio G, Jackson JD. Persistence with treatment for hypertension in actual practice. *Can Med Assoc J* 1999; **160**: 31–37.

Catalan VS, LeLorier J. Predictors of long-term persistence on statins in a subsidized clinical population. *Value Health* 2000; **3**: 417–426.

Cox, D. Discussion – The Limburg Compliance Symposium. *Stat Med* 1998; **17**: 387–390.

Cramer JA, Mattson RH, Prevey ML, Scheyer RD, Ouellette VL. How often is medication taken as prescribed? A novel assessment technique. *JAMA* 1989; **261**: 3273–3277.

Cramer JA, Scheyer RD, Mattson RH. Compliance declines between clinic visits. *Arch Int Med* 1990; **150**: 1509–1510.

Cramer JA. Microelectronic systems for monitoring and enhancing patient compliance with medication regimens. *Drugs* 1995; **49**: 321–327.

De Geest S, Abraham I, Moons P, Vandeputte M, Van Cleemput J, Evers G, et al. Late acute rejection and subclinical noncompliance with cyclosporine therapy in heart transplant recipients. *J Heart Lung Transplant* 1998; **17**: 854–863.

Delmas PD, Vrijens B, van de Langerijt L, Roux C, Eastell R, Ringe JD, et al. *Effect of reinforcement with bone turnover marker results on persistence with risedronate treatment in postmenopausal women with osteoporosis: improving the measurements of persistence on actonel treatment: the Impact study.* European Calcified Tissues Society Meeting. Rome, Italy; May 8–12, 2003.

Didlake RH, Dreyfus K, Kerman RH, Van Buren CT, Kahan BD. Patient noncompliance: a major cause of late graft failure in cyclosporine-treated renal transplants. *Transplant Proc* 1988; **20** Suppl 3: 63–69.

Eastell R, Garnero P, Vrijens B, van de Langerijt L, Pols HAP, Ringe JD, *et al. Influence of patient compliance with risedronate therapy on bone turnover marker and bone mineral density response: the Impact study.* European Calcified Tissues Society Meeting. Rome, Italy; May 8–12, 2003.

Efron B. Rejoinder. *J Am Stat Assoc* 1991; **86** (413): 25.

Efron B. Foreword – The Limburg Compliance Symposium. Stat Med 1998; **17**: 249–250.

Jones JK, Gorkin L, Lian JF, Staffa JA, Fletcher AP. Discontinuation of and changes in treatment after start of new courses of antihypertensive drugs: a study of a United Kingdom population. *BMJ* 1995; **311**: 293–295.

Kass MA, Gordon M, Meltzer DW. Can ophthalmologists correctly identify patients defaulting from pilocarpine therapy? *Am J Ophthalmol* 1986; **101**: 524–530.

Kastrissios H, Blaschke TF. Medication compliance as a feature in drug development. *Ann Rev Pharmacol Toxicol* 1997; **37**: 451–475.

Kruse W, Eggert-Kruse W, Rampmaier J, Runnebaum B, Weber E. Compliance with short-term high-dose oestradiol in young patients with primary infertility–new insights from the use of electronic devices. *Agents Actions* 1990; Suppl 29: Risk Factor for Adverse Drug Reactions: Epidemiological Approaches, 105–115.

Kruse W, Weber E. Dynamics of drug regimen compliance–its assessment by microprocessor-based monitoring. *Eur J Clin Pharmacol* 1990; **38**: 561–565.

Loeys T, Goetghebeur E. Causal proportional hazards estimator for the effect of treatment actually received in a randomized trial with all-or-nothing compliance. *Biometrics* 2003; **59**: 100–105.

Meier P. Discussion. *J Am Stat Assoc* 1991; **86** (413): 19–22.

Métry JM, Meyer UA. *Drug Regimen Compliance: Issues in clinical trials and patient management.* John Wiley & Sons Ltd: Chichester, UK, 1999.

Nevins E, Kruse L, Skeans MA, Thomas W. The natural history of azathioprine compliance after renal transplantation. *Kidney Int* 2001; **60**: 1565–1570.

Norell SE. Methods in assessing drug compliance. *Acta Med Scand* 1984; Suppl **683**: 35–40.

Pocock SJ, Abdalla M. The hope and the hazard of using compliance data in randomized controlled trials. *Stat Med* 1998; **17**: 303–318.

Psaty BM, Koepsell TD, Wagner EH, LoGerfo JP, Inui TS. The relative risk of incident coronary heart disease associated with recently stopping the use of beta blockers. *JAMA* 1990; **263**: 1653–1657.

Pullar T, Kumar S, Tindall H, Feely M. Time to stop counting the tablets? *Clin Pharmacol Ther* 1989; **46**: 163–168.

Pullar T, Feely M. Problems of compliance with drug treatment: new solutions? *Pharm J* 1990; **245**: 213–215.

Rovelli M, Palmeri D, Vossler E, Bartus S, Hull D, Schweizer R. Noncompliance in organ transplant recipients. *Transplant Proc* 1989; **21**: 833–834.

Rubin D. Comment: dose-response estimands. *J Am Stat Assoc* 1991; **86** (413): 22–24.

Rubin DS. More powerful randomization-based *p*-values in double-blind trials with non-compliance. *Stat Med* 1998; **17**: 371–386.

Rudd P, Byyny RL, Zachary V, LoVerde ME, Titus C, Mitchell WD, Marshall G. The natural history of medication compliance in a drug trial: limitations of pill counts. *Clin Pharmacol Ther* 1989; **46**: 169–176.

Sheiner LB. Learning versus confirming in clinical drug development. *Clin Pharmacol Ther* 1997; **61**: 275–291.

Urquhart J. The electronic medication event monitor – lessons for pharmaco-therapy. *Clin Pharmacokinet* 1997; **32**: 345–356.

Urquhart J. Pharmacodynamics of variable patient compliance: implications for pharmaceutical value. *Adv Drug Deliv Rev* 1998; **33**: 207–219.

Urquhart J. Pharmacoeconomic consequences of variable patient compliance with prescribed drug regimens. *Pharmacoeconomics* 1999; **15**: 217–228.

Urquhart J. Defining the margins for errors in patient compliance with prescribed drug regimens. *Pharmacoepidemiol Drug Saf* 2000; **9**: 565–568.

Urquhart J. Some economic consequences of noncompliance. *Curr Hypertens Rep* 2001; **3**: 473– 480.

Urquhart J. History-informed perspectives on the modeling and simulation of therapeutic drug actions. In: *Simulation for Designing Clinical Trials*, Kimko HC, Duffull S (eds). Marcel Dekker: New York, USA, 2002, 245–269.

Urquhart J, Chevalley C. Impact of unrecognized dosing errors on the cost and effectiveness of pharmaceuticals. *Drug Inf J* 1988; **22**: 363–378.

Urquhart J, de Klerk E. Contending paradigms for the interpretation of data on patient compliance with therapeutic drug regimens. *Stat Med* 1998; **17**: 251–267.

Vrijens B, Ringe JD, Watts NB, Pols HAP, Roux C, Eastell R, *et al. Electronic monitoring of adherence to therapy in postmenopausal osteoporosis: the Impact study.* European Calcified Tissues Society Meeting. Rome, Italy; May 8–12, 2003.

Vrijens B, Tousset E, Rode R, Bertz R, Mayer SL. *Within-patient variance reduced in an ARV PK study by switching from patient-reported to electronically-compiled dosing times.* Proceedings of the 2nd IAS Conference on HIV Pathogenesis and Treatment. Paris, France; July 13–16, 2003.

Wagner GJ. Predictors of antiretroviral adherence as measured by self-report, electronic monitoring, and medication diaries. *AIDS Patient Care STDS* 2002; **16**: 599–608.

Waterhouse DM, Calzone KA, Mele C, Brenner DE. Adherence to oral tamoxifen: a comparison of patient self-report, pill counts, and microelectronic monitoring. *J Clin Oncol* 1993; **11**: 1189–1197.

World Health Organization. *Adherence to Long-term Therapies*. World Health Organization: Geneva, Switzerland, 2004.

CHAPTER 31

Monitoring Drug Concentrations in Clinical Practice

Anthony W. Fox

EBD Group Inc., Carlsbad, CA, USA and Munich, Germany, and Skaggs SPPS, University of California, San Diego, USA

General principles of therapeutic monitoring

Clearly, all prescribing should be accompanied by some sort of therapeutic monitoring. Therapeutic monitoring comes in many guises, ranging from the absence of re-attendance of the patient with the same complaint (presumptive but not certain treatment success!), through various types of quantitative efficacy monitoring (e.g., activated prothrombin time and/or partial thromboplastin time for warfarin therapy; Nowak, 2001). Measuring drug concentrations, for example, in urine or blood is thus quite a small part of the general, laudable clinical goal of monitoring therapy. Although the pursuit of pharmacokinetic information is an obligatory part of drug development in general, this chapter focuses on the situation when drug concentration measurements become part of ordinary clinical practice and good product labeling will explain how.

Why monitor drug concentrations?

The following reasons can justify the need to monitor drug concentrations in plasma or urine:

- Avoidance of adverse effects for drugs with narrow "therapeutic windows."
- Maximizing probability of efficacy.

- Checking for compliance.
- Detection of exposure (e.g., environmental risk studies; Lange and Dietrich, 2002).
- Treatment decision-making.
- Avoidance of drug interactions.
- Dose adjustment for special populations (e.g., the elderly, children, renal failure).

Note that elderly patients and children have physiology that can lead to unexpectedly high serum concentrations after administration of standard doses of drugs in comparison with typical adults: lower renal and hepatic clearances, reduced volumes of distribution, and (for the elderly) an increased probability of concomitant therapies (Ohnishi *et al.*, 2003).

The drug concentration assays offered by most clinical laboratories are designed to fulfill one or more of these purposes: acetaminophen/paracetamol, digoxin, gentamicin, lithium, phenytoin, and salicylates are probably most common. It is useful to consider these same criteria during drug development. Should the product label carry information about, and should the risk management program include, plasma concentration monitoring? A few worked examples may be of use, with the general proviso that sample timing must be correct.

Narrow "therapeutic window"

Theophylline is a classic example. Its bronchodilator effects are related to plasma concentrations in the range of 5–20 mg l^{-1}. Monitoring plasma levels is helpful in avoiding the higher concentrations that are associated with tachyarrhythmias.

Principles and Practice of Pharmaceutical Medicine, 3rd edition.
Edited by L.D. Edwards, A.W. Fox, P.D. Stonier.
© 2011 Blackwell Publishing Ltd.

Maximizing probability of efficacy

Itraconazole is an antifungal agent of the triazole class (Buchkowsky *et al.*, 2005). This drug is commonly employed in immune-compromised patients with a substantial burden of disease and other concomitant therapies. Although the relationship between plasma concentration and efficacy is quite variable, levels above 250 ng ml^{-1} are more often associated with efficacy. However, itraconazole has several pharmacokinetic complexities making choice of dose difficult. There is substantial inter- and intra-patient variability in the dose–plasma concentration relationship, plasma protein binding is substantial, it has an active metabolite, it is a CYP 3A4 substrate, and it is compatible with P-glycoprotein transportation. This multiplicity of pharmacokinetic factors, some predictable and others idiosyncratic, is so great that it can be worth using a plasma concentrations to guide dose size.

Anti-epileptic drugs

Selective drug level monitoring reduces seizures and minimizes adverse events when using anti-epileptic drugs (AEDs). Glauser and Pippenger (2000) have enumerated the situations when this is useful:

• Evaluating lack or loss of efficacy.
• Evaluating intolerability.
• Finding a baseline efficacious concentration for comparison when things go awry later on, and understanding the scope for changing dose size.
• Judging when to change AED(s).

For example, for apparently clozapine non-responsive patients might benefit from a dose increase creating a plasma concentration that is greater than the "threshold" of 350–400 ng ml^{-1} (Bell *et al.*, 1998). Zonisamide has a therapeutic range of 10–40 μg ml^{-1}, although the dose required to achieve this plasma concentration varies with concomitant phenytoin or carbamazepine therapy (as well as *vice versa*; Mimaki, 1998).

Acetaminophen/paracetamol

In the European Community and North America, this is the most common of all drugs taken in overdose, and this over-the-counter drug thus causes a substantial public health burden. Among other things, this is the single largest demand for liver transplantation, and the shortage of donor livers means many patients die instead.

Jones and Dargan (2001) provide a definitive, condensed account of acetaminophen/paracetamol poisoning, and rightly label it a "deceptive" toxicity. Evidence of hepatic injury, sadly, may only arise 24 hours or more after ingestion, by which time opportunities to limit absorption of the overdose will have been lost. Renal injury can also occur.

The toxicity of acetaminophen/paracetamol is plasma concentration dependent. However, it should be remembered that plasma concentrations are dynamic, not static phenomena. Both plasma concentration and time elapsed since ingestion must be factored into predictions of degree of toxicity. Furthermore, the thresholds for time since ingestion and plasma concentrations are lower when the patient has also abused concomitant drugs or alcohol. The curvilinear nomogram indicating low or high risk of hepatic injury in patients generally starts at 100–190 mg l^{-1} (about 0.7–1.2 mmol l^{-1}) at four hours post-overdose. Plasma concentrations measured prior to 4 hours are probably a waste of time because measures to reduce absorption should take priority and, when low, such an early measurement provides no real estimate of the size of the exposure. The nomogram for high risk of liver injury falls to plasma concentrations of zero when measured 24 hours after the overdose. Thus, plasma concentration measurements a long time post-overdose are also pointless.

N-acetylcysteine is a relatively well-tolerated drug, providing a substrate that substitutes for endogenous glutathione. Its administration can be recommended on an "err on the safe side" basis, when time and concentration is near the thresholds shown on the nomogram found on the package insert. For the same reason, treatment decisions will be safely biased when dealing with overdoses taken in two parts, with some time interval in between them, by simply assuming that the whole overdose was taken on the first occasion. Anaphylactoid reactions can be treated by halting the infusion for half an hour and administering an antihistamine.

Oral methionine is probably now an anachronistic treatment even in the absence of peripheral venous access (intravenous drug abusers). The importance of treating acetaminophen/paracetamol overdose easily justifies the hazards of a subclavian cannula.

Salicylates

Mention of salicylate overdose is made here, even though its incidence is declining. Its treatment, presuming hemodialysis is not indicated, includes another classic type of beneficial drug interaction, that does not involve a specific antidote (cf. *N*-acetylcysteine, above). The combination of respiratory alkalosis with metabolic acidosis, and the nuances of promoting drug excretion by altering urine pH, have also long attracted Machiavellian examiners setting multiple choice questions!

Overdoses greater than 150 mg/kg (i.e., 20–40 tablets weighing 325 mg each) cause toxicity, although fatality is related not only to overdose size, but also to the patient's general condition. Children are sensitive to salicylates disproportionately to their body weight, and are also liable to more serious metabolic acidosis than adults.

Serious salicylate poisoning usually includes acute clinical signs and symptoms (complaints of tinnitus, hyperventilation, agitation, seizures, coma, abnormal arterial blood gases, etc.). Plasma salicylate concentrations become interpretable at about 4 hours post-overdose. Identifying the peak plasma salicylate concentration can be achieved with venous samples every 3 hours. There is a greater need to interpret these in the context of the clinical picture than when acetaminophen/paracetamol has been ingested (see Jones and Dargan, 2001); neurological signs of toxicity, in particular, indicate serious poisoning, regardless of the salicylate plasma concentration.

Forced diuresis by fluid loading is recommended in all salicylate overdoses. Urine alkalinization is generally recommended at plasma salicylate concentrations above 600 mg l^{-1}, or half that in children and the elderly. Even this, however, has its limits, and hemodialysis at salicylate concentrations of >800 mg l^{-1} in adults (half in children and the elderly), or regardless of plasma concentration

when there are signs of CNS toxicity, is becoming the treatment of choice.

The acid-base aspects to salicylate poisoning are as follows:
• Salicylate is an organic acid (as the suffix "-ate" indicates):
  – It is filtered through the glomerulus.
  – It is less ionized in acidic environments.
  – It is resorbed across the lipid membrane of the tubule of the nephron more easily when not ionized.
  – Therefore, acidic urine slows excretion.
• Moreover, acidosis must be aggressively treated because acidosis enhances CNS sequestration of salicylate. The blood gases indicate a mixed picture:
  – pH is low, and HCO_3^- is low, due to the direct acidotic challenge of the toxin.
  – pCO_2 is low due to hyperventilation (Kussmaul respiration, and also a direct effect of salicylate).
  – pO_2 is typically normal.
• Excretion of salicylate is principally in the urine and can be enhanced by alkalinization because
  – Salicylate is filtered in the glomerulus and this is pH independent.
  – The nephron is a lipid membrane; in an alkaline environment more salicylate is ionized and less able to be resorbed by the nephron.

Lastly, *vice versa*, remember that basic drugs are excreted more vigorously in urine that is acidified with oral ammonium sulfate. A common and popular drug of abuse at the moment in California is methamphetamine; the suffix again tells us it is a basic drug, and the same logic applies, but in reverse.

When is plasma concentration monitoring irrational?

Drugs for which concentration assays are clearly unsuited include acute therapies (i.e., not used at steady state), those with extraordinarily short half-times (e.g., injected or intranasal polypeptides), and those for which either treatment is indicated regardless (late acetaminophen/paracetamol overdose, see above) or when adverse events are almost automatic and should be monitored in other ways (e.g., CNS toxicity with salicylates (see above) or liability to bone marrow suppression with cytotoxic agents). Furthermore, the efficacy and tolerability of some drugs are known to be unrelated to circulating concentrations (e.g., the "type B" adverse event of penicillin anaphylaxis).

It is important to remember that just because a clinical laboratory offers a plasma level for a particular drug, this does not mean that it will be universally useful. For example, when monitoring for efficacy of antiviral drugs used in the treatment of HIV infection, plasma concentrations are inferior to CD4 lymphocyte counts and RNA measures of viral load (e.g., Back *et al.*, 2000). Another good example is the case of many antidepressant drugs. If the patient is also using a potentially interacting, concomitant therapy, if there is doubt as to treatment compliance, or if there is some other special clinical feature, a plasma level of, say, amitriptyline can be very useful. A plasma level might also be very useful in the Emergency Department for the diagnosis of an intoxicated patient. But studying lower concentrations of amitriptyline when treating depression is of almost no practical value in predicting efficacy (e.g., Orsulak, 1989). Although much is known about the pharmacokinetic interactions of selective serotonin reuptake inhibitors (and indeed some are even used as probes in clinical pharmacology studies), this does not extrapolate to their routine plasma level monitoring in the clinic (Sproule *et al.*, 1997). Thus, routine venesection of patients in psychiatric clinics is likely to have a relatively low yield of useful information and may not be cost-effective.

Concentration monitoring in other biological fluids

Urine

Urine is commonly screened for evidence of illicit drug use or alcohol consumption. This may be viewed as a drug concentration monitoring procedure, even if only of a qualitative type. It remains controversial whether poppy-seed bagels can lead to positive urine screens for opioids!

Materials such as radioactive sodium iothalamate or inulin can be regarded as drugs. These provide examples of quantitative urine concentration monitoring, and enable an assessment of the glomerular filtration rate (GFR). The GFR can measure renal injury with a greater degree of sensitivity than measuring serum creatinine or urinary protein excretion.

Cerebrospinal fluid (CSF)

It is a widely-held myth that drug in the CSF has crossed the "blood-brain barrier." This demonstrates an ignorance of basic anatomy and physiology. If a drug has appeared in the CSF it may have got there by filtration or secretion by the choroid plexi in the lateral ventricles, or by diffusion from the circulation directly. It is therefore rash to assume that drug concentration in the CSF is a good surrogate for actual brain exposure (Davson, 1967; de Lange and Danhof, 2002). *Vice versa* when a drug is not found in the CSF, to presume that it is not present in the brain parenchyma also presumes an absence of sequestration. Buprenorphine is a good example, where rapid disappearance of detectable drug in the CSF (and venous blood) is associated with a prolonged analgesic effect later on.

Quite apart from the so-called "blood-brain barrier" (and where it is lacking, e.g., some parts of the pituitary, hypothalamus, retina and brain stem, i.e., the chemoreceptor trigger zone), there are many other factors that govern equilibration of drug concentration between CSF and the parenchyma of the brain itself. The differential effects of P-glycoprotein saturable active transport can govern the CNS sequestration in a manner that is completely unrelated to relative lipophilicity or ambient drug concentration.

Lastly, there are, obviously, more technical and clinical obstacles to obtaining CSF for pharmacokinetic purposes than when sampling venous blood or urine. These illustrate the topographical complexities of measuring CSF concentrations. In animal studies, after systemic drug administration, drug concentrations in the CSF can be unequal between ventricles and the sub-arachnoid space. Clinically, CSF from the cisterna magna and from around the corda equina can also differ in drug concentration. It is for this reason that laboratory neuroscientists often resort to intracerebral microdialysis, and why magnetic resonance spectroscopy and positron emission tomography are now being pursued more commonly for drug studies. The scope for useful CSF concentration monitoring in the ordinary clinical situation, remains very small.

Summary

In this chapter, the measurement of drug concentrations in humans has been discussed in the context of ordinary clinical practice. This is therefore a chapter that impinges on product labeling and risk management plans, but not necessarily pharmacokinetics or the quantitation of drug interactions in normal volunteers. The general criteria for when plasma concentration monitoring may, and may not, be worthwhile have been reviewed. The essentially qualitative nature of urine monitoring, unless measuring GFR, and some fundamentals about CSF drug concentrations have also been reviewed.

References

Back DJ, Khoo SH, Gibbons SE, Barry MG, Merry C. Therapeutic drug monitoring of antiretrovirals in human immunodeficiency virus infection. *Ther Drug Monit* 2000; **22**:122–126.

Bell R, McLaren A, Galanos J, Copolov D. The clinical use of clozapine levels. *Aust NZ J Psychiatr* 1998; **32**:567–574.

Buchowsky SS, Partovi N, Ensom NH. Clinical pharmacokinetic monitoring of itraconazole is warranted in only a subset of patients. *Ther Drug Monit* 2005; **27**:322–333.

Davson H. *Physiology of the Cerebrospinal Fluid*. J&A Churchill: London, UK, 1967, *passim*.

De Lange EC, Danhof M. Considerations in the use of cerebrospinal fluid pharmacokinetics to predict brain target concentrations in the clinical setting: implications of the barriers between blood and brain. *Clin Pharmacokinet* 2002; **41**:691–703.

Glauser TA, Pippenger CE. Controversies in blood-level monitoring: reexamining its role in the treatment of epilepsy. *Epilepsia* 2000; **41**(suppl 8):S6–S15.

Jones AL, Dargan PI. *Churchill's Pocketbook of Toxicology*. Churchill Livingstone: London, UK, 2001, 69–76, 80–84, ISBN 0-4430-6476-8.

Lange R, Dietrich D. Environmental risk assessment of pharmaceutical drug substances-conceptual considerations. *Toxicol Lett* 2002; **131**:97–104.

Mimaki T. Clinical pharmacology and therapeutic drug monitoring of zonisamide. *Ther Drug Monit* 1998; **20**:593–597.

Nowak G. Clinical monitoring of hirudin and direct thrombin inhibitors. *Semin Thromb Hemostas* 2001; **27**:537–541.

Ohnishi A, Kato M, Kojima J, Ushiama H, Yoneko M, Kawai H. Differential pharmacokinetics of theophylline in elderly patients. *Drugs Aging* 2003; **20**:71–84.

Orsulak PJ. Therapeutic monitoring of anti-depressant drugs: guidelines updated. *Ther Drug Monit* 1989; **11**:497–507.

Sproule BA, Naranjo CA, Brenmer KE, Hassan PC. Sepective serotonin reuptake inhibitors and CNS drug interactions. A critical review of the evidence. *Clin Pharmacokinet* 1997; **33**:454–471.

CHAPTER 32

Generics

Gabriel Lopez[1] & Thomas Hoxie[2]
[1]Basking Ridge, NJ, USA
[2]Hoxie & Associates LLC, Millburn, NJ, USA

Generic drugs are drugs that are sold under their generic name rather than a particular brand name. Generic drugs are usually approved via an abbreviated approval process using a branded drug as a reference product. Rather than going through the long and expensive process of demonstrating safety and efficacy of the product in animal and human trials, the generic company simply needs to show that its product is identical or bioequivalent to the previously approved reference product. Generic approval and launch, however, are subject to patents and various regulatory exclusivity periods that provide incentives for innovator companies to develop new drugs.

Generic drugs have been with us for a long time. Aspirin is an example of a century-old compound for which basic patent protection has long expired and that has been sold generically ever since. The generics business rivals in size that of the branded drug business. Currently in the US, sales of generic drugs comprise about 40% of the market. In some countries, the percentage is much larger.

The great compromise: History of generics versus Big Pharma in the US

Excluding biotechnology, botanicals, "traditional medicine," and so on, the pharmaceutical industry can broadly be divided into "Big Pharma" and

Principles and Practice of Pharmaceutical Medicine, 3rd edition.
Edited by L.D. Edwards, A.W. Fox, P.D. Stonier.
© 2011 Blackwell Publishing Ltd.

generics. The business model for Big Pharma is the discovery of new medicines, the sales of which are protected by patents. Big Pharma can thus be interpreted here to include many start-up companies, which although small in market share, also rely on patent protection for their innovative concepts. During the life of the protective patents, the sale prices of these new medicines are well in excess of their manufacturing costs, which is justified by Big Pharma because of the need to reinvest these profits in the Research and Development needed to find the next new medicines. The business model for generics is to sell only medicines that are "off-patent." (Nevertheless, generics companies also seek patent protection for their innovations, although these patents protect a relatively small portion of their business.) Since the manufacturers' costs for generic medicines can be quite low, because the market has already been developed by the Big Pharma company that has been selling the medicine for years and there are virtually no advertising costs, the off-patent medicines can be sold at a considerably lower cost than the brand product (70–90% below is typical). The above description is painted with a broad brush, however; many variations and exceptions exist. Some companies have both generic and branded businesses, and some branded companies sell primarily off-patent drugs. This description is accurate enough, however, for the purposes herein.

In the late 1970s and early 1980s, these two sides of the pharmaceutical industry petitioned the US Congress for relief from two perceived injustices.

Big Pharma complained that what the government gave with one hand it took away with the other. Specifically, although an innovator company could get a patent on a new pharmaceutical invention, it was unable to profit from the invention and the patent because sales of the product were barred until regulatory approval was first obtained. The company had to file a New Drug Application (NDA), which contained proof in the form of the results of large-scale human studies that the new drug was both safe and efficacious for its intended use. The approval process could be quite lengthy, often taking many years. The regulatory agency involved is the US Food and Drug Administration (FDA), which is under no legal obligation to clear new drugs under a rigid timetable. Thus, after the innovator company had complied with all demands for data from the FDA, it then waited for the bureaucratic process to decide on approval, rejection, or a request for more data. All the while the life of the patent was ticking away. There was a solution to this "injustice," albeit not a satisfactory one. After FDA approval, innovator companies could petition the civil courts for relief and argue about their lost sales. In some cases this actually resulted in court-ordered patent term extension. However, it was an uncertain process because the court was not always convinced that any actual harm had befallen the company or, if relief was appropriate, how long the patent term extension should be.

Generics had a totally different complaint. Before they could bring their drugs to market, they also had to obtain FDA approval. Unfortunately for them, virtually none of the experimental work needed to file an NDA could be done prior to the expiration of the innovator's patent. Quite simply, they could not manufacture the compound needed for all the required testing because such manufacture would be an act of patent infringement. Thus, they argued, the patent owner was *de facto* getting a period of exclusivity far beyond that provided by the patent because of the need for FDA approval. Also, it seemed unnecessarily costly to regenerate all the safety and efficacy data, because these had already been obtained by the innovator and were already in the hands of the FDA.

The result of these competing petitions for relief was the Drug Price Competition & Patent Term Restoration Act of 1984, known simply as Hatch-Waxman.

Under Hatch-Waxman, Big Pharma received a guaranteed extension for its pharmaceutical patents if it could demonstrate that there were FDA delays in approving a new drug; that is, the FDA would now have certain time constraints put upon it and if these were exceeded the innovator was granted an extension on its patent term. The term of extension was fact-dependent for each drug approval, but could be as long as five years. The procedure is administrative; no civil court action is necessary.

Generics also received significant relief. Under Hatch-Waxman, a generics company now files an abbreviated NDA (ANDA). The ANDA requires no safety and efficacy data; it relies on the data already in the FDA's possession. What is required, however, are bioequivalence data; that is, proof that when the brand drug and the proposed generic drug are administered, the same amounts of active ingredient are available to the patient. These data are much less costly and time-consuming to generate than safety and efficacy data. The last major hurdle for a generics company is the "Certification."

A necessary part of the ANDA is a certification of one of four things, the first three of which are easy. The option is driven by the specific facts regarding the drug and the patent status. The first three options are certifications of the following: (i) there was never a patent on the drug; or (ii) there was a patent but it has expired; or (iii) the date on which the patent will expire and a request that the approval be given for the day after patent expiration. Clearly, in each of these cases there is no conflict between the patent owner and the applicant.

It is the Paragraph IV certification that is the most problematic. The generics company must certify that there is a patent but that either (i) the proposed drug will not infringe the patent or (ii) the patent is invalid. This certification is defined as an act of patent infringement and provides the patentee 30 days in which to defend its patent by suing for patent infringement. The lawsuit prevents the FDA from approving the generic drug for a period of time, pending resolution of the infringement action.

But what is the value obtained by the generics company from making a Paragraph IV certification, since it will certainly soon (within 30 days) be a defendant in a very costly lawsuit for patent infringement? It can be considerable. If it is successful and the patent is held to be invalid, the generics company is granted a period of exclusivity for six months to sell its drug, with competition only from the innovator company. When the period ends, other generics companies will undoubtedly enter the market and the drug's price will drop to about 10–30% of the brand drug price. However, during the period of exclusivity, the price drops to only about 70%, a handsome reward for invalidating the patent. These price drops are not dictated by law, just by the marketplace.

Success in court, however, is not always as rewarding for the generics company as indicated above. The innovator company has at least two techniques at its disposal following loss of patent protection. One is to obtain approval to market its product, or some formulation thereof, as an over-the-counter product. The lower price of such a product could immediately lower the price that the victorious generics company expected to charge. Another approach is to market a new version of its old drug. Such a product could be protected by patent and its sales bolstered by name recognition. If there is a competitive advantage to the new version, again the victorious generics company may not realize its projected profits.

It should be noted that since the patent in contention invariably protects a successful drug, the patentee can be expected to mount a vigorous defence thereof. The stakes for the generics company are also high since a loss in court not only means the loss of a potential product that has proven itself in the marketplace, but also puts it at risk for penalties for wilful patent infringement.

Although Hatch-Waxman is limited to the United States, laws in most other countries have some things in common with the US system: providing abbreviated approval processes for generic drugs, creating safe harbors from infringement to allow for development and clinical trials of generic drugs prior to patent expiry, and providing patent term extension and/or data exclusivity periods to ensure a reasonable period of exclusivity to the innovator company. The Paragraph IV challenge and pre-launch patent litigation process, however, is unique to the US. Consequently, outside the United States, the patent owner must usually wait until the launch of an infringing product to enforce its patents.

Seeking generic approval in the United States

In the US, there are two main routes to approval of a generic drug.

The more common route is via an ANDA. An ANDA requires that the generic product contains the same active ingredient and has the same dosage and route of administration as the reference drug. It must also be for the same indication. The applicant must show that the generic product is bioequivalent to the reference product, with respect to its pharmacokinetic and pharmacodynamic properties. Bioequivalence can be shown by demonstrating that the formulations are so similar that no difference would be expected, or by a small trial in healthy volunteers, measuring the blood levels of the active pharmaceutical in patients receiving the generic formulation compared to the reference formulation. Measuring blood levels to demonstrate bioequivalence is usually appropriate for oral formulations, but may be unsuitable for drugs that have a primarily local activity, such as inhaled or topical drugs, or for certain injectable drugs.

The second route to generic approval in the US is the so-called "paper NDA." This type of application is used when the product or its use is not the same as the reference drug. Although an ANDA is reviewed by the Office of Generic Drugs in the FDA, the paper NDA is treated as a regular NDA. The trials carried out by the applicant, which may include trials going well beyond simple bioequivalence in healthy volunteers, are supplemented by reference to a previously approved drug product or to published data. The exact nature of the data and trials required for approval is determined on a case-by-case basis. This type of application may be used by the originator company for line extensions as well as by generic companies. Drug products approved via this route may or may not be "AB-rated," that is they may or may not be considered bioequivalent, and thus fully substitutable for the reference drug.

Generic drugs are subject to quality assurance and manufacturing requirements similar to branded drugs, for example for approval, they must meet batch requirements for identity, strength, purity, and quality, and they must be manufactured in accordance with the FDA's good manufacturing practice (GMP) regulations.

Regardless of whether the generic applicant seeks approval via the ANDA route or the paper NDA route, it must provide the patent certification as described above. Moreover, approval of generic drugs is subject to registration data exclusivity periods. These periods are based on trade secret concepts; that is, the regulatory agency mandates that as a condition for drug approval the innovator must provide data that it would prefer to keep secret because the data are of commercial value to its competitors. The exclusivity periods provide some measure of protection to the innovator. No generic versions of a new chemical entity can be approved until after five years from the first approval of the new chemical entity. For new indications and new formulations of a previously approved active agent, the data exclusivity period is three years. These periods may be extended by six months when the drug has undergone additional FDA-requested trials for pediatric uses. Of course, data exclusivity periods are only applicable against a generic company that wants to rely on another company's drug as a reference; they do not apply when the generic company has generated a complete data package of its own.

The relevant data exclusivity periods for each approved drug product, as well as any applicable patents on the product or its use, are listed in the "Orange Book," which is published by the FDA and also available electronically on its website (www.fda.gov; accessed April 24, 2010).

Generic approval process outside the United States

In most countries, generic drugs may be approved via an abbreviated procedure similar to the ANDA procedure in the US. The applicant generally must show that the generic product has the same dosage of the same active substance and the same pharmaceutical form as the reference medicinal product. As in the United States, the applicant must demonstrate bioequivalence to the reference product.

All World Trade Organization (WTO) countries are required under the General Agreement on Tariffs and Trade (GATT) accords to provide some sort of registration data exclusivity periods. Europe has data and marketing exclusivity rules which, in their latest embodiment, preclude launch of a generic product until 10 or 11 years after first approval of the active substance. For products approved prior to the new rules, there are six or ten years of data exclusivity depending on the country. Approval may be either through the regulatory agencies in the individual countries or via a central procedure. In Japan, data exclusivity is normally six years for new chemical entities. The periods of exclusivity vary by country and may change over time. As in the US, clinical trials carried out by generic companies in support of regulatory approval are excluded from patent infringement in both the European Union and Japan. However, there is no procedure in Europe or Japan comparable to the US Orange Book listing and Paragraph IV challenge procedure described above. Consequently, patent holders must usually wait until launch of an infringing product to enforce their patents.

The relative strength of the generic industries in various countries is largely a function of differences in government regulation of prices and generic-for-branded substitution, as well as differences in the patent laws. In France and many southern European countries, there are strict price controls from the outset on the branded products, so that the branded products are already relatively cheap and there is less impact on price when the patent expires. Brand loyalty also tends to be relatively high, resulting in a large proportion of "branded generics" products, which are not patent protected but rather sold as branded products by a company other than the innovator. In Japan, the prices for branded products are initially relatively high, although prices are regulated down post-launch. As the higher-priced branded products are more profitable for pharmacists than generic drugs and there are few incentives to substitute generic drugs for branded drugs, the generic drug industry in Japan is relatively small. In northern Europe (e.g., the United Kingdom and Germany), there are no price caps as such, but pricing is strongly influenced by government reimbursement levels, which are reduced when generics become available, resulting in significant market share for generic companies. The US is the most open of the large markets, with very high prices for branded drugs, together with strong market incentives on the part of pharmacies and insurance companies to encourage generic substitution, resulting in potentially very large profits for the first generic on the market. Once there are multiple generic products in the market, however, the intense competition among generic companies results in rapid and dramatic price erosion. Finally, the generics industry is also strong in countries that have historically had weak patent protection for pharmaceuticals. Although these countries are typically poor and have low prices for branded and generic pharmaceuticals alike, limiting the value of the domestic market, these countries in some cases provide a manufacturing base and launching pad for products to be sold in countries with stronger patent protection.

Biopharmaceuticals

There is one type of medicine that does not fit into the regulatory schemes described above: biopharmaceuticals, also known as biogenerics or 'follow-on' biologics. Unlike the typical drug, which is of relatively low molecular weight (referred to as a "small chemical entity"), these massively large compounds are not easy to either synthesize or describe down to the individual atoms. They include compounds such as growth hormone, interferon, erythropoietin, and over 100 additional products, with a very tempting projected

generic market in the billions (US$). However, they present a twofold problem for the generics industry. First, unlike the Hatch-Waxman type of regulatory schemes, there is no generally agreed-upon approval process for biopharmaceuticals: specifically, what must be shown to prove bioequivalence. In the absence of a method to prove this, a generic company would be faced with the expensive task of running full safety and efficacy tests, the very thing that Hatch-Waxman and the similar non-US schemes were designed to eliminate. Second, the very high manufacturing costs associated with these drugs will preclude capturing market share by underpricing the brand drugs by 70–90%, as can be done with small chemical entities. Just these two hurdles will make inroads by the generics companies into this market slow for the foreseeable future.

There are currently legislative proposals intended to resolve the bioequivalence hurdle, which are intended to lead to the faster availability of biopharmaceutical drugs to the public. These proposals refer to "biosimilar" and "interchangeable" drugs. Approval for these drugs would require that the applicant demonstrate that there are no clinically meaningful differences between the new and the original product and that the one can be safely substituted for the other even though the two are not proven to be exactly identical in structure. This is an easier standard than that currently in effect. These proposals, if enacted, do not eliminate the high manufacturing costs of these new drugs and thus only provide some economic relief for the generics companies.

Blurring the lines

The pharmaceutical business is described above as being composed of generics and Big Pharma, each with its own business model. The distinction does not hold up in all cases. Although selling at a premium under the protection of a patent is Big Pharma's *modus operandi*, many patents are also obtained by generics companies. This is for two reasons, at least. First, because of the competition from all the other generics houses, a patent on a new formulation, manufacturing process, or polymorphic form of an old compound can potentially be quite valuable; clearly not as valuable as Big Pharma's original patent on the chemical entity itself but valuable enough in a very competitive marketplace. Of course, as with all patents, the value depends on whether or not they protect some economically desirable innovation. Second, some generics companies can be seen as having aspirations of becoming Big Pharma, or at least of developing and selling their own branded medicines; that is, they have research facilities to discover their own innovative medicines. Adding to the blur, Big Pharma has itself been in the generics business for some time, sometimes directly by owning generics subsidiaries. ("Ownership" must be viewed as taking various forms depending on the desire of the owning company and national law.) They have also entered into many types of partnering/licensing relationships with generics companies; that is, no actual ownership but a sharing of the sales of certain products. This can be useful, for example, if a product is about to go off-patent but the patentee does not wish to sell the product generically under its own name. If the patentee has valuable know-how relating to the product, it might license this knowledge to a generics company, which thereby gains an advantage over all its competitors.

The future

Many of the Big Pharma houses that were very well known for the past decades have now disappeared, their businesses having been consolidated by merger or acquisition into fewer and fewer, larger and larger pharmaceutical operations. This process continues to this day. A similar pattern has been emerging in the generics business. The reasons for this are undoubtedly the same as for other industries: economics of scale and the desire to expand both geographically and in breadth of product line. There is no reason to believe that this trend will stop anytime soon. Undoubtedly, one or more of these ever larger generics companies will become an acquisition target for a Big Pharma company in the future.

CHAPTER 33

Complementary Medicines

Anthony Fox

EBD Group Inc., Carlsbad, CA, USA and Munich, Germany, and Skaggs SPPS, University of California, San Diego, USA

Complementary medicines are very widely used. Their relevance to pharmaceutical medicine is the following:

- Many patients in clinical trials will be using complementary therapies (and we often omit to ask on the case report form).
- Many complementary medicines are pharmacologically active.
- Some complementary medicines risk well-described drug interactions or other adverse events.
- People uncritically pay for worthless therapies (e.g., the laetrile scandal).
- Clinicians are rarely trained in this area.

Geographical and cultural factors are as important as in any aspect of medicine; for example, there are especially strong complementary therapy traditions in places as different as Germany and the state of Utah. Furthermore, the popularity of drugs varies between places: for example, the United Kingdom apparently has the greatest faith in garlic. The market for complementary therapies is huge: The *Nutrition Business Journal* reported in 2007 that in the US alone, about US$39.5 billion of complementary therapies were sold, and that it is a growing market.

Historically, complementary therapies were the only therapies available. Some orthodox drugs have their origin in complementary medicine: Withering's discovery of digoxin was long after the gypsy had been using it for dropsy, and the Rev. Edmund Brown's willow bark extracts were the result of his belief in the doctrine of similari-

ties. Much of the Third World has little allopathic medicine available to it, and complementary therapies continue to be offered for a wide variety of diseases. Even in the developed world, most good hospices will have complementary therapists on staff.

The ethical aspects of this area of medicine are as varied as the therapies themselves, and could be debated almost *ad infinitum*. Thus, the purpose of this short chapter is to alert pharmaceutical physicians to this topic, discuss the most commonly encountered therapies (recognizing that this changes with time), and to describe their regulatory status (which is generally quite simple).

Terminology

The Cochrane Collaboration defines "Complementary Medicine" as follows:

> Complementary and alternative medicine (CAM) is a broad domain of healing resources that encompass all health systems, practices, accompanying theories and beliefs, other than those intrinsic to the politically dominant health system of a particular society or culture, within a defined historical period. CAM includes all such practices and ideas self-defined by their users for prevention or treatment of disease, or promotion of health and well-being. Boundaries within CAM and between the CAM domain and that of the dominant system are not always sharp of fixed.

The term "Alternative Medicine" is often now avoided in Western, developed countries, because it (often erroneously) suggested a mutual exclusivity between these therapies and conventional or *allopathic* approaches. Most of the diverse

Principles and Practice of Pharmaceutical Medicine, 3rd edition.
Edited by L.D. Edwards, A.W. Fox, P.D. Stonier.

disciplines now prefer the term "Complementary Medicine", so as to emphasize that the patient can benefit from a combination of orthodox and alternative approaches. There is no reason why complementary therapies may not be subject to evidence-based analysis, although there are very few such published examples, in comparison to orthodox medicine (see Critchley *et al.*, 2000).

The factor in common to all complementary therapies is that they are prescribed or recommended by practitioners who approach the patient as a whole (*holistic practitioners*). It might be said that so does any good general practitioner. However, the clinical variables used by complementary therapists are often unquantitated, may lack an orthodox clinical correlate, or occasionally, even defy translation into English (for example, the clinical variable "slipperiness" that is used in oriental medicine). Zollman and Vickers (1999) have pointed out that the same patient may be described with deficient liver Qi by an acupuncturist, as having a pulsatilla constitution by a homeopath, or having a peptic ulcer by a Western physician.

Complementary therapists may or may not be graduates of orthodox medical schools. Other complementary therapists are organized professionally, if separate from orthodox medicine (the United Kingdom operates a *General Chiropractic Council* that regulates chiropractors in a manner exactly analogous to the General Medical Council). Other complementary therapists are trained privately, or in more informal ways, such as by experienced older relatives. Chinese traditional medicine is codified and relies on the accumulated experience of both ancient and modern practitioners (Cheng, 2000).

The complementary therapies themselves also vary in their degree of characterization. Less well-characterized therapies include some forms of over-the-counter products (especially in the US), aromatherapies, crystal therapies, and various forms of psychotherapy. This is a book about drugs, and non-pharmacological therapies (e.g., the well-regulated areas of acupuncture and physiotherapy) are beyond its scope. *Herbal medicines* (a term widely used in the US) are basically unregulated pharma-

ceuticals; confusingly, materials that are not of vegetable origin (e.g., shark cartilage, oyster calcium, or selenates) are often included under the category of herbal medicines. *Alkaloid* is an older term referring to any drug with a plant origin (e.g., digoxin, aspirin, and warfarin), including both orthodox and complementary therapies. Incidentally, *opiates* are alkaloids (e.g., morphine, codeine) and *opioids* are semi-synthetic or synthetic drugs such as diacetylmorphine or pentazocine. *Pharmacognosy* is the science of plant-related, pharmacologically-active materials.

Homeopathy is the art and science of the treatment of disease using microscopical drug doses. *Homeopaths* believe that the most potent homeopathic products are those that have been most extremely diluted: in many cases, calculations based on Avagadro's number and the number of sequential dilutions suggest there may not be a single alkaloid molecule left in the administered dose. However, it is believed that the pharmaceutical method, which is at least as rigorous as for the manufacture of allopathic drugs, creates an emergent property in the administered vehicle that still has the therapeutic effect. Homeopathic medicines are available with and without prescriptions. Homeopathic prescribing resembles orthodox, if historical, prescribing. Homeopathic drugs are identified using the Latin terms for the (usually alkaloid) starting materials, and a set of apothecaries' symbols for dose size, dose frequency, and the number of dilutions required before dispensing.

In the United Kingdom homeopaths are regulated by law, and there is a *Faculty of Homeopathy* offering post-graduate examinations in the subject. Associate members of the Faculty of Homeopathy may include any clinician with statutorily registered qualifications; the *Licence* of the Faculty is available by examination, again to all clinicians, usually after study at any of five nationally-recognized homeopathic colleges. *Membership* of the Faculty is by examination and restricted to medical practitioners, and dental and veterinary surgeons; *Fellows* are selected from among the more prominent members. The Royal Household includes one or more homeopathic practitioners.

Common complementary medicines

The nine most commonly used complementary medicines that are in use in most of Europe and North America are derived from St. John's Wort, Saw Palmetto, *Gingko biloba*, Black Cohosh, glucosamine/chondroitin, SAM-e, Ephedra, Ginseng, and Kava. Although a certain amount of contemporary fashion seems to govern which products sell best, all have a long tradition in complementary therapy. These complementary medicines are not without adverse effects (Tomlinson *et al.*, 2000).

St. John's Wort

Extracts of St. John's Wort (*Hypericum perforatum*) are used for the prevention of migraine, depression, and anxiety. The clustering of indications for neurological purposes suggests that it contains an active alkaloid or alkaloid mixture. The remittent, relapsing nature of these diseases make assessment of the limited reports of its efficacy difficult, but there are one or two fairly sound papers concerning migraine and depression. Most formulations of St. John's Wort can reduce rates of absorption of antiviral drugs. Serotoninergic drugs (antimigraine agents, antidepressants, whether serotonin specific uptake blockers or not) ought to be most likely to interact with St. John's Wort, whereas on its own, St. John's Wort can cause photosensitivity. Pharmaceutical physicians should investigate herbal drug use whenever this unusual adverse event arises (see also Kava, below).

Saw Palmetto

Saw Palmetto (*Palmito caroliniensis*) is the State tree of South Carolina, being the only palm indigenous to the east coast of North America. Its seeds (which are used to derive the pharmaceutical) are rich in fatty acids, their esters, and sterols. The extract of these seeds is recommended for mild symptoms referable to the prostate, without any pharmacological rationale. A recent clinical trial has confirmed the uselessness of saw palmetto for this indication (Bent *et al.*, 2006), and furthermore, the danger is that patients will use the product to temporize for symptoms that could lead to an earlier diagnosis of malignancy. The doses administered are usually insufficient to reduce the absorption of oral fat-soluble drugs, but it would seem wise to separate the administration of vitamin D, warfarin, etc. and this lipophilic complementary therapy.

Ginko extract

The robust tree *Gingko biloba* has remained essentially unevolved for far longer than almost all other tree species. For this reason it is also known as the "Fossil tree" in the Far East, where most of its fossils are found. A specimen of *Gingko biloba* was the only living thing to survive at ground zero, Hiroshima, recovering its stature from the surviving root within about ten years. The product is used for memory loss and mental alertness, without good clinical trial evidence, but it has enjoyed this reputation for centuries in Asia, and now worldwide. Ginkaloids are antioxidant, but how this mechanism relates to its proposed neurological and cardiovascular effects is unclear. Some *G. biloba* extracts increase both the antiplatelet properties of aspirin and the anticoagulant properties of warfarin, perhaps suggesting that the interaction takes place at the level of plasma protein binding; which flavanoid or terpene lactone is responsible for this is unknown, and perhaps it is due to some other, unidentified component of these particular formulations. Hydrolyzed amino acids from cow brain are recommended for the same purpose in Central Europe (e.g., Cerebrolyticu® in Romania).

Black Cohosh

Black Cohosh (*Cimicifuga racemosa* or "Bugbane") is native to the Eastern United States and was first identified by the Algonquin tribes as an aid to inducing labor, and treating peri- and post-menopausal symptoms. Separation scientists have found no factors with known estragenic activity. It would be therefore be illogical to impute beneficial effects of this material on prevention of coronary heart disease or osteoporosis.

Glucosamine/chondroitin

Glucosamine/chondroitin combinations are promoted as "optimal support for joint health," and to "repair joint cartilage" in the US. Both materials may be prepared either from bovine or ovine sources, which reputable manufacturers usually obtain from herds that are free from scrapie or bovine spongiform encephalopathy prions. Glucosamines are also found in chitin (the material giving strength to insect exoskeletons and the shells of marine arthropods) and some plant cell walls. Patients with allergies to crabs and lobsters are also liable to be allergic to glucosamine formulations derived from these sources. Chondroitin is a sulfated mucopolysaccharide found in mammalian cartilage or tendons. Glucosamine, in large doses, can increase insulin requirements in diabetics. Chondroitin increases the likelihood of relative overdose with warfarin, probably by competition for plasma protein binding sites and increase in free warfarin concentrations.

SAM-e

SAM-e recently became popular in North America, although it has been used for much longer in Europe. It is recommended for the kindred syndromes of fibromyalgia and chronic fatigue syndrome, as well as unrelated diseases such as osteoarthritis and Parkinson's disease. SAM-e is also recommended for depression and anxiety, which can obviously be either primary or secondary to the other indications. Pure SAM-e is (usually) the S-isomer of adenosyl (L-) methionine, but it is often formulated with B vitamins; endogenous adenosyl methionine is found in the mammalian liver, and thus swallowing 200 mg per day (a typical dose) may not be able to change materially the biological economy of this substance. Perhaps by extrapolation from the known detoxicating properties of sulphydryl-containing amino acids, it is proposed that SAM-e removes "harmful metabolites" and that these in turn are responsible for the diseases for which the drug is indicated. It is also proposed that SAM-e can "optimize the synthesis of neurotransmitters, glutathione, and cartilage"; since glutathione is synthesized in many mammalian tissues at high concentration, always from glutamate, cysteine, and glycine, these claims cannot be entirely correct. One manufacturer's trademark for SAM-e is "Nature's Wonder®" and it

sells SAM-e formulated with unidentified "Methylation factors" as a "complete methylation support formula."

Ephedra spp.

Ephedra spp. (known as *"ma huang"* in Chinese medicine) is a large genus of woody, jointed, desert shrubs. These shrubs appear to be leafless from a distance, but on close inspection, possess scale-like leaf structures at the nodes. Ephedrine, pseudoephedrine, and related alkaloids are the active principles. Ephedra is marketed for many logical purposes, e.g., as decongestants, bronchodilation, etc. Less appropriate uses are to heighten awareness, remain awake when studying for examinations, and a street-sold alternative to illegal amphetamines. The predictable adverse events are hypertensive episodes, stroke, cardiac arrhythmias, and seizures, often in young people, and after doses as low as 1–5 mg, reported at a rate of about 100 per year to the US Food and Drug Administration (FDA). During general anesthesia, unexpected hypertensive problems occur due to supra-additive interactions. Renal stones have been reported to be associated with Ephedra use in one or two case reports, although a causal relationship must be viewed, at present, as uncertain. It would be illogical to recommend ephedra to patients with glaucoma, diabetes, hyperthyroidism, and any other condition that would usually cause contraindication of sympathomimetic agonists. In the US, Ephedra-containing food supplements were banned in 2005.

Ginseng

Ginseng is an extract of *Panax schinseng* (China) or *P. quinquefolius* (North America). It is a five-leaved herb with red berries. The part used for making complementary therapies is the aromatic root. Ginseng is recommended for holistic measures of good health, usually stated, at their most specific, as enhancing resistance to stress and improving sexual function. There are one or two case reports that ginseng can antagonize the effects of warfarin, but otherwise this herbal medicine appears to cause almost no adverse events. Ginseng is more widely used in North America and the Far East than in Europe.

Kava

Kava is an Australasian shrubby pepper (*Piper methysticum*). Amid much ceremony, its crushed roots have been made into an intoxicating beverage by the peoples of the Molucca Islands and the northern coast of Australia. Kava is usually recommended for anxiety. It has sedative and extra-pyramidal effects, in common with some anticholinergic and antidopaminergic drugs, and probably has synergistic sedative effects when administered with benzodiazepines, barbiturates (barbitals), alcohol, and some antiepileptic and antipsychotic drugs. Kava makes Parkinsonism worse, and can cause drug rash, photosensitivity, and itching.

Other complementary medicines

There are many thousands of other complementary medicines. These range from large doses of vitamins or minerals to extracts of many other plants and animals. Most are not characterized toxicologically or pharmacologically; the properties of the simplest may be anticipated with a good clinical biochemistry textbook at hand.

In Hong Kong, limited regulatory control of many traditional medicines has been found to be necessary due to their toxic nature. These regulations extend over root extracts from several *Aconitum spp.* (containing C_{19} terpinoid sodium channel blocking drugs), various herbs containing anticholinergic substances, toad venoms (which contain Na–K ATPase inhibiting bufotoxins), and even preparations from the more familiar genuses *Impatiens*, *Rhododendron*, and *Euphorbia* (Tomlinson *et al.*, 2000). The view through the window of a Chinese pharmacy, in the Chinatown of any city in Asia, Europe, or the Americas, may cause different emotions in the pharmaceutical physician and pharmacologist. While both may feel daunted, the true pharmacologist also beholds an almost inexhaustible new supply of drug development leads!

Adverse effects due to complementary therapies

It should be noted that almost all types of adverse event have been described above. These include agonist-antagonist interaction, protein binding competition, metabolic adaptation, and pharmacodynamic synergy.

The general public seems to have a preconceived notion that drugs with "natural" origins, or those that can be bought without prescription, are automatically safe (perhaps this notion complements the uncritical assumption that there is no need rigorously to prove efficacy). It is curious and illogical to assume that a complementary therapy has sufficient pharmacological activity to make an improvement in health (however imprecisely that may be defined), and yet insufficient properties to cause harm. Perhaps only the homeopathic medicines are safe in overdose.

Part of the problem is that adverse reactions to "natural" therapies are not reported in the same way as for orthodox drugs (Barnes *et al.*, 1998). Reporting bias also tends towards the association of adverse effects with the condition being treated rather than from the "harmless" over-the-counter or herbal remedy that has been administered.

Finally, "Ayurvedic" medicine in the US is often advertised in association with the use of a variety of herbs, essentially as prophylactic agents, to keep one's three "doshas" (energies) in appropriate equilibrium and to avoid disease. Slogans such as "just imagine only ever using drugs that are entirely natural" are used, presumably to attract converts. Lest we forget, Romeo's and Juliet's poison was natural.

Regulatory aspects

Homeopathic drugs are regulated in much the same way as allopathic drugs. There are some over-the-counter formulations, but most are prescribed and can only be dispensed by a pharmacist in the United Kingdom.

The UK Medicines and Healthcare product Regulatory Authority (MHRA) has recently issued its first public assessment report for a homeo-pathic product. Arnicare Arnica pillules have been approved without evidence of efficacy, and in pack-aging that falsely implies that the product contains an extract of *Arnica montana* (Wolf's bane or Moun-tain tobacco; MHRA 2009a, 2009b).

Traditional Herbal Registration

A new European Union category of product approval has been introduced, namely the Tra-ditional Herbal Registration (THR). This was in response to EU Directive 2004/24/EC, which basi-cally provided for marketing authorization of herbal products that do not fulfill the usual require-ments, especially the absence of any evidence for efficacy. The Directive accommodated the various approaches of EU Member States to such prod-ucts that had enjoyed long use and reputation; these approaches were ad-hoc country-by-country reflecting the wide variety of medical and cultural attitudes towards herbal products within the EU. The MHRA has issued a guidance addressing the change in status of some herbal products that already had a Product Licence in the UK (MHRA, 2009a).

The Directive did not distinguish between those products that were licensed or unlicensed in each Member State. The UK had an entirely unlicensed class of herbal remedies (under Section 12(2) of the Medicines Act, 1968), as well as some with Product Licences (PLs). Many of these PLs had been issued as of right following a review of herbal medicines in 1988–1990 by the then Committee on Review of Medicines, when it determined that the herbal remedy was for a minor disorder that was likely to be accurately self-diagnosed. In such cases, mere evidence of traditional use was accepted *in lieu* of pharmacology and clinical trials.

The new THR effort therefore had the primary goal of bringing those products that were entirely unlicensed into compliance with the Directive. Secondarily, where the THR would lead to a more streamlined review than for PLs, converting PL herbal products into THR products is being planned. This would create a single class of herbal remedy in the UK that cannot fulfill PL standards for purity, safety, and efficacy, and continued PL

status in the future will require orthodox demon-strations of efficacy, in particular.

The THR application in the UK focuses on prod-uct information. There will be a Quality Dossier, and an updated Module 1 for previous PL prod-ucts. The transfer of PL products into THR ones will take place over the next few years accord-ing to MHRA workload and with schedules pre-viously agreed with the herbal products' manu-facturers.

United States: "dietary supplements"

In the US, the euphemism "dietary supplement" is the preferred regulatory term for the sorts of prod-ucts that have become Traditional Herbal Remedies in Europe. The definition is broad, including vita-mins, minerals, herbs or other botanicals, amino acids, enzymes, tissues from organs or glands, concentrates, metabolites, constituents or extracts. These are regulated under the Dietary Supplement Health and Education Act (DHSEA), 1994.

The Act places the onus for the safety of the product on its manufacturer. It also requires that representations and claims should not be false or misleading. There is no requirement for the man-ufacturer to provide evidence on safety or effec-tiveness of these products, either before or after marketing.

Advertising claims are scrutinized not by the FDA, but by the Federal Trade Commission. In order to remain within the law, dietary supple-ment manufacturers are supposed to avoid mak-ing claims aligned with precise diagnoses. Thus to claim that a dietary supplement was useful "as a treatment for osteoarthritis" would make it into an unlicensed and illegal drug. But (as for a glucosamine/chondroitin combination product) to claim that it is a "joint soother" goes without regu-latory approbation. Yet, the current situation is that ludicrous claims of therapeutic benefit for various products are common in print and on television, and a gullible public pays up.

Chinese medicines

Chinese medicines are essentially unregulated everywhere. As in medieval Europe, these can be prescribed by both a Chinese medical practitioner and a Chinese pharmacist (using the term Chinese to describe their disciplines, not their nationality), and much responsibility rests on the pharmacist for identification of the correct plants, resisting the purchase of cheap materials from unreliable suppliers, and knowing what to look for in quality control. Other forms of herbal remedy (including all nine discussed above) are freely available in supermarkets and pharmacies in most jurisdictions. Mail order, using the Internet for advertising, is increasing, and will doubtless cause legal issues with cross-border commerce and transportation in the future.

References

Barnes J, Mills SY, Abbot NC, Willoughby M, Ernst E. Different standards for reporting ADRs to herbal remedies. *Br J Clin Pharmacol* 1998; **45**: 496–500.

Bent S, Kane C, Shinohara K, Neuhaus J, *et al.* Saw palmetto for benign prostatic hyperplasia. *New Eng J Med* 2006; **354**: 557–566.

Cheng JT. Review: Drug therapy in Chinese traditional medicine. *J Clin Pharmacol* 2000; **40**: 445–450.

Critchley JAJH, Zhang Y, Suthisisang CC, Chan TYK, Tomlinson B. Alternative therapies and medical science: Designing clinical trials of alternative/complementary medicines – Is evidence-based traditional Chinese medicine attainable ? *J Clin Pharmacol* 2000; **40**: 462–467.

MHRA. *Guidance on arrangements for the transfer of certain herbal products with a marketing authorisation to traditional herbal status*. Medicines and Healthcare Products Regulatory Agency: London, UK, 2009a.

MHRA. *Public assessment report Arnicare Arnica 30c pillules. NR 01175/1810 UKPAR* Medicines and Healthcare Products Regulatory Agency: London, UK, 2009b.

Nutrition Business Journal. NBJ's Complementary and Alternative Medicine and Practitioner Supplement Sales Report, 2007; http://nutritionbusinessjournal.com/ alternative-medicine/market-research/nbjs-complementary_alternative_medicine_practitioner_supplement_sales_2007/index.html; accessed April 24, 2010.

Tomlinson B, Chan TYK, Chan JCN, Critchley JAJH, But PPH. Toxicity of complementary therapies: An Eastern perspective. *J Clin Pharmacol* 2000; **40**: 451–456.

Zollman C, Vickers A. What is complementary medicine? *Br Med J* 1999; **319**: 693–696.

Further reading

Eisenberg DM, Kessler RC, Foster C, Norlock FE, Calkins DR, Delbanco TL. Unconventional medicine in the United States. Prevalence, costs, and patterns of use. *New Engl J Med* 1993; **328**: 246–252.

Ernst E. *Complementary Medicine: A Critical Appraisal*. 1996; Butterworth-Heinemann: Oxford, UK.

SECTION V
Drug Regulation

Introduction

Drug regulation is essential not only for public health, but also for the understanding of pharmaceutical medicine, which is practiced within what is widely acknowledged as the most highly regulated of all industries. Regulation is also a constantly changing field. In particular, it is anticipated that there will be major changes within Europe during 2010–2011, which will be within the currency of this edition of this book. The purpose here is simply to provide the practitioner of pharmaceutical medicine with a basic understanding, and conversancy with drug regulation. Needless to say, the editors would always recommend seeking specialist regulatory advice for any drug development program, and for all marketed products.

CHAPTER 34

United States Regulations

William Kennedy, with contribution from Lionel D. Edwards

The Food and Drug Administration: how we got where we are

Once upon a time ... there was no Food and Drug Administration (FDA). However, the history of food and drug regulation began well before any modern government administration, anywhere in the world. Drugs and foods have only become distinguished from each other in the relatively recent past, and it can be argued, as yet incompletely in the US.

The ancient Greeks, Romans, and Arabs all regulated food and drugs. Principally, their concern was with product purity, one of the three pivotal concepts that still form the basis for drug approval today. The typical penalty in ancient times for violating the standards was the loss of the dominant hand that had made the adulterated product. The Arabs were probably the most conscientious of regulators, with standards for about 2000 drug products, and like today's FDA, they were the first to establish a professional staff of food and drug inspectors. Their penalty for a baker of underweight loaves exceeded that of the drug adulterer: The bakers went summarily into their own ovens.

In 1202, the first English regulation was identified, traditionally, as the Assize of Bread. In fact, this assize had been held by manorial lords for a lot longer than this, and the lords were often also the exclusive owners of the ovens. To remedy this small aspect of local despotism, presumably with skepticism about self-regulation, the new national law forbade the incorporation of ground peas or beans in the flour meal. Meanwhile, the London Grocers had organized, and formed their own guild, again with self-regulation of a wider range of foodstuffs. In the 17th century, the London apothecaries (makers of medicines and also licensed medical practitioners in their own right) devolved from the Grocers. The Worshipful Society of Apothecaries of London still exists, can still award a medical license (although this is quite rare among British physicians), and is now the largest of all the London guilds.

What with 1776 and all that, the British jurisdiction of food and drug regulation ceased to apply in what was to become the United States. The apothecaries were still people who had trained mostly in London or Germany, or had graduated to professional status by apprenticeship. But there was a void in national regulation of food and drugs, and British patents, which had already been awarded to American drug recipes, also became null and void.

Over-the-counter (OTC) medicines (or "patent" medicines) thrived in this void. The American patent process was also undeveloped, and so these became what we would perhaps view as trade secrets held by named apothecaries and their apprentices. There were also no inspectors. Moreover, the British were not quickly mollified by the new political reality: European medicines were included in the embargo, and Yankee ingenuity began to be expressed to the full. The problem quickly evolved: Who was to say that the "eye of newt" in the Scottish witches' potion was not actually a bit of chicken?

Principles and Practice of Pharmaceutical Medicine, 3rd edition.
Edited by L.D. Edwards, A.W. Fox, P.D. Stonier.
© 2011 Blackwell Publishing Ltd.

It has been said that the drug law in the US developed in the 18th and 19th centuries with all the red, white, and blue of the anilene dyes that quickly became available. Regulations in the US rapidly developed in a characteristically idiosyncratic manner.

Sewers and food do not mix. This was the era of rapid expansion of Boston, Philadelphia, New York, Baltimore, and eventually Washington, DC itself. Massachusetts regulated food for the first time in 1784, but this again was a feeble attempt to control purity. No attempt was made to address the potions used to treat ineffectively the infectious diseases that were rampant.

"Dr Feel good" potions, typically named after the apothecary who compounded them, had eponymous effects. These potions usually contained alcohol and morphine, were used indiscriminately, and at least made people feel good. One of these survives, ironically enough in England, and is called "Dr John Collis-Brown's Compound".

The American geography constrained the regulatory environment. First, there was a lot of pioneer activity in the West: trained professionals were not the first to climb on the covered wagons. Second, new religions were being spawned at a rate far faster than had ever occurred in any European country. Third, worthless medicines were being distributed and used over millions of square miles with, at best, only rudimentary communications. The promotion of medicines became a form of entertainment, by bogus professors, showmen, fakers, and embezzlers in Desert Gulch! Meanwhile, little opportunity was taken to learn from the Native Americans, whose herbals were often quite well developed with active pharmacognosy. But the national government was not stirred into action until its own interests were directly affected: soldiers in the Mexican American War were poisoned by ineffective antimalarials south of the Rio Grande.

And so it was, in 1848, that the first drug regulation was established in the US. It simply banned the import of impure drugs. The medicine-man shows were left to local regulation (a legislative omission that is still with us today). And so it was that in 1850, the State of California became the first to enact anything resembling a comprehensive drug regulation.

By 1900, it is estimated that about US$40 million per annum was being spent on drug advertising. This was mostly in newspapers, which were thus only too happy to ally with potion makers in stirring up public opinion against the national regulation of their products. Medicines (some up to 50% alcoholic tinctures) became the only source of alcohol in some communities where religion forbade wine and whisky. For the more adventurous, morphine, opium, cannabinoids, and cocaine were available, even in some of the earliest formulations of Coca-Cola, although not, of course, today.

Harvey Wiley was a hero among the villains. He headed the Federal Bureau of Chemistry, and began calling for national regulation in 1890. His "poison squad," the forerunners of the Inspectorate Branch of the FDA today, began documenting and on occasion prosecuting the makers of fake and poisonous drugs. The convictions were usually for things that were very egregious, probably because Dr Wiley could only prosecute under the general laws. Unlike today's FDA inspectors, the members of this squad were expected to sample the questionable product themselves, and then give firsthand evidence of the adverse effects that they experienced!

Specific regulation began in 1902, and concerned the purity of serums and vaccines to be used in humans; The Center for Biologics Evaluations and Research (CBER) thus has a longer history than its colleague center for drugs (CDER).

Part of US food and drug regulatory lore includes, at this point, an unlikely convergence of two famous characters. One was President Theodore Roosevelt, nationalist ex-"rough-rider," soldier in Cuba, and hero of San Juan Hill. The other was Upton Sinclair, the United States' first published communist, and author of *The Jungle*, intended as an expose of North American capitalism at its worst. Sinclair's book was being serialized in the DC newspapers, which the President habitually read during his high-cholesterol breakfast, which always included sausages. In one daily episode of the book, Sinclair described the use of offal, floor waste, and other abominations at the end of the daily sausage run, in the attempt to maximize profits. Dr Wiley had his political ally, and the Pure Food and Drug Act (PFDA) and Meat Inspection Act were the result (1906).

The PFDA banned adulterated or misbranded drugs from interstate commerce, and this remains the legal basis for FDA actions to this day. Today's definitions of "adulterated" and "misbranded" are also those of nearly a century ago. The philosophy, however, has long been forgotten: if you made bad drugs, you had to sell them within your own community, and the local law enforcement people should have found you out fairly easily for themselves. This is, arguably, a survival of the Anglo-Saxon principle of frankpledge within the 21st century US laws.

From among the wide variety of dyestuffs available in the north-eastern factories before the First World War, just seven were authorized for human consumption by the Certified Color Regulations (1907). This brought dyestuffs within the canon of interstate commerce law. This is not as incongruent as it might seem because among these dyestuffs were the first, primitive antibiotics.

But then as now, the US Supreme Court was not averse to getting involved in unprecedented situations. In 1911, the Court held that the 1906 Act did not prohibit false or misleading therapeutic claims, but was strictly to be interpreted in terms of purity and composition. The PFDA was thus amended in 1912, to include specifically false therapeutic claims. However, the Act now required proof of intent to be fraudulent: it was essentially a criminal matter. This need for proof of intent made the Act hard to enforce, and few could be punished or made to change their ways. In 1914, a further amendment defined the presence of poisonous or adulterated substances to be specifically a violation of the Act, although the definitions of precisely what was a poisonous or adulterous substance would have to be developed on precedent.

It was not until 1924 that a further PFDA amendment made mere statements potentially a violation under the Act. For the first time, exaggerated claims of therapeutic effectiveness could be proscribed. This amendment went further to specify that even true statements that nonetheless deceive or misin-

form would henceforth fall foul of the Act (malt vinegar without any written claim to be apple cider vinegar, but with an apple depicted on the label, was cited as an example of how this situation could arise).

Ever since 1906, there had been many challenges to the Act and its amendments, and this consumed much administrative time and money. The innovation of 1930, expansion of the Bureau of Chemistry into a renamed Food and Drug Administration, was designed to relieve this administrative burden. The new Agency introduced a Bill into Congress, which was designed to invigorate and modernize the by-now patchwork and creaking amended PDFA.

Once again, there was resistance to the Bill. However, communications were modernized, and public opinion was molded not only by newspapers but also by radio: and radio could be heard hundreds of miles away. One small fly in the proverbial ointment, however, was that Teddy Roosevelt's nephew, Franklin Roosevelt, was now President; the President was wheelchair-bound due to polio, and believed in the therapeutic value of hot springs and other complementary therapies.

At about this time (1931), an OTC potion called "Jake" poisoned hundreds of people. It was probably a peripheral neurotoxin due to an adulterant in an extract of Jamaican ginger: "Jake-leg" became a recognized syndrome. While Jake "the Peg" with an extra leg (i.e., a crutch) became famous, it needed a much bigger disaster to move legislative and public opinion.

Domagk demonstrated in 1935 that sulfonamide-containing dyes could protect mice from infection; he became a Nobel laureate in 1938. The nostrum artists could hardly believe their luck: now they could peddle a drug that actually worked! The favored formulation at the time was an elixir, probably a holdover from evasion of alcohol restrictions due to religion, or the earlier flirt with prohibition. In any case, one company, supposedly laudibly, searched for a nonalcoholic solution for its sulfonamide. They chose diethylene glycol. In four weeks of marketing, the product was not a success: only 353 patients drank it; of these, 107 died. They were mostly children, and there was no renal dialysis in

1936. Thousands could have been killed had the company's market analysis been accurate.

But finally, there was sufficient groundswell, and the FDA obtained passage of the Food, Drug, and Cosmetic Act (FD&C Act) in 1938. Thus, the FD&C Act added safety as the second pivotal leg of drug approval.

There was still no requirement to prove product efficacy. But in 1941, with most of the world at war, an often overlooked piece of US legislation was passed. The FD&C Act was amended, to reflect an FDA proposal. Henceforth, the FDA was empowered to certify the potency of insulin. This required a bioassay, and for the first time the FDA was able to regulate pharmacodynamics. It was a short step to therapeutic efficacy.

In 1943, the Supreme Court again got involved. In an otherwise obscure case, it held that the FDA was empowered to establish standards for products labeling. The four principal arms of drug approval were finally concentrated in the hands of a single agency: purity, safety, efficacy, and labeling. To this day, much of the power of FDA is exercised by its control of what a label says, and not by the pharmacological characteristics of the particular drug in question. To Europeans this is sometimes a surprising concept, but in fact the principal extends to other areas of American commerce: for example, cars may be imported into California depending not upon whether the vehicle meets the emissions standards, but rather upon whether it is labeled as meeting those standards.

In the 1950s, the Delaney Amendment to the FD&C Act authorized an investigation into the new dyes, flavourings, and preservatives that were becoming available in an era of unprecedented chemical innovation. There was already a clear need to update the FD&C Act, and the Food Additive Amendment of 1958 was one result, which among other things, prohibited carcinogenic materials from foods and drugs. This required a method to establish carcinogenicity, which is now an important element in the toxicology package for an overwhelming majority of approved drugs. There are now exceptions. Antineoplastic drugs are often themselves carcinogenic, and the absolute restriction on such materials is somewhat tempered.

Furthermore, we now understand the dose relationships for chemical carcinogenesis, and how to measure it, very well; high-school exercises now routinely exceed limits of detection available in the 1950s. But the principle had been established in law. November 1958 saw the FDA recalling the entire cranberry crop, just before the Thanksgiving holiday, because there was a fear of weed-killer contamination, which it had established was a carcinogen in animals!

The other major piece of legislation in the 1950s was the Durham-Humphrey Amendment to the FD&C Act. Humphrey (unsuccessful Presidential candidate and later Vice-President) had been a pharmacist; he wanted to clarify what should and should not be an OTC drug. Hitherto, the only reason to get a prescription from a physician and have it filled by a pharmacist was because the patient did not know of an OTC drug to meet his or her need, and the prescription was one that needed to be compounded by a professional. The amendment provided, perhaps artificially, that when a disease or a drug side effect needed a physician's attention, any treatment required a prescription and only a licensed pharmacist could fill a prescription. Some view this as the genesis of general diagnostic education by the pharmaceutical industry, and in turn, the origins of direct-to-consumer advertising designed to drive patients into their doctors' offices.

In the late 1950s, there were also many other reasons to seek reform. The FDA's ability to regulate efficacy assessments was still restricted to a small number of highly specialized products, and modern advertising techniques were getting underway. As usual, there was public resistance, and it required a big disaster to get things done: to be precise, thalidomide.

Dr Frances Kelsey had the thalidomide application on her desk. She was busy and had simply not got around to it. Then from Europe she heard about a question of peripheral neuropathy, and possibly thyrotoxity; at that point she made an active decision to hold up the approval. It was an Australian dermatologist who identified drug induced phocomelia, and the rest is well known. Only nine cases of phocomelia were reported in the US, from an exposure of about 4000 women of childbearing potential, most of whom were pregnant. Kelsey received a medal from President Kennedy.

Amazingly enough, the 1962 amendments would still not have kept thalidomide off the market in the US. The precise strain of rodent that would have been required to identify the lesion was not in common use, and the adverse event frequency in neonates, in the average-sized New Drug Application (NDA) of the day, might not detect adverse events of such low frequency. However, the 1962 amendments required, in the general case, that drugs should be demonstrated to be effective prior to approval, for the first time.

The 1962 Kefauver-Harris amendments provided further capability to the FDA. They set forth the requirements of the Investigational New Drugs (IND) process. The FDA was empowered, for the first time, to seize a drug and cause it to be withdrawn. Adverse event reporting to the FDA became mandatory. Labeling and advertising requirements were clarified, and transferred that responsibility to the FDA from the Federal Trade Commission. Inspections of manufacturing sites were also facilitated by these far-reaching amendments.

In 1966, it was estimated that there were about 4000 drugs available that had been approved on pre-1962 criteria. The FDA commissioned the National Academy of Sciences/National Research Council (NAS/NRC) to review these "grandfathered drugs" against the modern standards. Some of the reviews lasted 15 years, and were contentious, while other drugs felt to be important had to be transferred to new manufacturing sites. The abbreviated NDA (ANDA; mostly thought of today in connection with generic drug approvals) was invented in 1970 for the latter purpose. The NAS review was extended to OTC drugs in 1972. Meanwhile, devices came under the FDA aegis in 1972, and biologics and vaccines were subsumed under the FDA umbrella in 1972.

As regulations increased, so did the risk of drug development. Complaints were loud that rare diseases, offering small potential markets, were increasingly ignored because the costs of drug development to address those markets had become so high as to deter research and development by the pharmaceutical manufacturers. After much debate,

a compromise was reached in the Orphan Drug Act (1983). If it could be demonstrated that the incidence of the disease in question was fewer than 200,000 persons per year in the US, Orphan Drug designation would be allowed. This provided tax credits and exclusivity guarantees, should an eventual NDA succeed. Currently, there is criticism that this absolute number of 200,000 patients has not been raised with time, because the US population is now greatly increased since 1983, and unless amended, this legislation will eventually become moot. Meanwhile, there is also often debate with the FDA on borderline cases of calculation of incidence. Several drugs that are in the market in Europe are denied to Americans by reason of the FDA not granting Orphan Drug designation, and there being no other method for gaining exclusivity for at least the seven years that the Orphan Drug Act provides.

The Waxman-Hatch Amendment (1984) traded off patent term restoration for innovative drug development with generic drug ANDA approval. The contents of the ANDA were clearly stated for the first time. Furthermore, FDA review times could be added to the patent-awarded period of exclusivity. Currently, the FDA compares these review periods in a highly conservative manner: the review period is compared to the period that the drug company has been conducting IND research, and the public is led to the view that FDA review is a trivial component of total development time. Furthermore, the FDA stops this artificial clock every time they send a question about the NDA back to the sponsor, even though review activities at the Agency continue. In one case, in the 1990s, when these procedures had been well established, 30 months elapsed between NDA submission and approval, but the patent term restoration was only nine months; no new clinical trials or toxicology studies were needed during this review.

The generic scandal of the 1980s involved pharmaceutical companies making, and FDA staff accepting, bribes in the interests of rapid generic drug approval. No new legislation resulted, even though two Vice-presidential commissions (one Republican, the other Democratic) inquired into the matter. Similarly, there was no new legislation following the massive Clinton initiative; drug pricing was probably the principal missed target on that occasion. It is arguable whether or not these events triggered the subsequent spate of mergers and acquisitions within the pharmaceutical industry.

The Prescription Drug Users Fee Act (PDUFA, 1992) traded off fees paid upon NDA submission for performance standards on the part of the FDA. This was the first time that any effective accountability had been applied to the FDA, somewhat reversing the orientation of the Agency. The PDUFA has now been reauthorized twice, and analysis of its effect is being conducted by several industry and government organizations.

A major revision of Food and Drug Law took place in 1997, coincident with the first reauthorization of PDUFA. The Food and Drug Administration Modernization Act (FDAMA) of 1997 was only the third major overhaul of the original 1906 Act. It was the first to occur without the impetus of a disaster or perceived disaster. After a troubled start in 1996, the FDAMA received overwhelmingly positive support in both houses of the US Congress, getting 98 of 100 votes in the Senate, and a unanimous vote in the House.

The perceived need for the FDAMA by Congress, the industry, and ultimately the FDA was the recognition that although the law and the regulations had changed little from the 1962 Amendments, the requirements made by the FDA of the industry had increased dramatically. Part was due to advances in technology and medicine, but part was due to the FDA reviewer preferences. Both of these contributed to the phenomenon known as "regulatory creep" that was demonstrated by wide variances across the FDA in requirements. Although there were some significant breakthroughs that advanced healthcare and the regulatory process, a major portion of the legislation focused on the formalization of "best practices" that existed within the FDA and making these the standard throughout the FDA.

Some of the major breakthroughs of the FDAMA included the following:
- formalization of the evidence needed from pharmacoeconomic studies;
- authorization and regulation of the dissemination of information on unapproved uses of approved products to healthcare providers by pharmaceutical companies;
- enhancement of the availability of labeling information for use in pediatric patients by recognizing the difficulties of developing drugs for this group and providing an incentive to undertake this work.

Examples of modernization that were the result of identifying "best practices" within the FDA and making them the standard include
- improvement of access to unapproved drugs;
- clarification of the definition of "substantial evidence of efficacy" to include only one pivotal study provided there is adequate confirmatory evidence (this had long been used for the approval of oncology drugs, but was now able to be applied more widely);
- formalization of various administrative aspects of the IND and NDA process.

Although the PDUFA and FDAMA offered significant opportunities to improve the drug development process and make more drugs available to more people, more quickly, for the most part the promise has yet to be fully realized. There are two reasons for this, both acknowledged before the legislative changes were initiated. The first reason is that the "regulatory creep" that was being corrected was something that took place over the period 1962–1997. It would be unrealistic, not to mention unsound, to expect 35 years of change to be corrected overnight, and at the same time, maintain a productive regulatory agency. Congress allowed for an implementation period. The second reason flows from the first. The drug development process is long and resource-intense. It is difficult to turn midstream. Once the FDA starts changing, the industry will have to respond with changes in the development process. This takes even more time. Simply stated, many of the changes have just not had sufficient time to get into the process.

Economic considerations

The FDA has jurisdiction over about 20–25% of the gross national product (GNP) of the United States.

In 1996, the FDA-regulated industries comprised about US\$1750 billion (i.e., US\$1.75 $\times$ 10^{12}), thus dwarfing the US Department of Defense budget by about a six-fold difference. This is about 150% of the entire GNP of the United Kingdom. These regulated industries include all medical devices, all drugs, many other OTC or *in vitro* diagnostic materials, and almost all food (meat is still the responsibility of the Department of Agriculture under Teddy Roosevelt's 1906 Act). These activities are all mandated by the FD&C Act and its various amendments.

In addition, FDA engages in various cooperative projects with organizations such as the National Institutes of Health, the Centers for Disease Control, the Drug Enforcement Agency, and the US Public Health Service (many of whose officers serve attachments to the FDA). A certain amount of independent research is supported in the FDA budget, as well as international liaisons. The FDA also conducts lobbying and legislative functions.

Organizational aspects

The FDA is part of the Department of Health and Human Services, which is represented at Secretary level within each President's cabinet. The secretary appoints a commissioner to head the FDA, and this is usually a political appointment (i.e., not held by a career civil servant). The commissioner appoints assistants or deputies to head the following centers or offices:
- CDER;
- CBER (now with a far smaller remit than previously);
- Center for Food Safety and Applied Nutrition;
- Center for Devices and Radiological Health;
- Center for Veterinary Medicine;
- Office of Regulatory Affairs;
- Office of Orphan Product Development;
- National Center for Toxicological Research.

The assistant and deputy commissioners might be either political appointees or career civil servants.

Each of these subdivisions is typically further subdivided. For example, the CBER has offices of Management, Compliance, Therapeutic Research and Review, Vaccines Research and Review, Establishment Licensing and Product Surveillance, Blood Products, and Communications and Training. Each are typically led by career civil servant Office Directors, although currently, the Office of Orphan Product Development is headed by a Rear-Admiral from the US Public Health Service.

The CDER has a larger product development responsibility than CBER, and thus has five Therapeutic Review Offices, each led by a career civil servant; in addition the lead review of Bioengineered medicines is now undertaken by the CDER. But the other divisions are similar to the CBER model, with divisions for Epidemiology and Statistics, Compliance, Pharmaceutical Sciences (including a specialized office of New Drug Chemistry), Biopharmaceutics, and Generic Drugs. A national center for Toxicology research is in place. Other offices, Counter terrorism and emergency coordination, Translational Medicine, and an organization called "The Critical Path" are now in place. An office of International Programs has been operating for some few years, the latter reporting into the Commissioner of Food and Drugs.

Most centers or offices have access to a network of field-based inspectors. These inspectors operate worldwide, and audit both animal and clinical studies, as well as manufacturing processes and premises. Such audits can be "for cause," for example a complaint from the public or an emergent safety issue, or "routine." Pivotal clinical trials in a submitted NDA or Biologics License Application (BLA) will usually garner an inspection of the clinical trial sites and statutory documentation.

This inspection process has recently been augmented with the establishment of an Office of the Inspector General (OIG), which reports at the level of the Secretary, not the FDA Commissioner. One of the first announced targets of the OIG, selected from the entire realm of foods and drugs that FDA regulates, is clinical trials. In particular, the OIG is actively investigating informed consent documents, and also has notified institutional review boards (the US equivalent of the ethics committee) that they are in for close scrutiny.

Make no mistake. One big difference between the European Medicines Agency (EMA) and FDA is that the FDA is also the police (and often the judge and jury, as well). Do not take lightly the appearance of your name on Form 1571.

Investigational new drugs (IND)

The student is urged to read the Code of Federal Regulations with this title, beginning at 21CFR310.

The legal basis for an IND was set up in the 1962 amendments. It is unlawful to transport an unapproved drug across state lines unless the FDA has issued an exemption. The IND is technically an exemption from the requirements of an NDA. Drugs labeled "Not for human use" are also exempt from the NDA requirements, before being transported, but carry regulatory restrictions. Note that technically and legally these regulations apply just as much to noncommercial research physicians, for example in universities, as to pharmaceutical companies.

The structure of an IND application is contained in the regulation and is quite easily followed. Almost all pharmaceutical companies, contract research organizations, and universities have templates for the writing of these documents. All the animal data, the proposed clinical study protocol, a clinical investigators' brochure, and the chemistry and manufacturing controls must be described. Once an IND is active, it can be amended with further clinical protocols, additional toxicology data and so on, as the development program proceeds.

The IND differs in a number of ways from its European counterparts. First, it is much longer; a typical IND is of at least 1000 pages, and for drugs with foreign human experience, often many multiples of this number. The UK Clinical Trials Certificate, was used very rarely for this reason. Now the Clinical Trial application under the European Directive 2001 is used. Second, an IND application is required for all human exposure to INDs and devices, and this includes normal volunteer studies. Third, all being well, there is only a 30-day wait between filing and commencement of the clinical study; no news from FDA after this time period has elapsed is presumptive evidence that the study may proceed (most FDA divisions will, in fact, issue

affirmative letters that this is the case, within 30 days). Fourth, once an IND has become active, there is no subsequent 30-day wait when further clinical protocols are submitted.

The FDA is at liberty to impose partial or total clinical holds on any protocols that it receives. Partial holds might limit, for example, the maximum dose that can be employed, prevent commencement until additional safety monitoring measures have been instituted, or restrict dose frequency.

It is no longer the case that an IND is needed merely for the export of an investigational agent to another jurisdiction, provided that the regulations that obtain in that jurisdiction are adhered to. This was one former peculiarity of the restriction on transportation of unapproved drugs across state lines.

There are variants of the IND process, which are described in Chapter 35.

Meetings with the FDA

Many Europeans are surprised at the access that pharmaceutical companies have to the reviewing divisions of the FDA. The typical investigational drug will be the subject of a pre-IND meeting, which the FDA will provide at its discretion and for which the agenda may be set by the prospective applicant. These meetings can also be held by telephone conference, and the FDA only accepts electronic files of data. An IND is, however, only allotted a number upon its submission.

It is fair to say that US companies differ in their approach to pre-IND meetings. Most companies probably view pre-IND meetings as desirable. However, under the law, proprietary information is only required to be kept confidential by the FDA when it is the subject of an IND. No known major disclosure has happened, but companies would have little recourse if the FDA leaked information following a pre-IND meeting. The other problem is that without an IND in place, the FDA has no obligation to meet with clinical trial sponsors: reviewers up against a PDUFA deadline on another project are unlikely to prepare thoroughly for a pre-IND meeting, and may entirely change their views after the IND, when they become obligated to adopt a position. Some companies file the IND first, with a simultaneous request for a meeting.

Typically, during Phase I and II development there will be sporadic communications between the IND sponsor and the FDA. These might be to clarify issues over post-IND clinical protocols, reach agreement on compatibility of toxicology data with clinical study design, carcinogenicity testing requirements (typically starting at this time due to their long duration and the necessity for their completion before filing the NDA), and the many technical matters associated with the scale-up of the chemistry and production processes.

It is typical to hold an end-of-Phase II meeting (EOP2). At this meeting, the FDA will review the current Phase I and Phase II clinical data, and the state of the toxicology program. The objective is to reach agreement on the design of the Phase III studies that will support NDA approval, as well as to identify any further problems that may be ameliorated without delaying the NDA. The FDA can also begin planning for the resources needed when the NDA arrives.

A pre-NDA meeting is typically held as the Phase III clinical trials are concluding. The principal objective is to check how the issues identified at the EOP2 meeting have been resolved. At this meeting, the entire structure of the forthcoming NDA can be agreed, and technicalities surrounding electronic submissions can also be arranged.

The new drug application (NDA)

The best NDAs have a table of contents before the EOP2 meeting, and are built as the various component nonclinical and clinical study reports become available. Most companies do this both electronically and as paper hard copy. Since 2002, the FDA was mandated by the revised PDUFA to accept electronic filings, and in turn it has required all NDAs to be submitted electronically and in the Common Technical Document format since January 2009. The structure is well described in the regulation, which the student is again urged to read.

On January 1, 2008, all NDAs or BLAs must be submitted in the electronic format of the Common Technical Document (CTD). This consists of five modules, Module 1 contains country- or region-specific administrative material, e.g., proposed package insert, "Expert Report," forms of application, etc. In this new format, the Integrated Safety and Integrated Efficacy summaries are to head up Module 5, the clinical reports section. See Chapter 37, page 477. The new drug must also be reviewed in comparison with the pharmacology and toxicology of kindred drugs. Justification for every statement in proposed labeling must also be provided. These integrated summaries, in contrast with a European expert report, are often 300–400 pages long.

Assembling a CTD is a long process. Usually there is a cut-off date for data that by then may be accruing from all over the world, but which are not pivotal for NDA approval.

The Integrated Safety Summary is then supplemented four months after NDA submission, and quarterly, during review, and for the next three years following approval. This usually provides a significant increase to the safety database either from ongoing studies that are rapidly accumulating patients in Phase IIIB or from marketing data from foreign countries where the drug may be already approved. The FDA requires updating on all safety information that has been gathered subsequent to the filing of the NDA.

Federal law requires that the FDA issues a notice of action within 180 days of filing the NDA. There are two forms of action: approval, or non-approvable. Non-approvable letters must indicate all the deficiencies that the FDA has identified that can, upon rectification, lead to approval. If such deficiencies require the submission of additional data, however slight, the FDA has another 180 days to review the application. If the deficiencies are administrative (e.g., debate over the precise wording in labeling), the FDA must act within 90 days of a resubmission. Lack of agreement on labeling is the most common cause of delays to an approval letter. Although most FDA reviewing divisions will only negotiate the proposed label, some companies have been able to go directly to an approval letter as the first action by a combination of good communication with the FDA and the submission of a realistic package insert. The labeling negotiation itself will often be done by fax and counter-fax, possibly culminating in a face-to-face meeting at FDA premises.

NDA approval is sometimes contingent on the sponsor making various commitments. Most recently, the company is being asked to conduct post-marketing surveillance studies for safety issues that may be more or less well defined. Post-NDA safety report frequency will also be agreed prior to approval. Occasionally, there may be a toxicology study that the FDA regards as outstanding but not crucial to drug launch. There may also be stated requirements for additional indications that have been refused by the company at the initial NDA approval.

Sources of guidance

Both the CDER and CBER have published a large number of guidance documents that are now also available at www.fda.gov. Some of these are simply ICH documents in English. However, the FDA has gone far beyond this, in supplying a large amount of valuable information. Guidances are not binding (on either sponsor or FDA), but it would be fair to say that clear reasons would have to be enunciated by the FDA when requiring the guideline to be exceeded, and by the sponsor when suggesting a variance from them.

One of the difficulties in dealing with the FDA is that reviewing divisions interpret these guidances differently. These differences can be profound. The term "adequate and well-controlled studies" is used to describe the requirement for complying with the need to demonstrate drug efficacy. Most reviewing divisions in CDER still tend to interpret this to mean at least two independent, large-scale Phase III clinical trials despite the clarification in FDAMA. Yet, CBER will approve drugs with a single Phase III study and some consistent Phase II data. Similarly, although the ICH guideline states that drugs used for intermittent, acute therapy do not need to

have lifespan carcinogenicity tests, there can still be different interpretations within the FDA regarding the definition of "intermittent." Anesthetic drugs are usually exempt from these long and resource intense animal studies; but should this apply to acute treatments for disease, labeled for a maximum of three doses per week, and with relatively short half-times of elimination, or not?

Another example relates to the pre-IND meeting. Some FDA divisions do not like them, and if reviewers attend, they have a tendency to provide less valuable information than they would for an EOP2 meeting or a pre-NDA meeting, the so called "entitled meetings." But within the industry, there are a number of companies who have similar attitudes about the value of pre-IND meetings. The notable difference is that the FDA has to go to the pre-IND meeting if scheduled. The companies who see little value merely do not schedule them.

The bottom-line is that guidances are merely that: guidances. Individual reviewers at FDA are unlikely always to agree with what are essentially consensus documents.

The CBER has innovated further with documents entitled "Points to Consider." These rank below guidances in terms of their gravity. These are designed to accommodate rapidly developing technologies, which, to be fair, is probably a greater challenge for CBER than CDER. These "Points to Consider" are almost completely outside the ICH process, and have been very well received by the regulated industries.

The FDA has also been keeping its eye on the public. Advisory committee hearings are typically held by the reviewing divisions prior to any significant NDA approval. These hearings are open to the public, and specifically include an agenda item that provides for public commentary, quite apart from the dialog that goes on between FDA staff, their recruited outside experts, and the NDA sponsor (again, all in public). The FDA has also begun to publish its policy statements. The AIDS community, in particular, has been especially effective in deflecting the FDA from its otherwise default-mode course in the review of investigational and new drugs.

Influences on FDA activities

The FDA, like any other branch of the US government, is subject to the oversight of Congress. It is Congress that writes the laws that the FDA must implement as regulations. The FDA must understand the Congressional intent in any law, or will find itself called before them to justify their actions. FDA is also dependent upon Congress for its budget, which it must get approved yearly. The court of public opinion has had more of an influence on the FDA in the past 20 years than during any other time in its history. This influence is directly focused at the FDA, or indirectly through interaction with Congress or the media. The AIDS community broke the ground in this arena in the 1980s when it demanded access to more drugs for this dreadful disease more quickly. Fueled by the success of its actions, other patient groups have challenged FDA authority since then: The American Association of Retired People voiced its concern on a wide range of activities and The American Academy of Pediatrics won its campaign of "more drugs for children." A number of cancer patient groups seek the ear of the FDA on a regular basis and pharmaceutical trade associations are also active voices.

Other recent regulatory developments, which are covered elsewhere in this book, include legislation regarding risk management as a forthcoming integral part of all NDA approvals (see also below), and new requirements for studying potential cardiotoxicity (which is the subject of a valuable ICH guidance).

Although the special nature of children in clinical trials is dealt with elsewhere in this book, it should not be forgotten that the FDA has been influenced to make regulatory changes specific to this age group as well. The victims of the sulfanilamide elixir tragedy that drove the 1938 Food, Drug, and Cosmetic Act were mostly children.

The Food and Drug Modernization Act (1997) again explicitly encouraged IND sponsors to study children earlier in their development programs than had been the case previously. A six-month extension of product exclusivity upon NDA approval was the incentive, and pediatric research guidelines were issued (see http://www.fda.gov/cder/pediatric; accessed April 24, 2010). In 1998, a mandatory rule requiring studies in children for certain therapeutic areas was introduced, and in 2002 the Best Pharmaceuticals for Children Act renewed these provisions as a matter of law, and expanded them on certain pharmacovigilance technical matters. The Pediatrics Research Equity Act (2003) constituted a separate Pediatric Advisory Committee within the FDA, and further codified the requirements for studies in children for almost all new molecular entities. European regulators have done likewise in 2005.

All these regulatory innovations have improved labeling for clinicians using drugs for children, and have increased the frequency of pediatric clinical trials many fold. By January 1, 2006, some 720 pediatric clinical trials had been specifically requested by the FDA in connexion with new product approvals, and of these 35% have been for efficacy and safety, 29% for pharmacokinetics and safety, 15% solely for safety, 9% for PK–PD assessments. and 12% for various others. These trials were reckoned to be in children with 117 different diseases, distributed among 15 specific therapeutic areas.

Developments from 2005

The year 2005 was tumultuous at the FDA for numerous reasons. However, there was one event that is likely to have a particularly long-lasting impact on researching investigational drugs and the approval of NDAs. This was the recognition by the FDA that certain cyclo-oxygenase-2 specific ("COX-2s"), non-steroidal anti-inflammatory agents (NSAIDs) carried an excess risk of cardiovascular adverse events in patients. In the case of rofecoxib (Vioxx), this led to its voluntary withdrawal from the market by its manufacturer.

Stereotypical behaviors resulted. Medical journal editors were prolix. Professional pharmaceutical industry bashers were given yet more cause for their wrath. Congress and the newspapers severely criticized the FDA. Plaintiffs' lawyers salivated.

This adverse event potential had been known for 2–3 years at least, judging by the publications in medical journals. But lost in the cacophony was that the underlying reason for this problem was the disappearance of an appropriate risk–benefit balance when prescribing such drugs. Undoubtedly, there are many patients with arthritis and other inflammatory conditions for whom other NSAIDs are either ineffective or intolerable. However, the volume of sales of the "COX-2s" would suggest that indiscriminate use of these agents as all-purpose analgesics had been taking place; famous, direct to consumer television and newspaper advertisements of these drugs by trade name undoubtedly increased this product demand.

The regulatory and industry responses to this crisis and the withdrawal of Zelnorm for Irritable Bowel Syndrome (similar cardiovascular increased events) have been numerous and include the following:
• a voluntary embargo by several pharmaceutical companies on advertising newly approved drugs (probably to be followed by regulations nonetheless);
• a vigorous debate on making risk management plans an intrinsic part of all NDA approvals and their continuing status;
• a reorganization and bolstering of FDA pharmacovigilance departments;
• an inordinate, in the opinion of some, new imbalance in regulators' practices, leading to evidence of intolerability excessively outweighing efficacy when making both IND study and NDA approval decisions.

Direct-to-consumer advertising of prescribed drugs by trade name now exists only in the US and UK (it was banned in May 2005 in its only other locale, New Zealand). In the UK this is limited to AIDs drugs, respiratory agents, and statins. Congressman Waxman, among others, is publicly opposed to this practice in the US. He now chairs the powerful House Energy Committee to which the Health and Environment Sub-Committee report, and serves on it in an *ex officio* capacity, and this debate will play out before the next edition of this textbook appears.

2007 to 2009: the Congressional Blitzkrieg, FDAAA

The political and public alarm to adverse drug events culminated in the passage of the Food and Drug Administration Amendments Act (FDAAA) in 2007, to be enacted starting in 2008, but not all to be completed in 2008. This Act greatly increased the responsibilities and authority of the FDA, and reauthorized several FDA critical programs as follows:
• PDUFA: The fee for filing an NDA with clinical data is, as of August 2010, US$1,405,500.
• Medical Device User Fee (MDUF).
• Pediatric Research Equity Act.
• Best Pharmaceuticals for Children (BPCA).

In addition, the following new legislation was introduced:
• Independent Review Boards to be registered with the Department of Health and Human Services. (This was postponed till September 2009, because the DHHS were not prepared to accept registration applications.)
• New requirements for additional bioequivalence studies for ANDAs.
• Modification for requirements for Supplemental NDAs (SNDAs).
• New pediatric medical device provisions, (the Pediatric Medical Device Safety and Improvement Act).
• Expanded clinical trials database enacted in Title VII for FDA involvement in the NIH run ClinicalTrials.gov database.
• Provision of extra funds to increase the FDA staff especially in the areas of pharmocovigilance, compliance, food, and manufacturing inspections to the tune of 2000 or more staff.
• Authorization of the Agency to require postmarketing studies, safety labeling changes, and Risk Evaluation.
• Mitigation strategies.
• Improvement of the information database across the whole Agency and interface with NIH for access.

This process was started in May 2008, with the "Sentinel Initiative," which ultimately is to create a nationwide electronic system for monitoring medical product safety, also assisting in satisfying section 905 that directs the FDA to obtain access to disparate data sources to establish a post-marketing risk identification and analysis system.

Summary

No apology is made for the extensive historical narrative that opens this chapter. Dealing successfully with the FDA requires an understanding of how the institution thinks, and how the individuals within it are constrained. The way the FDA thinks is predicated on its legislation—and how and why that legislation has evolved, mostly in reaction to crisis—but at last, recently, on progressive negotiations with the industry and patient groups to bring about change that is of mutual benefit. The FDA has a complicated structure, finds it hard to respond fast to change, and remains the most stringent regulatory authority in the world. We are likely to see yet further changes in the years to come. It remains to be seen how drug cost containment, healthcare reforms, higher development costs, higher regulatory hurdles, and even ever higher NDA/SNDA filing costs, will further impact on the industry's ability to innovate, thrive, and survive.

CHAPTER 35

Special US Regulatory Procedures: Emergency and "Compassionate" INDs and Accelerated Product Approvals

Anthony W. Fox

EBD Group Inc., Carlsbad, CA, USA and Munich, Germany, and Skaggs SPPS, University of California, San Diego, USA

Introduction

The special types of Investigational New Drugs (IND) and New Drug Applications (NDA) probably represent the greatest differences in regulatory practice between Europe and the United States. These differences reside not only in the particular procedures themselves, but also in the philosophy of regulatory authorities. Emergency INDs, Treatment INDs, and accelerated approvals are essentially of US interest, and the Code of Federal Regulations (1997), Title 21, Chapter I (21CFR), is where most of these rules are published (the Orphan Drug regulations may, perhaps, also be seen as a special type of IND or NDA, and are described in Chapter 22). It is probably fair to say that these procedures have created a quiet revolution in the US drug approval process, and have helped drug developers. Their careful and gradual introduction has not damaged the public health. This chapter covers the following topics:

- Emergency INDs;
- Expanded Access (or "Compassionate Use"): Treatment INDs;
- Accelerated approvals: serious and life-threatening diseases;
- Accelerated approvals: ANDAs and generic drugs.

Principles and Practice of Pharmaceutical Medicine, 3rd edition.
Edited by L.D. Edwards, A.W. Fox, P.D. Stonier.
© 2011 Blackwell Publishing Ltd.

It should be noted that an "investigator's IND," or "physician's IND," is not a specific practice defined by regulation, and that these are orthodox INDs. It is true, however, that these IND submissions are usually smaller than those from pharmaceutical companies (see the "Expanded access and the Treatment IND" section below).

Emergency INDs

The IND in the US is based legally on the notion that Food and Drug Administration (FDA) permission is needed to convey investigational (i.e., unapproved) drugs across state or international boundaries. This defines the jurisdiction of the Federal government in comparison to the state governments in all matters of commerce, not just drug development. The FDA imposes control over this process by requiring information of appropriate quantity and quality, before granting its permission. Much of the documentation is judged by how well it supports a proposed clinical protocol; the latter is one of the most important pieces of information that the FDA quite properly demands. Unapproved drugs in clinical research are termed *investigational drugs* or *biologics*.

Normally, a 30-day waiting period applies when an IND is submitted that describes the initial clinical study with an investigational drug or biologic. Thereafter, the FDA must be notified (by filing an IND amendment) of further clinical protocols, newly-developed toxicology information, and changes to the chemistry, manufacturing, or controls. However, there is no mandatory review period for IND amendments, and the changes to the IND that have been notified can usually be implemented immediately. Of course, the FDA may impose clinical holds on particular dosing regimes, patient populations, protocols, or entire projects, at any time when safety issues present themselves. For a detailed discussion of the typical IND, see Chapter 34 and Fox (1996).

The Emergency IND (21CFR para 312.36) is designed to permit a physician to treat a particular patient with an investigational drug with an urgency that precludes the writing and filing of an IND, or even of a clinical protocol. An emergency IND does not require the 30-day waiting period. Part of the philosophy behind the perceived need for this regulation is that the Federal government does not wish to interfere directly in the relationship between an individual physician and an individual patient. The emergency procurement of materials that are unapproved for human use would be illegal, without this regulation.

When the need for an investigational drug is too urgent for the filing of an IND, the procedure is for the patient's physician to identify a source of the desired compound, and then telephone the FDA for Emergency IND permission. For biologics, the telephone number is (301) 443-4864 (the Center for Biologics Evaluation and Research, HFB-230), and for all other drugs (301) 443-1240 (the Center for Drug Evaluation and Research, HFD-53; *note that the telephone number published in the 1995 Edition of 21CFR is out of date*). Out of ordinary office hours (0800–1600 Eastern Standard Time), the FDA's Division of Emergency and Epidemiological Operations maintains a 24-hour availability on (202) 857-8400. A confirmation will be provided to the requesting physician either with a number, or by a named FDA officer. The physician may then notify those details to the pharmacy or pharmaceutical company holding the investigational agent, and the drug may then be legally shipped. This information is also available from the website (www.fda.gov). It should be noted that this permission can only be obtained by the treating physician him- or her-

self; the pharmaceutical company cannot obtain an Emergency IND on behalf of a treating physician. It should also be noted that a paper IND must follow within reasonable time afterwards.

"Off-label" use of approved products (i.e., prescribing lawfully marketed products for indications other than those stated in their labeling) does not require an Emergency IND, under 21CFR paras 312.2(b)(i)–(v), provided that the intended use is as follows:

• It is not designed to support a forthcoming NDA or Supplemental NDA for a new indication.

• It is not designed to support promotional materials.

• It does not involve a significantly greater risk than the usual use of the agent (although not defined more precisely, large increments in dose, strange routes of administration, or special patient populations would all violate this provision).

• The ethical provisions of the Declaration of Helsinki still apply, and informed consent (which need not necessarily be in writing) has been obtained, i.e., the patient is fully informed of the unusual drug usage.

• No representations of safety or efficacy, and no monetary charges (ordinarily), are made (21CFR para 312.7).

• The usage is not prolonged beyond the period needed reasonably to ascertain its failure.

It may be noted that in anesthetics, pediatrics, and intensive care medicine, in particular, drugs are used "off-label" almost routinely, and in practice, it is doubtful that physicians in these specialties are even aware of these nuances in the IND regulations. Reimbursement systems in the US will, however, often refuse to pay for drugs used "off-label," and use these regulations as their justification.

The contrast in philosophy between these arrangements in the US and the emergency use of unapproved drugs in Europe was succinctly put by one German pharmaceutical physician recently: "We don't need any of that, I can prescribe cyanide if I want to!" Although an exaggeration, this comment is nonetheless telling. Compared to the US, there has always been a tendency for European regulatory authorities to place more discretion and responsibility on pharmaceutical companies and individual physicians when using investigational materials. For example, although recently changed by the Clinical Trials Directive, the former absence of the need for a Clinical Trials Exemption (CTX) for normal volunteer studies in the UK, and indeed the CTX procedure itself (in comparison to Clinical Trials Certification), as well as the limited review of investigational drug dossiers after filing in Germany, are examples of this difference in philosophy. In the United States, the regulatory process, like much else in other areas of government, is conceived in terms of full disclosure of data in their final form, enforcement, and affirmative acts of the granting of permission by the government.

"Expanded access" and the Treatment IND

Although the term is in common usage, the "Compassionate Use IND" does not exist. Patients have access to investigational drugs through only two pathways: a traditional IND protocol or what is termed "Expanded access." A guidance for the latter has published been published (Federal Register, 2009).

The Treatment IND aims to make an investigational new drug available to patients with a defined disease state that is serious (usually life-threatening), and for whom there is no alternative therapy. This application may be made whether or not an NDA is to be filed at a later date. Several criteria must be met for a Treatment IND to be acceptable to the FDA, under 21CFR paras 312.34(b)(i)–(iv). Within these criteria are several terms that further require definition or justification to the reviewers:
• The disease process must be serious or life-threatening.
• There must be no feasible alternative therapy.
• The drug is already under investigation in an orthodox IND.
• The sponsor of the drug must be actively pursuing marketing approval of the drug with all due diligence.

Treatment INDs are thus for pharmaceutical companies, not for individual physicians. All the usual clinical hold provisions apply.

There must already be information about the investigational drug supporting the proposed use, although this needs only to be "promising," and not as definitive as would be needed for an NDA. The judgment of what is and what is not "promising" is by the relevant reviewing division of FDA; in practice, it is usually the reviewers that have been responsible for an antecedent, ordinary IND that make this recommendation.

Frequently, circumstances arise during the interval between NDA submission and approval which make it desirable for the (as yet) investigational drug to be made more widely available. The Treatment IND or the Emergency Use IND (21CFR para 312.36, see above) generally accommodate this need (21CFR paras 312.34 and 312.35).

The stated objective of this section of the regulation, under 21CFR paras 312.34(a) and (b) can, however, often be achieved using an intelligently-designed ordinary IND. A seriously-interested physician can make this application for him- or herself. Pharmaceutical companies can cooperate by notifying the FDA that the physician may cross-refer to the chemistry and toxicology sections of their own ordinary IND. By quoting these cross-references, the physician's IND becomes abbreviated. The clinical protocol for the physician's IND need only use an open-label design, in pursuit of tolerability information. Inclusion and exclusion criteria can be kept broad and to the minimum needed to ensure patient safety.

These abbreviated INDs are otherwise of orthodox composition (21CFR para 312.23), and have the advantage that the complexities of the Treatment IND, demonstration "promising" efficacy, can be avoided. Furthermore, even with a rudimentary case report form, the pharmaceutical company can gather tolerability information by this means, even for products approved for other purposes, because the exemptions of 21CFR paras 312.2(b)(i)–(iv) have not been exploited (see above). Pharmaceutical physicians can use template word processing files for these physician's INDs, can complete the details for the particular physician over the phone, and mail it to him or her for signature and forwarding to FDA. The administrative burden, once this is set up, can be relatively light, and is often very much quicker and easier than navigating the complexities of a *de novo* Treatment IND. Although the 2009 guidance is reorganizing these paragraphs in the regulations, in practice they are going to survive elsewhere.

Accelerated approvals: Serious and life-threatening diseases

In the US there are numerous, active, non-medical communities that are interested in the treatment of human immunodeficiency viruses (HIV), age-associated or Alzheimer's syndrome, and to a lesser extent, emergency medicine and various rare genetic diseases. Another community has formed to support the availability of generic drugs, because of concern about healthcare costs (with drug prices as a small but highly visible part of this). These communities have accomplished a very rare thing: Using various parts of the political process, they have brought about change in the FDA, causing alterations, and acceleration, in the drug approval process.

The structure and format of NDAs that may be submitted under these regulations are the same as for ordinary NDAs (see Chapter 34). But the *reviewing practice* can be very different for these types of accelerated approvals.

Sub-Part H

The accelerated approval of new drugs for serious or life-threatening illnesses is provided for in 21CFR314. 500–560 ("Sub-Part H"). This new practice dates from 1992, and applies to all types of drug, including antibiotics and biologics. Under Sub-Part H, the following is stated:

> If the Secretary determines, based on relevant science, that data from one adequate and well-controlled clinical investigation and confirmatory evidence (obtained prior to or after such investigation) are sufficient to establish effectiveness, the Secretary may consider such data and evidence to constitute substantial evidence.

For example, zidovudine (azidothymidine) was approved under these regulations as a treatment for AIDS after an NDA that contained only one well-controlled trial in its support, and various

in vitro and uncontrolled human data as confirmatory; moreover, CD4 lymphocyte counts were accepted as a surrogate endpoint in the clinical trial.

Surrogate endpoints are not as new an invention as may first appear. Antihypertensive drugs are approved using blood pressure as the surrogate endpoint, and until recent huge studies, no approved antihypertensive had been demonstrated actually to reduce strokes or myocardial infarctions. This concept of surrogate endpoint should also be familiar to early-phase clinical trialists. The selection of development candidates at the IND stage, and assessing their worth during Phase I or II clinical investigation, often requires development decisions based upon surrogate endpoints, again because these are usually quicker to obtain than (for example) mortality data in support of the proposed indication for the drug. The current "biomarker" craze is really one of a new type of surrogate endpoint.

Thus, the differences in reviewing practice for accelerated approvals, in comparison to more typical NDAs, are that the regulations specifically permit the FDA to

- judge efficacy on the basis of surrogate endpoints;
- grant marketing permission on condition of greater degrees of monitoring for safety than the norm;
- to control promotional practices more stringently than usual.

It is also specified how the FDA may withdraw approval, which is usually threatened when the sponsor fails to conduct post-marketing research to which it committed as a condition of approval. Having said that, the requirements for validation of the surrogate endpoint, especially in the case of the treatment of diabetes (where short-term HbA1c evidence has been unpersuasive to the FDA and long-term cardiovascular adverse events still prevail for product approval) suggest that accelerated approval mechanisms are becoming redundant.

Sub-Part E

21CFR312.80–88 ("Sub-Part E") also provides for expedited approvals, when reviews can be accelerated for "Drugs intended to treat life-threatening and severely debilitating illnesses." This is generally understood to be disease states where there is no effective, alternative therapy. Sub-Part E anticipates flexibility, but continued observance of the statute, as for all drugs. Such products are officially termed "Fast Track Products." The target NDA review time is reduced from the ordinary ten months to six months under these provisions.

Within Sub-Part E, there is no specific anticipation of a relaxation of the requirement for two adequate and well-controlled studies. These regulations prescribe meetings and schedules, and simply suggest that there ought to be more flexibility in the application of the existing regulations to this type of drug.

What is "life-threatening" within the meaning of these regulations? This definition is not repeated in the accelerated approvals regulations. Thus, the presumption is that these definitions are similar to those provided elsewhere in the IND regulations (21CFR para 312.32(a), 21CFR para 312.34, and see Chapter 34). One problem that arises is in the interpretation of regulations couched specifically in terms of adverse events or justification of a Treatment IND, and how these apply to NDA approvability or the clinical definitions of a disease process. Usually, "life-threatening" is taken to mean that the patient's life is actually under threat by the currently observed disease process (or adverse event), and not that the same *type* of disease or adverse event, but to a worse *degree* than that actually observed in the patient, could be life-threatening. Clearly, the burden of proof for demonstration that a disease is serious or life-threatening, and thus that an NDA may be considered for accelerated approval, falls squarely with the pharmaceutical company, and the FDA will certainly need to be convinced of this as part of its judgment whether to accept the NDA under these regulations.

Post-marketing impact of accelerated approvals

Safety monitoring, after NDA approval, is required for almost all drugs in the US (21CFR para 314.98). The difference in practice with accelerated approvals is that almost always *specific* post-marketing safety studies (and sometimes efficacy studies) will be required as a condition of approval. These post-marketing safety studies range from agreement on drug surveillance procedures in detail, through the maintenance of patient registries, to specific studies with protocols.

Post-marketing safety studies are considered in Chapter 11 of this book. However, it should be noted here that patient registries have been associated with grave jeopardy of litigation in the US, and not necessarily on a sound scientific basis. On more than one occasion, pharmaceutical companies have been deterred from marketing new drugs when the FDA has required a patient registry as a condition of NDA approval.

The greater control over promotional practice, under the accelerated approval process, usually places less burden on an ethical company than the post-marketing safety requirements. Promotional materials must be submitted for review before NDA approval, with the obviously desirable intention that promotion should not be any broader than the approved indication, which under these special circumstances is likely to be narrower than usual. Furthermore, the package insert should usually quantitate how narrow or broad the tolerability experience with the drug might be; frequent labeling revisions and NDA supplements should be planned for.

These special arrangements create two unusual situations where withdrawal of an NDA approved on an accelerated basis is more likely than for an ordinary NDA. First, the approval may be conditional on further clinical studies; the FDA can withdraw NDA approval if these studies turn out to be inconsistent with that (those) in the original NDA. Usually, the interim reporting frequency for these studies will be agreed as part of the NDA pre-approval meeting. Second, as mentioned above, post-marketing research commitments must be pursued in good faith and with all due diligence. Regulators often have no experience of clinical study management, and the difficulties of studying the disease in question may be substantial. Thus, there can be controversy on what does and does not constitute due diligence under these conditions.

Failure to adhere to agreements over promotional materials can also lead to NDA withdrawal; this is under the pharmaceutical company's control, and is far more predictable than the results of post-marketing studies. All the usual reviewing and appeals processes are available to both FDA and pharmaceutical companies when NDA withdrawal becomes a possibility.

In practice, good NDA sponsors find that post-marketing studies lead to package insert changes much more often than withdrawal of the entire NDA. There is also no evidence, so far, that the accelerated approval process has led to any serious threat to the public health. This new reviewing practice appears to be working well.

The new guidance shows the FDA's intentions. Stop-gap open-label, uncontrolled studies are less likely to gain approval. Individual patient emergency INDs will survive more or less unchanged. Anything at a larger scale will be suppressed until a proper protocol is filed to the IND.

Accelerated approvals: ANDAs and generic drugs

The Abbreviated New Drug Application (ANDA) is another form of accelerated approval, for which the FDA is separately authorized under Section 505(j) of the Food, Drug and Cosmetic Act (as amended), which is reduced to regulation at 21CFR paras 314.3, and 314.92 through 314.99. This process applies to generic products that are bioequivalent to previously approved, innovative drugs. In this case, the submission document is not of the same structure as an ordinary NDA, and this is quite unlike the accelerated approval for serious and life-threatening diseases described above. Approval acceleration in this case is accomplished by a massive reduction in the documentation needed for FDA review and approval.

For all practical purposes, the generic equivalent will challenge a trademark drug, probably by price competition, in the market place. However, there are rare situations where a trademark drug may have been withdrawn from marketing for purely commercial reasons. Although absent from the market, such a drug could still be followed by an ANDA from another company. The most common case is where a large company withdraws an innovative, but off-patent drug due to insufficient market size. For strategic reasons, the innovator company may wish neither to license the product to some other company nor to continue its manufacture. The niche thus created can be filled by a small generic company for whom that small market size can still comprise a large fraction of their financial revenues.

The FDA publishes a current list of drugs that it considers suitable for ANDA applications. This may be obtained from the Superintendent of Documents, US Government Printing Office, Washington, DC, 20402, USA; telephone +1 (202) 783-3238, and will shortly be available on the Internet. This includes both antibiotics and orthodox drugs within the Center for Drugs Evaluation and Research (CDER).

Supporting information

An unusual aspect of the ANDA is that there are two ways to apply. The first is to file a straightforward ANDA, which describes a copy of an approved drug. The second way is to file a petition for a drug that is not identical but which may be sufficiently identical for the ANDA process to apply. The FDA is committed to reviewing complete ANDAs within six months.

The straightforward ANDA demonstrates that the generic drug is identical in its route of administration, active components, dosage form, strength, and stability. The previously approved drug must be identified specifically (21CFR para 314.93(d)), or exceptionally, the applicant can demonstrate that the new product falls within the range of previously approved specifications among several antecedent products. The Freedom of Information Act, which provides free access to the Summary Basis of Approval document for all approved drugs in the US, facilitates this exercise.

If one has a close, but not identical, copy of a drug, the second way to an ANDA is to file a petition under 21CFR para 314.93(b), identifying what the differences may be from the approved product, and making a case why the new drug should be the subject of a forthcoming ANDA. Successful examples have included differences in excipients, minor differences in *ex vivo* dissolution studies, and other matters that can be argued not to have much clinical impact. The FDA will rule on this petition, and there are various appeals procedures if the ruling is unfavorable. The checklist of matters to cover in the petition is as follows:

- Identity of active ingredients.
- Expectation of the same therapeutic effect.
- Failure of the new product to meet the definition of a "New Drug" under
- 21CFR para 314.1 and Section 201 (b) of the Federal Food, Drug, and
- Cosmetic Act (21USC, 301–392).

It should be noted that the therapeutic equivalence expectation is precisely that: no comparative clinical studies are required. A Phase I pharmacokinetic study, in support of the therapeutic equivalence, may be helpful but need not contribute any pharmacodynamic data. With a favorable ruling on this petition, the ANDA may then follow.

The overall structure of the ANDA is described in 21CFR para 314.94. Its component parts are as follows:

- application form;
- table of contents;
- basis of the ANDA, covering either the question of identity or the results of a petition, as described above;
- description of the conditions of use, and showing its similarity to the previously approved drug (usually best done simply by plagiarizing large sections of the previous package insert);
- description of the active ingredients;
- route of administration, dosage, and strength;
- bioequivalence data;
- previous drug's label and proposed labeling;
- chemistry, manufacture, and controls;
- samples for testing in FDA's own laboratories;
- other information;
- patent certification.

In practice, in comparison to an NDA, the chemistry, manufacturing, and controls section of an ANDA is just as long, but all the other sections are much abbreviated from an ordinary NDA. The issue of patents is covered in Chapter 56, but template wording for the certificates is provided, according to the various types of patent, in 21CFR paras 314.94–314.95.

At the time of writing (summer 2009), for reasons relating to manufacturing complexity, the FDA does not believe that it can approve an ANDA for a "generic" (or, more properly "follow-on") biologic. One product has been approved after litigation in the Federal Courts in 2008 after the submission of an abbreviated biologic application. Nonetheless, the FDA does not yet know how to approve products with comparable biological activity but with chemical structures that cannot be shown to be identical.

Post-marketing requirements for an ANDA are similar to those for an orthodox NDA, and not as stringent as for an accelerated approval for a serious or life-threatening disease (see above). The usual processes are available for amending ANDAs, either before or after approval.

The ANDA process has permitted large numbers of generic drugs to be provided to the general public at lower cost. The process was created at the same time as the Orphan Drug procedures, and the Waxman-Hatch Act in the US Congress. Many view the ANDA and the Orphan Drug initiatives as *quid pro quo*, and certainly both were the subject of negotiation with the US pharmaceutical industry.

Final comments

The intent of this chapter is to provide the context and philosophy behind these special procedures. All these special IND and NDA procedures are now widely used by pharmaceutical companies, and they have all been developed with a lot of industry input. By these measures, they can be judged to have been successful. It is a situation that is in flux: Practices with FDA are constantly evolving. Always check the current edition of the 21 CFR.

References

Code of Federal Regulations. 1997, Title 21, Chapter I, various paragraphs as mentioned in the chapter.

Federal Food, Drug, and Cosmetic Act. As amended, Title 21, sections 201–901.

Fox AW. The US IND: Practical aspects. *Reg Aff J* 1996; **7**: 371–377.

Federal Register 2009; **74**: 40900–40945 for expanded access.

Further Reading

Federal Register 2009; **74**: 40872–40900 for charges applicable to investigational drugs.

CHAPTER 36

The Development of Human Medicines Control in Europe from Classical Times to the 21st Century[1]

John P. Griffin
Asklepieion Consultancy Ltd, Welwyn, Hertfordshire, UK

The evolution of human medicines control from a national to an international perspective

"The past shapes the present." It is this fact that justifies the study of history, because without it we cannot truly appreciate the present or shape the future.

From classical times to the end of the eighteenth century

The privilege of being credited with the invention of a medicinal formulation that has endured the test of time for 2000 years belongs to few people. Belong it does, however, to Mithridates VIth, King of Pontus, surnamed Eupator (Geddie and Geddie, 1926). He succeeded to the throne in about 120 BC as a boy of 13 years, had received a Greek education, and it was claimed could speak 22 languages. He subdued the tribes who bordered on the Euxine

as far as the Crimea and made incursions into Cappadocia and Bithynia, which were then in the Roman sphere of influence. In the First Mithridatic War, he defeated the Romans and occupied Asia Minor, but in 85 BC he was defeated by Flavius Fimbria and compelled to make peace with Sulla, giving up all his conquests in Asia Minor, surrendering 70 war galleys and paying 2000 talents in reparations. In the Second Mithridatic War, which endured from 83 to 81 BC, Mithridates was wholly successful.

In the Third Mithridatic War, 74–64 BC, Mithridates VI was finally defeated on the banks of the Euphrates by Pompey the Great. New schemes of vengeance by Mithridates upon the Roman Republic were frustrated by his son's rebellion in 63 BC. When he found himself under siege by his own son, he killed his wives and concubines and then committed suicide.

Pontus abounded in medicinal plants, and Mithridates acquired considerable knowledge of them. Like every despot of that period, Mithridates lived in fear of being assassinated by poisoning, in consequence of which he sought the universal antidote to all poisons. Mithridates proceeded along a simple line of reasoning. Having investigated the powers of a number of single ingredients, which he found to be the antidote to various venoms and poisons individually, he evaluated them experimentally on condemned criminals. He then compounded all the effective substances into one antidote, hoping thereby to produce universal

---

[1] This chapter is an adapted and expanded update of the chapter on drug regulation in Europe, published in Griffin JP, O'Grady J, D'Arcy, PF (eds). 1998. *Textbook of Pharmaceutical Medicine*, 3rd edn. The Queen's University of Belfast Press: Belfast. The author retains sole copyrights on this chapter.

Principles and Practice of Pharmaceutical Medicine, 3rd edition.
Edited by L.D. Edwards, A.W. Fox, P.D. Stonier.
© 2011 Blackwell Publishing Ltd.

protection. A daily dose was taken prophylactically to provide the immunity he sought.

After Mithridates VI's defeat by Pompey, a store of his writings containing detailed information on medicinal plants was captured. Pompey instructed a freed slave, Lenaeus, to translate these writings into Latin. It was said that Pompey did a greater service to the Roman Republic by the value of these writings than by his military prowess. Our knowledge of these writings of Mithridates (Watson, 1966) has come down to us in the writings of Pliny and Galen, as the translation by Lenaeus has been lost.

Pliny writes:

> By his unaided efforts Mithridates devised the plan of drinking poison daily after first taking remedies in order to achieve immunity by sheer habituation. He was the first to discover the various antidotes, one of which is even known by his name.

So effective was Mithridates' formulation that he tried unsuccessfully to commit suicide by poisoning, and finally killed himself with a "Celtic sword." Galen, writing in the second century AD at a time when he was physician to the Roman Emperor, Marcus Aurelius, refers to "mithridatium" and a formulation derived from it by one Andromachus, Nero's physician. It is said that Andromachus removed some ingredients from Mithridates' formulation and added others, particularly viper's flesh. To this new product he gave the name "galene," which means "tranquillity." Galene became known as theriac. Details of various theriacs, including mithridatium and galene, were given in Galen's "Antidotes I" and "Antidotes II." In Galen's "Antidotes I," he distinguishes three kinds of antidote, those that counter poisons, those that counter venoms and those that counter ailments. Some antidotes will counter all three, and Galen claimed that to this class belong mithridatium and galene. According to Galen, mithridatium contained 41 ingredients and the galene of Andromachus 55 components.

The preparation of galene was simple, in that its ingredients were free of fractional measures. Four vipers, cut down small, were placed in a solution of sal ammoniac, about 1 gallon, to which were added nine specified herbs and Attic wine, together with five fresh squills, also cut down small. The pot was covered with clay and set upon a fire. When the vapor came out of the four small holes left in the clay seal, dark and turgid, the heat had reached the vipers and they were cooked. The pot was left to cool for a night and day. The roasted matter was taken out and pounded until all was reduced to powder. After ten days, the powder was ready for the next stage of manufacture. At the final stage, the prescribed quantities of 55 herbs, previously prepared by various processes, along with the prescribed quantity of squill and viper flesh powder (48 drachms), were added to hedychium, long pepper, and poppy juice (all at 24 drachms); 8 herbs including cinnamon and opobalsam (all at 12 drachms); 18 herbs including myrrh, black and white pepper, and turpentine resin (at 6 drachms); 22 others and then Lemnian earth and roasted copper (at 4 drachms each); bitumen and castoreum (the secretion of beaver); 150 drachms of honey and 80 drachms of vetch meal. The concoction took some 40 days to prepare after which the process of maturation began. Twelve years was considered by Galen the proper period to keep it before use. Galen records that Marcus Aurelius consumed the preparation within two months of its being compounded without ill effect.

Mithridatium was similar, but contained fewer ingredients and no viper, although it did contain lizard! The other differences were that the opium content of Andromachus' theriac was higher than that of mithridatium, which also differed in containing no Lemnian earth, copper, or bitumen and 14 fewer herbal ingredients.

Both mithridatium and galene were taken orally with water or wine, but were also used topically on the skin, or even in the eye. The theriac, galene, was also used by Galen to treat quartan fever (malaria), which was prevalent in the Pontine Marshes near Rome. Aetius (first century AD) stated that beyond question the best remedy for venomous bites is theriac of Andromachus, applied as a plaster: "The patient should also drink this theriac or mithridatium or some similar compound."

Paul of Aegina was the last of the physicians of the Byzantine culture to practice in Alexandria, which fell to the Arabs in his professional lifetime in

AD 642. He refers to both mithridatium and theriac. Paul of Aegina was a link between Greek medicine and Mohammedan medicine. His book was used by Rhazes (AD 854–930), one of the greatest of the Arab physicians. Avicenna (AD 980–1037) approved of mithridatium as an antidote to poisons, and Maimonides, a Jew born in Moslem Spain, was also familiar with mithridatium. Mithridatium re-entered Western medicine culture by two routes. A Saxon leechbook of the 11th century records that Abel, the Patriarch of Jerusalem, sent mithridatium or theriac to King Alfred the Great, who died on October, 26 899 (Stenton, 1947).

The Leechbook of Bald (Rubin, 1975) is the most important piece of medical literature to have survived from the Saxon period. The document is in two parts or leechbooks; the first contains 88 chapters and the second 67 chapters. They were written circa AD 900–950 from an earlier 9th century Latin text. Following them is a third book, consisting of 73 sections, written in the same hand, but which is nevertheless a separate and additional work. It, too, is of similar age and likely to be a copy of earlier material. A verse at the end of the second leechbook suggests that these books belonged to a physician or leech called Bald, and were written down by a scribe called Cild.

These three leechbooks were obviously intended as manuals of instruction for the treatment of a variety of illnesses, injuries, and mental states, together with instructions for the preparation of herbal mixtures. Interspersed with these remedies are sections dealing with rites, charms, and invocations. Christian and residual heathen practices are represented, the latter including Greek and Roman traditions in addition to Germanic and Celtic folklore, which the Saxons had either brought with them from their homeland or found persisting on their arrival in Britain. There can be no doubt that these leechbooks were intended to be consulted in the physician's everyday practice. Certain phrases and remedies can be traced to classical times, for example the 6th century Alexander of Tralles, and the 5th century Marcellus Empiricus. A most important passage is contained in the second leechbook and concerns King Alfred. It refers to his request that the Patriarch Elias of Jerusalem

send him remedies that the prelate had found to be effective. A theriac formulation appears in this leechbook.

The second route by which mithridatium entered Western medicine culture was when the works of the Greek and Roman medical writers again became available in Italy, possibly via Spain or through the university at Salerno. Theriac appears to have been more greatly favored than mithridatium as a remedy for poisons. In the 12th century, theriac was being manufactured in Venice and widely exported. In England it became known as "Venetian treacle" (the word treacle is a corruption of theriac). Theriac became an article of commerce, with Venice, Padua, Milan, Genoa, Bologna, Constantinople, and Cairo all competing. The manufacture of these theriacs took place in public, with much pomp and ceremony.

It was commonly thought by those in authority that if mithridatum or theriac did not produce the desired cure, this was due to incorrect preparation (perhaps with adulterated or poor-quality materials) or incorrect storage after use. As the only cause for therapeutic failure therefore lay with the pharmacist who compounded the mixture, the remedy lay in careful scrutiny of manufacture, which should be in public. Any misdemeanor should then be detected and immediately punished. The earliest written code of quality control in Britain seems to be the *Ordinances of Guild of Pepperers of Soper Lane* in 1316. The Pepperers in the 12th century took over the distribution of imported drugs and spicery (which includes spices, sugar, confections, and fruit). They were not always easy to distinguish from the Spicers, who themselves became intermingled with or perhaps succeeded by the Grocers. The Ordinances of 1316 possibly included the Apothecaries and the Spicers and forbade the mixing of wares of different quality and price, the adulteration of bales of goods, or falsifying their weight by wetting.

For the next several hundred years, the story is a confused one, containing the roots of the later separation of the Apothecaries as a craft guild and their emergence, first as compounders of medicine and then as a division into those who ultimately became general medical practitioners and those who, together with the emergent chemists and druggists, founded the pharmaceutical society and became the pharmacists as we know them today. The Apothecaries were originally part of the Guild of Grocers and unsuccessfully petitioned Elizabeth I in 1588 for a monopoly of selling and compounding of drugs. It was not until 1607, however, that James I was to grant a Charter to the Grocers, who recognized the Apothecaries as a separate section. Ten years later, in 1617, James gave the Apothecaries a Charter to separate them from the Grocers as "The Worshipful Society of the Art and Mistery of Apothecaries."

The story over this period and for much later is that of a long fight with the physicians, and as early as 1423 the "Commonalty of Physicians and Surgeons of London" appointed two apothecaries to inspect the shops and their colleagues and bring any who offended in the quality of their wares before the Mayor and Aldermen.

The College of Physicians was founded in 1518 by Henry VIII, and in 1540 one of the earliest British statutes on the control of drugs was passed (32 Henry VIII c.40 for Physicians and their Privileges), which empowered the physicians to appoint four inspectors of "apothecary wares, drugs and stuffs." Section 2 of the Act gave the physicians the right to search Apothecaries' shops for faulty wares, with the assistance of the "Wardens of the said mysterie of Apothecaries within the said City." If the search showed drugs that were "defective, corrupted and not meet nor convenient to be ministered in any medicines for the health of man's body," the searchers were to call for the Warden of the Apothecaries and the defective wares were to be burnt or otherwise destroyed. The right of the Royal College of Physicians to conduct visitations of apothecaries' premises was withdrawn at the time of the implementation of the Food and Drugs Act 1875.

This Act of Henry VIII was obviously incorrect in defining the Apothecaries as a separate body, and was corrected later in the reign of Queen Mary by an Act of 1553 (1 Mary sess 2 c.9), in which it was enacted:

for the better execution of the searche and view of Poticarye Wares, Drugges and Compositions accord-

ing to the tenour of a Statue made in the Two and Thirtieth yeare of the Reigne of the said late King Henry Eighth That it shall be lawfull for theWardeins of the Grocers or one of them to go with the say'd Physitions in their view and search.

It is revealing that, whereas the penalty for refusing to have wares examined was 100 shillings in Henry's day (of which he took half), by Mary's day this had been raised to £10. The wording of the Act was also changed slightly, in that under Henry the Wardens were to be called for, but under Mary they had to go. Henry was also determined that the 1540 Statute would be obeyed and an errant apothecary punished and not allowed to make excuses:

... in the Kings Court ... no wager of law, esoin [excuse] or protection shall be alloweth for ... apothecaries to sell or prescribe any poisonous substance or drug ... to the body of any man, woman or child save on the written prescription of a physician or upon a note in writing from the purchaser.

The Apothecaries hotly disputed this Order and there is no record of any action being taken on it. They asked the physicians to tell them of specific abuses and that they would then cooperate in reforming them. The Apothecaries said that others, such as druggists, grocers, and chandlers, could sell poisons quite freely and many craftsmen used them daily. The Apothecaries further said that to restrict them to providing poisons solely at the request of the physicians would take away their livelihood and interfere with the liberty of the subject to have free use of all medicines.

In England, after the founding of the Royal College of Physicians in 1518, the making of theriac and mithridatium was made subject to supervision under the Pharmacy Wares, Drugs and Stuffs Act of 1540. In the reign of Elizabeth I, the making of theriac was entrusted to William Besse, an apothecary in Poultry, London. He had to show the finished product to the Royal College of Physicians. In 1625, three apothecaries made respectively 160, 50, and 40 lbs of mithridatium when London was stricken with plague.

Another technique to control the quality of drugs is the issue of a pharmacopoeia (from Greek "pharmakon," a drug; "poiia," making). The official and obligatory guide for the apothecaries of Florence was published in 1498 and is generally regarded as the first official pharmacopoeia in Europe in the modern sense, that is of a specific political unit. Other cities soon followed in the publication of obligatory formularies: for example, Barcelona in 1535 (*Concordia Pharmacolorum Barcinonesium*) and Nuremberg in 1546 (*Dispensatorium Valerii Cordis*). Similar compilations were also issued in Mantua in 1559; Augsburg, 1564; Cologne, 1565; Bologna, 1574; Bergamo, 1580; and Rome, 1583. Britain was somewhat slower, and it was not until Elizabethan times that it became obvious that there was a need for such a pharmacopoeia or formulary. This was first considered by the College of Physicians in 1585. However, work proceeded very slowly and the *Pharmacopoeia Londinensis* was not published until 1618. There were two issues: one on May 7, and the first "official" edition on December 7. This latter was by no means a reprint of the earlier one and was substantially enlarged and changed. The publication of this *London Pharmacopoeia* in December 1618, setting out detailed formulations of theriac and mithridatium, had made supervision easier and the manufacture was clearly no longer entrusted to a single apothecary.

Nicholas Culpepper, in his *Dispensatory* (1649), refers to both mithridatium and "Venetian treacle." References in English literature to theriac always refer to it as treacle. Miles Coverdale translated balm as treacle in his Bible of 1538. This was repeated in the Matthew Bible and Bishops' Bible of 1568. Jeremiah 8 v 22 therefore reads: "Is there no treakle in Gilead? Is there no physician there?"

In 1665, the Great Plague of London broke out and Charles II turned to the Royal College of Physicians for advice. It was eventually published as "Advice set down by the College of Physicians (at the Kings Command) containing certain necessary directions for the cure of the Plague and preventing infection." The streets were to be kept clean and flushed with water, in order to purify the air, fires were to be lit in streets and houses and the burning of certain aromatic materials, such as resin, tar, turpentine, juniper, cedar, and brimstone, was enjoined. The use of perfumes on the person was recommended. Special physicians, attended by apothecaries and surgeons, were appointed to carry this out. The main internal remedies for the plague that were recommended were London treacle, mithridatium, galena, and diascordium, a confection prepared from water germander. Victims of the plague who developed buboes were treated with a plaster of either mithridatium or galene, applied hot thrice daily.

Inspection in the 18th century extended to all manufacturers

In December 1720 The College of Physicians of London approved the President's draft of a petition to Parliament regarding the difficulties that the servants of the College met when they collected, at the place of execution, corpses of malefactors to which their Elizabethan Charter gave them a right. On June 25, 1723, Sir Hans Sloane, as President, proposed that a Bill should be promoted to make the procuring of bodies easier: but the College was then led by the President and Censors to combine this with clauses about searching apothecaries' shops. The Bill was drafted by Mr Mead, the College attorney, who worked in the new point that the censors were empowered to search shops of all persons selling medicines, as they already did for apothecaries' shops, and the right of search was to be extended from the City of London, to which it had hither to been confined, to an area of 7 miles radius around the City. Various attempts were made to insert other clauses to the Bill. The Apothecaries wished to require that the concurrence of the Apothecaries would be necessary before any medicines were destroyed. Other attempts to exempt warehouses from the search were unsuccessful. However, all medicines made by virtue of letters patent were exempted. This exemption was made because of a clause submitted by a Licenciate of the College, Dr Joseph Eaton, who had patented a styptic and who wished it to be exempt from search. Another clause exempted any physician from search. The physicians' self-interest thrived! The Bill became Law in April 1724 as 10 Geo 10 c 20, but strangely the original purpose of the Bill—the procurement of corpses for dissection—was lost.

Records of "visitations" of apothecaries shops and premises from which medicines were sold exist in The College Library for the years 1724–1754. It is clear from these records that the College Censors wasted no time in enforcing their new powers outside the City of London. The following is a synopsis of their visitations over this period:

On 27 May 1724, 28 premises in the Strand, Pall Mall, St James, and German (Jermyn) Street were inspected. Mr James Goodwin of Haymarket was found to have manufactured Venetian treacle which was described as "almost very indifferent – reprimanded." The Censors were back on 7 June 1724 and several medicines condemned to be burnt in public before the doors of Mr Goodwin's shop. Goodwin had two shops, one in the City and the other in Haymarket – the latter was searched the second time in the owner's absence, two assistants being in charge. Goodwin claimed that the censors behaved with ferocious violence and had condemned five lots of his medicine including his stock of Venetian treacle. Mr Goodwin was not a Freeman of the Worshipful Society of Apothecaries and was clearly targeted by the College and the Society. Goodwin, however, took advantage of new appeal procedures, but at a special meeting of the full Comitia of the College the Fellows compared specimens of the condemned medicines with type-specimens from Apothecaries Hall and they upheld the decision of the Censors unanimously. A few days later the Censors destroyed the condemned medicines before his door, and continuing their visitation found and destroyed several more medicines.

James Goodwin nursed his grievance and made representation to the House of Lords in a pamphlet "Brief for James Goodwin, Chymist and Apothecary, upon his Petition to the House of Lords" in 1725, but his protests came to nothing.

The College Censors were diligent in their extended powers. On June 22, 1724, they conducted 15 visitations in the Borough, Southwark, and London Bridge area and destroyed Venetian treacle confiscated from the shops of Mr Snaggs and Mr Thomas Pont. The visitations of July, 20, 1724 record the inspection of 18 premises in the same area, eight of which belonged to surgeons. One of these surgeons, Mr J. Wood, was found to be in possession of defective Venetian treacle.

The 1724 Act was originally drafted to run for three years; its scope was extended in 1727 for a further three years. After 1731 the Act was not extended and the Censors had to operate within the terms of the Acts of Henry VIII and Mary I, but with their area of inspection extended beyond the City.

In the 30 years of visitation for which records exist, only two apothecaries raised objection to being inspected.

Also, Sir George Clark in his *History of the Royal College of Physicians of London* (1966) records that the Worshipful Society of Apothecaries tested the strength of the College by a calculated defiance. Robert Gower, a trainband colonel, and Master for the second time, refused to show his medicines to the Censors. The College comitia of 1727 was informed and sought Counsel's opinion. No opinion has been found in the College archives, and so no further light can be obtained from the Society's history. The answer probably lies in the fact that the joint inspections by the College Censors and the Society's Wardens continued for another 150 years until these powers were revoked under the Food and Drugs legislation of 1872, although the last joint visitation had taken place in the 1850s. In the 10-year period from May 27, 1724, to July, 30, 1734, 791 shops were visited in the course of 37 inspection days, giving an average of 21 premises per day's inspection. In subsequent decades the College Censors were not quite so active (see Table 36.1).

Table 36.1 Analysis of visitations by decade 1724–1754 (source: Griffin (2004))

Years	Number of visitations	Number of premises visited (average per visitation)
1724–1734	37	791(21)
1734–1744	22	384(17)
1744–1754	18	325(18)
1756–1757	4	56(14)

At this period the Julian Calender, with New Year's Day 25 March, was in use. From visitation of *Apothecary, Chyrnist and Druggist Shoppes*, College of Physicions of London, in three volumes: Vol. 1 1724–1731; Vol. 2 1732–1747; Vol. 3 1748–1754. The final volume also contains records of four visitations for April 14, 1756, June 21, 1756, and August 10, 1756, at which Willom Heberden was one of the four Censors, and the last recorded visitation of 9 June 1757.

On a typical visitation day, the four censors of the College of Physicians and two Wardens of the Society of Apothecaries assembled at 10.00 hours. After their round of inspections the group retired to a hostelry where at 16.00 hours they sat down to dinner, at the College's expense, with the President, Registrar, and Treasurer of The College of Physicians.

Inspections were as frequently commenting on products absent from premises as products that were defective. Products frequently reported as defective were Venetian treacle/Mithridatum/Theriac Andromachus, Tincture of Rhubarb, cinnamon, helleboris niger, absinth, aloes, jalop, and most frequently, Peruvian bark.

Three areas were noted where apothecaries' premises were most likely to be the source of problems. The Southwark/Borough/London Bridge, Whitechapel/Houndsditch/Aldgate, and Clerkenwell areas seem to have figured large as areas of poor-quality shops. Surgeons' premises were frequently described as very bad, particularly in Southwark!

Mr Bevan's shop in Plough Court, the predecessor of Allen and Hanbury's (now part of Glaxo SmithKline), was singled out for very favorable comment on several inspections. For example, September 11, 1728, it was described as "extra ordinary good." The College of Physicians exerted their privilege to search apothecary shops up to the early 19th century. It is interesting to note that when the Censors visited Allen and Hanbury's (then William Allen and Co.) in the 1820s, they noted it was "an excellent house."

Doubts as to whether theriac and mithridatium were the universal panacea had been voiced by Culpepper and other physicians such as Dr John Quincy, who died in 1722. The real attack on these two long-standing remedies came from Dr William Heberden (1745) in a 19-page pamphlet entitled *Antitherica: Essay on Mithridatium and Theriac*. Heberden concludes his attack on the lack of efficacy of these products with words:

> Perhaps the glory of its [mithridatium's] first expulsion from a public dispensary was reserved to these times and to the English nation, in which all parts of philosophy have been so much assisted in asserting their freedom from ancient fable and superstition, and whose College of Physicians, in particular, hath deservedly had the first reputation in their profession. Among the many eminent services which the authority of this learned and judicious body hath done to the practice of Physic, it might not be the least that it had driven out this medley of discordant simples...made up of a dissonant crowd collected from many countries, mighty in appearance, but in reality, an ineffective multitude that only hinder one another.

In William Heberden's entry in Munk's (1878) Roll it is stated that he was always ready to attack the "idle inventions of ignorance and superstition." Heberden was born in 1710, entered St John's College, Cambridge University, in 1724 at the age of 14, graduated BA in 1728, became a Master of Arts (MA) in 1732, and obtained his MD in 1739. He published his *Essay on Mithridatium and Theriac* in the same year as he obtained his FRCP. Heberden founded the *Medical Transactions of the Royal College of Physicians* in 1767 and in the first three volumes, 1768–1785, he published 16 papers. Heberden is known for his description of Heberden's asthma (cardiac asthma) and Heberden's nodes, which are calcipic spurs on the articular cartilage at the base of the terminal phalanges in osteoarthritis. He made the clear point that they had no connection with gout, which was the main and highly fashionable arthritic ailment of his time. Heberden died in 1801 and was buried in Windsor Parish Church, where there is a memorial plaque to him and his son William Heberden Junior, who was physician to George III during his years of insanity, which we now believe was due to porphyria.

The 1746 *London Pharmacopoeia* was the last in which mithridatium and galene appear; they were absent from the 1788 edition. The *Edinburgh Pharmacopoeia*, first published in 1699, dropped mithridatium and galene from the 1756 edition. Not all Western European countries were so quick to expunge these formulations, for galene with its vipers appears in the *German Pharmacopoeia* of 1872 and in the *French Pharmacopoeia* of 1884. With the disappearance of mithridatium from the French

Pharmacopoeia, the long-used complex remedy attributable to an experimental toxicologist from the 1st century BC came to an end.

Prior to the doubts on the efficacy of mithridatium raised by a number of English physicians, including Culpepper and Quincy, and culminating in William Heberden's attack and condemnation of these products, there had been occasions when these formulations had been noted to be ineffective. In all these circumstances, it was believed that the formulations had been inadequately compounded; or that the quality of the ingredients was suspect (the quality of cinnamon was frequently raised); or even the species of viper used in theriac was questioned. These concerns to maintain the quality of mithridatium and theriac led to the introduction of strict controls over the quality of ingredients and blending. For example, the manufacture had to be done in public in Venice and the ingredients had to be open to inspection. Pharmacopoeias were produced, which laid down standards, not only for mithridatium and theriac, but also for other therapeutic substances. Perhaps, in the final analysis, the contribution of mithridatium and theriac to modern medicine was that concerns about their quality stimulated the earliest concepts of medicine regulations.

The *Medical and Physical Journal*, one of the earliest to supply regular information on new work in medicine, pharmacy, chemistry, and natural history, suggested in its first volume in 1799:

> ... we would submit to the legislature the propriety of erecting a public board composed of the most eminent physicians for the examination, analysation and approbation of every medicine before an advertisement should be admitted into any newspaper or any other periodical publication and before it should be vended in any manner whatsoever.

By the end of the 18th century all the ingredients for an efficient regulation of medicines had been conceived, but in a piece-meal fashion (see Table 36.2). What was missing was the integration into a single scheme. This would have to wait until the passing of the Medicines Act (1968) and its implementation on September 1, 1971.

Table 36.2 The development of concepts of medicines regulation in England as illustrated by the history of mithridatium and theriac (source: Griffin (2004))

Regulatory measure	Date
Quality and inspection	1423, 1540, 1723
Fines for breach of regulations	1540, 1553, 1617
Specified composition	1586
Licensing of specific manufacturer(s)	1586, 1625
Destruction of faulty product	1540, 1723
Pharmacopoeial monograph	1619, 1650, 1721, 1746, 1788
Fraud prevention	1688
Multidisciplinary scrutiny	1723
Appeal procedures	1723
Exemptions from legislation	1723
Efficacy	1745
Ideas of regulatory scrutiny prior to marketing	1799

The 19th and 20th centuries to the Medicines Act 1968

Compulsory vaccination against smallpox was established by the Vaccination Act of 1853, after the report compiled by the Epidemiological Society on the state of vaccination following the first Vaccination Act of 1840. The 1840 Act had provided free vaccination for the poor to be administered by the Poor Law Guardians.

Under the Vaccination Act of 1853, all infants had to be vaccinated within the first three years of life, default of which meant the parents were liable to fine or imprisonment. New legislation incorporated in the Vaccination Act of 1867 made it compulsory for children under the age of 14 years to be vaccinated, and encouraged the notification of default by doctors by providing financial inducements for compliance and penalties for failure.

The law was further tightened in 1871, when the appointment of vaccination officers was made compulsory for all local authorities. A House of

Commons Select Committee, set up in 1871 to investigate the efficacy of the compulsory system, was concerned by a report by Dr Jonathan Hutchinson, who gave an account of the transmission of syphilis in two patients by arm-to-arm inoculation of the material from the pustule of one patient to the arm of another. The use of calf lymph vaccine did not become standard until 1893, when a commercially available preparation was introduced. Prior to this, it had been impossible to standardize the material used for vaccination.

In 1858, the Medical Act created the General Medical Council, one of whose duties was to compile an official pharmacopoeia for the whole of the United Kingdom to supersede the three current ones for London, Edinburgh, and Dublin. The first *British Pharmacopoeia* was published in 1864 (the 1958 and 1993 editions were published by the Health Ministers on the recommendations of the Medicines Commission; see below).

It has to be acknowledged that there was little momentum during the 19th century concerning the general requirement for scrutiny of medicines for safety and efficacy, in addition to the quality requirements already in existence, before products were marketed in Britain. A few attempts were made to do this and, as far back as 1880, a British Medical Association (BMA) working party investigating sudden deaths occurring in chloroform anesthesia had suggested the establishment of an independent body to assess drug safety. Chloroform was first used as an anesthetic in 1847 and, as its use increased, it was found that occasionally people died unexpectedly during the induction of anesthesia. In 1877, the BMA appointed a committee to investigate this and the final report was published in 1880. They found that chloroform not only depressed respiration but had a deleterious effect upon the heart in very small doses and could cause cardiac arrest. This was the first major collaborative investigation of an adverse reaction to a drug ever carried out.

This study had very little impact on generating public or political concern to set up a regulatory authority. However, the appearance of two publications by the BMA concerning certain proprietary medicines, entitled *Secret Remedies* (1909) and *More Secret Remedies* (1912), caused a Parliamentary Select Committee on Patent Medicines to be set up. This Select Committee reported in 1914, but World War I intervened and all the proposed legislation was shelved. It is worth listing several of the recommendations of this Committee, some of which had to wait until the Medicines Act (1968) controlled and kept standards under review, and many of these became internationally recognized:
- *Recommendation 56(1).* That the administration of the law governing the advertisement and sale of patent, secret, and proprietary medicines and appliances be coordinated and combined under the authority of one Department of State.
- *Recommendation 56(5).* That there be established at the Department concerned a register of manufacturers, proprietors, and importers of patent, secret and proprietary remedies. . .
- *Recommendation 56(6).* That an exact and complete statement of the ingredients . . . and a full statement of the therapeutic claims made . . . be furnished to this Department. . .
- *Recommendation 56(7).* That a special Court or Commission be constituted with power to permit or prohibit . . . the sale and advertisement of any patent, secret, or proprietary remedy. . .
- *Recommendation 56(12).* That inspectors be placed at the disposal of the Department . . .
- *Recommendation 58(2).* That the advertisement and sale (except the sale by a doctor's order) of medicines purporting to cure the following diseases be prohibited: cancer, consumption, lupus, deafness, diabetes, paralysis, fits, epilepsy, locomotor ataxy, Bright disease, rupture.
- *Recommendation 58(3 and 4).* That all advertisements . . . [of] diseases arising from sexual intercourse or referring to sexual weakness . . . [or] abortifacient . . . be prohibited.

Still, little attention was paid to the efficacy of drugs and treatment. The Venereal Disease Act of 1917 and the Cancer Act of 1939 prevented the public advertisement and promotion of drugs for these conditions, to prevent sufferers from inadequate or unsuitable treatment and from fraudulent claims. It was necessary to wait until the Medicines Act was in force before further consideration was given to efficacy (but see the Therapeutic

Substances Act below), but it may be noted here that this was a foretaste of control of advertisement and promotional literature for medicines.

The antisyphilitic drug arsphenamine (Salvarsan) had been discovered in Germany in 1907 and was imported into Britain until the outbreak of World War I, when the Board of Trade issued licenses to certain British manufacturers to make it. Each batch had to be submitted to the Medical Research Council for approval before marketing. The problem was that, although synthetic, and hence the chemical identity of the product was known, highly toxic impurities could only be detected by biological testing.

It began to be realized also that the increasing use of potent biological substances and the extension of immunization were raising new questions of proper standardization of such preparations and of the competence of manufacturers. The only law at this time concerned with the purity or quality of drugs was the Food and Drugs Act of 1875, and this had a very limited application.

Control of biological substances was difficult to contain within a pharmacopocial monograph, for it demanded the use of biological standardization, because the purity and the potency of these substances could not be measured by chemical means. The Therapeutic Substances Act (TSA) aimed to regulate the manufacture and sale of such substances and to provide standards to which they must conform, to regulate their labeling and, to a certain extent, their sale. The principal substances to which the Act applied were vaccines, sera, toxins, antitoxins, antigens, arsephenamine, and related substances, insulin, pituitary hormone, and surgical sutures. Certain suture material had been found to be contaminated with *Clostridium welchii*, and this was the reason for inclusion of sutures under the TSA. It provided for a licensing system, with the Minister of Health as the Licensing Authority for England and Wales, the Department of Health for Scotland, and the Minister of Home Affairs for Northern Ireland. The TSA also recognized that the competence of the employees of the manufacturer and the conditions under which they worked were equally as important as the tests applied to the end products. Factory inspections

and in-process control therefore played a large part in supervision by the Licensing Authority. Records of sale also had to be kept by the manufacturer, and the container had to identify both the manufacturer and the batch.

This Act began modern concepts of safety. Further regulations issued between 1925 and 1956 brought more substances under control and kept standards under review, and many of these became internationally recognized. The whole TSA was revised and consolidated in 1956, but has now been superseded by the Medicines Act (1968).

The Biological Standards Act (1975) established the National Biological Standards Board. This Board, appointed by the UK health ministers and funded by the Health Department, is responsible for standards and control of biological substances, that is substances whose purity and potency cannot be adequately tested by chemical means, such as hormones, blood products, and vaccines. The Board operates through the executive arm, the National Institute for Biological Standards and Control.

Thalidomide and its aftermath

The story of thalidomide is too well known to bear much repetition here, but it was the stimulus that laid the ground rules on which the Medicines Act in the United Kingdom and most other modern European states' legislation, including the European Community's Directive 65/65EC, was built, and therefore it is relevant to summarize these events. Thalidomide first went on sale in 1956 in West Germany and enjoyed good sales, both there and in other countries, as a sleeping aid and as a treatment of vomiting in early pregnancy, because of its prompt action, lack of hangover, and apparent safety. Adverse reports of peripheral neuropathy and myxoedema appeared in the literature in late 1958 and 1959, associated with thalidomide. In 1961, reports began to be made of a remarkable rise, in West Germany since 1959, in the incidence of a peculiar malformation of the extremities of the newborn. This condition was characterized by the defective long bones of the limbs, which had normal to rudimentary hands or feet. Owing to its external resemblance to a seal's flipper, it was given the name "phocomelia." This condition had previously been very rare in West Germany but whereas no cases had been reported in the ten years 1949–1959, there were 477 cases in 1961 alone. In the UK, 400–500 cases were reported during 1959–1961. The public and government were not prepared for these unforeseen consequences of the therapeutic revolution that had been taking place for 30 years. This complacency was now shattered, public concern was vocal, and the government was galvanized into action.

The joint subcommittee of the English and Scottish Standing Medical Advisory Committees, under the chairmanship of Lord Cohen of Birkenhead, made recommendations regarding future legislation for the control of medicines, in addition to the immediate establishment of the Committee on Safety of Drugs, which came into operation in 1963 and whose function was to review the evidence on new drugs and offer advice on their safety. The Committee consisted of a panel of independent experts from various fields of pharmacy, pathology, and so on. The Committee was serviced by a professional secretariat of pharmacists and medical officers, who undertook the assessment of the submissions and presented these to the committee and various subcommittees.

The Committee on Safety of Drugs was set up in June 1963 by the Health Minister, in consultation with the medical and pharmaceutical professionals and the British pharmaceutical industry, with the following terms of reference:

1. To invite from the manufacturer or other person developing or proposing to market a drug in the United Kingdom any reports they may think fit on the toxicity tests carried out on it; to consider whether any further tests should be made and whether the drug should be submitted to clinical trials; and to convey their advice to those who submitted reports.

2. To obtain reports of clinical trials of drugs submitted thereto.

3. Taking into account the safety and efficacy of each drug, and the purposes for which it is to be used, to consider whether it may be released for marketing, with or without precautions or restrictions on its use; and to convey their advice to those who submitted reports.

4. To give to manufacturers and others concerned any general advice they may think fit.

5. To assemble and assess reports about adverse effects of drugs in use and prepare information thereon which may be brought to the notice of doctors and others concerned.

6. To advise the appointing ministers on any of the above matters.

The Committee had no legal powers, but worked with the voluntary agreement of the Association of British Pharmaceutical Industry and the Proprietary Association of Great Britain. They promised that none of their members would put on clinical trial or release for marketing a new drug against the advice of the Committee, whose advice they would always seek. The joint English and Scottish Standing Medical Advisory Committee also recommended that there should be new legislation regarding many aspects of drug safety, and after a review and consultation, a White Paper, *Forthcoming Legislation on the Safety, Quality and Description of Drugs and Medicines* (Cmnd 3393), was published in September 1967, and the Medicines Act, based on these proposals, received the Royal Assent in October 1968. The Act is a comprehensive measure replacing most of the previous legislation on the control of medicines for human use and for veterinary use. The first provisions laid down in the Act, regarding licensing of medicinal products and other aspects of control, came into effect on September 1, 1971. The Act was administered by the health and agriculture ministers of the UK, acting together or in some cases separately, as the health ministers or the agriculture ministers in respect of human and veterinary medicines, respectively.

The Medicines Commission was appointed by ministers to give them advice generally relating to the execution of the Act. A number of expert committees with specific advisory functions were appointed by ministers after considering the recommendations of the Commission, as proposed in Section 4 of the Medicines Act.

Under the Medicines Act (1968), the Licensing Authority consists of the Secretaries of State for Health and Social Services, the Secretary of State for Agriculture, and the Secretaries of State for Wales, Scotland, and Northern Ireland. The Medicines Act (1968) was implemented to operate from September 1971. The day-to-day administration of the Act for human medicines was conducted by the Medicines Division of the Department of Health and Society Security (DHSS) and was managed jointly by an under-secretary and the professional head of the Division, who held the rank of Senior Principal Medical Officer.

In 1988, the DHSS was split into two departments, the Department of Health (DoH) and the Department of Social Security (DSS). Following the Evans–Cunliffe report, from April 1989, the Medicines Division of the DoH became the Medicines Control Agency (MCA) under a director, and was expected to self-fund its operation from fees commensurate with the services provided. The UK MCA in 1997 had 458 staff, of whom 150 approximately worked in licensing, 130 in post-licensing, including pharmacovigilance, 75 in licensing inspection of manufacture and enforcement, and 28 on the *British Pharmacopoeia* and the United Kingdom contribution to the *European Pharmacopoeia*. This increased to 600 staff in 2002.

On September 12, 2002, the then Health Minister, Lord Philip Hunt, announced that the MCA would merge with the Medical Devices Agency (MDA) with effect from April 1, 2003. The merged agencies became known as the Medicines and Healthcare Products Regulatory Agency (MHRA).

The Licensing Authority is advised by expert committees, appointed by ministers, as advised by the Medicines Commission under Section 4 of the Medicines Act. These advisory committees consist of independent experts, such as hospital clinicians, general practitioners, pharmacists, and clinical pharmacologists, not the staff of the DoH, and are appointed by ministers on the advice of the Medicines Commission. Since 1971, the relevant advisory committees have been: the Committee on Safety of Medicines (CSM); the Committee on Review of Medicines (CRM), which was set up in 1975 and disestablished on December 31, 1994; the Committee on Dental and Surgical Materials (CDSM), which was established in 1975

and disestablished on March 31, 1992; the British Pharmacopoeia Commission (BPC); and the Veterinary Products Committee, which is administered through the Ministry of Agriculture, Food and Fisheries (MAFF).

In February 2004 the MHRA issued a consultation letter (MLX No. 300) seeking wider views on the amalgamation of the Committee on Safety of Medicines (CSM) and the Medicines Commission (MC). In summary, from Autumn 2005, the new advisory structure comprised:

• A new Commission on Human Medicines (CHM) that amalgamates the responsibilities of the former MC and the CSM, which will advise Ministers directly on matters relating to medicines for human use.

• A number of other committees established by Ministers which will be able to advise Ministers directly on issues for which they are responsible. These are: The Advisory Board on the Registration of Homeopathic Products (ABRH); a new Herbal Medicines Advisory Committee (HMAC); and the British Pharmacopoeia Commission (BPC).

• A number of Expert Advisory Groups (EAGs) that will advise the Commission, ABRH, HMAC and the BPC on specific and technical matters.

• A panel of experts (including toxicology and statistics) to provide specialist advice to the above bodies and EAGs if required.

• A panel that brings together the Lay (Patient and Consumer) representatives on the various bodies and EAGs.

The cynically minded might believe that these changes were an attempt to pre-empt the **"House of Commons Select Committee Report March 2005"**. The MHRA was the subject of serious criticism in this very detailed Select Committee Report entitled **"The Influence of the Pharmaceutical Industry"**. The Select Committee states that "this is the first major study of the pharmaceutical industry by a Select Committee since the Select Committee on Patent Medicines reported on 4th August 1914."

In its general Summary the following criticisms were leveled at the MHRA:

"The regulator, The Medicines and Healthcare Products Regulatory Agency (MHRA), has failed to adequately scrutinise licensing data and its post-marketing surveillance is inadequate."

"The consequence of lax oversight is that the industry's influence has expanded and a number of practices have developed which act against the public interest".

"We are concerned that a rather lax regime is exacerbated by the MHRA's need to compete with other European regulators for licence application business."

In Para 280 the Report states:

"In its own interests the Agency (*MHRA*) needs to keep a close eye on its market share of regulatory business: increasingly it competes with other European drug regulatory agencies to scrutinise drug licence applications."

The licensing of new medicines

The UK joined the European Community (EC) in 1973, but the data requirements for granting Marketing Authorizations (MAs) has, as the implementation of the Medicines Act (1968), been in accordance with *EC Directive 65/65* and the subsequent *Directive 75/318*, which elaborated on the requirements for preclinical testing, pharmaceutical quality, and manufacture. Both these Directives and the Medicines Act (1968) envisaged that MAs issued on the basis of these requirements would be valid for five years and subject to review and/or renewal.

During the period 1971–1981, after the implementation of the Medicines Act (1968), the Licensing Authority granted 204 MAs for new chemical entities (NCEs), 3665 marketing approvals for new formulations, and 6898 variations of marketed formulations (Griffin and Diggle, 1981). In the period 1971–1994, there were 525 NCEs approved for marketing, 30 new biological entities (NBEs), and 28 products of biotechnology (Jefferys *et al.*, 1998). Of these new active substances, 35 product licenses were surrendered by the manufacturers and a further 22 were withdrawn for safety reasons.

National MAs were intended to be phased out after January 1, 1998, but national approvals for marketing continued beyond that date. The future foresees that all MAs within the European Union (EU) will have been issued under the rules governing medicinal products in the EC by virtue of the centralized procedure or the so-called "mutual recognition" or "decentralized procedure" (see below).

Controls on conduct of clinical trials in the United Kingdom

In the United Kingdom, when the Medicines Act (1968) came into operation, all clinical trials in patients had to be covered by a clinical trial certificate (CTC). Under the Medicines Act, studies on normal healthy human volunteers (Phase I studies) were exempt prior to later EU directives.

A clinical trial in the terms of the Medicines Act (1968) is an investigation, or series of investigations, consisting of the administration of one or more medicinal products, where there is evidence that they may be beneficial to a patient by one or more doctors or dentists for the purpose of ascertaining what effects, beneficial or harmful, the products have. The Licensing Authority does not lay down rigid requirements concerning the data, which must be provided before authorization can be given for the clinical trial of a new drug. It issues guidelines for applicants.

By the late 1970s, it had become apparent that the need to apply for a CTC and the regulatory delay that this caused was driving clinical research out of the United Kingdom. The Secretary of State for Social Services approved the introduction of a new scheme in 1981, the details of which were announced by Griffin and Long (1981). The new procedures allowed for a clinical trials exemption (CTX) from the need to hold a CTC; the applicant company was required to produce a certified summary of data generated to support the proposed clinical studies, signed by a medically qualified advisor or consultant to the company. The regulatory authority had 35 days to respond to the notification, but could in exceptional circumstances require a further 28 days to consider the notification. If the CTX was refused, the applicant could apply for a CTC, in which circumstances complete data had to be filed. If the CTC application was refused, the statutory appeal procedures came into play if the applicant company wished to avail itself of this provision. These appeal procedures are identical with those for marketing applications.

The basis of the CTX scheme was that, together with a detailed clinical trial protocol, summaries of chemical, pharmaceutical, pharmacological, pharmacokinetic, toxicological, and human volunteer studies may be permitted instead of the additional details normally required for a CTC or product license application. This CTX scheme is based on the requirement that (i) a doctor must certify the accuracy of the data; (ii) the supplier undertakes to inform the Licensing Authority of any refusal to permit the trial by an ethical committee; and (iii) the supplier also undertakes to inform the Licensing Authority of any data or reports concerning the safety of the product.

Speirs and Griffin (1983) described the effect of the CTX scheme in attracting clinical studies on NCEs in the first year of operation of the scheme. In 1980, there were 87 applications for CTC; in 1981, the first year of the CTX scheme, there were 210 applications for CTX, of which 79 were for NCEs. Speirs *et al.* (1984) studied the effects of the CTX in encouraging inward investment into research in the UK: 23 companies had increased their research investment by 100%.

Doctor's and dentist's exemption

This is an exemption that is available to doctors or dentists who are undertaking clinical trials initiated by them but not at the request of a pharmaceutical company. Outline information about the trial is required and a decision is made by the Licensing Authority within 21 days. Where the product to be used is unlicensed or is complex, further information may be requested and the 21-day time period is extended.

Clinical trials on marketed products

Where a clinical trial is proposed with a marketed product, the applicant can submit a copy of the trial protocol, provide information on the investigators, and depending on whether or not the applicant is the MA holder, information on the procedures for reporting adverse drug reactions (ADRs). It is only possible to use this procedure for UK-marketed drugs. It does not apply to unauthorized products manufactured specifically for trial, nor to products that may be licensed in other countries but are not in receipt of a MA in the United Kingdom.

The various member states of the EU were surveyed by Griffin (1987); the United Kingdom, Eire, The Netherlands, and Italy did not have legislation requiring regulatory approval for studies affecting human (non-patient) volunteers; in Germany, Denmark, and Sweden, legislation did impose controls on such studies. This survey indicated that a clear definition of what was meant by a "human volunteer" was also lacking between national regulatory authorities in Europe. As clinical trial provisions varied greatly between EU member states, therefore the EC, in accord with their prevailing philosophy of "harmonization," wished to change this situation.

With a view to harmonizing the conduct of clinical trials across the EU, Directive 2001/20/EEC was finally agreed on 14 December 2000, and was formally adopted in May 2001 with a three-year transition for its implementation.

The EU Clinical Trials Directive contains specific provisions regarding the conduct of clinical trials, including multicenter trials, on human subjects. It sets standards relating to the implementation of good clinical practice and good manufacturing practice (GMP), with a view to protecting clinical trial subjects. All clinical trials, including bioavailability and bioequivalence studies, must be designed, conducted, and reported in accordance with the principles of good clinical practice.

The Directive defines "clinical trial" as any investigation on human subjects intended to discover or verify the clinical, pharmacological and/or other pharmacodynamical effects of one or more investigational medicinal product(s), and/or to identify any adverse reactions to one or more investigational medicinal product(s), and /or to study absorption, distribution, metabolism, and excretion of one or more investigational medicinal product(s) with the object of ascertaining its (their) safety and/or efficacy. It defines "subject" as an individual who participates in a clinical trial as a recipient of either the investigational medicinal product or a control. Thus, healthy volunteer studies are included.

Member states have 60 days to consider a valid request from an applicant to conduct a clinical study; in the case of trials involving medicinal products for gene therapy or somatic cell therapy or medicinal products containing genetically modified organisms, an extension of a maximum of 30 days may be allowed. If the request to conduct a study is refused by the competent national authority, the sponsor may, on one occasion only, modify or amend the protocol to take account of the objections raised. No further appeal mechanism is provided.

Premises where clinical studies are to be conducted are open to inspection by the GCP Inspectorate set up by the MHRA in accordance with the EU Directive on good clinical practice. The inspectorate is required to give a preliminary oral report at the conclusion of the inspection and a written report within 30 days.

Various sectors of the pharmaceutical industry lobbied hard against the Clinical Trial Directive; particularly, the industry based in the UK objected to the inclusion of Phase I studies involving healthy volunteers being brought under legislation. These objections are based on the negative effects on research conducted in the UK by the CTC scheme introduced by the Medicines Act 1968, and the subsequent deregulation achieved by the CTX scheme.

A negative effect on Phase I clinical research was reported in the UK by Clinical Research Organisations (CROs) and Academic University Departments in the autumn of 2004.

The review of products on the market pre-1971

At the start of product licensing in the United Kingdom in 1971, products already on the market were granted Product Licences of Right (PLRs), which were subject to review. Between 1971 and 1982, 22,376 PLRs lapsed or were revoked or suspended, and 598 had been converted to full product licenses. The Committee of Review of Medicines was deemed to have completed its work in 1991 and was disestablished on 31 March 1992.

All member states of the EC were similarly required to review the quality, safety, and efficacy data of products on their market. Various

dates were set for the completion of such national reviews, and the time schedule had to be revised on a number of occasions due to slow progress of the exercise. The various national review processes have not led to harmonized marketing approvals for these older products within Europe.

Pharmacovigilance and the adverse reactions voluntary reporting system

One of the most important aspects of the UK regulatory system is the scheme provided by the voluntary reporting of adverse reactions to a marketed drug. As most serious ADRs are rare events, they are unlikely to be detected in early clinical trials. The problem is essentially one of numbers, because relatively small numbers of patients are exposed to a new drug before it is released on to the market. Marketing may, therefore, be the first adequate safety trial. The main functions of the adverse reactions reporting system are as follows:
• to provide an alerting signal of a risk due to a particular drug;
• to provide confirmation of an alert detected by some other method;
• to provide data to assist in the evaluation of comparative risks of related drugs.

The spontaneous adverse reaction reporting system in the UK is based on the submission of ADR reports by doctors and dentists by means of reply-paid "yellow cards." The system was introduced in 1964 by Professor Witts, the first chairman of the Adverse Reactions Subcommittee of the original Committee on Safety of Drugs (CSD). The system has continued unchanged to the present time, and the number of reports and fatal reactions each year of the scheme's operation is shown in Table 36.3.

Membership of the EU and the establishment of the European Medicines Agency (EMA) has imposed a European dimension on ADR monitoring and given it a new title: "pharmacovigilance." The requirements of the European dimension can be summarized as obligations for Regulatory Authorities and obligations for the pharmaceutical company holding a MA, as described in the next two sections.

Table 36.3 Annual input of adverse reaction reports to CSM and total number of fatal reports

Year	Total ADR reports	Total deaths	Fatal reaction as a percentage of total ADR reports
1964	415	86	5.9
1965	3987	169	4.2
1966			
	2386	152	6.4
1967	3503	198	5.7
1968	3486	213	6.1
1969	4306	271	6.3
1970	3563	196	5.5
1971	2851	203	7.1
1972	3638	211	5.8
1973	3619	224	6.2
1974	4815	275	5.7
1975	5052	250	4.9
1976	6490	236	2.6
1977	11,255	352	3.1
1978	11,873	396	3.3
1979	10,881	286	2.6
1980	10,179	287	2.9
1981	12,357	303	2.5
1982	14,701	340	2.3
1983	12,689	409	3.2
1984	12,163	340	2.8
1985	12,652	348	2.8
1986	15,527	403	2.6
1987	16,431	390	2.4
1988	19,022	410	2.2
1989	19,246	475	2.5
1990	18,084	377	2.1
1991	20,272	541	2.7
1992	20,155	478	2.4
1993	18,066	480	2.7
1994	17,546	412	2.3
1995	17,668	467	2.6
1996	17,191	393	2.3
1997	16,637	455	2.7
1998	18,062	529	2.9
1999	18,505	560	3.0
2000	33,094	610	1.8
2001	21,467	650	3.0
2002	17,622	666	3.8
2003	19,257	737	3.8
2004	20,206	861	4.3
2005	21,831	NA	NA
2006	21,426	NA	NA
2007	21,464	NA	NA

Agency granted under the centralized procedure (the Agency referred to is the EMA) and member state responsibilities

• Receive all relevant information about suspected adverse reactions to medicinal products authorized by the centralized procedure.

• MA holders and member states are required to provide such information to the Agency.

• Member states must record and report to the Agency within 15 days all suspected serious adverse reactions.

• The Agency is responsible for informing national pharmacovigilance systems and the establishment of a rapid network for communication.

• The Agency shall collaborate with WHO on international pharmacovigilance issues and submit information on community measures that are relevant to public health protection in Third World countries.

MA holder's responsibilities

• To have a qualified person responsible for pharmacovigilance.

• Establishment and maintenance of a system for collection, evaluation, and collation of all suspected adverse reaction information so that it may be accessed at a single point in the community.

• Preparation of six monthly scientific reports and records of all suspected serious adverse reactions for the first two years after marketing, annual reports for the next three years, and thereafter at renewal of the authorization.

• Reporting to the member state concerned within 15 days of receipt information on all suspected serious adverse reactions within the community.

• Reporting to member states and the Agency within 15 days of all suspected serious unexpected adverse reactions occurring in Third World countries.

Good Manufacturing Practice (GMP)

Manufacturers' licenses were issued by the UK Licensing Authority from the inception of the Medicines Act to cover all manufacturing operations, including those previously embraced by the TSA. The Medicines Inspectorate laid down standards in its *Guide to Good Manufacturing Practice*, otherwise known as "The Orange Guide;" the most recent edition was issued in 2007. Although the issue of manufacturers' licenses remains a national regulatory function, it is governed by the standards set in EC Commission Directive 91/356 EEC, which can be summarized as follows.

The Directive lays down the principles and guidelines of GMP to be followed in the production of medicines, and requirements to ensure that manufacturers and member states adhere to its provisions. Manufacturers must ensure that production occurs in accordance with GMP and the manufacturing authorization. Imports from non-EC countries must have been produced to standards at least equivalent to those in the EC, and the importer must ensure this. All manufacturing processes should be consistent with information provided in the MA application, as accepted by the authorities. Methods shall be updated in the light of scientific advances, and modifications must be submitted for approval.

Principles and guidelines for GMP

• Quality management: implementation of quality assurance system.
• Personnel: appropriately qualified, with specified duties, responsibilities, and management structures.
• Premises and equipment: appropriate to intended operations.
• Documentation.
• Production: according to pre-established operating procedures with appropriate in-process controls, regularly validated.
• Quality control: independent department or external laboratory responsible for all aspects of quality control. Samples from each batch must be retained for one year, unless not practicable.
• Work contracted out: subject to contract, and under the same conditions, without subcontracting.
• Complaints and product recall: record keeping and arrangements for notification of competent authority.
• Self-inspection: by manufacturer of its own processes with appropriate record keeping.

Good manufacturing standards are enforced by the Medicines Inspectorate of the Medicines Control Agency. The UK has been involved in the Phar-

maceutical Inspection Convention since its inception and, through the Orange Guide, set standards that are now reflected in the EC Directives.

Wholesale dealers' licenses

This activity, established under the Medicines Act 1968, still remains wholly within the remit of national regulatory authorities, but in accordance with Directive 92/25 EEC on the wholesale distribution of medical products for human use (*Official Journal* L113/1–4 30 April 1992).

Routes of sale and supply

In the United Kingdom, the Medicines Act 1968 assumes that all medicinal products will be sold through a pharmacy unless it is decided by the Licensing Authority that supply of the product should be limited to being dispensed only on a registered medical practitioner's prescription. Such products appear on the Prescription Only Medicines List and their packaging is marked "POM." Certain products are also available through outlets other than pharmacies and are designated as General Sales List (GSL) products and listed as such. Additional restrictions on supply are imposed by the Misuse of Drugs Act 1971, and the Misuse of Drugs Regulations substances that have a potential for abuse are scheduled under three categories: classes A, B, and C:

• Class A includes alfentanil, cocaine, dextromoramide, diamorphine (heroin), dipipanone, lysergide (LSD), methadone, morphine, opium, pethidine, phencyclidine, and class B substances when prepared for injection.
• Class B includes oral amphetamines, barbiturates, cannabis, codeine, ethylmorphine, glutethimide, pentazocine, phenmetrazine, and pholcodine.
• Class C includes certain drugs related to the amphetamines, such as benzphetamine and chlorphentermine, buprenorphine, diethylpropion, mazindol, meprobamate, pemoline, pipradrol, and most benzodiazepines.

The Misuse of Drugs Regulations 1985 define the classes of person who are authorized to supply and possess controlled drugs while acting in their professional capacities, and lay down the conditions under which these activities may be carried out. In the regulations, drugs are divided into five schedules, each specifying the requirements governing such activities as import, export, production, supply possession, prescribing, and record keeping that apply to them:

- Schedule 1 includes drugs such as cannabis and lysergide, which are not used medicinally. Possession and supply are prohibited, except in accordance with Home Office authority.
- Schedule 2 includes drugs such as diamorphine (heroin), morphine, pethidine, quinalbarbitone, glutethimide, amphetamine, and cocaine. They are subject to the full controlled drug requirements relating to prescriptions, safe custody (except for quinalbarbitone), the need to keep registers, and so on (unless exempted in Schedule 5).
- Schedule 3 includes the barbiturates (except quinalbarbitone, now in Schedule 2), buprenorphine, diethylproprion, mazindol, meprobamate, pentazocine, phentermine, and temazepam. They are subject to the special prescription requirements (except for phenobarbitone and temazepam) but not to the safe custody requirements (except for buprenorphine, diethylproprion, and temazepam) nor to the need to keep registers (although there are requirements for the retention of invoices for two years).
- Schedule 4 includes 33 benzodiazepines (temazepam is now in Schedule 3) and pemoline, which are subject to minimal control. In particular, controlled drug prescription requirements do not apply, and they are not subject to safe custody.
- Schedule 5 includes those preparations which, because of their strength, are exempt from virtually all controlled drug requirements other than retention of invoices for two years.

There is no "harmonized "comprehensive legislation to control drugs of abuse under an EU Directive.

The European controls of medicinal products

Directive 75/319 laid down the legal basis for the establishment of the Committee on Proprietary Medicinal Products (CPMP). This met for the first time in November 1976, at which time there were nine member states in the EC. Each member state was represented at the CPMP by its named representative and specified alternate.

At this time, a procedure was laid down in Directive 75/318, a scheme for "mutual recognition "of MAs. Article 9 of this Directive envisaged that

The member state which has issued a marketing authorization for a proprietary medicinal product shall forward to the Committee a dossier containing a copy of the authorization, together with particulars and documents specified in Article 4 second paragraph of Directive 65/65, if the person responsible has requested the forwarding to at least five other Member States.

This was later changed to "at least two other member states" in Directive 83/570 to encourage the use of the procedure, which was initially very slow in taking off.

This "mutual recognition procedure," initially called the "CPMP procedure," has had several other names attached to it, for example the "multistate procedure" and the "decentralized procedure." Manufacturers could choose the country that they would wish to be the initiating or reference country to forward their dossier into the multistate procedure. Some countries were more popular than others (see Table 36.4).

In December 1986, the Council Directive on the approximation of national measures relating to the placing on the market of high-technology medicinal products, particularly those derived from biotechnology (87/22/EEC), was published. This Directive introduced the concept of two classes of high-technology medicinal product.

Annex A concerns medicinal products developed from the following biotechnological processes:

- Recombinant DNA technology.
- Controlled expression of genes coding for biologically active proteins in prokaryotates and eukaryotates including transformed mammalian cells.
- Hybridoma and monoclonal antibody methods.
    Annex B covers the following:
- Other biotechnological processes.
- Medicinal products administered by means of a new delivery system which, in the opinion of the competent authorities, constitutes a significant innovation.

Country	CPMP procedure		Multistate procedure	
	Country of origin	Recipient country	Country of origin	Recipient country
Belgium	5	33	14	147
Denmark	7	26	27	106
Germany	5	25	17	195
Greece	–	12	0	124
Spain	–	–	0	144
France	7	15	51	101
Ireland	–	24	32	87
Italy	–	38	16	142
Luxembourg	–	37	0	139
The Netherlands	–	35	20	131
Portugal	–	–	0	38
UK	16	18	75	82
Total dossiers/applications	41	263	252	1436

Table 36.4 The distribution of work to the rapporteur countries under the former CPMP procedure (*Directive 75/319/EEC*) 1978–1986, and the multistate procedure (*Directive 83/570/EEC*) 1986 to October 1992

- Medicinal products containing a new chemical entity.
- Medicinal products based on radioisotopes.
- Medicinal products the manufacture of which employs a significantly novel process.

This Directive required that products covered by the Annex classification had to be referred to the CPMP for an opinion before a MA could be granted in any member state. This process became known as the "concertation procedure" or the "central procedure." Products covered by Annex B could, at the request of the manufacturer, be dealt with by the concertation procedure or by an individual national authority, and then achieve entry into other EU member states markets if requested by means of the multistate procedure. In the concertation procedure, the opinion given by the CPMP was not binding on the member states.

Directive 2309/93 introduced further changes. It established a new body that is based in London, established on January 1, 1994, and two procedures for obtaining entry to the markets of the member states, namely the "multistate or decentralized or mutual recognition procedure" and the "centralized procedure;" see Figures 36.1 and 36.2, which show schematically the procedures that became operative on 1 January 1995.

Under the mutual recognition procedure, the applicant company would receive a number of national MAs from national drug regulatory authorities. Under the centralized procedure, the applicant company would receive a single marketing approval from the EMA, valid in all EU countries.

Centralized procedure

In the centralized procedure, products falling within Annex A have to be processed by this route; products in Annex B may be processed by this route at the discretion of the manufacturer. Applicants using the centralized procedure may nominate a member of the CPMP to act as rapporteur and co-rapporteur. However, the final choice of rapporteur and co-rapporteur remains within the remit of the CPMP. The membership of the CPMP has been made so that it is now a technically expert committee that advises the EMA. The opinions of the CPMP are referred to member states, who have a period of time to comment back to the CPMP. Thereafter, an opinion is issued, which is binding on the member states.

Tables 36.5 and 36.6 show the work of the EMA in terms of centralized procedure applications dealt with since the inception of the scheme on January 1, 1995, to December 19, 1999. Table 36.5 shows the new applications submitted to the EMA under the centralized procedure, and Table 36.6 shows the number of variations to MAs

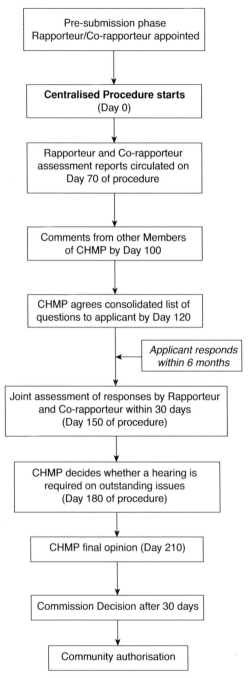

```
┌─────────────────────────────────┐
│      Pre-submission phase       │
│  Rapporteur/Co-rapporteur       │
│          appointed              │
└─────────────────────────────────┘
                │
                ▼
┌─────────────────────────────────┐
│   Centralised Procedure starts  │
│            (Day 0)              │
└─────────────────────────────────┘
                │
                ▼
┌─────────────────────────────────┐
│   Rapporteur and Co-rapporteur  │
│   assessment reports circulated │
│         on Day 70 of procedure  │
└─────────────────────────────────┘
                │
                ▼
┌─────────────────────────────────┐
│    Comments from other Members  │
│       of CHMP by Day 100        │
└─────────────────────────────────┘
                │
                ▼
┌─────────────────────────────────┐
│  CHMP agrees consolidated list  │
│  of questions to applicant by   │
│            Day 120              │
└─────────────────────────────────┘
                │
                ▼
           ┌─────────────────────┐
           │ Applicant responds  │
           │ within 6 months     │
           └─────────────────────┘
                │
                ▼
┌─────────────────────────────────┐
│  Joint assessment of responses  │
│  by Rapporteur and Co-rapporteur│
│        within 30 days           │
│      (Day 150 of procedure)     │
└─────────────────────────────────┘
                │
                ▼
┌─────────────────────────────────┐
│ CHMP decides whether a hearing  │
│ is required on outstanding      │
│ issues (Day 180 of procedure)   │
└─────────────────────────────────┘
                │
                ▼
┌─────────────────────────────────┐
│  CHMP final opinion (Day 210)   │
└─────────────────────────────────┘
                │
                ▼
┌─────────────────────────────────┐
│  Commission Decision after 30   │
│            days                 │
└─────────────────────────────────┘
                │
                ▼
┌─────────────────────────────────┐
│    Community authorisation      │
└─────────────────────────────────┘
```

Figure 36.1 Centralized procedure for biotech (mandatory) and high-tech (optional) medicines (from 1 January 1995) (source: Griffin and O'Grady (2009)).

granted under the centralized procedure. It can be envisaged that variations are going to comprise the major part of EMA's workload, in the same way as it does for national drug regulatory authorities.

The MCA (now the MHRA) has remained the dominant regulatory authority regarding the share of work conducted under the two revised community procedures, for example in March 1996, the Annual Report of the MCA for 1995/96 states: "The MCA was responsible for eight of the 21 mutual recognition procedures that had been successfully completed (38%) and was the reference member state for 10 of the 23 procedures in progress at that date." The UK was also the rapporteur or co-rapporteur for 19 of 81 applications made to the centralized procedure in 1997 (European Agency for the Evaluation of Medicinal Products, Third General Report, 1997). The distribution of work on centralized applications by the member state is shown in Table 36.7. The processing times for centralized applications is shown in Table 36.8.

Decentralized or mutual recognition procedure

Table 36.9 shows the use of the "decentralized" (or "multistate" or "mutual recognition") procedure during 1997. In this procedure, the initial or reference member state that granted marketing approval forwards the necessary documents for registration to the other member states where the manufacturer wishes to market its product, and a copy is also sent to the EMA/CPMP. If one or more member states raise objections, the applicant had the right, until 31 December 1997, to withdraw the request for a MA in that member state. Thereby, the applicant avoided the application being forwarded to the CPMP for arbitration (see Table 36.10).

Application for marketing approval

Application for marketing approval, using either the centralized or decentralized procedure, has to be accompanied by three expert reports, which cover: (i) chemistry, pharmacy, and manufacturing route; (ii) preclinical aspects, including pharmacology, safety pharmacology, pharmacokinetics,

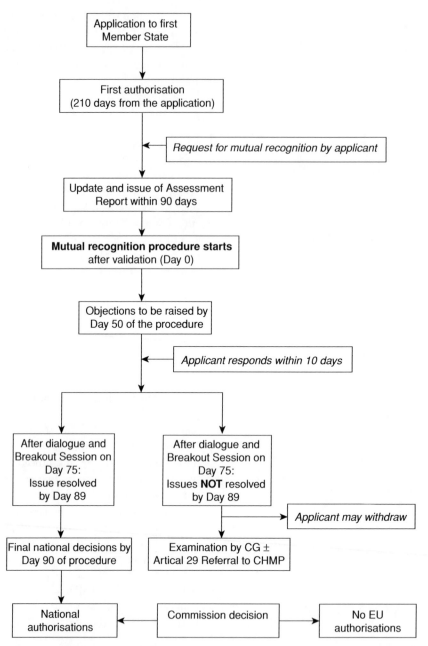

Figure 36.2 Mutual recognition procedure for all products except those of biotechnology (source: Griffin and O'Grady (2009)).

Table 36.5 Centralized marketing applications to EMEA

Centralized procedures	1997	1998	1999	Total 1995–1999
Applications received				
Part A	20	12	18	224
Part B	40	33	29	
Withdrawals				
Part A	3	8	1	38
Part B	4	12	7	
Opinions adopted by product				
Part A	6	11	9	133*
Part B	19	30	17	
Opinions adopted by substance				
Part A	6	11	8	105*
Part B	13	19	15	

*These figures include negative opinions given for seven products (representing four substances), and for two variations

single and repeat-dose toxicological evaluation, reproduction studies, and mutagenic potential and carcinogenicity; (iii) clinical studies covering Phase I– III studies and ADRs notified to the company

Table 36.6 Variations and line extensions to marketing applications processed by centralized procedures

Centralized procedures	1997	1998	1999	Total 1995–1999
Type I variations				
Part A	57	50	68	569
Part B	52	108	207	
Type II variations				
Part A	19	26	48	239*
Part B	28	40	61	
Extension and abridged applications				
Part A	32	11	6	73
Part B	2	4	13	

*These figures include negative opinions given for seven products (representing four substances), and for two variations

Table 36.7 Distribution of work on centralized procedure applications among EC member states

Country	Number of times a country has been rapporteur or co-rapporteur
Belgium	17
Denmark	25
Germany	34
Greece	2
Spain	19
France	37
Ireland	25
Italy	18
Luxembourg	6
The Netherlands	33
Austria	12
Portugal	12
Finland	15
Sweden	36
UK*	36

*UK has been rapporteur for 21 applications

during clinical studies. If the product has been marketed, all post-marketing experience should be assessed. Expert reports are not a promotion platform for the product but an assessment of the data generated: an explanation of the results and an interpretation. An expert report should not normally exceed 25 pages of A4 size. The expert reports should also make clear whether or not the studies submitted have been conducted according to GLP standards and whether the clinical studies have been conducted to GCP principles and in accord with the Declaration of Helsinki. A statement of the environmental effects of the product is also necessary.

DG XXIV Scientific Committee on medicinal products and medical devices

In a communication to the Council and European Parliament on "Consumer Health and Food Safety" (*COM(97) 183 Fund*), the European Commission emphasized that high-quality scientific committees are an essential foundation for EC rules in this area.

It was decided in August 1997 that DG XXIV Consumer Policy and Consumer Health, now

Year	Assessment phase	Decisions process	EMEA post-opinion phase	Company clockstop	Total
1995	189	45	119	59	412
1997	169	40	79	119	407
1997	178	32	86	139	435
1998	185	42	83	109	419
1999	183	38	70	148	439

Table 36.8 Processing times (days) of centralized applications to EMEA, 1995–1999

Table 36.9 Total number of finalized mutual recognition procedures by type, August 1995–December 1997*

	Number	Percent
New active substance	77	31.5
Generics	45	18.4
Line extensions	29	11.9
Fixed combination	20	8.2
OTC	6	2.6
Herbal	2	0.8
Others	65	26.6

*The number includes multiple procedures (total = 244)

renamed the Health Directorate in 1999 Protection, should set up eight new advisory committees, including a Scientific Committee on Medicinal Products and Medical Devices. These committees expected to meet ten times per year, and the Committee on Medicinal Products and Medical Devices met for the first time on November 10–14, 1997. The *European Drug and Device Report* stated that feathers were ruffled in the EU's Committee for Proprietary Medicinal Products, because up to now, the CPMP has largely held a monopoly on scientific opinion.

The Commission said that the new Scientific Committee will not overlap with the CPMP and there does appear to be a role for both panels. Unlike the CPMP, its minutes would be public. Drug companies have feared that the committee would lean more toward consumers than industry.

The interaction between the CPMP (which reports to the Enterprise Directorate, formerly the Commissions DG III Industry Affairs) and the new Medical Products and Medical Devices Committee, which reports to the Health Directorate, formerly DG XXIV Consumer Policy, is very uncertain. It has to be borne in mind that the objective of Directive 65/65 was to advance the free movement of goods within the EC, that is, an industrial/commercial objective. In the future, it might be more logical for the functions of the EMA to be the responsibility the Health Directorate rather than the Enterprise Directorate.

The CPMP and European harmonization of data requirements and ICH

It might not be immediately apparent that the drive toward "harmonization" of regulatory requirements had its birth at the first meeting of the CPMP in November 1976. The CPMP at that juncture had

Mutual recognition procedure	Total submitted in 1999*	Under evaluation in 1999	Ended positively in 1999	Arbitrations in 1999
New applications	275	48	210	2
Type I variations	695	90	625	0
Type II variations	254	109	292	2

Table 36.10 Mutual recognition procedure and arbitrations for 1999

*The number includes multiple procedures

been established to operate a "mutual recognition" procedure, laid out in Directive 75/318, but it had no work to do initially. It was, however, immediately clear to the CPMP that the data requirements laid down for registration were being interpreted differently by the regulatory authorities of individual member states. For example, there was no agreement on requirements for reproduction studies, carcinogenicity, studies, and so on. At that first meeting, two expert working groups on safety and efficacy were established to draw up guidelines (later, other expert working groups were established). A great deal of international harmonization of requirements and thought was achieved, and this could clearly be extended beyond the confines of the EC.

By June 1984, the EC Commission decided that a meeting with the Japanese authorities, attended by Mr Fernand Sauer and the Chairmen of the Safety and Efficacy Groups J.P. Griffin and J.M. Alexander should take place in Tokyo. As a result of this, a second meeting with the Japanese authorities (the JPMA), the EC Commission, and EFPIA representatives took place. This was the stimulus for the EFPIA, JPMA, and PMA, as it then was in the United States, to press for wider consultation. From such a start, the International Conference on Harmonization (ICH) was born. The ICH Steering Committee established expert working groups (EWG) to discuss areas where harmonization was possible and to produce universally acceptable guidelines. Thus, under the auspices of the ICH, a considerable number of guidelines have been issued in the areas of quality, safety, and efficacy, with the objective of achieving harmonization of requirements for registration between regulatory authorities, and thus reducing the need for duplicating studies. It must be made clear that these documents should be regarded as *guidelines*, not requirements. These guidelines are not at the cutting edge of science but represent acceptable compromises. Guidelines will need updating, and this must be coordinated, otherwise there will be "regulatory drift" toward disharmony.

If harmonization can be achieved, as it has been, across sufficiently broad areas of quality, safety, and efficacy, there is no logical reason why a

common technical document (CTD) or dossier cannot be prepared that would be acceptable to all drug regulatory authorities. Movement to a CTD would appear to be the next step toward further internationalization.

The ICH guidelines and details of their evolution can be obtained in the Proceedings of the First, Second, Third, and Fourth International Conferences on Harmonization, held in Brussels, Belgium (1991), Orlando, FL, USA (1993), Yokohama, Japan (1995), and Brussels, Belgium (1997), published by the Queen's University of Belfast and obtainable from the IFPMA Offices, 30 Rue du St Jean, P.O. Box 9, 1211 Geneva 18, Switzerland. The clinical guidelines applicable to the EC may be obtained from the MHRA, EuroDirect Guideline Service, Room 1615, Market Towers, 1 Nine Elms Lane, London SW8 5NQ, UK. Tel.: +44 (0) 171 273 0352/0228.

Mutual recognition of established products and line extensions

The bulk of national licensing activities relates to new formulations of older products, generics, and line extensions. However, over the years, the indications, contraindications, warnings, dosages, and so on of even well-known products differ significantly from member state to member state. The national reviews required of older products that were conducted by each member state of the EC were not accompanied by any international concentration of effort and did not lead to harmonization within the EC. This has made it difficult for companies to use the mutual recognition procedure for the introduction of generic products, because the summary of product characteristics (SPC) differs between member states. The same problem can affect the originator of an established chemical entity when the company wishes to introduce a line extension, because even under the operation of the mutual recognition procedure, where the CPMP opinion was not binding, there were differences in dosages, indications, contraindications, and warnings between member states.

In 1996, the Swedish government proposed a solution to the impasse affecting the use of the mutual recognition procedure for generic products. This would have allowed generic companies to apply for recognition only of the quality and bioequivalence data. The rest of authorization to market, that is, indications, contraindications, and warnings, would be decided by the national authorities, bearing in mind these factors as they applied to the originator's product in each member state.

In April 1997, the EC Commission announced that, rather than change the Directives to allow the "core SPC idea" as advanced by Sweden, it would "reinterpret" them. In practice, this means that generic companies would, from January 1, 1998, be able to use the mutual recognition procedure only when the originator's SPC was identical in all member states, that is, the originator's product had mutual recognition status or a centralized license. In practice, this means that generics will have to use national procedures "which were due to be phased out on December 31, 1997." Line extensions of existing products, that is, new dosage forms and so on, would logically be caught in the same net as generics if the initial product did not have an identical SPC in all member states. Currently, some companies are withdrawing products from the market and replacing them with a new salt of the same active substance in an attempt to thwart generic products entering the market.

Changes ahead for European regulation?

Possible changes to the centralized procedure
In view of the increased membership of the EU, in future years, if standards of granting MAs for medicines are not to decline, measures will have to be taken to preserve the standards that operated in Northern Europe prior to 1994. It could be conceded that all NCEs should be handled through the centralized procedure. This could only be acceptable in terms of consumer safety if the competence of advice available to the EMA was increased. EMA staff themselves must be technically competent to do the assessment work currently done by those national drug regulatory authorities, appointed to act on behalf of the rapporteur and co-rapporteur.

The use of national drug regulatory authorities to do the work of rapporteur and co-rapporteur would cease. The staff recruited to the EMA to do this expert work should be recruited on the basis of quality, rather than having regard to the adherence of "national quotas" of staff. The CPMP, currently composed of one member from each of the 25 member state's regulatory authority, should be disbanded. The technical advisory committee serving the EMA should be served by expert panels, covering chemistry and pharmacy, pharmacology, and toxicology, and multiple clinical panels of experts, covering for example cardiovascular, respiratory, diabetic and endocrine disorders, oncology, and so on, on the pattern used by the US Food and Drug Administration (FDA). This would be a way forward, with synthesis of an overall view done by a standing expert committee. It would have to be recognized that not all EU member states would be involved in every committee or expert panel. Although attempts should be made to involve all member states at some level in the procedure, it must be accepted that, in the public interest, expertise should predominate over national representation. The role of selection of the experts to serve on this standing committee and expert panels should be the role of the EMA Management Board, and nominations should be made by the Ministers of Health of the member states of the EU, on a similar basis to the way the membership of the British Committee on Safety of Medicines is drawn together.

Possible changes to the decentralized or mutual recognition system
The current mutual recognition system is cumbersome and could be improved. A true mutual recognition system for marketing applications that did not involve a NCE could be devised, drawing on the system operating in the medical devices area, where authorization by one regulatory agency leads to an EU-wide approval, provided that marketing in all EU member states is identical with the approval granted in the reference member state. A single chemical entity MA number would be used to cover the authorization in all member states of the EU. Applicant companies would be wise to

select a credible national drug regulatory authority to process such a mutual recognition. In fact, it might be better if the scheme were to designate competent national authorities to operate such a procedure, and laid down strict criteria for delegating such authority to competent national regulatory bodies (not all national authorities would necessarily qualify).

Single assessment/single marketing approval
Both systems, modified as outlined, would lead to a single EU-wide marketing approval, following a single assessment.

Conclusion

The European system for granting MA for medicinal products will continue to evolve and change; however, like the advice given to the person seeking directions (I would not start from here if I were you), we do not have an option. Finally, it has to be understood that the EU is not a country—it is a collection of member states, and there continues to be much fertile ground for continuing debate and dissent.

References

Geddie WM, Geddie JL. Chambers Biographical Dictionary. *The Great of All Nations and All Times*. WR Chambers: London, UK, 1926, 662.

Griffin JP. An international comparison on legislation regarding human volunteer studies. *Int Pharm J* 1987; **1**:57–60.

Griffin JP. Venetian treacle and the foundation of medicines regulation. *Br J Clin Pharmacol* 2004; **58**(3):317–325.

Griffin JP, Diggle GE. A survey of products licensed in the United Kingdom, 1971–1981. *Br J Clin Pharmacol* 1981; **12**:453–463.

Griffin JP, Long JR. New procedures affecting the conduct of clinical trials in the United Kingdom. *Br Med J* 1981; **283**:477–479.

Griffin JP. *The Textbook of Pharmaceutical Medicine*, sixth edition. Blackwell BMJ Books: Boston, MA, USA, 2009.

Heberden W. Antitherica: Essay on mithridatium and theriac. London, UK, 1745.

Jefferys DB, Leakey D, Lewis JA, *et al.* New active substances authorized in the United Kingdom between 1972 and 1994. *Br J Clin Pharmacol* 1998; **45**:151–156.

Munk W. *The Roll of Royal College of Physicians of London, Vol. II (1701–1800)*. Royal College of Physicians: Pall Mall East, London, UK, 1878, 159–164.

Rubin S. *Medieval English Medicine*. David & Charles: Newton Abbot, UK, 1975, 43–128.

Stenton FM. Anglo Saxon England. In *Oxford History of England*, second edition. Oxford University Press: Oxford, UK, 1947, 266.

Speirs CJ, Griffin JP. A survey of the first year of operation of the new procedure affecting the conduct of clinical trials in the United Kingdom. *Br J Clin Pharmacol* 1983; **15**:649–655.

Speirs CJ, Saunders RM, Griffin JP. The United Kingdom Clinical Trial Exemption Scheme – its effects on investment in research. *Pharm Int* 1984; **5**:254–256.

Watson G. *Theriac and Mithridatium. A Study in Therapeutics*. The Wellcome Historical Library: London, UK, 1966.

Recommended information sources

European Agency for the Evaluation of Medicinal Products (EMEA). First, Second and Third General Reports. *EMEA*: 7 West Ferry Circus, Canary Wharf, London E14 4HB, UK, 1995, 1996, 1997.

European Commission. *The Rules Governing Medicinal Products in the European Community, Vols I–IV*. Commission of the European Communities: Brussels, Belgium.

Medicines Control Agency. *Annual Report and Accounts*, 1994/5, 1995/6, 1996/7. HMSO: London, UK, 1995, 1996, 1997.

CHAPTER 37

Medicines Regulation in the European Union

Anne-Ruth van Troostenburg[1] & Giuliana Tabusso[2]
[1]Takeda Group R & D, London, UK
[2]Milan, Italy

List of abbreviations

ABPI	Association of British Pharmaceutical Industry
CAT	Committee Advanced Therapies
CEP	European Pharmacopoeia Certificate of suitability
CHMP	Committee for Human Medicinal Products
CIOMS	Council of International Organizations of Medical Sciences
CMC	Chemistry, Manufacturing & Controls
CMD(h)	Coordination Group for MRP and DC (human)
CMS	Concerned Member State(s)
COMP	Committee for Orphan Medicinal Products
CP	Centralized Procedure
CPMP	Committee for Proprietary Medicinal Products
CTA	Clinical Trial Authorization
CTD	Common Technical Document
CVMP	Committee for Veterinary Medicinal Products
EEA	European Economic Area
EFPIA	European Federation of Pharmaceutical Industries' Associations
EMA	European Medicines Agency
EPAR	European Product Assessment Report
EU	European Union
FDA	Food and Drug Administration
GCP	Good Clinical Practices
GLP	Good Laboratory Practices
GMO	Genetically Modified Organism
GMP	Good Manufacturing Practices
GSL	General Sales List
HCMP	Committee for Herbal Medicinal Products
ICH	International Conference of Harmonization
IM	Intra Muscular
IMP	Investigational Medicinal Product
IV	Intra Venous
MA	Marketing Authorization
MAA	Marketing Authorization Application
MAH	Marketing Authorization Holder
MedDRA	Medical Dictionary of Regulatory Activities
MRFG	Mutual Recognition Facilitation Group
MRP	Mutual Recognition Procedure
MS	Member State(s)
P	Pharmacy
PA	Protocol Assistance
PAGB	Proprietary Association of Great Britain
PDCO	Pediatric Committee (of the EMEA)
PIL	Patient Information Leaflet
POM	Prescription Only Medicine
PIP	Pediatric Investigation Plan
PSUR	Periodic Safety Update Report
QP	Qualified Person (for GMP)
QPPV	Qualified Person for Pharmacovigilance
RA	Regulatory Authority

Principles and Practice of Pharmaceutical Medicine, 3rd edition.
Edited by L.D. Edwards, A.W. Fox, P.D. Stonier.
© 2011 Blackwell Publishing Ltd.

REC	Research Ethics Committee		
RMS	Reference Member State		
SAWG	Scientific Advice Working Group		
SPC	Summary of Product Characteristics		
SUSAR	Serious Unexpected Suspected Adverse drug Reaction		
TAG	Therapeutic Advisory Group		
TSE	Transmissible Spongiform Encephalopathies		
USP	US Pharmacopoeia		

The European Regulatory Framework

In 1957, the Treaty of Rome established a community of European countries with different cultures and history. This began, among other things, a process of harmonization of Regulations and technical requirements for the Marketing Authorization (MA) of medicines, within a European Common Market. By 1975, the fundamental Directives concerning medicines had been issued. The European Union was formalized by the treaty of Maastricht in 1992. As a political union of sovereign, independent nations, the European Union comprises today 27 Member States (MSs), with 20 official languages and a population of over 300 million (see Figure 37.1).

The European legislative mechanism

The European Communities and the European Union have been established by Treaties. Treaties

Belgium	Denmark	Sweden	Malta
France	Ireland	Cyprus	Poland
Italy	Greece	Czech Republic	Slovakia
Luxembourg	Spain	Estonia	Slovenia
The Netherlands	Portugal	Hungary	Bulgaria
Germany	Austria	Latvia	Romania
United Kingdom	Finland	Lithuania	

Figure 37.1 The 27 EU Member States (as of June 2010).

are written agreements between MSs, subject to ratification by National Parliaments. Treaties define the role and responsibilities of European Institutions and bodies involved in decision-making processes as well as the legislative, executive, and juridical procedures of community law and its implementation.

The European law is an independent legal system that takes precedence over national legal provisions.

There are three different but interdependent types of legislation:
• primary legislation constituted by treaties and other agreements such as treaties amendments;
• secondary legislation, derived from treaties, which takes the form of regulations, directives, and decisions;
• case law, which includes judgements of the European Court of Justice.

The instruments of the EU to achieve legal, technical, and administrative harmonization are Regulations, Directives, decisions, opinions, communications, and finally guidelines.

Directives are issued by the European Commission, the Council, and the Parliament and are binding as to their objectives and results. MSs are obligated to transpose these into national law according to a preset timeline. In the case of medicines Regulation, this happens not only in the 27 countries of the EU, but also, on a voluntary basis, in the additional countries of the European Economic Area (Norway, Liechtenstein, Iceland).

Regulations are laws of immediate application for all MSs and overrule national law.

EU Decisions are binding for a named addressee. Addressees can be individual MSs, particular economic sectors, or even single organizations and physical persons.

In Europe, Opinions and Communications are not legally binding. However, these do enunciate governmental views and attitudes, and they are often the basis for the future issuance of Decisions, Regulations, or even Directives. An important tool to achieve harmonization is represented by the guidelines, which provide a technical interpretation of the law, thought to be acceptable to Regulatory Authorities (RAs). In the field of medicines

Regulation, guidelines can be issued by individual scientific committees (e.g., the Committee for Human Medicinal Products; CHMP), and although they are not binding, they constitute an official reference or precedent. Any deviation from such guidelines must usually then be explained with sound scientific justification.

Unlike the informal status of guidances in the United States, it is important to know that in the European Union guidelines can have legal status. Those guidelines relating to a formal request laid down in a Directive or Regulation are published by the European Commission and are legally binding (e.g., the Notice to Applicants and the labeling guideline)

The legal basis for medicinal product marketing authorization

In the effort to harmonize medicine Regulations across MS, many Directives and Regulations have been issued over the years. These aim to achieve uniform requirements and decision-making criteria for MA and post-marketing surveillance processes throughout the EU.

The very first Directive issued was Council Directive 65/65 concerning "The approximation of provisions laid down by law, Regulation or administrative action relating to proprietary medicinal products," and it was a milestone on the path to a pharmaceutical Europe, which could extend the same opportunities in pursuit of health to all EU citizens, through the removal of legal, technical, and regulatory barriers within the framework of the Common Market.

Directive 65/65 defined Quality, Safety, and Efficacy as the sole criteria for approval of medicines in the EU. The principle is that products that are awarded MA must demonstrate conformity with these three criteria. Approval are thus granted on a purely technical basis, without political or economic implications.

Directive 75/318 defined testing and protocol standards, whereas Directive 75/319 introduced the Committee for Proprietary Medicinal Products and what is now known as the "mutual recog-

nition procedure" for MA (see below). The Committee for Proprietary Medicinal Products (CPMP) was restructured in compliance with Regulation 726/2004 to form the CHMP (see below). The above three Directives represent the basis of pharmaceutical Regulation that is common to the whole of Europe, and culminated in the creation of the EMEA in 1995 by Regulation 2309/93. Note, however, that according to this Regulation a different "centralized" procedure is used to authorize biotechnological and certain other innovative products. Regulation 726/2004 actually allows licensing of generic products, under specified conditions relating to the interest of the EU citizens.

All these relevant legal requirements for human medicines other than those foreseen by Regulation 2309/93, currently replaced by Regulation 726/2004, have been collected together in Directive 2001/83 entitled "Community code relating to medicinal products for human use." This, together with Directive 2003/63, defines the requirements for each technical section of the marketing application dossier for different product categories such as chemical synthesis products, biologics, plasma derivatives, fixed combinations, radiopharmaceuticals, vaccines, homeopathic, herbal, and orphans medicinal products.

As statutory requirements, manufacturing and control data must comply with GMP (Good Manufacturing Practices), nonclinical toxicological data with GLP (Good Laboratory Practices), and clinical data with GCP (Good Clinical Practices). These requirements have been set up in Directives and extensively described in the relevant guidelines (see Figure 37.2).

The International Conference on Harmonization (ICH) process

In recent years, the pharmaceutical industry has displayed an increasing tendency to globalize the market, particularly for innovative medicines. The differences of requirements in different geographical areas often caused duplication of experiments, with consequent waste of time and resources, adding to the escalating costs of research &

Vol 1 Pharmaceutical legislation (human)

Vol 2 Notice to Applicants (human)

Vol 3 Guidelines (human)

Vol 4 Good Manufacturing Practices (human and veterinary)

Vol 5 Pharmaceutical legislation (veterinary)

Vol 6 Notice to Applicants (veterinary)

Vol 7 Guidelines (veterinary)

Vol 8 Maximum residue limits (veterinary)

Vol 9 Pharmacovigilance (human & veterinary)*

Vol 10 Clinical Trials (human)

*Since February 2007, a revision has separated human and veterinary pharmacovigilance: human pharmacovigilance regulations are found in Volume 9A (latest version September 2008), while Volume 9 remains valid for veterinary products.

Figure 37.2 European Regulations and guidelines that support the European pharmaceutical legislative framework are collected in the ten volumes of "The Rules governing medicinal products in the European Union", edited by Eudralex.

development. Uniformity of approach across the EU has the potential to minimize redundancy and reduce development costs and time.

It was quickly realized that even wider international harmonization could benefit pharmaceutical research and development. This led to the collaborative project involving Europe, Japan, and the USA known as the "International Conference on Harmonization of Technical Requirements for Registration of Pharmaceuticals for Human Use" (ICH). The ICH aims to provide harmonized guidelines acceptable in all three regions.

The main scopes of ICH can be summarized as follows:
• harmonize technical requirements for marketing approval;
• contribute to protection of public health from an international perspective;
• maintain a forum for dialog;
• avoid duplications and divergent requirements;

• facilitate adaptation to scientific and technical progress;
• facilitate dissemination and communication on harmonized guidelines and their use.

Both national RAs and industry participate in the ICH process. The parties form Steering Committees to address issues identified by industrial and RA experts (often in working parties). Many tripartite guidelines have now been issued on matters of drug quality, safety, and efficacy. Some of these have led to precisely-designed working tools, for example, the Medical Dictionary for Drug Regulatory Affairs (MedDRA), and the Common Technical Document (CTD), a guideline for the structure, format, and content of the dossier (the documents to be submitted to the RAs for product license approval), which has been mandatory in the EU since 2003.

The ICH is also harmonizing many monographs of the *European Pharmacopoeia* and the *USP*, so that such monographs can be referred to in both regions.

In this chapter we give an overview of current regulatory procedures in Europe. We address the practical aspects of drug development Regulation, the MA processes, and other activities, such as advertising Regulations in the EU.

The European Medicines Agency (EMA)

The EMA is an advisory body reporting directly to the European Commission and is located in London. From 1995 to 2004 the agency was known as the "European Medicines Evaluation Agency" (EMEA). Currently its name is the "European Medicines Agency", but the abbreviation EMEA was retained for a transition period and for old documents published before December 2009. The agency is launching a new visual identity with a new logo incorporating a new slogan—Science, Medicines, Health—that is, the three words representing the expertise, focus, and purposes of the Agency. The new name in fact reflects the wider responsibilities attributed to the Agency according to Regulation 726/2004, which go beyond the mere evaluation of drugs.

Actually, Regulation 726/2004 defines its structure and responsibilities as primarily protecting and promoting public and animal health through coordination of the existing resources put at its disposal by the MSs for the evaluation, supervision, and pharmacovigilance of medicines for human and veterinary use.

Within this framework the main tasks are as follows:

• provide MSs and the Community institutions with the best possible Scientific Advice on questions concerning quality, safety, and efficacy of medicinal products for human and veterinary use (note that this does not include medical devices);

• establish multinational scientific expertise through mobilization of existing national resources;

• organize rapid, transparent, and efficient procedures for the authorization, surveillance and, when necessary, withdrawal of medicinal products in the EU;

• provide Scientific Advice to the sponsors of pharmaceutical research;

• draw up scientific opinions concerning evaluation of medicinal products or of the starting materials used in their manufacture at the Commission's request;

• reinforce the supervision of existing medicinal products by coordinating national pharmacovigilance and inspections activities;

• improve cooperation between the EU government, MS, international organizations, and third countries;

• provide assistance on information of medicinal products to physicians and the public;

• create and maintain a European database of medicinal products accessible to the general public;

• transmit and make publicly available assessment reports, Summaries of Product Characteristics (SPC), product labeling, and package information leaflets for medicines subject to Community procedures;

• coordinate verification of compliance with Good Manufacturing, Good Laboratory, and Good Clinical Practices guidelines (GMP, GLP, and GCP, respectively);

• facilitate availability of drugs intended for rare diseases (orphan drugs).

Thus, the fundamental objectives of the EMA are to:

• protect and promote public health by mobilizing the best scientific resources in the EU;

• promote healthcare through effective Regulation of medicines and better information for users and health professionals;

• facilitate quicker access and free circulations of medicines within the EU;

• collaborate in harmonizing scientific requirements to optimize pharmaceutical research worldwide;

• develop efficient, effective, and responsive operating procedures;

• stimulate innovation and research in the pharmaceutical sector.

The EMA comprises (see Figure 37.3):

• a Management Board that approves the Agency's work programme and approves the budget;

• an Executive Director, legal representative of the Agency and responsible for the overall working of the Agency;

• a Secretariat that provides technical, scientific, and administrative support to the Scientific Committees;

• the Scientific Committees, responsible for the scientific opinions delivered by the Agency:

   – Committee for Human Medicinal Products (CHMP)

   – Committee for Veterinary Medicinal Products (CVMP)

   – Committee on Orphan Medicinal Products (COMP)

   – Committee on Herbal Medicinal Products (HCMP)

   – Pediatric Committee (PDCO)

   – Committee for Advanced Therapies (CAT)

Standing working parties and ad-hoc expert groups support these committees. Some 4500 European experts have been listed and will support on request the scientific work of the Committees. The list is published on the EMEA website (www.ema.europa.eu).

The EMA peer review evaluation system works through a network of European experts made

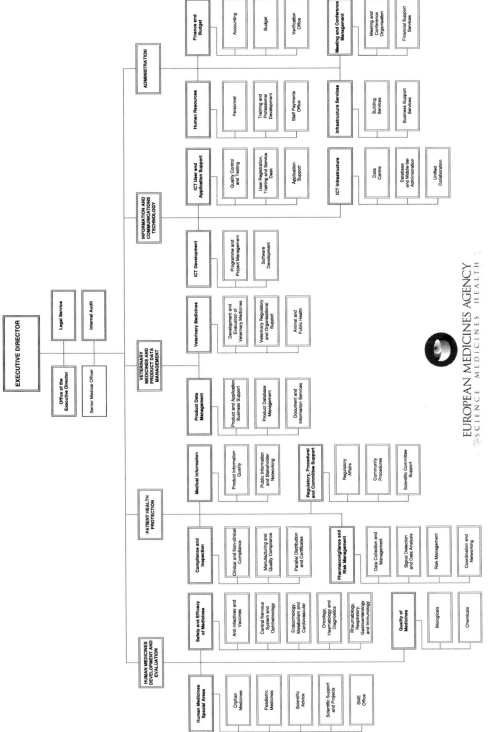

Figure 37.3 The organizational structure of the EMA. Copyright – European Medicines Agency, 2009.

Human Medicines Development and Evaluation

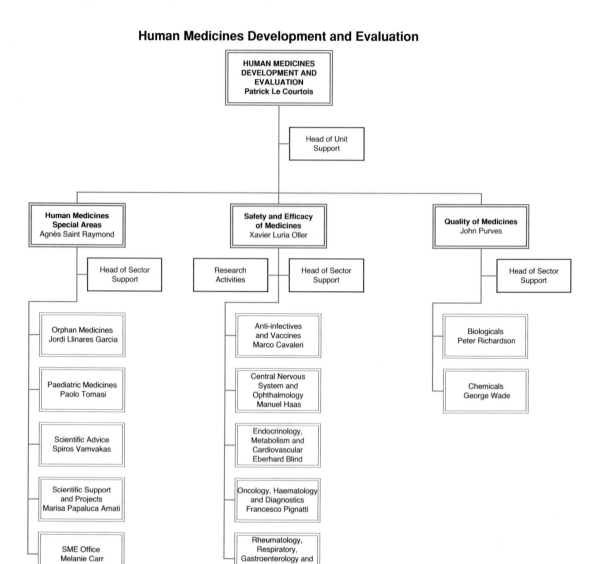

Figure 37.3 (*Continued*).

available to the Agency by the national competent authorities of the 27 European Union MSs and of the 3 EEA-EFTA States Iceland, Liechtenstein, and Norway. These experts serve as members of the EMA Scientific Committees, of the working parties, or as part of the scientific assessment teams.

Current European regulatory practice

Clinical trials: Directive 2001/20

This Directive came into force on May 1, 2004. Approval of clinical trials was no longer based on the national law of each MS, but rather on

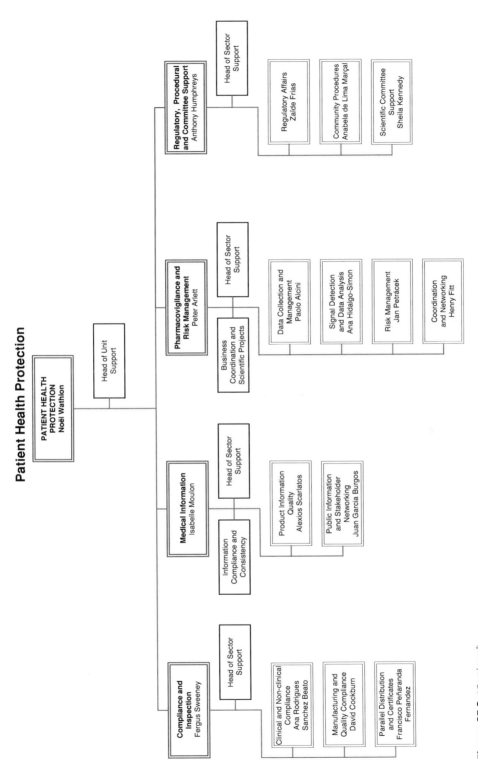

Figure 37.3 (*Continued*).

Veterinary Medicines and Product Data Management

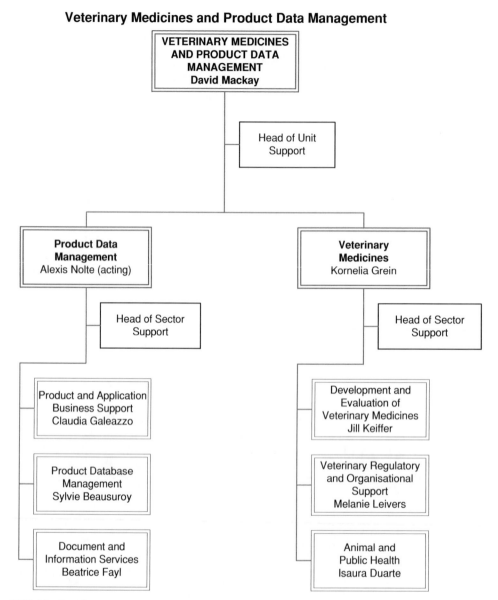

Figure 37.3 (*Continued*).

how each state has implemented the Directive. The scope of the Directive is broad. All clinical studies of medicinal products involving human subjects, whether they are patients or volunteers, are within its remit, unless the trial is merely observational and noninterventional. This applies equally to the pharmaceutical industry, academia, government research institutes, and all others.

The Directive

• sets standards for the protection of study subjects, including especially vulnerable groups such as children and incapacitated adults;

Information and Communications Technology

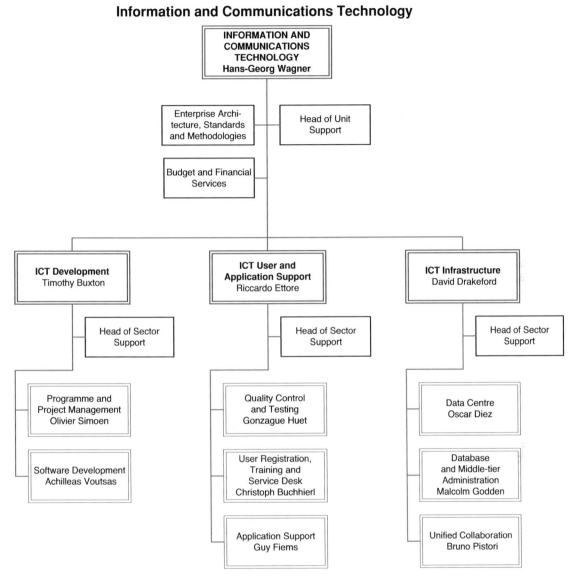

Figure 37.3 (*Continued*).

- requires every MS to have a central governing body that oversees Ethics Committees;
- mandates that national licensing authorities must now affirmatively permit clinical trial initiation;
- prescribes standards for the manufacture, import, and labeling of all investigational medicinal products (IMP);

- establishes an inspection system to ensure compliance with GMP and GCP;
- focuses particularly on the safety monitoring of participating subjects in trials and sets out procedures for safety reporting to a pan-European pharmacovigilance database (Eudravigilance, Clinical Trial module).

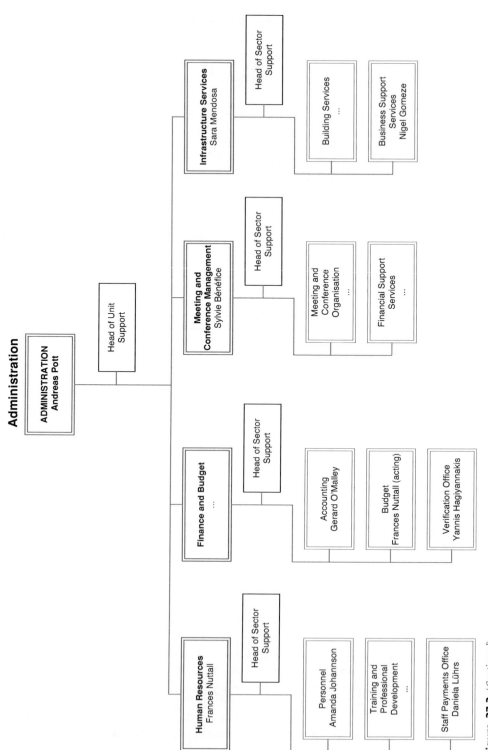

Figure 37.3 (*Continued*).

Directorate

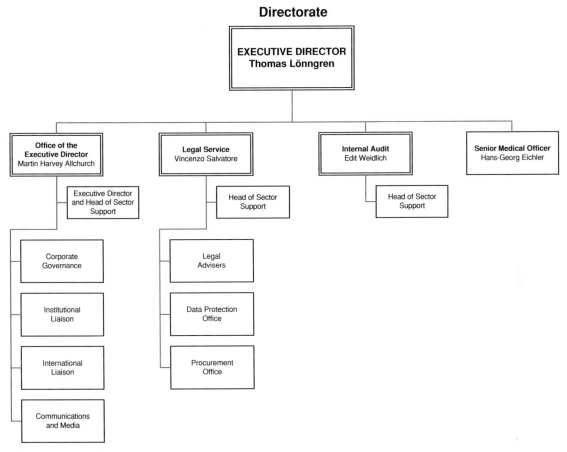

Figure 37.3 (*Continued*).

The competent RA in each MS reviews the proposed clinical trial and if satisfied with the information notifies the sponsor that it has no grounds for objection. The Directive sets a timeline for review of up to 60 days for most trials, but there are options to extend this timeline under special circumstances. There is no time limit for review of gene therapy protocols. The authorization granted by the RA—the Clinical Trial Authorization (CTA)—is study-by-study, and not per IMP (an important difference from the United States Investigational New Drug (IND) exemption).

The EU Directive requires the integration of GCP into national law of all MSs and local RAs have to inspect for compliance with both GCP and GMP; inspections take place at both spon-sor's facilities and clinical trial sites. A further update to GCP requirements in the EU was issued through the Good Clinical Practice Directive (Directive 2005/28/EC).

All research involving human subjects (apart from wholly noninterventional, observational studies), including academic research and clinical pharmacology studies in healthy volunteers, has to provide the same amount of information and be subject to RA review.

The European Commission issued a set of detailed guidelines on the requirements for clinical trial application to competent authorities and Ethics Committees, also providing the application forms. Directive 2001/20 required every applicant for a CTA) in any EU MS to have a legal representative in Europe, through which all activities and communications are executed. Non-European applicants for a CTA must name a representative, resident in the EU (a similar requirement exists in the US).

EudraCT

The pan-European clinical trial database (EudraCT) enables the various European RAs to track all clinical trials taking place anywhere in the community at a single source of information. Every clinical trial in the EU must be registered with this database, which issues a unique registration number for each trial, even when held in multiple EU countries (the EudraCT trial number). The EudraCT database is for the sole use of RAs and cannot be accessed by trial sponsors or the general public beyond the registration of a clinical trial. Efforts to link the EudraCT number to the Adverse Events database Eudravigilance and thus facilitate the Agencies' efforts at monitoring the safety of subjects participating in clinical trials are underway.

Sponsors must have a system in place to guarantee that duplicate EudraCT numbers are not requested for the same trial.

The information to be provided about the clinical trial at time of registration is similar to, but less extensive than, that provided in the CTA and must contain the following:
- the identity of the trial;
- the identity of the applicant;
- the type of application;
- the trial monitoring and central facilities;
- information about the IMPs;
- information about the placebo;
- the manufacturer or importer of the IMPs;
- information about the trial;
- details of the trial subjects;
- information about the REC.

The applicant has no access to the information, once it has been registered with the database: only the RA can make changes.

Ethics Committees

Directive 2001/20 has also led to a set of detailed Guidance documents, to help MSs interpret the Directive and implement appropriate systems. The "Detailed Guidance on the Application Format and Documentation to be Submitted in an Application for an Ethics Committee Opinion on a Clinical Trial for a Medicinal Products for Human Use" (October 2005) is self-explanatory. This document includes a table that collates each MS's special requirements, and it is designed to be used with the national guidances, where they exist.

All proposed clinical trials in Europe have to receive an affirmative favourable opinion from a properly constituted Ethics Committee, before commencement. In the case of multinational, multicenter trials, only a single Ethics Committee opinion is needed per MS, although various exceptions in individual MSs exist. There remains the capability for individual sites, with additional Ethics Committees to reject a clinical trial. But a negative opinion from the local Ethics Committees would only stop the trial at the particular site, and not affect the overall approval given from the lead Ethics Committee in the relevant MS.

Both sponsors and investigators are empowered to apply for Ethics Committee opinion. The Directive states that the applicant can choose to make parallel applications to the competent authority and the Ethics Committee or do it sequentially. However, in practice national preferences vary in whether sequential applications are preferred. It is important to make sure that the version of the reviewed documents at the Ethics Committee and the RA match.

The RA and Ethics Committee initially validate the application and the sponsor is informed that the application is valid (i.e., complete and accurate). Ethics Committees have the same review clock as RAs, including the special situations with extended or eliminated timeframes (see above). Note that the guidance foresees the possibility for sponsors to supply further information once without extension of the review timeframe (under ideal circumstances).

Any clinical trial can only commence after both the favorable opinion of the Ethics Committee has been received in writing as well as the RA's notification of no grounds for objection (see above).

Usually, if, in the course of a trial, a substantial amendment to the protocol becomes necessary, a repeat opinion of the Ethics Committee must be sought before implementing any change. Substantial amendments are defined as amendments to the terms of the Research Ethics Committee's application, or to the protocol, or any other supporting documentation that is likely to affect to a significant degree any of the following:

- the safety or physical or mental integrity of the subjects of the trial;
- the scientific value of the trial;
- the conduct or management of the trial;
- the quality or safety of any investigational medicinal product used in the trial.

Note, however, that amendments that are made to reduce an immediate clinical hazard to the trial participants may be implemented immediately, and remains the primary responsibility of the designated medical monitor for the study, without prior written approval from the Ethics Committee. However, the investigator is under obligation to inform the Ethics Committee and the sponsor must inform the RA, both as soon as possible and in any case within 72 hours.

Minor amendments, also called "administrative amendments," do not have to be approved by the Ethics Committee or RA, although most research sites choose to notify the Ethics Committee of those changes on a periodic basis. These would include, for example, typographical errors, amended contact information, appointment of new support staff, and changes in the logistical arrangements for storing or transporting samples.

Finally, the Guidance also lays out the procedure of informing the Ethics Committee at the termination of a trial, and lists the required documentation to be submitted.

Clinical Trial Authorization (CTA) by member states' competent authority

The relevant Guidance is the "Detailed guidance for the request for authorization of a Clinical Trial on a medicinal product for human use to the competent authorities, notification of substantial amendments, and declaration of the end of the trial" (February 2007). Although existing trial authorizations from the pre-Directive period (e.g., in the UK

a CTX, CTC, DDX, or CTMPs) retained their validity, automatically becoming CTAs, the new process became mandatory for any trial commencing after May 1, 2004.

The CTA application process is a relatively straightforward, written procedure. It does not require extensive preparatory meetings with the regulators. The information on the IMP is necessarily not as complete as in a MA. The extent of information is proportional to the clinical phase of the protocol and must comply with the Guidance document for GMPs as they apply to IMPs (Annex 13, Rev 1 of the document) and the guideline on the requirements to the chemical and pharmaceutical quality documentation concerning IMPs in clinical trials.

The core of a CTA application in all MSs includes the following, which is submitted both to RAs and Ethics Committees:

- covering letter;
- EudraCT number;
- application form;
- investigator's brochure;
- protocol and amendments;
- protocol summary;
- list of competent authorities to which the application was submitted, and their decisions.

The supporting documentation, submitted only to the RA, comprises

- IMP dossier or simplified IMP dossier for known products;
- Summary of Product Characteristics (SPC)*;
- Ethics Committee approval*;
- outline of all active trials with the same IMP;
- IMP manufactured in EU: copy of manufacturer authorization;
- IMP not manufactured in EU: QP statement that site complies with EU GMP (or at least equivalent to EU GMP);
- IMP not manufactured in EU: copy of importer authorization;
- certificate of analysis for test product where impurities are not justified by the specification*;
- examples of IMP label;
- viral safety studies;
- authorization for GMO, radiopharmaceuticals (in the UK: ARSAC approval)*;

- TSE certificate* (Transmissible Spongiform Encephalopathy);
- declaration of GMP status of active biological substance;
- manufacturing license (on request);
- authorization for Contract Research Organization to represent sponsor*.

(* indicates if applicable and/or available)

Documents that need to be submitted to the Ethics Committee only are as follows:

- informed consent form;
- subject information;
- recruitment procedures, including advertisements, etc., and informed consent;
- all information to be provided to the subject, e.g., questionnaires, diaries etc.;
- peer review of trial*;
- ethical assessment made by the principal investigator;
- suitability of site and adequacy of facilities;
- suitability of investigator and key staff; résumés (CVs); name and address of investigator; information on key staff;
- funding and possible conflicts of interest;
- compensation;
- sponsor indemnity;
- investigator's insurance;
- payment to subjects;
- agreement between sponsor and investigator;
- publication policy and investigator's access to data, if not in protocol.

(* indicates if applicable and/or available

After receipt of the application, the submission is first validated, and then the review clock starts. The review clock stops when a query is raised, and begins again with the sponsor's response. The procedure will end with an affirmative decision (one way or the other). Sponsors *cannot*, however, presume CTA approval in the absence of receiving objections within the 60 days specified by the Directive. The review schedule for different products is identical for Ethics Committees and RAs. Many RAs have responded to the needs of the industry to shorten the review times and have agreed to review trials in shorter time periods, e.g., MHRA in the UK aims to review all CTA applications for Phase I trials within 14 to 21 days.

Radioactive IMPs

In this special case, additional approval is needed from the national authorities controlling radiation safety. For example, in the UK this is the Administration of Radioactive Substances Advisory Committee (ARSAC). Application to the ARSAC only requires a summary of the study protocol, but must include a careful scientific justification of the amount of radiation employed and the number of subjects exposed. The EU Directive 97/43/Euratom sets dose limits for healthy subjects and patients.

Good Clinical Practice (CLP)

The European Clinical Trial Directive has the central objective of protecting subjects taking part in medical research. The principles within the Declaration of Helsinki (as amended) are now integrated into the legal framework in GCP (and GMP, see next section). Briefly, these principles are as follows:

- Clinical trials should be conducted in accordance with the ethical principles that have their origin in the Declaration of Helsinki (as amended), and that are consistent with GCPs and the applicable regulatory requirements.
- Before the trial is started, foreseeable risks and inconveniences should be weighted against the anticipated benefit for the individual trial subject and society. (However, the Declaration has a central tenet that civilians must not be subjected to undue clinical hazards, without any potential for benefit themselves but in order to benefit society at large.)
- The rights, safety, and well-being of the trial subjects are the most important considerations and should prevail over interests of science and society.
- The available nonclinical and clinical information on an IMP should be adequate to support the proposed trial.
- Clinical trials should be scientifically sound and described in a clear, detailed protocol.
- The trial should be conducted in compliance with a protocol that has received Ethics Committee(s) and competent authority's approval.

• The medical care given to, and medical decisions made on behalf of, subjects should always be the responsibility of a qualified physician or dentist.

• Each individual involved in conducting a trial should be qualified by education, training, and experience to perform his or her respective tasks.

• Freely given informed consent should be obtained from every subject prior to clinical trial participation.

• All clinical trial information should be recorded, handled, and stored in a way that allows its accurate reporting, interpretation, and verification.

• The confidentiality of records that could identify subjects should be protected, respecting the privacy and confidentiality rules in accordance with the applicable regulatory requirements.

• Investigational products should be manufactured, handled, and stored in accordance with applicable GMP. They should be used in accordance with the approved protocol.

• Systems with procedures that ensure the quality of every aspect of the trial should be implemented.

For a fuller discussion of CLP, please see Chapter 13 of this book.

Good Manufacturing Practice (GMP)

Directive 2001/20 required that GMP was introduced into national law of MS. GMP inspections have long been standard for all companies at the time of a MAA, but there had previously been no such requirement for IMPs. This gap was thus closed.

Briefly, the components of GMP are as follows:

• A quality assurance system (Article 6).

• Appropriately qualified personnel with training documentation, organizational charts, and job descriptions that define roles, responsibilities, and hierarchy (Article 7).

• Premises and equipment appropriate and documented (Article 8).

• Documentation system for all processes with appropriate record keeping; up to date and free of errors (Article 9).

• Production to pre-established Standard Operating Procedures (SOP) and appropriate, validated in-process controls (Article 10).

• A quality control system and independent audit staff. Samples from each batch must be retained for testing and archiving, if at all practicable (Article 11).

• Any out-contracted work is subject to the same conditions and cannot be further delegated; precise contracts must define roles and responsibilities (Article 12).

• A system must be in place for complaints and product recall and notification of the Regulatory Authority (Article 13).

• Self inspection by the manufacturer with appropriate record keeping (Article 14).

Directive 2001/20 also requires that any site where IMPs are manipulated (other than pure administration to the trial subjects) should have a valid Manufacturer's License for GMP-compliant IMP preparation. Hospitals, health centers, or registered pharmacies are exempt from needing an IMP Manufacturer's License, provided that changes to the IMP are done under the supervision of a doctor or pharmacist for use at that site. A further exemption is when manipulation of the IMP is simply a reconstitution activity directly prior to drug administration (e.g., adding diluent to a lyophilized injectable). Contract Research Organizations (CROs) and commercial Phase I units are not exempt from these requirements, but can apply for a Manufacturer's License and are subject to inspection. The RAs issue IMP Manufacturer's Authorizations after a comprehensive GMP inspection of the applicant.

Importation of IMPs from non-EU countries is also strictly regulated by Directive 2001/20. The Community Code (Directive 2001/83) defines rules and circumstances under which re-testing or re-certification of both European-manufactured products and imported goods have to be performed.

Qualified persons (QPs)

A holder of a Manufacturer's License must have a QP. The QP's central role is to authorize batch release. The QP must be qualified by training and experience and the manufacturer must notify the competent authority of the name of the QP with supporting documentation for his or her qualification to fulfill this role.

Scientific advice and protocol assistance

Scientific advice

Scientific advice (SA) is provided by RAs so that sponsors can design drug development plans that, eventually, are likely to satisfy the reviewers for MA. The national authorities in Europe offer SA, on written request, and so does the EMA through the CHMP. Requesting SA from the CHMP can be sought irrespective of a product's eligibility for the centralized approval procedure. SA can be provided whenever no guidance or consultation document is available for a specific development plan. Which authority to approach with a request for SA is a sensitive case-by-case corporate decision with many considerations.

Scientific advice can be requested on Chemistry, Manufacturing, and Control (CMC), preclinical, and clinical development of a medicinal product, wherever issues are not covered by existing guidelines, or if a sponsor wishes to deviate from published guidance. SA should not be regarded as a pre-submission review. The advice given by the RAs is not binding on either the Regulatory Authority or the sponsor.

The timing of a SA request should be carefully planned. The CHMP and national authorities recommend that SA requests are best when made early in the development of a drug; follow-up questions on the advice provided, and renewal of questions throughout the development process are possible and encouraged.

Application procedure for SA

Scientific advice from the EMA

According to Regulation 726/2004, the CHMP established a permanent working party, the SAWP, with the sole remit of providing SA and Protocol Assistance (PA) to applicants. The mandate, objectives, and rules of procedure of SAWP are reported in EMEA/CHMP/SAWP/69686/04 Rev 7.

EMEA/H/4260/01/Rev.5 outlines the procedure to obtain the SA or PA and provides guidance for preparing the request. The highly structured, formal procedure does not necessarily include a face-to-face meeting between the company and the SAWP. Final advice is given in writing. It is binding for the applicant, not for the RA. Therefore any change introduced by the company must be scientifically justified. There is a substantial fee, although this varies according to the nature and extent of the questions on which the advice is sought. The procedure provides for follow-up requests after the original written SA response has been issued.

The SAWP is a multidisciplinary group with wide scientific expertise. It comprises one Chair and 27 members including 1 vice-chair person, one member of CAT, and 3 COMP members. The Chairperson of the SAWG is nominated by the CHMP for a term of three years, renewable. The Chair may or may not belong to the CHMP. The Vice-Chairperson is elected by and from among the SAWP members for a term of three years, renewable. The CHMP appoints the members for a term of three years. SAWP members may be CHMP members of EMA experts. In the nomination a fair representation of the following expertise needed for SA and PA is ensured: pharmaceutical development, toxicology, methodology and statistics, pharmacokinetics, and other therapeutic fields as appropriate. (The EMA publishes its list of European experts.) SAWP meets 11 times a year at the Agency, and these are advertised on the EMA website. The EMA is encouraging discussion without fee, before the official SA request is submitted.

A detailed description of the exact procedure, and the fees to be paid, can be found in the Scientific Advice Guidance Document on the EMA website. Applicants should inform the EMA Secretariat of the intention to submit a SA request about two months before start of the procedure through a formal letter of intent. The Agency will issue an invoice when the application is validated and fees will be payable within 45 calendar days of notification. The final, written SA response is issued within 40 to a maximum of 70 days, when it is formally adopted by the CHMP.

Scientific advice from national RAs

Scientific advice from individual national authorities, instead of the EMA, is also available. Applicants contact the national authority prior to sending the formal request, and the rest of the procedure, in most MS, is similar to that in the EMA procedure. With less administrative effort and more frequent presence of key members at the national authorities, SA at the national level is often quicker to obtain, and the costs are considerably less than that for the CHMP. However, national authorities will decline to give SA when it has also been requested from the CHMP, viewing the effort as duplication and redundant.

Protocol assistance

Protocol Assistance is a possibility offered to sponsors of orphan drugs. Its legal basis is laid down in article 6 of Regulation 141/2000 of December 16, 1999, on Orphan Medicinal Products. A sponsor may request PA from the EMA after the European Commission has granted the sponsor the designation of orphan drug status for a medicinal product. Although it is usually subject to payment of fees, there is an exception for orphan products. As in the case of scientific advice, PA may be given where no guidance is available in the form of adopted guidelines or consultation documents.

The SAWP is in charge of PA: EMEA/CHMP/SAWP/69686/04 Rev. 7 provides the framework and responsibilities of the working group. The SAWP may consult relevant working parties or Scientific Advisory Groups in relation to issues presented.

PA can be requested at any stage during initial development of the orphan medicinal product, but also during the post-authorization phase, on issues related to the therapeutic indication for which orphan state has been granted. However it cannot be used as a pre-submission consultation on data supporting a MAA application. Hence, a request for PA will not be accepted shortly before submission or during assessment of a MAA. PA is not binding, either on EMA/CHMP or on the sponsor.

The procedure for requesting PA and the timetable to be followed are basically the same as those defined for SA.

The request for PA should refer to prospective questions relating to the proposed development of the orphan product. The questions may concern the following:

- demonstration of significant clinical benefit of the orphan drug for the chosen indication;
- demonstration of clinical superiority over similar orphan products authorized for the same indication;
- problems relating to clinical plans and design of the trials.

Demonstration of clinical superiority over an already authorized product may involve methodological problems linked to the rarity of the disease, and may require alternative designs that emphasize the importance of the PA.

A follow-up PA may be expedient, to reconsider advice already provided, in the light of new information that may have become available.

The EU pediatric regulation

A new Pediatric Regulation 1901/2006 entered into force on January 26, 2007. The background of the Regulation is based on the consideration that a child is not a small adult. Most studies are performed in young adults, not in children, and suitable formulations are necessary.

The objective of the Regulation is to improve the health of children in Europe by

- facilitating the development and availability of medicines for children aged 0 to 17 years;
- ensuring that medicines for use in children are of high quality, ethically researched, and authorized appropriately;
- improving the availability of information on the use of medicines for children, without subjecting them to unnecessary trials or delaying the authorization of medicines for use in adults.

The Pediatric Regulation changed the regulatory environment for pediatric medicines in Europe substantially.

The pillars of the regulation are as follows:

- an expert committee, the pediatric committee (PDCO);
- an agreed pediatric investigation plan (PIP);
- a set of rewards and incentives;
- tools for information transparency and stimulation of research.

Pediatric Committee of the EMA (PDCO)

The main responsibility of the PDCO is to assess the content of pediatric investigation plans and adopt opinions on them in accordance with Regulation (EC) 1901/2006 as amended. This includes the assessment of applications for a full or partial waiver and assessment of applications for deferrals.

Other tasks of the Pediatric Committee include the following:

• Assessing data generated in accordance with agreed pediatric investigation plans and adopting opinions on the quality, safety or efficacy of any medicine for use in the pediatric population (at the request of the Committee for Medicinal Products for Human Use or a competent authority).

• Advising MSs on the content and format of data to be collected for a survey on all existing uses of medicinal products in the pediatric population.

• Advising and supporting the EMA on the creation of a European network of persons and bodies with specific expertise in the performance of studies in the pediatric population.

• Providing advice on any question relating to pediatric medicines (at the request of the EMA Executive Director or the European Commission).

• Establishing and regularly updating an inventory of pediatric medicinal product needs.

• Advising the EMA and the European Commission on the communication of arrangements available for conducting research into pediatric medicines.

The PDCO is not responsible for MAA for medicinal products for pediatric use. This remains fully within the remit of the CHMP. However, the CHMP or any other competent authority may request the PDCO to prepare an opinion on the quality, safety, and efficacy of a medicinal product for use in the pediatric population if these data have been generated in accordance with an agreed PIP.

The Pediatric Committee is composed of:

• five CHMP members with their alternates, appointed by the CHMP itself;

• one member and one alternate appointed by each MS (except MSs already represented through the members appointed by the CHMP);

• three members and alternates representing healthcare professionals, appointed by the European Commission;

• three members and alternates representing patients' associations, also appointed by the European Commission.

Members of the PDCO are appointed for a renewable period of three years.

Pediatric Investigation Plan (PIP)

Any new MAA or important variation of an existing MA requires that the applicant has agreed with the authorities a pediatric development program prior to submission of the application. The PIP is a development plan aimed at ensuring that the necessary data are obtained through studies in children, when it is safe to do so, to support the authorization of the medicine for children. The plan is submitted to the Pediatric Committee, which is responsible for agreement or refusal of the plan.

The PIP includes a description of the studies and of the measures to adapt the way the medicine is presented (formulation) to make its use more acceptable in children. For example, children cannot swallow big tablets, and so a liquid formulation may be more appropriate. The plan should cover the needs of all age groups of children, from birth to adolescence.

The plan also defines the timing of studies in children compared to adults. In some cases, studies will be deferred until after the studies in adults have been conducted, to ensure that research with children is done only when it is safe and ethical to do so. As some diseases do not affect children (for example, Parkinson's disease), the development of medicines for these diseases should not be performed in children, and so the requirement for a PIP will be waived in these cases. A list of class waivers has been published.

Products specific waivers may be requested, with appropriate justifications, in compliance with Art. 11 of the pediatric regulation. Applicability of a class waiver would require confirmation from the PDCO. This would facilitate future validation of the marketing application. If the PDCO considers class waiver not applicable, a product specific waiver or formal application for PIP should be submitted.

Even for products intended exclusively for use in adults, the PDCO is interested in being informed about the product to decide whether the it might fill a therapeutic need in another condition. This would be communicated and would allow submission of a PIP.

Following its assessment of any application for a PIP, including deferral, waiver, or modification of an agreed PIP, the PDCO formulates an opinion, which is delivered to the applicant. The applicant is then given an opportunity to request a re-examination of the opinion. In this case, the PDCO will consider the grounds for a re-examination of the opinion and will adopt a "definitive opinion" on the application. The EMA then adopts a decision, based on the definitive opinion of the PDCO, which the Agency communicates to the applicant. All decisions of the EMA on PIPs, deferrals, or waivers of the pediatric development are published.

Note that there is only one opportunity for re-examination of a PIP. In practice, the need to agree a PIP prior to an application submission has been an effective means to increase the systematic study of medicines for use in children.

A pediatric scientific advice may be requested. This would be given free of charge and may be requested prior to submission of PIP or during PIP implementation and may include advice on pharmacovigilance and risk management systems. The advice would not be binding on the Pediatric Committee.

All clinical trials, performed anywhere, should be included in the EudraCT database.

The European Commission issued a Guidance (2009/C 28/01) on the information concerning pediatric clinical trials to be entered into the EU database on clinical trials (EudraCT) and on the information to be made public by the EMA, in accordance with Art. 41 of Regulation 1901/2006.

The regulation also introduces a new type of MA: the Pediatric Use Marketing Authorization (PUMA).

This authorization can be applied for a medicine already authorized, but no longer covered by a patent, and to be exclusively developed for children. The development must follow an agreed PIP.

It can benefit from the centralized procedure (CP) and will be given ten years of market protection.

A number of scientific guidelines relating to pediatric development is available on the EMA website.

Marketing authorization

European controls on medicinal products were originally laid out in Directive 65/65, but it was Directive 75/319 that established the Committee for Proprietary Medicinal Products (CPMP) as the pivotal European medicines review committee. With the major revision of the medicines Regulation and the enlargement of the EU to today 27 MSs, the CPMP has been restructured and renamed as the Committee for Human Medicinal Products (CHMP), and it now comprises one representative from each MS (and often MSs co-opt a second representative and an alternative, to alleviate the requirement of presence for every one representative), as well as non-voting representatives from the European Economic Area countries (Norway, Iceland, and Liechtenstein). Currently, the CHMP meets during the third week of each month at the EMA headquarters in London.

There are two types of authorizations in the European Union:
- national authorizations;
- community authorizations.

National authorizations are granted by the competent authorities of the MSs. They concern products intended for a single national market and products authorized through the mutual recognition procedure (MRP) or decentralized procedure.

Community authorizations are granted to products filed through the centralized procedure, according to Regulation 726/2004. Such procedure leads to a single authorization valid throughout the EC: it cannot be revoked or changed at national level.

There are also two types of applications:
- complete;
- abridged.

Complete applications include all data foreseen by regulatory requirements, that is manufacturing and control data, pharmacological and toxicological tests, and clinical trials. There are three types of complete applications:

- full, independent applications including original data;
- mixed data applications, composed of both original tests and trials integrated by published scientific literature;
- biobliographical reference applications, where results of toxico-pharmacological tests and clinical trials are provided by published scientific literature: This type of application is governed by the requirements relating to well established constituents, as detailed in Art. 1 of Directive 2001/83 as amended.

Abridged applications are not required to include the results of toxico-pharmacological tests and clinical trials, because they refer to a product authorization through a full dossier.

These applications are foreseen in two cases:

- *Informed consent applications:* The Marketing Authorization Holder (MAH) of the original product has consented that reference is made to the nonclinical and clinical data contained in his original dossier.
- *Generic applications:* The medicinal product is a generic of a reference product authorized within the EU, whose patent is expired.

Since an abridged application does not contain all the data foreseen in a full application, reference cannot be made to another abridged application, but only to a full dossier.

In any case, and for all types of applications, manufacturing and control data must be fully developed and submitted.

The Common Technical Document (CTD)

The format of the submission dossier and the technical requirements are the same in all cases: the CTD has been compulsory in Europe for all submissions since 2003. The CTD format is described in ICH Guidance M4, and is organized in five modules (see also Figure 37.4):

- *Module 1* is specific to the region in which the application is made (the EU in this case) and is, technically, not part of the CTD. It contains regional administrative information, a comprehensive table of contents, the Summary of Product Characteristics (SPC; i.e., the draft package insert), the labeling, environmental risk assessment, information relating to market exclusivity for orphan drugs, forms with the experts' signature and their résumés (CVs), information relating to pharmacovigilance and to clinical trials conducted outside the EU, and pediatric information.

- *Module 2* contains the CTD Summaries. These are introduced with a table of contents for Modules 2–5 and an introductory document. The Summaries cover Manufacturing and Quality Control presented as "Quality Overview," nonclinical information, presented as a nonclinical overview and a nonclinical written and tabulated summary, clinical data presented as a clinical overview, and a clinical summary. Overviews are relatively short critical documents, comparable to the "expert reports" in previous forms of European submissions.
- *Module 3* contains the detailed manufacturing and quality data: it starts with its own table of contents, and then continues with the organized body of data and any applicable literature references.
- *Module 4* contains the nonclinical study reports. Like Module 3, it has its own table of contents, and then all the study reports and relevant literature references.
- *Module 5* contains the clinical study reports, again starting with a table of content for the module. A tabular summary of the studies is useful when inserted before the study reports themselves.

For most applications, English can be used for Modules 2–5. However, for national applications, some authorities require a national language and this should be checked with the RA well in time before submission. The EMA website provides administrative details concerning submissions, such as formats for electronic submission, which is practically the only format currently accepted.

Requirements for marketing authorization

Directive 65/65 established that a medicinal product can only be marketed after being authorized by the competent authority. Such obligation is reiterated in article 6 of Directive 2004/27 and article 3 of Regulation 726/2004.

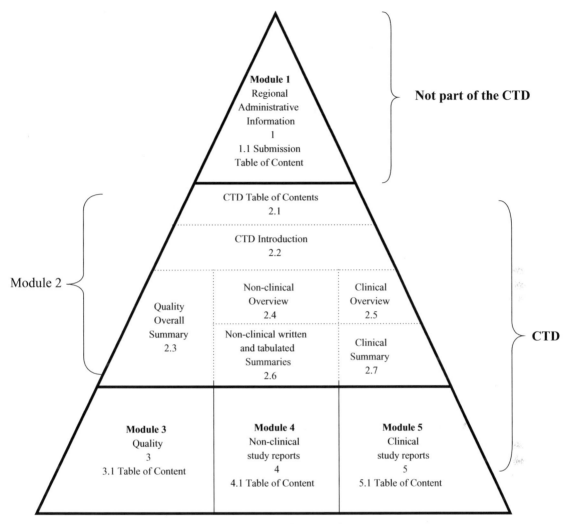

Figure 37.4 The organization of the ICH Common Technical Document (CTD).

Regulation 726/2004 covers biotech products and other innovative products as specified in the relevant annex; The main consequences of the changes of this Regulation will be introduced in the later section relating to the centralized procedure (CP).

Article 2 of Directive 2004/27 states that "this Directive shall apply to medicinal products for human use intended to be placed on the market in MSs and either prepared industrially or manufactured by a method involving an industrial process," whereas, according to Article 3, the following products are not included in the scopes of the Directive:

• Any medicinal product prepared in a pharmacy in accordance with a medical prescription for an individual patient (commonly known as the magistral formula).

• Any medicinal product that is prepared in a pharmacy in accordance with the prescription of a pharmacopoeia and is intended to be supplied directly to the patients served by the pharmacy in question (commonly known as the officinal formula).

- Medicinal products intended for research and development trials, but without prejudice to the provisions of Directive 2001/20/EC.
- Intermediate products intended for further processing by an authorized manufacturer.
- Any radionuclides in the form of sealed sources.
- Whole blood, plasma, or blood cells of human origin.

Criteria for granting a MA refer to quality, safety, and efficacy, which according to the new law "should enable the risk–benefit balance of all medicinal products to be assessed both when they are placed on the market and at any other time the competent authority deems this appropriate."

In fact a MA shall be refused if (Article 26)

- the risk–benefit balance is not considered to be favourable;
- the therapeutic efficacy is insufficiently substantiated by the applicant;
- the qualitative and quantitative composition is not as declared.

Authorization shall likewise be refused if documents submitted in support of the application do not comply with Directive requirements.

Article 26 of the Directive and Article 17 of the Regulation also state that "the applicant or holder of the MA shall be responsible for the accuracy of the documents and of the data submitted," which strengthens and formalizes the close relationship that must exist between Regulatory and Quality Assurance

A MA may be renewed after five years, based on a re-evaluation of the risk/benefit ratio, and after that the MA "shall be valid for an unlimited period, unless the competent authority decides, on justified grounds relating to pharmacovigilance, to proceed with an additional renewal."

An authorization will cease to be valid if the authorized product is not put on the market within three years after the authorization been granted, or if an authorized product is not present on the market for three consecutive years. Exemptions may be granted where justified.

Global marketing authorization

When a product has been granted an initial MA, any additional strength, dosage form, administra-

tion route, presentation, as well as any variation and extension shall be considered as belonging to the same, global MA. Thus the global MA contains the initial MA and all variations and extensions thereof authorized through separate procedures and also under a different name, granted to the MAH of the initial authorization. Where a product is initially authorized nationally and subsequently an additional strength or dosage form or route of administration is authorized through the centralized procedure, this shall also be part of the same global MA and multiple applications of the same MA are also covered by the notion of global MA.

Note that the term "global" refers to the dossier for European MA.

National application procedure

To obtain a national MA, an application is submitted to the competent authority of the MS. The documentation is the same as required for the MRP and the technical assessment should be completed within 210 days.

Since January 1998 independent national applications are limited to products that are to be authorized in not more than one MS, or to the initial phase of the MRP and decentralized procedure.

Mutual recognition procedure (MRP)

The legal basis for the procedure is Directive 2001/83, as amended by Directive 2004/27. The procedure requires MSs to recognize assessments done by any other of them, provided that no risk to the public health can be identified. Risk to the public health is a broad term, and can include any quality, safety, or efficacy issue within a particular national context. The MRP cannot be used for products falling under the mandatory scope of the centralized procedure (see the later section):

- The MRP is based on the principle of recognition of the technical assessment of an approved dossier, by the competent authorities of other MSs.
- The MRP can be used more than once for subsequent applications (repeat use).
- The MS that made the assessment is called the "Reference Member State" (RMS).

- The MSs where recognition of the MA is requested are called "Concerned Member States" (CMS).
- The RMS is chosen by the applicant and it is responsible for preparing an assessment report to be circulated to the CMS.
- The CMS must receive a dossier identical to that evaluated by the RMS.

The procedure is coordinated by the Coordination Group for the MRP and the decentralized procedure, the CMD(h) where "h" stands for human.

Following the initial approval by the RMS, the RMS will then facilitate communication between the applicant and the CMS. The CMS are not expected to conduct another assessment of the dossier, but rather declare whether they are in agreement with the assessment report and the SPC. The CMS may offer comments and suggestions for changing the SPC. When there are opinions that diverge between the RMS and the CMS, and if efforts to compromise fail, arbitration may be requested by CMS, or even (rarely) by the applicant. All CMS must check the correct translation of the SPC and labeling in their national language. The CMD(h) refers an application to arbitration by the CHMP if needed. The RMS later handles all post-marketing issues, such as variations and renewals.

The decentralized procedure

The decentralized procedure allows the applicant to submit an identical dossier for a new application, before any MA has been granted, in selected MS, asking the RMS to prepare a draft assessment report, a draft SPC, label, and package leaflet, and forward them to the CMS and applicant within 120 days after receipt of a valid application. Thereafter the procedure will not be different from the MRP and should be completed within 90 days, totaling the 210 days as foreseen for all national applications.

Both, the MRP and decentralized procedure can be used for full-length and abridged applications. Variations to an authorization obtained through the MRP or the decentralized procedure follow the same regulatory pathway. The MRP cannot be used for products that have received a negative opinion

in the CP or have been withdrawn from the CP (see below), except by submitting a completely new dossier.

Figure 37.5 provides a flowchart and timelines for the MRP (see also: *Notice to applicants: Procedures for Marketing Authorization Application, Vol. 2A*, Chapter 2, Mutual recognition, Revision 5, Feb 2007), and Figure 37.6 provides the same for the decentralized procedure.

To start an MRP, the applicant requests an assessment report of the dossier on which the MA has been granted, or the updating of an existing report from the licensing authority. Then the applicant requests the RMS to send the report to the CMS; the assessment report should be made available within 90 days. Possible changes and additions to the original dossier should be processed through the variation procedure. If a large volume of data is involved, a suitable timetable should be agreed with the competent authority of the RMS.

The applicant then submits the dossier to the CMS. The application must be accompanied by a declaration that all the dossiers filed as part of the procedure are identical, including the SPC. The SPC is the fundamental document on which mutual recognition is based. The applicant also informs the EMA that MRP is started, but a full dossier is only sent to the EMA in case of arbitration.

In all cases, the appropriate fees for the national applications must be paid and all necessary translations provided, at the time of the MRP submission. Chapter 7 of the *Notice to Applicants* provides, for each MS, the administrative details such as number of hard copies of the dossier, specified languages, samples of active substance and finished product, electronic formats, etc.

Each CMS submits the application to a check-in validation procedure and the MRP starts when the dossier is found valid and the assessment report has been sent to CMS. The MA granted by the RMS should be recognized within 90 days.

By day 50 of the procedure, CMS must communicate any objections to the RMS and the applicant. The applicant is allowed to discuss its position verbally or in writing. Objections are only permitted for major concerns for public health, and arbitration to the Community should be an exception to

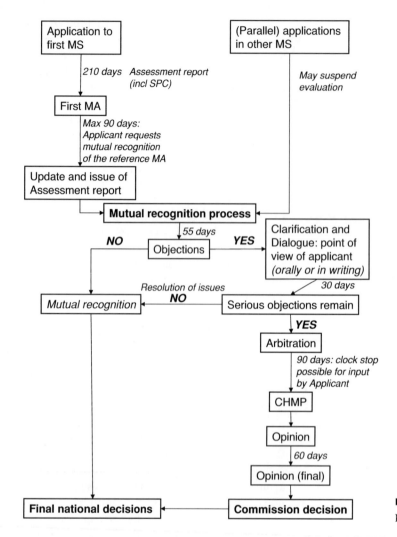

Figure 37.5 Mutual recognition procedure.

the general rule of mutual recognition. The MS who fails to recognize the MA must provide an in-depth justification of its position, also indicating what could be done to correct the identified deficiencies. The applicant is not allowed to present additional studies during the procedure, however it is acceptable to present additional analyses from studies already included in the dossier.

If by day 90, disagreements have still not been resolved, the matter may be referred to the EMA for arbitration.

The applicant is entitled to withdraw the application in any particular MS, and so avoid arbi-

tration. It must be noted though, that after withdrawal of the application from a CMS, no independent national application in that MS is permitted.

Whenever an arbitration procedure is initiated, the result is a decision by the European Commission, with the same pathway as for the CP (see below). The CHMP reaches its opinion, and if negative, the applicant has the opportunity to present an appeal, after which the Commission makes the final decision. The Commission's decision is binding on the RMS and all the CMS involved, and must be implemented within 30 days

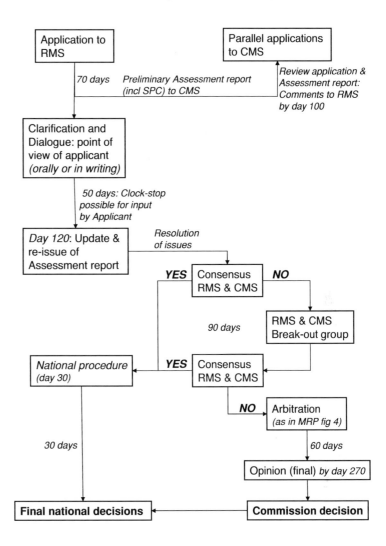

Figure 37.6 Decentralized procedure.

of issuance. These Commission decisions are made publicly available. Any CMS that had previously approved the RMS assessment report, the SPC, and the labeling can, at the request of the applicant, authorize the product within its territory without waiting for the outcome of the arbitration procedure. Nonetheless, if the arbitration procedure leads to a negative outcome, this national approval must be revoked within the 30 day implementation period.

MSs should set off the MRP on receipt of a national application for a product that has already been approved in another MS (Article 18, Directive 2004/27).

After the 90 days, the CMS should grant the national registration within 30 days. Experience shows that there are delays.

The MRP has several advantages. The processing time for applications is relatively rapid, and there are several elements of flexibility for the applicant (choice of RMS and CMS, provision of draft report). The MRP also allows for approvals to include different trade names for the same product, unlike the CP (see below). The MRP can be used many times, gradually including all MSs of the European Union.

An important exception from mutual recognition is the classification for supply; different MSs may decide to classify the same product differently.

Coordination group

The formally instituted coordination group, the CMD(h), replaced the informal Mutual Recognition Facilitation Group (MRFG), which had been active since 1995. This group issues guides, SOPs, recommendations, and position papers to help initiation and development of the MRP and decentralized procedure. The Coordination Group is composed of one representative per MS and is entitled to examine any question relating to MA of a medicinal product in two or more MSs.

Centralized procedure (CP)

The CP provides for a single application to result in a MA decision for the entire European Union. The CP concerns itself purely with the scientific and technical assessment of quality, safety, and efficacy of the product. Pricing, classification for supply, and marketing aspects (e.g., advertising) are left to the individual MSs. Thus, starting from an approved pan-European SPC, for each MS MAH may select from the approved indications, pack sizes, patient information leaflets, and so on, that fit the national health system. The main objective of the CP is that of creating a harmonized European environment for innovative products, through a highly qualified single assessment made on a single dossier, resulting in the same recommendations for use of the product throughout the EU, and thus ensuring the same safeguard for all EU citizens.

The CP is *compulsory* for products, which are (Regulation 726/2004):
- manufactured using recombinant DNA technology;
- synthesized through controlled expression of genes coding for biologically active proteins in prokaryotes and eukaryotes (including transformed mammalian cells);
- produced by hybridoma or other monoclonal antibody biosynthesis;
- veterinary products, intended primarily for use as performance enhancers in order to promote the growth of treated animals or to increase yields from treated animals;
- containing a new active substance(s) intended for the treatment of

- AIDS
- cancer
- neurodegenerative disorder
- diabetes
- auto-immune diseases, other immune dysfunction, and viral diseases;
- orphan medicinal products (see below).

Any medicinal product not included in the above list *may* use (but not compulsorily so) the CP if
- "the medicinal product contains a new active substance which, on the date of entry into force of the Regulation, was not authorized in the community; or
- the applicant shows that the medicinal product constitutes a significant therapeutic, scientific, or technical innovation or that the granting of authorization in accordance with this Regulation is in the interest of patients or animal health at Community level."

Abridged applications are possible for products that have previously been approved through the CP.

Generic applications of centrally-authorized products may be authorized by the competent authorities of MSs through the national, MRP, or decentralized procedures, provided they retain the same SPC and the same name in all MS.

The CP is divided into the following phases:
1. Pre-submission;
2. Submission and validation of the dossier;
3. Payment of fees;
4. Scientific evaluation;
5. Decision-making process;
6. Commission decision;
7. Post-authorization provisions.

Pre-submission activities

Four to six months before a planned CP submission, the applicant has to notify the EMA of the intention to file an application and provide an estimate for the date of submission. The notification should include information on the product (a draft SPC), the legal basis for the application (whether complete or abridged), proposal for classification for supply, justification for request of MA using the CP, information on manufacturing and batch release arrangements that may be linked to pre-authorization inspections, and the proposed product trade name.

Only one trade name can be proposed within the CP (unlike for the MRP), although a second may exceptionally be permitted when there is good reason to show that a single name cannot be used throughout the EU. Trade name proposals can be submitted to the EMA even 12 months before filing the application, in case of any doubt on this point, where they are evaluated by the Name Review Group (NRG), which will check with national authorities whether the name may be misleading for its therapeutic use or could otherwise generate confusion, create safety problems, or offend against local anti-promotional Regulations. The NRG ignores any aspect relating to intellectual property rights. CP applications without suitable trade names can be filed using a generic or chemical name, together with the name of the manufacturer.

Pre-submission meetings are held with the Agency, primarily to receive advice on preparing a submission in compliance with procedural, regulatory, and legal requirements. These meetings are also an important opportunity to establish a good working relationship with the personnel who will handle the application, and in particular, the project manager who will coordinate all the review activities.

Next, three to four months before submission, the CHMP will appoint the Rapporteur and Co-rapporteur. These are the members of the CHMP who will be responsible for the scientific assessment of the dossier. The specific expertise of CHMP members and the overall workload distribution among the CHMP members are taken into account for the appointment of the Rapporteurs. The applicant cannot appeal these appointments.

Submission and validation of the dossier

The submission date should be agreed with the EMA and planned in such a way as to match, following the predefined review schedule, with CHMP meetings. Since January 1, 2009, the EMA has recommended electronic only submissions, either e-CTD or non-e-CTD, and commencing July 1, 2009, e-CTD only submissions are strongly recommended. Paper and other electronic formats would

now be an exception. Similarly, Rapporteurs and CHMP member should receive e-CTD documents.

The Agency sends an acknowledgment of receipt of the dossier and starts the validation process. In the event the EMA requires additional data or clarifications to complete the validation, the additional data will be provided within a specified time limit. Copies of any additional information should also be sent to the Rapporteur and Co-rapporteur. In the case of positive outcome of the validation, the applicant is notified in writing including the timetable for the evaluation. If the dossier is found severely deficient or the applicant fails to provide the required information, the validation will be failed and thus the submission rejected for review.

Payment of fees

The EMA will issue an invoice on the date of notification of validation and fees are payable within 45 days of notification.

If the application cannot be validated, the EMA will issue an invoice to charge the administrative cost of non-validation

Submission of dossier (continued)

The Agency will also set up a Product Team, consisting of a Product Team Leader (PTL) and product team members. The team will be responsible for the handling of all the procedural aspects of the application and acts as a liaison between the EMA and the applicant. It will be involved in all phases of the evaluation and participates in all discussions with the applicant.

Applicants for a MA must have a legal representative resident within the EU. Furthermore, the application must identify persons with the following responsibilities (including relevant addresses and phone numbers):

- QP for pharmacovigilance;
- responsible person for scientific communications, and in overall charge of the information on the product;
- QP responsible for batch release and contact person for product defects and recalls.

If the application is for a product containing or consisting of genetically modified organisms

(GMO), it is also required to provide:

- evidence that the relevant competent authorities approve of the use of the GMO for this research and development purpose; and
- the complete technical dossier for the GMO itself (per Directive 2001/18) together with the environmental risk assessment.

The applicant may be requested to submit to inspections to verify compliance with GMP, GLP, and GCP. The responsibility for performing inspections rests with the inspection services of the competent authorities of the EU MSs or the countries of the EEA. On advice of the Rapporteur/Co-rapporteur, the inspection team may include scientific experts and/or a Rapporteur. Inspections are carried out on behalf of the EU and are coordinated by the EMA.

Scientific evaluation

The CHMP renders its scientific opinion with an overall deadline of 210 days. The Rapporteur and Co-rapporteur prepare draft assessment reports during the first 80 days, and send them to the CHMP and the EMA secretariat, who in turn send them to the applicant. After exchange of comments and opinions between the Rapporteurs and the CHMP, a collated list of questions is sent to the applicant by day 120. The review clock is stopped at this point, and restarts with the applicant's response. If the applicant believes that more than six months are needed to answer the list of questions, the application should be withdrawn.

On the day when written responses are received, the review clock restarts with day 121. The Rapporteurs assess the responses, and submit their final assessment report by day 150. The final assessment is again sent to the CHMP, the EMA, and the applicant. CHMP members have until day 170 to file any comments. Outstanding issues are discussed at a CHMP meeting by day 180.

If any unresolved issues remain at this stage, the CHMP or the applicant can request a meeting for oral explanation. The review clock is stopped (usually not for more than a month), so that the applicant can prepare for this meeting.

After the oral explanation, the clock is restarted at day 181. The applicant sends the final draft SPC, package leaflet, and labeling (revised as needs be) to the Rapporteurs, the CHMP, and the EMA. The CHMP adopts a final opinion, either positive or negative, by a single majority vote at a CHMP meeting on or before day 210.

In case of a positive opinion, between days 210 and 240 the applicant prepares the final SPC and labeling in all the 22 required languages. Between days 240 and 300, the EPAR (European Public Assessment Report) is finalized in agreement with the applicant. The EPAR is published, after the Commission decision, on the EMA website. Similarly, where the MA is refused, which constitutes a prohibition to market the product throughout the Community, the EMA makes the reason for refusal publicly available through a "refusal EPAR" following the Commission decision.

A negative opinion may be subject to appeal. The EMA informs the applicant of the reasons for an unfavorable conclusion and provides details on the divergent opinions of the CHMP members (if any). The applicant then has 15 days within which to notify an intent to appeal to the EMA. The detailed grounds for the appeal must then be provided within 60 days, and the applicant may also request a meeting at the CHMP to provide justification for the appeal. The CHMP would appoint new Rapporteurs, and within 60 days of the receipt of the grounds for appeal will consider whether the opinion can be revised. No meeting is granted within this 60-day time frame. During the appeals process, no new study can be presented, and a revised opinion may only be issued concerning the same data as originally presented.

Decision-making procedure and Commission decision

The EC or where relevant the Council converts the scientific opinion of the EMA into a legally binding decision for MSs. In this phase of the centralized procedure, the Commission is assisted by its Standing Committee of Medicinal Products, whose members, appointed by MS, receive the documents. The draft decision must occur within 15 days of receipt of the EMA opinion (ref Regulation 726/2004), and is forwarded to MSs and the applicant. Verification of the draft decision must then be completed in 22 days.

A MS may still raise objections to the Commission's draft decision, and ask for a meeting of the Standing Committee of Medicinal Products. If the objections identify important issues not addressed in the EMA opinion, the decision-making procedure is suspended and a new opinion is requested of the EMA. A further Standing Committee review follows the EMA reply. A favorable opinion of the Standing Committee is adopted as a decision within 15 days and is published in the Official Journal.

Very rarely, the Commission, being politically and legally responsible for the approval decision, may disagree with the scientific opinion adopted by the EMA even after Standing Committee review. In this case, the decision is submitted to the Council. If within three months of submission the Council has not made a decision, the Commission will adopt its own proposed decision.

Post-authorization provisions

Marketing authorizations may contain commitments of the applicant to the EMA for various actions, which have to be fulfilled and reported to the EMA in order to maintain the validity of the granted MA. These provisions are frequently related to risk management of the newly approved product and will be laid out in the Risk Management Plan with a timetable for reporting of the measures taken. Post-authorization Safety Studies (PASS) are a typical post-authorization commitment, and fall under special regulations provided in Volume 9A (see later in this chapter).

Application withdrawals

Applicants withdrawing their dossiers do so at some cost. An explanation why the dossier is being withdrawn must be provided to the EMA, and this information will be published. The EMA will also publish assessment reports if prepared at this time.

Expedited reviews

The new Regulation foresees the possibility of an expedited procedure of only 150 days duration, for products of major interest for public health that are addressing an unmet medical need. Also a conditional approval may be granted, which would be reviewed yearly.

Conditional MA

A conditional MA is a MA based on incomplete data, usually, clinical data. It may be granted for products intended for seriously debilitating or life-threatening diseases. It will be valid for one year on a renewable basis, but will not remain conditional indefinitely. The applicant is required to submit a plan for data completion, which shall be made publicly available.

MA under exceptional circumstances

In special cases, when for instance the indication is so rare that the applicant cannot be expected to provide comprehensive evidence, or in the current state of scientific knowledge comprehensive information cannot be provided, or it would medically unethical to collect such information, a MA under exceptional circumstances may be granted. It will be submitted to annual reassessment of the conditions.

Exclusivity

All medicines approved through the CP will be granted an eight-year period of data protection and a ten-year period of marketing protection (see below). This period can be extended to 11 years if during the first 10 years a major new indication is developed.

Once a product has been approved through the centralized procedure, all further regulatory activities, such as license variations, labeling changes, new indications, and so on must be CP submissions.

Community referral

The European pharmaceutical legislation includes mechanisms whereby a Community arbitration may be triggered on the basis of specific articles of Directive 2001/83, as amended. The arbitration ends up in a binding decision, issued after a scientific evaluation of the matter involved. The CHMP is responsible for the evaluation and will endorse the referral as admissible when the issue to be discussed can be framed in the relevant articles of Directive 2001/83 EC.

A referral may be started not only for a particular medicinal product, but also for a specific class of products. Community referrals are contemplated in cases foreseen by the following articles of Directive 2001/83 EC:

• *Article 29—Mutual recognition referral:* This applies whenever a concerned MS, during a Mutual Recognition Procedure, considers that a product may present a risk to public health. Rules and procedures involved are described in the earlier section, Mutual Recognition Procedure.

• *Article 30—Divergent decisions referral:* This article applies whenever divergent national decisions are taken by MSs concerning authorization, suspension, or withdrawal of a medicinal product. The procedure covers purely national MAs or MAs issued following a MRP, in cases, for example, where:

   – indications significantly diverge in different MS;

   – a product is suspended or withdrawn in one or more, but not all, concerned MSs;

   – a national authorization is varied, introducing a divergence versus other national authorities.

   The referral may be started by any MS, the Commission, or the MAH.

• *Article 31—Community interest referral:* This article applies to conditions where the interest of the Community are involved. This may especially refer to public health issues related to a product marketed in the EU, in the light of new data emerged on quality, safety, efficacy, or pharmacovigilance. The referral may be started by MSs, the Commission, or the applicant/MAH.

• *Articles 35, 36, 37—Follow up referrals:* These articles refer to arbitration mechanisms aimed at resolving divergences after harmonization has been achieved on a particular product already submitted to a community procedure and a MS considers that a change/variation, suspension, or withdrawal of a harmonized MA may become necessary for protection of public health. Likewise, by reference to article 5(11), 6(12), 6(13) of Regulation 1084/2003, one or more MS may not recognize a draft decision of the Reference MS on a variation. In this case, therefore the CHMP will issue an opinion on the variation to the terms of a MA, its suspension or withdrawal, where such actions are justified by public health issues. These referrals may be started by the MS or the MAH.

Procedure

To start a referral procedure different forms must be used, according to the type of referral; such forms are annexed to the Guideline included in the Notice to Applicant Volume 2A, Procedures for Marketing Authorization, Chapter 3, Community Referral, February 2004.

Before starting a referral procedure, a notification should be sent to the EMA, stating

• the intention to submit a referral;

• information on the medicinal product concerned;

• clear and concise formulation of the questions to be discussed;

• proposal on the documentation to be provided;

• where appropriate, request for a meeting with the EMA to deal with issues linked to the referral.

The scientific opinion on the referral questions will be provided by the CHMP and all the pertinent documentation should be submitted by the MS or applicant/MAH.

Where the referral follows the suspension or withdrawal of a product from the market in a MS, this MS should immediately inform the CHMP members, the authorities of the other MSs, and the EMA of the action taken.

If the referral is started by an applicant/MAH, the documentation submitted should include the expert reports updated with the data supporting the reasons for referral.

Timeframe for the referral

The CHMP issues a reasoned opinion within 90 days of the referral. This period may be extended to 180 days in case of Article 30, 31, 36, and 37 referrals.

The timetable is described in detail in Volume 2a of the above guideline.

The clock of the procedure may be stopped to allow the applicant to prepare explanations, to be submitted or discussed in a hearing.

The opinion of the CHMP may be subject to appeal; the intention to appeal should be notified to the EMA within 15 days after the opinion has been issued and within 60 days the detailed grounds for appeal must be forwarded to the EMA. A final opinion will be adopted by the CHMP within the following 60 days, together with an assessment report, stating the reasons for the conclusions reached. In the event of an opinion in favor of granting or maintaining a MA the opinion will include a draft SPC, the proposed labeling, and any condition deemed to be relevant for the safe and effective use of the product. This opinion will be sent within 15 days to MSs, the Commission, and the applicant/MAH.

The subsequent Commission's decision-making procedure is essentially the same as for the centralized procedure. But the decision is not only addressed to the applicant, but also to the MSs concerned in the referral, who are required to take actions, such as grant, suspend, or withdraw a MA, as established in the decision within 30 days following its notification. The MSs are also required to inform the Commission and the CHMP of the measures taken.

Consequences of the decision

The decision following a referral is only applicable to the products and MSs involved in the procedure.

In the case where an Article 29 referral (mutual recognition referral) relates to a product with MA in MSs other than those involved in the procedure, a new Article 30 referral can be triggered for those MAs to pursue harmonization of the SPC. This is also applicable to cases where a MA is pending for the product submitted to referral: the MSs are obliged to grant or reject the MA in conformity with the Community decision.

Subsequent applications for the same medicinal product, must follow the community decision, and use the harmonized SPC.

Stopping of the referrals

In the case of an Article 29 (mutual recognition) referral, an application may be withdrawn by the applicant at any time in any MS where it has been submitted. This action may avoid the referral. However if an issue of Community interest is identified,

MSa or the Commission may start an Article 31 referral.

For referrals relating to Articles 30, 31, and for follow-up referrals, the procedure can only be stopped if the applicant/MAH withdraws the concerned product from all the EU markets. In such a case, the CHMP may decide to close the referral procedure, or to proceed in spite of the withdrawal, where public health issues are considered to need continuing discussion.

Unilateral actions by MSs in urgent cases

MSs may take unilateral urgency measures, such as suspending the marketing and use of a medicinal product, whenever such action is deemed necessary to protect public health, and until a final decision is adopted. The EMA must be informed on the following working day, and the matter is discussed in the following CHMP meeting. A referral procedure, where appropriate, may be triggered by either a MS or the Commission.

Overall, these procedures have not been extensively used; as to Article 29 referral, applicants have preferred, in most cases, to withdraw the application in the countries unwilling to accept the mutual recognition, rather than go through the CHMP arbitration and face possibly unfavorable consequences.

However, it should be reminded that such procedures have to be regarded in the perspective of the general scope of achieving the highest possible degree of harmonization within the Community.

Orphan medicinal products

Orphan medicinal products are defined as those diagnosing, treating, or preventing life-threatening or very serious conditions that affect no more than 5 per 10,000 persons in the European Union.

Regulation EC 141/2000 established the Committee for Orphan Medicinal Products (COMP) formed by one representative from each MS, three from various patients groups, and three from the EMA to liaise with CHMP. The role of COMP is to

- help sponsors to prepare orphan designation applications through free pre-submission meetings;
- provide SA on the development of the product after orphan designation has been granted;
- examine applications for designation of orphan drug status;
- assist the European Commission on development of orphan drug policies.

The incentives for orphan products are: market exclusivity for ten years after the MA, even if a previously authorized product is now developed for a new orphan indication; protocol assistance (SA on development and dossier preparation); access to the centralized registration procedure; fee reduction for all types of regulatory activities (applications review, inspections, variations, SA, etc.); and provision of a limited amount of EU-funded research grants for orphan products.

Orphan designation can be applied for at any stage of the development with appropriate scientific justification. The designation of an orphan product is preliminary to application for a MA, and entitles the sponsor to the above-listed incentives for development of the drug.

Sponsors need to notify the EMA of the intent to file an application for orphan designation. A pre-submission meeting with COMP will be arranged, if viewed as desirable. The submission is usually validated within 10 days of receipt, and then the COMP will assess the submission within a further 60–90 days. When the COMP has adopted an opinion, it is send to the European Commission, whose binding decision is issued within a further 30 days. Orphan drug designations are published in the Official Register on the EMA website, after applicants have had the opportunity to review a draft and redact proprietary information.

Generic medicinal products

Directive 2004/27 provides the following definition of generic medicinal product (Article 10, 2. (b): "generic medicinal product shall mean a medicinal product which has the same qualitative and quantitative composition in active substances and the same pharmaceutical form as the reference pharmaceutical product, and whose bioequivalence with the reference medicinal product has been demonstrated." As a result of various recent treaties, Europe, like the rest of the world, recognizes patent protection on all new inventions for 20 years after the patent application is filed. However, in the special case of medicinal products, where the long development cycle allows a product onto the market only late in the life of the patent, a supplementary patent protection for a maximum of five years can be applied for, under certain circumstances. While detailed discussion of European patent law is outside the scope of this chapter, we shall adopt a general definition for a "generic drug" as one that is approved as a bioequivalent product after the innovator's patent has expired.

Nomenclature

Dossiers for generic products must be as complete for all quality and manufacturing aspects as any innovator product. However, a generic drug dossier can merely reference an innovator's dossier for data concerning product safety and efficacy. For this reason the application for a generic product is also known as an "abridged" application.

The innovator's product is termed a "reference medicinal product" for the same reason. This is a product that has a legally valid MA in a (some) MS(s), which was granted on the basis of a full-length dossier.

Application to market a generic medicinal product can be made in one MS even when the reference product is only authorized in a different MS. In this case, the MS in which the reference product is marketed can be asked to transfer a copy of all the relevant documents by the MS holding the generic application. There is a one month deadline for this.

Quite apart from patent protections, innovator products are granted eight years of data protection and ten years of market exclusivity (see above), plus a further year of market exclusivity if a major new indication is registered. This means that a generic medicinal product can be placed on the market only 10 (or 11) years after the original authorization, although experimental activities to prepare the dossier, in particular to conduct bioequivalence studies, can start two or three years earlier.

Following the CTD format, a generic application must contain

- Module 1 (administrative information);
- Module 2 (overviews and summaries);
- Module 3 (quality).

Bio-equivalence data, since they refer to clinical experimentation, are submitted in a separate binder, following the numbering system of Module 5 (Section 5.3.1.2).

Drug substance

Different salts, esters, ethers, and derivatives of the same active moiety will not be considered different active substances if they have the same characteristics of safety and efficacy. Proof of absence of significant differences must be supplied by the applicant through appropriate studies, the extent and content of which has to be decided on a case-by-case basis.

Different manufacturers may follow different synthetic pathways, which may originate different impurity profiles. It is the generic applicant's responsibility to define the impurity profile, provide impurity levels, their characterization, and biological qualification according to current guidelines. Presence of a toxic impurity, or an impurity endowed with a particular biological activity, not present in the reference product, make the latter an inappropriate reference; this may drive the decision to change the reference product. Toxicity of impurities should be discussed in the nonclinical overview, with cross-references to the quality overview.

Whenever an active substance is the subject of a pharmacopoeia monograph, suitability of the monograph for the substance must be controlled. On request of the active substance manufacturer, the *European Pharmacopoeia* issues Certificates of Suitability (CEP), which replace the information of the corresponding sections and allows reference to the pharmacopoeia monograph. Any technical characteristics not covered by the certificates must be supplied as additional information.

Drug product

A generic product should comply with the following characteristics:

- Same qualitative–quantitative composition of the active ingredient as the reference product.
- Known excipients of established use.
- Same pharmaceutical form. Oral solid pharmaceutical forms of immediate release, such as tablets and capsules. are regarded as the same dosage form.
- Bioequivalence with the reference product.

The note for guidance CPMP/EWP/QWP/1041/98 on investigation of bioavailability and bioequivalence sets the criteria for showing pharmacokinetic equivalence and thus permit waiver of extensive clinical trials for demonstration of efficacy.

Two products are considered bioequivalent when the drug substance, in the same molar concentration, is absorbed at the same rate and extent. Authorization of a generic product is essentially based on demonstration of identical bioavailability that is defined as the rate and extent at which an active ingredient is absorbed and becomes available at the site of action.

In the great majority of cases, medicines are intended for a systemic therapeutic activity. Therefore, being difficult or impossible to measure the quantity of active substance at the site of action, it is accepted that equivalence of levels in the systemic circulation, or other biological fluids, are accepted as surrogates of therapeutic equivalence.

For the typical generic application, a bioequivalence study against a reference product in a crossover, single, and/or multiple dose design in healthy volunteers (or patients wherever appropriate) is used to demonstrate bioequivalence. The CPMP "Note for Guidance on Investigation of Bioavailability and Bioequivalence" provides details on design and conduct of studies, statistical and analytical aspects, selection of subjects, and conditions for study standardization. The number of subjects to be included depends on many factors, such as the variability of the primary characteristic to be assessed, the predetermined significance level, and the required power. In any case not less than 12 subjects should be used. Clinical therapeutic bioequivalence must always be documented for oral modified release and transdermal dosage forms.

Rarely, waivers from human bioequivalence can be granted, although these are only under the most straightforward situations imaginable. The commonest case is that of a generic, intravenous, aqueous solution containing the same active drug at the same concentration. The same concept can be extended to intramuscular and subcutaneous injectables, when the test and reference products consist of the same type of solution with the same or comparable excipients. This does not extend to topical products, however, when a bioequivalence study must always be carried out if a systemic action is expected.

Different problems are encountered for approval of "copies" of biotechnologically derived products. The issue is of practical relevance since the patent of many biological products has or is going to expire. Biotechnology derived products may represent a scientific and regulatory challenge, insofar as the synthetic process takes place inside a living organism. The synthetic process cannot be controlled directly and this fact alone introduces a series of aspects linked to factors, which are certainly more difficult to control and standardize. Years ago the regulatory thinking for biotech products was based on the paradigm "the process defines the product"; implying that changes in manufacture could result in changes in the product difficult or impossible to detect, with the risk of non-therapeutic biological responses. This excluded, in practice, the possibility of generic applications for biotech products.

Now there has been a substantial change in attitude toward biotech products: technological improvement and higher sophistication of analytical methodology make it possible to design integrated control strategies allowing physicochemical characterization to begin to shift the focus from the process to the product.

In any case, Article 10 of Directive 2004/27 introduces the concept of "similar products" as follows:

> Where a biological medicinal product, which is similar to a reference biological product, does not meet the conditions in the definition of generic medicinal product, owing to, in particular, differences relating to raw materials or differences in manufacturing process of the biological medicinal product and the reference biological medicinal product, the results of appropriate preclinical tests or clinical trials relating to these conditions must be provided. The type and quantity of supplementary data to be provided must comply with the relevant criteria stated in Annexe 1 and the related detailed guidelines. The results of other tests and trials from the reference medicinal product's dossier shall not be provided.

Note that the Directive makes two important points: (i) similar biological products are legally admitted and (ii) at least partial reference to the originator dossier is acceptable, making it possible to prepare a dossier based on "bridging studies," to be decided on a case-by-case basis. A corresponding Guidance has also been published (EMEA/CPMP/BWP/3207/00/Rev.1, EMEA/CPMP/3097/02/final).

When considering how extensive the comparative studies must be, the following factors are relevant:
- stage where the manufacturing change is introduced;
- potential impact of the change on product characterization;
- suitability of analytical techniques to detect potential modifications;
- relationship between established quality criteria with safety and efficacy results, based on the overall preclinical and clinical experience.

Where similarity to an already authorized product is claimed, the nonclinical and clinical data to be submitted will probably be decided on the basis of the following considerations:
- the extent to which the product may be characterized;
- the nature of the changes in the new product compared to the reference product;
- the observed/potential differences between the two products;
- the clinical experience with the particular class of products.

One critical issue may be that of immunogenicity. This must always be investigated, and a plan for a post-marketing monitoring must be included in any "generic biological product" application.

Herbal medicinal products

Herbal medicinal products represent a large market in the EU, although unevenly distributed across MSs. Although there is a separate chapter on Complementary Medicines in this book (Chapter 33), we must here consider the special regulatory approach that is taken towards these distinctive products within the European Union. The following definitions are from the Guidance CPMP/QWP/2820/00:

• *Herbal medicinal products* are medicinal products containing exclusively herbal drugs or herbal drug preparations as active substances.

• *Herbal drugs* are mainly whole, fragmented, or cut plants, part of plants, algae, fungi, or lichen, in an unprocessed state, usually in dried form but sometime fresh. Certain exudates that have not been subjected to a specific treatment are also considered herbal drugs. Herbal drugs are precisely defined by the botanical scientific name according to the binomial system (genus, species, variety, and author).

• *Herbal drug preparations* are obtained by subjecting herbal drugs to treatments such as extraction, distillation, expression, fractionation, purification, concentration, or fermentation. These include comminuted or powdered herbal drugs, tinctures, extracts, essential oils, expressed juices, and processed exudates.

Differences in criteria and methods of assessment of the characteristics and properties of herbal products may represent a risk for consumers and an obstacle to their free circulation within the Community. Therefore, in 1997, an *"ad hoc* working group" was established at the EMA, which was tasked with addressing the problems of demonstration of quality, safety, and efficacy. Subsequently the group became a permanent Working Party of the CPMP and developed a set of guidelines on the requirements and assessment of herbal medicines.

The revised legislation (Regulation 726/2004) established a new committee within the structure of the EMA named the Committee on Herbal Medicinal Products (HCMP). This committee has the task to provide "the MSs and the institutions of the Community with the best possible Scientific Advice on any question relating to the evaluation of the quality, safety and efficacy of medicinal products," as well as advising interested parties on the conduct of the various tests and trials necessary to demonstrate quality, safety, and efficacy.

The complex composition of herbal medicines makes quality a fundamental and critical aspect, that have been dealt with in two guidelines:

• *Note for Guidance on Quality of Herbal Medicinal Products*: CPMP/QWP/2819/00;

• *Note for Guidance on Specifications: Test Procedures and Acceptance Criteria for Herbal Drugs, Herbal Drug Preparations and Herbal Medicinal Products*: CPMP/QWP2820/00.

The first guideline addresses special quality issues of herbal products because of the difference to products containing chemically pure, well-defined active substances. This document, should be read in conjunction with Annex 7 "Manufacture of Herbal Medicinal Products" of Volume 4 of the Rules governing Medicinal Products in the EU. GMP recommendations should be respected and consistent quality can only be ensured when

• starting materials are defined in a rigorous and detailed manner, including the specific botanical identification, geographical origin, and the conditions under which the herbal drug is obtained;

• the manufacturing process of the finished product, starting from a herbal drug or a herbal drug preparation, is described in a detailed manner, including in-process controls with details of test procedures and limits, as defined in the "Note for Guidance on Manufacture of the Finished Dosage Form" (Vol. 3 of the Rules governing Medicinal Products in the EU).

The second guideline provides the general principles for setting specifications for herbal drug preparations, as required to build up an application for a MA of a herbal medicinal product. The document therefore defines the criteria to be followed and reports a list of physicochemical and biological tests relevant for an overall quality control strategy and consistency of quality and characteristics of herbal drugs, herbal drug preparations, and herbal medicinal products.

Traditional herbal medicinal products

A MA for a herbal medicinal product may be submitted, as for any medicinal product, through a full application with new tests and trials, whenever the application refers to a new product or a therapeutic innovation. Alternatively, for a well-established drug (defined in Directive 99/83) a bibliographic application may be submitted, when safety and efficacy for a given indication, dose, and patient population are satisfactorily described in the published literature.

There is, however, a large number of herbal products that in spite of having been used for a long time are not supportable by data that qualifies for well-established use with recognized efficacy and acceptable safety. The political decision was made that, within limits, the public interest in keeping these products on the market could outweigh imposing a burden of clinical experimentation, while also eliminating differences in requirements and Regulations in different MSs that could cause distortions in commerce. Thus, Directive 2004/24 was issued, which amends Directive 2001/83 and the Community Code relating to medicinal products for human use. This new Directive creates a category of "Traditional Herbal Medicinal Products" as well as provides for a simplified procedure for their MA. Even when the definition of herbal medicinal product/herbal drug/herbal preparation is actually the same as those mentioned above, the Directive also allows the presence of vitamins and minerals, if of well-documented safety, in the composition of herbal products, provided that their action is ancillary with respect to the herbal ingredient.

A "traditional herbal medicinal product" should comply with the following characteristics:
• indication does not require the supervision by a medical practitioner for diagnostic purposes or for prescription or monitoring of treatment;
• administration according to a specified strength and posology;
• administration exclusively by oral, external, and/or inhalatory route;
• bibliographical or expert evidence to the effect that the product itself, or a corresponding product, has been in medicinal use throughout a period of at least 30 years preceding the date of the application, including at least 15 years within the Community;
• data on the traditional use are sufficient to prove that the product is not harmful in the specified conditions of use and the pharmacological effects or efficacy are plausible on the basis of long-standing use and experience.

The simplified procedure for registration of traditional herbal medicinal products includes full administrative information and a complete pharmaceutical dossier on the assumption that the quality of the product is independent of its traditional use. Nonclinical data are not necessary where information on the traditional use proves that the product is not harmful in the specified conditions of use. However, where concerns are raised with regard to the product's safety, the competent authorities may ask for additional data necessary to assess safety. The dossier will therefore include a bibliographic review of safety data, and additional data where required, together with an expert report.

No clinical data is required provided that efficacy is at least plausible on the basis of long-standing use and experience. The dossier will also include information on any authorization obtained in another MS or in a third country, and details of any decision to refuse to grant an authorization.

The labeling must state that the product is a traditional medicinal product for use in specified indications exclusively based upon long-standing use. The same statement must also accompany any advertisement. Furthermore, the labeling must indicate that the user should consult a doctor if symptoms persist or if adverse effects not mentioned in the labeling occur.

The HCMP has been given the task of preparing a list of herbal substances, herbal preparations, and combinations thereof to be used in traditional herbal medicinal products. The list will contain for each substance the indication, strength, posology, route of administration, and any information necessary for the safe use of the traditional herbal medicinal product. Where an application will refer to a product included in that list, it will not be necessary to provide proof of long-term use, or evaluation of safety data.

The new Directive became effective on March 31, 2004, and had to be implemented by MSs by October 30, 2005. For traditional herbal medicinal products already on the market, these new provisions become effective March 31, 2011, thus providing a seven-year transitional period for manufacturers to comply with the minimal regulatory requirements of the Directive.

Labeling

Summary of product characteristics (SPC)

The Summary of Product Characteristics is among the most crucial documents in the MA application, because it forms the basis of the MA and consequently is the basis for the labeling of the product. Any statement in the SPC must be supported by experimental data in the dossier. It is defined during the development of the drug and finalized through a scientific discussion with the RA, and therefore constitutes a reference that cannot be changed, unless new experimental data are made available, approved, and authorized. The SPC represents the basic element of communication for the company: in fact any information on the drug, including labeling and advertising, is bound to this document, which also plays a fundamental role in the MRP.

Directive 2001/83/EC as amended by Directive 2004/27, specifies the required information for the SPC and the patient information leaflet.

In the guideline on SPC the exact layout and the contents are defined. Additional guidelines issued by central bodies as well as national RAs provide recommended wording for specific text in various different classes of medical products in the jurisdiction of the RA (e.g., the MHRA document "generic" overdose sections for selected SPCs, February 2004).

Separate SPCs for each pharmaceutical form and strength of a medicinal product are required. Reasonable merging of multiple SPCs into one for advertising of a single product is permitted.

The headings in the SPC are as follows:

1. Name of the medicinal product (trade) name of product, strength, and pharmaceutical form.

2. Qualitative and quantitative composition for the active substances.

3. Pharmaceutical form (standard terminology per the *European Pharmacopoeia* and Section 1 of the SPC).

4. Clinical particulars:

4.1. Therapeutic indications.

4.2. Posology and method of administration, including advice on pediatric experience, or lack thereof with reference to Section 5.3; dose adjustments (e.g., in renal insufficiency).

4.3. Contraindications (pregnancy only to be mentioned if actually contraindicated).

4.4. Special warnings and precautions for use (in the order: relative contraindications, warnings. and precautions) including special populations at risk. Warnings about excipients and hypersensitivity are mandatory in this section. However, interactions, pregnancy, lactation. and ability to operate machines do not belong in this section

4.5. Interaction with other medicinal products and other forms of interactions, with recommendations for contraindication of concomitant use, mechanism of interaction (if known).

4.6. Pregnancy and lactation. It must be made clear what extent of experience in pregnancy or lactation, or the lack of experience, exists. Relevant preclinical details should be given in Section 5.3. Further recommendations about women of childbearing potential and lactation.

4.7. Effects on ability to drive and use machines.

4.8. Undesirable effects. The precise wording prescribed for expression of frequencies of adverse effects is given in the guideline.

4.9. Overdose.

5. Pharmacological properties:

5.1. Pharmacodynamic properties.

5.2. Pharmacokinetic properties.

5.3. Preclinical safety data.

6. Pharmaceutical particulars:

6.1. List of excipients.

6.2. Incompatibilities.

6.3. Shelf-life—as packaged for sale, after reconstitution (if applicable), after first opening of packaging container.

6.4. Special precautions for storage.

6.5. Nature and contents of container.

6.6. Instructions for use and handling, and disposal.

7. Marketing authorization holder.

8. Marketing authorization number(s).

9. Date of first authorization/renewal of authorization.

10. Date of revision of the text.

Products authorized through the centralized procedure carry a "blue box" on the package label, containing information specific to the MSs in which the product is marketed. This is the only part of the label that can vary for those products, and is the result of retained national authority for decisions on package size, pricing, and classification of centralized, authorized products.

Package labeling and patient information leaflet

The patient information leaflet and the label of the drug container itself are as precisely regulated as the SPC. Changes in any of these documents have to be approved by the RA (see license variations below).

Directive 2001/83, the Community Code, sets the standard for labeling and the patient information leaflet (PIL).

Investigational Medicinal Product (IMP) labeling is regulated by the GMP guidelines. These labels should include the following:
- name of the sponsor;
- pharmaceutical dosage form, route of administration, quantity of dosage units, (and name/identifier of the product and strength/potency in the case of an open trial);
- the batch and/or code number to identify the contents and packaging operation;
- the trial subject identification number, where applicable;
- directions for use;
- "for Clinical Trial use only";
- the name of the investigator (if not included as a code in the trial reference code);

- a trial reference code allowing identification of the trial site and investigator;
- the storage conditions;
- the period of use (use by date, expiry date, or retest date as applicable) in month/year;
- "keep out of reach of children," except when the product is for use only in hospital.

If the outer packaging of the IMP contains all the above listed items, the immediate packaging needs to carry only the first five items; there are further specifications on the labeling of various immediate packages (addressing blister packs, ampoules, etc.).

Marketing authorization variations, renewals, and reclassification

License variations

Most of the work of the national RAs concerns license variations, line extensions, and license renewals. The application will follow the same approval procedure in which the original authorization was obtained. As many products currently licensed have been licensed through national procedures, before the mutual recognition or centralized procedures were available, many of the applications are still undergoing the national approval process in each MS separately.

In Oct 1, 2003, the new European Variations Regulations came into force, introducing a newly revised Annex I to Directive 2001/83. The relevant Commission Regulations 1084/2003/EC and 1085/2003/EC concern mutual recognition and centralized procedures, respectively. The Mutual Recognition Facilitation Group (MRFG) has issued a Best Practice Guide, which implements the Directive and gives guidance to MAHs on how to apply for the variations under national or mutual recognition procedure. Guidance on variations in the centralized procedure can be found in the CPMP document on post-authorization guidance (Human medicinal products), February 2004.

License variations are divided into three main categories termed "Type I variation," Type II variation," and "extensions." The main changes introduced by the new legislation are as follows:

• a new category of minor variation (Type IA notification) with a 14-day timeline and requiring only scientific validation;

• the former revised Type I minor variation categories are now classed as Type IB notifications, and have a 30-day review timeline;

• reference MSs act on behalf of all CMSs for products approved by the MRPs for Type I minor variations;

• flexibility of timelines for Type II variations (extension for new indications and reduction for safety variations);

• introduction of a process of appeal by MAHs when Type IB and Type II variations are rejected;

• streamlined decision-making for centralized notifications;

• new Annex II of the Variations Regulations and definition of extension applications.

Frequently, MAHs find it difficult to classify the requested labeling change into Type IA, IB, and so on. The "Notice to applicants of the EU Commission—Guideline on the categorization of new applications versus variations applications, January 2002" aimed to clarify these issues, and was supplemented (in July 2003) by the "Guidance on dossier requirements for Type IA and IB notifications," which lists of all foreseen variations, their classification, and the documentation required. Revisions for the former were issued in late 2009.

In general, Type IA and IB variations are, for example, changes of an administrative nature: such as the address of the MAH; changes in batch sizes within limits; and minor changes in test procedures. These contrast with "Extension" applications, which are necessary when the following has occurred:

• changes to the active substance(s);

• changes to the indications;

• changes to strength, pharmaceutical form, and route of administration;

• changes specific to veterinary medicinal products.

Any of these changes has to undergo a full scientific evaluation as for any new marketing application. An exception to this rule is the annual human influenza vaccine, which, although a change to the

active substance, can be applied for as a Type II variation.

In the UK, variation applications are sent to the MHRA Variation Processing Division. The application and supporting data should be submitted in a clearly laid out dossier applying the headings and numbering of the CTD format. There is a reduction in fees for bulk applications, incorporating multiple changes (fees are published on the RA's website).

The application documents for any variation are as follows:

• Cover letter, clearly stating the Product License numbers involved, the reason for the change, for example, if it has been requested or is as a result of harmonization, and whether the application is national or mutual recognition variation.

• The list of dispatch dates, for mutual recognition applications where the UK is the Reference MS.

• Confirmation that the appropriate fee has been paid.

• Table of contents.

• The variation application form, dated and signed by the official contact person. All changes proposed should be clearly explained in the scope of the variation.

• Supporting data relating to the proposed variation.

• Update or Addendum to quality summaries, nonclinical overviews, and clinical overviews (the former "expert reports") as may be relevant. When nonclinical or clinical study reports are submitted, their relevant summaries should also be included in Module II.

• In cases where the changes affect the SPC, labeling, and/or PIL the revised product information must be submitted. Mock-ups are required of proposed labels and PILs, and both annotated, old as well as the proposed, final versions of the labeling are required.

"Complex" Type II variations require a higher fee, because the review involved is more extensive; the timeline is also longer. The following changes are usually regarded as "complex":

• Reformulation of the product introducing a novel excipient that has previously not been included in medicinal products.

• A new route of synthesis that has not previously been assessed and a Ph Eur Certificate of Suitability is not available.*
• New method of sterilization of a product.*
• New container materials for a sterile product.*
• New active ingredient manufacturer, not previously approved to manufacture the active ingredient concerned, and who does not hold a Ph Eur Certificate of Suitability for the substance concerned.
• Flu Vaccine: new manufacturer or process.
• Reformulation of a product that is supported by bioavailability studies.
• Change in the product's preservative system.
• Change in excipients that significantly affect the pharmaceutical or therapeutic properties.
(* indicates specific to the active ingredient)

If a company submits a variation application that needs to be newly assessed because it is supported by the results of clinical trials or other data (including pharmacological and toxicological tests as well as extensive evidence from post-marketing experience or publications), the RA will classify it as a Type II complex variation. The calculation of fees is complicated.

License renewals

MAs are granted for five years in the first instance, after which a renewal is necessary. This requires submission of a review of all the product experience since the drug was first marketed. Essential parts of this review are the periodic safety update reports (PSURs), required every six months during the first two years of marketing, and annually thereafter. Normally, after the MA renewal, further PSURs are required every three years. Under special circumstances, more frequent PSURs may be required for products that the authorities wish to keep under closer review. There is never any relaxation of the requirement for expedited reporting of serious, unexpected, adverse events.

For most products, the revised Regulation foresees only one renewal based on a re-evaluation of the risk/benefit balance, after which the validity of the MA is unlimited. However, at its discretion, national RAs can still require subsequent renewals

(Article 24 of Directive 2004/27 and Article 14 of Regulation 726/2004).

Reclassification

Reclassification (e.g., an "over-the-counter switch") remains the responsibility of each national RA. The EU guideline on changing legal classification for the supply of medicinal products (the rules governing medicinal products in the European Community – Volume IIIb) sets out the standards that must be fulfilled in order to change the legal classification of a medicinal product.

New products, when first licensed, are usually approved as "prescription only medicine" (POM). With increasing experience in the use of the medicine, it might seem likely that a medication is safe for use with pharmacy supervision only; then, the national competent authority may remove the prescription requirements and allow sale or supply from a pharmacy without prescription, that is, the medicinal product is reclassified as Pharmacy (P). If further experience shows that access to professional advice is not required for safe use of the medicine, it may finally be reclassified as General sale list (GSL) to allow sale from a wider range of retail outlets on an over-the-counter basis.

In the UK, the post-licensing division of the MHRA deals with all reclassification requests. By law, all medicines are P unless they meet the criteria for POM or GSL. Pack size restrictions for GSL products are listed in the "Medicines (Sale or Supply) (Miscellaneous provisions) Regulations, 1980." For all licensed medicines, legal status is ultimately determined by the MA.

Directive 2001/83 provides that prescription control is applied to any product that
• is likely to present a direct or indirect danger to human health, even when used correctly, if used without the supervision of a doctor or dentist; or
• is frequently and to a very wide extent used incorrectly, and as a result is likely to present a direct or indirect danger to human health; or
• contains substances or presentations of substances of which the activity requires, or the side effects require, further investigation; or
• is normally prescribed by a doctor or dentist for parenteral administration.

Exemptions from prescription control may be made with regard to
- the maximum single dose;
- the maximum daily dose;
- the strength of the product;
- its pharmaceutical form;
- its packaging; or
- other circumstances relating to its use that would be specified when reclassification is determined.

After the national RA has received and validated an application, it classifies the application into one of three types: standard, complex, or "me-too" applications not supported by full data.

Complex applications require initial committee referral and therefore the procedure takes 180 days; a full fee is charged for review.

Standard applications are generally reviewed within 120 days, and this timeline will only be lengthened if issues arise that require referral to a full committee review; the applicant may also be approached to clarify details of the application. An initial full fee has to be paid by the applicant; if the procedure passes without referral to the full committee, the RA will refund half of the fee to the applicant.

A "me-too" application, for a product, which has analogous products with the classification applied for already on the market, is handled as standard Type II variation, and the corresponding fee is charged.

After an application has been filed, it is published for consultation with interested parties for a 4–6 week period: immediately in the case of a standard application (based on the Reclassification summary), or after the committee's advice for reclassification in the case of a complex procedure. The consultation period is not included in the timelines for approval.

The documentation necessary for a valid reclassification application is listed below:
- reclassification application form;
- reclassification summary—a comprehensive summary in a set format, which will form part of the information, provided for the public consultation (2 pages A4);
- safety and efficacy summary—supporting safety and where necessary efficacy data;

- patient information—full details of leaflets and labels and an indication of the advertising plans;
- training and education—a summary of what provision has been made for appropriate education and training;
- clinical expert report—a critical evaluation of the proposed pharmacy product demonstrating that none of the prescription criteria (see above) apply.

Crucial issues that must be addressed in the expert report of the application are: the ease of self-diagnosis of the target disease; whether the substance is a narcotic or a psychotropic substance; if there is a risk of abuse leading to addiction; and whether the substance has a potential for misuse for illegal purposes.

If the maximum dose is restricted when the medicine is supplied P or GSL to protect against adverse effects from correct or incorrect use of the medication, it is important to prove that the restricted dose is still as effective and keeps the same benefit–risk relationship as the original full dose.

GSL can be considered for those medicines, which can with reasonable safety, be sold or supplied without the supervision of a pharmacist. The following classes of products are excluded from GSL:
- anthelmintics;
- parenterals;
- eye drops;
- eye ointments;
- enemas;
- irrigations used wholly or mainly for wounds, bladder, vagina, or rectum;
- aspirin or aloxiprin for administration wholly or mainly to children.

Product recall

The GMP Directive requires each manufacturer to have a system for complaints and product recall readily in place. Section 8 of the Directive requires review of any complaint about potentially defective products following a written procedure and if necessary the effective and prompt recall of defective products from the market. It is a requirement to inform the Qualified Person (QP) and the Quality Control department during the review and analysis of all product complaints that need to be thoroughly investigated.

In order to allow effective tracking of products, record keeping of product distribution is necessary. Sufficient information on wholesalers and/or directly supplied customers with precise batch numbers and quantities supplied together with contact numbers and addresses must be available and up-to-date. The process of the recall must be recorded including reconciliation between delivered and returned quantities of the products.

A designated person in the company needs to be responsible for execution and coordination of product recalls. This person should be independent from the sales and marketing personnel. The QP of the company must be made aware of the product recall. Furthermore it is required to inform the RAs of any recall action.

Safety reporting and pharmacovigilance

The assessment of safety in the use of medicinal products starts before the first administration to humans and continues throughout the development of the medicine to the MA for the lifetime of the drug. It is governed by a set of comprehensive rules, which are published in Volume 9A of the rules governing the use of medicinal products in the EU, Notice to Applicants (see earlier Figure 37.2; last update September 2008) for post-marketing activities and post-authorization studies, and in ENTR 3 and 4 of Volume 10 for clinical trials. These rules have seen several major updates in the time since the first publication in 1986, and a comprehensive review is currently ongoing, which is expected to change the post-marketing pharmacovigilance regulations is Europe substantially. The nonclinical aspects of product safety are discussed elsewhere in this book.

Directive 2001/20 had a major impact on pharmacovigilance in Europe because it demanded the creation of a pan-European safety database for all medicinal products on the market and extending to investigational medicinal products (IMPs). The system was named EudraVigilance. The EudraCT system (clinical trials registration, see above) was created as part of it. The detailed guidance about reporting of adverse reactions to investigational medicinal products, whether licensed or not, was issued in April 2004.

Safety monitoring in clinical trials

The sponsor of an IMP or the MAH in the case of a clinical trial using a licensed medicine, is responsible for the ongoing safety assessment, compliance with reporting timelines, and distribution of reports to all concerned parties. Furthermore, the sponsor of a trial now also has the responsibility to report Serious Adverse Drug reactions occurring in the use of active comparator products, even if the sponsor of the trial is not its MAH. The guidelines recommend that the sponsor also inform the MAH about the reported case.

An adverse event (AE) is defined as follows: Any untoward medical occurrence in a subject or clinical investigation subject administered a pharmaceutical product and which does not necessarily have to have a causal relationship with this treatment.

An AE can therefore be any unfavorable and unintended sign (including an abnormal laboratory finding, for example), symptom, or disease temporally associated with the use of a medicinal product, whether or not considered to be related to the medicinal product.

A serious adverse event (SAE) is defined as any untoward medical occurrence that at any dose:
- results in *death*;
- is *life threatening**;
- requires in-patient *hospitalization* or prolongation of existing hospitalization;
- results in persistent or significant *disability/incapacity*;
- is a *congenital anomaly/birth defect*;
- is an *important medical event* that may require intervention to prevent the above five conditions or may expose the subject to danger, even though the event is not immediately life-threatening or fatal or does not result in hospitalization.

(* "life-threatening" refers to an event in which the patient was at risk of death at the time of the event;

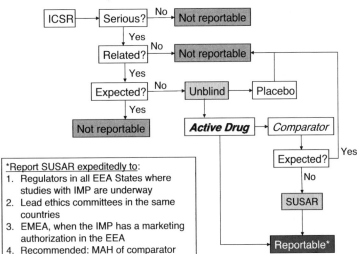

Assessment of expedited reportability in blinded trials

Figure 37.7 Assessment of expedited reporting from blinded clinical trials in the EEA.

it does not refer to an event that hypothetically might have caused death if it were more severe)

In clinical trials of IMPs without a MA, sponsors must report all suspected unexpected serious adverse reactions (SUSARs) within eight calendar days if they were fatal or life threatening, and within 15 days for other serious cases. The initial report has to be followed up within seven days for fatal or life-threatening cases, within 15 days for other serious reports. These expedited reporting requirements mean that the treatment code in blinded trials must be broken, because it is otherwise impossible to decide which treatment the patient received and therefore impossible to determine whether an event could possibly be a reaction: if a patient received placebo, there is no suspicion of a possible adverse reaction to the IMP and authorities do not require expedited reporting (unless the adverse event could have been a reaction related to an excipient present also in the placebo).

"Expected" adverse drug reactions in clinical trials—even if serious—are not reported in an expedited fashion. An "Expected" adverse drug reaction is one that is mentioned in the SPC (in the case of a licensed product) or in the Investigator's Brochure in the case of an IMP. It is important to understand that expectedness is solely refer-

ring to experiences made with a given individual product—class reactions, if not observed with an individual medicinal product or reactions relating to the underlying disease, are not "expected" for the given product and if considered possibly related to the medicinal product, must be reported in an expedited fashion, if fulfilling the criteria for expedited reporting. Figure 37.7 illustrates the evaluation of a case (ICSR) for expedited reporting when arising from a blinded clinical trial with sites in the EEA.

Clinical trial sponsors also have the obligation to report safety information to investigators and Ethics Committees in a timely fashion. Ethics Committees are informed in an unblinded fashion within the same timeframe as the RAs. The investigators can be updated periodically in a blinded fashion, provided that no compelling safety reason to unblind has emerged.

Annual update reports for all clinical trials are required to be sent to regulators and Ethics Committees. For short trials (up to six months), or trials involving less than 50 subjects, this can be combined with the notification of end of trial.

Clinical trials constitute well-monitored environments, in which most events (whether related to the IMP or not) can be collected and added to a database that will gradually outline the safety profile of the drug, allowing for a risk–benefit assessment that will form the cornerstone of any marketing application. After MA has been granted, the population exposed to the drug usually increases exponentially, while the conditions of product use become suddenly less well-controlled. Thus, new safety issues often surface immediately after MA.

The MAH is therefore required to provide with the application for MA a EU-risk Management Plan, including a pharmacovigilance plan, outlining the intentions and systems in place to further evaluate and strengthen the risk–benefit analysis of the medicinal product under review. During the early phases of drug development, safety assessments in clinical trials are generally viewed as "hypothesis forming"—broadly applied systems to collect as much useful data, that might help to identify special issues or problems with a given drug. In later development, the profile of the product must be investigated more in depth in those areas that previously might have given rise to attention (e.g., hepatic issues, gastric bleedings, or other special issues that a drug might present during initial clinical trials). The pharmacovigilance plan aims at outlining the risk management procedures planned and will usually contain a series of planned studies or observations, preclinical or chemical test programs, aimed at characterising the drug further and to help understand the true risk–benefit profile of the medicinal product.

Post-marketing pharmacovigilance

Pharmacovigilance in the post-MA period is tightly regulated and published in Volume 9A (September 2008). Pharmacovigilance obligations do not depend on a product being actively marketed in the EU. Case collection, literature searches, expedited and periodic reporting, and all other pharmacovigilance requirements are obligatory from first MA and until even after removal of a product from the market. As in North America and Japan, Europe has adopted the ICH guidelines with a few, relatively minor additions. The MAH must have systems and qualified personnel in place to fulfill all its obligations for the monitoring of the safety of its medicinal products.

Within Module I of the MA application, the applicant is required to submit a detailed description of pharmacovigilance systems (DDPS; section 1.8.1); any changes to the DDPS after initial authorization is obtained will constitute a variation to the MA and has to be submitted for review by the authorities as a Type II variation. The MAA further contains the EU-Risk Management Plan (EU-RMP; section 1.8.2) in a proscribed template describing the safety specifications, pharmacovigilance plan, and risk minimization measures proposed for the product under review. The EU-RMP contains in Annex 1 an electronic summary of the suspected adverse reactions, both potential and identified, which will be used by the RAs to link with the EudraVigilance database and conduct signal detection activities.

The qualified person for pharmacovigilance

Similarly to the QP for GMP, MAH are required to identify to the authorities an individual to take the role of the qualified person for pharmacovigilance (the "EU QPPV"). The qualified person must be fully versed in all aspects of pharmacovigilance and carries personal responsibility for compliance with all applicable regulations and must reside within the EU.

The QPPV is responsible for (Volume 9A)
• establishing and maintaining/managing the MAH's pharmacovigilance system;
• having an overview of the safety profiles and any emerging safety concerns in relation to the medicinal products for which the MAH holds authorizations;
• acting as a single contact point for the Competent Authorities on a 24-hour basis.

The QPPV should have oversight of
• the establishment and maintenance of a system, which ensures that information about all suspected adverse reactions that are reported to the personnel of the MAH, and to medical representatives, is collected and collated in order to be accessible at least at one point within the EU;
• the preparation of
  – Individual Case Safety Reports (ICSRs);
  – Periodic Safety Update Reports (PSURs);

– Company-sponsored post-authorization safety studies (PASS);

• the conduct of continuous overall pharmacovigilance evaluation during the post-authorization period;

• the ensuring that any request from Competent Authorities for the provision of additional information necessary for the evaluation of the benefits and the risks is answered fully and promptly (including volume of sales or prescriptions, post-authorization studies, and data from other sources).

The oversight should include quality control and assurance procedures, standard operating procedures, database operations, contractual arrangements, compliance data (e.g., in relation to the quality, completeness, and timeliness for expedited reporting and submission of PSURs), audit reports, and training of personnel in relation to pharmacovigilance.

The EU QPPV is therefore responsible for ensuring that the MAH is diligently collecting safety information on all its marketed products and adheres to obligations taken with the RAs (e.g., commitments made in the pharmacovigilance plan at time of the MA). Regular surveillance over many different sources of information must be maintained (e.g., medical journals, spontaneously reported cases, "Yellow Card" schemes, safety data from clinical trials, observational trials, market research, and so on) and reportable information identified and processed in a timely fashion.

Pharmacovigilance inspections by RAs

The competent national authorities have established inspectorates for pharmacovigilance systems of any MAH, similarly to the GMP and GCP inspectorate, and are equipped with considerable power extending from re-inspection over fines to MA suspension and criminal prosecution of the qualified person, if critical findings are identified and not sufficiently addressed. Pharmacovigilance inspections are conducted to verify the adherence to Volume 9A. Inspections are the responsibility of national authorities and usually conducted by the authority within whose territory the EU QPPV resides, and can also be conducted upon request and in participation with the EMA.

Expedited reporting

In addition to the periodic reports (see above), all serious adverse drug reactions reported spontaneously, identified in the worldwide scientific literature (literature screening is mandatory at least weekly, both local and global publications) or through post-marketing safety studies have to be reported in an expedited fashion. Of any serious reactions (SADR) arising from within the EEA and cases arising from outside the EU, only the unexpected serious (SUSAR) cases must be reported in an expedited fashion. Timelines for expedited reporting of post-marketing cases are within 15 days; there is no requirement for eight-day reporting of life-threatening or fatal reactions as there is in for cases arising from clinical trials. Figure 37.8 illustrates the assessment of expedited reporting for products with a MAH in the EEA. Clinical trial cases from such drugs were illustrated in the earlier Figure 37.7 and will be sent to the clinical trial module of EudraVigilance, whereas all other cases are reported to the post-marketing module.

There are additional requirements for expedited reporting depending on the license type of the product, such as additional requirements to report to the Reference MS all EU SADRs for products licensed through the MRP or Black Triangle reporting requirements in the UK for products newly put on the market. These special requirements are detailed in Annex 2 of Volume 9A and must be observed.

Licensing agreements

Companies with co-licensing agreements have to prepare detailed contracts about exchange of safety information and reporting responsibilities, because duplication of reports is unacceptable to the RAs. Responsibilities and oversight of EU QPPVs must be carefully laid out, because these are subject to intense scrutiny during pharmacovigilance inspections.

Periodic safety update reports

As described earlier in this chapter, the MAH is required to submit regular safety updates to the competent authorities for each licensed product. Combination products can either be submitted as

Assessment of expedited reportability in EEA for products with MAH

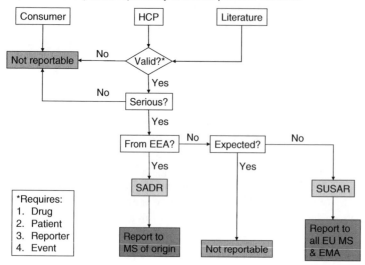

Figure 37.8 Assessment for expedited reporting for spontaneous ICSRs for products with MA in the EEA.

separate PSURs or enclosed in one PSUR covering all indications, strengths, and license variations of a given medicinal product. The PSUR reports licensing and marketing status of the product, and estimates exposure during the reporting period and cumulatively since first launch of a product. Any regulatory action or changes to the Core Company Safety information on the compound (CCSI) must be listed in detail. All reported adverse reactions from any source are listed; serious and nonserious reactions of special interest for a given compound, overdoses, congenital abnormalities, interactions, and newly received clinical trial data must be presented in detail and discussed.

Most companies elect to prepare six-monthly reports and when the reporting intervals to the RA prolong, to submit a number of reports together with a brief bridging report. Please note that data is always presented for the reporting period and cumulatively since launch of a product.

The timing of the PSUR is governed by its international birth date: the date of first launch of the product. Expectations of PSURs and standard format are laid down in Volume 9A.

Individual case safety reports (ICSR)

The basis for all expedited, and also cumulative or periodic, reports are individual case reports.

The accepted reporting format for individual case reports is the CIOMS I form. However, all other forms are in principle acceptable as long as they contain the necessary information. Cases must fulfill minimum requirements to qualify for reporting: a reporter, an event, a drug, and a patient must be identifiable. In the EU, the reporter can only be a healthcare professional, unlike in the USA, where the FDA accepts reports from consumers. Various pilot programs are underway to investigate the value of consumer reporting in the EU.

All European RAs have access to the EudraVigilance database. Electronic transmission of ICSRs to the EMA has been mandatory since 2004, and electronic reporting to national authorities and electronic receipt of case reports from any authority have been mandatory since November 20, 2005. RAs and pharmaceutical companies alike have set up electronic gateways to exchange safety information and compile it in EudraVigilance in the standard E2B format (referring to the ICH E2B guideline, identifying standard data elements for case safety report electronic transmission—these standards are currently undergoing review and are expected to change in the near future).

It is important to be aware of the requirements for expedited reporting in the EU and the national requirements, which also must be observed and are outlined in Volume 9A Annexes. For example, in the UK products within two years of initial MA or otherwise identified by the MHRA as being under heightened surveillance, are indicated by a black triangle in the prescribing information and subject to additional reporting requirements in the UK. In France, all cases must be subjected to additional causality assessments in compliance with the French method of imputability. It is thus critical that each MAH has within its pharmacovigilance system a mechanism in place, by which to ensure full awareness of all regulations as pertaining to pharmacovigilance and be able to respond to changes in a timely manner.

In 2010, new issues connected with the EU pharmacovigilance regulations are expected and will bring with them major changes for RAs and MAHs alike.

Regulation of advertising and promotion

Advertising and promotion are again covered in detail elsewhere in this book. Here we shall just briefly discuss some of the European regulatory aspects.

Directive 2001/83 sets the framework for the Regulation of promotion and advertising in the EU. The European Federation of Pharmaceutical Industries' Associations (EFPIA) has produced the European Code of Practice for the promotion of medicines and requires each MS to establish a committee to deal with complaints. This committee must include independent members. Despite the Directive and the European Code, the Regulation of promotion and advertising of medicinal products is still not harmonized throughout the EU. Every MS can make individual additions to the code and, as always, the Directive gives only general guidance with room for individual interpretation.

Voluntary codes of practice have been in use in many MSs for many years. For example, in the UK, the "ABPI Code of Practice" is applicable to prescription medicines, as is the Proprietary Association of Great Britain (PAGB) "Code of Standards of Advertising Practice" for over-the-counter medicines.

The general principles of advertising and promotion are as follows:

- It is an offense to issue a false or misleading advertisement or representation about a medicinal product; in particular the advertisement has to comply with the approved SPC.
- The product must be presented objectively and without exaggeration, to encourage its rational use.
- It is an offense to issue an advertisement about a nonauthorized indication and no promotion of a medicinal product is permitted before it is granted MA.
- The advertising of prescription only medicines to the consumer (the patient) and thus the general public is prohibited.

In the UK, copies of all advertisements must be submitted to the RA every 12 months. Furthermore, it is a requirement that the approved SPC is supplied within 15 months of an advertisement. Meanwhile the British pharmaceutical industry provides a compendium of SPCs to every practicing physician and pharmacist in the country as one mechanism to comply with the Regulation.

Many of the promotional activities of the pharmaceutical industry are directed at professionals in the healthcare market (doctors, pharmacists, hospitals, etc.), because advertising POM medications directly to the patient is prohibited. However, companies are receiving an increasing number of enquiries directly from patients about their products. This has necessitated the provision of a regulatory Guidance for companies on how to answer such direct requests for information from the general public.

Pharmaceutical companies are now permitted to answer general inquiries in a nonpromotional way. However, promotion to the public is specifically permitted *only* in the case of P (Pharmacy) or GSL (General Sales list) medicinal products.

Disease awareness campaigns are a recognized and approved way for pharmaceutical companies to communicate with the general public. Disease awareness campaigns may make reference to treatment options, but need carefully to avoid highlighting any specific medicinal product, because this would be viewed as promotional. Any promotion of a particular medicinal products will bring the campaign within the scope of the Community Code (Directive 2001/83), and violate the law.

Promotional aids, gifts, hospitality, supply of free samples, and the conduct and training of medical representatives all fall as squarely within the Regulations as printed and audio-visual promotional materials.

Prospective of EU medicines regulation

A major revision of the European medicines regulation is underway at the time of writing of this chapter. It is expected to pass the EU parliament in 2010. Although it can be assumed that the current proposals will still undergo numerous changes prior to being adopted and transferred into Regulations and Directive, the foreseeable impact on all aspects of EU medicines regulations will be very substantial.

Medicines Regulation in Switzerland

Switzerland is a federation of cantons. Each canton governs its own regional issues, while the Swiss government is concerned with national matters. Democracy extends to a yet smaller scale in Switzerland because, even within the cantons, individual villages or cities retain varying degrees of independence. The result is a fascinating legal mosaic: a system of great diversity within the national borders of a relatively small country.

Switzerland lies outside both the EU and the EEA. Nevertheless the Swiss Regulatory Authority has adopted all the ICH guidelines and requires MA applications in the Common Technical Document format. Modules 2–5 can be submitted in English, although the country-specific Module 1 has to be submitted in one of the Swiss languages (German, French, Italian, or Romantsch; however, informally, the RA discourages the last of these). The SPC and patient information leaflet must provide information in German, Italian, and French,

unless for some peculiar reason, the product will only be distributed in cantons using just one of these languages. Switzerland does not automatically ratify European MA but will grant "fast-track" reviews for products with an EU MA.

Although Swissmedic functions as a RA for all Switzerland, there are nonetheless parts of Medicines Regulation that are governed by cantonal laws, and not centrally harmonized across the whole country. For example, the GMP and GCP inspectorate and distribution of medicines is a cantonal, not national, responsibility, even though the GMP and GCP Guidances are issued nationwide by Swissmedic. It is advisable to talk to the relevant personnel (e.g., the cantonal pharmacist for GMP and medicines distribution issues) at the cantonal administration, when applying for MA.

As in the EU, an inland legal representative is needed for all non-Swiss applicants. These legal representatives are as valuable to sponsors for navigating this complicated situation as to Swissmedic, as a point of contact and communication.

Medical devices and drug/device combinations

All medical devices are subject to regulatory review and MAs similar to medicinal products. In the UK, the national RAs for devices and medicinal products were merged in 2003. However, note that the EMA, CHMP, and COMP do not regulate medical devices, unlike their US equivalents.

The Medical Device Directive 93/42 defines medical devices and products, which combine a drug with a device. For regulatory purposes, the latter are subdivided and dealt with as follows:
- Where device and drug are supplied separately (e.g., syringes marketed empty), the device is subject to devices controls and the medicine is subject to medicines control.
- Integral, non-reusable products intended solely for use in the given combination (e.g., syringes marketed pre-filled) are subject to medicines control, but the device feature must satisfy the relevant essential requirements of the Directive relating to safety and performance.

- Devices incorporating a drug where the action of the drug is ancillary to that of the device (e.g., anticoagulant-coated catheters) are subject to devices control, but the drug must be verified by analogy with medicines control criteria and the medicines licensing authority must be consulted.

Further reading

Order of listing:
- Declaration of Helsinki;
- EU Directives, Patent convention;
- ICH documents;
- EMEA and CPMP and COMP Regulations, guidelines, and SOPs;
- UK regulatory bodies (MHRA, DoH, COREC, ARSAC);
- BfArM;
- Voluntary organizations (CIOMS, ABPI);
- Presentation notes;
- Websites.

1. World Medical Association Declaration of Helsinki. Ethical principles for medical research involving human subjects. As amended.
2. Pharmacos 4—Eudralex: The rules governing medicinal products in the European Union. http://ec.europa.eu/enterprise/sectors/pharmaceuticals/documents/eudralex/index_en.htm; accessed April 21, 2010.
3. Regulation 726/2004 of March 31, 2004, laying down Community procedures for the authorization and supervision of medicinal products for human and veterinary use and establishing a European Medicines Agency.
4. Council Directive 65/65/EEC of January 26, 1965, on the approximation of provisions laid down by law, Regulation, or administrative action relating to proprietary medicinal products (requirements for medicinal products on quality, efficacy, and safety).
5. Council Directive 75/318/EEC on the approximation of the laws of MSs relating to analytical, pharmaco-toxicological, and clinical standards and protocols in respect of the testing of proprietary medicinal products (OJ L 147, 9.6.1975), as last amended by Directive 93/39/EEC (mutual recognition).
6. Council Directive 75/319/EEC on the approximation of provisions laid down by law, Regulation or administrative action relating to proprietary medicinal products (OJ L 147, 9.6.1975), as last amended by Directive 93/39/EEC (CPMP).
7. Directive EEC/2001/20 of the European parliament and of the Council of April 4, 2001, on the approximation of the laws, Regulations, and administrative provisions of the MSs relating to the implementation of good clinical practice in the conduct of clinical trials on medicinal products for human use (the new Clinical Trial Directive).
8. Directive 2001/83/EC of the European parliament and of the Council of November 6, 2001, on the Community code relating to medicinal products for human use (Classification of Medicines).
9. Directive 2001/83 Annex I of June 20, 2002 (License variations).
10. Directive 2004/27/EC of March 31, 2004, amending Directive 2001/83/EC on the community code relating to medicinal products for human use.
11. Directive 2005/28/EC (Good Clinical Practice Directive).
12. Directive 92/27/EC (labeling and Patient Information leaflet).
13. Directive 91/356/EEC of June 13, 1991, laying down the principles and guidelines of good manufacturing practice for medicinal products for human use (GMP).
14. Directive 2003/94/EC of October 8, 2003, laying down principles and guidelines of good manufacturing practice in respect of medicinal products for human use and investigational products for human use.
15. Directive 87/22/EEC (centralized procedure).
16. Directive 97/43/Euratom "Medical Exposure Directive."
17. Directive 92/28/EC (advertising and promotion).
18. Medical Device Directive 93/42/EEC.
19. Directive 89/105/EEC of December 21, 1988, relating to the transparency of measures regulating the pricing of medicinal products for human use and their inclusion within the scope of national health insurance systems (transparency of price and reimbursement).
20. European Patent Convention Part II, 11th edition, July 2002.
21. EC commission: detailed guidance on the application format and documentation to be submitted in an application for an Ethics Committee opinion on the Clinical Trial on medicinal products for human use; October 2005.
22. EC commission: detailed guidance for the request for authorization of a Clinical Trial on a medicinal product for human use to the competent authorities, notification of substantial amendments. and declaration of the end of the trial; February 2007.

23. EC commission: detailed guidance on the collection, verification. and presentation of adverse reaction reports arising from Clinical Trials on medicinal products for human use; April 2004 revision 1 (Brussels ENTR/CT3).

24. The Common Technical Document for the registration of pharmaceuticals for human use: organization of common technical document (CPMP/ICH/2887/99), ICH M4 guideline.

25. ICH E6 Guideline for good clinical practice (CPMP/ICH/135/95).

26. ICH Topic E2B (M) Clinical safety data management: data elements for transmission of individual case safety report.

27. ICH Topic E2C Clinical safety data management: periodic safety update reports for marketed drugs.

28. Council Regulation (EEC) No 2309/93 of July 22, 1993, laying down Community procedures for the authorization and supervision of medicinal products for human and veterinary use and establishing a European Agency for the Evaluation of Medicinal Products. Amended by Commission Regulation (EC) No 649/98 of March 23, 1998, amending the Annex to Council Regulation (EEC) No 2309/93 (EMEA).

29. European Pharmacopoeia document "Standard Terms," January 2000.

30. Commission Regulation (EC) No 1084/2003 of June 3, 2003, concerning the examination of variations to the terms of a MA for medicinal products for human use and veterinary medicinal products granted by a competent authority of a MS (mutual recognition variations).

31. Commission Regulation (EC) No 1085/2003 of June 3, 2003, concerning the examination of variations to the terms of a MA for medicinal products for human use and veterinary medicinal products falling within the scope of Council Regulation (EEC) No 2309/93 (centralized procedures variations).

32. Orphan designation: Regulation (EC) no 141/2000 and No 847/2000, ENTR/6283/00.

33. Detailed guidance on the European Clinical Trial database (EUDRACT database) ENTR/F2/BL D (2003).

34. Regulation 540/95 arrangements for reporting suspected unexpected adverse reactions which are not serious.

35. The European Commission: notice to applicants, a guideline on Summary of Product Characteristics, December 1999 (included in the Rules governing medicinal products in the European Community Volume 2A and 2B).

36. Summary of Product characteristics for benzodiazepines as anxiolytics or hypnotics (Eudralex Vol III BC1A).

37. Summary of product characteristics for ACE inhibitors (Eudralex Vol III BC2A).

38. User leaflet for oral contraceptives (Eudralex Vol III BC3A).

39. Summary of product characteristics for antimicrobial medicinal products (Eudralex Vol III BC4A).

40. Summary of product characteristics for antibacterial medicinal products (Eudralex Vol III BC5A).

41. CPMP/108/99 SARG role and responsibilities.

42. SOP 2072/99 on Scientific Advice by the CPMP.

43. Council Regulation (EC) No 297/95, of February 10, 1995, on fees payable to the European Agency for the Evaluation of Medicinal Products. Amended by Council Regulation (EC) No 2743/98 of December 14,1998, amending Regulation (EC) No 297/95 on fees payable to the European Agency for the Evaluation of Medicinal Products. Council Regulation 2743/98 (fees for Scientific Advice).

44. Notice to MAHs—Pharmacovigilance guidelines no. PhVWP/108/99.

45. CPMP Note for Guidance on Electronic Exchange of Pharmacovigilance Information for Human and Veterinary Medicinal Products in the European Union, August 1999.

46. CPMP Joint Pharmacovigilance plan for the Implementation of the ICH E2B M1 and M2 requirements related to the electronic transmission of individual case safety reports in the community.

47. Conduct of pharmacovigilance for medicinal products authorized through the mutual recognition procedure EMEA June 1997.

48. Conduct of pharmacovigilance for centrally authorized products EMEA, April 1997.

49. CPMP SOP 986/96 Rev 1 (trademark review).

50. Commission Regulation (EC) No 847/2000 of April 2, 2000, laying down the provisions for implementation of the criteria for designation of a medicinal product as an orphan medicinal product and definitions of the concepts "similar medicinal product" and "clinical superiority."

51. Quick-Look Leaflet: "Orphan Medicinal Product Designation in the European Union" (EMEA/COMP/661801), updated October 2003.

52. CPMP note for guidance (CPMP/EWP/QWP/1401/98) on the investigation of bioavailability and bioequivalence.

53. CPMP/3097/02 Guidance on the comparability of biotech derived proteins as active substances in medicinal products.

54. Notice to applicants of the EU Commission—Guideline on the categorization of new applications versus variations applications, 2003.

55. EMEA CPMP: post-authorization guidance (human medicinal products) February 2004 Document reference: EMEA/H/19984/03/Rev 2.

56. "Changing the legal classification in the United Kingdom of a medicine for human use" guidance booklet, MCA 2002.

57. The Prescription Only Medicines (Human Use) Order 1997 (The POM Order).

58. The Medicines (Products other than Veterinary Drugs) (General Sale List) Order 1984 (the GSL Order).

59. The Medicines (Pharmacy and General Sale—Exemption) Order.

60. The Medicines (Sale or Supply) (Miscellaneous Provisions) Regulations.

61. The Medicines Act 1968 (as amended).

62. MHRA document "generic" overdose sections for selected SPCs, February 2004.

63. MHRA: best practice guideline on labeling and packaging of medicines. Guidance note no. 25, June 2003.

64. Promotion of Medicines in the UK, Guidance notes on the Medicines (Advertising) Regulations 1994 (as amended): the Medicines (Advertising) Regulations 1994, SI No. 1932; the Medicines (Monitoring of Advertising) Regulations 1994, SI No. 1933; the Medicines for Human Use (Marketing Authorizations etc.) Regulations 1994, SI No. 3144; The Medicines (Advertising) Amendment Regulations 1996, SI No. 1552.

65. The Medicines (Advertising and Monitoring of Advertising) Amendment Regulations 1999, SI No. 267.

66. Department of Health. GAfREC: http://www.dh.gov.uk/en/Publicationsandstatistics/Publications/PublicationsPolicyAndGuidance/DH_4005727; accessed April 21, 2010.

67. MHRA: Disease awareness campaigns guidelines. Guidance note no. 26, June 2003.

68. COREC New Operational procedures for NHS RECs Guidance for applicants to Research Ethics Committees.

69. Notes for guidance on the Clinical Administration of radiopharmaceuticals and use of sealed radioactive sources, ARSAC, December 1998.

70. The ionising Radiations Regulations 1999 SI no 3232 and the ionising radiation (medical exposure) Regulations 2000.

71. "Guide to Good Manufacturing Practice," The Orange Book, 1997.

72. Guidance for notified bodies. Devices, which incorporate a medicinal substance—consulting the MHRA. MHRA Guidance note no. 18, revised June 2003.

73. Supplementary remarks of the BfARM in addition to the Joint Notification by BfARM, BgVV, and PEI of 4 Sept 1998—Guide for applicants (national Scientific Advice).

74. CIOMS IV form for reporting of serious unexpected suspected adverse drug reactions: www.cioms.ch; accessed April 21, 2010.

75. ABPI Code of Practice, 2003; http://www.abpi.org.uk; accessed April 21, 2010.

76. ABPI Guidelines, 4th edition, draft 2004 (written and compiled by MJ Boyce); http://www.abpi.org.uk; accessed April 21, 2010.

77. Prescription medicines code of practice authority, constitution and procedure, operative from July 1, 2001.

78. EMA website: www.ema.europa.eu; accessed April 21, 2010.

79. EudraCT database homepage: https://eudract.emea.europa.eu; accessed April 21, 2010.

80. ICH website: www.ich.org; accessed April 21, 2010.

81. BfArM (Bundesinstitut für Arzneimittel und Medizinprodukte) (Federal Institute for Drugs and Medical Devices) website: www.bfarm.de; accessed April 21, 2010.

82. Swissmedic website: www.swissmedic.ch; accessed April 21, 2010.

83. MHRA website: www.mhra.gov.uk; accessed April 21, 2010.

84. Centre of Research Ethical Campaign (COREC) website: www.corec.org.uk; accessed April 21, 2010.

85. The ABPI website: www.abpi.org.uk; accessed April 21, 2010.

86. EMEA. Procedure for European Guidelines and related documents within the pharmaceutical legislative framework. London: June 20, 2005. Doc. Ref. EMEA/P/24143/2004.

87. European Commission. Detailed Guidance on the European Clinical Trials database (EUDRACT Database). April 2003, and successor documents CT 5.1 Amendment describing the development of EUDRACT-Lot 1 (May 1, 2004) and CT 5.2 EUDRACT core dataset.

88. European Commission Directive 2003/94/EC. Principles and Guidelines of good manufacturing practices in respect of medicinal products for human use and investigational medicinal products for human use.

89. European Commission Directive 2005/28/EC. Principles and detailed guidelines for Good Clinical Practices for good clinical practices as regards investigational medicinal products for human use as well as the requirements for authorization of the manufacturing or importation of such products.

90. EMEA. Guidance for companies requesting Scientific Advice and protocol assistance, June 2008. EMEA/H/4260/01/Rev.2.

91. European Commission. Proposal for a guideline on the definition of a potential serious risk to public health, November 2005.

92. European Commission. Procedures for MA: Chapter 3. Community Referral, February 2004.

93. Regulation (EC) No 1901/2006 of the European Parliament and of the Council of December 12, 2006, on medicinal products for pediatric use.

94. Regulation (EC) No 1902/2006—an amending regulation to the above pediatric regulation in which changes to the original text were introduced relating to decision procedures for the European Commission.

95. "Guideline on the format and content of applications for agreement or modification of a pediatric investigation plan and requests for waivers or deferrals and concerning the operation of the compliance check and on criteria for assessing significant studies." Commission Communication (2008/C 243/01), September 24, 2008.

96. MHRA: (the "Purple guide"): Good Pharmacovigilance Practice Guide, 2010.

CHAPTER 38

Japanese Regulations

Etienne Labbé
UCB S.A., Brussels, Belgium

Japan is a country of 128 million inhabitants, compared to the 305 million of the United States, and covers a geographical area equivalent to the size of California. It had 270,000 medical practitioners as of 2004, and is the third largest drug market in the world. Although economically very attractive, it remains for Westerners a difficult country to understand and communicate with. A strong Dutch and then German influence during the 18th and 19th centuries, respectively, opened Japan to Western medicine; it then developed its own techniques to become internationally recognized as one of the most advanced countries in the world of biological and medical sciences, with an average life expectancy of 82 years. However, Japan, a land of contrast, also preserved its traditional therapies of Chinese origin: herbal medicine ("kampo") is still popular and commonly co-prescribed with ethical drugs. Such co-prescription seeks to add different pharmacological effects at low doses without inducing adverse drug reactions (ADRs). It is unethical for a physician to be responsible for iatrogenic incidents, and drug safety has long been a priority to the detriment of efficacy. Japanese regulators developed the most severe guidelines regarding drug safety studies in animals and, paradoxically, clinical development remained, until recently, a pragmatic approach totally in the hands of medical doctors, at times hierarchical for clinical drug investigation. Nowadays, the rules regulating clinical trials recommend the use of international standards, and Japan became

the leader of several topics at the International Conference on Harmonization (ICH). It has been a full member since 1991. This chapter will present the main preclinical and clinical regulations governing drug development on Japanese territory.

Organization of Japanese health authorities

General organization

Under the authority of the Minister and the Vice-Minister, the Ministry of Health, Labor, and Welfare (MHLW or Koseirodosho in Japanese) is responsible for social security, public health, and the promotion of social welfare. For such purposes, the organization includes (see Figure 38.1) the following:
- A main body (central offices).
- An external bureau: the Social Insurance Agency.
- An advisory body: the Pharmaceutical Affairs and Food Sanitation Council (PAFSC), involved in New Drug Application (NDA) review.

The main body of the MHLW is divided into three branches:
- The *core administration*, which consists of the Secretariat (including the Statistics and Information Department), and the following bureaus: Health Policy Bureau; Health Service Bureau; Social Welfare and War Victim's Relief Bureau; Health and Welfare for Elderly Bureau; Equal Employment, Children and Families Bureau; Insurance Bureau; Pension Bureau; the Pharmaceutical and Food Safety Bureau (PFSB), which plays a major part

Principles and Practice of Pharmaceutical Medicine, 3rd edition.
Edited by L.D. Edwards, A.W. Fox, P.D. Stonier.
© 2011 Blackwell Publishing Ltd.

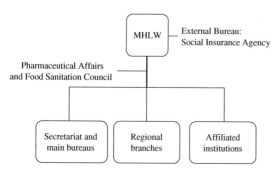

Figure 38.1 General organization of the Ministry of Health, Labor, and Welfare.

in drug regulations; and the Director-General for Policy Planning and Evaluation. Around 2000 officials work full-time in the central offices.

• *Regional branches*. Each prefectural government (47 prefectures) offers a local branch of the Health Authorities and Labor Bureaus: the Regional Medical and Pharmaceutical Affairs offices, and the District Narcotics Control offices. NDAs are made through the regional office of the prefecture where the company is situated.

• *Affiliated institutions*. In the present organization, national hospitals such as the National Cancer Center and three affiliated institutions operate under MHLW supervision:

– The National Institute of Health Sciences, performing tests and research on drugs, food, and chemical substances.

– The National Institute of Infectious Diseases, conducting research on pathogenicity, etiology, prevention of certain diseases, and tests and research on vaccines and blood products.

– The National Institute of Population and Social Security Research, training public health technicians, conducting surveys related to public health, and so on.

More than 50,000 officials work for the MHLW general organization.

Pharmaceutical administration

The PFSB, the Health Policy Bureau, with the assistance of the PAFSC, and the Pharmaceuticals and Medical Devices Agency (PMDA or Kiko in

Japanese) represent the managing authorities of Japanese pharmaceutical administration, in charge of reviewing drug application for approval, re-examination, or re-evaluation.

The PFSB

The PFSB consists of a Secretary General, five divisions, and one office. It ensures safety and efficacy of drugs, quasi-drugs, and medical devices, editing as well policies regarding blood supplies, blood products, narcotics, and stimulants.

General Affairs Division

This division coordinates all activities of the PFSB, enforces the Pharmaceutical Affairs Law (PAL), manages questions related to the PAFSC, and provides guidance and supervision to the PMDA. Two offices attached to the Planning Division are as follows:

• The Office of Access to Information, ensuring publication of information held by administrative organization.

• The Office of Drug Induced Damages, which supervises the PMDA and the administration of work related to ADRs damages.

Evaluation and Licensing Division

This division surveys and coordinates regulation of production, research, and trade of drugs, quasi-drugs, and medical devices. Many other services are provided by this division: licenses for manufacturing or import of drug and medical devices; designation of orphan drugs and medical devices; guidance to the PMDA; supervision of standards and specifications for drugs, quasi-drugs, and cosmetics; guidance for the Japanese Pharmacopoeia (JP); re-examination and re-evaluation of drugs and medical devices.

Safety Division

The responsibility of this division is to ensure the safety of drugs, quasi-drugs, medical devices, and cosmetics. The Office of Appropriate Use of Drugs, attached to this division, collects and evaluates information related to ADRs and promotes the appropriate use of drugs.

Compliance and Narcotics Division

The role of the division is to control and inspect, looking for quality issues, faulty labeling, and unlicensed drugs, quasi-drugs, medical devices, and cosmetics. It gives guidance for advertising, testing, official certification. and good manufacturing practice (GMP). It supports the enforcement of the Narcotics and Psychotropics Control Law, Cannabis Control Law, Opium Law. and Stimulants Control Law.

Blood and Blood Products Division

This division regulates blood collection, proper use of blood products, and production and distribution of biological products.

The Health Policy Bureau

The Health Policy Bureau handles promotion of R&D, drug, quasi-drugs, medical devices, and sanitary materials production and distribution policies. It is divided into two divisions: the Economic Affairs Division and the Research and Development Division, both having a relationship with the pharmaceutical industry.

The PAFSC

The PAFSC, an advisory organ of the MHLW, investigates and discusses important matters related to pharmaceutical affairs and food sanitation. The PAFSC members are experienced specialists in the field of medicine, pharmacy, biology, dentistry, and veterinary medicine, coming from universities, public hospitals, and research institutes; there are 55 permanent members and about 400 specialty non-staff reviewers whose function is to address the relevant subject under discussion. Major subjects treated by the PAFSC include the following:

- revision of the JP;
- determination of standards for drugs;
- evaluation of the relevance of allowing import or manufacturing of drugs;
- review of NDA;
- designation of drugs to be submitted for re-examination and re-evaluation;
- judgments concerning the payment of relief funds under the provisions of the ADR Relief and Research Promotion Fund Law.

For such purpose, the PAFSC is organized into 16 committees and 21 subcommittees.

The Pharmaceuticals and Medical Devices Agency (PMDA)

In 2005, there were significant revisions to the Japanese PAL, requiring Third Party certification systems for new low-risk and priority high-risk medicines and devices.

In preparation for these changes, in April 2004, the Pharmaceutical and Medical Device Evaluation Center (PMDEC), the Japan Association for the Advancement of Medical Equipment (JAAME), and the Organization for Pharmaceutical Safety and Research (OPSR) were merged and integrated in the National Institute of Health Sciences. This consolidated a unified organization for the regulation of pharmaceuticals, and biological and medical devices, and thus became the Pharmaceuticals and Medical Devices Agency (PMDA) (see Figure 38.2).

The main activities of the PMDA are to offer the pharmaceutical industry consultations with regard to clinical trial protocols and drug and medical devices development plans, to conduct new drug application review, and to confirm the quality of the submitted data. The PMDA, or Drug Agency, is composed of 15 offices to conduct different services (see Figure 38.3).

Main offices related to new drug application, approval review, drug safety issues, re-examination and re-evaluation are as follows.

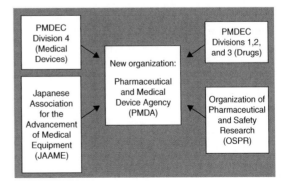

Figure 38.2 Birth of the PMDA.

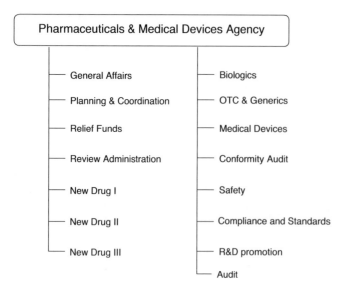

Figure 38.3 Organization of the PMDA.

Office of New Drug I
This division takes in charge anti-HIV agents, anti-malignant tumor agents, anti-bacterial agents, and related drugs.

Office of New Drug II
This division operates review of cardiovascular drugs, metabolic disease drugs when in combination with other drugs, reproductive system drugs, anal and urogenital drugs, and diagnostics and radiopharmaceuticals for *in vivo* use.

Office of New Drug III
This division takes care of hormonal agents, metabolic disease drugs when not in combination with other drugs, dermatologic agents, gastrointestinal tract agents, central and peripheral nervous system drugs, sensory organ agents, anti-allergy drugs, respiratory tract drugs, and narcotics. Office of Biologics. This department reviews files for biological products, and cell- and tissue-derived products. It is also involved in agents used in gene therapy.

Office of OTC and Generics
This division reviews applications for approval of generics, non-prescription drugs (OTC), quasi-drugs, and cosmetics.

Office of Medical Devices
Medical devices and *in vitro* diagnostics are reviewed by this department.

Office of Safety
This office collects, organizes, and analyzes safety information from drugs and medical devices, in collaboration with some other offices from the ministry, and participates in the dissemination of the safety information.

Office of Compliance and Standards
In this department, data compliance to good laboratory practice (GLP), good clinical practice (GCP), and good post-marketing surveillance practice (GPMSP) is carefully controlled. Applications are checked to determine whether they were prepared according to the Criteria for Reliability of Application Data.

The PMDA covers a wide range of other services, such as guidance for the development of orphan drugs, communication with drug consumers, and guidance on the necessity of different types of certificates. One of the most important services is the "Kiko consultation." Starting April 1, 1997, with the Drug Organization, PMDA carries on today several types of consultations (19 subtypes) for the

pharmaceutical industry. The main consultations for drug development are as follows:
- on initial plans for clinical trials (Phase I);
- at the end of Phase IIa and at the end of Phase IIb;
- before filing (dealing with long-term trials or pre-NDA consultation, checking the acceptability of the NDA);
- on protocols: Fees of ¥0.5–3.3 million are charged for consultation services; records of the guidance and advices are kept and can be used as attached data for a new drug application.

Japanese pharmaceutical laws

Japanese pharmaceutical administration has a long history; it started during the reign of Emperor Meiji, a period during which Japan reopened its frontiers to Western countries. The first law, enacted in 1874, dealt with pharmaceutical sales and handling, but it was limited to three areas (Tokyo, Osaka, and Kyoto). Fifteen years later, the law covered the whole country and was merged with another law, the Patent Medicine Law, in 1925; it was then renamed the "Pharmaceutical Affairs Law" in 1943.

The Pharmaceutical Affairs Law (PAL)

The first "modern" law was born in August 1960, when it was split into the PAL and the Pharmacists' Law. The original goal of the Law was to ensure the quality and safety of drugs. Following the evolution of medicines, technique, quality standards, and so on, the Law was revised and amended several times in order to incorporate new regulations, such as the GCP. Nowadays, the PAL and the Enforcement Regulations of the PAL regulate drugs from production and development to marketing and distribution, its scope covering new drugs, quasi-drugs, cosmetics, and medical devices. It was further revised in 1996, and the first physician was appointed to the Regulatory Authorities in 1997. Last amendments were made in 2002 mainly to improve post-marketing surveillance (PMS) policy and revision of the approval and licensing systems; it includes provisions for safety measures for bio-

logical products, investigator-initiated clinical trials, a rationalization plan to establish the PMDA and revision of the review system, and provisions related to manufacturing and distribution business.

The Law contains 11 chapters and 89 articles. A survey of this Law in brief, and chapter contents are described below:
- Chapter 1. *General provisions.* Purpose of the Law and definitions of drug, quasi-drug, cosmetic, medical device, orphan drug, and pharmacy.
- Chapter 2. *Pharmaceutical Affairs Council.* The PAFSC is established, as well as local prefectures councils.
- Chapter 3. *Pharmacies.* Defines license standards and supervision of the pharmacies.
- Chapter 4. *Manufacture and import of drugs and so on.* Here it is specified that import or manufacture of a drug needs official review by the PMDA and approval, and that the drug should be re-examined and then re-evaluated after a certain period of marketing.
- Chapter 5. *Selling drugs and medical devices.* Deals with licenses for sales and restrictions.
- Chapter 6. *Standards and tests for drugs and so on.* Establishes the JP and other standards.
- Chapter 7. *Handling of drugs and so on.* Specifies the handling of poisonous and powerful drugs, drugs requiring prescription, package inserts, containers, labeling, sales, and manufacturing restrictions.
- Chapter 8. *Advertising of drugs and so on.* Regulates advertising of drug and handling of biological products.
- Chapter 9. *Supervision.* Defines on-site inspection and potential sanctions, orders for improvement, cancellation of approvals and licenses, and so on.
- Chapter 9.2. *Designation of orphan drugs and orphan medical devices.*
- Chapter 10. *Miscellaneous provisions.* Deals with data submission and the handling of clinical trials, and so on.
- Chapter 11. *Penal provisions.* Defines and fixes the penalties for violation of different articles of the Law.

The Law generally describes the frame of the regulations; for most of the articles, more details and complementary information are provided by the Enforcement Regulations of the PAL, which regulates most of the drug development. These regulations will be reviewed in the next sections.

Other pharmaceutical laws

Separated from the main Law in 1960, the Pharmacists' Law deals with the activities of pharmacists, examination, licensing, and duties; the Law concerning the Organization for Pharmaceuticals and Medical Devices was revised a few years ago. Several other laws are involved in pharmaceutical administration. Their scope is restricted to limited areas and most of them aim at preventing drug abuse and health damages. They are the Poisonous and Deleterious Substances Control Law, the Narcotics and Psychotropics Control Law, the Cannabis Control Law, the Opium Law, the Stimulants Control Law, and the Blood Collection and Blood Donation Services Control Law.

Drug development regulations overview

In order to clarify the following sections, some regulations have been artificially separated. For Western people not familiar with Japanese regulations, these rules, delivered through hundreds of notifications from the Pharmaceutical Affairs Bureau, are a huge maze. We have tried to simplify this review, and we apologize for the lack of precision consequently induced.

Generalities

Marketing approval, manufacturing, and import approval

To be authorized to market a new drug in Japan, it is necessary to obtain a drug approval and a manufacturing or import approval for the drug. Drug Approval is an official confirmation, based on scientific data, that the drug is effective and safe. The Approval is granted for a drug to a person or a juridical person. The manufacturing or import approval for a given drug is granted after ensuring that the applicant is healthy and sane, legally competent, and that the personnel, facilities, and

equipments comply with the Pharmaceutical Law requirements and quality standards in order to be able to manufacture or import the approved drug properly. The manufacturing approval is granted for a specific drug to the facilities where the drug will be manufactured. Manufacturing approval can be transferred to legally authorized manufacturers, for example, through contracts or mergers.

In-country caretaker system

Approval can be obtained by either a domestic company or directly by a foreign company settled abroad, since the revision of the PAL in May 1983. However, clinical data establishing efficacy and safety should be generated in Japanese patients, on Japanese territory; therefore, if the foreign company has no means of conducting these clinical trials on its own, it should appoint an in-country caretaker, domiciled in Japan. A clinical research organization (CRO) is allowed to perform such clinical development in respect to the PAL; the CRO may be subject to spot inspections or other specific requests from the MHLW, such as report submission regarding ADRs. The CRO should be able to take necessary measures to prevent the occurrence or spread of health damages induced by the drug under investigation (for more information about CROs in Japan, please refer to Bentley, 1997).

Substances and devices regulated by the PAL

Main groups defined by the law

Four groups are defined, which usually need an Approval to be marketed in Japan, unless specifically designated by the MHLW:

• Drugs, including substances listed in the JP, substances for diagnosis, treatment, or prevention of human and animal diseases, and substances affecting any structure or function of the human or animal body. Apparatus or instruments are, of course, excluded. This group can be divided into prescription drugs (or ethical drugs) and nonprescription drugs.

• Quasi-drugs are substances that exert a mild action on the body, such as drugs used to prevent

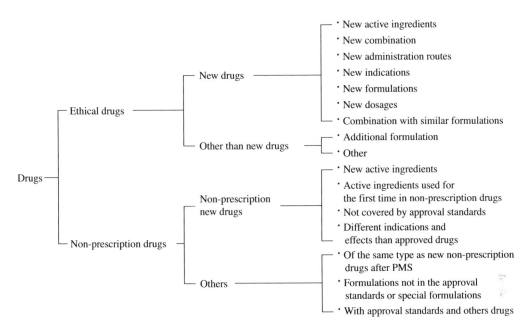

Figure 38.4 Classification of drugs, function of the data to apply.

nausea, bad breath, body odor, hair loss, heat rash, and so on.

• Cosmetics are substances also having a mild action or no action on the body, but are for external use, applied by rubbing or spraying on the skin or hair, and are used for cleaning or beautifying.

• Medical devices are instruments or equipment used for the diagnosis, treatment, or prevention of human or animal diseases. They are designated by ministerial ordinance.

Drug classification

The four groups above include numerous subclasses, which vary according to the function of different parameters: for example, approval procedures, approval authorities, handling of standards, and list of data to be submitted. Regarding drugs and data to be submitted for approval, Figure 38.4 gives a good example of a possible classification.

Orphan drugs

Within the ethical drug class, a particular group should be distinguished: orphan drugs. Orphan drugs status was originally defined in 1993 as fol-

lows: a drug is designated as orphan by the MHLW after recommendation by the PAFSC, when efficacy is scientifically established and when it can benefit less than 50,000 patients. Orphan drugs are subject to financial aid, priority review, and extension of the re-examination period from 6 to10 years.

Data required for a NDA

According to Notification 481 from the PMSB, dated April 8, 1999, the whole original list of data required for a NDA should include from April 2000:

• Data on origin, details of discovery, use in foreign country, and so on: 1. Data on origin and details of discovery. 2. Data on use in foreign countries. 3. Data on characteristics and comparison with other drugs.

• Data on physical and chemical properties, specifications, testing methods, and so on: 1. Data on determination of structure. 2. Data on physical and chemical properties, and so on. 3. Data on specifications and testing methods (standards).

• Data on stability: 1. Data on long-term storage test. 2. Data on severe test. 3. Data on acceleration test.

• Data on acute toxicity, sub-acute toxicity, chronic toxicity, teratogenicity, and other toxicity studies in animals: 1. Data on single dose. 2. Data on repeated dose. 3. Data on mutagenicity. 4. Data on carcinogenicity. 5. Data on reproduction. 6. Data on local irritation. 7. Other safety data.
• Data on pharmacological action: 1. Other safety data. 2. Data on efficacy (mechanism of action). 3. Data on safety (general pharmacology). 4. Other animal pharmacology data.
• Data on pharmacokinetics (PK): 1. Data on absorption. 2. Data on distribution. 3. Data on metabolism. 4. Data on excretion. 5. Data on bioequivalence. 6. Other PK data. 7. Data on the results of clinical trials.

Some of these requirements are omitted when applying for a new dosage, a new indication, a new route of administration, or a new formulation with regard to a drug already approved, or may vary according to drug classification, non-prescription drug (Notification 0827003 from PSFB, August 27, 2003), quasi-drug, or cosmetic.

Quality standards

Quality standards for substances and devices regarding properties, technical specifications, and test methods

1. The Japanese Pharmacoepia (JP). The main and the oldest document specifying standards for drugs is the JP, first published in 1886. The JP is established by law (Article 41). It aims at regulating quality for important drugs used in healthcare and specific standard test methods. The JP is revised by law every ten years; but in practice, the revision is carried out every five years. The 14th edition was published in 2001 and already contains some monographs harmonized with the US and European Pharmacopoeias. The 15th edition was issued in 2006.

2. For drugs not mentioned in the JP, Article 42 of the PAL indicates that the MHLW can lay down necessary standards for drugs and so on, requiring particular cautions. The following standards for drugs have been gazetted through ministerial ordinance:

(a) Standards for Biological Materials (MHLW Notification 210, 2003).
(b) Minimum requirements for biological products.
(c) Minimum requirements for blood grouping antibodies.
(d) Radiopharmaceutical standards.

Other standards were published for quasi-drugs (e.g., sanitary products standards), cosmetics (e.g., standards for the quality of cosmetics), and medical devices (e.g., standards for blood donor sets, cardiac pacemakers, and medical X-ray apparatus).

3. For substances not mentioned in the JP and not covered by Article 42 of the Law, additional standards were notified by the MHLW, for example, the Japanese standards for pharmaceutical ingredients, standards for crude drugs, standards of raw materials for clinical diagnostics, and so on.

4. Finally, for drugs having particular manufacturing technology and test methods, such as biotechnological products, a government certification based on "batch tests" is necessary.

Quality standards for data, facilities and functional organizations

These standards cover different fields describing "good practices" ensuring the quality of the drug, the quality and reliability of the data generated with the drug, and finally, warrant the efficacy and safety of a given drug for a given disease, with respect to scientific and ethical considerations for both humans and animals.

GMP

Enforced in 1976, GMP establishes the requirements ensuring drug production of a high and constant quality. Ordinances 92 and 95, revised in May 2003, contain guidance on the following:
• Manufacturing control and quality control (GMP software).
• Duties of the Control Manager (self-inspection, education and training, etc.).
• Standards for buildings and facilities for manufacturing plants (GMP hardware).

In 1988, GMPs for medical devices were also enforced. A group of inspectors attached to prefectural government perform regular on-site inspections of manufacturers, importers, and distributors in order to check their compliance to GMP.

GMP compliance certificates for Japanese drug plant have been issued since 1982; today bilateral agreements have been signed with the United States and the EU since May 2003, with regard to GMP compliance recognition.

Regulations for Imported Drug Management and Quality Control

Also related to drug quality, the standards for Quality Assurance of Imported Drugs and Medical Devices were notified in 1993, establishing basic quality assurance requirements with which the drug importer should comply. The MHLW ordinance 62 of June 1999 today regulates drug import to Japan.

GLP

In order to ensure the reliability of animal data, GLP standards were published by the PAB in March 1982, enforced one year later, and revised in October 1988. GLP describes standards for personnel and organization (management, quality assurance unit, etc.) for animal care facilities and equipment, standard operating procedures for the operation of testing facilities, test and control articles, the conduct of a study, the study report, and the storage of the raw data.

These standards originally concerned animal safety studies; today, they are applied to all animal studies, for example, toxicology, pharmacology, and animal PK. GLP was legalized as an MHLW Ordinance in 21 March 1997, requiring in particular to establish Standard Operating Procedures (SOPs) and the preparation of protocols and study reports. The PMDA is conducting GLP compliance reviews and on-site inspections of testing facilities.

GLP applies to foreign data when attached to the NDA. Mutual GLP agreements have been signed between Japan and the United States, EU, and Switzerland.

GCP

Written in 1985, Japanese GCP standards were notified by the MHLW in 1989 for a general appli-

cation from October 1990. They laid down rules for conducting a clinical trial properly from an ethical and scientific standpoint:

- Definition of the respective role and responsibilities of the sponsor, the investigator, and the medical institution.
- The contract for a clinical trial between the sponsor and the hospital conducting the study.
- The institutional review board (IRB) in each medical institute, its role, and organization.
- The informed consent of the patient to participate into the trial, which was not originally a "written" consent.
- The storage of the study records (source data) during a certain period of time.

These rules, however, were to be applied to a clinical development organization specifically in Japan, and were very different to Western ones (see the section on "Clinical Development," below). Within the framework of the ICH, GCP were discussed for several years and finally concluded in 1996. New harmonized GCP standards are now applicable to the United States, Europe, and Japan as well, but they require profound changes of the Japanese system to be fully applied; the PAL had to be amended in order to permit the enforcement of the new GCP from April 1997. These had a major impact on new study starts, the need for informed consent being the largest reason.

The main changes for the Japanese clinic (Takahashi and VandenBurg, 1997) include the following:

- New obligations for the sponsor, such as the preparation of the clinical protocol and the writing of a clinical study report.
- The abolition of the "chairman" of the investigator steering committee (see Figure 38.5).
- The designation by the medical institution of an IRB, which can be outside the hospital, such as an academic society, and which will compulsorily have a member from outside the institution.
- The sponsor must establish an independent monitoring system in order to conduct an adequate evaluation of progress of the clinical trial, safety information, and efficacy endpoints. This means that Japanese companies will now have to hire medical doctors to handle medical matters.

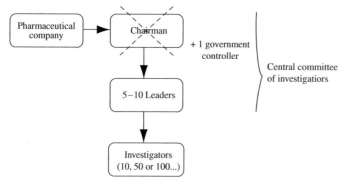

Figure 38.5 Clinical trials in Japan.

• The informed consent becomes a written consent and necessitates true and complete information for the patient, including risk and compensation for damage to the health of subjects.

The new GCP standards are, of course, similar to those of the US and European GCP, to which the reader should refer for detailed regulations.

The GPMSP

The PMS system is a well-established system in Japan for collecting safety data in order to prepare the documentation requested for re-examination, which will be described in the section on "Post-approval activities", below.

GPMSP standards were enforced in April 1994 after revision of the text published in May 1993. It became a law in 1997, and was further revised in 2000, to add the "Early Post-Marketing Surveillance," applying to new drug in the first six months of marketing. These standards specify the rules to be observed by the manufacturer in order to ensure the reliability of the PMS data, mainly the following:

• The manufacturer shall establish a PMS department independent of the marketing division and shall employ sufficient staff.

• PMS managers shall prepare standard operating procedures for PMS in order to collect information on drug use, assess this information and take appropriate measures, undertake surveys and special surveys when necessary, perform post-marketing clinical trials, conduct self inspections, train and educate PMS personnel, contract-out PMS works, and store the information records properly.

• Serious unexpected ADR and Infections Reporting System are to follow ICH rules for reporting within 7, 15 and 30 days. From October 2003, it became mandatory to use MedRA for individual adverse event report.

Specific guidelines for drug development

In addition to the Law and Quality Standards, specific guidelines have been notified for both preclinical and clinical studies. They regulate the preparation of the data to be submitted for approval by the authorities and they should generally be strictly followed. These guidelines explain what kind of data have to be produced and indicate the methodology to generate these data; many of these guidelines were discussed at the ICH, and most of them are already harmonized and implemented on Japanese territory.

Other guidelines or recommendations regulate the administrative procedures surrounding development works, such as the import or labeling of the study drug. The PAL directly describes the procedures for notifying clinical trials in its section "handling of clinical trials." These regulations will be reviewed with the next section.

Drug development procedures

After the chemical research and screening test periods, the development of a new chemical entity (NCE) follows preclinical and clinical steps similar to Western ones. It takes 8–10 years to establish the efficacy and safety for a new drug and to prepare the documentation required for a NDA.

Regarding the development of a new drug in Japan that is already approved in a foreign country, even if preclinical data were harmonized up to 95%, six to eight years are still necessary in order to conduct clinical development on Japanese territory on Japanese subjects and patients from Phase I to Phase III. New regulations, such as "ICH E5" implementation in Japan, offer potential strategies to reduce the development time, using foreign data; however, in practice, acceptable cases are rather limited.

Preclinical studies

Physicochemical properties, specifications, and test methods

Basic chemical data, identification, purity, and test methods should follow the Guidelines "Setting Specifications and Test Methods of New Drugs," notified in May 2001. Several others dealing with analytical validation, impurities, or residual solvents were established on the basis of ICH agreements. When available, standards published in the JP or other quality standards (see the earlier section on "Quality standards") represent the references for specifications and test methods.

Stability studies

Stability data on the active principle and on the formulation(s) are required on three batches, according to the Stability Test Guidelines issued in April 1994. These guidelines are now harmonized between the three ICH regions, implemented in Japan with the New Stability Test Guidelines, June 2003. Long-term data and tortured conditions test data should be submitted for new drug application; accelerated conditions tests only are necessary for applications regarding new dosages or new indications of a drug already registered.

Animal safety data

In May 1980, Notification 698 from the MHLW specified the type of data required for the evaluation of safety in animals and Guidelines for Toxicity Studies were subsequently established in 1984. It is necessary to generate data on acute, sub-acute, and chronic toxicity, and effect on reproduction, dependence, antigenicity, mutagenicity, carcinogenicity, and local irritation.

After several revisions, including ICH agreements in 1993 and 1999, the present Guidelines for Toxicity Studies cover almost all these items, describing the tests methods to be conducted for the following:

- single-dose toxicity study;
- repeated-dose toxicity study, 1 or 3 months and 6 or 12 months administration, and guidance for toxicokinetics;
- reproductive and developmental toxicity studies;
- drug dependence studies were notified in 1975 by the Narcotic Division (for drugs having a pharmacological effect on the central nervous system);
- antigenicity studies;
- skin sensitization and skin photosensitization for dermatological preparations;
- genotoxicity studies;
- carcinogenicity studies (requirements and dose selection for carcinogenicity study has been harmonized).

All toxicity studies supporting a new drug application should comply with GLP standards.

Pharmacology

Pharmacological data should include two different types of data:

- "Specific pharmacology" data provide information regarding the main effects on the target disease in animal models and try to clarify the mechanism of action as far as possible. There are no guidelines for specific pharmacology.
- "General pharmacology" studies are conducted to assess the overall pharmacological profile and to obtain information about the effects on the main physiological functions and potential adverse events. Three dose levels are studied (low, intermediate, and high or very high doses) in a battery of tests exploring the main body functions. General pharmacology studies are regulated by guidelines notified in January 1991.

In 2001, general pharmacology data were classified in "efficacy pharmacology, secondary/safety pharmacology, and other pharmacology." All pharmacological studies should also comply with the GLP standards.

Animal PK

Data on absorption, distribution, metabolism, and excretion in animal are necessary to clarify the drug's biological fate in the body and to establish an appropriate dose regimen in animal studies, and ultimately in humans.

The guidelines for nonclinical PK studies were notified in January 1991. They request those studies to be performed after single and repeated administration. Japan was traditionally the only country systematically to conduct a two- or three-week administration test in order to detect tissue accumulation.

Recently, the ICH-harmonized tripartite guideline, Guidance for Repeated Dose Tissue Distribution Studies, opened the door for such repeated dose studies, but recognized that there was no consistent justification to conduct these tests systematically. In June 2001, new guidelines on nonclinical PK studies were notified.

Clinical development

Efficacy and safety data supporting a NDA approval do not differ fundamentally from the Western clinical data package. They are generated through similar phases, which are
• human pharmacology studies (Phase I);
• therapeutic exploratory studies (dose determination studies, Phase II);
• therapeutic confirmatory studies (safety and efficacy studies versus a reference drug, Phase III).

However, Japanese clinical trials show some differences in their organization and methodological approaches, which are still in practice in spite of regulations requesting the application of internationally validated standards.

Clinical trials regulations

The PAL and its Enforcement Regulations establishes some basic rules for clinical trials; that is, in summary, it is necessary to
• conduct preclinical tests (toxicity, pharmacology, etc.) before starting human administration;

• request in writing to an adequate medical institution to conduct a clinical trial;
• inform the patient before his/her enrollment into the trial;
• submit to the MHLW information regarding the clinical protocol for each study, along with information concerning the study drug and a summary of the preclinical tests.

Each change in the study course should be notified to the authorities by filling specific administration forms (protocol modification, study suspension, study completion).

Notification 698 of May 1980 does not provide much more information regarding clinical trials, requesting to submit "at least 150 cases in at least five institutions" for a new ethical drug application for approval.

Two guidelines notified in 1992 brought more detailed guidance on the purpose, methodology, and assessment of the three clinical development phases:
• Guidelines for the Statistical Analysis of Clinical Study Results (May 1992);
• General Considerations for the Clinical Evaluation of New Drugs (June 1992);
• General Considerations for Clinical Studies, including ICH standards (April 1998).

Phase I should estimate a range of safe dose levels up to a maximum tolerated dose, and characterize the PK profile of the study drug in humans. Generally, a single-dose study and a one-week repeated-dose study are conducted in a small number (six to eight) of healthy male volunteers. Food effects, drug interactions, and bioequivalence studies nowadays belong to this clinical pharmacology phase, as well as PK in the elderly and studies in subjects with poor kidney or hepatic function.

Phase II is traditionally divided in two sequences: Phase IIa or early Phase II; and Phase IIb or late Phase II. Phase IIa is generally an open study with three or four arms, performed to explore efficacy and safety of three or four doses in patients, and it should also bring supplementary information regarding PK parameters. This is different from conventional Phase IIa, which is Proof of Concept Study (POC). Phase IIb is a double-blind study comparing the effects of two or three doses to placebo effects, aiming at the determination of the optimal dose and dose regimen for a specific indication. It should be noticed that placebo use is not mandatory, but is used "if necessary." The final galenic formulation and dosage forms of the study drug are required for the conduct of Phase IIb.

Phase III should confirm the efficacy and safety of the optimal dose and dose regimen in a large group of patients under the usual therapeutic conditions. A large randomized double-blind trial should be conducted versus a reference drug (traditionally, a reference drug in Japan has been marketed for at least six years, and its efficacy and safety has been confirmed through the re-examination procedure).

Long-term trials have now to be conducted and meet international standards, the Extent of Population Exposure to Assess Clinical Safety (it was difficult in the past to obtain long-term data). Some open Phase III trials might be added to study particular patient subgroups, for example, the elderly or a specific subgroup of the disease.

The guidelines on statistics indicate how to analyze the study results properly and introduce international and validated standards for the statistical evaluation.

Specific guidelines

With regard to certain pharmacological or therapeutic classes, several specific guidelines have been published since 1980, describing the type of data necessary for a NDA and how to generate these data. Twelve guidelines have been published, in different clinical fields; guidelines for clinical trials on urinary tract infections and on dysuria are to be announced soon; other therapeutic fields should be covered in the coming years.

ICH guidelines

In addition to these Japanese original guidelines for clinical development, internationally harmonized guidelines are now implemented in Japan, as follows:
• Clinical Trials in Special Population (Geriatrics);
• Dose–Response Information to Support Drug Registration;
• The Extent of Population Exposure to Assess Clinical Safety;

• Clinical Safety Data Management (Definition and Standard for Expedited Reporting);
• Clinical Study Reports: Structure and Content;
• Clinical investigation in Pediatric population;
• Choice of Control Group and Related Issues in Conducting Clinical Studies;
• Ethnic factors in the acceptability of foreign clinical data.

International GCPs

All clinical studies supporting a drug registration should comply with the harmonized Good Clinical Practices, which were enforced in April 1997.

Other development rules and practices

Regarding the clinical development organization, by tradition some aspects were unique to Japan (Labbé, 1995). Traditionally, an investigators' committee took full charge of the clinical development from Phase I or Phase IIa through Phase III. The committee consisted of a chairman, a senior leader in his or her specialty, chosen by the pharmaceutical company. The chairman recommended key investigators and well-known experts to the sponsor (see the earlier Figure 38.5).

Each of the five or eight key investigators recommended several medical institutions, public or private, where the investigators performed the clinical trial. The investigators' committee was supposed to: write the clinical protocol, follow the study progress, and propose action when something wrong happened (serious adverse events, for instance); decide whether to keep or reject a case report form before statistical analysis; and write the clinical study report. They met and worked under the supervision of a government controller (often a clinical pharmacologist).

There is usually, for one indication, one study per phase from Phase IIa, and all trials are multicenter studies. Regulations require around 100 patients for Phase II and 200 for Phase III; however, 1000–1500 cases are commonly submitted in the NDA; because one investigator may produce only one, two, or three case reports, 30, 80, or more investigators may consequently be involved in a Phase II or III trial.

Clinical development has to progress step by step, according to the general guidelines; after each phase, the steering committee of investigators decided whether the study results justified whether or not to proceed to the next step. It was surprising to notice that the placebo was not considered as mandatory in dose determination studies (always mentioned in the protocols as "placebo if necessary"), and it was never used in phase III studies, for ethical reasons, unless no reference treatment is available. This is still true today.

These specificities and many others, however, are changing with the implementation of the ICH guidelines, for example, the enforcement of the new GCP abolishes the traditional Steering Committee of Investigators, the "controller" is only responsible to warrant the "blindness" of the trial. However, it generally takes a long time in Japan to modify such strong traditions, and they will probably still be in practice for some years more.

2. Foreign data could be helpful to reduce the six to eight years necessary for clinical development in Japan. However, the clinical development of a foreign drug has to be duplicated in Japan from Phase I to Phase III, because of potential genetic, diet, and medical practice differences. Key data in the NDA are Japanese data; the foreign clinical data package is considered as complementary information, only used when safety issues are raised during the approval process.

Some clinical pharmacology studies only can be accepted as key data, such as drug interaction studies or kinetic studies in renal or hepatic insufficiency. The topic "Ethnic factors in foreign data acceptability" (E5) was passed in 1998 in Japan after six years of discussion; it is now recognized that cultural factors are far more important than genetic differences (ICH 2 Proceedings, 1993; ICH 3 Proceedings, 1995). This allows for a regulated mutual recognition of clinical data, which should significantly reduce the number of useless duplications of clinical studies and consequently save development resources (see Chapter 19).

3. The import of a foreign study drug is strictly regulated: imported amount of bulk and/or pharmaceutical form should be clearly justified and limited to the exact quantity necessary for the development. When a clinical trial protocol is available, a copy has to be submitted for approval by a customs officer with a Drug Import Report Slip (Form 12) and a copy of the invoice. When the protocol is not available, a certificate from the Inspection and Guidance Division must be obtained after submission of the following documentation: an Import Report Form (Form 1), a Drug Import Report Slip (Form 13), a Memorandum (Form 2), a protocol outline, a Memorandum stating that the protocol will be submitted within three months, and a copy of the Drug Import business license.

The labeling of the study drug should mention, on the drug packaging, container, or wrapper, the fact that the drug is for study purposes, the name and address of the institution, the chemical name or symbol, the manufacturing code number, storage instructions, and expiry date.

The anticipated brand name, indications or effects, and directions for use and doses of the trial drug should not be mentioned on the drug container or wrapper or on any document attached to the trial drug.

New drug approval process

Content of the NDA

Once the clinical development is completed, four to six months are necessary to prepare the presentation of the NDA, which should be as perfect as possible. The content of the NDA is defined by the notification of April 1999, "Approval Application for Drugs." The ICH agreement induced several revisions in July 2001 and June 2003, to describe the preparation of the Common Technical Document (CTD), enforced in April 2005, and later electronic CTD.

Module 1

Module 1 contains regulatory information such as application forms and information on attached documentation. Module 1 is region specific. For Japan this contains:

1. Table of content.
2. Approval application (copy).
3. Certificates.
4. Patent situation in Japan and abroad.

5. Background of origin, discovery, and development.

6. Data related to conditions of use in foreign countries.

7. List of related products: comparison of the main characteristics of the drug with those of similar drugs already registered in Japan.

8. Draft Package Insert.

9. International Non-proprietary Name (INN) and Japanese Accepted Name (JAN) publications.

10. Data for review as powerful, poisonous drug, and so on.

11. Draft plan and protocol for PMS.

12. List of attached documentation.

13. Other documents.

Other modules

Module 2 (Data Summaries; the GAIYO in Japanese), Module 3 (Quality), Module 4 (Safety), and Module 5 (Efficacy) are common to the ICH Regions. Please refer to the ICH M4 guidelines.

Foreign data attached to the NDA are not necessarily translated into Japanese. They may be submitted in English, with a Japanese summary; this is not mandatory however, for original English entries of the CTD.

Review process

Before submission of the NDA to the Authorities, the dossier is carefully checked because no other data, unless specifically required by the MHLW, can be added after submission. No clinical trial with the study drug is allowed on Japanese territory once the review process has started, unless authorized by the Authorities.

The application for approval is submitted to the Health Authorities through the prefectural branch of the MHLW (see Figure 38.6). The 2006 total application fees (MHLW PMDA fees) were ¥16,881,800 (around US$140,000) for the first dosage of a new ethical drug and ¥4,235,300 for each further dosage (about US$35,000); ¥12,018,400 (around US$100,000) for the first dosage of an orphan drug and ¥3,011,100 (around US$25,000) for each further dosage; ¥44,300 to 655,300 (around US$4500) for a generic drug; and ¥129,600 (around US$1000) for a non-prescription drug.

The NDA is transmitted to the PMDA which first conducts reliability and GLP compliance reviews. When the data quality is confirmed, specialized team of experts review the NDA data and prepare a list of requests and questions addressed to the

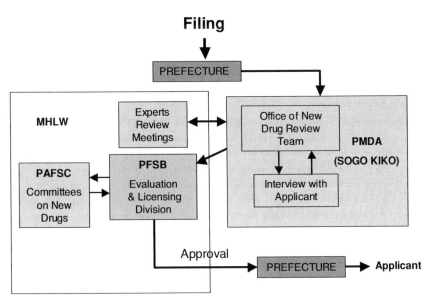

Figure 38.6 Approval process overview.

applicant. After receiving the answers from the applicant, a review report is prepared. Samples of the active principle might also be requested, for analytical control by the National Institute of Health Sciences.

A meeting with Clinical Experts is then organized with the review team members of the PMDA (Specialists Meeting) to discuss key issues of the NDA. At this stage, within six months after application, a hearing is generally held between the reviewers and the sponsor, which may today be accompanied by its own experts.

Another "follow-up" meeting is organized between the reviewers and the specialists, and a second review report is finalized. The report is transferred to the Evaluation and Licensing Division of the PFSB. After a careful reading, the report will be circulated to the Committee on New Drugs of the PAFSC.

When the subcommittees are satisfied with the review report, the dossier goes back to the PFSB with a recommendation for approval. The minister will officially grant the New Drug Approval to the pharmaceutical company, through the prefecture. Around 18–24 months are necessary to obtain a new drug approval if there are no special issues, 6 months for a quasi-drug, 3 months for cosmetics, and 12 months for a medical device.

A New Drug Approval Information Package is prepared from this report, and is published, and is available to medical institutions.

Summary of the product characteristics

The data sheet is called the "package insert" in Japan, because it can be found in the drug packaging. The data sheet is drafted by the company and checked and completed by the authorities after the NDA review and the recommendation for approval. The content has been defined by the MHLW notification, and was revised in May 1997. Besides general information on the product, the most important entries are warnings, precautions, and contraindications, and a list of adverse events quantitatively reported. These entries will be revised if necessary, with the safety data regularly analyzed for the periodic safety update report;

however, an *ad hoc* revision is made at any time in case of serious events.

NHI price fixing

Prescription drugs are listed on the National Health Insurance Drug Price List in order to be reimbursed under the National Health Insurance Program. The price is fixed by a commission, including medical doctors, consumers, and Central Social Insurance Medical Council representatives ("Chuikyo" in Japanese). Recent available treatments serve as price references and premiums of 3–100% are added to compensate for novelty and clinical advantages. The NHI price needs two to three months after the drug approval to be listed on the drug tariff. The product can be launched the following day.

Post-approval activities

From the first day of its launch, the drug enters the PMS period until the end of its marketing life cycle. Besides Phase IV trials, the regulation of which are under reorganization and which should meet GCP standards, post-approval activities mainly aim at ensuring the new drug safety and efficacy. For such purposes, a surveillance system has been settled by the PAL. It consists of three different types of investigations: the ARD collecting system; the Re-examination; and the Re-evaluation. Quality standards for those three activities are defined in by GPMSP (see the earlier section in this chapter).

PMS organization

Several systems allow the collection of drug adverse events and their assessment by the MHLW as shown in Figure 38.7:

• *ADR Monitoring System.* Voluntary reports on ADRs are sent to the MHLW from around 3000 facilities designated by the MHLW, including national hospitals, and university and municipal hospitals; it is also called the "hospital monitoring system."

• *Pharmacy Monitoring System.* This is a similar system, collecting ADRs related to non-prescription drugs, by designated pharmacies. Around 2800 pharmacies report ADRs to the MHLW.

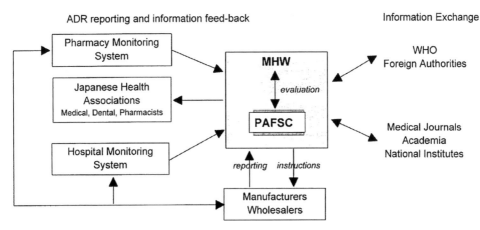

Figure 38.7 The Japanese post-marketing surveillance system.

• *Medical Device Monitoring System.* Another similar system reports to the MHLW the problems encountered with medical devices.

• *Manufacturers (and wholesalers).* These should also report ADRs to the MHLW, according to the Law.

The type of ADR to report and the time limits are defined by the international guidelines on Safety Data Management. In addition, periodic safety update reports are sent to the MHLW with respect to these international standards. Traditionally, in Japan, ADRs are classified into three grades (mild, moderate, severe), according to severity criteria, and into function of the body apparatus.

The MHLW collects and exchanges ADR information through other sources:

• WHO International Drug Monitoring Program.

• Relations with foreign health authorities, such as the FDA in the United States and the EMEA in the European Union.

• Survey of medical journals.

• Relations with universities and national institutes, and so on.

The safety information collected on a drug is assessed by the PAFSC (subcommittee on ADRs evaluation), and when necessary, the MHLW instructs the manufacturer to take measures such as follows:

• the revision of the data sheet (warning, dose, etc.);

• to conduct new investigation in animals or in humans;

• to discontinue import or manufacturing;

• to recall drugs from the market.

Re-examination

The re-examination system is part of, and complementary to, the PMS. After a certain period of marketing, safety and efficacy data are re-examined in the light of data collected during this period, which is

• six years for new drugs (extension up to eight years upon discussion), combined drugs, and new administration route;

• four years for a new indication, or a new dosage;

• ten years for orphan drugs.

Re-examination aims at confirming the conclusions from the drug approval and particularly the daily recommended dose, treatment duration, safety in long-term use, and so on. The manufacturer should apply a re-examination file three months before expiration of the six-year period for a new drug.

The dossier contains data from case report forms collected from hospitals. The number of cases is around 3000–4000 observations, reporting prescriptions on a routine basis (survey of use). Safety information comes from this particular survey and from spontaneous ADR reporting (serious events reports and the synthesis of the periodic safety update reports). Of course, information on

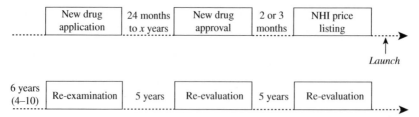

Figure 38.8 Flow chart of the regulatory process after new drug application.

measures taken during the period should be added (modification of the data sheet, etc.), as well as updated information regarding approval of the drug in foreign countries.

The Safety Division is in charge of reviewing the application; subcommittees and committees of the PAFSC will carry out the scientific assessment of the data and will either confirm the usefulness of the drug or ask for modification of the data sheet.

Re-evaluation

The spirit of the re-evaluation system is different from that of re-examination. Here, the efficacy and safety are reconsidered in the light of the evolution of medical sciences and regulatory progress. The re-evaluation is nowadays periodical, that is, every five years after the re-examination (see Figure 38.8); however, *ad hoc* re-evaluation can occur at any time upon request of the MHLW, when efficacy or safety is questioned for some therapeutic groups. Re-evaluation is done for each drug designated by the MHLW; drugs are usually grouped by therapeutic categories for re-evaluation; consequently, it may happen that for a given drug, re-evaluation is performed just before the re-examination, because re-evaluation is not directly dependent on the approval date. Additional studies might be requested by the MHLW to keep the drug on the market if the available data are not consistent with the present regulations and/or medical knowledge. If a drug designed by the MHLW does not undergo re-evaluation or does not show evidence of usefulness, the drug approval is cancelled.

So, from approval to market withdrawal, the drug dossier is a "living document," regularly completed by the pharmaceutical company and periodically revised by the health authorities.

Conclusion

Japanese regulations regarding drug development and PMS were recently amended, because of the progress of the ICH program, and for other reasons; recent incidents related to contaminated blood infusion and a fatal interaction between an antiviral and an anticancer drug most probably prompted the changes. However, there is a strong will from the Japanese authorities to apply international standards to drug development, particularly in the clinical field. The introduction of new GCP and GPMSP rules deeply modifies the background of the traditional Japanese R&D: the industry has to modify its structure and take over new responsibilities, hiring medical doctors in order to organize medical departments for clinical R&D and to assess ADRs. The predominant role of the investigators will decrease. The drug evaluation system by the authorities will have to be modified as well; it already shows, however, a strong will to a more scientific evaluation with the creation of the Japanese Drug Agency (PMDA).

The move is not limited to drug R&D. Many other fields are involved in this general evolution of the Japanese healthcare system: for example, the separation of prescription from dispensing ("bungyo") made recent progress; also, an important NHI price reform is under discussion, which could be a step toward a large change of the health insurance system.

Finally, the rapid evolution of the drug regulations may invalidate this chapter within a few years, but it is important for the pharmaceutical industry to understand that the whole drug environment is moving toward international standards under the pressure of scientific progress, quality requirements, and economical issues. This situation represents a chance to integrate Japan into the conception of the global dossier, for which the ICH has already laid the foundations.

References

Bentley S. Clinical research and CROs in Japan. *Appl Clin Trials* 1997; **8**(4):30–34.

Japanese Pharmacopoeia and Supplement 1 and 2, fourteenth edition. Yakuji Nippo: Tokyo, 2001.

Labbé E. Clinical trials in Japan: overcoming obstacles. *Appl Clin Trials* 1995; **4**(1):22–32.

Takahashi Y, VandenBurg MJ. Implementing the ICH GPC guideline in Japan. *Appl Clin Trials* 1997; **8**(4): 22–28.

Further reading

Drug Registration Requirements in Japan, fifth edition. Yakuji Nippo: Tokyo, 1993.

Guidelines for Clinical Evaluation of New Drugs. Yakugyo Jiho: Tokyo, 1986.

Guidelines for Clinical Evaluation of New Drugs (II). Yakugyo Jiho: Tokyo, 1988.

Japanese Guidelines for Nonclinical Studies of Drugs Manual. Yakuji Nippo: Tokyo, 1995.

Japanese GMP Regulations, third edition. Yakuji Nippo: Tokyo, 1988.

Japanese Pharmaceutical Manufacturers Association, Center For Pharmaceutical Publications. *Data Book,* 2006.

Japan Medical Products International Trade Association. *Japan Pharmaceutical Reference,* fifth edition. Japan Medical Products International Trade Association: Tokyo, 1999.

Pharmaceutical Administration in Japan, seventh edition. Yakuji Nippo: Tokyo, 1996.

Pharmaceutical Affairs Law, Enforcement Ordinance and Enforcement Regulations. Yakugyo Jiho: Tokyo, 1996.

Society of Japanese Pharmacopoeia. 1995. *Drug Approval and Licensing Procedures in Japan.* Yakugyo Jiho: Tokyo, 1995.

The Japan Federation of Medical Devices Associations. *The Pharmaceutical Affairs Law – New Regulations Effective in 2005.* Yakuji Nippo: Tokyo, 2004.

CHAPTER 39

Drug Registration and Pricing in the Middle East

Edda Freidank-Mueschenborn[1] & Anja König[2]
[1]Bungalowsiedlung 1 B, D-17406 Rankwitz, Germany
[2]Engelhard Arzneimittel AG, 61138 Niederdorfelden, Germany

The market

Commercial and Cultural Background

The Middle East is comprised of 14 independent countries located on or near the Arabian peninsula, which is bound by three bodies of water: the Mediterranean Sea to the north, Red Sea to the west, and the Arabian Sea to the east and south. The nations in this region are Bahrain, Kuwait, Oman, Qatar, Saudi Arabia, United Arab Emirates (UAE), Yemen, Syria, Lebanon, Israel, Jordan, Egypt, Iraq, Turkey, and the Palestinian Territories.

The region is not homogeneous. Individual countries differ significantly in government, economics, per capita income, size, population, and religion. Saudi Arabia is the largest country with 2 million square kilometres and Bahrain is the smallest with only 711 square kilometres. Yet Bahrain is the most densely populated country (917 people per square kilometre) with Oman at the other extreme (9 people per square kilometre). Absolute monarchy is found in Kuwait and complete democracy Lebanon. The distribution of Islam, Christianity, and Judaism will be familiar, with some countries almost totally one or other, while others are more mixed (e.g., 40% of the Lebanese population is Christian).

In many Middle-Eastern countries, the economy pivots on the sale of oil. However, phosphate pro-

duction and tourism (Jordan), aluminium and textiles (Bahrain), citrus growing (Israel), etc., are also major products, if less well-known. Gross domestic product (GDP) per capita per year ranges from US$1,527 in Yemen to more than US$26,000 in the UAE. The UAE is heterogeneous within itself: it was created as a Federation of seven states in 1971–1972 (formerly the "Trucial States"), each of which has considerable economic autonomy. Oil-rich Abu Dhabi is the capital and dominates the country economically; Dubai rose within the UAE on service industries, shipping, and real estate, but at the time of writing (November 2009) is deeply in debt. The remaining five emirates are small and relatively poor.

Arabic is an official language used by all regulatory authorities in the Middle East. However, some will also accept documents in English or French, and Israel also accepts documents in Hebrew.

Most of these countries have health systems that are very modern and up-to-date. There is an average of one physician for every 500 people in the region as a whole, and in some countries, especially the wealthier oil states, medical services and pharmaceuticals are free to the public. There are exceptions however, usually being in the poorest and least peaceful states in the region.

In general, the methods of diagnosis and treatment in the Middle East are very similar to those in Europe. However, there are large differences in epidemiology because *only 30% of the population in the Middle East is over 30 years of age.* This contrasts with the inverted age "pyramids" found in Europe

Principles and Practice of Pharmaceutical Medicine, 3rd edition.
Edited by L.D. Edwards, A.W. Fox, P.D. Stonier.

and North America, where the diseases of old age are slowly predominating in the capacity to deliver healthcare.

Important authorities/organizations

Authorities

The national competent regulatory authorities in the Middle East region are each country's Ministry of Health (MoH). These control the whole process of product approval from application formats to product pricing. In Egypt, the Ministry of Health and Population (MoHP) sub-divides its regulatory division into the National Organization for Drug Control and Research (NODCAR; which works together with the Central Administration for Pharmaceutical Affairs; CAPA) and the Drug Policy and Planning Centre (DPPC).

Realizing the benefits of harmonization, the following countries now accept a standard format marketing application: Saudi Arabia, Bahrain, Kuwait, Oman, Qatar, and the UAE. These are coordinated by a Gulf Central Committee for Drug Registration (GCC-DR). By 2006, submission of applications to the GCC-DR had become mandatory for most pharmaceutical classes, although older licenses within the GCC-DR territory are still amended nation-by-nation. Most companies taking this regulatory route actually model their dossiers on the long-standing requirements of Saudi Arabia, which has always had the most rigorous review system in the region (see also the Appendix at the end of this chapter).

Other organizations involved in regulatory affairs and health policy

The Levant Industry Group, founded in 1995, is headquartered in Amman, Jordan. Its objective is to represent the pharmaceutical industry in dialog with governments in healthcare issues. Its membership includes pharmaceutical companies that are active in Cyprus, Jordan, Lebanon, and Palestine.

The Pharmaceutical Research and Manufacturing Affiliates (PhRMAG) was founded in 1999, and is based in Dubai (in the UAE). Its objective is to represent the pharmaceutical industry in discussions with governments in healthcare issues, and to communicate the value of innovation and research. Its membership is mainly the Middle East affiliates of European and American pharmaceutical companies that are active in the five Gulf States (Kuwait, Bahrain, Qatar, UAE, and Oman).

The Middle East Regulatory Conference (MERC) was founded in 1995 by the pharmaceutical industry. Meeting annually in different countries by rotation, the objectives of the MERC are to facilitate communication between the regulatory authorities and the industry, to understand and discuss registration requirements and their relevance, to provide updates on new trends and concepts, to align perceptions of both the industry and authority, to facilitate discussions on current and key issues, to seek solutions, and generally to continue to build trust and partnerships between industry and authorities.

Company and product registration

The registration process of pharmaceutical products in the Middle East countries depends on two licenses: one for the company as a whole and the other specific to the product. The company registration includes documentation for each manufacturing site and all the relevant subsidiaries. In some countries, this company registration must be approved prior to product registration (Saudi Arabia, Bahrain, Oman, Syria, Iraq, and Yemen), while elsewhere company and product registration applications can be filed in parallel (Egypt, Kuwait, Qatar, UAE, Jordan, and Lebanon). Some countries (e.g., Saudi Arabia, Yemen) make inspections during or after the company registration process. Applicants in these countries can expect to pay the costs for two or three inspectors for the duration of that inspection, which usually lasts for about a week. The general description here is supplemented by details in the Appendix.

General requirements for company registration

The required documentation is as follows:
• Application form/questionnaire, which is country specific: information pertaining to the company size, staff, equipment, production, quality control.

• Company profile.
• Good Manufacturing Practice (GMP) compliance.
• Research & Development (R&D) activities.
• Product information.

There are no time limits for the review of company registrations by the regulatory authorities, and long delays are common (up to three years, especially in Turkey and Oman). Furthermore, the bureaucratic process is not streamlined. Legalizations by the equivalent of a Notary Public are obligatory for many certificates, confirmations, and leaflets. Sometimes it seems that no piece of paper moves without a rubber stamp.

Drug Registration (see Figure 39.1)

Product classification

As a first step, the relevant MoH classifies the new drug into one of the following groups:
• Prescription only medicine (POM), for e.g. new chemical entities or narcotics.

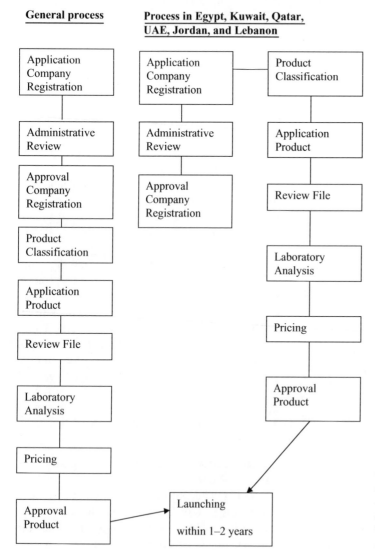

Figure 39.1 Flowchart for the company and product registration process in the Middle East. During examination of the application, many interim responses are usual to meet the requests of the Ministry of Health (MoH) concerned.

- Pharmacy only, and there are differences (with sub-classes for over-the-counter (OTC) products and herbal medicines).
- Food supplements or cosmetics.

The regulatory application requirements are different for each category, with the most needed for POM products, and the least for food supplements or cosmetics. Line extensions, for example an alternative route of administration, are approved with similar requirements as regards documentation to primary applications for new chemical entities.

General requirements for product registration

The required documentation for submission is as follows:

- A country specific application form.
- Certificate of a Pharmaceutical Product (CPP) according to the format issued by the World Health Organization (WHO).
- Dossier with administrative data, pharmaceutical, pharmacological-toxicological, and clinical documentation. The latter dossier should include:
  - Documentation similar to that specified in the Notice To Applicants (NTA).
  - Stability data (which are probably more stringent than elsewhere in the world); three batches must be tested at three different temperatures/humidities for the complete shelf life: 25°C/60% and 30°C/70% relative humidity (RH). Additionally six months, 40°C / 75% RH, must be studied.
  - Pharmaceuticals containing alcohol, or even where ethanol has been used in the production process but is absent in the finished product, usually run into great difficulty during the registration process (especially in Saudi Arabia).
  - Similarly, porcine products are a complete anathema (heparins, collagen, chondriotin, lung surfactants, and, mostly now historically, insulins). Special declarations, confirmations, and statements of interest are usually necessary to convince authorities who require absolute bans on alcohol- and porcine-derived products.

  - Expert reports on pharmaceutical, pharmacological-toxicological, and clinical data.
  - Supporting literature from any source.
- Price certificate, which is country specific, sometimes in three forms, Cost Insurance Freight (CIF) price, wholesale price, retail price.
- Finished product samples with Certificate of Analysis (CoA).
- Packaging (leaflet has to be part of the CPP for some countries, e.g., Jordan, Israel).
- Reference substances with CoA.

Pricing and economics

The Middle East is a high-import region. It is estimated that of all pharmaceuticals sold in the region, the proportion that are imported into each country ranges from 60% (Israel) to 94% (Saudi Arabia). Pharmaceutical manufacturing in the region is limited to generics, including the largest generic company in the world, situated in Israel. Pricing is part of the registration process in all countries. Some countries will only approve product prices tied strictly to some external factor, such as the lowest price available in Europe or elsewhere in the Middle East (see also Appendix). Currency exchange rates for exporters to the Middle East thus have a double-complexity in that product price is fixed at the exchange rate of the day permanently, whereas future revenues will fluctuate thereafter.

Product launch

After approval, launching of the registered product must be made within a certain time period—usually one to two years. At the time of launch, in most countries the product supply must meet a definition of "fresh," that is, at least two-thirds of the product's shelf-life must be remaining. Usually, the product must also be registered and sold in the country of origin. It should have the same trade name, composition, shelf life (confirmation often required as an attachment to CPP, e.g., UAE), and leaflet. Exceptions are possible; often it depends on good contact with the partner in the country.

Labeling

The package insert must be like the leaflet of the country of origin, pending an officially approved translation in some countries (Saudi Arabia, UAE, Jordan, and Oman). Otherwise, the language can be English and/or Arabic. Nonetheless, inadvertent offence must be avoided in these religious countries. Objections to labeling can come from unexpected quarters in a region where there are cultural obstacles to the use of terms such as "naturally powerful" or "uses the knowledge of nature" in advertising. These will not be acceptable, for example, in Saudi Arabia (and some other countries) because of a societal presumption that only Allah is all-knowing and therefore only Allah is powerful.

Summary

The Middle East is a complicated region for regulatory professionals who are outsiders and inexperienced. A local affiliate, who will act as an intelligent professional partner, and who can manage the product registration details with the Ministries of Health, is a major advantage for doing business in this region. Business plans and financial models must anticipate the possibility of long approval times. Direct contact between applicant and regulatory authority, or between Ministry and Marketing Authorization Holder (MAH), is unlikely in a region where there is little governmental transparency in general. Finally, during Ramadan (currently mid-November to mid-December on the European calendar), most regulators' offices, pharmaceutical companies, and distribution channels operate with minimal activity.

Appendix: application processes

New application
This requires classification as to prescription-only, etc.

"Variation"
The documentation depends on the kind of change (see the following table):

Change	Requirements
Composition	CPP, updated documents, stability, samples
Shelf life	CPP, stability data, samples
Leaflet	CPP, updated leaflet
Pack size	CPP, stability data, samples
Price	Price certificate
Analytical methods	Updated pharmaceutical documents

CPP = Certificate of a Pharmaceutical Product

Renewal

Most countries have a re-registration system. Approvals are valid for five years. Three to six months before the expiration date of the marketing authorization, an updated file must be submitted. In some countries, it is sufficient to submit only a new CPP, such as in Lebanon.

Certification/legalization procedures

As mentioned earlier in this chapter, legalizations or notarizations play a major role in the registration process in Middle-Eastern countries. Even if, as a premise, a relationship based on trust and honor exists between the authority, partner, and applicant, ministries still insist on several confirmations, certifications, declarations, and so on; additional legalization may also be required from the Embassy of the product's origin. A common request for a declaration is to give a statement that the product does not contain any substances from animal sources (especially pork) or that products are alcohol-free.

Difficulties also arise in unexpected quarters. Regulatory authorities may have a particular respect or regard for some forms of notarization and not others. Thus, the identity of the notarizing entity can count for as much as the notarization itself. Furthermore, even when the notarizing entity is well-respected, the very form of the notarization can cause concern. For example, Jordan only accepts documents from the German regulatory authority (BfArM) when they bear the old-fashioned rubber stamp with its image of an eagle. Personal contacts and people with deep local experience become mandatory under such conditions.

Pricing

For pricing, the classification is necessary to determinate whether the product fits into a category that needs price fixation or not. Normally, for all prescription products and some OTC products, a price fixation is obligatory. For OTC products, it depends on the active substance and the indications mentioned for the product itself. No price fixation is necessary for products that are herbals and food supplements, nor for cosmetics.

For pricing, the process starts by submitting a legalized certificate for the specific product with the following information:

• name of the manufacturer or marketing authorization holder;
• name and address of the local partner;
• wholesale price in the country of origin;
• registered price in neighboring countries (if available);
• suggested CIF in the specific country.

Such a certificate has to be signed by the manufacturer and must be legalized by the Chamber of Commerce and the Embassy of the concerned country. Innovative products will generally receive a price that is higher than for a follow-on product with the same, or similar, active ingredient. Generics must accept a lower price. The basis for price-finding is always evolving, and an average price, using the three lowest prices from the region itself, is a recent development.

The time needed to obtain a price is usually about six months, depending on the MoH.

Saudi Arabia has a separate pricing committee, which considers ex-factory wholesale price, public price in the source country, export price to Saudi Arabia, and export price of some 30(!) other countries. Normally, the lowest price found will then be awarded.

Tender

Governmental companies or institutions, for example army or hospitals, offer tender business throughout the Middle East on an *ad hoc* or annual basis. It is even possible that unregistered products can be tendered for, especially when serious diseases or the need of huge amounts of medicines exist. Every company can apply for a tender; the government will choose the most appropriate one, depending on quality and price.

The Gulf Central Committee for Drug Registration (GCC-DR)

The member states of the GCC-DR are as follows:
➢ Saudi Arabia;
➢ Kuwait;
➢ UAE;
➢ Oman;
➢ Bahrain;
➢ Qatar.

The executive office for the health ministers is located in Riyadh, Saudi Arabia. The committee consists of a chairman, two members of each of the six member states, and a secretariat. The responsibilities of GCC-DR are as follows:
• registration of pharmaceutical companies;
• registration of pharmaceutical products;
• inspection of pharmaceutical companies concerning GMP compliance;
• approval of quality control laboratories;
• review of technical and post-marketing surveillance reports;
• responsible for the program of bio-equivalence studies as part of quality assurance.

The aim of the GCC-DR is to harmonize company and product registrations between the member states.

Applications to the GCC-DR for Company registration (original plus six copies) must include the following:
➢ application form;
➢ GMP certificate (needs legalization, preferably from Saudi Arabian Embassy, but the other member states are also accepted);
➢ manufacturing license;
➢ product information table;
➢ research summary;
➢ certificates issued by the parent company, in case of subsidiaries;
➢ confirmation of payment of fee.

After a positive evaluation, the company must prepare for the three-person inspection from the authority.

Documents that have to be submitted for the GCC-DR Product registration (original plus six copies) include the following:

➢ application form;
➢ Certificate of Pharmaceutical Product (CPP);
➢ dossier;
➢ 15 finished product samples (with CoA);
➢ 15 samples of packaging material (labeling needs health authority approval, leaflet should be in Arabic and/or English);
➢ animal source information, percentage of alcohol (if applicable);
➢ list of countries in which the product is registered;
➢ confirmation of payment of fee.

The GCC-DR review of the dossier

At the first stage, two member states make a review and compile an evaluation report, which is then reviewed by the committee. Afterwards, the preliminary technical and pricing approval follows.

The second stage includes the laboratory analysis (only performed in Saudi Arabia, Kuwait, or the UAE). Then a GCC-DR registration certificate is issued. Thereafter, each member state issues its own national license, usually after receiving payment of fees.

Further reading

Deutsche Gesellschaft für Regulatorische Angelegenheiten e.V. Auswaertiges Amt, Deutschland, July 2009, www.auswaertiges-amt.de; accessed November 12, 2009.

Executive Board of the Health Ministers' Council for the GCC States. www.sgh.org.sa; accessed November 27, 2009.

Gihan T. Registration of medicinal Products in Egypt. *Reg Affs J* 2000; **11**:318–329.

Kukhun SR. Product registration in Saudi Arabia. *Reg Affs J* 2001; **12**:645–665.

CHAPTER 40

China's Regulated Pharmaceutical Market

*Yan Yan Li Starkey**

GlaxoSmithKline Consumer Healthcare, Parsippany, NJ, USA

*The opinians expressed by YY Li Starkey in this chapter are her own and do not necessarily reflect the views of GlaxoSmithKline—Consumer Healthcare.

Introduction

China's pharmaceuticals market is growing rapidly along with its economy in general. According to *Business Monitor International*, China's pharmaceutical market will post a double-digit growth rate through 2013, which is the fastest growth rate of any country in the world; it is already the fourth largest market. The key drivers are robust economic growth, a growing non-communicable disease burden, an ageing population, and urbanization. Also middle class growth (a more affluent population), government spending on healthcare, and medical reform are stimulating the growth of the pharmaceutical industry in China. This has made China a most attractive destination for worldwide pharmaceutical companies in last two decades.

Good clinical practice (GCP) was officially introduced in China in 1998 by the Ministry Public Health (MPH), and as a result more robust clinical trial activities have been conducted in recent years. China began to play an extremely important role in drug development for global pharmaceuticals initially due to cost savings and globalization of drug development. Later, other advantages of doing clinical research in China become increasingly important including large patient pools for many diseases, a centralized healthcare system, and a fast growing Contract Research Organization (CRO) industry that provide an ideal clinical research environment to allow for faster patient recruitment and easy patient monitoring.

A lesser known advantage is the fact that Chinese investigators and research sites are especially qualified and licensed by the State Food and Drug Administration (SFDA). The majority of clinical research staff including study coordinators, Clinical Research Associates (CRAs), and study trial managers have MD or PhD degrees not only at investigational sites but also in CROs and the pharmaceutical industries as well. Disadvantages for an international company operating in China are the different regulatory environment and intelligent propriety rights (IPRs). These issues have been steadily improving since the implementation of a regulatory system modeled after international standards such as that of US FDA and ICH in 2003 and the participation of the World Trade Organization (WTO) in 2001

Advantages

Here is a summary of the advantages of China as regards the pharmaceuticals market:

- robust economic growth;
- lower cost of drug development and clinical trial;
- top pharmaceuticals R&D centers set up;
- rich disease resource provides large patient pools;
- healthcare system centralization provides easy and fast enrollment;
- CRO industries in fast growing track;
- plentiful, trained human resource;
- government spending on healthcare increase and medical reform.

Principles and Practice of Pharmaceutical Medicine, 3rd edition.
Edited by L.D. Edwards, A.W. Fox, P.D. Stonier.
© 2011 Blackwell Publishing Ltd.

Disadvantages

Here is a summary of the disadvantages of China as regards the pharmaceuticals market:

• lengthy regulatory process for Investigational New Drug (IND) (CTA) and New Drug Applications (NDA);
• IP protection issues not fully resolved;
• lack of domestic funding resources and venture capital;
• most CROs have less capability for global trials management;
• insufficient communication platform;
• laboratory facilities tends to be less advanced.

China has become the fastest growing pharmaceutical market

The global pharmaceutical market is expected to grow 4.5–5.5% in 2009 (IMS Health, 2008). The report predicts that global pharmaceutical sales will exceed US$820 billion in 2009. This includes more established markets such as the USA with a slow 1–2% growth rate that will reach US$297 billion. The top five European Union countries (France, Germany, Italy, Spain, and the UK) are forecast to grow 3–4%, reaching sales of US$172 billion. Japan, the world's second-largest single country market, is expected to see higher growth of 4–5%, reaching about US$85 billion. The key emerging markets of China, Brazil, India, South Korea, Mexico, Turkey, and Russia are expected to show sustained double-digit growth of 14–15% to around US$110 billion (see Table 40.1).

China has become the fasted growing pharmaceutical market driven by robust economic growth and a demographic shift to an ageing, urban, middle class population. According to *Business Monitor International* (BMI, 2009), China's US$37 billion pharmaceutical market will post a compound annual growth rate (CAGR) of about 13% through to 2013, when combined sales of prescription drug and over-the counter (OTC) medicines will have reached US$68 billion, which is the fastest growth rate of any country in the world. Already the fourth largest market, China will become the second-largest single country pharmaceutical market by 2020.

Government support to develop infrastructure and the healthcare system

The Chinese government has been working actively on the reform of its healthcare system. At one time, only government employees and those working at the numerous state-owned enterprises had nearly free access to medical care for the whole family. China has the world's largest urban population exceeding half a billion people. This entire urban population has received the benefit of at least basic health issuance since 2007. A new urban medical insurance system was introduced in 2000. Supplementary private insurance can also be obtained for more extensive coverage. In addition, the great majority of China's rural population has some kind of basic insurance although this is currently quite limited.

Table 40.1 Pharmaceutical market forecast in 2009

Market	Annual growth rate (%)	Market size (US$ billions)
Global	4.5–5.5	820
USA	1–2	297
France, Germany, Italy, Spain, and the UK	3–4	172
Japan	4–5	85
China, Brazil, India, South Korea, Mexico, Turkey, and Russia	14–15	110

China's currently medical resources and infrastructure are limited on a per capita basis. With the government's strong support for basic medical care China's Healthcare Environments is becoming more structured and is moving in the right direction and benefits multinational companies. China's investment in hospital construction has increased by about 20% annually during the past decade. In 2005, China had about 2 million physicians (~1.5 per 1000 persons) and about 3 million hospitals beds (~2.4 per 1000 persons). The government plans to improve 80% of China's existing hospitals over the next decade (BUYUSA, 2009). Currently there is a focus on rebuilding and improving in areas such as infectious disease, emergency medicine, family healthcare, and chronic diseases. For example, in terms of overall sales of medical devices for care and rehabilitation, China is the fastest growing market in Asia. China is rapidly increasing its support for hospital construction and medical equipment in both urban and in rural areas. The government target for 2020 is to achieve universal access to good quality and affordable medical care.

Ageing and urbanization with a shift to non-communicable diseases provide large patient pools

Urban-affluent consumers are the main target for global companies. The ratio of population living in urban/rural has been dramatically increased. As of 2008 China has 22 cities with more than 2 million people and 33 cites with 1–2 million people. By 2030 there will be 1 billion people living in China's cities of which 221 cities have more than 1 million people. During the next 20 years a huge middle class will emerge with increased incomes and changing spending patterns, which will also provide vast opportunities for core-consumer segmentation and post many challenges for pharmaceutical industries to develop more innovative drugs in China (Diana *et al.*, 2006).

The ageing population is growing with 100 million people >65 years today and this group will

be 24% of the population by 2050. Under these demographic changes the disease burden will further shift to chronic and non-communicable diseases, which now account for 80% of all deaths. Infectious diseases and water born disease were the major cause of death in the 1950s, 1960s, and 1970s, but today a surge of diseases of affluence such as cancers, diabetes, hypertension, hyperlipidemia, asthma, COPD, and CNS diseases are among the unfortunate side effects of a booming economy and pharmaceutical clinical research. For example, in the last three years three of the largest worldwide drug companies (Novatis, Astra-Zeneca, and GSK) have invested millions of dollars to set up CNS R&D centers in China to study diseases including dementia, Parkinson's disease, schizophrenia, and Alzheimer's disease that have become common illnesses in China. Dementia is predicted to be the third major chronic condition in China by 2050 after lung cancer and CV diseases.

The population in China is currently 1.3 billion; cancer is the leading cause of death followed by CV disease. Approximately 2.5 million cases of cancer are diagnosed in China every year; 1.8 million people die from cancer in China every year. Among men, the most common cancers (around 40/100,000 men) are lung, stomach, and liver, which are the top three causes of cancer deaths. In women, the cancers with the highest incidence are breast, lung and stomach each occurring in almost 20/100,000 females. By 2012 there will be around 250,000 cases each for lung and gastric cancers just in urban areas (see Figure 40.1 based on Globocan 2002 database, IARC. WHO).

The high prevalence of some types of cancers provides large patient pools with especially large numbers of treatment-naïve patients for clinical studies. In general, clinical trial endpoints in oncology are based on survival rates and this can make oncology studies very long and extremely costly. Therefore pharmaceutical companies are looking to the Orient to obtain tremendous cost reductions, such as the Philippines, South Korea, and China. Since 2004 the number of oncology trials conducted in China has doubled, while oncology trials done in Western Europe showed a decrease (Alice, 2008).

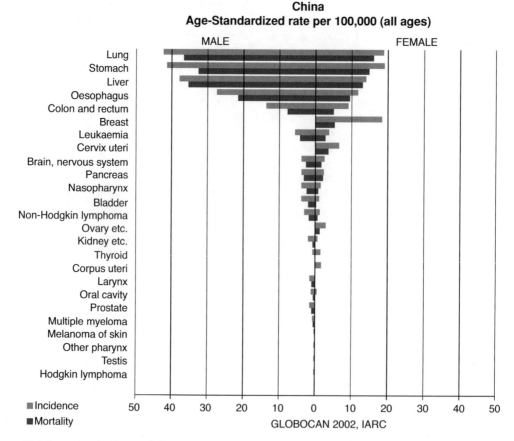

Figure 40.1 Increasing incidence of all major cancer types in China: overall forecast number of cases in urban area (000). Source: Globocan 2002, IARC. Courtesy of the World Health Organization.

Attractive cost/quality mix

Lower cost for labor and clinical procedures

The cost of conducting a clinical trial has risen dramatically in recent years. The cost in developed countries has increased many fold more rapidly than for other aspects of drug development. Typically pharmaceutical companies achieve commercial success with only a small faction of the compounds they evaluate in clinical trials. This presents a significant problem for the sponsors of clinical trials, especially for pharmaceutical companies who are in need of a lower cost venue and are looking to the lower cost countries to achieve this. The aver-

age drug now costs approximately US$1.5 billion to develop from a candidate molecule to a commercial product. The advantage of using China as the R&D site for clinical research is not only the low cost of clinical trials done there but also the high quality. Conducting clinical trials in China costs about 50% less than the same trial run in the US or many European countries. Indeed in Germany the costs are three times as great (see Figure 40.2, based on *Fast Track Systems Global Cost Databases*, 2006). For example, the routine automated CBC costs about US$13 in China, which is a 75% cost reduction compared to the US$51 in the US. The cost for a routine ECG with at least 12 leads including tracing interpretation and report is US$50 in China

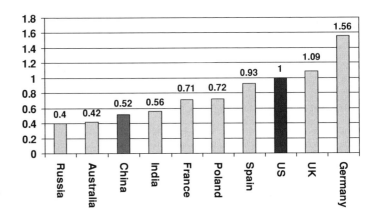

Figure 40.2 Clinical study cost comparisons by country clinical trial cost ratio.

compared to US$120 in the US (a 58% of reduction) (see Table 40.2).

Another good example for cost saving is conducting a Phase I PK bioequivalence study for an OTC analgesic in 24 subjects with 4-way crossover design, which normally costs about US$50,000 to US$80,000 in China but is much more costly in the US (about US$150,000) and in the UK (US$210,000). In addition the Chinese government provides tax incentives for domestic R&D and gives preferential loans for the construction of R&D facilities. Overall the cost of bringing a new drug to market through research, development, and com-

mercialization in China is dramatically less than in the US.

Hospital centralization for reducing monitoring costs

As previously mentioned, China has large patient populations, a fact that allows for rapid and easy enrollment of patients and an increase in patient quality since the investigator can be very selective in enrollment. This is especially helpful when studying relatively uncommon diseases where sufficient patients may be hard to find in other countries. In China the medical system is organized

Table 40.2 The cost comparison of clinical procedures between the US and China

Item	USA (US$)	China US$	% reduction of China versus US
Screen or based line visit: includes vital sign, physical examination, comprehensive medical history, or other outpatient examination (around 60 minutes)	250~210	120~100	52~43
Urine pregnancy, gonadotropin chorionic(hCG) (betah CG), qualitative	41	10	76
Blood count: complete (CBC), automated (Hgb, Hct, RBC, WBC, and platelet count), and automated differential WBC count	51	13	75
Inclusion/exclusion criteria	52~57	30	42~47
Electrocardiogram, routine ECG(EKG) with at least 12 leads, includes tracing, interpretation, and report	120	50	58
Physician per visit (initial visit, final visit)	175~140	130~110	26~21
Study coordinator per visit (initial visit, final visit)	125~115	65~60	48
Hospital EC (IRB) submission	2500~1200	700~550	72~54

around large centralized comprehensive hospitals in major cities rather than small clinics and independent offices such as in the US. This speeds up the conduct of clinical trials because the patients are centralized and pooled in these large hospitals and this makes it very easy to enroll patients within short periods. In addition all the necessary diagnostic and ancillary facilities are in one place. The patient does not have to be sent to scattered facilities to carry out protocol required tests. Due to investigational site centralization in large cities, it is very cost effective to monitor and clean data at these sites.

FDA accepted data to open a door for China to participate in global R&D

Due to its high efficiency and cost savings the number of international multicenter trials and also local clinical trials conducted in China has been growing dramatically. The quality of the work done can be good to excellent as evidenced by the decision of the US FDA to accept data from clinical trials conducted in China in applications for product approval. The study (Karlberg, 2008) analyzed trials registered in the US (www.clinicaltrials.gov) since July 2008. The results showed that greater China (including China, Hong Kong, and Taiwan; see Table 40.3) contributed more multinational sponsored clinical trials ($n = 377$) than other Asian countries. More than 50% of all the sites in mainland China are located in three major cities in

China: Beijing (351 sites), Shanghai (286 sites), and Guangdong (130 sites). The majority of the trials conducted in China are Phase III trials.

SFDA-accredited clinical research sites

Clinical trials in mainland China can only be conducted at SFDA-accredited sites. According to the SFDA guideline: "to accredit a clinical trial site is to safeguard that all clinical trials-related activities are properly conducted, study results are scientifically reliable, and all rights of study subjects are fully protected". Normally these centers are located in top university hospitals with comprehensive facilities or specialized hospitals in major cities such as Beijing, Shanghai, and Guang Zhou. The sites need to be trained and then qualified by the SFDA with a special certification. In other words, without SFDA permission, the investigator and center have no right to conduct clinical drug trials.

According to the SFDA website, as of April 2007, 251 sites (either hospitals or academic university centers) were permitted by the SFDA to conduct clinical trials. Each site is required to have an ethics committee. Split by disease populations, cardiology, GI, and RT are becoming predominately therapeutic areas in these sites. But early stage research sites such as PK Phase I units are very few (see Figure 40.3, Karlberg, 2008).

Highly educated clinical research staff

Clinical trials sites in China are required to meet ICH GCP standards. Principle investigators are

Table 40.3 The number of industry sponsored trials and study sites registered with clinicaltrials.gov between October 2005 and July 2008 for the most active countries/regions in Asia

Country/ region	Local Prot. n	Local Sites n	Multinational Prot. n	Multinational Sites n	Total Prot. n	Total Sites n	Sites/Prot. n	Prot. Local %	Sites Local %
China	121	618	134	787	255	1,405	5.5	47.5	44.0
Hong Kong	13	16	193	314	206	330	1.6	6.3	4.8
Taiwan	65	190	260	802	325	992	3.1	20.0	19.2
Total	**199**	**824**	**377**	**1,903**	**576***	**2,727**	**4.7**	**34.5**	**30.2**
Japan	367	5,751	56	710	423	6,461	15.3	86.8	89.0
South Korea	106	493	285	945	391	1,438	3.7	27.1	34.3
India	45	174	344	2,075	389	2,249	5.8	11.6	7.7

Source: Karlberg. *Clinical Trial Magnifier*, 2008 **1**(8). Reproduced with permission.

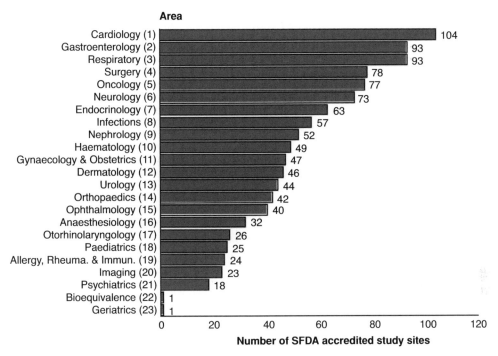

Figure 40.3 SFDA accredited investigational sites. Source: Karlberg. *Clinical Trial Magnifier*, 2008 **1**(8). Reproduced with permission.

generally well known academic scientists with extensive clinical practicing in their specialty area and a lot have received training abroad. Study coordinators are nurse or clinicians who can be completing their early resident period. Recently a survey (Fan, 2008) was conducted to show the current CRA capacities in China. The survey covered 229 CRAs from 31 cities in China. 61% worked at pharmaceuticals, 29% in CROs, and 11% in biotech companies.

The majority of CRAs are very young, often in their twenties. This young age provides a benefit in that young people are well suited for the extensive travel required of a CRA. Despite their young age, 61% of the CRAs had a medical doctor's degree. As physicians, many of these CRAs have practical experience in hospital medicine. This is very helpful for them in understanding the needs of the study and the issues that investigators face. About a quarter of CRAs have pharmacy degrees but only 3% are nurses. This background makes Chinese CRAs especially suited to writing protocols and understanding the underlying logic of clinical trials

as well as interpreting and filing adverse reaction reports. However, their young age and brief experience with managing multicenter clinical trials can be a weakness and require appropriate supervision and training during the early stages of their careers.

China's impressive cost/quality mix presents a great opportunity in the current global marketplace. China is able to produce clinical trials at costs 50–70% less than other countries. China could leverage this cost leadership to establish itself as a key player with a more broad-based presence in the global pharmaceuticals market.

Integrated R&D centers in China facilitate innovation in drug development

With the rapid growth of the pharmaceutical market in China, in the last couple of years most pharmaceutical companies have been prompted to set up their own R&D centers. Pfizer, Roche, J&J,

Merck, AstraZeneca, Novatis, Ely Lilly, GSK, Bayer Schering, and others have each invested hundreds of millions of US$ to set up their R&D centers in China. Initially, R&D activities focus on addressing urgent medical needs in China and Asia, but later on they can become part of a global strategy to developing and emerging innovation products. One disease is liver cancer caused by the hepatitis viruses. Some one-third of the 400 million people infected with the hepatitis B virus live in China, with experts estimating that the virus kills 300,000 people in mainland China each year.

Novartis opened a new R&D center in Shanghai investing US$100 million in 2006. This is a very large center with more than 400 scientists. The great majority of the researchers were recruited in Shanghai's central academic, biotech, and pharmaceuticals research institutions. Daniel Vasella, the chief executive of Novartis, said that

> the level of scientific expertise in China is rising rapidly. At the same time, the healthcare needs of the Chinese are growing, primarily the result of urbanization, lifestyle changes, and associated chronic diseases … The Shanghai center will allow us to combine modern drug discovery approaches with those of traditional Chinese medicine that have been used to treat patients in China for thousands of years. This new research center will help Novartis contribute to the needs of patients in China and elsewhere and has the potential to become a global center for biomedical innovation.

This new center will enable Novartis to increase its global capability for innovative drug research and will especially provide it with a capability to develop medicines for the Asian market in Asia.

GSK opened a CNS R&D center (US$100 million) in Shanghai in 2007 aiming for a staff of 1000 by 2010. The center is focused on drug development for neurological degeneration (Alzheimer's, Parkinson's disease) and multiple sclerosis. Moncef Slaoui, the Chairman of R&D for GSK, described the Shanghai center as a "one-stop shop" that will do research on drugs for neurodegenerative disease. Neural stem cell research and natural product compounds will be particular areas of expertise

for this center. It is planned that the Shanghai center will eventually become GSK's chief center of excellence in neurodegenerative disease research.

GSK considers that China is an excellent location for this center not only because of the low research costs, but also due to the large amount of scientific talent now becoming available in China. Many scientists who have been trained in the US and Europe are now returning to China to take advantage of opportunities for university positions and government-supported businesses of their own, which are now being offered in order to develop the Shanghai area into a cutting edge research environment (named the Shanghai Zhangjiang bio-pharmaceutical park) comparable to that in the Boston area.

According to IMS Health, Bayer was the number one healthcare company in China with the annual growth rate around 43% in 2007. Currently China is the third largest market for Bayer. Bayer Schering Pharma is aiming to develop China to be its third global R&D center in addition to Germany and the US. Therefore, in 2009 Bayer Schering Pharma AG, the pharmaceutical division of Bayer Healthcare (BHC) decided to establish a global R&D center in Beijing with the investment of 100 million euros over the next five years. Similar to the Shanghai high-tech environment, Beijing is also a center with a highly talented scientific team focusing on development of innovative medicines (named the Beijing Zhonguancun Life Science Park). "We are continuously increasing our presence on the Asia pacific Region where China is our key growth driver. In our new R&D center in Beijing, we will establish a world class R&D team extending our global R&D expertise and capabilities. Beijing will be an important site for our global innovative drug development," said Andreas Fibig, Executive Committee member of BHC and Chairman of Bayer Schering Pharma AG's board of Management.

CRO industries are on a fast-growth track in China

The worldwide CRO market maintained an annual growth of 20–25% in recent years. This market is expected to achieve a total value of US$36 billion by 2010 with a yearly growth of 16%. Following the trend of the global CRO market, the Chinese CRO market has been rapidly expanding over the last few years. This was mainly stimulated by rapid global pharmaceutical R&D growth, which greatly elevated the demand for outsourced research. In fact, in 2007 the Chinese CRO market was estimated to be around US$200 million and to account for only 2.3% of the global CRO market.

In 2009, China listed 138 CROs with the capability of conducting R&D studies (*Business Wire*, 2009). Of these, only about 7% had international capability and 52% had domestic capability only. The remaining 41% are principally Chinese CROs with limited foreign capability. The young global CRO business in China is challenged in trying to meet the robust growth of the pharmaceutical R&D industry, which is becoming a disadvantage and slowing down China in merging into the global clinical research stream. CROs in China are located primarily in two large biotech parks: Shanghai Zhangjiang bio-pharmaceutical park (part of the Zhangjiang high-tech Park) and Beijing Zhonguancun Life Science Park.

Chinese central labs are fully outsourced by the pharmaceutical industry, and so central labs are expanding considerably in China and India and are mostly set up by major global CROs. Either by establishing new labs or partnering with local labs in the region, CROs are rapidly responding to set up central labs to meet the global market demand: MDS Pharma Service developed the first central lab operations in Beijing, where the business recently tripled and the testing capacity was increased five fold. Following this MDS, PPD, Covance, and Icon expanded their Global Central Lab services in Shanghai. Central labs no longer only provide safety, hematology, and chemistry testing services, but also provide more complex testing such as biomarker and bioanalysis, PK, PD, genomic biomarker, and so on.

A major regulatory hurdle in China is that whole blood cannot be taken out of the country, which therefore requires local lab support. When the central lab and CRO work together as one unit it can bring benefits to the client not only financially as a one-stop-shop, but also operationally with time gains and communication efficiency with one point of contact for the sponsor.

Overview of regulatory IND and NDA in China

Here is a summary of the position in China:
- *National laws:*
  - Drug administration law;
  - Implementing regulation of the drug administration law.
- *Regulations:*
  - Drug registration regulation for chemical, biological, traditional Chinese medicine (TCM), and herbal drugs;
  - Regulations for the supervision and administration of medical devices.

China has different requirements and a considerably longer duration for proceeding CTA (IND) and NDA review and approval compared to the US and EU. This has been a major concern and a significant hurdle for global drug development. Overall drug development and registration in China is under the national laws including the *drug registration law*, the *implementing regulation of the drug administration law*, and *drug and medical device registration regulation*.

The drug administration law of China was established by the People's Congress in 1984. Originally new drug and import drug approval in China were administered by the MPH. The focus of domestic drugs (mostly generic drugs) or drug approval at that time was the adoption of well established foreign drugs for use in the Chinese market. A separate bureau, called the State Drug Administration (SDA) was formed in 1999. The agency's name was changed in 2003 to the State Food and Drug Administration (SFDA), which replaced the MPH in order to allow for the review of a full range of drug research (Phases I to IV) and approval of new chemical entities.

Recognizing the limitations of the 25-year-old Drug Administration Law and the complex procedures required for its update, the SFDA has in recent years taken a number of important actions within its authority at the normative level to improve the regulatory framework in order to meet the need of the changing industrial landscape worldwide in an era of regulatory, R&D, manufacturing, and supply network all at a global scale. The number of trials submitted and number of drugs approval has grown at a 40% annual rate since the modernization of regulatory process in SFDA. The registration process became more transparent and the approval process for fast track opportunities, such as for oncology products, has been emerging. Despite this improvement a number problems remain in optimizing IND/NDA regulatory process.

Similar to the US FDA of the 1970s and 1980s, the current SFDA is significantly under-funded and under-staffed. The SFDA consists of only about 200 hundred people including Center for Drug Evaluation (CDE) members (see Figure 40.4) to handle more than a thousand applications annually. This results in a very long time for CTA (IND)/NDA approval and a huge backlog of applications. In 2003, the SFDA improved the implementation of the regulatory system modeled after international standards such as that of the US FDA and ICH, with the issuance of provision for drug registration in October 2007 and the requirements for Special Approval of New Drug Registration (the requirements) in January 2009 to encourage the innovative drug development and to give priority during the review at CDE.

The review by the CDE was reduced from 120 to 80 working days. However the approval duration for CTA (IND) still takes on average 135 working days (at least six months). Figure 40.5 presents the special review process of CTA (IND) in China. One unusual aspect of the Chinese process can result in substantial delays in obtaining CTA approval: This is a requirement of the SFDA to repeat the chemical analyses of the clinical samples (normally three batches from original manufacturers) to meet standard specifications in the Chinese national institutional centers of pharmacologic bio-analytical products (NICPBP) authorized by the SFDA. This process normally takes about 85 days and sometimes even requires shipment of analytical instruments, and reference standards from the original company and training the laboratory technicians

in the validated analytical methods. This analytical result will be needed as a part of the CTA/IND submission dossier for CDE review. However it is not required for chemical drugs' global study application. After 80 days of CDE review, one can obtain a verbal approval which allows to submission to the ethics committee (EC). The EC approval timing is quite similar or even shorter than in the US/EU. Once a CTA is issued by the SFDA, the final study protocol, ICF, EC approval letter, and investigational site's information can be submitted to the SFDA and the clinical trial can be started.

If the drug has been approved and extensively marketed in developed countries and is now to be marketed in China, a bridging registration trial is required. A mandatory Phase III efficacy and safety study in Chinese population is required (minimum samples size: 100 patients in each study arm: testing product versus existing active product). In many cases a PK/BE study is also required (minimum sample size: 20~30 subjects). The CTA submission is same as the above (120~135 days). The final study report included in the NDA dossiers needs to be submitted as an NDA in order to obtain an import drug license. Generally the review needs at least 215 working days to obtain the final NDA approval (see Figure 40.6).

The SFDA may implement special review and approval in the process of drug registration for drugs specified in the following categories:

• active ingredients extracted from plants, animals, and minerals, etc. and their preparations not yet marketed in China, and newly discovered Chinese crude drugs and their preparations;
• chemical drug substances and their preparations and biological products not yet approved for marketing in China or abroad;
• new drugs for the treatment of diseases such as AIDS, malignant tumors, and rare diseases, etc. with significant clinical advantage;
• new drugs for the treatment of diseases, for which effective therapeutic methods are not available.

The CDE of the SFDA then organizes expert meetings to discuss and determine whether or not to conduct special review and approval for the drug.

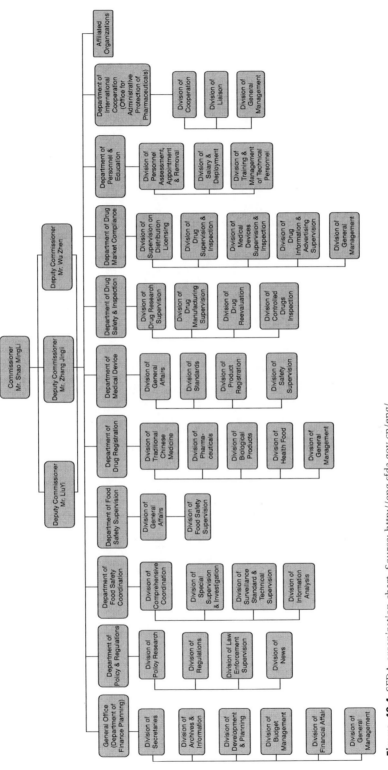

Figure 40.4 SFDA organization chart. Source: http://eng.sfda.gov.cn/eng/

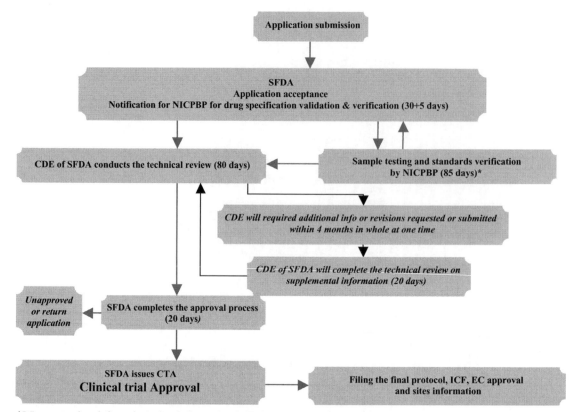

*Not required for chemical drugs' global study application

Figure 40.5 IND (CTA) Special Review Process (~135 working days): (Import drug registration 1).

Document requirement for IND/NDA registration

Additional documentary requirements vary with different reviewers, and the rapidly changing regulatory requirements often delay approval time. The Requirements for Special Approval of New Drug Registration (the Requirements) issued in 2009 allow for early intervention, priority review, multi-channel communication, and dynamic data supplement to encourage innovation and risk control. The most important element of the Requirements is perhaps the attempt to create a separate system for the approval of IND application that differs from the approval process for NDAs, a distinction unrecognized by the Provision for Drug Registration. Previously, to gain an approval to conduct an IND-type clinical trial in China, a sponsor needed to submit data to the SFDA that were equivalent to the full NDA in such areas as pharmacology, toxicology, chemistry, manufacturing, and control. This was a great burden for the sponsors and was a key reason why China lagged behind South Korea and Chinese Taiwan in the participation of simultaneous global drug development. The new Requirements also allow the SFDA to offer new communication opportunities for sponsors via a meeting on schedules that is equivalent to the US FDA pre-IND and end of clinical phase meeting.

Among the emerging top five global pharmaceutical markets, the China regulatory environment drives toward international standards by increasing ICH guideline compliance and frequency of

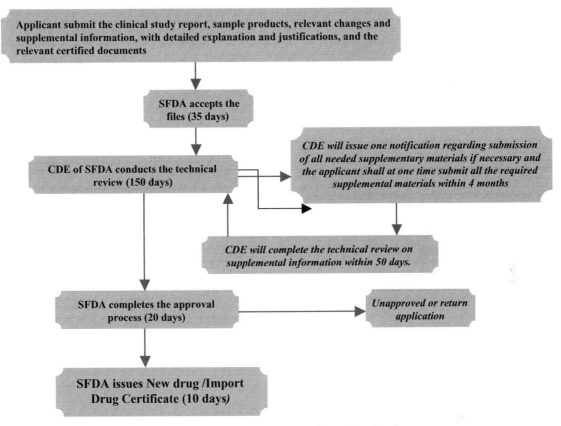

Figure 40.6 NDA approval process (~215 working days): (Import drug registration 2).

communication and more transparency; it is felt that the sample test of chemical drugs for global study application is not required. Thus some of the long lead times for CTA and NDA approval and the huge backlog at the CDE is expected to be shortened. OTC regulatory process will be established separately. The time-line is expected to be shortened in 2010: (i) the CDE hoped to complete the review for all backlog applications that have already been delayed by the end of 2009; (ii) applications for generic products will have been significantly reduced; (iii) a new infrastructure of the CDE will have been implemented; and (iv) experienced reviewers are being encouraged to focus on data review. CMC documents review, however, will be more strict than before. As at the time of writing (November 2009), the review time is still six months.

In order to compensate for this challenging regulatory environment, a few recommendations are offered:

• Consult frequently with the SFDA not only in pre-submission and but also during review stages; this can help to ensure that clinical program and submission dossiers meet its needs.

• Share regulatory experience and knowledge.

• Engage early with clients or headquarters of the regulatory department to advise the requirement to plan the IND submission to meet the global trials time-line.

• Use reliable translation vendors and SOPs to shorten the time on dossier preparation and ensure the consistency and accuracy of the submission file.

• Prepare clear summaries to support the authority's review.

- Ensure important support from a third party of technical experts
- Ensure a rational regulatory strategy.

The following is a list of the basic requirements of CTA (IND)/NDA submission dossiers:

- **Volume I: Summary Information**
  1. Name of the drugs
  2. Certified Documents
  3. Objectives and basis for R&D
  4. Summary of study result
  5. Sample of leaflet
  6. Design of packaging and labeling
- **Volume II: Pharmaceutical Data**
  7. Summary of Pharmaceutical Study
  8. Research information and relevant literature of the production process of the drug substance; research information and relevant literature of formula and process of the preparations
  9. Study information and relevant literature for the chemical structure and components determination
  10. Study information and literature for quality specification
  11. Draft of quality specification and notes, and providing reference standard
  12. CoAs
  13. The source, CoAs, and quality specification of drug substance and recipients
  14. Stability study and relevant literature
  15. Selection basis and quality specification of immediate packing material and container
  16. Summary of pharmacology and toxicology study
  17. Primary pharmacodynamic study and literature
  18. General pharmacology study and literature
  19. Acute/single dose toxicity study and literature
  20. Repeated dose toxicity study and literature
  21. Special safety study and literature of hypersensitive (topical, systemic, and phototoxicity), hemolytic, and topical irritation (blood vessel, skin, mucous membrane, and muscle) reaction related to topical and systemic use of the drugs
- **Volume III: Pharmacological and Toxicological data (continued)**
  22. Study and relevant literature on pharmacodynamics, toxicity, and pharmacokinetics

change caused by the interactions among multiple components in the combination products
  23. Study and literature of mutagenicity test
  24. Study and literature of reproductive toxicity
  25. Study and literature of carcinogenicity test
  26. Study and literature of drug dependence
  27. Study and literature of preclinical pharmacokinetics
- **Volume IV: Clinical Study Information**
  28. All clinical study information (used during the application for marketing in the local countries or region where the manufacturer is located)
  29. Clinical study protocol
  30. Investigator's brochure
  31. Draft of Informed Consent Form, approval of the Ethics Committee
  32. Clinical study reports

Note that clinical information items 31–32 will be added with the completion of clinical studies in the final NDA submission dossier. So the NDA dossier will include the previous IND dossier, clinical study reports, sample product, relevant changes, and supplement information, with detailed explanation and justification, and the relevant certified document among other items.

Intellectual property rights are improving

China has had patent laws since 1984. They were modernized in 1992 and again in 2000. One of the concerns of multinational companies in penetrating China's pharmaceutical market is the protection of intellectual property rights (IPR). In the past many multinational pharmaceutical companies have struggled with IPR protection in China. This is a concern mainly because generic medicine occupies such a large proportion of the market with very competitive low prices and efficient distribution channels. Global companies' imported products often compete against local generics that have already won Chinese regulatory approval. In many cases companies obtained patent registration for their products in China before marketing, and yet local generic companies in China still mimicked their products regardless of the patent.

Under the pressure of participating in the World Trade Organization (WTO) in 2001 and a government commitment to adhere to IPR protection in China, the situation has improved. This is largely due to great government efforts from both the Ministry of Public Security and the SFDA who have taken serious actions:

• They have stringently limited phony drug makers including some well-known large companies that do not respect patent rights strictly.

• In 2006 the SFDA shut down over 1200 drug and medical-device makers for producing fake or low-quality goods

• The Chinese government significantly reduced the approval rate for generic products where patented molecules were already on the market

• The Chinese government is increasingly concerned about the needs of foreign investors and pharmaceutical companies. It has proposed a third revision of China's patent laws to be finalized by the State Intellectual Property Office (SIPO).

In spite of the fact that ensuring drug safety and effectiveness for human beings is a key SFDA role, this agency is fully committed to take responsibility for the facilitation of pharmaceutical IP protection in four aspects:

• provide administrative protection for pharmaceuticals, which it has done in 155 instances;

• abide by the promises made by the Chinese government regarding the accession to the WTO;

• engage in active collaboration with the IPR authorities, strengthen international exchange and cooperation, introduce, apply, and reference internationally accepted rules and advanced experience overseas and implement pharmaceutical IPR protection;

• conduct early intervention in innovative drug R&D, and guide and standardize the R&D of innovative drugs with self-owned IPR.

OTC market

The impressive growth of the Chinese market will be underpinned by a continuing rise in disposable incomes of the Chinese people, which have increased significantly in recent years due to the robust growth of the economy. Rising disposable incomes and the ageing of the population have stimulated substantial demand for nutritional products. Increasing awareness of personal healthcare will be the key driver of the market in the future. Chinese people will no longer take drugs only when they are unwell: they will pay much more attention to illness prevention with a focus on nutritional products. Increasing demand for healthcare products, especially health food, has also favored the expansion of OTC business. Chinese consumers are thus able to spend more on healthcare. Sales of basic OTC products, such as analgesics, and cough, cold and allergy remedies, have increased as not only people in urban but also those in rural areas are now more able to afford these medicines. Life in urban areas is becoming more stressful in China. Long working hours can cause problems for the digestive system and headaches, generating demand for digestive remedies and analgesics.

With its robust growth, China is going to be the largest OTC market in the world by the mid-21st century. China's OTC market ranked as the fourth largest in 2005, with a total of US$4.2 billion sales, behind only the US, Japan, and Germany. China sold OTC drugs worth US$7.3 billion in 2007, surging approximately 11% from a year ago, and the growth was faster than the average global growth of 5.4%, according to statistics from OTC consulting company Nicholas Hall & Company (NHC) and Jowin Communication Co., Ltd. In addition, sales of vitamin, mineral compositions, and food supplements amounted to US$2.6 billion, accounting for nearly 40% of the total OTC drugs sales. Sales of drugs for treatments of cough, cold, and allergy reached US$2 billion, ranking second among OTC drugs. The sales of digestive drugs, dermatology drugs, and antipyretic analgesics were also robust. The Chinese OTC drugs market is estimated to hit US$16.3 billion in 2017 (COMTEX, 2009).

Summary

The Chinese pharmaceutical industry is being pressured in its new endeavor by the Chinese government and by the opportunity in global markets to become a key player in the global pharmaceutical world, not only importing pharmaceuticals but also as a major source and exporter. This will require cutting edge drug development, improvements in the regulatory environment, and a highly talented research community. Today, multinational companies are addressing the challenge of entry into this emerging market by investing time and money to establish their foundations in China. Now and in the future China will be an excellent destination for Western pharmaceutical companies and their products.

References

Alice NF. Oncology clinical trials-journey to the East. *GCP Journ* 2008; August:29–31.

BMI, China pharmaceuticals and healthcare report, *Business Monitor International* 2009; **3**:19.

Business Wire. China CRO: Lays out the landscape of the Chinese CRO industry for international drug and medical device developers (industry overview). *Business Wire* 2009; May.

BUYUSA US. China, healthcare product and services. Commercial service, 2009.

COMTEX. China pharmaceutical CRO market fast grows. SinoCast Daily Business Beat via COMTEX, February 2, 2009.

Diana F, *et al.* The value of China's emerging middle class. *The McKinsey Quarterly; special edition*: serving the new Chinese consumer. 2006; 60–69.

Fan J. Clinical research associates in China. *GCP Journ* 2008; August:22–24.

Fast Track Systems Global Cost Databases, 2006.

Globocan. *Database: International Agency for Research on Cancer*. World Health Organization, 2002.

IMS Health. Global Pharmaceutical and Therapy Forecast, October 30, 2008.

Karlberg JPE. Industry sponsored clinical trials in China. *Clinical Trial Magnifier*, 2008; **1**(8).

Further reading

Cyranoski D. Pharmaceutical futures: Made in China? Published online. *Nature* 2008; **455**:1168–1170.

Le Deu F. Seizing China's pharma opportunity. *The McKinsey Quarterly* 2008; 1–10.

Mao DL, Zheng Q. Encouraging an environment for pharmaceutical R&D in China. *Journ Pharm Innov* 2009; **4**(3):152–154.

Medcof JW. Pharmaceutical R&D in China by Western MNC's. *China R&D IAMOT* 2006; 04 25.doc.

Pharma China. weekly e-alert-June 18, 2009. WiCON news. www.pharmachinaonline.com; accessed April 15, 2010.

Pharma Marketletter, November 10, 2008. http://eng.sfda.gov.cn/eng (in English); www.sfda.gov.cn (in Chinese); accessed April 15, 2010.

Zhou YB. Contract research drives China's pharma sector. August 2006; http://www.pharmamanufacturing.com/articles/2006/158.html; accessed April 15, 2010.

CHAPTER 41

India's New Era in Pharmaceuticals

Darshan Kulkarni
The Kulkarni Law Firm, Philadelphia, PA, USA

Introduction

Despite being only slightly larger than one third the size, India has a population nearly four times as large as the United States.[1] Of this population, 63.6% are between the ages of 15 and 64. Linguistically, despite being made up of many peoples and cultures and more than 200 spoken languages and/or dialects, English has emerged as a unifying language and has become the language of government, science, law, and medicine.

Domestic pharmaceutical industry

The Indian pharmaceutical market is the fourth largest in the world by market size and 15th largest by sales.[2] As of 2008, the industry had an impressive annual growth rate of 13% for the previous six years.[3] The domestic pharmaceutical

industry has grown at a rate 1.5–1.6 times the GDP growth rate. This growth rate is projected to continue due to several factors in its favor. Several multinational pharmaceutical companies (MNPCs) have already joined hands with local companies like Aurobindo, Dr Reddys, and Claris Lifesciences to create generics.[4] However, several factors may slow such growth, including the following:

- inadequate rural penetration of distribution channels;
- insufficient regulatory and intellectual property infrastructure;
- uncertainty of pricing policies.

Legal background

The Drugs and Cosmetics Act, 1940 (the "Drugs Act") is the backbone of the legal structure that governs the Food and Drug Administration in India. The Drugs and Cosmetics Rules, 1945, provides rules for the Drugs Act.[5] The Act and Rules, together, came into effect in 1947. The Drugs Act controls the manufacture, sale, and distribution of drugs.[6] Schedule Y to the Act also covers various issues affecting clinical trials. Pharmaceutical laws that directly affect the industry include: The Pharmacy Act, 1948; The Drugs and Magic Remedies Act, 1954; The Narcotic Drugs and Psychotropic

---

[1] CIA Factbook, https://www.cia.gov/library/publications/the-world-factbook/geos/in.html (last accessed November 24, 2009)

[2] Budget 2009 Snapshot: Specific Proposals for Pharmaceutical Sector, http://www.pwc.com/en_IN/in/assets/pdfs/pharma.pdf (last accessed November 24, 2009)

[3] Pharmaceutical Distribution in India: Drug manufacturers in India are struggling to improve a highly fragmented domestic distribution network. *BioPharm International*, **21**(10) (also at http://biopharminternational.findpharma.com/biopharm/India+Today/Pharmaceutical-Distribution-in-India/ArticleStandard/Article/detail/557245) (last accessed November 24, 2009)

Principles and Practice of Pharmaceutical Medicine, 3rd edition.
Edited by L.D. Edwards, A.W. Fox, P.D. Stonier.
© 2011 Blackwell Publishing Ltd.

[4] Pharma Summit 2009: India Pharma Inc: Overcoming Challenges to Maximise Potential, http://www.in.kpmg.com/TL_Files/Pictures/Pharma_2009.pdf (page 3, last accessed November 24, 2009)

[5] Manual on Drugs & Cosmetics, Ram Avtar Garg (Introductory)

[6] Indian Chemical and Pharmaceutical Works v. State of Andhra Pradesh AIR 1966 SC 713. (Manual on Drugs & Cosmetics, Ram Avtar Garg (page 2))

Substances Act, 1985; The Medicinal and Toilet Preparations Act, 1956; and the Drugs (Price Control) Order, 1995 under the Essential Commodities Act. Finally, The Industries (Development and Regulation) Act, 1951; The Trade and Merchandise Marks Act, 1958; The Indian Patent and Design Act, 1970; and the Factories Act all play a valuable role in the manufacture and trade of pharmaceuticals in India.

Intellectual Property Rights (IPRs)

The first Indian Patents Act[7] was drafted and enacted in or around 1856. After many versions and modifications, the Patents Act of 1970 was passed that embodies the foundation of modern Indian patent law. The Act:[8]

- Decreed that patents not be granted on important matters to prevent monopolies in such matters.
- Recognized that there were two types of patents: (i) process patents and (ii) product patents. Generally speaking, process patents allow a patent for a way of making a product while product patents allow a patent for the product itself.
- Required that no product patents be granted for medicines, food items, and chemicals except to their manufacturing process.

The Trade Related Aspects of Intellectual Property Rights (TRIPS) Agreement, to which India is a signatory, requires that patents be available for both products and processes, in all fields of technology, if such inventions are (i) new, (ii) involve an inventive step, and (iii) are capable of industrial application.[9] A review of the Patents Act of 1970 demonstrated that several provisions in the Act did not comply with the TRIPS agreement.[10] The Act was hence subsequently amended multiple times.

One of these amendments, the Amendment Act, 1999, allowed for product patents in the fields of pharmaceuticals, agriculture, and biotechnology.[11] As a result, MNPCs are less reluctant to enter the Indian market because they are less worried that their IPRs may be violated.

Indian drug organizations

The Indian FDA has a decentralized administrative structure. This structure, as it presently exists, is described in Figure 41.1. There is at present a bill in parliament to transform this decentralized structure into a centralized structure, modeling the US FDA, by or around 2015.[12]

Indian Drugs Standard Control Organization (IDSCO)

IDSCO consists of two separate organizations each with its own duties: (i) the Central Drugs Control Organization (CDSCO) and (ii) the State Drugs Standard Control Organization (SDSCO).

CDSCO

Headed by the Drug Controller General of India (DCGI), the CDSCO is responsible for functions including, but not limited to, regulating the marketing and authorization of new drugs, regulating clinical research in India, and publishing the Indian Pharmacopoeia. It is also responsible for arranging meetings of the Drug Technical Advisory Board (DTAB) and Drug Consultative Committee (DCC).

Drug Technical Advisory Board (DTAB)
The DTAB is an advisory board that counsels the central and state governments about drug control technicalities. For example, the DTAB was asked, by the DCGI, to re-examine drugs that are banned in other countries due to potential health hazards, but are widely available in India. Some specific

---

[7] *Intellectual Property Rights*, J.K. Das (first edition, page 251)

[8] *Intellectual Property Rights*, J.K. Das (first edition, page 33)

[9] *Intellectual Property Rights*, J.K. Das (first edition, page 33)

[10] The WTO's Agreement on Trade-Related Aspects of Intellectual Property Rights (TRIPS), negotiated in the 1986–94 Uruguay Round, introduced intellectual property rules into the multilateral trading system for the first time. (http://www.wto.org/english/thewto_e/whatis_e/tif_e/agrm7_e.htm; last accessed November 23, 2009)

[11] *Intellectual Property Rights*, J.K. Das (first edition, page 33)

[12] Taking Wings: Coming of Age of the Indian Pharmaceutical Industry, http://www.indiaoppi.com/OPPI%20-%20EandY%20Report%202009.pdf (page 61, last accessed November 29, 2009)

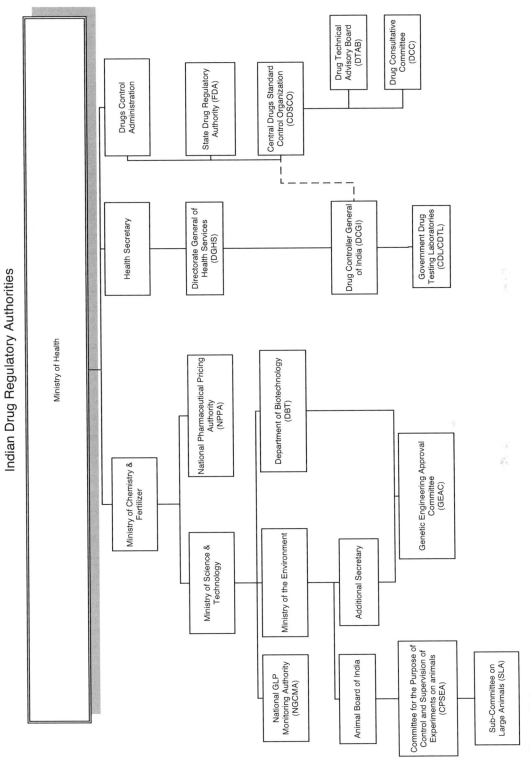

Indian Drug Regulatory Authorities

Figure 41.1

drugs under scrutiny include Nimesulide, Phenyl-propanolamide, Gatifloxacin, and Deanxit.[13]

Drug Consultative Committee (DCC)
The DCC consists of two representatives of the Central Government and one representative of each State Government to be nominated by the State Government concerned. The DCC enforces drug control measures in the various states and frames the rules of nationwide implementation. Among its other functions, the DCC issues licenses to import biological and other special products

SDSCO
Headed by the State Drug Controller, the SDSCO is responsible for functions including licensing drug manufacturing and sales organizations, pre- and post-licensing inspections, and recalling drugs in their respective territories.[14]

National Pharmaceutical Pricing Authority (NPPA)
The NPPA, a part of the Indian Government, was established to address the prices of controlled bulk drugs and formulations, and to enforce the pricing and availability of medicines under the Drugs (Prices Control) Order, 1995. In addition to controlling the prices of controlled drugs, the NPPA also monitors the prices of decontrolled drugs to keep their prices at reasonable levels.[15]

Biosimilars
Presently, the Institutional Bio Safety Committee, the Review Committee on Genetic Manipulation, the Recombinant DNA Appraisal Committee (RDAC), the DCGI, the Central Drug Standards Control Organization, and the Genetic Engineering Approval Committee (GEAC) are all involved in the approval of biosimilars. A single umbrella organization, the National Biotechnology Regulatory Authority, is currently being set up to assist and streamline the biosimilars approval process.[16]

Price controls
The NPPA was established in 1997 as an independent body of experts to be the primary determiner of prices and margins of drugs for the wholesaler and the retailer.[17] The price of a finished product, as determined by the NPPA, is primarily dependent on the active ingredients in the product. Depending on whether a constituent ingredient is considered a scheduled or non-scheduled drug, price caps may apply. The NPPA also monitors the prices of non-scheduled drugs to ensure availability and compliance with the Drugs (Price Control) Order, 1995. A scheduled drug is price-controlled, while a non-scheduled drug is not. At present, there are 76 scheduled drugs[18] including certain insulin preparations, antibiotics, and certain antihypertensive medicines.[19]

According to the draft of the National Pharmaceuticals Policy of 2006, it is expected that all patented products launched in India after 2005 would be subject to mandatory pricing negotiations before granting such products marketing approval.[20]

---

[13] DTAB to re-examine the controversial drugs widely distributed in India, http://www.pharmabuzz.org/news.php?news_id=1883 (last accessed December 6, 2009)

[14] Central Drugs Standard Control Organization, http://cdsco.nic.in/html/Drugs_ContAd.html (last accessed November 27, 2009)

[15] National Pharmaceutical Pricing Authority, http://nppaindia.nic.in/index1.html (last accessed December 6, 2009)

[16] *Bridges that Indian Biosimilar Makers Must Cross to Prosper in International Markets*, http://www.genengnews.com/specialreports/sritem.aspx?oid=59809892 (last accessed December 2, 2009)

[17] National Pharmaceutical Pricing Authority, http://nppaindia.nic.in/index1.html (last accessed November 27, 2009)

[18] Pharmaceutical Distribution in India: Drug manufacturers in India are struggling to improve a highly fragmented domestic distribution network. *BioPharm International*, **21**(10). (Also at http://biopharminternational.findpharma.com/biopharm/India+Today/Pharmaceutical-Distribution-in-India/ArticleStandard/Article/detail/557245) (last accessed November 24, 2009)

[19] Compendium: National Pharmaceutical Pricing Authority, http://nppaindia.nic.in/index1.html (page 4, last accessed December 4, 2009)

[20] National Pharmaceuticals Policy, 2006 (Draft), http://pib.nic.in/archieve/others/2005/documents2005dec/

Innovative small molecules

It was argued, at the time India was being made TRIPS compliant, that product patents would cause India to become an incubator country for innovative new products. While this has largely been true in the biotechnology arena, and for service provider industries like the preclinical and clinical research industries, no noteworthy breakthrough small molecules have resulted due to the change in the patent regime. Work done by governmental institutions, private companies, and combinations thereof may eventually lead to this goal, but so far India has remained a powerhouse, in the small molecule arena, primarily in the generic industry.

Medical device regulations

India's medical device industry has largely been unregulated. At present, the term "medical device" is not even specifically defined.

Recently, a task force consisting of various trade and advisory groups such as the Indian Chamber of Commerce (ICC), the Confederation of Indian Industry (CII), the World Health Organization (WHO), and the United States Food and Drug Administration (US FDA) devised a new set of regulations applicable to medical devices that were approved by the DCC and DTAB. The proposal included:

• The recently approved schedule M-III will contain a specific definition for medical devices as separate from drugs.

• The proposed Central Licensing Approval Authority (CLAA) will assume primary responsibility for regulating medical devices. The CLAA's functions may include:

– Classification, conformity assessment, and post-market surveillance of medical devices.

– Ensuring that all medical devices imported into or exported out of India conform with the new regulations.

There are, at present, two other proposals pending with the central government:[21]

• The 2006 Medical Device Regulations Bill (MDRA), originated by the Department of Science and Technology, proposed the establishment of a Medical Devices Regulatory Authority (MDRA) as an independent government ministry to regulate medical devices.

• The 2007 Drug and Cosmetics Amendment Bill (DCAB) proposed the creation of a central drug authority (similar to the US FDA) with a separate division responsible for the regulation of medical devices. DCAB failed to pass before the parliamentary elections of 2009.

In June, 2009 the proposed regulations, approved by the DCC and DTAB, were forwarded to the health ministry for its approval.[22]

Generics

India has continued to be a leader of generic medications produced not only for the Indian consumer, but also for consumers across the world. Prior to 2005, before the Indian Patent Act recognized product patents, most MNPCs were reluctant to enter the Indian market for fear that their IPRs would be violated. However, since 2005, once India began recognizing product patents, large MNPCs have begun recognizing the value proposition offered by Indian pharmaceutical companies (IPCs), which not only offer a foothold in a country of 1.13 billion people, but also offer recognized mastery in generic manufacturing. Accordingly, large MNPCs such as Pfizer and Daiichi Sankyo have begun partnering with and/or acquiring such IPCs.

Biosimilars/Biogenerics

Indian companies have been acclaimed leaders in small molecule generic manufacturing. Indian scientists are now trying to replicate this success in the large molecule/biologics space. The "Made-in-India" biosimilars market, which includes both

---

documents2005dec_chemfert.pdf (page 11, last accessed December 1, 2009)

[21] Asia/Pacific: Formal Notification Imminent for Medical Device Regulations in India, http://www.devicelink.

com/consultants/archive/09/09/gross.html (last accessed December 6, 2009)

[22] India's DCC and DTAB Approve New Regulations for Medical Devices, http://www.pacificbridgemedical.com/newsletter/article.php?id=414 (last accessed December 6, 2009)

domestic sales and exports, was around US$200 million in 2008.[23] This market is expected to expand to about US$580 million by 2012. The Indian biosimilars industry has seen this significant growth due to several factors:

• The Indian price control act does not cover most biotechnology drugs, with the exception of insulins. Biotechnology manufacturers can therefore potentially enjoy greater profit margins.

• Internationally, almost US$26 billion worth of biologics are expected to go off patent over the next ten years.

• Indian firms may be able to manufacture biosimilars patented prior to 2005 without violating the TRIPS Agreement.

• Biotechnology companies have access to space via numerous biotechnology parks, some of which is publicly funded.

• Healthcare professionals in India have been readily prescribing locally manufactured biosimilars.

There are, however, several factors that may limit India's success in the biogenerics space:

• *Price:* The Indian pharmaceutical market is very price sensitive. Biogenerics do not offer the same pricing discounts, compared to their respective branded products, as small molecules do. This lack of substantial discounting may affect the large-scale adoption of biogenerics in India. In effect, competition to biogenerics may come not only from their respective comparator brands, but also small molecule generic and brand molecules that may be able to replicate substantially similar clinical effects.

• *Infrastructure:* At present, even though there are large numbers of Indians who get their PhDs (equivalent to the numbers in the US and slightly less than the number of PhDs that graduate from Chinese universities) in the biological sciences, better infrastructure and employment opportunities often lure these experts to migrate to Western countries. This accounts for a significant "brain drain." To stem this tide of departing experts, the Indian government and the private industry must improve their existing biopharmaceutical infrastructure, and expand employment opportunities in India.

• *Regulatory pathways:* At present, the biosimilar regulatory pathway is an *ad hoc* system that is applied on a case-by-case basis. For example, although the DCGI does not typically require Phase I and II trials for biosimilar drugs, it does sometimes require extensive clinical trials in some situations. This lack of a clear pathway to biosimilar approval makes business planning uncertain. Such uncertainty is not conducive for long-term business planning and growth. The central government is therefore working to create a predictable biosimilars regulatory pathway and aims to introduce it by 2010.

• *Distribution infrastructure:* The Indian pharmaceutical distribution network is uneven and unreliable. Many medications, including biologics, are temperature and pressure labile and can be easily denatured due to temperature variations and physical acts as simple as shaking. Due to unreliable distribution networks, temperature variations and/or physical shaking while traveling from the site of manufacture to the site of patient use are commonplace. Accordingly, implementing a cold chain infrastructure for Indian conditions can become increasingly problematic. Although the infrastructure in so called "tier-1 cities," such as Mumbai and Delhi, is significantly better than that available in the rest of India, optimization of the entire distribution infrastructure is necessary for the growth of the Indian biosimilars industry.[24]

International potential

The global generics market is expected to grow at a Compounded Annual Growth Rate (CAGR) of about 10.5% between 2007 and 2012, driven by various factors including (i) the impending "patent

[23] Bridges that Indian Biosimilar Makers Must Cross to Prosper in International Markets, http://www.gene-ngnews.com/specialreports/sritem.aspx?oid=59809892 (last accessed December 2, 2009)

[24] Bridges that Indian Biosimilar Makers Must Cross to Prosper in International Markets, http://www.gene-ngnews.com/specialreports/sritem.aspx?oid=59809892 (last accessed December 2, 2009)

cliff" where several blockbuster drugs are expected to go off patent, (ii) governments encouraging the use of generics, and (iii) tougher economic conditions that encourage the use of generics.[25] IPCs are acknowledged to be one of the leading producers of low-cost, high quality generic small molecules. The IPCs are therefore now using this existing infrastructure to leverage their assets not only in generic manufacturing, but also throughout the pharmaceutical development chain.

Contract research organizations (CROS)

Introduction

When contract research work is outsourced, it can be accomplished in one of at least two ways: (i) a MNPC opens open a local facility; or (ii) a MNPC partners with existing local vendors. While the first method requires significant capital investment and commitment to the area, the second requires trust in the ability of the local vendor to deliver. Work done in India tends to be primarily setup through partnerships, joint ventures, and other alliances with local vendors who are considered to be "abundant, nimble, and resourceful."[26] MNPC investments in pharmaceutical outsourcing along the entire pharmaceutical development chain provide MNPCs with both near and long-term efficiency and productivity boosts.[27]

Preclinical research organizations outsourcing
Introduction

There are two major types of preclinical assignments that can be outsourced: (i) chemistry-based preclinical assignments; and (ii) biology-based preclinical assignments. While chemistry-based assignments look at issues such as stability, biology-based

assignments look at elements such as animal trials. Although India is already proficient in chemistry based-drug development, it is still developing its infrastructure in biology-based drug development.

General GLP monitoring

The Organisation for Economic Co-operation and Development (OECD) is an international organization that recommends the use of Good Laboratory Practices (GLPs) to help companies establish data that their products, including pharmaceuticals, do not pose a human health hazard. The Indian Government's Department of Science and Technology realized the importance of preclinical development of drugs and established the National GLP Compliance Monitoring Authority (NGCMA) in April 2002 to advance its goals. At present, the NGCMA offers industries, testing facilities, and laboratories voluntary GLP certification if (i) they manage chemicals and (ii) desire approval from the appropriate regulatory authorities.[28,29]

Although India is an observer to the OECD working group on GLP, other OECD member countries do not currently recognize an Indian GLP certification because India does not share Mutual Acceptance Data (MAD) status with OECD nations. India hopes eventually to obtain MAD status with OECD nations. India is promoting its cause by transitioning, by late 2010, to a mandatory GLP program.[30]

[25] Pharma Summit 2009: India Pharma Inc: Overcoming Challenges to Maximise Potential, http://www.in.kpmg.com/TL_Files/Pictures/Pharma_2009.pdf (page 3, last accessed November 24, 2009)
[26] Looking Eastward: tapping China and India to Reinvigorate the Global Pharmaceutical Industry, *BCG Report* 2006: 9
[27] Looking Eastward: tapping China and India to Reinvigorate the Global Pharmaceutical Industry, *BCG Report* 2006: 9

[28] National Good Laboratory Practice Compliance Monitoring Authority, http://indiaglp.gov.in/index.htm (last accessed November 30, 2009)
[29] To be GLP certified, the relevant facility must fill out the appropriate documentation and submit it to the NGCMA. At such point, GLP inspectors conduct a pre-inspection of the laboratory and then conduct a final inspection. During an audit multiple facets of the organization including facility, personnel, equipment, documentation, and audits and inspections are evaluated. The resultant report by the GLP inspectors is reassessed by the Technical Committee that makes its recommendation to the NGCMA Chairman. Once obtained, a GLP-compliance certification is valid for a period of three years. Periodic re-evaluation is required to maintain certification.
[30] Preclinical CRO Markets: China v. India, http://www.croasia.net/resources/preclinical_cro_markets:_india_vs_china.html (last accessed November 30, 2009)

Animal protection bodies

In addition to organizations, such as the NCGMA, that promote GLPs, several organizations are primarily dedicated to monitoring testing performed, on animals. The Prevention of Cruelty to Animals Act (PCAA) was enacted in 1960 to (i) prevent the infliction of unnecessary pain or suffering on animals, and (ii) to amend the laws relating to the prevention of cruelty to animals. The Animal Board of India was formed to advance the purpose of the PCAA.

In June 2005, India amended Schedule Y of the Drugs Act to provide clear guidelines on the use of animals in preclinical tests. This amendment aimed to prevent animal rights lobbyists from predominating an institution's animal ethics committee. It hoped, instead, to provide a stronger voice to neutral scientists and experts who served on such committees.

Current core strengths

India is currently known to have strong capabilities in areas such as assay development, high throughput screening, computer aided drug design, structural drug design, structural chemistry, combinatorial chemistry, focus libraries, analytical chemistry, and analog preparation. MNPCs can hence increase productivity and efficiency by outsourcing these and other functions to India. Several advantages to performing work in India are listed in the following sections.

Chemistry research

Due to a historical focus on generics manufacturing, Indian-based, chemistry-focused research scientists are plentiful, abundantly qualified, and available for a relatively low cost. These scientists often performed work in reverse engineering and alternative process development that did not violate pre-existing process patents, but still resulted in similar products with substantially similar safety and efficacy profiles.

Regulatory advantages

A regulatory system, though not fully established, allows for predictable trial approval timelines from the associated authorities and hence makes planning and conducting preclinical trials easier.

Through the amendments to Schedule Y and to the rest of the Drugs Act, India has positioned itself to be a leader in the preclinical research industry.

Impending changes such as FDA centralization, mandatory GLP requirements, MAD status with OECD nations, and giving more power to scientists and regulators in organizations such as the NCGMA and the Animal Board will enhance the predictability of drug development in India and make it a more desirable location to do outsourced work.

Information Technology (IT) infrastructure

India's core competence in IT, combined with its access to cost effective, well educated, plentiful graduates in the biological sciences allows it potentially to play a role in the rapidly evolving fields of bioinformatics and computational biology. Bioinformatics explores the use of information technology to create a "global perspective from which unifying principles in biology can be discerned."[31] The data acquired using bioinformatics data acquisition processes are processed and analyzed in a field referred to as computational biology.[32] Although there have already been instances where such complementary skill sets have been used, it is expected that the rate of using such skill sets will increase over time.[33] Recent transactions between IBM and Indian vendors, and Astra Zeneca's captive R&D facilities are examples of MNPCs maximizing the efficiencies inherent in using such crossover knowledge.[34]

---

[31] Just the Facts: A Basic Introduction to the Science Underlying NCBI Resources http://www.ncbi.nlm.nih.gov/About/primer/bioinformatics.html (last accessed December 6, 2009)

[32] Just the Facts: A Basic Introduction to the Science Underlying NCBI Resources http://www.ncbi.nlm.nih.gov/About/primer/bioinformatics.html (last accessed December 6, 2009)

[33] Looking Eastward: Tapping China and India to Reinvigorate the Global Pharmaceutical Industry, *BCG Report* 2006: 12

[34] Looking Eastward: Tapping China and India to Reinvigorate the Global Pharmaceutical Industry, *BCG Report* 2006: 13

Investigator access

Preclinical trial organizations in India have access to large numbers of investigators, often qualified with doctorates and/or masters degrees in the relevant chemical or biological sciences, who can conduct trials in accordance with the latest GLPs. These investigators have often been trained, or are under the guidance of individuals who have been trained, in Western countries. These scientists are often abreast of the latest research and can therefore work to further existing work. These advantages bode well for the expansion and growth of the Indian preclinical market.

Management philosophy

The management philosophy of Indian managers, as part of the world's largest democracy, is similar to the management philosophy in Western countries.[35] Although cultural differences may make interactions more complex, the similarity in management styles makes working in India easier for most Westerners. MNPCs often find it easier to partner with local partners to increase efficiency and productivity immediately and yet demonstrate long-term cost savings.

Limitations

IPR protection concerns

MNPCs continue to remain cautious about entering the India market because of data privacy and data protection concerns. These concerns have been largely addressed by Indian vendors who have taken a variety of measures to stem the loss of information, including the following:

• maintaining strict standards of confidentiality;

• walling off a MNPC's research from in-house R&D programs to prevent data crossover;

• splitting a project into multiple subdivisions and assigning separate groups of scientists to each individual subdivision;

• maintaining a client's name in confidence.[36]

These steps have significantly addressed MNPC fears of IPR loss.

Animal rights concerns

Most Indian preclinical providers companies are set up to provide preclinical trial studies in small animals, such as mice and rodents. Some even offer limited capabilities in large animals such as dogs. However, most Indian companies have almost no capabilities in primates.[37] This is problematic in the case of disease states where studies may require the use of primates. MNPCs desiring the use of Indian facilities may find that they can do some work in India, but must perform work on primates in other countries. Some MNPCs may not want to use this piecemeal approach to conduct trials in multiple countries and may hence choose to avoid entering the Indian market altogether for preclinical work.

Limited opportunities

At present, there are only 13 GLP certified facilities in India.[38] This limited scope, to work in preclinical facilities, feeds into the cycle of producing fewer individuals with the appropriate experience, who can do preclinical work. This therefore limits the type of individuals who can teach and mentor a new preclinical workforce.

Biology research

Due to a historical focus on small molecule generics, Indian scientists tend to be weaker in the biological research areas. This is changing over time, with several companies poised to take on roles in biologics development and the impending biosimilars regulation in the US market. Considering the focus on biotechnology, Indian scientists are already set to make strides in the local and EMA-based biosimilars markets.

---

[35] Preclinical CRO Markets: China v. India, http://www.croasia.net/resources/preclinical_cro_markets:_india_vs_china.html (last accessed November 30, 2009)

[36] Looking Eastward: Tapping China and India to Reinvigorate the Global Pharmaceutical Industry, *BCG Report* 2006: 14

[37] Looking Eastward: Tapping China and India to Reinvigorate the Global Pharmaceutical Industry, *BCG Report* 2006:9

[38] Lab Next: Next Generation GLP guidelines, http://www.expresspharmaonline.com/20091130/retrospective 200908.shtml (last accessed December 1, 2009)

Lack of GLP facilities and MAD status

Without Indian laboratories being provided MAD status, MNPCs are reticent to conduct preclinical research in India. Without MAD status, they often doubt the veracity and dependability of Indian lab results. It is expected that by late 2010 India will move to a mandatory GLP program. This will increase the trustworthiness of results from the country and therefore increase the inflow of pre-clinical work to India.

Clinical research organizations outsourcing
Introduction

As drug development costs have continued to rise, and world economies have simultaneously stumbled, limited budgets, and a desire for increased efficiencies, have encouraged MNPCs to leverage international efficiencies beyond traditional Western countries to provide value all along the pharmaceutical development chain. Such efficiencies include conducting clinical trials. India is one of the countries where such efficiencies are often realized. Although the US FDA has accepted Indian data, submitted as part of the clinical database, no pivotal clinical studies totally conducted in India have been the basis of a US approval. As of 2009, despite advantages in costs, patient recruitment, facilities, investigator pool, trial experience, and regulatory environment, India accounted for only 2% of the global clinical trials market.[39] This section explores why India only has such a limited portion of the market and why the market is expected to expand dramatically in the coming years.

Clinical trial applications

Multiple parts of a clinical trial must be registered before initiating a trial. For example, not only must a trial itself be registered, but also components such as importation of the requisite drug substance. Applications to conduct clinical trials in India, for new or investigational new drugs, require the express permission of the statutory Licensing Authorities prior to starting the trial.[40] The fee due to the Licensing Authority is dependent on the phase of the trial that must be conducted.[41]

Importing a new drug, to be used in clinical trials, also requires the Licensing Authority's permission. The requirements, to import a new drug, may be relaxed if

• the new drug has been approved and marketed for several years in other countries; and

• there is adequate published evidence regarding the safety of the drug.

Alternatively, such requirements may be waived on a case-by-case basis, in the case of a demonstrated overriding public interest.[42]

Advantages
Cost advantages

Due to the lower cost and easy availability of a well-qualified, English-speaking labor force in India, it is often advantageous to conduct clinical studies in India. This lower cost of labor also manifests in lower patient recruitment costs. It is important to note that it is customary for potential subjects to bring family members during a consent meeting. Accordingly, the costs associated with bringing such family members may need to be included in calculating trial costs. Despite the additional travel costs of an extra person, it is often substantially cheaper than conducting similar experiments in Western countries. Additionally, the use of a support system, such as an extra person, provides greater assurance of truly obtaining informed consent because this trusted person allows for a meaningful conversation, with the patient, in which the risks and benefits of participation in the trial are discussed.

---

[39] Pharma Summit 2009: India Pharma Inc: Overcoming Challenges to Maximise Potential, http://www.in.kpmg.com/TL_Files/Pictures/Pharma_2009.pdf (last accessed November 24, 2009)

[40] Rule 122 DA of Drugs and Cosmetics Rules, 1945
[41] Import or Manufacture of New Drug for Clinical Trials or Marketing, http://cdsco.nic.in/html/Sec_122_A.htm (Section 122DA: Application for permission to conduct clinical trials for New Drug/Investigational New Drug, last accessed December 1, 2009)
[42] Import or Manufacture of New Drug for Clinical Trials or Marketing, http://cdsco.nic.in/html/Sec_122_A.htm (Section 122DA: Application for permission to conduct clinical trials for New Drug/Investigational New Drug, last accessed December 1, 2009)

Availability of trained investigators

At present, there are over 1000 physicians and 800 hospitals in India who have conducted, or are capable of conducting, clinical trials in accordance with US FDA and International Committee on Harmonization (ICH) guidelines.[43] Additionally, many of India's thought leaders, in the healthcare industry, have been trained in Western countries such as the US and the UK. Such training allows these investigators to better adhere to GCPs as proposed by members of the ICH in general and the US FDA and EMEA in particular. Quite often, these investigators also speak both English and local languages, and can hence communicate and obtain informed consent from potential subjects. These appropriately qualified, multilingual investigators are often boons for sponsors and CROs looking to conduct large multinational clinical trials where patients may often only be able to speak local languages.

Patient population

India's 1.16 billion population has significant numbers of drug-naïve patients. The major diseases presently prevalent in India include HIV/AIDS, tuberculosis, and malaria. Other prevalent diseases include 8 million epileptics, 5 million rheumatoid arthritis patients, 34 million diabetics, 1.5 million Alzheimer's patients, 40 million asthmatics, and 2 million patients suffering from cardiac-related diseases. Additionally, several disease specific populations that may be rare across the world are often plentifully found in India.

The combination of drug naïvety with potentially large numbers of patients makes India a valuable country in which to conduct clinical trials.

Regulatory infrastructure

It is assumed that the regulatory approvals required to conduct research in India are both time consuming and bureaucratic. Surprisingly, quite the reverse is true. The Indian approval process is considered to be both predictable and among the fastest in the world.

Category A clinical trials. For global clinical trials whose protocols were approved by drug authorities in the US, UK, Switzerland, Australia, Canada, Germany, South Africa, Japan, and/or the EMEA, which are using India as a location, the typical DCGI approval time is aimed to be between 2–4 weeks. Practically, however, it takes between 4–6 weeks for a Category A approval.[44]

Category B clinical trials. For trials, other than Category A trials, the typical approval time, from the DCGI's office was expected to take between 8–12 weeks, but can take as long as 12–16 weeks.

Clinical Data Management (CDM)

CDM is the use of IT to collect and analyze information accumulated during clinical trials. The primary method of data collection is often case report forms. India has a strong existing infrastructure supporting IT. As previously explained, India also has a significant workforce specializing in the biological and chemical sciences. The combined use of the IT and biological/chemical sciences backgrounds has proved to be a boon for the Indian CDM industry because it creates a fertile ground for developing crossover knowledge. At present, despite paying above average salaries for the IT sector, the cost of maintaining the salary bill in India is approximately one-third the cost of an equivalent CDM center in the US.

International Committee on Harmonization (ICH)

Since Indian GCPs are strongly aligned with those promulgated by the ICH, studies conducted in India are therefore often ICH compliant. There remain, however, significant differences between the ICH and Indian GCPs in certain situations. It is important that a review of the differences be conducted before performing any clinical trial in India.

---

[43] Demystifying India: Understanding Common Myths and truths surrounding one of the fastest growing clinical trial markets. http://appliedclinicaltrialsonline.findpharma.com/appliedclinicaltrials/article/articleDetail.jsp?id=615145&sk=&date=&pageID=2 (last accessed November 29, 2009)

[44] Drug Controller General Minutes, http://cdsco.nic.in/Global_Clinical_Trials.htm (last accessed November 29, 2009)

Potential limitations

Short supply of GCP trained investigators

Despite the availability of a large number of trained investigators, the demand for such investigators often exceeds the supply. At present, there are several institutions that offer to train potential investigators in GCP and teach them to conduct clinical trials in India. These efforts will result, in the near future, in more available GCP investigators.

Inadequate infrastructure

Due to bad roads and unreliable public transportation, the transfer of people and clinical trial materials can be difficult in India. This becomes especially true in the case of labile drugs, such as several biologics, which must often be maintained as part of a cold supply chain. This inadequate infrastructure may inordinately affect transportation of subjects, the trial team, and clinical trial materials and hence cause higher transportation costs. The uncertainty associated with such variables can dissuade sponsors from conducting clinical trials in India.

Intellectual property rights

Though the Patents Act of 1970, and the Amendments thereto, have allowed for product patents, the delays inherent in the Indian legal system and the resultant delays in patent rights enforcement have resulted in suboptimal IPR protection. Such delays have previously dissuaded, and continue to play a role in scaring, MNPCs from investing in the India. Although it is expected that these cultural and administrative issues will be resolved eventually, MNPCs and local vendors have already set up alternative ways to maintain data security and protect IPR. Measures taken include maintaining data on US-based servers, and using confidentiality agreements whose jurisdictional clauses use the US as the site of litigation. Vendors have even taken steps like restricting computer functions such as printing and saving options.

Data exclusivity laws

Data exclusivity refers to a practice whereby, for a fixed period of time, drug regulatory authorities do not allow the registration files of an originator to be used to register a therapeutically equivalent generic version of that drug.[45] Data exclusivity is completely separate from patents.[46] At present, there are no Indian laws that prevent data obtained during clinical trials for one drug to be used, by the DCGI, for the approval of other drugs. Such laws would be considered to be "TRIPs Plus."

The MNPCs see the lack of data exclusivity laws as worrisome because they believe that the lack of such laws provides their competitors with an unfair advantage potentially to copy their research. These proponents, of data exclusivity, argue that data exclusivity is an expression of trade secrets, and that as such, should be independent of patents. Opponents of data exclusivity argue that if data exclusivity is a form of trade secrets, it is protectable beyond the term of the patent effectively extending the patent, for an infinite period of time. These opponents therefore argue that in the case of a country that provides unlimited data exclusivity, all data provided to its drug regulatory agencies, by an originator company, is a trade secret and therefore protectable until the earlier of

- an infinite period of time;
- or until another company reinvents the same or similar data.

Accordingly, a generic company would be unable to introduce a generic until such time as it reinvents the product and reproduces similar requisite submission data, but no earlier than until the relevant patents expire.[47]

First-in-human trials

Prior to 2005, clinical studies in India of "non-Indian" origin could only be tested at an earlier phase of development than in the rest of the world. Thus, if Phase II studies were completed in the rest of the world, Phase I was required to be repeated

---

[45] Data Exclusivity: An Indian Perspective, http://www.ipfrontline.com/depts/article.asp?id=12300&deptid=6 (last accessed December 6, 2009)

[46] Data Exclusivity: An Indian Perspective, http://www.ipfrontline.com/depts/article.asp?id=12300&deptid=6 (last accessed December 6, 2009)

[47] Taking Wings: Coming of Age of the Indian Pharmaceutical Industry, http://www.indiaoppi.com/OPPI%20-%20EandY%20Report%202009.pdf (page 61, last accessed November 29, 2009)

in India. Similarly, if Phase III studies were being undertaken elsewhere, India could only conduct Phase II studies. This was largely abolished starting in January 2005.

However, after 2005, the Indian government does not allow first-in-human Phase I drug studies for drugs discovered outside India to protect Indian patients from effectively becoming human guinea pigs.[48] MNPCs, of non-Indian origin, that want to conduct clinical trials in India would not be able to conduct Phase I studies in India. This forces these MNPCs to either use multiple CROs in multiple countries or conduct all trials in countries that allow Phase I, first-in-human trials. There may hence be reluctance in MNPC engagement of local CRO service providers to conduct clinical trials in India, to avoid a potential lack of continuity.

Generics and Contract Manufacturing Organizations (CMOs)

Setting up a pharmaceutical manufacturing unit in India is up to 30% cheaper than setting up a similar plant in the US.[49] India's pool of trained chemists and pharmacists is six times larger than in the US and is available at 10% of the cost. The cheap cost of setting up a pharmaceutical unit, combined with access to trained chemists and pharmacists, has resulted has resulted in India having the largest number of "FDA approved" facilities outside the US.[50] These advantages position Indian companies to become prominent players in the international pharmaceutical market as both contract drug manufacturers and generic companies in their own right. Indian companies have traditionally been very good at generic small molecule manufacturing. They have now extended these skill sets to

produce drugs not only for themselves but also for their international partners.

MNPCs have previously been reluctant to enter markets such as India because of previously listed concerns including potential issues of reliability and acknowledged expertise in reverse engineering and generic manufacturing. These issues concern innovator companies who worry that they may lose their IPRs, and volatility of the local currency.[51, 52]

Generics
Indian production of antiretrovirals
Several Indian companies, which have traditionally participated in generic manufacturing, have contributed to saving lives that could potentially have been lost to diseases such as HIV/AIDS. IPCs such as Ranbaxy and Cipla manufactured low-cost antiretroviral (ARV) drugs that competed directly against large multinational companies. As a result of this direct competition, the cost of providing ARVs dropped precipitously from US$8000 per year to under US$200 per year. These low-cost ARVs, though manufactured in India, were distributed not only in India but also exported to countries in Africa such as Nigeria. Prior to 2005, Indian manufacturers were required to adhere to process patents but not product patents, because such patents did not exist in India. Since 2005 product patents were allowed. Accordingly, to avoid violating the TRIPs agreement, any ARVs patented after 1995 could not be legally manufactured and/or sold in India. This has resultantly put an end to the Indian cottage industry of manufacturing low-cost ARVs for domestic and international use.

Big pharma–Indian pharma partnerships
Despite the previously acrimonious relationship between MNPCs and Indian pharmaceutical

[48] Demystifying India: Understanding Common Myths and truths surrounding one of the fastest growing clinical trial markets. http://appliedclinicaltrialsonline.findpharma.com/appliedclinicaltrials/article/articleDetail.jsp?id=615145&sk=&date=&pageID=2 (last accessed November 29, 2009)

[49] http://www.indiaoppi.com/OPPI%20-%20EandY%20Report%202009.pdf (last accessed April 12, 2010)

[50] Pharma Summit 2009: India Pharma Inc: Overcoming Challenges to Maximise Potential, http://www.in.kpmg.com/TL_Files/Pictures/Pharma_2009.pdf (page 27, last accessed November 24, 2009)

[51] Pharma Summit 2009: India Pharma Inc: Overcoming Challenges to Maximise Potential, http://www.in.kpmg.com/TL_Files/Pictures/Pharma_2009.pdf (page 29, last accessed November 24, 2009)

[52] Pharma Summit 2009: India Pharma Inc: Overcoming Challenges to Maximise Potential, http://www.in.kpmg.com/TL_Files/Pictures/Pharma_2009.pdf (page 31, last accessed November 24, 2009)

companies, the two factions have now found common ground. Some of the largest MNPCs have, as a result of several factors including the impending patent cliff of 2012, started partnering with IPCs to produce generic versions of their products. Such companies include Pfizer, which has struck a deal with Aurobindo Pharma Ltd, and Daiichi Sankyo Co, which bought a majority stake in Ranbaxy Laboratories Ltd. Products of these acquisitions and ventures are expected to be sold not only in regulated markets like the US and EU countries, but also emerging and semi-regulated markets (for example, India, China, and Russia).[53]

Manufacturing/Contract Manufacturing Organizations

In 2003 the central government required the Indian pharmaceutical industry to comply with WHO Good Manufacturing Practices (GMP). As a result of this requirement, contract manufacturers had to ensure that not only the parent unit but also their loan licensees were compliant with WHO GMP if their product was being exported. The cost of converting a non-WHO GMP unit to a WHO GMP compliant facility varied between approximately US$35,000 to approximately US$225,000 per unit. In certain situations it even resulted in moving facilities altogether. The WHO GMP requirement spelt the death knell for several small drug manufacturers who could not afford the cost of compliance. The survivors of this fallout were companies that made significant capital investments and demonstrated a strong commitment to quality products.[54]

Current topics

FDA office

The US FDA regulates a large number of the approximately US$2 trillion worth of products that enter the US. This number has roughly doubled between 2003 and 2008. Accordingly, the FDA initiated the "Beyond Our Borders" Initiative. The goal of this Initiative was to allow the FDA to better address international challenges to public health and national security by

- increasing collaboration with its foreign counterparts;
- learning more about foreign exporters and their products;
- providing technical assistance to foreign regulators and industries;
- establishing overseas offices within some foreign countries.[55]

As part of this Initiative, the US FDA opened its office in India in January 2009. It is presently planned that when fully staffed, the FDA will have 12 staff members in India split between Mumbai and New Delhi. The staff is expected to be based out of the US Embassy in New Delhi and the US Consulate General in Mumbai.[56] Secretary Mike Leavitt announced that the goal of the Indian office was to enhance the safety of food and medical products in both countries.[57]

USP office

In September 2005, the United States Pharmacopoeia (USP) announced its intention to set up a wholly owned subsidiary in Hydrabad, India. The facility in India includes a business office and testing laboratories featuring state of

---

[53] Pfizer pins hopes on Aurobindo, does not rule out Indian buys, http://www.livemint.com/2009/11/26233806/Pfizer-pins-hopes-on-Aurobindo.html (last accessed December 4, 2009)

[54] Impact of Product Patent on FDI in Indian Pharmaceutical Industry, http://ezinearticles.com/?Impact-of-Product-Patent-on-FDI-in-Indian-Pharmaceutical-Industry&id=89594 (last accessed December 4, 2009)

[55] FDA Beyond Our Borders, http://www.fda.gov/ForConsumers/ConsumerUpdates/ucm103036.htm (last accessed December 6, 2009)

[56] India, http://www.fda.gov/AboutFDA/CentersOffices/OC/OfficeofInternationalPrograms/ucm115258.htm (last accessed April 12, 2010)

[57] HHS Preparing to Open FDA Offices in China, India, Europe, and Latin America This Year, http://www.hhs.gov/news/press/2008pres/10/20081016a.html (last accessed November 27, 2009)

the art instrumentation including HPLCs and gas chromatographs. The facility will be responsible for evaluating reference standards on collaborative testing and establishing reference standards used by industry throughout the world. The facility's initial project focused on the quality of dietary supplements and ingredients and is expected to grow to include APIs and excipients in the near future.[58] According to John Fowler, the USP's Chief Business Officer and Senior Vice-President, the standards setting organization chose India because it was "the right place to go because of the significant growth and the number of companies that are exporting to other parts in the world."[59] According to Fowler, "India is a great and growing market, and half of the generic drugs today use Indian-manufactured APIs. There is a huge need for standards, which are vitally important to protecting consumers." He continued, "Our operations in India will help ensure the safety of India's domestic drug supply as well as what is shipped outside of India."[60]

Clinical trial registry

The clinical trials registry of India was set up in July 2007.[61] The goals of the registry are to
• improve transparency and accountability;
• improve validity of trials;
• conform trials to accepted ethical standards;
• report all relevant results in the area.

While registration itself was voluntary at first, the Directorate General of Health Services, Office of Drugs Controller General (India) (New Drug Division) recently announced that all clinical trials

initiated after June 15, 2009, would be required to be mandatorily registered in the clinical trial registry.[62] It is expected that the mandatory registration will promote the goals of the registry.

Ranbaxy: issues resolved

The Indian Pharmaceutical Industry is represented by a handful of big players. These players include Ranbaxy, Cipla, Dr Reddys, and Wockhardt. These players dominate the Indian landscape and are also stalwarts in the US generic industry. As stalwarts, these companies represent, in many ways, the best and brightest of the Indian drug industry.

In February 2009, the US FDA "announced that a facility owned by . . . Ranbaxy Laboratories falsified data and test results in approved and pending drug applications."[63] As a result of the FDA audit conducted, the FDA
• asked Ranbaxy to cooperate with the agency to resolve the questions of data integrity and reliability;
• stopped all substantive scientific review of any new or pending drug approval applications that contained data generated by the relevant facility;
• issued two warning letters;
• instituted an Import Alert barring the entry of all finished drug products and active pharmaceutical ingredients from multiple Ranbaxy facilities (into the US), alleging violations of US current GMP requirements.

Since then, and as of November of 2009, Ranbaxy had settled out of court and used its first-to-file status to bring generic valaciclovir to the market.[64]

---

[58] USP India's New Facility Opens its Doors, http://www. pharmamanufacturing.com/articles/2006/066.html (last accessed November 27, 2009)

[59] US Pharmacopeia sets up subsidiary here, http://www. thehindubusinessline.com/bline/2005/09/15/stories/ 2005091501540300.htm (last accessed November 27, 2009)

[60] USP India's New Facility Opens its Doors, http://www. pharmamanufacturing.com/articles/2006/066.html (last accessed November 27, 2009)

[61] Clinical Trials in India: ethical concerns, http://www. who.int/bulletin/volumes/86/8/08-010808/en/index. html (last accessed November 27, 2009)

[62] Central Drugs Standard Control Organization, http:// cdsco.nic.in/CTRegistration.doc (last accessed November 29, 2009)

[63] *FDA Takes New Regulatory Action Against Ranbaxy's Paonta Sahib Plant in India*, http://www.fda.gov/NewsEvents/ Newsroom/PressAnnouncements/ucm149532.htm (last accessed December 2, 2009)

[64] Ranbaxy launches new drug in the US: PharmAsia News, http://www.moneycontrol.com/news/business/ ranbaxy-launches-new-drugthe-us- pharmasianews_427536.html (last accessed December 2, 2009)

The resolution of these issues bode well, not only for the narrow issue of Ranbaxy US FDA relations, but also for broader relations between Indian and US companies who want to establish partnerships to develop products, not only for emerging, semi-regulated countries but also regulated markets such as the US and EU.

Indian IP Developments

The Indian Utilization of Public Funded Intellectual Property Bill (IUPFIP), 2008, is the Indian equivalent of the US Bayh-Dole Act. The IUPFIP provides for the protection and utilization of IP originating from governmental funding. It has currently been approved by the Union Cabinet and is under consideration by parliament.

Presently, academic institutions whose inventions originate from governmental funding cannot commercialize their inventions. Under the proposed law, academic inventors could patent their inventions and would receive a portion of the royalties and licensing fees resulting from the invention. Supporters of the Act applaud the use of governmental funding since it may result in commercially viable inventions. However, detractors to the Act state that it is not optimized to Indian realities, citing the following:

• allegations that the Act has been hastily drafted without an assessment of how the US Act has impacted the US industry;

• there has been an inadequate assessment of the official draft of the bill, which was neither released nor publicly debated;

• allegations that the bill would only advance the cause of scientists who were well connected to the industry and also had a commercial acumen.

This Act may severely impact research conducted, for the Indian pharmaceutical industry, with Indian academic researchers and may have a fallout beyond what is currently projected. However, it is too soon to tell if and whether any of these projected doomsday or paradise scenarios play out.[65]

---

[65] The Indian Version of the Bayh-Dole Act, http://www.iam-magazine.com/issues/article.ashx?g=af438a8b-2c

Patent linkage

Patent linkage, is a system whereby marketing approval for generic medicines is linked to the patent status of the comparator brand product. Accordingly, patent linkage requires that if a brand drug is patented, and such patent is valid, a generic version of the drug cannot be approved by the DCGI until such time as the original patent on the branded product expires.

Most legal commentators agree that India is not obliged by international law, including that of the WTO, to introduce patent linkage. Some countries, including the US, China, Canada, and Australia, have incorporated patent linkage into their law. The US controls its patent linkage system by using a database that tracks patents (commonly referred to as the orange book.) Conversely, other countries, including the EU, have not incorporated patent linkage, and have done so without violating their obligations under WTO laws, including the TRIPS Agreement. The EU Directorate General for Competition (DGC) stated, in relevant part, that "patent linkage is considered unlawful under the applicable EU regulations" and cited the Bolar exception.* India, like the EU, amended its IP laws to make them TRIPs compliant. However, like the EU, India cited the Bolar exception and did not recognize patent linkage.

US-based pharmaceutical giant Bayer through its Indian subsidiary (collectively, "Bayer"), challenged the position of the Indian government in not recognizing patent linkage. Bayer filed a writ petition in the Delhi high court against the Union of India, DCGI, and Cipla Ltd (Cipla). Bayer hoped to prevent the DCGI from accepting Cipla's application for a generic version of its patented drug, Sorafenib Tosylate, a treatment of kidney cancer. In making its case Bayer asserted that the generic

---

4e-4771-b573-32171a1c4c65 (last accessed December 4, 2009)

*Note: The Bolar exception provided in Article 30 of the TRIPS agreement, allows governments to make limited exceptions to the rights of patent holders in the "legitimate interest" of third parties, provided such exceptions do not "unreasonably" conflict with the patent holder's right to "normal" exploitation of the patent.

drug proposed to be manufactured by Cipla would be a "spurious drug" under section 17B of the Drugs Act. Bayer further asserted that a government authority, such as the DCGI, cannot grant marketing approval where this would affect patent rights.

The court initially, in November 2008, enjoined the DCGI from processing Cipla's application. However, in August 2009 the court dismissed Bayer's writ petition, and held that there was neither a parliament-mandated "drug-patent linkage" system in India nor any legislative intent to place patent policing powers with agencies such as DCGI. The court further rejected Bayer's assertion that Cipla's drug would be a "spurious drug" under the Drugs Act. The court lastly rejected Bayer's argument that the DCGI cannot grant marketing approval where this would affect patent rights.[66]

---

[66] Storm over drug-patent linkage after court rejects Bayer petition, http://www.livemint.com/2009/10/11205401/Storm-over-drugpatent-linkage.html (last accessed December 5, 2009)

Bayer is currently appealing the decision. Until then, like the EU and unlike the US, India does not recognize patent linkage.

Conclusion

India is a country of many talents and tremendous potential. Domestically, its 1.13 billion people are underserved due to the lack of cheap available drugs. Internationally, MNPCs are beginning to understand the efficiencies and potential productivity increases they can realize by using Indian pharmaceutical outsourcing providers. As these trends mature, more MNPCs, not only in the US but also the EU and Japan, will enter India to contribute to its growth and experience its advantages.

SECTION VI
Medical Services

Introduction

Medical Services (or "Medical Affairs" in some pharmaceutical companies) comprises some of the less tangible aspects of pharmaceutical medicine.

First, the term is somewhat of a misnomer. An effective medical services department does a lot of things that are not strictly "medical," and without any, even slightly tangential, clinical implication. These may include imagining new development ideas for old drugs, attending to post-marketing commitments for newly approved products, pharmacovigilance "data-mining," reviewing marketing materials and promotional activities, providing scientific input to price negotiations, and so.

Second, these diverse tasks bring diverse responsibilities. Very often, those working in medical affairs departments will find themselves in the role of an in-house ombudsman. Ebullience in the marketing department might need to be tempered by the realities of product labeling. Pharmacovigilance signals usually need sifting for decision about which to investigate. Corporate responses to technical inquiries must be properly designed. Manufacturing deviations must be assessed from both clinical and legal viewpoints. If the company must defend itself in litigation (almost inevitable in the USA today), it is the medical affairs specialists that must ensure that the defense lawyers are properly briefed on the technical issues. This role as an ombudsman can sometimes be lonely: insistence on what is right can often be counter to short-term financial aspirations elsewhere in the company.

The best medical affairs specialists are those with long experience. Although these chapters contain a useful knowledge base, nothing can replace several years' experience "in the trenches" of a vigorous medical affairs department. The cross-disciplinary role can also be the most stimulating of any in the industry for a versatile generalist.

CHAPTER 42

Medical Affairs

Gregory P. Geba

Clinical Development, MedImmune, LLC, One MedImmune Way, Gaithersburg, MD 20878, USA

Introduction

The role of clinical trials in evaluating efficacy and safety of drugs extends well beyond the confines of the registration package submitted to health authorities. Due to the increasing costs and time associated with drug development, a strategy often pursued in drug registration is one that takes the most direct route to answering specific clinical efficacy and safety questions required to judge the benefit– risk profile of a drug to secure marketing approval for specific indications. This approach permits the most expeditious drug development, which can bring therapeutics to areas of unmet medical need. This is counterbalanced by the additional requirement to assess most thoroughly the long-term tolerability of medicaments, whether they are small or large molecules, for specific indications, in more narrowly defined cohorts of patients. It is rare that a drug has only one use, and almost every new medicine can be employed in different clinical scenarios, in different patient populations, be studied using different clinical outcomes, and be compared to other drugs of the same or other classes in already approved indications. Such studies are usually the focus of clinical research departments that are organized under the rubric of *Medical Affairs*, to distinguish them from *Clinical Development* departments, which are focused on the submission of the New Drug Application (NDA).

Medical Affairs divisions are usually fully capable research organizations, housed within large phar-maceutical companies, which consist of medical, clinical, and managerial staff (usually healthcare-oriented clinical staff including physicians, pharmacists, public health experts, and statisticians). In addition, they contain very extensive support staff that facilitate the implementation of clinical trials, which includes clinical research associates (in-house or field-based personnel who are the direct contacts for investigational site interactions and communications), scientific liaisons, data analysis, medical writing, regulatory, and legal personnel. The goal of such organizations is to allow pharmaceutical companies most effectively to conduct clinical trials or statistical analyses and prepare and submit data and claims to regulatory authorities. In some companies, safety monitoring for marketed drugs is housed in these divisions, in others, pharmacovigilance is a separate function reporting to the Chief Medical Officer. Additional roles of such organizations include the dissemination of information via meetings and symposia, and peer reviewed journals of high scientific value, enhancing understanding and potential public health impact of marketed medicines.

Medical Affairs departments are frequently capable of conducting various types of clinical research. The type of research culminating in the further categorization of the efficacy and safety of a new medicine can take the route of conventional Phase III clinical development, sometimes conducted by a Medical Affairs division, whereby a new indication is sought. In the US, these studies, commonly categorized as Phase IIIb if conducted after dossier submission and prior to full marketing approval, lead to a supplementary new drug application (sNDA), extending the data package and

Principles and Practice of Pharmaceutical Medicine, 3rd edition.
Edited by L.D. Edwards, A.W. Fox, P.D. Stonier.

indications of the original drug approval. Another goal of the research supported by these groups is to perform necessary clinical trials and seek approval to promote features of benefit–risk that are supported by clinical data, that may lead to change in registered label use.

Other approaches include the design and execution of clinically important trials whose results are disseminated principally via their scientific publication to more or less targeted, broader clinical audiences. These approaches have in common the necessary requirements to adhere to principles of good clinical practice (GCP) and clinical trial ethics. Clinical trials performed for any reason, in any phase, need to comply with the principles outlined by the Belmont Report, the Declaration of Helsinki, and the International Council for Harmonization (ICH) guidelines, and thus need to be hypothesis-driven studies that appropriately take into consideration the risk and benefit of clinical trial participation, and ensure adequate statistical power to maximize the likelihood of obtaining a result that is scientifically rigorous and interpretable.

Other objectives of later phase clinical research include addressing health authority commitments after the drug has been approved (Phase IV commitments), which can focus either on safety or efficacy questions that were not fully addressed in the registration package. This can take the form of additional clinical trials focused on endpoints different from those addressed in the NDA, or in the form of patient registries to address the possibility of rare adverse events that require a large population-level exposure to assess. Clinical trials of this sort, in the Phase IV environment, are pursued to provide further information to health authorities and clinicians as to the long-term safety and efficacy of drugs that otherwise have been demonstrated in earlier clinical research phases in trials of generally shorter duration. An additional purpose of studies in the Phase IV environment may be to provide data showing efficacy and safety in pediatric populations, if this had not been the focus of the original registration of the drug. The overall process, thereby, may accelerate the availability of valuable new medicines, while at the same time fostering design and execution of addi-

tional research to further categorize the drug via the conduct of these later stage clinical trials or monitored-use programs.

Additional research efforts conducted by many Medical Affairs divisions of pharmaceutical companies include the study of Health Economics and Clinical Outcomes Research, to provide information on the effect of drugs in the setting of healthcare delivery systems, such as patient-reported outcomes information, or data that address quality of life. This information is often considered critical for healthcare reimbursement groups, whether in the private sector (as is common in the US), or in the government (more typical of organization such as NICE in the UK), allowing such groups to assess their impact on distribution of healthcare funds, to maximize the ability to provide the highest level of healthcare within the limitations of available resources. Because of the importance in securing formulary inclusion and reimbursement, the activities of health outcomes and pharmacoeconomics groups in some cases have been folded into earlier stage research groups, exemplified by clinical development, which permits earlier incorporation of critical measures of patient-reported outcomes in the clinical development plans conducted to support initial drug approval. Finally, useful summaries of efficacy and safety often result from data mining of pooled databases, conducted by clinical and statistical personnel in Medical Affairs divisions, often in collaboration with internal and external scientific advisors, to provide further information, based on progressively larger databases, concerning the safety and efficacy of marketed drugs.

Phase III and Phase IIIb studies

Clinical trials falling under the rubric of Phase IIIb are those that are performed with the rigor of the Phase III registration program, but for a different purpose. Most commonly, such studies, designed while the Phase III program is nearing completion and often initiated prior to NDA submission and conducted during agency review, are performed for the purpose of new data dissemination during or just after launch of the new drug. The type of study that is often performed is a randomized double-blind comparator study to assess the safety or efficacy of a drug, compared to another of its, or another, class that is indicated for a specific medical condition. Hence, these trials usually employ outcome measures that were used in the Phase III program, and often also employ additional endpoints, which due to the evolution of science, or that of the medical practice, at regional or international levels, may be useful to assess its efficacy and/or clinical effectiveness. Many other types of designs can be employed including, but not limited to, single-blind studies, open-label trials, crossover studies, and other types of clinical trials that aim to provide additional efficacy or safety information that would assist clinicians in assessing the value of the new drug in their medical practice. Importantly, this is not the same as increasing potential market uptake of pharmaceuticals through "experience" or "seeding" trials that are not scientifically driven, have no hypothesis, and do not provide important new information, but rather represent hypothesis-driven clinical trials with clear scientific rationale that are pre-specified and adequately powered for, and documented in, study protocols.

In the past, the form of planned data dissemination often determined the type of trial conducted. Such choices could have included methods of communication from simple data sharing at invited scientific symposia, to disclosure of research via publication in peer-reviewed scientific journals. As a response to the increasing scrutiny of medical research at all levels, the approach currently is much more robust and defined, driven by industry- and health authority-initiated efforts to make access to clinical trial results more transparent. As this is now mandated by Federal laws, and has been guided by trade (PRMA), regulatory, journal-based, and academic groups interested in effective communication of randomized clinical trials and clarity about the roles of all authors on manuscripts (i.e., Consolidated Standards of Reporting Trials (CONSORT) statement and International Committee of Medical Journal Editors (ICMJE) guidelines), the approach can vary slightly from company to company, but takes the form

of both online communication via the clinicaltrials.gov website as well as disclosure by publication in abstract form with presentation at national scientific meetings. The attention to real or perceived conflict of interest and disclosure of study funding, remuneration for participation in scientific advisory committees, ownership of equity, and so on, is now appropriately required of industry, as well as of academic authors.

Because the publication of a paper describing the results of a clinical trial is not guaranteed by journals, which accept papers for publication based on interest to the readership as well as their scientific value, the full communication of trial results in the form of a peer-reviewed manuscript may be delayed for some time after receipt of the final statistical report. Moreover, once data are available, the focus is commonly on preparation of abstracts for scientific meetings, which need to be submitted often one year or more prior to their ultimate presentation, and on the preparation of a detailed clinical study report (not uncommonly several hundred pages in length), containing all data from the trial, which are incorporated into the dossier submitted to regulatory agencies. Thus, communication in the form of abstracts and online publications, as well as the full disclosure of clinical trial results to regulatory agencies, has acquired increasing importance in the process of data communication. In addition the use of public websites to provide access to additional trial information, implemented nearly a decade ago, has become common practice for most large companies, which stipulate strict timelines for updating of these databases.

In addition to such forms of publication, it should be noted that health authorities in the US and other regions are also informed as to the design and goals of all clinical trials. Trials are usually approved at the level of company-based protocol review committees, which often include independent, outside experts, before internal approval and submission to regulatory authorities for comment, or revision, prior to the study initiation. Finally, during investigator meetings, protocols undergo another level of scrutiny in the setting of the full complement of trial investigators, which can result in amendments that need to be approved in final form by regulatory authorities prior to study start or continuation. If health authorities do not approve of changes, studies can be placed on "clinical hold" subject to resolution of issues and final approval. These are designed to protect study subjects, ensure appropriateness of study design, and allow the necessary time for health authorities to suggest final modification of clinical studies, if needed, based on study-specific scientific goals.

Communication of safety information from clinical trials beyond Phase III by clinical development or medical affairs groups, or by independent investigators, under individual- or university-sponsored Investigational New Drugs (INDs), are incorporated into Annual NDA Safety Updates, which are also submitted to health authorities for the purposes of ongoing safety monitoring of newly marketed drugs.

Another purpose of conducting clinical trials in Phase IIIb is to provide practicing physicians with information concerning efficacy or safety of drugs soon to be on the market relative to other drug comparators, some of which are available for comparison later in a drug development. Trials of this sort, if performed with pre-specified aims, outlined in a clinical study protocol, conducted via GCP standards, and meeting pre-specified study hypotheses relevant to the disease state being treated, can be submitted to a division of the FDA that has responsibility for drug promotion—the Division of Drug Marketing, Advertising and Communications (DDMAC)—often in consultation with clinical divisions of CDER/FDA. The DDMAC also regulates direct-to-consumer advertising of biopharmaceuticals and the clinical trial data related to those products via promotional materials.

One procedure for obtaining additional regulatory approval for the dissemination of promotional material that can be presented by sales associates directly to physicians is for these types of clinical trial results to be submitted to DDMAC along with all proposed language, advertisements, or detail aids describing study results. Such descriptions need to demonstrate balanced presentation of the efficacy and safety in treatment of indicated medical conditions. Analogous to the registration

of drugs for marketing approval, the process can be lengthy and requires careful review of the dossier, often with input from the division originally responsible for approval of the NDA, supplemented by interactions in the form of discussions among scientific, regulatory, and commercial associates and DDMAC. The final output usually takes the form of promotional materials that can be left with the physician by the sales or marketing personnel, which detail the clinical trial results. Alternatively, trial results can be incorporated into direct-to-consumer advertising efforts, as appropriate, involving television, radio, or web-based promotion. If compliance with these requirements is incomplete, FDA can also take various types of action to correct promotional efforts deemed noncompliant. This can take the form of sanctions and letters that are directed to consumers or to practicing physicians, developed in order to provide the necessary clarification and may include additional corrective action.

Phase IV studies

Clinical trials conducted by Medical Affairs divisions that are categorized as Phase IV studies are those that are conducted while the drug is already in the market. This can include safety and efficacy questions that arise on further experience with the drug, or the pursuit of clinical trials to examine the efficacy of the drug relative to newer agents entering the market. The two main types of studies that are performed are those that are pursued to respond to specific requests of health authorities that were stipulated in the initial approval of the drug (Phase IV commitments), and those studies conducted to answer medical questions that are raised while the drug is being used in the clinic. The former are studies analogous to Phase IIIb studies, which are conducted at a different time point in the product cycle, whereas the latter are usually the results of extensive discussion with health authorities aimed to answer specific questions raised by the agency itself or by members of advisory committees responsible for providing guidance to the health authority at the time of initial evaluation of drugs for approval.

Phase IV commitments can be varied in aims and scope. In order to expedite the market availability of novel drugs that can improve human health, health authorities make qualitative assessments of the value of delaying approval versus requesting more efficacy or safety information. A process that allows novel drugs to enter the market while assuring further safety and efficacy monitoring is to approve drugs with stipulations as to the types of additional studies a company will commit to performing within a stipulated time period after drug approval. These Phase IV commitments generally take the form of longer trials assessing safety, or trials that address efficacy in specific patient populations that may be at greater risk of side effects or have the potential to experience a greater degree of efficacy, but were not studied in the program designed for original registrations; the latter usually focuses on patient populations in which the drug would most likely be used. Detailed pharmacovigilance plans are often provided before, or at the time, of dossier submission in the form of Risk Evaluation and Mitigation Strategies (REMS), which are prepared under newly available FDA guidance. These plans can include a component managed by Medical Affairs divisions. If approved REMS plans are not followed by sponsors, very substantial penalties can be levied.

The design of Phase IV commitments can include the traditional approach of a randomized, double-blind, placebo-controlled study, an open label trial, or can be approached via the establishment of patient registries. In the case of comparative trials in a Phase IV environment, drugs are much more commonly compared to other approved therapies. The use of placebo arms is much less common due to the desire to allow the most "real-world" use of the drug (where placebo is not given). The vast majority of such trials are conducted randomized and blinded to study drug allocation to reduce the chance that identification of study drug biases the perceived benefits in favor of the novel medicine. There are, however, examples of Phase IV studies that are conducted as "open-label" trials, whereby both drugs can be identified by both patients and treating physicians. The advantage of such trials is that they mimic more closely real-world exposure, where knowledge of the drug taken is the norm. However, the ability to make definitive conclusions concerning relative safety and efficacy can be compromised by the potential for bias, particularly if the outcome measures chosen are patient or physician-reported. Thus the randomized, blinded trial remains the method generating the highest level of evidence. Nevertheless, an open label design can be effectively conducted in evaluating therapy using more robust outcomes that would not be affected necessarily by patient or investigator knowledge of drug allocation, typified by objective measurements such as blood chemistry results, radiographic assessments, time to objective, well-defined clinical outcomes, and so on.

Often the size of clinical trials in a Phase IV environment needs to be large, to provide sufficient power to assess outcomes between two drugs shown previously to be effective. Thus, in this setting, perhaps more than any other, patient recruitment and retention are key to the successful enrollment and ultimate interpretability of trial results. Pharmaceutical, governmental (i.e., NIH), and academic groups sponsoring such Phase IV studies often require additional staff to resource these trials adequately. Various organizations have been established to assist sponsors in the conduct of clinical trials, and can be of particular benefit to smaller companies that do not have the internal resources to conduct clinical trials on their own, or by larger companies whose resources are occupied in other on-going trials. These include Contract Research Organizations (CROs), which can design, implement, analyze, and report the results of clinical trials, and Site Management Organizations (SMOs), which assist in the recruitment and monitoring of randomized patients at individual investigator levels, or small groups of clinical research centers, which do not have the staff necessary to implement clinical trials adequately.

Phase IV studies can also take the form of patient registries to determine the effect of a new drug on very rare outcomes. Such studies can be regarded as a form of industry-sponsored prospective cohort study. Generally these registries are established to exclude the possibility of rare adverse events and hence require very large sample sizes for reliable signal detection. Registering users of new medications while on the market and following outcomes as they occur with simple questionnaires is one way such research can be conducted. Within the cohort being followed, "nested" case control studies can also be conducted to understand the association of very rare outcomes with drug exposure, adjusting for factors that could theoretically influence outcomes.

The size of Phase IV studies, particularly those focused on adverse events, means that some special form of safety monitoring is generally necessary. This often is the responsibility of external data safety monitoring boards (DSMBs) and/or internal pharmacovigilance groups (safety monitoring committees or signaling committees) that have routine and regular access, and if and when needed, can unblind treatment allocation in order to ensure protection of subjects in these trials. The potential for a large number of adverse effects is especially important to account for in structuring plans to assess medicaments that will have particularly rapid uptake, exemplified by vaccines. The potential exists for a large number of adverse events to occur prior to planned full analysis of the data, which would otherwise provide a signal as to a side effect meriting further evaluation. If trials are especially large or are enrolled very rapidly, or there is concentrated use of a novel biologic or pharmaceutical, substantial resources need to be applied to ensure most rapid acquisition and analysis of safety data. The use of electronic databases and application of state-of-the-art computational methods can help ensure that this is possible.

The creation of DSMBs has become routine in pharmaceutical and government-sponsored trials. The responsibilities of DSMBs are generally documented in a charter that stipulates the leadership and members, as well as their roles and responsibilities. The main reason to establish a DSMB is to determine whether any safety signal is sufficient to change the course of a clinical trial. Other reasons can include assuring independent perspective via the establishment of a committee not directly connected to the study to assess trial

progress in regard to outcomes such as efficacy or safety endpoints that could lead to a sample size recalculation or protocol amendments. Usually these boards are comprised of prominent clinicians and clinical trialists in the field, epidemiologists, and statisticians. There is usually also at least one "unblinded" statistician with knowledge of treatment allocation, allowing analysis of data based on the treatment allocation, in order to ensure that any adverse reactions can be reported to the DSMB, unblinded to treatment if requested and as appropriate. The DSMB is led by a Chairperson who organizes the board and establishes a schedule of meetings based on clinical trial metrics or time intervals. Decisions of the DSMB are communicated to those clinicians primarily responsible for trial conduct, and the sponsor, and generally consist of approving continuation of the trial, modifying it via amendment, or even potentially halting it.

Data mining in the Phase IV environment

Phase IV studies can also take the form of retrospective pooled analyses, which are designed to reflect the totality of clinical research experience with a new drug that is usually obtained via analysis of pooled clinical trial databases. Such "data-mining" efforts should not be considered inferior to data obtained from an individual clinical trial. In fact, such approaches, leading to the generation of meta-analyses of multiple individual clinical trials, can lead to the highest level of scientific evidence. There are substantial benefits of such an approach, as the results of a given trial, especially if the endpoint is not pre-specified to be primary because of power limitations, can be a function of chance. To ensure that the results obtained from pooled analyses are not biased, a pre-specified data analysis plan is often formulated as the first step, outlining the clear goals of the proposed analysis as well as its methodology. Key to this type of analysis is the definition of the outcome measure. Both efficacy and safety measures can be the focus of these types of analyses. Pooled analyses are commonly used to assess the safety of drugs that have been already evaluated on an individual subject level by adjudication committees. Such committees are usually comprised of a combination of clinicians, epidemiologists, and statisticians, who meet to discuss the specifics of pre-specified, suspected adverse events, in order to provide the greatest precision in diagnosis. Typically if an adjudication committee is established to evaluate safety outcomes, detailed information concerning the adverse event of interest is requested of the clinical investigator shortly after the event occurs to ensure that the necessary, most accurate, and complete clinical information is available for each event, which allows the committee to assess and categorize adverse events.

Thus pooled analyses of data that are adjudicated across a large clinical program can provide the most robust assessment of drug safety and efficacy. The strength of the approach lies in increasing the sample size available for the analysis, which increases substantially the ability to make more definitive statistical inferences. Because the sample size and, hence, power of the analysis is substantially greater, this approach can replace large clinical trials that would be very costly and time consuming. If the analysis is performed according to rigorous statistical methodology, the results can sometimes serve as a substitute for specific Phase IV commitments. For more information, see Chapter 44 on data mining.

Practitioner and investigator interaction

Medical information and communications unit

Another major function of the Medical Affairs department is that of providing information about a company's products. Their customers range from fellow healthcare professionals to the public and internal company clients. The frontline is usually comprised of nurses and registered pharmacists who respond to telephone and written requests for medical information about products, spanning clinical safety and efficacy questions. Companies commonly offer this service as needed and most

can respond to clinical questions within 24 hours of a request with specific and detailed information. A frequently-asked-questions document is prepared to enhance rapidity of response. If this document does not provide the needed information, further research by Medical Information specialists, often in collaboration with internal clinical staff, is pursued to yield the necessary response.

Callers are frequently retail pharmacists and physicians who ask about potential drug–drug interactions. In addition, Medical Information Units, housed in Medical Affairs departments, often receive unsolicited requests for information on "off-label" use, which may have been described in a medical journal or at a medical meeting. Medical Information staff often provide articles that describe results from clinical trials, or information from studies to response to such queries. Procedure requires that there be no confusion as to the indicated use of a product and that "off-label" use implied by any materials provided in this setting, be clearly marked so as not to misrepresent the intended use of the medicament.

Medical writing unit

The Medical Information department may have its own medical writers dedicated to Phase IV (post-approval) publications, booklets, and pamphlets. Many large companies have a specific Medical Writing department usually reporting into the research department, which assists in writing clinical reports and publications in conjunction with the Investigator authors, and helps prepare the clinical investigational brochure or NDA annual safety reports. These associates usually have science degrees and have been trained in technical and medical writing.

Drug safety unit

In many companies, depending on the mission and functions supported by it, this unit reports to the Chief Medical Officer as a stand-alone department, or is housed in Clinical Development, or placed in Medical Affairs. This unit is responsible for tracking the safety record of drugs, in many smaller companies both those in development as well as those that are already on the market. Since the largest use of a new drug or device is usually after it is marketed, the Medical Affairs department often has primary responsibility for overseeing this function. Rare serious adverse events occurring at the incidence of one in 10,000 patients will not be found in the average NDA database of 2000–3000 patients. In this instance 30,000 patients would be required for a 95 % confidence level of one event being reported. This is known as the rule of 3. A clear "signal" may not emerge until many thousands of patients have been exposed, allowing discrimination from "background" incidence of rare clinical adverse events. The mechanism of safety monitoring usually takes the form of adjudication of adverse events that occur in the setting of ongoing clinical trials by a blinded (usually external) committee and compilation of adverse events from pooled databases or by analysis of MedWatch reports provided via the Adverse Events Reporting System (AERS) of the FDA, which also continuously assesses the safety of marketed drugs. This is often supplemented by internal safety databases that are maintained by pharmaceutical companies separately from governmental databases.

Advertising, promotion, and training overview

Medical Affairs is a critical component for the review of promotional materials. The review of this type of material, whether detail pieces provided in person to physicians in practice, slide sets for speakers on behalf of the company, or general promotional material disseminated via print, radio, TV, or web, is performed by company committees comprised of Medical Affairs staff, regulatory and legal personnel.

In addition to the company review, this material must be sent to the FDA for review. These materials should be available for FDA review at least by day of first use. Review by the FDA's DDMAC should be sought for TV advertisements. In addition, any Field Sales instructions, Public Relations, Financial Analysts Statements, and Press Releases should be reviewed for appropriateness and approved or modified by the Medical Affairs Department. Such review will also be coordinated with review by both the Legal and Regulatory Affairs departments. Moreover, materials for medical liaison activities, communications to third party insurers, and responses to other inquires, are reviewed and typically need medical approval prior to release. Specific to launch materials, it is recommended that these be submitted to the Advertising and Promotional Branches (APLB), which recommend a 120 day review prior to intended use. This approval therefore is usually submitted during the pre-approval period. All of these materials, whether submitted to DDMAC or APLB, must disclose appropriate language that makes clear the approved indications and balances efficacy claims with full transparency regarding safety. Thus the review of materials for potential use in promotion is an extremely important function of the Medical Affairs department.

Medical science liaison (MSL) function

MSLs were introduced by the Upjohn Company in the 1970s, initially as a scientific communication tool to academia. The function has subsequently been refined and now incorporates the dual functions of scientific communication to key opinion leaders (KOLs) and interaction with the same, facilitating more direct and consequential interaction of the scientific community with pharmaceutical companies. KOLs can be recognized on an international, national, regional, or district basis and their involvement in increasingly earlier stages of development enhances the relevance and focuses the direction of pharmaceutical research.

MSLs are scientists with MD, PhD, or PharmD qualifications. They may be specialists in an area of research, and thus are often experts in their own fields. Because they are usually Medical Affairs employees, they do not report to Sales and their job metrics are not determined by commercial success. The separation of Marketing and Sales departments and their budget from MSL activities, housed in Medical Affairs departments, first outlined in 2002 by the Pharmaceutical Research and Manufacturers Association (PhRMA) and shortly after by the Health and Human Services Office of the Inspector

General in 2002, is now the standard that has been implemented by most companies, due to this guidance.

Continuing medical education (CME) activities

CME and associated credit requirements have to be earned by health practitioners in many countries with modern medical systems to ensure that physician knowledge and practice are up to date. The providers of this education may be universities, professional associations, or not-for-profit firms or departments that are separate from sales organizations within pharmaceutical companies. Pharmaceutical manufacturers may provide funding for these events, but may not be involved in other aspects of the programs. In the US, the courses must comply with the relevant accrediting bodies, and are subject to scrutiny and monitoring.

Pharmaceutical companies are often requested to support these programs financially. These monies must not be disbursed by the company to a given individual, but to the organization responsible for the CME program (though this is often administered by a third party, independent of either provider or sponsor). In order to maximize independence, often the budgets have been taken out of Marketing and Sales and placed in the Medical Affairs department, with an oversight committee that ensures appropriateness of the grants. Speakers at meetings are required to disclose any real or potential conflicts of interest, including financial relationships with commercial entities, required for full transparency.

Access to ongoing clinical trial information

Increasing scrutiny of clinical trial data emanating from the industry, academic, and government sectors has led to an important evolution in access to information concerning ongoing clinical trial data and knowledge of the status of publication of completed clinical trials. Dialog among the three major entities involved in these types of studies has led to new processes that have been established by pharmaceutical companies to ensure increased transparency of clinical trial conduct and communication of results. This has taken the form of three related methods of communication of trial metrics.

A website was established by FDA (and managed by NIH), whose informational and timing provisions were outlined in Section 113 of the Food and Drug Administration Modernization Act (FDAMA). It provides continuously updated information concerning the existence and purpose of Federally and privately supported clinical trials, such as those conducted at pharmaceutical companies (www.clinicaltrials.gov). The trials listed are those that are ongoing or had been completed since January 2004. Information available includes the name and purpose of the study, brief entry or exclusion criteria indicating who may participate, and participating investigative sites including contact information and status of enrollment.

A second source of information regarding clinical trials was established with a different goal by PhRMA. In 2004, PhRMA launched a Clinical Results Database (www.ClinicalStudyResults.org) to provide a central repository for clinical trial results, positive or negative, of "hypothesis testing" clinical trials involving marketed drugs. The goal of this industry-initiated effort was to have substantial information available via electronic database concerning all studies completed after October 1, 2002. As full publication clinical study results may be delayed by the complicated process of manuscript acceptance by journal editorial boards, the purpose of this repository database was to enhance the transparency of clinical trial results and expedite their communication. As of July 1, 2005, all new studies meeting the criteria established by PhRMA had to be listed, and by September 13, 2005, all ongoing clinical trials as well.

PhRMA subsequently updated its guidance to increase transparency of clinical research via the publication of revised PhRMA Principles. These were issued in April of 2009 to take effect by October 1, 2009. The new principles addressed clinical trial design, selection and training of investigators, institutional review board approval and informed consent, clinical trial and safety monitoring, privacy, confidentiality, and quality assurance, as well as the conduct of trials in the developing world. To ensure objectivity of research, PhRMA outlined principles and objectives related to independent review and safety monitoring via DSMBs, payment schedules for patients and investigators participating in sponsored research, and disclosure of conflicts of interest. Further guidance was also provided concerning clinical trial registration, authorship on study result dissemination (to follow the International Committee of Medical Journal Editors and the major journal guidelines for authorship) as well as the role of contributors and their acknowledgement in a publication, full disclosure to investigators of all summary trial information (in the form of a final statistical report, slide presentation or clinical study report), research participant communication of study results, sponsor review prior to journal submission, and the provision of the study protocol, if requested, by the journal considering submission of a manuscript communicating study results (http://www.phrma.org/news_room/press_releases/revised_clinical_trial_principles_reinforce_phrma).

A final source of information for the public concerning the status of clinical trials was established by individual pharmaceutical companies to allow prospective patients' access to knowledge concerning the availability of clinical trials. The exact web addresses can be obtained by searching company-specific web pages. Such websites fill a third need: to help an individual patient make an educated decision about participating in a clinical trial. Usually these websites include a listing by disease and study number of ongoing clinical trials, a brief description of the precise disease category being studied, the purpose of the trial, the key entry and exclusion criteria, and the treatment arms and duration. In addition links are provided to study specific websites, and supplemental information about the disease being studied, its manifestations, and how it is diagnosed are included. Questionnaires are also often available, which can be completed by patients to identify eligible patients and provide information concerning the nearest location of a clinical trial site.

Summary

Medical Affairs departments have multiple functions, spanning comparative Phase III and later clinical trials, monitoring of post-marketing safety, and headquarters, as well as field-based informational support of product-related queries. The design and conduct of creative clinical trials is central to providing important later phase data about soon-to-be-marketed or already marketed drugs with respect to efficacy when compared to other products targeting similar disease states and related indications, as well as to supplying additional information that supplements the core dataset leading to original drug approval. This additional information, often obtained in a more real-world setting, can have extremely high public health value and can inform further clinical development in later phases of the product's life cycle. Finally, the ability to pool data sets, conduct specific outcomes research, and progressively assess benefit–risk and pharmacoeconomics in an evolving healthcare environment, is critical for formulary and access decisions, and calculating the ultimate public health value of pharmaceuticals, making these departments indispensable to pharmaceutical companies and clinicians who depend on an ongoing stream of clinical data.

The content contained herein reflects the experience and personal opinion of the author only, and does not necessarily reflect the position or view of MedImmune.

Further reading

Anderson DL. *A Guide to Patient Recruitment and Retention.* Thompson Centerwatch: Boston, MA, USA, 2004.

Food and Drug Administration. *Code of Federal Regulations (21 CFR), Parts 11, 50, 54, 56, 312, 314,* first edition, 2001; http://www.accessdata.fda.gov/scripts/cdrh/cfdocs/cfcfr//CFRsearch.cfm; accessed April 11, 2010.

Friedman LM, Furberg CD, DeMets DL. *Fundamentals of Clinical Trials,* third edition. Springer-Verlag: New York, USA, 1998.

Hulley SB, Cummings SR, Browner WS, Grady D, Hearst N, Newman TB. *Designing Clinical Research: An Epidemiologic Approach,* second edition. Lippincott Williams & Wilkins: New York, USA, 2001.

International Conference on Harmonization (ICH). *ICH Harmonized Tripartite Guideline for Good Clinical Practice*, second edition, 1997. http://www.ich.org/LOB/media/MEDIA482.pdf; accessed April 11, 2010.

Meinert CL, Tonascia S. *Clinical Trials. Design, Conduct and Analysis, Vol* 8. Oxford University Press: New York, USA, 1986.

Munro Hazard B. *Statistical Methods for Health Care Research*, fifth edition. Lippincott Williams & Wilkins: Boston, MA, USA, 2005.

Piantadosi S. *Clinical Trials: a Methodologic Perspective*, second edition. John Wiley & Sons Inc: New York, USA, 2005.

Spriet A, Dupin-Spriet T. *Good Practice of Clinical Drug Trials*, third edition. Karger: Basel, Switzerland, 2004.

Stephenson H. *Strategic Research, a Practical Handbook for Phase IIIB and Phase IV Clinical Studies*. Quintiles Transnational Corporation: Research Triangle Park, NC, USA, 2005.

Useful websites

http://www.fda.gov/downloads/Drugs/Guidance-ComplianceRegulatoryInformation/Guidances/UCM184128 .pdf; accessed April 11, 2010.

http://www.fda.gov/BiologicsBloodVaccines/DevelopmentApprovalProcess/AdvertisingLabelingPromotionalMaterials/ucm118171.htm; accessed April 11, 2010.

www.oig.hhs.gov/; accessed April 11, 2010.

CHAPTER 43

Drug Labeling

Anthony W. Fox

EBD Group Inc., Carlsbad, CA, USA and Munich, Germany, and Skaggs SPPS, University of California, San Diego, USA

Introduction

The purpose of the drug label is stated succinctly in the Japanese guidelines:

> Package insert statements should generally contain information essential to using the specified drug for approved indications and within the range of approved dosage and (route of) administration. However, other important data regarding any use of the drug should also be evaluated and described.
>
> (PAB Notification, 1997)

In other words, the drug label is the summary of all that is learned during drug development plus that which is inevitably discovered during post-marketing surveillance. The terms "drug label" and "package insert" (the former in common use in North America, the latter in Europe and Japan) are used interchangeably in this chapter. The "Summary of Product Characteristics" (SpC; 2009) is the European equivalent.

The intent of this chapter is to review drug labels in North America, Europe, and Japan. The philosophy of these differing types of labeling will be explored. The reader can easily access local examples of current, approved labeling (*Compendia* in the United Kingdom, *Rote Liste* in Germany, *Physicians' Desk Reference* in the USA, etc.). These will not be reproduced here because they could become rapidly out of date. Much of the content of drug labeling is the subject of other chapters in this book, and so the approach here will avoid redundancy.

Principles and Practice of Pharmaceutical Medicine, 3rd edition.
Edited by L.D. Edwards, A.W. Fox, P.D. Stonier.
© 2011 Blackwell Publishing Ltd.

Drug labeling in Japan

(with acknowledgment to Dr. Hiroko Sakai, Yamanouchi Pharmaceuticals, Tokyo, Japan)

The Ministry of Health and Welfare has a subordinate organization known as the Pharmaceutical and Medical Safety Bureau, which supervises drug labeling in Japan. This bureau has prescribed a standard set of subtitles for drug labeling, which must always appear (see Table 43.1).

As Table 43.1 shows, the structure of a Japanese drug label is a standard format whose content, if not typographical arrangement, would be familiar to physicians in Europe or North America.

The one major difference, however, is that a separate regulation (PAB Notification no.607, April 25, 1997) governs how precautions should be displayed in drug labels, and this is quite elaborate in comparison to European or North American counterparts. The Warnings and Contraindications sections of the drug label (items 6 and 7 in Table 43.1), are required to contain, under this regulation, the subsections shown in Table 43.2).

Although most of the subtopics shown in Table 43.2 would have stand-alone counterparts in drug labeling elsewhere in the world, this regulation emphasizes drug tolerability, consistent with the approach taken with much of regulatory affairs in Japan (albeit a chronologically increasing emphasis in the rest of the ICH regions since about 2007). The visual presentation of the precautions subsections goes further to make this point: In Japan, Warnings are printed in red within a red box, while contraindications are printed in black, again within a red box. Finally, contraindications

Table 43.1 Subtitles that must appear in Japanese drug labeling, and the order in which they appear (after Article 52, Item 1 of the Pharmaceutical Affairs Law).

1. Date of preparation or revision of label	11. Precautions
2. Japanese Standard Commodity Number	12. Pharmacokinetics
3. Therapeutic category (e.g., bronchodilator)	13. Clinical studies
4. Regulatory Classification (e.g., "Designated Drug")	14. Pharmacology
5. Brand name	15. Physicochemistry
6. Warning(s)	16. Precautions for handling
7. Contraindications	17. Conditions for approval
8. Composition and description	18. Packaging
9. Indications	19. References and how to order
10. Dosage and administration	20. Identity of manufacturer, etc.

for coadministered drugs must be printed as a table within a red box.

Japanese labeling regulations require that animal data and data from other members of the same chemical or pharmacological class of drugs should be included, even when these allude to adverse effects that have not actually been observed for the product that is labeled. So-called class labeling is following this lead within the US Food and Drug Administration (FDA). When direct drug attributability of an adverse event has not been established, it remains a requirement that other indirectly obtained information must still be included; this would include epidemiological information or pharmacodynamic effects observed in normal volunteer studies. Adverse event frequencies may be presented in a table, usually containing all adverse event types reported with frequencies >5%, between 0.1–5 %, and <0.1 %.

Drug labeling in the United States

The US FDA is, among other things, probably the most stringent controller of drug labeling of all the world's regulatory authorities; the world's longest package inserts are the result. Typically, drug labels are agreed with pharmaceutical companies at meetings shortly before product approval, where the proposed label is debated line by line. Such meetings often include not only the reviewing Division Director, but also his or her superior, the Center Director. The relevant parts of the Code of Federal Regulations (CFR) are authorized by the Food, Drugs and Cosmetics (FD&C) Act (21 United States Code 321). Although the licensing of drug products (21CFR310 & 314) and biologicals (21CFR601) are different, their labels are governed in a similar manner. It should be noted that promotional materials are considered to be a form of labeling in the United States, and the

Table 43.2 Subsections of "precautions" in Japanese drug labeling.

1. Warnings	6. (i) Clinically significant adverse events
2. Contraindications (do not administer to the following types of patients)	(ii) Other adverse events
	7. Use in the elderly
3. Careful administration (Administer with care to the following patients)	8. Use in pregnancy, delivery, and lactation
4. Important precautions	9. Pediatric use
5. Drug interactions:	10. Effects on clinical laboratory tests
(i) Contraindicated coadministrations	11. Overdosage
(ii) Precautions for coadministration	12. Precautions concerning use
	13. Other precautions

FDA regulates these as stringently as the package insert (21CFR201.1). All magazine advertisements and so on have to be accompanied by a complete copy of the approved package insert adjacent to the published promotional materials. A recent label for an injectable treatment for rheumatoid arthritis (etanercept; Enbrel®; Amgen and Wyeth) can only be described as a poster, being 58 by 63 cm, and filled with print on the whole of both sides in mostly 10- and 11-point font!

The general principles that apply to all US drug labeling (whether a package insert or an advertisement) are as follows:
- consistency with approved package insert;
- absence of misleading information;
- fair balance;
- absence of relevant omissions;
- defensibility from the clinical trials database.

A specific division of FDA (the Division of Drug Marketing, Advertising, and Communications; DDMAC) reviews all promotional materials prior to product launch and must be provided with all subsequent advertising. Companies can (and frequently are) ordered to recall promotional materials, as well as being required to take corrective measures after promulgating advertising that the FDA views as misleading.

The FDA uses black boxes around the text in labeling to indicate major hazards associated with marketed products. Most drugs that are "black-boxed" in the US usually remain on the market pending the sponsor's compliance not to engage in any further promotion of the product. However, this does not apply to certain opioids, muscle relaxants, and cytotoxic drugs, all of which are black-boxed, when these are promoted to specialist physicians (in these cases, anesthesiologists/anesthetists, and oncologists, respectively).

The format of US package inserts has recently been revised (21CFR 201.56–201.57 and subparts). Probably as a response to voluminous package inserts that are unlikely to be read, the modern product label now contains an initial "highlights" section. It is then followed by a full length package insert as before. Patient information leaflets are then reproduced after that. These regulations became permanent in the spring of 2008, having had a staged roll-out since 2006 (FDA, 2006). The same rule change was applied to biologics at the same time (FDA, 2006).

The components of US package inserts are provided in 21CFR201–202. Related matters (e.g., imprinting of tablets, labeling of controlled drugs, use of official and trade names, etc.) are governed by regulations scattered between 21CFR206–299. Spanish translations of drug labels are permitted (especially for products sold in California, Florida, New York, and Puerto Rico), and some mandatory, equivalent Spanish vocabulary appears in the regulations (e.g., 21CFR201.16). Most European physicians comment on the greater technical detail and length of US labels, in comparison to those in Europe, and the improbability of prescribers studying them.

Labeling of non-prescription drugs brings an additional complexity. Here the target audience is not a "learned intermediary" (e.g., pharmacist or physician) but a member of the public of supposed ordinary understanding; "the man on the Clapham omnibus" is the somewhat-dated British term for this. An average reading age of 14 years is one American standard for the same thing (for which 52% of California high school students met this definition, by the age of 18 years, in the summer of 2009). In any case, a Draft Guidance on the care that must be taken in label language for non-prescription drugs in the US was issued in the Spring of 2009 (FDA, 2009).

Drugs that are extemporaneously compounded from legally-obtained starting materials, by pharmacists according to a physician's (frankly) idiosyncratic prescription, are not subject to the same regulations (see 21CFR216). Among other things, these regulations nonetheless contain a list of drugs that are prohibited from compounding, usually in response to corresponding product withdrawals under the orthodox regulations (e.g., dexfenfluramine, chlorhexidine, tetracycline, for any, topical, and pediatric uses, respectively). This relatively anachronistic part of pharmacy practice is also prohibited from engaging in widespread promotion.

A central legal term in the United States is "misbranding" of an approved drug, meaning that the provisions of the New Drug Application (NDA) (as it might have been amended) have been breached. Such breaches may include: (i) when the FDA has determined that the drug is being promoted for indications, dose sizes, or routes of administration that are outside the approved labeling; (ii) unapproved ingredients have been used in the manufacture; (iii) approved ingredients have failed some quality control that is specified in the NDA; or (iv) the sponsor has violated some previous agreement with the FDA about how the drug product should be marketed. Almost any infraction perceived by the FDA will be termed misbranding. Comparative statements ("Drug X was better than Drug Y") and active comparator clinical trials data in a proposed package insert, are especially likely to meet with disapproval by the FDA.

FDA enforcement actions may be listed in escalating order of severity:

1. Warning letter from the FDA to the manufacturer, requiring a specified corrective action within a reasonable time frame.

2. Mandatory issuance of a "Dear Doctor" letter to the medical profession.

3. Black boxing of drug product (usually with agreement not to promote).

4. Product recall (although, in practice, most of these are voluntary on the part of the sponsor).

5. NDA withdrawal.

6. Product seizure and establishment closure.

The FDA can take these actions independently. For example, although a product seizure can be appealed against in Federal Court, the product remains seized from the outset, and sales remain halted while the legal process takes place, usually over at least several months. This prolonged period *per se* is often sufficient to kill the product in the market place, even if agreement for its reintroduction is eventually reached. The more serious enforcement actions are also punishable with prison terms and fines under the FD&C Act. A large, de-centralized inspectorate is distributed throughout the US and around the world as part of the FDA's enforcement arm.

Typically, the FDA requires that post-marketing surveillance of new drugs is reported at less than annual intervals. Usually, after three- or four-years market experience, annual reports can then be agreed. A review of the labeling is made on each of these occasions, which, for non-urgent matters, is when a sponsor or the FDA might suggest amendments to it. All advertising materials that have been used during the year must be filed with these annual reports, even though they were sent to DDMAC at the time of their introduction. Risk Management Action Plans (RiskMAPS) may have to be re-filed on all of these occasions.

It is surprising that these strict regulations and their energetic enforcement apply only to approved drugs. The US currently has a vigorous market in so-called "natural products." Thus, oral proteoglycans "to repair joint cartilage," *Gingko biloba* extracts "to improve memory," or the "anti-aging effect" of oral, powdered shark cartilage, may yet be advertised to the general public with impunity, and purchased by the general public without prescription. Legally, this creates a paradox because manufacturers want people to believe that these drugs are effective, and yet therapeutic effectiveness is tantamount to one criterion for bringing drugs within the jurisdiction of the FD&C Act. However, at present, there is strong political support against extending FDA jurisdiction over such products.

European labeling

There is reasonable similarity across the countries of the European Union, and these labels are collated into national compendia such as the *Rotte Liste* in Germany or the *Data Sheet Compendium* in the United Kingdom, to which the reader is referred. Consistency between countries is likely to increase now that drug licensing has been centralized at the European Medicines Agency (EMEA). Many of the headings within European labeling correspond to those shown for Japan (see the earlier Table 43.1), and the United States.

American or Japanese physicians are frequently surprised at European drug labels. Their brevity, and the relative scarcity of quantitative data, reflects a very different philosophy. Such labels arise from a regulatory milieu which itself has a different philosophy, expecting product manufacturers to assume responsibilities that would be accepted by the regulatory authorities in the US and Japan; this in spite of a stronger clinical pharmacology tradition in Europe and Japan than in the US. There is no European equivalent of the worldwide enforcement arm of the FDA.

There can be no doubt that the principles that underlie European labeling are the same as those enumerated in other jurisdictions. Consistency of promotional material (and especially the SpC) with the approved package insert, the absence of misleading information in package inserts, fair balance, absence of relevant omissions, and defensibility of all statements from the clinical trials database are also characteristic of good European labeling.

However, there is a sentiment widely expressed in Europe that the long and technical labels promulgated by FDA are unlikely to be read (nor understood) by the ordinary generalist prescriber. Thus, European labeling aims for concise and well-balanced summary information. For this reason, European labels are usually more difficult to write than, say, American labels, and are much more likely to be debated among the physicians in a company's medical affairs department, and between the company and the regulatory authority on subjective, interpretative grounds.

These fundamental differences between European and American drug labels also lead to unexpected, tangential difficulties, especially for international corporations. Corporate lawyers in the US live in a more litigious environment than their European or Japanese colleagues. Plaintiffs' litigation often makes the claim that a patient has experienced an adverse event that had not been disclosed in the package insert. Companies are sued in America for adverse events that occur in Europe, and plaintiff's counsel will often exploit the differences that exist in drug labels between different jurisdictions. Thus the company lawyers in the US would usually like two things: (i) any and all adverse event types to appear in labeling, so that the company cannot be accused of failing to disclose any relevant information; and (ii) consistency of such information in all drug labels around the world so that a picture cannot be painted suggesting to a jury that the company was willing to warn

Americans but not Europeans of a particular adverse event type. Given the typical inability to assign drug attributability to low-frequency adverse events, and the philosophy of European labeling, foreign subsidiaries often object to the inclusion of (probably irrelevant) minutiae in their labeling.

Final words

The real key to understanding drug labeling is to work with it, for real. Almost all entry-level medical affairs positions can provide this if the post-holder expresses appropriate interest. Similarly, almost all successful drug development (i.e., Phases 1–3) positions are guided by draft labeling. When writing labeling, the first thing to do is to seek out a recent model, for a drug that is already approved (indeed, such models can also serve as guides to clinical development plans at the very start of drug development). When making judgments about how to amend labeling and what may or may not be an acceptable précis when converting a US label to a European label, remember to seek the advice of those with experience, both within the medical, regulatory and legal departments.

References

EMA Guidance on Summary of Product Characteristics, Annex 1, version 7.2, 10/2006; 2009.

FDA. *Federal Register* 2006; **71**:3922–3997.

FDA. *Draft Guidance for Industry: Label Comprehension Studies for Nonprescription Drug Products*. US Dept of Health and Human Services, CDER, 2009.

PAB Notification No. 606, April 25, 1997.

Further reading

http://www.fda.gov/NewsEvents/Newsroom / PressAnnouncements/2006/ ucm108579.htm, for the revisions to US package insert format; accessed August 18, 2009.

http://www.accessdata.fda.gov/scripts/cdrh/cfdocs/cfcfr/ CFRSearch.cfm, for revisions to 21 CFR 201.56 and 201.57; accessed August 18, 2009.

CHAPTER 44

Data Mining

Mirza I. Rahman[1] & Robbert P. van Manen[2]

[1]Health Economics & Reimbursement, Evidence Based Medicine, Ortho-Clinical Diagnostics, Inc., Rochester, NY, USA
[2]Health Economics and Clinical Outcomes Research, Medical Affairs, Centocor Inc., Horsham, PA, USA

Data mining has been defined as "The nontrivial extraction of implicit, previously unknown, and potentially useful information from data" (Frawley *et al.*, 1992). However, an easier way to grasp the concept of data mining is to think of it as a process that uses automated, analytic tools to search large databases, in order to discern useful information.

Introduction

The goal of data mining in the pharmaceutical industry is to simplify the process for sorting through vast amounts of data to generate valuable and actionable information in support of a business proposition. Given the large volume of data that is collected in a variety of industries and the speed with which it is being accumulated, digging through those databases to get to the kernels of knowledge may be impossible if done manually. The development of powerful computers, along with software that contains data mining algorithms, provides the individual with an additional tool to better do their job.

Some common uses of data mining are in the marketing of specific products to customers who show a propensity for purchasing a particular product. Although it may be intuitive that customers who buy a particular product may be more apt to purchase a similar type of product if it is marketed to them, searching for hidden correlations between disparate products (e.g., soap and tea purchases) may generate new avenues to co-market or at least place products in close proximity to one another. Additionally, high-value customers can be segmented from the general customer population to allow for a more focused marketing approach to them.

Data mining has been used in several industries and in many different ways, including in banking to detect credit card fraud, by retailers in direct mail marketing campaigns, and in the sales of goods from wholesalers to retailers. In the pharmaceutical industry, data mining has been used in sales and marketing to focus on the types of customers the company wants to focus on, in reviewing sales force performance, in examining clinical and nonclinical toxicology data for potential claims to pursue, and now in the review and assessment of post-marketing safety surveillance data. This last topic will be discussed in depth, later in this chapter.

As important as it is to define what data mining is, it is equally important to state what it is not! Data mining is not a panacea for business problems. It is simply another tool to be used in seeking solutions to business problems. There will still be a need for analysts and healthcare professionals with the ability to assess the validity of the results generated by a data mining algorithm. Additionally, data mining is not data dredging, which is a pejorative term used to imply the repeated evaluation of a dataset, usually involving multiple comparisons with no prior defined method, to find some "statistically significant" event. Given the statistical problems associated with conducting multiple comparisons,

Principles and Practice of Pharmaceutical Medicine, 3rd edition.
Edited by L.D. Edwards, A.W. Fox, P.D. Stonier.

such a "statistically significant" event may merely be a random finding that only gets noted due to the multiple comparisons, or data dredging.

For post-marketing safety surveillance, a range of spontaneous adverse event (AE) reporting databases are available for analysis. Under the Freedom of Information Act, the US Food and Drug Administration (FDA) Center for Drug Evaluation and Research (CDER) publicly makes available the database contents of the Spontaneous Reporting System (SRS), which was used to collect spontaneous AE reports from 1968 to 1997, and the Adverse Event Reporting System (AERS), which has been in use since 1997. The FDA Center for Biologics Evaluation and Research (CBER) publishes the data from the Vaccine Adverse Event Reporting System (VAERS) in the same way.

Medical device adverse event information from the Manufacturer and User Facility Device Experience database (MAUDE) is made available publicly by the FDA Center for Devices and Radiological Health (CDRH). However, unlike the AERS and VAERS databases, the public version of the MAUDE database does not contain AE terms, only a flag about whether a product complaint was associated with an AE or not, making it very difficult to use this database for safety signal detection.

The database most commonly used for signal detection is the FDA AERS database; therefore the rest of this chapter will focus primarily on this database. Additionally, research using longitudinal healthcare databases as sources of safety signals is becoming more common (Curtis *et al.*, 2008).

Methods

Before any data mining algorithms or models are used on a database, it is important to first make sure that the data have been collected appropriately and that they have been organized and checked for accuracy. Subsequently, there is a choice from among multiple data mining methods that can be used. Among these are the Multi-Item Gamma Poisson Shrinker (MGPS) algorithm, which generates an Empirical Bayesian Geometric

Mean (EBGM) score, the Proportional Reporting Ratio (PRR) method, and the Bayesian Confidence Propagation Neural Network (BCPNN) approach. For large numbers of case reports the Bayesian methods (MGPS and BCPNN) will provide scores very similar to the PRR, but for smaller numbers of case reports they will "shrink" the resulting score towards the neutral value of 1.

EBGM is a statistical measure of disproportionality, comparing the observed and expected reporting frequency within a database (see Figure 44.1 for a list of EBGM terms). The determination of the expected reporting frequency assumes complete independence of cases associated with either a drug or an event. Thus, in a hypothetical database of 100 cases, if Drug Z represented 20 cases in the database and there were 10 cases of rhabdomyolysis, the expected reporting frequency would be 20/100 (probability of Drug Z) × 10/100 (probability of rhabdomyolysis) × 100 cases (total database size) = 2 expected cases. If the observed number of drug–event cases was 8, then the Relative Reporting Ratio (RR) would be $8/2$ (N/E) $= 4$ and the EBGM would be between 4 and 1, depending on the amount of "shrinkage" that occurs based on the model.

The larger the number of AE reports for a particular drug (for a drug that has been on the market for a long time may have a lot of AE reports in the database) and/or the larger the number of cases of a particular AE (a common AE), the larger the expected "E" will be. The larger that "E" is, the smaller the EBGM will be. A new drug or a very rare AE would represent lower proportions of the total database and thus the expected "E" would be lower.

The disproportionality methods described above are all based on the extraction of individual drug–event pairs from spontaneous AE reports. This approach has a number of disadvantages; for example, if two drugs are often administered together and one drug causes a specific AE, the other drug will also appear to be associated with this AE—the so-called "innocent bystander effect." On the other hand, if a certain AE is common in the background, a drug causing this AE may not generate a signal—so-called "masking" or "cloaking."

- *N* is the observed number of cases with the combination of items.
- *E* is the expected number of cases with the combination. Calculated as:

$$E = \frac{\text{Observed \# cases with DRUG}}{\text{Total \# cases}} \times \frac{\text{Observed \# cases with EVENT}}{\text{Total \# cases}} \times \text{Total \# cases}$$

RR	Relative Reporting Ratio (the same as N/E). Observed number of cases with the combination divided by the expected number of cases with the combination. This may be viewed as a sampling estimate of the true value of observed/expected for the particular combination of drug and event.
EBGM	Empirical Bayesian Geometric Mean. A more stable estimate than RR; the so-called "shrinkage" estimate.
EB05	A value such that there is less than a 5% probability that the true value of observed/expected lies below it.
EB95	A value such that there is less than a 5% probability that the true value of observed/expected lies above it.
90% CI	The interval from EB05 to EB95 may be considered to be the "90% confidence interval".

Figure 44.1 Empirical Bayesian Geometric Mean (EBGM) terms.

The occurrence of AEs may also be influenced by factors such as age, gender, and time (for example, an increase in reporting after a Dear Doctor letter had been issued by the FDA). In some cases, such effects can be addressed through stratification, the calculation of individual expected values for specific cross-sections of the population followed by summation for the whole population. A more powerful approach, called logistic regression, makes it possible to identify the specific relationship between a single medical product and a single AE, while eliminating the effect of external factors such as concomitant medication, demographics, or timing.

Safety surveillance

The safety surveillance mission is to implement the systematic review of spontaneous post-marketing data for proactive risk identification and assessment. In general, signal generation is done using clinical trials data, the medical literature, knowledge of class effects, and spontaneous reports.

There are numerous challenges with spontaneous reports databases, including the fact that they are numerator based, that they are subject to many reporting biases, that they can be hard to place in population context, that they are clearly dependent on coding practices, and given the granularity of the Medical Dictionary for Regulatory Activities (MedDRA), there can be a dilution of the signal.

Additionally, spontaneous post-marketing safety surveillance databases were developed for regulatory reporting, and as such, differences that exist with the national reporting requirements can alter the type, frequency, and number of post-marketing safety surveillance reports that get entered into a database. Also, different companies may interpret the regulations differently, resulting in differential reporting of post-marketing safety surveillance reports. Furthermore, changes take place over time with dictionary versions, with reporting standards, and with product labeling. Data migration may cause sufficient changes to take place so that data conversion and legacy data can be lost. Moreover, causality assessment is rarely consistent.

There are several factors that affect both the quality and quantity of post marketing reports. One of these is sometimes referred to as the "Weber Effect," where the newness of a drug to market results in a peak in post-marketing reports during the second year of being marketed. Additionally, if a drug is the first in its class to market, as opposed to being the second or third drug in a class to be marketed, there can be higher reporting rates of post-marketing safety surveillance reports. In addition, items such as publicity, whether it is from a regulatory action such as a Dear Doctor letter, litigation, or coverage in the media, can all result in increased post-marketing reports.

In addition, there are some countries, such as the United States, which allow for consumers to report AEs, whereas other countries only allow healthcare professionals to make such AE reports. This can result in higher numbers of reports, though the information that is received may not be completely valuable or beneficial when searching for safety signals. Consumer reports can also be increased as a result of direct-to-consumer advertising, especially when consumer hotlines are published.

There are two key approaches to safety surveillance. The first is the intra-product signaling, which seeks to identify changes in the overall AE pattern for specific products over time. This monitors selected AEs for a specific product over time to determine changes in the frequency and severity of AE reports. The second type of approach is the inter-product signaling, which compares a specific product with all products in the database.

This inter-product signaling is usually based on data mining and essentially it determines a disproportionality score to detect drug–event combinations that are distinct or stand out from the background rate. Both approaches should be used systematically to screen large data sets to identify and analyze drug–event associations. These are, however, hypothesis generating approaches and the idea is to search for new, preventable, serious AEs with potential public health importance. In addition, the surveillance program should be set up to evaluate new and emerging safety issues.

Intra-product signaling essentially looks at a company's own database to determine whether the frequency of a particular AE has been increasing, after appropriately adjusting for sales. Inter-product signaling uses computer-assisted application of statistical algorithms to measure disproportionality. It tries to identify drug combinations that occur more frequently than expected. It is

important to remember that such signal scores are measures of statistical associations and do not necessarily imply a clinical or a causal association.

There are several disproportionality analyses that can be conducted, but essentially an observed rate is compared to an expected rate. Following the calculation of an EBGM or a PRR, there is an ability to generate a case series and then to characterize that case series. As a result of the surveillance process, hypotheses are generated. These hypotheses may then need to be evaluated using additional quantitative methods as appropriate, looking at the company's database, or requiring stimulated reporting, or enhanced surveillance, or epidemiological studies to try and evaluate these hypotheses.

Thus, it is clear that the safety surveillance process is an iterative one. It looks at multiple data sources, whether screening large regulatory databases, looking at company databases, or looking at lot-related AEs for manufacturing problems. The surveillance process screens the data using both the intra-product and the inter-product methods. The object is to identify topics for further review to develop case definition, to compile a case series, and then to characterize that case series.

Data mining in safety surveillance

Data mining is used in the review of safety surveillance data to try and detect strong, consistent associations that occur at higher than expected frequencies. Data mining usually uses AE safety databases that lack denominator data. It detects frequency of drug event combinations in post-marketing reports. It also determines the relative frequency that the drug event combinations are reported for drug X than for any other drug. Data mining attempts to quantify the strength of potential drug–event association, whereby signal scores are calculated and represent the relative reporting rate for AEs.

As stated, data mining does not equal data dredging. Instead, it is a systematic screening for drug–event combinations that are being reported disproportionately. It is essentially a quantitative signal detection method. The data mining method that is currently being used widely in the US, by both the FDA and the pharmaceutical industry, is the MGPS, which adjusts disproportionality scores based on the number of case reports from which they are derived. The MGPS generates an EBGM, which is an estimate of the relative reporting ratio. It is the ratio of the observed over the expected counts. A 90% confidence interval is calculated around the EBGM covering the lower 5% and the upper 95% of the confidence interval.

Among the major challenges that data mining has had, is the belief that this is simply data dredging and that this is not a worthwhile scientific endeavor. However, data mining is a scientific, statistically valid method that encompasses a quantitative computer-assisted method of trying to determine safety signals.

Two of the FDA's post-marketing safety surveillance databases, the AERS and VAERS, are used in safety signaling and data mining, along with the World Health Organization's Vigibase adverse events database. A third, MAUDE, in its currently public form, is not useful for safety surveillance or data mining, because it lacks the adverse event terms associated with the report. However, the FDA can and does perform both safety surveillance and data mining on the MAUDE database because it has all the reported information available. The FDA's databases contain all US reports along with serious, unlabeled reports from outside the United States. The WHO database contains reports from more than 82 national authorities, including the FDA's database.

The FDA's SRS was in operation from 1968 to October 1997. The reports were transitioned to the AERS, which has been used from October 1997 to the present. A publicly-released version is made available on a quarterly basis, although there is a five to six month lag time between submitted reports and their availability. It is a passive surveillance system in which direct volunteer reporting accounts for 10% of reports from healthcare professionals and consumers. Ninety percent of reports in the FDA's post-marketing safety surveillance database come from pharmaceutical companies, because they are mandated by regulations to report AEs that they receive. The combined SRS+AERS

database currently contains approximately 3.8 million reports and is growing rapidly, at over 525,000 reports annually. The number of reports has more than doubled in the last ten years and because the FDA is interested in serious, unlabeled reports, that figure has grown as a percentage of the total number of reports submitted to the FDA.

Some of the limitations of the FDA's AERS database are that the lag time can be several months, there is under-reporting, and there can be increased reports as a result of stimulated reporting. Additionally, there can be biased reporting due to a number of factors, including publicity, regulatory letters, and so on. and because of the differential interpretation of the reporting regulations, reports may differ by country and company. Additionally, duplication, quoting errors, variable historical data, poor quality of information, and changes over time are all limitations to information recorded in the AERS database.

The data mining output is similar to the safety surveillance output in that hypotheses are generated and these may need to be evaluated with additional quantitative analyses as appropriate using the company database, stimulated reporting, or enhanced surveillance, or they may require the conduct of epidemiological studies.

Case study

Rhabdomyolysis and statins

Introduction
In this case example, the FDA's SRS+AERS database, through the end of the fourth quarter of 2008, was data mined to determine the lower 95% confidence interval limit of the Empirical Bayesian Geometric Mean scores (denoted as EB05), a measure of disproportionality, for rhabdomyolysis associated with the use of statins. The drugs of interest were: atorvastatin, cerivastatin, fluvastatin, lovastatin, pravastatin, rosuvastatin, and simvastatin.

EB05 guideline
A guideline that has been used for identifying a signal score for pair-wise combinations as

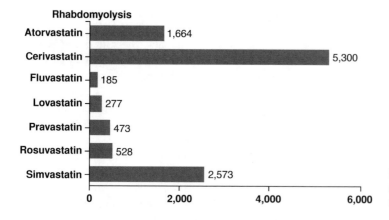

Figure 44.2 The number of cases of rhabdomyolysis in the AERS database associated with statins.

higher-than-expected is an EB05 ≥ 2. This criterion ensures with a high degree of confidence that, regardless of count size, the particular drug–event combination is being reported at least twice as often as it would be if there were no association between the drug and the event (Szarfman *et al.*, 2002).

Data source

This case study is based on cumulative data from the FDA SRS+AERS database through the end of the fourth quarter 2008.

This database contains approximately 3.8 million patient records. It includes branded and generic prescription products that are marketed in the US. The database contains both US reports (including consumer reports) and a subset of non-US reports (AEs that are both serious and unexpected, that is, not contained in the US package insert).

All data were retrieved utilizing Empirica™ Signal 7.0 from the Phase Forward Lincoln Safety Group, which is a data mining application used in post-marketing safety surveillance to support product risk management. Unless specified, individual case reports were not specifically checked for duplicate reporting. However, the vendor does implement an algorithm to screen the database for duplicates as part of standard data cleansing. Searches were conducted based on "drug mentions within a report." This means that all case reports where the selected drug is classified as either a concomitant or suspect drug are included.

Data output

Figures 44.2 to 44.5 show the frequency and EB05 scores, both total and cumulative by year, of rhabdomyolysis associated with the use of the statins. AEs in the FDA database are codified using MedDRA. It is important to note that a single case report may contain more than one preferred term.

For disproportionality scores, the color of the bar represents a measure of disproportionality, that is "how disproportionate" is the observed report frequency of the AE–drug combination compared to what might be expected, if all AE–drug combinations in the database were independent. The color scale ranges from light gray, which represents low disproportionality— that is, the observed frequency is not substantially different from the expected—to darker gray, representing AE–drug combinations with higher measures of disproportionality.

The sector map shown in Figure 44.6 represents the "safety fingerprint" of a product, highlighting areas of interest, spatially organized by system organ class. The shading in this diagram represents disproportionality scoring. Various strengths of association between a product and adverse event type(s) appear as different shades. The shades can also mark inverse relationships between a product and one or more adverse event type(s), as well as no relationship between them (i.e., mutual independence between product use and an adverse event type that has been reported).

The boxes in Figure 44.6 represent adverse events, represented by individual MedDRA

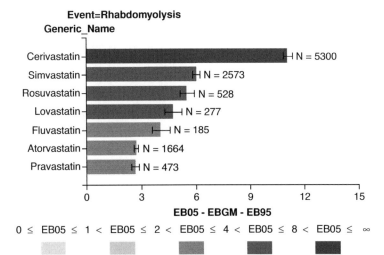

Figure 44.3 The disproportionality score (EB05) of cases of rhabdomyolysis in the AERS database associated with statins.

preferred terms, arranged according to the MeDRA hierarchy and with their relative size calculated on the basis of the public health impact of the associated adverse event, based on the combined frequency of occurrence and severity of the event.

Drug interactions can be represented as the confidence interval of the disproportionality score for each drug individually (see Figure 44.7), compared to the confidence interval for both drugs jointly. If the individual and joint confidence intervals do not overlap, this can be interpreted as a signal for a drug interaction.

Interpretation

Figures 44.2 to 44.5 show the frequency and EB05 scores, both total and cumulative by year, of rhabdomyolysis associated with the use of the statins. Although all the statins have an EB05 $\geq$ 2 for rhabdomyolysis, and this is a well-recognized AE associated with the use of statins, both the frequency (5,300) and the EB05 (10.85) noted with

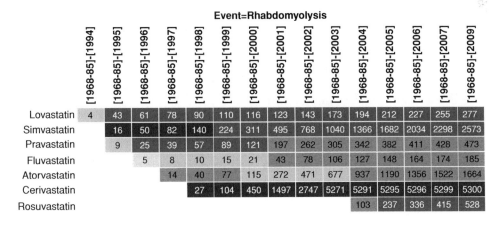

Figure 44.4 The cumulative annual number of cases of rhabdomyolysis in the AERS database associated with statins.

Event=Rhabdomyolysis

	[1968-85]-[1994]	[1968-85]-[1995]	[1968-85]-[1996]	[1968-85]-[1997]	[1968-85]-[1998]	[1968-85]-[1999]	[1968-85]-[2000]	[1968-85]-[2001]	[1968-85]-[2002]	[1968-85]-[2003]	[1968-85]-[2004]	[1968-85]-[2005]	[1968-85]-[2006]	[1968-85]-[2007]	[1968-85]-[2009]
Lovastatin	1,013	7,144	6,875	6,811	6,553	6,533	5,946	4,611	4,322	4,208	4,25	4,78	4,06	4,222	4,301
Simvastatin		8,491	10,255	10,324	9,22	6,262	5,608	4,628	4,517	4,306	4,805	5,09	5,488	5,704	5,857
Pravastatin	1,875	5,721	6,486	5,409	5,61	4,721	3,949	2,964	2,441	2,406	2,41	2,401	2,364	2,479	
Fluvastatin			0,964	1,312	1,335	1,484	1,657	2,318	2,97	3,026	3,238	3,399	3,479	3,516	3,597
Atorvastatin				2,17	3,041	2,193	1,665	1,711	1,824	1,819	2,188	2,414	2,463	2,567	2,626
Cerivastatin					34,054	40,343	38,728	27,321	17,398	10,823	10,85	10,849	10,846	10,851	10,852
Rosuvastatin											3,331	5,119	4,983	5,068	5,121

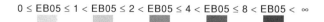

0 ≤ EB05 ≤ 1 < EB05 ≤ 2 < EB05 ≤ 4 < EB05 ≤ 8 < EB05 < ∞

Figure 44.5 The cumulative annual disproportionality score (EB05) of cases of rhabdomyolysis in the AERS database associated with statins.

cerivastatin are significantly higher than any of the other statins. This clearly suggests an association between cerivastatin and rhabdomyolysis that requires further investigation, with possible regulatory action.

The cerivastatin sector map in Figure 44.6 shows a variety of areas that have a strong association of adverse events, in particular, the hepatic, musculoskeletal, and renal areas. Additionally, the drug interaction graph in Figure 44.7 demonstrates several known drug interactions with statins, because the confidence intervals of the disproportionality score for each drug, compared to the confidence interval for both drugs, do not overlap, indicating a possible signal for a drug interaction.

The clinical importance of these observations could have been explored through other informational sources as needed. A case series of rhabdomyolysis associated with cerivastatin could have been constructed and analyzed to evaluate the company's post-marketing experience, and clinical trial data could have been examined if additional follow-up was required.

Summary

An evaluation of the FDA's SRS+AERS database, through the end of the fourth quarter 2008, showed that there was an increased risk of rhabdomyolysis associated with the use of all the statins. The frequency and EB05 was significantly higher for cerivastatin, compared to the other statins. On August 8, 2001, the FDA announced that cerivastatin was being voluntarily withdrawn from the US market by its manufacturer, because of reports of sometimes fatal rhabdomyolysis.

Caveats

Data source caveats

Reports may be submitted using either a drug's generic or brand name. Since brand names may differ among countries, all standard signaling activities are performed using the generic drug name, as it appears coded in the database. Reconciliation among different names/formulations does not occur on a routine basis.

Important limitations of this regulatory database include general under-reporting of post-marketing events and reporting bias. Factors such as publicity, length of time the drug is on the market, and regulatory action can influence the rate of reporting as well as the types of events reported. In addition, this database can contain duplicate reports because of multiple potential reporters, and the same case may come from different reporters. Also, a single

Drug=Cerivastatin

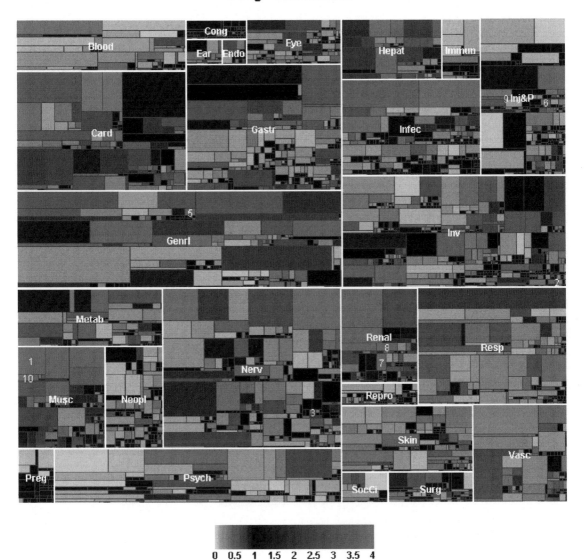

Figure 44.6 The sector map for cerivastatin.

case report may contain more than one preferred term.

Data interpretation caveats

Phase Forward's Lincoln Safety Group, the company that prepared the data, prepares it for Empirica™ Signal without making changes to the original reports.

Signal scores are generated by computer algorithms based on relative ratio, the ratio of the observed event for the specific drug as compared with the expected occurrence based on other drugs within the database. A potential signal is generated when an AE–drug combination has a disproportionately high occurrence compared with the background. It is important to stress that an elevated

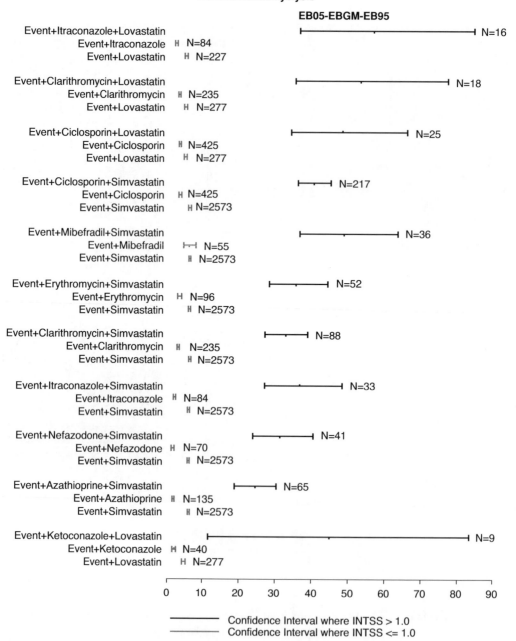

Figure 44.7 A graph of confidence intervals showing possible drug interactions with statins.

ratio is a measure of statistical association and not a clinical association between an AE and a drug.

These identified AE–drug combinations are hypotheses for further testing; follow-up may be necessary to determine whether they represent a real drug safety issue. Further evaluation may include a query and review of the company's safety database, review of the scientific literature and preclinical data, and consultation/discussion with internal and external experts. If a product safety issue were identified, next steps would include the development of a risk management and risk communication plan.

It is important to note that the numerator reflects only reports in the database. The actual number of patients exposed to the drugs is generally not known, and so it is not possible to calculate the true incidence of an adverse event from this database. Thus, comparing EB05 scores across drugs should not be done as a surrogate calculation for incidence. Incidence data are not available from this database; there are too many factors that could influence the EB05 in an asymmetric manner, for example, coding and the lack of ex-US serious labeled reports, making this an invalid comparison.

Since the signaling data source are post-marketing reports, factors that influence reporting will affect the signaling output. With rarely reported AEs, a disproportionality may become magnified since even one reported case against an expected background of zero may be statistically significant even though its clinical significance may be unknown.

Special caution should be exercised with any comparison of reporting ratios across different products, for example, comparison with competitor drugs. Differences in company interpretation and applications of the international health authority regulations, coding and case processing standards and practices, and factors such as time on the market, labeling, product publicity, and total patient exposure may be important factors in explaining apparent differences. The latency between agency receipt of data and public availability of the data may obscure differences between older and newly marketed products.

Data obtained by proportional reporting evaluations or EB05 scores should be reviewed in light of clinical experience with the product, and in general should be validated using an external source of data such as exposure estimates, clinical trial results, review of the scientific literature, and clinical and epidemiological studies.

For all of these reasons, these types of reports should be used solely for the purpose of initial signal identification. Causality cannot be determined using this instrument, and its primary utility is for generating hypotheses for further evaluation. These data cannot be used alone to make safety decisions or recommendations about safety issues, because signal analysis cannot prove or disprove a causal association between a specific drug and an adverse event, in the absence of other compelling evidence. Appropriate regulatory and legal guidance should be sought concerning other uses of these types of reports.

Regulatory guidance

According to two FDA Guidance documents issued in 2005 (FDA, 2005a, 2005b), and presented in synoptic form below, applying data mining techniques to large AE databases, such as FDA's AERS or VAERS, can enhance risk identification and assessment. Data mining, by systematically examining reported AEs, may be able to provide additional information about the existence of an excess of specific adverse events reported for a product, warranting further investigation.

This technique can be used to supplement existing signal detection strategies, but does not establish a causal association between the drug–event pairs being studied. However, it can be used for assessing patterns, time trends, and events associated with drug interactions. Data mining can be improved by adjusting for aspects of reporting (e.g., cumulative reporting by year) or characteristics of the patient (e.g., age or gender), or limiting the analysis to drugs of a specific class or for those used to treat a particular disease. The score generated by data mining quantifies the disproportionality between the observed and expected values for a given product–event combination

Although it is recognized that all these approaches are inherently exploratory or hypothesis generating, they may provide insights into the patterns of adverse events reported for a given product relative to other products in the same class or to all other products. The FDA urges caution when making such comparisons among products, because voluntary adverse event reporting systems such as AERS or VAERS are subject to a variety of reporting biases.

As of now, the use of data mining techniques is not a required part of signal identification by regulatory authorities, however, if data mining results are submitted to the FDA, it is expected that they will be presented in the larger appropriate clinical epidemiological context, to include the following:

• A description of the database used.
• A description of the data mining tool used (e.g., statistical algorithm, and the drugs, events, and stratifications selected for the analyses) or an appropriate reference.
• A careful assessment of individual case reports and any other relevant safety information related to the particular drug–event combination of interest (e.g., results from preclinical, clinical, pharmacoepidemiological, or other available studies).

Data mining techniques should always be used in conjunction with, and not in place of, analyses of single case reports. Data mining techniques facilitate the evaluation of spontaneous reports by using statistical methods to detect potential signals for further evaluation. This tool does not quantify the magnitude of risk, and caution should be exercised when comparing drugs. Further, when using data mining techniques, consideration should be given to the threshold established for detecting signals, because this will have implications for the sensitivity and specificity of the method (a high threshold is associated with high specificity and low sensitivity). Confounding factors that influence spontaneous AE reporting are not removed by data mining.

Privacy

Privacy concerns are becoming more important as data mining becomes more common. Besides issues of data ownership, there are questions that abound

on who has access to the data, the amount of identifying information that is present in the database, and how the results of the data mining will be used.

Furthermore, there are laws both in the US and Europe that regulate data privacy, and in addition the FDA has separate rules on data integrity and traceability. All these issues will have an impact on the way data are collected, data mined, and how those results are used.

The European Union's Directive on Data Protection bars the movement of personal data to countries that do not have sufficient data privacy laws in place. Additionally, the US's Health Insurance Portability and Accountability Act (HIPAA) set national standards for the protection of health information, as applied to the three types of covered entities: health plans, healthcare clearinghouses, and healthcare providers who conduct certain healthcare transactions electronically. This law was enacted in recognition of the fact that advances in electronic technology could erode the privacy of health information.

The discussion about data mining and privacy is just beginning. There will be increased scrutiny of data mining and its impact on privacy in the years to come. This is especially true as consumers and lawmakers become more aware and concerned about the potential for data mining, if used improperly, to violate the privacy rights of individuals. At the same time, however, governments are actively engaged in data mining for national security and law enforcement purposes, as they too begin to recognize the tremendous value of using this powerful technique. Nevertheless, as long as the data that are collected contain any potentially identifying information, legal, ethical, and privacy questions will need to be addressed.

Limitations

The biggest limitation with data mining is the quality of the data. Simply put, the results of the analyses are only as good as the data from which they are derived. The best databases are those that are relevant, complete, have rich quality data, are large, and get updated frequently. Unfortunately, many databases are designed for purposes entirely different than what they are being used for, when they are data mined.

Additionally, as errors can easily occur in databases, it cannot be assumed that the data they contain are entirely correct. Even after "data cleaning" a process to remove obvious errors and duplicates, there may be inherent errors or misclassification in the data being collected, particularly if there is subjectivity involved in the measurement that is used. Furthermore, in large, constantly changing databases, there must be rules in place for the data mining algorithm to capture the most current data.

Finally, because the results obtained from the data mining process can be difficult to interpret, it is extremely useful for the results to be presented in a graphical form that allows the user to interact with both the data and results. This allows the end user to further explore and better understand the results obtained. By being able to go from a broad perspective to a fine focus, this ability for users to "drill down" to the level of detail in which they are interested can be helpful. Furthermore, a graphical display of the data can help to identify data problems, provide insights not achievable with mere tables, and demonstrate new relationships.

Summary

Data mining does not supplant traditional pharmacovigilance methods. Instead, it supplements safety surveillance methods and allows a systematic identification of potential safety signals. The promise of data mining using large regulatory safety databases is that the huge size and diversity are primary advantages, because they enable multiple comparisons and provide valuable information whether one is looking in groups of events or classes of drugs. Essentially it allows the review of all the data and is very sensitive in detecting safety signals.

In 2009, the FDA requested proposals to build a "sentinel" system for AEs, to supplement its data mining efforts with its own databases. This sentinel system will potentially be able to identify AEs faster and more powerfully. It will be vitally important to ensure that the threshold for reporting is just right; not too low, which could lead to excessive warnings, many of which will turn out to be spurious associations, nor too high, which could lead to too few warnings and subsequently, a failure to report real signals (Avorn, 2009).

Once information is generated using data mining tools, regulators and manufacturers will require additional decision-analytic tools to help discern the potential clinical utility of the new information. As is evident, the interpretation of data mining results needs the expertise of safety reviewers and medical officers to analyze and interpret the output appropriately. Data mining signals by themselves are not indicators of problems, but are indicators of possible problems. Moreover caution must be exercised with any comparison of disproportionality ratios across different products, for example, comparison with competitor drugs because of the various limitations that exist when making these kinds of comparisons.

Finally, all signals should be evaluated, recognizing the possibility of false positives. In addition, the absence of a signal does not necessarily indicate the absence of a problem!

References

Avorn J *et al.* Managing drug-risk information: What to do with all those new numbers. *N Engl J Med* 2009; **361**(7):647–649.

Curtis J *et al.* Adaptation of Bayesian data mining algorithms to longitudinal claims data: Coxib safety as an example *Medical Care* 2008; **46**(9):969–975.

FDA Guidance for Industry. Good Pharmacovigilance Practices and Pharmacoepidemiologic Assessment, 2005a; http://www.fda.gov/downloads/RegulatoryInformation/Guidances/UCM126834.pdf; accessed April 12, 2010.

FDA Guidance for Industry. E2E Pharmacovigilance Planning. Step 4 of the ICH process, November 2004, 2005b; http://www.fda.gov/downloads/RegulatoryInformation/Guidances/UCM129423.pdf; accessed April 12, 2010.

Frawley W *et al.* Knowledge discovery in databases: An overview. *AI Magazine* 1992; Fall:213–228.

Szarfman A *et al.* Use of screening algorithms and computer systems to efficiently signal higher-than-expected combinations of drugs and events in the US FDA's spontaneous reports database. *Drug Safety* 2002; **25**(6):381–392.

Further reading

Colman E *et al.* An evaluation of a data mining signal for amyotrophic lateral sclerosis and statins detected in FDA's spontaneous adverse event reporting system. *Pharmacoepidemiology and Drug Safety* 2008; **17**(11):1068–1076.

HHS OCR HIPAA Privacy. General Overview of Standards for Privacy of Individually Identifiable Health Information, 2003; http://www.hhs.gov/ocr/hipaa/ guidelines/overview.pdf; accessed April 12, 2010.

Norén N *et al.* A statistical methodology for drug–drug interaction surveillance. *Statistics in Medicine* 2008; **27**:3057–3070.

Woo E *et al.* Effects of stratification on data mining in the US Vaccine Adverse Event Reporting System (VAERS). *Drug Safety* 2008; **31**(8):667–674.

CHAPTER 45

Risk Management in Product Approval and Marketing

Anthony W. Fox

EBD Group Inc., Carlsbad, CA, USA and Munich, Germany, and Skaggs SPPS, University of California, San Diego, USA

What is risk management?

Risk management is both a philosophy and a good practice. There are three major components. At its core is a philosophy or attitude willing to seek, anticipate, or otherwise identify clinical hazard associated with a medicinal product. This then guides some sort of intervention, which is designed to reduce that hazard. Finally, and *sine qua non*, there is review to see whether that designed intervention has been effective in reducing patient risk. This three-step process is an extension of the practice of pharmacovigilance, and translates the observations of that discipline into actions that reduce clinical hazard. This is the art and science of getting the right drug to the right patient at the right time.

Note that clinical hazard has two aspects. The most obvious is avoiding the inappropriate exposure of a patient to a potentially harmful drug. But let us not forget that clinical hazard can also be created by restrictions on product distribution channels; if these are too rigorous, the drug might never reach a patient who could experience benefit beyond that from any alternative therapy.

This chapter begins with the regulatory basis for risk management programs, as far as is needed beyond the information contained in Chapters 34 to 37 on European and American regulations. Practical examples will then be considered.

Principles and Practice of Pharmaceutical Medicine, 3rd edition.
Edited by L.D. Edwards, A.W. Fox, P.D. Stonier.
© 2011 Blackwell Publishing Ltd.

Regulatory frameworks

Of all areas of regulatory science, the regulations concerning risk management programs (RMPs) are among the least internationally-harmonized (EMEA, 2005, 2008; FDA, 2005). It can be argued that this is good. As we shall see below, special RMPs work best when tailored to the specific characteristics of the product, its indication, *and the venue of its use*. Flexibility of approach may be required to adapt a RMP to different geographical and cultural contexts, even when the same product and indication are under consideration.

The ordinary case

All sponsors/Marketing Authorization Holders are required to implement pharmacovigilance programs for all marketed products. Reports to regulatory authorities of the findings of these programs are usually required more frequently in the early part of the product life cycle than later on. The least restrictive ordinary situation is when clinical hazard is seen as being so slight that prescription is judged unnecessary. Products can then be licensed for over-the-counter use, with or without pharmacist-oversight. In the opposite direction, "Black box" labeling might recommend restriction of the distribution of the product to practitioners with specific training (e.g., in the United States, neuromuscular junction blocking drugs to anesthesiologists, and cytotoxic agents to oncologists and rheumatologists). "Black box" warnings might also draw attention to particularly serious adverse event types, and restrictions on advertising and marketing can thereby also be attached.

These common situations are discussed in the previous chapters on regulatory affairs in Section V. They can be viewed as the default set of RMPs, to be implemented in the absence of any special clinical hazard.

The earliest RMPs in the US

Sub-chapter D of the *Code of Federal Regulations* (CFR) authorizes the US Food and Drug Administration (FDA) to approve new drug products on an accelerated basis, provided that the indication is for a serious or life-threatening condition (see: 21*CFR* 314.500-560, also known colloquially as "Sub-part H" because of where it resides in the sub-chapter). This regulatory innovation took place in 1992, with a minor amendment in 1999. The candidate new drug product *must also* offer "meaningful clinical benefit" to be approved under these provisions; the FDA must be able to anticipate that there are patients for whom alternative treatments are clearly inferior, either through lacking efficacy or risking substantial intolerability.

Accelerated, Sub-part H, approvals rely on less clinical data than an ordinary approval. On the efficacy side, this might include, for example, the use of a surrogate endpoint instead of a disease outcome (for example, an antihypertensive drug can be approved without a p value for reduction of stroke). On issues of tolerability, an accelerated approval almost always means a database with fewer patients than would be otherwise desirable. It is in this latter case that the FDA will mandate a special risk management action program (RiskMAP). The Agency will review and approve a specific program design, to which the sponsor must agree, before issuing the product approval.

The design of these special risk management programs may involve one or more components. In general, these components fall into the following categories:
• Restriction in product distribution (location, medical procedure, or quantity of dispensing).
• Need for special training of prescriber or pharmacist before authority to prescribe or dispense.

• Need for special education of patient prior to dispensing.
• Specific clinical tests prior to patient eligibility.
• Documentation of patient's informed consent prior to dispensing.
• Mandated patient registries.
• Targeted post-marketing clinical studies.

The term "access program" is often used when publicizing these special measures. The sponsor's performance according to the agreed plan becomes a condition for the approval to remain active; however, if the FDA does wish subsequently to withdraw approval for failure to follow a post-marketing RMP, the sponsor is entitled first to a hearing.

Modern extensions of the US RiskMAP practice

Although the Guidance states that it is hoped that sponsors will identify products that merit RiskMAPs for themselves, the Agency is also authorized to ask for them as part of a drug approval or post-marketing action (without any consideration of "Sub-part H"). By 2009, RiskMAPs have become routine for long-acting oral opioids, all teratogenic products, and products for degenerative neurological diseases with rare adverse event types.

Special regulatory provisions: European Economic Area (EEA)

The components of RMPs in Europe have been similar to those listed above. Pan-Community, both the European Commission and the European Medicines Agency (EMA) have interests in RMPs for pharmaceutical products. Both organizations are interested in the safety of the general public, and also in ensuring equal access to pharmaceutical products across the Community. The Commission tends to take a more economic view; for example, it has expressed concern about special programs that drive product costs upwards and when these costs are absorbed by the health systems more easily in large countries than in small ones.

Within the EMA, there are multiple departments and divisions with responsibilities that impinge on different aspects of RMPs. The Committee for Proprietary Medicinal Products (CPMP) maintains a Pharmacovigilance Working Group. The Committee for Orphan Medicinal Products (COMP) wants to ensure access to drugs for patients with rare diseases, and is motivated to document product tolerability in what are necessarily small databases. Labeling groups have the daunting task of ensuring that written descriptions of how to mitigate drug hazards mean the same thing in more than 20 languages.

European National Competent Authorities (NCAs)

Ultimately, the NCAs are at the forefront of post-marketing surveillance and product safety. Each NCA can mandate product withdrawal within its boundaries, albeit with a responsibility to notify other NCAs about its concerns. But such a decision is never binding in any other part of the EEA, and there is no obligation for one member state to implement a RMP that has been mandated at the national level elsewhere.

Academic, cultural (including religious), ethical, and medical attitudes also diverge within the EEA. For example, with the exception of clinical trial participation, in many European countries, a requirement for written informed consent for a marketed product is seen as unethical. The corollaries foreseen are that no informed consent would mean no therapy. Therefore the patient may be under duress to provide informed consent, or simply provide uninformed "consent," in order to gain access to medical treatment. Additionally, it is suspected that some of the burden of responsibility for drug exposure would then have shifted to the patient, this being construed as an abrogation of the responsibility of the prescriber or pharmacist.

Patient registries and databases can also run into problems within the EEA. Regardless of whether or not these rely on public funding, they are seen as potential violations of patient confidentiality. In some European countries, this is emphasized by national privacy legislation. The entry of an identifiable patient into a registry, as a condition of drug supply, can be seen as a situation where it is a registry administrator, checking inclusion and exclusion criteria, that ultimately decides whether a patient is treated; this is again seen as *de facto*

interference with the clinician–patient relationship. For all these reasons, it can be impossible to operate the same RMP in every European country.

Practical examples

What sorts of drugs and indications have special clinical hazards and need special risk management programs? At the pan-European level, the EMA now considers RMPs more or less routinely prior to Marketing Authorization; every Type A license amendment must also include a revision of the RMP. But in general, the products for which detailed risk management plans are almost always be required are as follows:

- biological products;
- new chemical entities with novel mechanisms of action;
- significant changes in indication for older products;
- new target populations;
- major issues of intolerability;
- products undergoing the prescription-only to over-the-counter "switch";
- orphan medicinal products (where clinical trials patients are automatically few).

Although most of the "Sub-part H" examples in the US fall into these same categories, these are good, general criteria that should stimulate sponsors to consider implementing detailed RMPs, regardless of whether or not this is being mandated by a regulatory authority.

Abuse liability

Psychotropic drugs with abuse and dependence potential, and the associated restrictions on product distribution (i.e., "scheduling" under a Controlled Substances Act or equivalent) form a well-established system of RMPs. Most countries recognize the need for four or five degrees of scheduling with graded increases in product restrictions, thus forming a usefully flexible system. This is also now harmonized internationally by the signatories to the United Nations Psychotropic Drugs Convention, which covers opioids, thebaine-derivatives, barbitals (barbiturates), amphetamines, the natural and semi-synthetic products of *Erythoxylon coca* and *Ephedra spp.*, as well as other drugs with both medical purposes and abuse liability.

Even in the most extreme case of RMP, where the risk–benefit assessment is deemed to be so hopeless that a drug is absolutely banned, there can be a lack of international harmonization. The easy illustration within this class of drugs is diacetyl-morphine (diamorphine, "heroin"). In the US, this is a Schedule 1 controlled substance, defined as being without any medical value; prescribing and dispensing is absolutely prohibited. In contrast, several European countries value this drug for the treatment of pain in terminally-ill patients, and for its greater solubility than morphine (making large doses of opioid easier to swallow). In the EEA, this is achieved by a lower grade of "Scheduling" than in the USA, although prescription, storage, and dispensing nonetheless requires greater storage security and accountability than for ordinary prescription-only medicines.

Note, too, that this well-established type of RMP has indirectly led to competitive advantage in at least one case. One manufacturer of a modern product for insomnia advertises in the US that this drug "is not a narcotic." Simplicity in prescribing and dispensing, and a perception of the relative safety of an unscheduled product, is attractive to physicians, pharmacists, and patients with insomnia, alike.

Major issues of toxicity: thalidomide

The story of thalidomide in the 1960s is too well-known to need much repetition here. The full spectrum of its pharmacology and toxicology is still not fully understood, but in addition to its supposed anti-emetic effects during pregnancy, this drug is also immunomodulatory. In the 1990s, interest in this latter property grew, and thalidomide (often in combination with dapsone) was found to be effective for erythema nodosum in patients with Hansen's Disease (leprosy) and without peripheral neuritis. What has been the response, in terms of RMPs, to allow patients to have access to this teratogenic drug?

In the US, thalidomide was approved in 1998 under the "Sub-part H" provisions. The product

label carries no fewer than seven different "Black Box Warnings," some of which appear twice. These describe precisely the teratogenicity and RMP associated with this drug. More or less every component from the list above is deployed, in what is known as the System for Thalidomide Education & Prescribing Safety (the "STEPS Program"), including the following:

- Product supply chain to a small number of registered pharmacies (fewer than an average of one per State).
- Dispensing permitted against prescriptions written by only a small number of named, specially-registered physicians.
- Requirements for special training of these registered physicians and pharmacists.
- Documented informed consent by patients, emphasizing contraception and pregnancy testing, along with the risks of teratogenicity.
- Documented informed consent for minors, from parents or guardians.
- Mandatory regular pregnancy testing for women of child-bearing potential.
- Maximum one-month supply per prescription, with no refills permitted.
- Mandatory patient registration by name and location prior to dispensing.
- Close pharmacovigilance of all registered patients with frequent FDA reporting.

Erythema nodosum associated with Hansen's Disease is a rare disorder in the US, and the manufacturer of thalidomide enjoys the exclusivity provided by orphan drug status. This might be a rare situation where the toxicology of an orphan drug product is well-known due to its severity, relatively high incidence, and prior exposure to a larger patient population for a previous, failed indication. But, thus far, there have been no reported disasters.

European views about STEPS-type programs are very different (see also above). First, there is conflict between patient (and probably clinician) registration and privacy laws in many countries. Second, the patient registers and documentation of informed consent is seen as interfering with the doctor–patient relationship. Third, there is the potential for iniquity of drug distribution; some of

Europe, including areas where leprosy is to be found, is only sparsely provided with physicians and pharmacists, and those that are unregistered for this special purpose effectively block access for a proportion of the EU population. Fourth, for the cultural reasons described above, the patient registries would probably have to be at the national level; the cost–benefit ratio of these schemes might be less attractive to smaller countries than large ones, again creating iniquity. Fifth, there is skepticism that the required documentation can automatically correspond with the quality of education imparted to clinicians and patients alike (this concern applies more widely to many matters of continuing medical education and revalidation in Europe). Finally, the STEPS program can be seen as one where the Marketing Authorization Holder actually decides whether a patient is eligible to receive the treatment, and whether a doctor is qualified to prescribe it, thus pre-empting those who would otherwise be duly empowered to do so, either by reason of ethics or by law. In Europe, no RMP has been implemented, and there is no marketing authorization for thalidomide.

Major clinical hazard: mifepristone

This prostaglandin analog is capable of inducing abortion of a uterine pregnancy of less than 49 days duration when administered orally. In 2000, it was approved in the US amid controversy associated with the cultural aspects of pregnancy and its termination.

The RMP that has been deployed for mifepristone is less restrictive than that for thalidomide. The use of the product is restricted to those physicians who are capable of determining the duration of pregnancy, and who can identify ectopic implantation. Availability and training in the use of ultrasound is therefore required. Doctors who prescribe the drug must also be able to provide surgical intervention in cases of incomplete abortion or severe bleeding, although it is unclear whether this includes (for example) the situation of an endocrinologist prescriber who works with a gynecologist in a closely coordinated environment, or whether the prescriber and the surgeon-in-reserve has to be the same person.

At the time of writing, about nine years have elapsed since product launch. The most widely reported serious adverse events during this period have been four cases of fatal sepsis, a clinical hazard that is much smaller than the general risks associated with pregnancy to full term. There has been no epidemic of hemorrhage.

This is an example of a RMP that currently appears to have been scaled appropriately for the minimization of direct clinical hazard. Cultural aspects of this form of therapy continue to provoke protest at product availability, and reported adverse events are also used to keep these protests in the public eye.

Examples of international disharmony

The examples of diacetylmorphine and thalidomide (see above) are examples of pharmaceutical products that are available either only in Europe or only in the United States, respectively. Within Europe the existence of National Competent Authorities (NCAs) provides further scope for non-uniform RMPs.

A good example is cisapride, a propulsive gastrointestinal drug that was found (especially in the context of drug interactions) to cause prolongation of the QT interval and predispose to *torsades de pointes* ventricular tachyarrythmia. This information caused some of the NCAs in Europe to suspend marketing authorization for this drug. The (then) CPMP within the EMEA subsequently reviewed the pan-European pharmacovigilance data on this product. Cisapride has now been returned to the marketplace with various restrictions having been placed on national authorizations, including a variety of non-harmonized RMPs.

A similar situation applies to sertindole. In this case, the marketing authorization for this antipsychosis agent was initially suspended by a single member state (some would claim with too little advance notice). This was followed by complete withdrawal of the product, on a voluntary basis, by the Marketing Authorization Holder. Again, an EMEA pan-European review took place for all the pharmacovigilance data that were available. Again, the product has now been reintroduced, albeit with RMPs of different designs in various European countries.

Intra-county (*sic*) problems implementing RMPs

If there was ever a need to emphasize the need for flexibility of approach in RMPs, no better illustration can exist than dealing with problems that can arise within a single county! San Diego County is the most south-western within the 48 contiguous US, bordering on Mexico and the Pacific Ocean. It is quite a large county (about the size of the country of Lebanon) and has substantial Spanish-speaking, Italian-speaking, Mandarin-speaking, Anglophone, Roman Catholic, Protestant, Buddhist, Iraqi, and non-religious communities.

Pity, then, the San Diego pediatrician trying to cope with the nationally-designed RMP for isotretinoin, when used in adolescent girls with acne vulgaris. Advice to avoid sunlight, given the local climate and architecture, might be somewhat *pro forma*. But the ability to hold effective discussions about contraception and repeated pregnancy-testing with supposedly under-aged, tattooed, Californian surfers, as well as conservative, teenage Latinas accompanied by their mothers, can only inspire awe.

Summary

RMPs are not a new invention (e.g., "scheduling" of drugs with abuse liability). There are classes of drugs for which RMPs are clearly indicated beyond those that are routinely required for product approval and marketing. The menu of measures that can be used is long, and should be scaled against the clinical hazard that has been identified or is suspected. Political, national, and cross-cultural factors have a large impact on the success of RMPs; the most effective ones are likely not to be internationally-harmonized.

Acknowledgments

For this chapter, much is owed to the analysis offered by the following experts at the 5th Scripps-

BIO Drug Development Conference (La Jolla, California, February 2003): Rear-Admiral Marlene E. Haffner USPHS MD MPH FRCP (US FDA); Professor P. Kurki MD (National Agency for Medicines, Finland); M. Toivonen MD PhD (EMEA); H. Greenaway MD (Scripps Clinic, California); and R. Wagner PharmD (Kaiser Permanente, USA). The views expressed at that conference were those of the experts themselves, and were not necessarily those of their employers; nor should anything in this chapter be inferred as being the opinion of these experts.

References

EMA (European Medicines Agency). Committee for medicinal Products for Human Use: Guideline on risk management systems for medicinal products for human use. London: 2005; EMEA/CHMP/96268/2005.

EMA (European Medicines Agency). Committee for medicinal Products for Human Use: Guideline on safety and efficacy follow-up risk management of advanced therapy medicinal products. London: 2008; EMEA/149995/2008.

FDA (United States Food and Drug Administration). *Guidance for Industry: Development and Use of Risk Management Action Plans*. Rockville, MD, 2005.

Further reading

Daniel DG, Wozniak P, Mack RJ, McCarthy BG. Long-term efficacy and safety comparison of sertindole and haloperidol in the treatment of schizophrenia. *Psychopharmacol Bull* 1998; **34**:61–69.

Honein MA, Moore CA, Erickson JD. Can we ensure the safe use of known human teratogens? Introduction of generic isotretinoin in the US as an example. *Drug Safety* 2004; **27**:1069–1080.

Kartzinel R. Guyidelines for scheduling drugs under the Controlled Substances Act [Proceedings]. *Psychopharmacol Bull* 1981; **17**:40–42.

Mechcatie E. Risk management program for IBS drug on track: Alosetron was reintroduced to the market in 2002 with a few caveats, including a narrower indication. *Clin Psychiat News* 2004; **32**:78–81.

Schaefer C, Hannemann D, Meister R. Post-marketing surveillance system for drugs in pregnancy—15 years' experience of ENTIS. *Reprod Toxicol* 2005; **20**:331–343.

Stang PE, Gardner J. Epidemiology and pharmacoeconomic research. In *Principles of Pharmacoeconomics*, Bootman JL, Townsend RJ, McGhan WF (eds). Harvey Whitney Books: Cincinnati, OH, USA, 1996. ISBN 0-929-37517-3.

Uhl K, Kennedy DL, Kweder SL. Risk management strategies in the *Physicians' Desk Reference* product labels for pregnancy category X drugs. *Drug Safety* 2002; **25**:885–892.

Waller P. Dealing with uncertainty in drug safety: lessons for the future from sertindole. *Pharmacoepidemiol Drug Safety* 2003; **12**:283–287, 289–290.

Weatherby LB, Nordstrom BL, Fife D, Walker AM. The impact of wording in "Dear doctor" letters and in black box labels. *Clin Pharmacol Ther* 2002; **72**:735–742.

Wehnert A. The European Post-marketing observational Serdolect (EPOS) project: increasing our understanding of schizophrenia therapy. *Int Clin Psychopharmacol* 1998; **13**(suppl 3):S27–S30.

Wilkinson JJ, Force RW, Cady PS. Impact of safety warnings on drug utilization: marketplace lifespan of cisapride and troglitazone. *Pharmacotherapy* 2004; **24**:978–986.

World Health Organization. WHO Expert Committee on drug dependence: Thirty-second report. *WHO Tech Rep Ser* 2001; **903**:i–v, 1–26.

CHAPTER 46
Publishing Clinical Studies

Anthony W. Fox

EBD Group Inc., Carlsbad, CA, USA and Munich, Germany, and Skaggs SPPS, University of California, San Diego, USA

Introduction

This chapter has three objectives. First, it is necessary to discuss the ethics and desirability of publishing clinical trials, and the biases that may be involved with that process. Second, younger clinical trialists may benefit from some discussion of classic parts of an orthodox clinical trial report in a peer-reviewed journal, and some clues for effective oral presentations. Third, alternative forms of publication are discussed, including isolated abstracts and posters, electronic publication, and press releases; the clinical trials registry (now mostly mandatory) is considered as one of these special forms. The scope of this chapter is strictly about publications: regulatory documents (which are typically not published and are a different form of clinical trials reporting) and marketing materials are dealt with elsewhere (Section V and Chapter 54, respectively). In addition, although the term "publishing" is used to describe electronic submissions to regulatory authorities, these are also not within the subject area of this chapter. A summary and prospectus closes the chapter.

Ethics in publishing clinical trials

For all forms of publication, the objective usually goes beyond the mere reporting of clinical trials data. In some way or another, the clinical trialists will interpret their data to reach conclusions, and

Principles and Practice of Pharmaceutical Medicine, 3rd edition.
Edited by L.D. Edwards, A.W. Fox, P.D. Stonier.
© 2011 Blackwell Publishing Ltd.

will want to urge some change in the behavior of the target audience. These changes might include prescribing habits, healthcare resource utilization, public health policy, or regulatory practices.

Whatever the form of publication, the only tools available to persuade people to make these behavioral changes are the data; these must be converted into a well-created document, audiovisual presentation, press release, and so on. The dissemination of these materials might be repeated, and can take place at a time or place remote from the author's immediate supervision. Publications must be well-made for stand-alone use.

Conclusions that extrapolate beyond the range of available data are inappropriate in scientific publications (and nor do they belong in regulatory documents or marketing materials). Omissions of details in methods and results pursuant to a concise presentation will always be subjective. While the traditional advice has always been to provide as much methodological detail so as to permit replication of the experiment, we all know that the probability of that is miniscule in the realm of clinical trials.

The pressures on the clinical trialist, whether writing him- or herself, or when guiding specialist medical writers, are many, and sometimes contrary to common standards of integrity because they often emanate from powerful people who lack the training needed to assess data objectively. Such people will include journalists who oversimplify or sensationalize, marketing department staff wanting to amplify positive messages and silence negative ones, and corporate officers who want to use publications as vehicles for enhancing the company's share price or negotiating better financial arrangements on Wall Street. Rarely, even government politicians get involved, whose tactics include those used by journalists, the diligent application of complete ignorance, and the forced fit of technical information to a predetermined political position (e.g., rosiglitazone and cardiovascular hazard, during the summer of 2007).

The publication of clinical trials, therefore, is one example where the clinical trialist (acting as publicist or medical writer) may become an agent for social change (Gray, 1994). Even when he or she acts solely as a medical writer, authors must understand their ethical responsibility to represent the material in a fair, balanced, and, above all, accurate manner. While an ombudsman-like role may help in finding compromise among the various pressures that are applied to this process from diverse outside parties, the author of a clinical trial report may inevitably (but hopefully only occasionally) find him- or herself as the sole repository of integrity in this process; this can feel lonely, but nobody else is going to fulfill this role.

Desirability of, and biases, in the publication of clinical trials

Everybody finds the publication of an *ideal* clinical trial to be highly desirable. Clinical development departments find it efficient to mail out reprints in response to clinicians' inquiries and to append them to Investigators' Brochures and Investigational New Drug (IND) amendments. Regulators controlling promotional practices need only satisfy themselves that the publication accurately reflects the Clinical Study Report that has been submitted to the approved Marketing Authorization Application (MAA) or New Drug Application (NDA). Marketing departments can use these publications for promotional purposes, knowing that the data are cast-iron, the message is unarguably positive, and that the self-evident benefits of the drug will be understood when the most skeptical clinician meets the least adept sales person. Lastly, senior management can bask in the glory of its contribution to the public health, and direct observers on Wall Street will appreciate the appearance of its

investments in the world's most respected medical journals. For small companies, this might even be life-saving. How on earth could such a laudable activity go wrong?

The answer, of course, lies in the fact that many clinical trials are less than ideal. These poor publication candidates may not have resulted in a positive outcome for the active treatment group, or may have only generated prosaic tolerability data in a special patient population. Studies that are not original, for example, where replicating a previous positive finding may have been a regulatory necessity, but nonetheless leading to a me-too paper, do not find homes in eminent journals. Also, some good studies are less than ideal publication candidates solely because the manuscript has been drafted badly.

Negative trials are rarely accepted for publication by good journals unless their results dispel some important previously-held dogma. Some areas of therapeutics are notorious for the high proportion of negative clinical trials results (e.g., pharmacological treatments for depression). However, the majority of negative clinical trials are those where either drug efficacy is simply not evident or where no difference is found between two active treatments; sometimes the latter will be published as a less-than-spectacular non-inferiority study (provided the statistics were done right). Negative data are the inevitable result of conducting clinical trials that are true experiments; there is nothing dishonorable in such a result, even if it is disappointing. However, the inability to publish such studies risks redundancy of further resources and duplication of the patient hazard when another, independent study group sets out to discover later the same negative result. While Chalmers (1990), somewhat hyperbolically, has actually characterized under-reporting of clinical trials data as scientific misconduct, this is what clinical trial registries may improve upon (see below).

If this underreporting is suboptimal, then those who publish clinical trials must take their share of the blame. Incongruously, it is those same journal editors who are least likely to publish negative data that make the most noise about how unsatisfactory is the performance of the pharmaceutical industry in failing to publish it (e.g., Horton and Smith, 1999; Tonks, 1999). This author cannot agree with Dickersin *et al.* (1992) who wrote: "Contrary to popular opinion, publication bias originates primarily with investigators, not journal editors"; the busy clinical trialist is unlikely to waste his or her time writing a paper that he or she knows has little chance of publication. Rarely, journal editors themselves have recognized their complicity (de Angelis *et al.*, 2004).

The establishment of clinical trials registries may be one way to overcome the bias against reporting of negative clinical trials. This is not a new idea (e.g., Simes, 1986) and several worthwhile attempts have been made to accomplish this end. The National Health Service (NHS) in the UK (Peckham, 1991) has initiated, and an amnesty for the publication of clinical trials offered by some journals (Roberts, 1998) and specialized databases (especially in the areas of malignant disease and AIDS) have been, partial responses to the many pleas for registration of clinical trials. Two large pharmaceutical companies have taken an initiative to register their own clinical trials (e.g., Sykes, 1998), but have been ungratefully criticized both for doing too much and for doing too little: some think that the registered information is insufficient, while others believe that this creates a commercial disadvantage (Horton and Smith, 1999).

Government and quasi-governmental clinical trial registries also now exist. The United States National Institutes of Health (NIH) operates www.clinicaltrials.gov (with 88,775 registered trials as at April 26, 2010) for their own studies and for privately-sponsored clinical trials that others may wish to contribute voluntarily. An alternative venue is www.controlled-trials.com, which offers searches both within its own and other clinical trial registries, including both those within the NHS of the UK and the NIH.

A further bias in clinical trials publishing is the selective reporting of subsets of secondary endpoints. This is usually associated with active-comparator trials having a primary objective of demonstrating the superiority of one treatment over the other. All too often the primary objective of the trial is not achieved: the authors then selectively publish a few of the many secondary endpoints that did support their hypothesis. The "if you have 100 endpoints and $\alpha = 0.05$, then at random five endpoints will be statistically significant" principle supervenes; fallacious treatment differences are claimed after reporting only those five endpoints and neglecting to mention the 95 unspectacular results. Solutions to this problem could include an independently-prepared summary of the protocol, with its prospective objectives and complete list of endpoints, perhaps in mini-type, at the end of such papers, as well as sensitization of reviewers to this potential problem. Journal editors sometimes approach this ideal by asking for protocols to accompany the submitted manuscripts; some companies view their protocols as confidential, and one wonders whether this is one of the reasons why. Results modules in www.clinicaltrials.gov became compulsory in September 2009, and these include both efficacy and adverse event data.

Thus, there are multiple ways in which publication bias may be created by study sponsors, publicists, medical writers, and those who control journal content. Those constructing meta-analyses from published studies should beware.

The classic components of a clinical trial report in a peer-reviewed journal

The publication of clinical trials in peer-reviewed journals normally follows the same format as for any other paper: title, authors, sponsorship, abstract, introduction, methods, results, discussion, concluding paragraph, acknowledgments, references, tables, and figure legends, with each figure attached on a separate sheet labeled on the reverse. It is beyond the scope of this chapter to teach how to write a scientific paper: there are many other books, manuals, and journals that devote enough space for this purpose (succinct examples include Skelton, 1994; Bonk, 1997; Fromter *et al.*, 1999).

All journals publish guidelines describing the formats for the often diverse types of article that will be considered. The corollary is that the writer should identify the target journal before putting pen to paper, and judge whether the quantity of material supports a whole paper, a brief report, or even more than one paper.

Authorship on papers is a matter of substantial debate. Under some circumstances, literally dozens of coauthors will clamor to be listed, and this phenomenon is not restricted to the publication of huge multicenter clinical trials. Clinical trials are a specific case of this general, perennial problem, to which Rafal (1991) has provided a somewhat humorous guide. There are two solutions.

The first solution is the prospective promulgation of a set of criteria that every author must meet. Many journals publish their own specific guidelines or criteria, and these do not differ greatly in qualitative terms. In the practicality of publishing clinical trials, the following would be typical:

• The principal investigator(s) is/are authors unless so numerous as to require a team designation (see below).

• The statistician(s) who personally accept(s) responsibility for the statistical analysis in the corresponding document(s) that is/are submitted to regulatory authorities should sign off on the paper and be named as author(s).

• Key members of the clinical team within the pharmaceutical company may (but do not necessarily need to) be authors.

• All named authors should be able to personally defend the paper after publication, and be familiar with (but not necessarily have personally performed) all the methods employed in the clinical trial.

• There should be no circumstances where "guest authorship" or "gratitude authorship" is awarded; all authors' participation must have been fundamental to the conduct and success of the clinical trial.

• All authors should be prepared to disclose all conflicts of interest and the sources of financial support for the clinical trial.

Many good clinical protocols now include publication plans. Part of this will be the rules as to who will appear as an author on the paper, and in which order. Often these are defined by a minimum patient recruitment and a rank order of

numbers of patients recruited, with a limit of two authors at each study site, commonly the principal investigator, one or two associate investigators, and the study site coordinator.

The second solution is to publish the paper under the name of the team that conducted the trial, rather than the personal names of the participants. The acknowledgments can then list all those who took part (e.g., The Subcutaneous Sumatriptan International Study Group, 1991). A hybrid variant is also sometimes used, where a one (or a few) lead author(s) are named and stated to represent the rest of the team (e.g., Cady *et al.*, 1991). The advantage of this tactic is that at least one person accepts responsibility for defense of the paper after publication. A further advantage is that this can be used to motivate investigators in multisite studies: the protocol can state that the investigator who recruits the most completed patients, without violations, will be the named first author in any publication (and get the phone calls from the journalists!).

Isolated abstracts and posters

An argument can be made that the isolated abstract format is not a good vehicle for the publication of clinical trials. Indeed, the inclusion and exclusion criteria in most clinical protocols alone exceed the word limit of most scientific meeting abstracts. Too often, the publication of an abstract or poster is a criterion used by companies to justify the time and expense of sending staff to a conference: authors then generate and submit unimportant abstracts, principally for use as tickets to venues that attract them for ulterior reasons.

There are a few exceptions to this generalization, however. Legitimate retrospective analysis of the database of a clinical trial that has been previously published in full sometimes can make an isolated abstract, provided the full reference is provided, and an educated audience at, say, an academic conference, will be aware of the potential biases of this technique. Similarly, the open-label tolerability extension to a previously published controlled trial might be usefully published as a poster. But these are minor exceptions to the general principle that in order to assess the validity of a clinical trials report, far more detail is needed than can be published in the small spaces of isolated abstracts and posters.

Audiovisual presentations at academic meetings

It is amazing that apparently intelligent people routinely attempt to speak to large numbers of their peers at academic meetings with (i) disorganized speech (due to disordered thought processes and/or acute episodic dysarthria) and (ii) an inability to control a Powerpoint® projector that should (by now in the developed world) have universally replaced the chaos of 2-x-2-inch photographic slides. Such ineptitude is displayed without insight by all medical specialties (including clinical trialists). One's amazement is all the greater because these incompetent speakers must often have heard equally bad productions, and today's projector controls are simpler than an hotel alarm clock.

The most important time when making oral publications is before you even begin to talk. You should have the following three things *sine qua non*:

• An understanding of the audience and the vocabulary needed to communicate with them (the general public, a patient advocacy group, an academic society, and an in-house department seminar all require very different approaches).

• A slide set that is cogent, organized, and familiar/

• A look at the venue and the various pieces of equipment that will be at your disposal; think about how to match your speaking volume to the open-air or to the microphone (if any), where to stand so that you can see your slides without having your back to the audience, and how to use a laser pointer without imitating a demented firefly.

For the talk itself, one useful checklist is as follows:

• What is the take home message, in one simple sentence of the language of the conference (e.g., "Drug X was superior to placebo in treating disease Y, in a patient population with characteristics A, B, and C, i.e., like the known epidemiology of the disease")?

• State the purpose of the talk at the beginning: Usually this will be to explain how one will defend the take-home message (e.g., "This talk is to describe the clinical trial that has led us to conclude that drug X is effective for disease Y in a patient population that is representative of the known epidemiology of this disease").

• Organize one's slides in a manner that would be used sequentially to illustrate a written paper in a peer-reviewed journal (see above).

• Make sure all slides are legible (e.g., a minimum of bold 24 point text for a Microsoft Powerpoint® presentation).

• Avoid tables of data in slides; if you cannot graph it, it is probably not worth showing at all; 24 × 12 lines of data in a table might as well be a micrograph of a small part of the surface of a spiky-state platelet.

• Make the text of each slide concise (e.g., maximum of 30 words per slide).

• Create slides to be self-supporting: If you gave your set of slides to someone else, could that person, without any further explanation, more or less work out your subject, principal conclusions, and give the talk?

• Plan to use about one slide per minute of time allotted.

• If you are a troglodyte iconoclast, and still using photographic slides, at least number your slides with bright labels on the plastic holder (so that you can see or feel the bright label in near-darkness). Use a consistent location for your label, and then use that label to orient the slide when loading the carousel. Usually, but not always, this is "right way round, wrong way up." Practice showing one slide before wrongly loading all of them.

• Relate the middle part of your talk to your take-home message (e.g., if disease Y is type I diabetes, then "As shown in this slide, the patient population included 30% adolescents because this group represents a relevant fraction of the whole population with type I diabetes").

• At the end, repeat the scientific conclusions, briefly review the data that you have presented in their support, and then interpret these conclusions, once again, into your take-home message.

In short, tell them what you are going to show them, then show them, then tell them what you showed them!

Most people are in an altered psychological state shortly after giving a talk, whether or not it seemed to go well. In this psychological state, they gladly accept thanks and congratulations, but are incapable of hearing constructive feedback. Feedback is essential to either improve the talk the next time round or to improve one's presentation skills in general. Seek out this learning opportunity from friends, and tell them in advance that you will be asking for this feedback, probably a few days after the event.

Newer forms of clinical trials publication

Electronic publishing is relatively new and is not yet in any standardized form. It is important to understand, however, the main classes of electronic publication, before taking the big step of committing your clinical trial report to it. Only then can the central question be answered for that clinical trial: Would electronic publication make these data more easily available to the audience that can best use them (Geddes, 1999)?

The CD-ROM versus the textbook is probably the most primordial form of the digital versus analog debate. This battle has probably now been fought to a standstill, with winners and losers on both sides. Example replacements include the approximately two dozen annual volumes of *Index Medicus*, or both 37 annual volumes of *Headache* and 17 annual volumes of *Cephalalgia*, by single CD-ROM disks. This replacement saves trees, speeds search times, and has lower production and shipping expenses, but requires readers to have access to a computer at the same place as the disk; many readers will nonetheless print out the papers that they want to read. Clinical trial databases can be usefully placed on CD-ROM, and this can facilitate explorations beyond the prospective trial objectives. Epidemiological studies, in which huge numbers of patients are often studied, may be especially suited to this form of publication.

Many traditional journals have sprouted electronic limbs. The most common form at present is probably the distribution of electronic facsimiles of printed papers, usually in .pdf format, which can be read using Adobe Acrobat® software that can be downloaded without charge. Access to these fac-similes is usually restricted to those who also have a subscription to the paper version of the journal and thus represents a duplication of or extension to paper publication, rather than its replacement. In some cases, journals publish electronically a wider selection of submitted papers than can be accommodated in their paper versions, or restrict new electronic material to correspondence that does not appear in print (Chalmers, 1999; Delamothe and Smith, 1999; McConnell and Horton, 1999).

Song *et al.* (1999) have suggested that electronic journals can reduce publication bias (see above) principally by accommodating and providing access to greater quantities of published materials. Chalmers (1999 and see above) is an enthusiast, and so presumably this is correct. Chalmers and Altman (1999) have even proposed that not only will publication bias be reduced but also the intrinsic quality of clinical trials themselves could be improved as a result of electronic publication; this is unproven at present. However, this enlarged volume of publications also mandates a different peer-review system, or even no peer-review at all. It is possible that electronic publications may come to be suspected as both providing higher quantities of information but possibly with lower quality than more orthodox publications. The non-profit Public Library of Science (PLoS; www.plos.org) has developed this idea with several online journals that share the principles of open access, scientific integrity and excellence, cooperation, community engagement, internationalism, and avoidance of narrow specialism.

Press releases

Clinical trialists in large pharmaceutical companies might only very rarely be exposed to the need for press releases concerning their clinical trials. In contrast, the small entrepreneurial pharmaceutical company may live or die on the outcome of a single clinical trial, and the rapid dissemination of the results of such a clinical trial to the appropriate audience (shareholders and investment community) is legally required when material to the prospects of a small, public company. The press release then becomes an important tool for publishing clinical trial results.

When writing press releases, absolutely no technical knowledge can be assumed on the part of the recipient. Often the investors' questions parse simply to "Did the drug work or not?". Extended detailed explanations can actually create the false impression that the drug did not work, when in fact the trial outcome was quite satisfactory for continued product development purposes. Equally, when clinical trials fail, ingenious but scientifically meaningless explanations by corporate officers can create the false impression that the outcome was better than it was. A good example is the often used: "We still have confidence in our ability to register Drug X; Drug X performed as we expected, but it was just that the placebo response rate in this (pivotal) study was unexpectedly high."

Clinical trialists may often want to avoid involvement in the drafting of press releases altogether. However, this creates a liability that one's independent comments may not then dovetail with the company's press releases, causing harm not only to the company but also to one's longevity within it!

The best advice on press releases may be twofold. First, avoid scientific nuance and technical detail. Second, state clearly whether or not the primary objective of the clinical trial was met. Whichever the case, state clearly the implications of these data to the clinical development plan: if it needs redirection, state what that redirection is, and the implication for the registration timeline.

Copyright

Copyright exists to prevent the exploitation of a publication (or trademark) by anyone other than the publisher. This protection of the right to exploit a publication is central to the promotion of publishing *per se*, and thus an incentive to disseminate free speech.

In most developed countries, copyright can exist in two forms. First, for a fee, the protected publication can be registered with the national office of copyright. Second, the copyright holder can simply assert in the publication ownership of copyright under the Common Law. Both forms may use the familiar © symbol. The registered copyright is easier to enforce in court because the date of registration and priority of first publisher are on independent record and can be compared to the behavior of the alleged infringer. The Common Law alternative can also be legally enforced, but requires the development of a set of evidence; an infringer usually has at least an initial defense that due search of the national register failed to locate the alleged infringed copyright.

It is a peculiar and remarkable aspect of academic journals that their publishers make a profit while receiving almost all their copy entirely for free. Almost all journals require transfer of copyright from authors to publisher upon acceptance of submitted manuscripts. Technically, this requires that authors need specific permission from the publisher to use their own manuscripts later; in practice this permission is routinely granted upon written application. A few journals now seek only exclusive licenses from authors, one condition of which preserves the authors' right to personally use their own work, and which leaves copyright ownership with the author(s); the license can also become void if the publisher fails to exploit it, and can yield royalties to the authors. In practice, this license removes the administrative burden of granting routine permissions by the publisher, and royalties on journal reprints are either nominal or absent.

But there are exceptions. Copyright for publications is not universal. In the US, manuscripts from Federal employees cannot be claimed as proprietary because their work product is deemed always to belong to the general public, whether published or not. Most journals operate a copyright exemption system for this purpose. In many countries outside of North America, Australasia, or Europe, copyright, if it exists at all, is unenforceable.

Reprints disseminated for medical information or marketing purposes should be those purchased from the publisher. Alternatively, photocopying license fees can be paid, and in the US a national clearing house exists for this purpose. Direct purchase of .pdf copies of published papers from publishers is now also common online.

Every website page can potentially be copyrighted. Few are actually registered, although assertion of Common Law copyright is common. So far, there has been insufficient litigation to delimit the copyright aspects of electronic publishing.

Summary and prospectus

In summary, the construction of a clinical trial report for use in the peer-reviewed literature is much like that for any other scientific paper; it must contain most of the things that would appear in the executive summary of a clinical report used for regulatory purposes. Clues for effective oral presentations are also provided. Systems for publication of clinical trials are currently neither comprehensive nor universally available to the relevant target audiences. Pharmaceutical companies and journal editors both introduce publication bias; the former is likely only to expend resources in reporting, and the latter is likely only to publish, clinical trials with positive outcomes. Registration of clinical trials should be routine. Electronic publications are making the publication of every clinical trial easier, whether positive or negative.

References

(Note: all the websites cited in this chapter were accessed April 24, 2010.)

Bonk RJ. *Medical Writing in Drug Development*. Pharmaceutical Products Press/Haworth Press: Binghamton, NY, USA, 1997, 77–81. ISBN 0-7890-0174-8.

Cady RK, Wendt JK, Kirchner JR, Sargent JD, Rothrock JF, Skaggs H. Treatment of acute migraine with subcutaneous sumatriptan. *JAMA* 1991; **265**:2831–2835. (See especially the footnote to the first column on page 2831, and the acknowledgments).

Chalmers I. Underreporting research is scientific misconduct. *JAMA* 1990; **338**:367–371.

Chalmers I. A symbiosis of paper and electronic publishing, serving the interests of the journal's readers. *Br J Psychiatr* 1999; **175**:1–2.

Chalmers I, Altman DG. How can medical journals help prevent poor medical research? Some opportunities

presented by electronic publishing. *Lancet* 1999; **353**: 490–493.

De Angelis C, Drazen J, Frizelle FA, *et al*. Clinical trial registration: a statement from the International Committee of Medical Journal Editors. *New Eng J Med* 2004; **351**:1250–1251.

Delamothe T, Smith R. The joy of being electronic. The BMJ's website is mushrooming. *Br Med J* 1999; **319**: 465–466.

Dickersin K, Min YL, Meinert CL. factors influencing publication of research results: follow-up of applications submitted to two institutional review boards. *JAMA* 1992; **267**:374–378.

Fromter E, Brahler E, Langenbeck U, Meenen NM, Usadel KH. Das AWMF-Modell zur Evaluierung publizierter Forschungsbeitrage in der Medizin. *Dtsch Med Wochenschr* 1999; **124**:910–915.

Geddes JR. The contribution of information technology to improving clinicians' access to high quality evidence. *Int J Psychiatr Med* 1999; **29**:287–292.

Gray BS. Health communicators as agents for social change. *Am Med Writers Assoc J* 1994; **9**:11–14.

Horton R, Smith R. Time to register randomised trials. *Br J Med* 1999; **319**:865–866.

McConnell J, Horton R. Lancet electronic research archive in international health and eprint server. *Lancet* 1999; **354**:2–3.

Peckham M. Research and development for the National Health Service. *Lancet* 1991; **338**:367–371.

Rafal RB. A standardized method for determination of who should be listed as authors on scholarly papers. *Chest* 1991; **99**:786.

Roberts I. An amnesty for unpublished trials. *Br Med J* 1998; **317**:763–764.

Simes RJ. Publication bias: the case for an international registry of clinical trials. *J Clin Oncol* 1986; **4**:1529–1541.

Skelton J. Analysis of the structure of original research papers: an aid to writing original papers for publication. *Br J Gen Pract* 1994; **44**:455–459.

Song F, Eastwood A, Gilbody S, Duley L. The role of electronic journals in reducing publication bias. *Med Inform Internet Med* 1999; **24**:223–229.

Sykes R. Being a modern pharmaceutical company. *Br Med J* 1998; **317**:1172–1180.

The Subcutaneous Sumatriptan International Study Group. Treatment of migraine attacks with sumatriptan. *New Eng J Med* 1991; **325**:316–321.

Tonks A. Registering clinical trials. *Br Med J* 1999; **319**: 1565–1568.

CHAPTER 47

Organizing and Planning Local, Regional, National, and International Meetings and Conferences

Zofia Dziewanowska[1] & Linda Packard[2]
[1]New Drug Associates, Inc., La Jolla, CA, USA
[2]American Academy of Pharmaceutical Physicians, Research Triangle Park, NC, USA

Using scientific meetings appropriately can be one of the most powerful tools for the promotion and Phase IV development of corporate assets. Other types of meeting, crucial in the development process, are investigators' meetings, pan-corporate international staff meetings, and conferences to resolve issues of harmonization or standardize clinical trial methodology. Almost all clinicians working in the industry will, from time-to-time, find themselves taking part in such meetings, whether as speaker, attendee, reporter, or chairperson.

Most clinicians lack formal training in meeting planning. Hands-on experience is always the best tutor, but perhaps here we can provide some clues and frameworks for how meetings take place.

In this chapter, we concentrate on large meetings. Small meetings will obviously only require a subset of this information.

Goals, types of meetings, and participants

It is usually best to start with the goals of the proposed meeting. This will dictate the type of meeting, its duration, and participants. Organizational approval of these goals is a *sine qua non* and

should be obtained early. Table 47.1 provides some examples.

With the goals of the meeting in place, the format and content of the meeting can then be designed. Usually, this works best if a meeting chairperson or central organizer can be identified. This should be a person experienced in the type of meeting that is envisaged, one who can clearly enunciate a vision for the future meeting to the many and varied people who will eventually have to implement the plan. In the case of large meetings (see Table 47.2) there may be separable parts, and desirable chairpersons for each part may well differ in their background and experiences (see Table 47.3).

Large meetings inevitably require professional organizers, while small ones might simply use volunteers. One way or the other, these people deserve good leadership, and it will be your meeting that suffers if those deployed are not put to good use. Professional organizers will obtain the relevant physical space for the meeting, get the meeting advertised (if appropriate), coordinate the preparatory materials and their distribution, handle the catering contract(s), manage registration, handle the social and companion programs, and basically do everything that you do not want to do. Getting a local meeting professional is always best: they will know the management of the facility itself, as well as the potential for local tours, activities, and so on.

Principles and Practice of Pharmaceutical Medicine, 3rd edition.
Edited by L.D. Edwards, A.W. Fox, P.D. Stonier.
© 2011 Blackwell Publishing Ltd.

Table 47.1 Typical goals of conferences and meetings

To exchange scientific opinion and information
To educate a target audience
To secure consistency of clinical trial conduct and evaluation
To obtain peer/opinion leader review input
To obtain drug recognition among relevant clinicians
To launch a new drug with a sales force
To promote a new drug, or a newly-approved indication for an old drug

Table 47.3 Leadership of separable components of large meetings

Chairperson of the scientific program
Chairperson of the social program
Collaborators and Advisory Board members
Moderators of individual sessions
Speakers and panelists
Judges of presentations
Poster display organizer
Organizers of registration and attendees' services
Audiovisual coordinator
Director of supply and serving food and beverages
Partnering meetings coordinator

The schedule of the scientific program is usually pivotal in a large meeting, and everything must fit in around it. It goes without saying that the scientific chairperson must be a thought-leader in the meeting's topic(s). However, another vital qualification is that this eminent person must also be somebody who is willing to cooperate with lesser mortals, and who is decisive, consistent, and communicative. The advisory board, if there is to be one, should generate comments on a draft of the scientific program that the scientific chairperson provides early. With that advice the scientific chairperson can finalize the program, and then recruit the speakers and moderators.

The key word for speaker and moderator recruitment is balance. Balance should be sought not only in diverging scientific opinion, but also in the geographical origins of the speakers and moderators. The latter must be people who can broach no subversion of accurate time keeping, and yet impose that discipline on speakers politely. In preparation and in the conduct of international meetings, especially multicenter investigators' meetings, one

Table 47.2 Types of meeting depending upon meeting goals

Multicenter investigators' meeting
Advisory board/consultants' meeting
Intra-company product launch meeting
Satellite symposia at meetings of academic societies
Regulatory presentations
Therapeutic review conferences
International Conference on Harmonization (ICH) subcommittees

has to be particularly sensitive to the difficulties of the attendees in understanding presentations in the foreign languages. More extensive use of audiovisual tools may be very helpful. While the investigators are usually very familiar with English, their coordinators and the other staff may be much less so.

Time and place

For a large-scale conference, if you start less than 18 months in advance you are usually headed for disaster. Every effort must be made at this early stage to avoid dates that conflict with other conferences that may attract the same audience, and thus compete, with yours. This planning interval can become smaller as meetings become smaller, but a multi-investigator protocol meeting can usually not attract all the required participants with less than three or four months notice.

Constructing (or purchasing) a mailing list should be the next early step. Contact details for known participants, and a set of characteristics for desirable unknown participants, should be defined. For the latter, until registrations are received, advertising in relevant journals may be the only way to contact them.

Geographical location for the meeting is the next decision. This can be an iterative process when it turns out that there is no suitable meeting facility in the place that would minimize the aggregate travel time and costs for the participants: again, the larger the facility required, the longer the lead time.

Convention halls in major cities are often booked years in advance; one general rule is to start booking one year ahead of the event for every 100 attendees expected, up to a maximum of five years. Small meetings in university towns can often collide with events such as graduations or (in the USA) sporting events, and accommodations in even small hotels may be unavailable or highly expensive. When the location is known and the facility is booked, this is material for a press release and another round of conference announcement mailings if it is a large, commercial meeting.

Budgets

If the meeting is purely company-sponsored, the meeting organizer should determine the size and location of the meeting, calculate the costs, and present the budget for approval. If that budget is cut back, the number of attendees, duration of the meeting, and/or social program can be adjusted downwards accordingly. If there would appear to be no compromise between a budget that is too small and the number of attendees desired, do not forget to consider breaking the meeting into two smaller ones at different geographical locations; reductions in travel costs can compensate for the economy of scale that might be achieved with a single large meeting. Sometimes the location of two meetings may be determined by the primary language of the area, for example, English versus Spanish speaking continents.

Satellite symposia usually come with fixed price-tags payable to the sponsoring academic society. If the budget will not support it, shop around; almost every discipline has more than one annual meeting of interest. Furthermore, contracting for a satellite symposium at each annual meeting for the next three years can obtain a volume discount, but you should reserve the right to retail those that you have paid for, just in case you do not need them.

Some professional academic organizations specifically prohibit a concomitant yet conflicting meeting, especially sponsored by the industry, and so specific permission should be sought.

There has recently been a lot of adverse publicity pertaining to the symposia sponsored by the pharmaceutical industry, accusing the sponsoring industry of unfairly promoting its product and/or unapproved indications. The meeting organizer has to be particularly sensitive to this fact and has to review the current regulations and restrictions, specific often to a particular country and/or regulatory agency, prior to arranging the meeting.

If the meeting planned includes paid registrations, seek professional help with the budget. The process will be much more complicated, and dependent upon the rates of registration, both actual and projected, in order to trim the meeting expenditures where it may be necessary, and avoid going broke!

Promoting the meeting

The mailings, fliers, e-mail reminders, and press releases should begin 8–12 months before the event. A schedule for regular promotions should be set out at the beginning of the planning process.

Licenses and permits

Usually, the facility that you have chosen will be able to tell you whether any of these are needed. Usually, applications made six months before the event are sufficient.

Registrations

Opening early-bird registration five months before the event is usually effective, and a motivating discount is usually good for early cash flows. The outline program should be ready at this point, even if some of the participants have either not yet replied to the invitation or are to be determined. Calls for papers and abstracts can also begin at this time. Both early-bird registrations and scientific submissions should have deadlines, and it is best if these are rigidly adhered to. Otherwise you will be bombarded by supplicants for exceptions and special treatment!

One month before the event

All the programs should be finalized, and the definitive version printed. All audiovisual bookings and menus should be contracted. The remnants of the hotel room reservation block can then be released (those registering at the door can fend for themselves). This is a good time to send out reminder postcards with basic information: where and when registration is, location and directions to the facility, and the name of the nearest airport or railway station. The publication plan should also be agreed at this point.

Two weeks before the event

Most caterers will want final numbers on food and beverages being served. The meeting staff should be taught how to find their way round the facility, and where, nearby, such things as business services, restaurant advice, and traveling essentials can be obtained.

Half a day before the event

Train the registration desk staff, make friends with the audiovisual people, and test all their systems. Set up the message board and signage to all the conference rooms.

Feedback

During the conference ask the attendees what they think about it. In some cases, for example where medical education credits are offered, there will probably be a formal mechanism required for the scientific content. However, even a small meeting might engender unexpected opinions on the hotel rooms, the food, or the travel arrangements, and these can only add to your own experience as well as contribute to the success of the next meeting you are planning.

The first to arrive and the last to leave

The meeting staff will probably be required to remain at the facility for at least a day and a half after the final gavel. Dismantling display materials, finalizing invoice arrangements with vendors, and getting the proceedings publication started are common tasks. There should also be a time for general recovery and celebration; the latter will enhance morale, and, if you can retain them, make next year's conference easier.

Summary

Arranging and running large meetings are tough and time-consuming. Patience, ability, decisiveness, and good communication under pressure are essential. Review of current regulatory and/or academic regulations regarding industry sponsored meetings needs to be followed, but the rewards, both personally and professionally can be great, and the payback for the sponsor will make it all worthwhile.

CHAPTER 48

When Things Go Wrong: Drug Withdrawals from the Market

Ronald D. Mann

Professor Emeritus, University of Southampton, UK

Introduction

From the point of view of a pharmaceutical company, the worst way in which things can go wrong is when the marketing authorization for a major product is threatened with revocation or suspension due to reports of serious or fatal adverse drug reactions.

The losses involved in such a disaster can be so sudden and so damaging that the threat polarizes the Managing Director, the Medical Director, the Marketing Manager, and the rest of the executives, and sets them apart from one another. In most cases it also bewilders them, for it is highly unlikely that any of them will have previously faced such a situation.

The relevant literature that might provide useful examples and guidance is pretty sparse. Micturin (terodiline hydrochloride) was withdrawn from sale in 1991 after it was discovered that its use was associated with serious cardiac arrhythmias, most notably a rare and sometimes fatal form of ventricular tachycardia known as *torsades de pointes*. As we shall shortly see, other drugs have been withdrawn for the same reason but the story of terodiline was written up by the physician who was Medical Director of the relevant company at the time. This account (Wild, 2002) should be read by anyone who may become involved in a sudden drug withdrawal due to toxicity, for it represents one of the few such firsthand accounts in the literature.

A comparable account of the withdrawal of nomifensine due to the unexpected occurrence of hemolytic anemia has also been published (Stonier and Edwards, 2002) and, again, this account records the views and experience of the physician who was Medical Director of the relevant company at the time of the crisis and drug withdrawal.

It is a staggering fact that in the present state of scientific knowledge we cannot prevent the loss, after marketing, of licensed pharmaceuticals that are found to produce unexpected grave toxicity. This has been known for virtually 40 years and yet the pharmaceutical industry has not seen fit to organize itself collectively to protect companies that suffer these unexpected and damaging drug withdrawals.

Drug regulatory bodies were set up in Europe in response to the thalidomide disaster of the very early 1960s. In the United Kingdom, drug regulation began with the Committee on Safety of Drugs, which was chaired by Sir Derrick Dunlop. This Committee (the forerunner of the Committee on Safety of Medicines) functioned from January 1, 1964, until it provided its last report for the combined years of 1969 and 1970. The experience of those six or seven years led the Committee to make the following quite remarkable statement in its final report (Committee on Safety of Drugs, 1971):

> *No drug which is pharmacologically effective is entirely without hazard. The hazard may be insignificant or may be acceptable in relation to the drug's therapeutic action. Furthermore, not all hazards can be known before a drug*

Principles and Practice of Pharmaceutical Medicine, 3rd edition.
Edited by L.D. Edwards, A.W. Fox, P.D. Stonier.
© 2011 Blackwell Publishing Ltd.

is marketed: neither tests in animals nor clinical trials in patients will always reveal all the possible side effects of a drug. These may only be known when the drug has seen administered to large numbers of patients over considerable periods of time.

Thus, we can try to prevent these drug disasters to the maximum extent possible, we can try to identify and diagnose them at the earliest possible date (and so minimize the number of patients hurt or disadvantaged), but in the present state of scientific knowledge we cannot eliminate drug withdrawals due to unexpected toxicity.

A list of 39 drugs withdrawn due to major safety concerns in the UK between 1975 and 2005 has been published (Mann, 2005) and the list is summarized in Table 48.1.

It is notable that 11 (28%) of these withdrawals were due to causes that appeared only once in

Table 48.1 Reasons for 39 drug withdrawals: UK 1975–2005

Reason for withdrawal	Number of drugs withdrawn
Hepatotoxicity[1]	9
Cardiovascular[2]	5
Arrhythmias[3]	4
Skin and mucus membrane lesions[4]	4
Gastrointestinal lesions[5]	2
Blood disorders[6]	2
Anaphylaxis[7]	2
Others (singles only)[8]	11
Total	39

Key:
1: benoxaprofen, clomacran phosphate, perhexiline, dilevalol, pemolin, troglitazone, tolcapone, trovafloxacin, kava-kava.
2: fenfluramine, dexfenfluramine, droperidol, amfepramone phenteramine, rofecoxib.
3: terodiline, sertindole (license restored), grepafloxacin, cisapride.
4: practolol, fenclofenac, feprazone, valdecoxib.
5: indoprofen, Osmosin.
6: nomifensine, remoxipride.
7: zomepirac, Althesin.
8: polidexide, zimeldine, suprofen, metipranolol eye drops, triazolam, temafloxacin, remoxipride, mibefradil, pumactant, cerivastatin, coproxamol.

the 30 years considered in the table. Examples are polidexide, withdrawn in 1975 because the formulation contained impurities, and coproxamol, withdrawn in 2005 because it was frequently used in suicides. The most common single cause of withdrawal was hepatotoxicity (nine drugs withdrawn), but adverse cardiovascular events, if grouped with arrhythmias, were equally conspicuous. Drugs that challenge liver function would seem poor candidates for development and it seems reasonable to suggest that prolongation of the QTc interval clearly needs to be carefully excluded before new drugs move very far along their path of development.

Prevention is better than cure

It is now well understood that post-marketing surveillance (PMS) must be undertaken when newly licensed drugs enter everyday clinical usage. The data available at the time of marketing speak far more fully to the efficacy and quality of the drug than they speak to its safety. This is because the number of patients included in the clinical trials is small compared with the number of patients who can be exposed once the drug is available for prescription; additionally, the populations are very different, because the prelaunch program will have been conducted in patients with only one disease, whereas the drug, once licensed, will often be used in an older population of patients with more than one disease. Thus, the PMS program should emphasize populations covering the age ranges appropriate to the indications for the drug; it should also include appropriate drug–drug interaction studies and studies in any special populations, such as children, who may receive the drug once it is in everyday clinical usage. Clearly, the PMS program needs to include studies intended to resolve any queries or questions that have been noted in the animal safety evaluation studies or the earlier studies in humans.

A great deal of guidance is now available and is, in its essentials, common to all areas of the developed world. The fundamentals are given in the *Guidance for Industry—Good Pharmacovigilance Practices and Pharmacoepidemiologic Assessments*

(http://www.fda.gov/Drugs/GuidanceCompliance
RegulatoryInformation/default.htm; accessed April
24, 2010). This document outlines the methods
of obtaining and assessing observational data
regarding drugs; it considers the methods of
detecting signals of adverse effects, assessing and
interpreting these signals, and planning effective
PMS. A second similar document is entitled
*Guidance for Industry—E2E—Pharmacovigilance
Planning*. This is available on the same website
and is, in essence, concerned with the generation
and review of a formal plan for the conduct of
a well thought out PMS or pharmacovigilance
program. The third document in this series is
entitled *Guidance for Industry—Development and Use
of Risk Minimization Action Plans*. This document,
like those of other regulatory authorities, has
arisen from discussion over recent years and it
accepts that there is a risk, and plans to discuss the
risk and minimize it. Not to plan and conduct an
effective pharmacovigilance and risk minimization
program is clearly negligent.

"When the balloon goes up"

The threat to the marketing authorization usually
develops very rapidly and often in response to an
event that grossly biases the data. Typically, a few
worrying reports have been trickling in and then
one of the regulatory bodies makes an announcement seeking additional data—and this produces
a flood. Doctors and other reporters remember a
case they could not make up their minds about,
but the announcement, however gentle, makes up
their minds for them and they report. The trickle
becomes a flood and the company is put on notice
that action of some sort is likely to have to be
taken. There is no sacred text that tells the officers
of a company what to do, but the following steps
should, experience suggests, be considered:

1. Organize a task force of appropriate in-house
experts and specialists supported by outside consultants who have lived through the presenting
kind of problem before. Support the task force
by obtaining the advice of two or three national
specialists whose expertise is directly relevant to the
problem. The task force should be chaired by the
Chief Executive Officer and contain the Research
Director, Medical Director, Legal Advisor, Head of
Regulatory Affairs, and the Principals dealing with
the product in question. It should meet frequently,
have an organized agenda, and record minutes.

2. Advise the regulatory authority who is on the
task force and who is its Technical Secretary and
contact point. This will reassure the regulatory
people with whom it is essential to establish professionally trustworthy relationships.

3. If any information has leaked out (e.g., by
requests for additional data), prepare a sensible and
comprehensive press release. This should emphasize that these problems cannot be prevented as
rare events but they can and are being controlled.
Have one Press Liaison Officer and allow no other
press contacts. Any evidence of a "cover-up" provides the press with a story in its own right and this
is best avoided by openness.

4. In an organized way, re-examine the molecular
structure of the drug and the known adverse effects
of related molecules. In the same way, revisit the
animal safety evaluation data and the clinical trials
data to make sure, in the light of the new suspicion,
that nothing has been missed.

5. Get full but anonymized copies of the suspected
Adverse Drug Reaction (ADR) reports in the hands
of the regulatory authority. Eliminate duplicate and
triplicate reports (as these can swell the numbers in
an alarming way). Do everything possible to ensure
that the reports have been followed up properly
and the final diagnosis established. Make sure that
patients suffering from inborn errors of metabolism
are not being included just because they are receiving the drug in question. Look for clustering, for
example, several reports coming from the same
doctor or practice (is the so-called hepatotoxicity
really a local outbreak of viral hepatitis or due to
some strange doctor still giving aspirin to children
and causing Reye syndrome?).

6. Carefully reassess the balance of benefit and
risk and determine if this has changed and, if
so, in what way. The ADR data (yellow cards
in the UK) form the numerator. The company
is in the best position to know the number of
patients treated (the denominator). Has the ratio

changed? What is the indication for the drug (rare, severe adverse effects may be acceptable in an effective anticancer agent, whereas almost total safety would be demanded for an oral contraceptive used in fit, healthy people early in adult life). If the drug is withdrawn, what remedies remain for the management of the indication—and what is the picture of their comparative toxicity? Make quite sure that the problem is not arising from some new, previously undescribed iatrogenic disease (e.g., the oculomucocutaneous syndrome with practolol); in a similar way, rule out long latency adverse reactions (e.g., sclerosing peritonitis—again with practolol). Be careful to determine what other drugs the patients were receiving (is the problem a drug–drug interaction?).

7. Consider whether the current pharmacovigilance program is adequate to deal with the new issues arising. The situation may have greatly changed—new data may focus attention on one specific adverse effect and, for example, a case control study on that reaction might need to be established with the General Practitioner Research Database (GPRD), or some other database, as a matter of extreme urgency. It is now known what the cases must be in such a study and that changes the picture completely. Any such study must almost always need to be conducted in an existing database as time and the urgency of the situation will not permit any study that requires the prospective acquisition of data.

Escaping from the maze

Although escape may be impossible, and the drug has to be withdrawn in the best interests of the patients, there have been survivors. The techniques used have included the following:

1. *Focused surveillance*: The classic example is clozapine and the Clozaril Patient Monitoring Service. Clozapine is a valuable antischizophrenic agent used in patients unresponsive to other antipsychotic agents. Its side effect profile includes fatal agranulocytosis, myocarditis, and cardiomyopathy. Because the drug can be effective in severe schizophrenia when other remedies have failed it was desired to maintain it in clinical use despite the known incidence of uncommon blood dyscrasias and cardiac adverse reactions. This was accomplished by establishing the Clozaril Patient Monitoring Service with which the patient, prescriber, and supplying pharmacist must be registered before the drug will be supplied. The monitoring service ensures that leukocyte and differential blood counts, plus other observations, are undertaken at suitable intervals. The scheme has been highly effective and similar schemes have been established by other pharmaceutical houses supplying the drug. Clearly, this kind of intense focused management can be used only when it will prevent withdrawal of a uniquely valuable therapeutic agent active against life threatening disease.

2. *Contraindication in a susceptible subpopulation*: Aspirin (acetylsalicylic acid) has been associated with the occurrence of Reye syndrome and, as a result, the Committee on Safety of Medicines has advised that aspirin containing preparations should not be given to children and adolescents under 16 years of age unless specifically indicated, for example for Kawasaki syndrome. Establishing this contraindication, relating to what is probably the most widely used medicine known, involved educating the whole community and represented one of the most remarkable therapeutic achievements of the late 20th century. The literature on the difficulties that are encountered in getting doctors to observe new contraindications is very extensive and it is clear that this procedure is not to be lightly undertaken.

3. *Consider the formulation*: Osmosin was a modified release preparation of indomethacin. It was designed to release the active drug under osmotic control. Instead it allowed its potassium content to be released in a way that caused perforation of the small bowel distal to the duodenum. The drug provides an example of the formulation causing the problem, and the drug serves as a reminder that consideration needs to be given to the formulation as a possible cause of trouble, which can be remedied by reformulation.

4. *Get the dose right*: Problems readily arise if the development program gets locked into the wrong dose range early on. It is important to titrate dose ranges down to lessen Type A side effects and to make sure that domiciliary patients are not treated with a dose that is appropriate for seriously ill, hospitalized subjects.

5. *Consider the indication*: Very little will be tolerated, in terms of side effects, for oral contraceptives or other drugs to be used in young, fit people early in life. The situation is different in respect of anticancer drugs used late in life in patients who have a disease with a poor prognosis. Trimming down the indications and claims made for the drug can materially affect the benefit-to-risk ratio. In assessing this ratio, consideration has to be given to the treatability of any side effects, the drugs available to treat the indication if the suspect drug is withdrawn, and the fate of those many patients using the suspect drug with benefit and without complaint.

6. *The availability of additional data*: The first year after launch can be a difficult time because very few of the important data sources are fully functional apart from the ADR data. Thus, the Medical Department needs to monitor the Drug Analysis Print (DAP) very carefully and review all ADR reports received by the company with equal diligence. One cannot set up case control or similar studies until one knows what cases are relevant. Even then it needs to be remembered that the GPRD covers only a minor proportion of the population, and so cases may be few and far between in the first months of the life of the drug. Prescription-Event Monitoring (PEM) also tends to start fairly slowly because there is a delay before the Prescription Pricing Authority (in the UK) sends out the first batches of prescriptions; then there will be a delay of perhaps six months before the first batches of the green form questionnaire are sent out to general practitioners (again, in the UK).

Doctors in Scotland tend to be cautious about prescribing new drugs and so the record-linkage programs of the Medicines Evaluation and Monitoring Organization (MEMO) also tend to get off to a slow start. The point is that the ADR data and the DAPs need to be watched like a hawk. It has been suggested that the DAP data should be reanalyzed to make their clinical significance easier to understand and this exercise may well be worth the time devoted to it (Mann, 2005). In respect of matters in the UK, the GPRD is of special value, and one needs to know, at reasonably short intervals, the number of reports of the new drug on the database and what those reports comprise. It is a major feature of the database that its data were collected before any alert appeared—the data can be divided into two: before and after the alert, that is, before and after gross bias distorted the picture.

7. *Consider the legal position carefully*: The tests are now onerous, because one must consider not only negligence but also the Product Liability Directive and the Consumer Protection Act with its requirement that the product must be as safe as the consumer might reasonably expect it to be. Among others, the medical people need expert and objective legal guidance. If one reads nothing else in preparation for dealing with responsibilities in this area, it is wise quietly to read through the approved judgment of Mr Justice Mackay in the oral contraceptive litigation (Mackay, 2002).

References

Committee on Safety of Drugs. *Report for 1969 and 1970*. HMSO: London, UK, 1971.

Mackay, The Honourable Mr Justice. Neutral Citation No: (2002) EWHC 1420 (QB). In the High Court of Justice, Queens Bench Division, Approved Judgment. Case No: 0002638, 2002.

Mann RD. A ranked presentation of the MHRA/CSM Drug Analysis Print (DAP) data on practolol. *Pharmacoepidemiol Drug Safety* 2005; **14**:705–710.

Stonier PD, Edwards JG. Nomifensine and haemolytic anaemia. In *Pharmacovigilance*, Mann, RD, Andrews EB (eds). John Wiley & Sons Ltd: Chichester, UK, 2002, 155–166.

Wild RN. Micturin and torsades de pointes. In *Pharmacovigilance*, Mann RD, Andrews EB (eds). John Wiley & Sons Ltd: Chichester, UK, 2002, 129–134.

CHAPTER 49

International Trials: Successful Planning and Conduct

Katie P.J. Wood
Foster City, CA, USA

In the past decade, just as science has progressed immeasurably, so too have the complexities of planning and executing clinical trials. Conducting an international clinical trial is now extremely complicated, with multiple organizations, people and functions, and a myriad of activities, all of which need to be coordinated in a timely and efficient manner. Clinical operations, as a specialty, has come a long way since 1747 when James Lind FRCS of the Royal Navy proved the effectiveness of citrus juice in preventing scurvy in the first controlled, parallel group clinical trial!

In the ever-changing climate that is our world today, the importance of always checking local regulations and relying on local expertise cannot be underestimated. Regulations and local laws and policies are in a constant state of flux and what works in one country one day may not necessarily be the same even just one or two months later. Ignorance is not bliss when defending oneself against the regulatory authority or ethics committee in a foreign country where a clinical trial is being conducted, and the national competent authority wants to conduct an inspection.

Why do international studies at all?

With all the complexities involved, the first question to ask is why global studies are even con-

ducted. Apart from the obvious examples of diseases that exist with clearly uneven geographical prevalences (malaria, tuberculosis, Chagas disease, etc.), the advantages are often substantial:

- Access to patient populations with differential epidemiological and genetic composition, so as to assist in understanding whether the drug's mechanism of action can be truly generalized.
- Opportunity to develop a local base of experience and support that can guide larger studies and/or marketing the drug in the region.
- The opportunity to obtain parallel registration in many countries and thus early market support.
- Economies of time, and (less commonly, see below) cost in recruiting large studies.
- Capability to study diseases that are relatively uncommon in substantial patient numbers.

The Tufts Center for the Study of Drug Development analyzed the Bioresearch Monitoring Information System Files. This showed that, in 1997, of all the FDA Form 1572s, 86% were from the USA, 9% from Western Europe, and 5% from the rest of the world (ROW). Ten years later, in 2007, these figures were 57% from the USA, 14% from Western Europe, and 29% from the ROW. This demonstrates clearly that the clinical research industry has globalized.

Populations and their clinical behaviors

The first questions to ask when planning any clinical study in any indication are medical: One must analyze the required patient population in all its aspects. Are there potential population/genetic

Principles and Practice of Pharmaceutical Medicine, 3rd edition.
Edited by L.D. Edwards, A.W. Fox, P.D. Stonier.
© 2011 Blackwell Publishing Ltd.

differences that may alter recruitment rates or pose clinical hazards? Moreover, if it is an anti-infective study, this applies to the microorganism too, for example, is hepatitis C mostly genotype I in both Italy and the United Kingdom? There may also be a need to study a particular route of drug delivery or device because different countries have varying medical practices: Is a suppository study really going to find patient acceptance outside of France? There are also huge differences in "standard of care" between countries, and these need to be considered when conducting active comparator trials.

Infrastructures available

The next thing to investigate is the infrastructure of the countries in which you are proposing to work. This again varies hugely, and usually (but not always) in line with the degree of economic development; when selecting clinical trial sites, there may also be large differences from region-to-region within a single country, and these need to be taken into account. It is the standard of infrastructure (or the lack of it) that will drive the resources needed at each clinical trial site, and in some cases eliminate that site from consideration.

Clinical endpoint complexities

Next, clinical endpoints (disease indexes, measurement scales, and laboratory units) vary widely around the world. All this should be addressed at the outset of any project planning regardless of whether it is for a single country, single center, small number of subjects study, or a large, multinational Phase III or IV study involving hundreds or thousands of subjects.

Database management

Any Central Laboratory used needs to have the capability to convert and do data transfers of US and ex-US data in the same format. It is important to consider that when conversion of units from SI to Conventional or vice-versa occurs, occasionally this can cause a value to fall outside the normal range causing a high or low flag. A good example is the counting of large numbers (white and red blood cell counts) in India and Iran by Crore (in India one crore = ten million, but in the Persian numbering system one crore = 500,000, thus even defeating a conversion by a factor of ten). This can therefore require database checks that are more sophisticated than usual, so as to avoid querying data erroneously. Rules need to be put in place to avoid immense frustration when trying to lock the database at the end of the study!

Concomitant therapies

Another important goal at the early planning stage should be to find out what other drug or non-drug treatments are commonly used and how these might differentially bias the outcome of the clinical trial. In the Far East, for example, herbal treatments are widely prescribed and used: Can the case report form capture these? Moreover (particularly in Europe) the use of placebo is becoming increasingly less accepted; placebo controlled trials are less likely to receive ethics committee approval than standard of care active-comparator studies. Can the study design tolerate different comparator treatments in different countries? This may well be the case if they are all thought genuinely to be without effect.

Quality analysis

Why is it that many international clinical protocols never specify precisely who is responsible for the quality of what? The *Good Clinical Practices* (GCP) guidelines know no national boundaries, and state unambiguously:

> *The sponsor is responsible for implementing and maintaining quality assurance and quality control systems with written SOPs to ensure that trials are conducted and data are generated, documented (recorded) and reported in compliance with the protocol, GCP, and the applicable regulatory requirement(s)* (ICH/GCP 5.1; ICH, 2002).

> *A sponsor may transfer any or all of the sponsor's trial related duties and functions to a CRO, but the ultimate responsibility for the quality and integrity of the trial data always resides with the sponsor. The CRO should implement quality assurance and quality control* (ICH/GCP 5.2.1; ICH, 2002).

The fundamental point is that responsibility for quality is a three-way partnership between the sponsor, the CRO, and the study site. However, ultimately it is people and office-holders who are responsible for this role, and not the less tangible notion of an entire organization.

Documentation, Standard Operating Procedures (SOPs), and globalization

Documentation is particularly important because clarity of processes and conduct make for a quality trial. When preparing trial documentation, particularly SOPs, we would do well to heed the words of Rudyard Kipling who reminds us (*The Elephant's Child* anthology):

> I had six honest serving men,
> They taught me all I knew
> Their names were *what* and *why* and *when*
> And *how* and *where* and *who*.
> I send them over land and sea,
> I send them east and west;
> But after they have worked for me,
> I give them all a rest.

Documentation is the pivotal tool for the principles of GCP (see Chapter 13). SOPs provide the framework for work of the same quality as might be performed in the USA, Europe, or Japan, and are now widely accepted in most countries of the world. Understanding of the SOPs used by the sponsor and a Contract Research Organization (CRO), and determining which shall apply, is a key early decision, just as it is when using a CRO in one's own country. This is essential to withstand regulatory authority audit, which is inevitable for a pivotal study in a New Drug Application (NDA).

Protocol adherence

Study site monitoring is the skill and art of ensuring that the protocol is, in fact, being followed. The clinical research associates who perform this function are essentially the eyes and ears of the medical monitor. But more importantly, they are the first, and most important, guardian of the sponsor's resources; money and time is wasted if the exercise becomes "garbage in, garbage out." In the international situation this role requires tact, and avoidance of misunderstandings due to cross-cultural differences or language barriers. Major cross-cultural differences exist in the identification of technical error. Take the instance of a simple case report form error, for example, an inconsistency of birthdate and age in years. Simply correcting it at the site so as to prevent yet another database query at the end of the study would seem to be a straight-forward, practical, and completely blameless thing to do. However, in some cultures that are more perfectionist, it can also needlessly be inferred as indicating some sort of inadequacy of the site staff with embarrassment and administrative slowing down as a result.

Trial monitoring

Medical monitors can encounter cross-cultural problems in much the same way as clinical research associates. For some reason, those with medical degrees are held in such high regard in some countries that doctors assume an aura of infallibility. Questioning whether an inclusion/exclusion criterion has been interpreted correctly by the principal investigator (PI) at the site thus becomes an act of heresy and poisons the working relationship forever afterwards. It is for this reason that clinical site monitors (especially in Eastern Europe, Russia, and some parts of the Far East) often hold medical degrees themselves, so that such discussions take place on a more collegial, and less ego-threatening manner.

CRFs and information flow

This uniformity ensures consistency of data and thus knowledge that it can be reproduced again with the same results. Given the many factors discussed above, it is sometimes necessary to handle the data in two stages, first collating at the regional level, before then merging the regions into a single database.

Research in developing countries—controversial?

The Council for International Organizations of Medical Sciences (CIOMS) guidelines state that

No research is to be carried out in developing countries unless it could be carried out in developed countries, and it should be responsive to the health needs and priorities of the country in which it is to be conducted.

By *developed countries*, Europe, most of the Asia-Pacific region, and North America is clearly meant; arguably there are also countries in sub-Saharan Africa, the Caucases, the Indo-Chinese peninsula, India, and most of South America that are now falling within the definition, too. Presuming the relevant biological substrate, CIOMS then recommends that Phase I drug and Phase I and II vaccine studies should be conducted only in the developed communities of the sponsor's country. Phase III vaccine and Phase II and III drug trials should be conducted simultaneously in the sponsor's country (again presuming some prevalence of the appropriate disease there), as well as in developing countries.

The CIOMS 2002 Revisions addressed the wider aspects of labor and medical responsibilities in developing countries. When necessary for the conduct of research, sponsors should provide facilities and personnel to make healthcare services available to the population from which research subjects are drawn. This avoids the diversion of labor, which may be in very short supply, to the clinical trial and away from the ordinary medical services of the clinical trial country.

Consideration should be given to maintenance of the patients that have been studied within the host country after research completed. The National Bioethics Advisory Committee (NBAC, 2001) recommended that researchers and sponsors should make reasonable efforts before study initiation to secure that, at conclusion, continued access to the test medication for all participants should be available in the event that the experimental intervention proved effective. Thus, research proposals should include explanation of how new interventions proven to be effective will be made available to some or all of the host country population beyond research participants

How does the FDA view global trials?

The US FDA has always accepted foreign studies, provided they meet the usual standards of design, conduct, and investigators qualified by experience and training, and are conducted in accordance with ethical principles acceptable to the world community. 21 CFR 312.120 (FDA, 2005) emphasizes that foreign clinical research is required to have been conducted in accordance with the ethical principles stated in "Declaration of Helsinki" and/or the laws and regulations of the country in which the research was conducted, whichever represents the greater protection of the individual.

The ruling replaces the requirement that these studies be conducted in accordance with ethical principles stated in the Declaration of Helsinki issued by the World Medical Association, specifically the 1989 version with a requirement that the studies be conducted in accordance with good clinical practice, including review and approval by an independent ethics committee.

Essentially the FDA will now allow the pharmaceutical industry to run international clinical trials in which patients in the control group can be treated with placebos. The change will have important practical implications as more and more medical research is being done overseas. Doing research in poorer countries offers several benefits for the industry including lower costs and, now, the possibility to use placebos in control groups.

And what, exactly, might Europe be?

Europe is an ever-growing region officially recognizing at least 26 different languages, not to mention regional dialects. Associated with all these languages and dialects are differing cultures. Although the EU has set up common institutions to which it delegates some of its sovereignty, each country is still governed by its own laws many of which impact the conduct of clinical trials and recruitment to those trials.

Licenses for transportation

Import licenses are often required for investigational drug products, and in some countries an export license for trial materials will also be needed (including not only drug but also and laboratory supplies). Practices are highly variable from country-to-country, including licenses for separate shipments, "umbrella licenses," to whom fees are paid, and so on. Seek local expert help.

Drug supplies and the European qualified person (QP)

Article 13 of the EU Directive sets new regulations for the role of the QP with respect to the manufacturer and import of Investigational Medicinal Product. The importance of establishing a *drug supply management and accountability plan* at the study outset cannot be underestimated. Major decisions include establishing whether patient enrollment and drug supply allocation will be managed by an automated or in-house manual method.

Other parts of the study drug management plan include management of drug accountability, return of supplies, and their destruction. These decisions will be dictated in the most part by the type and packaging of the drug under investigation and local rules and regulations (both pharmaceutical and environmental). In Europe, the QP will be held personally liable for any breach of the plan.

Labeling

Annex 13 to *Good Manufacturing Practices* (GMP) guidelines provides detailed guidance on labeling. This includes a statement that the cumbersome details of the address and telephone number of the emergency contact to obtain more information on the clinical trial may be omitted if subjects have been given a leaflet or card that provides these details and they have been instructed to keep this in their possession at all times. The trick is then to comply not only with GMP, but also the additional requirements of the country where the trial is taking place, *and* to arrive at something that is of practical use to the study site and the patient. If the patients will be taking their drug home, it is imperative that the tablet bottle, enema, and so on is labeled in the local language on the bottle,

enema, itself. If medication is to be administered solely in hospital then usually local language labeling is required on the outer packaging only.

Extension of expiry dates

If this is likely to occur in any study, it is necessary to check who can perform this function and when. In some cases the CRO—as sponsor representative—and the pharmacist can do this, whereas other countries may mandate that this be done by the QP. In some places the PI is expected to act as his or her own pharmacist, with the dual set of responsibilities.

Budgeting for drug supply management

This aspect therefore goes beyond just supply, labeling, and shipping. Extra costs of which one should be aware are those involved in any destruction process—especially if destruction has to be done locally. Also to note are the storage costs at any central drug depot both of ready-to-ship supplies and also of returns, which more often than not can only be destroyed in batches rather than as returns are made. Sites may often charge extra for any re-labeling, which is necessary especially if regulations state that this should be done by a local qualified person.

Translations

Translations are never easy. Even English comes in many forms: US, British, Australian, Caribbean, and so, and what is considered to be a 12-year-old reading age in one place may not be the same in another. Spelling and punctuation can change the meaning of words and sentences and it is important to be consistent in the choice of US or British spellings and grammar and to be as concise and clear as possible when detailing protocol definitions and procedures. There is an increasingly standardized language called "Simple English"; the website of the British Broadcasting Corporation (www.bbc.co.uk) includes this as one of the languages its news pages are translated into, and may offer good precedents.

Next, the frequent debate: Which documents require translation and who is going to translate them? There are many commercial organizations that offer these services. One helpful tip is to take the translation provided, and give it to a second, independent translator to convert back into (presumably) English; this process is called *double-translation*. The sponsor should be sure that it can live with the result. The EU is currently working on standardizing the requirements for translations; the European Medicines Agency (EMA) website (www.emea.europa.eu) is expected to furnish further details on this area in mid-2010.

Contracts and finance

Contracts and budgets are an important part of the clinical trial set-up. Their set up and negotiation can affect both the timelines and the overall study budget. The Tufts Center for the study of Drug Development recently reported that of the causes of delay experienced by US sponsors of foreign clinical trials, 52% were due to contract and budget issues and 24% due to slow legal review.

Beware the boilerplate! Contractual boilerplate is among the least negotiated, but most important aspects, of the clinical trial agreement. Many reviewing parties focus on the terms that are directly related to contract performance and just skim over the provisions they have seen so many times before. This is a dangerous practice because "standard" boilerplate is anything but standard. There are often subtle differences that can have a great impact on dispute resolution and the rights or obligations of the party. One of the most common problems is that, by local law, parties may be prevented from stipulating that the contract is governed by a foreign jurisdiction. Delays to timelines can be avoided by resolving that issue at the outset of contract negotiations, although often unspoken is the question of whether a local jurisdiction can rule over some foreign entity. Occasionally, contracts are required to be in the local language and in some countries there needs to be separate contracts for the PI and the institution, as well as for subinvestigators. Double-translation (see above) is again recommended. Contract and budget negotiations are inevitably slower for international studies than for national ones, and room for this needs to be built into the project plan.

It is a common myth that conducting clinical trials outside the "developed" world leads to significant cost savings. Although this may be true in terms of one part of the budget, it may be compensated for in another. For example, there may be economies in study-site grants, but telecommunications costs arise when meetings are not being conducted face-to-face (as do costs for international travel of study staff). Courier costs for shipping samples to central laboratories in another continent, and the shipping supplies, are another expensive item. A budget item that is also often forgotten are the costs of transferring and converting currencies, *per se*, and the inconstancy of conversion rates during studies that last for considerable periods of time. Moreover, where is the helpline for any electronic data capture based? If not in the country, it should at least be within the same continent if not time-zone. Even 24/7 coverage from a distant continent has not always proved effective, and is almost always more expensive than for a study conducted within a single country. These can all add substantial line items to any budget that is supposedly for an economical foreign study.

Disclosure of financial terms is mandated under the EU Clinical Trials Directive (see Chapter 37). This includes the details on proposed financial transactions with the institution/investigator and subject/investigator compensation will need to be provided to the ethics committee. In some EU Member States, responsibility for reviewing this is also scrutinized by the National Competent Authority. Again this adds time and yet more complexity to a process and often underestimated in its impact on the overall study timelines and budget. Under the EU Directive, ethics committees are also required to review the provisions for insurance and indemnity. In addition a statement is often requested regarding the differing sponsor and investigator liabilities.

Insurances

Insurance requirements are in constant flux; costs can change hugely and rapidly in response to natural and unnatural disasters around the world. Many countries require a local insurance as well as a global certificate. Experience has found that it is much quicker to have a local expert address this issue. Indemnity/Liability and Insurance verbiage in contracts needs to account for local requirements and local law. Some countries require that the amount of coverage per patient as well as per the study overall is stipulated. It is very important however to check that the coverage offered is appropriate for the needs of the sponsor as well as the clinical trial site.

Postal systems and avoiding them

Size of paper/envelopes varies internationally and this is important to note if a US sponsor decides to ship binders and paper case report forms to the site. The sizes and types of binders also differ, that is, generally in the EU paper is 2 hole-punched, or sometimes 4-hole punched, but never 3! As the trial progresses and the amount filed in the binders grows, the papers will be harder to keep neat and clean if they are hanging out of a binder into which they do not fit properly! Whose shelf heights must we meet?

With more and more reliance on e-mail and the ability to scan documents rather than fax, it must be remembered that in many countries the ability to do this is limited due to the lack of availability of scanning equipment at study sites.

It is worth noting, however, that although the quality and age of imaging or other machines may be a concern in some countries, it is not correct to assume that those countries in "emerging markets" have worse machines or technology than the Western world. This applies not only to commonly used technologies—the computer, scanner, fax, and so on—but also to specific and highly specialized machines used in the different clinical studies—medical imaging, for example, as well as the various arthro/endo/gastro and other scopes and so on. I recall visiting a site in a little known town in the Czech Republic when the physician with whom I was traveling fell silent with awe at the advanced nature of the endoscopy suite that we were visiting as part of our site qualification process. It does happen that occasionally the hospital buildings themselves may seem to be falling down but the care given inside and the quality of the machinery used is top notch!

Different voltage and thus different plugs/adaptors are required across continents. Do not send electronic equipment without checking local country requirements. It may well be cheaper and logistically simpler to have anything electronic purchased locally (this also applies to infusion pumps).

Patient confidentiality

There are varying regulations regarding the use of patient identifiers. Some countries have gone as far as to no longer allow the patient's initials and date of birth to be used together as an identifier. As these regulations are in a state of flux, it is always advisable to check the local regulations on data protection for any country in which a trial is to be planned.

Miscellanea

Clinical trial materials fall foul of national laws in unexpected ways. Although materials of bovine origin must be certified BSE-free in some countries, they have always been broadly illegal for religious and cultural reasons in others. Pharmaceutical formulations containing ethanol (even in microscopical amounts) are automatically illegal in almost all Islamic countries, as are almost all materials of porcine origin (the sole domestic pig in Iran is a specimen in the Tehran zoo).

Transportation of clinical supplies and laboratory specimens are usually under conditions of greater stress in international studies than within a single country. Study sites in Singapore, for example, will receive supplies that have spent several hours at low temperature in an aircraft hold, only to be then exposed suddenly to an ambient temperature that may exceed body temperature and a thorough soaking by condensation. Moreover, international customs authorities tend to work at their own pace, and will have no concern whatever about leaving your lab samples to bake nicely on the airport apron, not to mention the intense infrared and ultraviolet irradiation. Ask your local sites about couriers that are effective, which is much more important than the place of consignment.

Recruitment

The most important success factor in clinical research subject recruitment is good and timely planning! Going global does have advantages especially for large studies and for rare subject populations.

First, varying demographics create less healthy populations—for example, patterns of smoking and alcohol consumption. A study excluding smokers will go much more slowly at sites in Russia or Germany than in Colorado.

Second, differences in the healthcare environment may create interest in trial participation. Medically underserved populations may view trial participation as a way to improve on otherwise limited access to medication. It requires careful judgment whether this can become a form of duress and thus counter to the notions of autonomy and properly informed consent.

Recruitment strategies to adopt outside of the US are very different to those within. For one thing, the EU directives are explicit that this is within the purview of the ethics committee; arguably, that should be true everywhere.

Culture/local regulations/language and the legal frameworks play a large part in what is and is not allowed to encourage recruitment. Thus it is not really possible or feasible to make standard global recruitment campaigns. Any campaign has to be tailored to the local site needs and capabilities. TV/radio/newspaper advertising will almost always be found unacceptable in less-developed countries. Gifts/gift certificates are also often regarded with suspicion as coercive: "small" gifts by Western standards are large gifts to poor people.

But, on the bright side, international clinical trials may find that there are fewer competing trials in relatively less-developed countries. Moreover, the large medical centers that do exist can serve relatively large catchment areas, and thus provide a higher concentration of candidate patients per study site than is possible in North America or Europe. Also on the bright side, most staff enjoy visiting a place that they consider to be exotic.

Direct communication from the sponsor or CRO by e-mail, letter, or telephone is by far the most successful medium: The relationship between the sites and the sponsor is a critical one and sites expect, and are please to have, direct contact with the sponsor. Newsletters are not taken seriously in some countries, or are even regarded as impolite as an appropriate communication medium—often PIs readily admit that they throw them away! Particularly in emerging markets, a visit by the sponsor is taken very seriously and is generally highly regarded.

Educational grants can be successful. These might allow study staff to attend conferences/seminars. In some countries where clinical research is relatively new, it can also be helpful to offer free, comprehensive, GCP training in the local language as a general educational resource. Purchase of equipment is also usually well-accepted and appreciated—this might include infusion pumps, fax machines, photocopiers, glucometers, and so on.

Communication/cultural diversity in the research team

A multicultural workforce is obligatory for international studies. It is crucial for the members of the clinical trial team to perceive and understand the nature of cultural differences. Always consider the following:
- How am I being perceived?
- How am I best able to communicate?

By taking a little time to understand the culture, history, politics, and socio-economic climate of the countries in which we work, conflict really can be avoided. One also has conversation for those less formal moments, over meals and in work-breaks, which can contribute so much to within-team harmony. It also costs little, except a bit of personal effort.

It is beyond the scope of this chapter to go into the theory and practice of cross-culturalism. However, it is the telephone, of all mediums, that usually causes the most trouble. Telephone tactics must also be super-sensitive in the absence of the body language to go with it. Try to say what you mean as clearly and as simply as possible. Keep language simple and courteous at all times; avoid slang, colloquialisms, and elaborate sentence structures. Repeat, paraphrase, and confirm understanding, and make allowances for the other party to do the same. Misunderstandings can be costly in terms of time and money. Common, if not excessive, courtesy can go a long way in cross-cultural relations, even if it does take a bit of time.

And finally, remember the words of Lord Byron: "Always laugh when you can—it is cheap medicine."

References

FDA. 21 CFR 312.120, 2005; http://edocket.access.gpo.gov/cfr_2009/aprqtr/pdf/21cfr312.120.pdf; accessed April 12, 2010.

ICH (International Conference on Harmonization). *Good Clinical Practices*, 2002; http://ichgcp.net/?page_id=116; accessed April 12, 2010.

NBAC (National Bioethics Advisory Commission). *Ethical and Policy Issues in International Research: Clinical Trials in Developing Countries*, 2001; http://bioethics.georgetown.edu/nbac/clinical/Vol1.pdf; accessed April 12, 2010.

Further reading

CIOMS (Council for International Organizations of Medical Sciences). *International Ethical Guidelines for Biomedical Research Involving Human Subjects*, World Health Organization, 2002. ISBN 0-9290360-7-5-5.

Craig A. *The Interpretation of Clinical Laboratory Data in Safety Studies*. Institute of Clinical Research Publishing, 2004, Version 1.0.

Good P. *A Manager's Guide to the Design and Conduct of Clinical Trials*, second edition. John Wiley & Sons Inc.: New York, USA, 2006. ISBN 978-0-471-78870-6.

Hedgecock A. *Insurance in Clinical Trials*. Institute of Clinical Research Publishing, 2005. Version 1.0. ISBN 0-9549345-6-3.

Jacobs D. *Patient Recruitment in Clinical Research*. Institute of Clinical Research Publishing, 2005. Version 1.0. ISBN 0-9549345-3-9.

Meeson J. *A Pocket Guide to the EU Directive*. Institute of Clinical Research Publishing. 2005. Version 1.0. ISBN 0-9549345-1-2.

Raven A. *Consider It Pure Joy – An Introduction to Clinical Trials*, third edition. Cambridge Healthcare Research: Cambridge, UK, 1997.

Useful websites

(Note: as with all websites cited in this chapter, the following were accessed April 24, 2010.)

www.cioms.ch
www.icr-global.org
http://csdd.tufts.edu
www.bioethics.gov

SECTION VII

Legal and Ethical Aspects of Pharmaceutical Medicine

Introduction

Ethical conduct in both drug development and ordinary clinical practice is obviously *sine qua non*. This section brings together aspects of this essential prerequisite with some of the mechanisms that are used to enforce it.

In drug development, the rare clinical disasters that are well-publicized almost always turn out to have an ethical component during the investigations that follow. Although it is the pharmaceutical industry that usually garners most negative press, the fact is that neither academic institutions nor governments are free of ethical lapses during clinical trials. Some of the most egregious examples of ethical violations that are known to the general public (e.g., the yellow fever study in Panama 1899–1902, the atrocities of the Third Reich, and the Willowbrook and Tuskeegee experiments after the Second World War) were those of governments, not the pharmaceutical industry.

Although, on its face, this book does not seem to be about clinical practice, let us also not forget that pharmaceutical companies, disease management enterprises, economists, third-party payers, regulators of formularies, whether local committees or national bodies such as the National Institute for Health and Clinical Excellence (NICE) in England and the Scottish Medicines Consortium, and politicians, among many others, all have an indirect hand in shaping that ultimate clinical activity: prescribing. Arm's-length influence over clinical practice is no excuse for ignoring the ethical implications of one's actions, however indirect they may be.

The law, it can be argued, is the inefficient enforcement of ethics. Respect for intellectual property (seen especially in Japan where patent litigation is almost unknown), appropriate prescribing, and the detection and punishment of those who unethically invent "paper" patients or alter research data, are the subjects of other chapters in this section. This may seem pessimistic. However, there is a yet stronger argument to be made: the law can be a rather blunt tool for dissecting ethical issues, and may not be able to right a wrong when it is somebody's personal health that has been damaged. Moreover, if we did not exercise our best ethical judgment at all times then the law, in any case, could only ever address a small minority of cases that would arise.

Clearly, other chapters in this book could have appeared in this section. An early chapter in this book (Chapter 8) is on Informed Consent; its location is designed to indicate the supervening importance of that particular application of autonomy, beneficence, and equipoise in clinical trials. But ethical behavior is also at the very center of Good Clinical Practices. Chapter 46 on Publishing Clinical Trials also examines some of the ethical aspects of that activity. Dr Belsey also enters into this area with his chapter on Advertising and Marketing (Chapter 54). Ethics and the law are therefore presented in conjunction in this section.

CHAPTER 50

Introduction to Bioethics for Pharmaceutical Professionals

Andrew J. Fletcher
Temple University School of Pharmacy, PHARM-QA/RA, Philadelphia, PA, USA

Introduction

Discourse on ethics dates back at least as far as the Ancient Greeks and Romans and undoubtedly has much earlier origins, in both religious and secular systems of thought. Bioethics may be viewed as a subdivision of ethics, from which it borrows most of its tools and concepts, albeit with refinements. Bioethics developed rapidly during the 20th century, paralleling the recent era of growth in medical technology and research, and has been defined as follows:

A discipline dealing with the ethical implications of biological research and applications, especially in medicine.[1]

The study of moral issues in the fields of medical treatment and research.[2]

The study of ethical issues concerning the life sciences and the distribution of scarce medical resources.[3]

The branch of ethics that studies moral values in the biomedical sciences.[4]

Most people in clinical research and medicine tend to assume that they have a good grasp on ethics and ethical principles, and that acting ethically is simply a matter of doing "the right thing." Thus, those with little formal training in bioethics (probably most people) feel perfectly capable, most of the time, of making appropriate ethical decisions in the conduct of pharmaceutical medicine. Personal and professional ethics probably derive from a variety of sources, for example:

- one's personal beliefs;
- one's professional code of practice;
- state or federal law;
- intuition—one's innate sense of "the right thing."

Most bioethical decisions are of the straightforward "right versus wrong" type. These decisions usually require no formal tools of bioethics. But decisions are more difficult when they involve "right versus right" (dilemmas). Parsing the notions of "right" and "wrong," four broad categories of bioethical dilemma have been identified:[5]

- self or small-group interest versus community or large-group interest;
- short-term interest versus long-term interest;
- loyalty versus truth;
- mercy versus justice.

In the highly regulated environment of the pharmaceutical industry, "ethical" approaches often seem to be predetermined by local legislation and regulation (or "fiat"). Additionally, we are

---

[1] Merriam-Webster at www.m-w.com; accessed April 15, 2010
[2] Many sources, including www.bioethics-singapore.org; accessed April 15, 2010
[3] Adapted from the University of Penn, Center for Bioethics, www.bioethics.upenn.edu; accessed April 15, 2010
[4] WordWeb Online: www.wordwebonline.com; accessed April 15, 2010

Principles and Practice of Pharmaceutical Medicine, 3rd edition.
Edited by L.D. Edwards, A.W. Fox, P.D. Stonier.
© 2011 Blackwell Publishing Ltd.

---

[5] Kidder RM. *How Good People Make Tough Choices*. Fireside: New York, USA, 1996

guided by voluntary national guidelines, as well as by international codes of practice (see below). Nonetheless, merely relying on these alone is dangerous. A decision may be within the letter of the law, covered by all such voluntary codes, and yet still be arguably unethical. Shannan Muskopf has written:[6]

- Science asks *"Can we?"*
- Law asks *"May we?"*
- Ethics asks *"Should we?"*

Thus, although regulations help ensure minimum ethical standards, they do not necessarily ensure the highest ethical standards. Increasingly, therefore, the medical and pharmaceutical research and practice environments face a growing need for a formal approach to ethics, and particularly to bioethics.

Basic tools of bioethics

The process of analyzing and solving ethical problems involves the following:

- recognizing the relevant ethical issues;
- analyzing the subcomponents of these ethical issues;
- finding appropriate tools to help solve these issues and their subcomponents;
- applying those tools;
- checking that the selected tools have indeed met the recognized bioethical need.

The two fundamental types of bioethical tools are deductive and inductive reasoning. There are, however, complexities and adaptations for both of them. Let us first consider the two fundamental systems and then examine their complexities.

Deductive reasoning

Deductive reasoning is the process of concluding that something must be true because it is a special case of a general principle that is known to be true. It relies on the establishment of laws or rules that are generally applicable. It can be summed up as

---

[6] http://www.biologycorner.com/quests/bioethics.html; accessed April 15, 2010

top-down reasoning: one moves from the general to the specific(s). Much of medicine uses deductive reasoning: a general law, such as a fractured tibia heals best when immobilized in the correct position, is applied frequently to individual patients in the Emergency and Accident departments.

Emmanuel Kant (1724–1804) can probably be credited with enunciating best the classic approach to deductive reasoning. Kant believed that the moral worth of an action was based not on the ultimate outcome of the action, but rather on the motive behind that action. Kant described morality as being governed by universal laws that he termed *categorical imperatives*—these are duties that are inescapable. Perhaps the most famous of his categorical imperatives is that one has a duty always to tell the truth. Kant took the hypothetical example of a would-be murderer seeking to kill one's friend. If the friend is hiding in one's house, when the murderer knocks on the door one has an absolute duty to answer truthfully his inquiry whether the friend is inside. This truthfulness, according to Kant, might not, however, preclude shouting the answer loudly, thus giving the friend the chance to escape. There was no such thing as a "white lie" for Kant.

Inductive reasoning

Inductive reasoning is the process of concluding that a general principle is true because the special cases you have seen are true. This is the opposite of deduction, and may be thought of as bottom-up reasoning. One moves from the specific(s) to the general. Clearly, the likelihood that inductive reasoning is "correct" improves with the cumulation of larger numbers of special cases. Inductive reasoning can thus generate the general laws that can later be applied deductively.

One might assume that deductive reasoning is superior—as it would appear to offer mathematical style "proof." But a "law" is only as good as the premise on which it is based. Virtually, all scientific laws are derived inductively—from observation. But once the "law" is established, it is then applied deductively. However, when the original "law" turns out to be flawed it has usually been disproved inductively. Thus, in bioethics (as in science), the best approach is often a mixture of deductive and inductive reasoning.

Utilitarianism

Utilitarianism is a doctrine, enunciated by Jeremy Bentham (1748–1832) and John Stuart Mill (1806–1873): it is the search for "the greatest happiness for the greatest number"[7] or, more eloquently, the "quantitative maximization of some good for society or humanity . . . a form of consequentialism." *Consequentialism* is the belief that what ultimately matters in evaluating actions or policies of action are the consequences that result from choosing one action or policy rather than the alternative.[8] Thus, utilitarianism is a direct counter to the motivation-based categorical imperatives (essentially a deductive approach) of Kant.

Casuistry

Casuistry is an inductive method: it is the task of deriving principles from cases. Moral dilemmas can be addressed by comparing them with "agreed responses to pure cases." Its main weakness is that there can be inadequate selection of suitable comparative cases, which may be by omission or commission (the latter being especially common among politicians). Occasionally, there is also obscurity concerning the specifics of what the "agreed responses" might be.

Feminist bioethics

Feminist bioethics deals with bioethical issues that particularly affect women and/or with issues seen from a classically female perspective. Controversially, it has been asserted by some that women approach ethical dilemmas differently to men, because of dissimilar contexts. The ethic of care (Sherwin, 1989) is proposed as a "female" trait, while the ethic of justice or rights (Gilligan, 1982) is supposedly more "male." A common illustration of this is when a married couple is asked to include a clause in their wills concerning the disposal of property in the case of their simultaneous deaths: the wife will often propose a scheme dividing joint property unequally and according to need and number of all their relatives; the husband frequently sees the situation as requiring a simple 50–50 split between their two families.

The golden rule

Another important principle is "The Golden Rule," which states "Do unto others as you would have others do unto you." This is also called the Ethic of Reciprocity. Note that this is *not* the same as "tit-for-tat" or "an eye for an eye," which describes post hoc responses and vengeance, rather than prospective guidance of behavior by an ethical, golden rule standard. Again, this is principally a deductive approach, and not very far from Kant's categorical imperatives.

Objectivism versus subjectivism

A final consideration is whether ethical principles are relative or absolute. *Ethical objectivism* (Kant's categorical imperatives fall under this heading) asserts that ethical solutions are always absolute. In contrast, *ethical subjectivism* maintains that ethical solutions are never absolute. *Ethical relativism* (*cultural relativism*) provides a compromise, which may or may not be "correct," that ethical behavior should be judged relative to the norms of one's culture: what may be wrong for one society may be right for another, and this is clearly a utilitarian principle; an example may be the difference between civilian and military healthcare. In the civilian world, "every patient deserves the very best treatment" is the ideal, and is an absolute ethical objective. At a field dressing station, where medical staff and their equipment may be suddenly overwhelmed, triage is practiced with the aim of providing the greatest benefit for the greatest number. Thus, on the battlefield it will not be the case that every wounded soldier gets the best medical care, and this is an example of utilitarianism and ethical relativism. Both medical practices are ethically sound (or "correct"), and the term *universal prescriptivism* was formulated by R.M. Hare (1919–2002) to describe such combinations of Kantianism and utilitarianism.

---

[7] http://www.wordwebonline.com; accessed April 15, 2010

[8] http://en.wikipedia.org; accessed April 15, 2010

Four basic principles

When using these formal tools, there are four basic domains of bioethics wherein they are applied. These are the following:

- *Beneficence:* Providing individual benefit—is every action oriented toward the benefit of the individual?
- *Nonmaleficence:* Avoiding harm—is any action likely to harm the individual? (Note that nonmaleficence is included under "beneficence" in the Belmont Report.)
- *Autonomy:* Free participation, without external influence—does every individual agree with every action applied to him or her?
- *Social justice:* A fair distribution of scarce resources across societal groups—is every action consistent with this approach?

Although these principles are particularly relevant to the conduct of clinical studies (see below), they also apply to the ordinary practice of medicine and, indeed, all situations where one human being has a responsibility to care for another human being. Let us not forget the old maxim that the fundamental goals of healthcare, even in this age of rapid technological progress, are to "cure sometimes, relieve often, and comfort always," and this should not be violated in the context of clinical studies.

Ethics of human experimentation

Protection of the research subject in clinical trials poses a number of bioethical questions. We have already mentioned beneficence (the anticipation of some benefit), nonmaleficence (freedom from harm), autonomy (free participation without coercion), and social justice (for instance, whether or not there is a duty for people to participate in clinical studies, as benefactors of those who have previously volunteered). Each of these needs further discussion. These domains were egregiously violated by various governments during the 20th century (German Nazis, Tuskegee, etc.). It was the Nuremberg code that first provided for the protection of the research subject, and the Declaration of Helsinki, as amended, is its successor.

Above all, the rights of the individual must be seen to trump any need or possibility of scientific advance. The duty toward the individual must always have a far higher priority than some intangible benefit that might attach to the population as a whole in the future. In protecting the research subject, the first principle is "informed consent."

Informed consent

As the term implies, subjects must be fully informed about the nature of the experiment, the known benefits and risks, and the possibilities of unknown risks to which they will be exposed. Consent must be given *autonomously* and obtained *without any coercion*—direct, indirect, or perceived.

Already, a number of problems are evident. Fully informing a patient as to the nature of an experiment and its attendant risks, known and unknown, is an arduous task. The language used must lack ambiguity, and understanding must be real—even for those who cannot fathom the technical issues.

It has been shown repeatedly that humans are notoriously bad at assessing personal risk. As Henry Beecher (1904–1976) has suggested, (Beecher, 1966) although many patients are willing to help their doctors, their fellow humans, and science to improve medical care, most are not willing to assume significant risk in this endeavor, and few would be willing to risk serious injury or death. Yet, such outcomes nonetheless continue to occur, and analysis of recent disasters has often centered on whether subjects have fully understood the nature of their consent, rather than on the actual clinical procedures being implemented.

Beecher discussed the key concepts in human research of consent and autonomy, and the inherent difficulties in achieving these. People in positions of dependency may be termed "vulnerable groups"; these can include minors, prisoners, employees, and family members (Beecher, 1966). Conversely, Beecher established that there is no duty to participate in clinical research—an example in which public or societal good cannot outweigh personal risk (Beecher, 1966).

The primacy of truly informed consent is such that it deserves its own chapter (see Chapter 8).

Clinical equipoise

Benjamin Freedman (1951–1997) defined clinical equipoise as "a state of genuine uncertainty on the part of the investigator [or—present or imminent controversy in the clinical community] regarding the comparative therapeutic merits of each arm in a trial." Freedman continued that "at the start of the trial, there must be a state of clinical equipoise regarding the merits of the regimens to be tested, and the trial must be designed in such a way as to make it reasonable to expect that, if it is successfully conducted, clinical equipoise will be disturbed." Clinical equipoise and informed consent raise issues of beneficence and nonmaleficence, both of which may be violated by participation in the trial. However, if there is intent to do good and to avoid harm, arguably these concerns are satisfied.

Ethical behavior by study subjects

Concern about ethical conduct in clinical trials applies not only to investigators, but also to their subjects. In the early 1960s, Stanley Milgram, a Yale psychologist, carried out a number of "Studies of Obedience," examining how far subjects would go in carrying out "orders." One famous study[9] involved the delivery of "electric shocks" of increasing intensity to subjects who chose incorrect answers. Similar studies have examined the behavior of "guards" and "prisoners" in simulated prison conditions (Phillip Zimbardo in the Stanford Prison Experiment[10]; Haslam and Reicher in the BBC Prison Study[11]). In these and similar studies, a substantial proportion of subjects (typically exceeding 60%) performed actions they believed to be harmful to other subjects, apparently under the presumption that they were merely carrying out orders and were therefore not directly responsible for any resulting harm. The dangers of such reasoning, in a corporate or academic environment for example, are very clear.

---

[9] http://en.wikipedia.org/wiki/Milgram_experiment and http://www.videosift.com/video/The-Original-Milgram-Experiment-1961; accessed April 15, 2010

[10] www.prisonexp.org/; accessed April 15, 2010

[11] www.bbcprisonstudy.org/; accessed April 15, 2010

Ethics of animal experimentation

Public disagreement surrounds the use of animals in research—which occurs primarily to benefit humans, although some agricultural and veterinarian studies are carried out to benefit animals themselves. Three distinct approaches are offered here:

- "Duties Toward Animals" (Kant, 1963)
- "A Utilitarian View" (Bentham, 1999)
- "All Animals Are Equal" (Singer, 1974)

Kant argues that we do not have a direct duty to animals, and therefore killing them for food is acceptable. On the other hand, being cruel to animals is undesirable because it diminishes us morally.

Bentham argues that use of animals for human good, if carried out as humanely as possible, is justified if it results in an overall benefit to humans. Thus, harm inflicted to one species is justified if it results in overall benefit to another. This justification assumes an inherent moral superiority of humans over the animals being experimented upon. Such arguments meet their greatest challenge when the test subjects are necessarily primates (e.g., HIV research); a degree of self-awareness can be deduced in these species, and yet their consent is obviously absent.

Singer, in contrast to Bentham, believes all animals (humans included) are morally equal, and that Bentham's arguments are "speciesist" (although Bentham does question the inherent superiority of humans, tending toward Singer's viewpoint).

Further issues of concern to the pharmaceutical industry and medical research

Ethical violations in human experimentation

There is a long history of unethical human experimentation. King George I of England offered pardons to inmates of Newgate Prison (London), in return for inoculation with smallpox, as part of a variolation experiment—an enrollment approach that would now be considered coercive (Huth, 2005). We delude ourselves if we assume that such ethical violations are now a thing of the past. In 1966, Beecher reviewed a series of unethical medical experiments (Beecher, 1966). These included problems with consent, the withholding of known effective treatment, and studies to improve medical knowledge but without obvious benefit (and with inherent risk) to the participants. A sample of more such studies is offered here, in addition to those of the egregious government of Nazi Germany, mentioned above.

In 1932, the Tuskegee Syphilis Study[12] began, sponsored by the US Health Service. Over the next 40 years, 399 rural African American men, living in Tuskegee, Alabama, were enrolled in the study. The study participants received regular medical examinations, but were not told they had syphilis, and were left untreated. The unethical aim of the study was to observe the natural history of the disease, and the study continued until 1972—long after the discovery of a proven treatment, penicillin, in the early 1940s.

In 1996, Nicole Wan, a student at the University of Rochester, underwent bronchoscopy as a healthy volunteer. She collapsed at home shortly afterwards and died at home two days later. The cause of death was an excessive dose of lidocaine administered to help the procedure. An investigation determined a failure to establish safe dosage guidelines for lidocaine administration during these procedures.

In 1996, an antibiotic study of bacterial meningitis was conducted in children in the city of Kano in Nigeria—a strife-torn city suffering an epidemic of bacterial meningitis.[13] In a study organized by a pharmaceutical company, 100 children received the antibiotic trovafloxacin (which had not yet been approved for use in children), and another 100 children received ceftriaxone (a well-established antibiotic). Eleven children died—five taking trovafloxacin and six taking ceftriaxone. Subsequent investigations suggested that the study had not been properly approved, that the dose of ceftriaxone was too low, that informed consent had not been obtained, and that families were not told that an alternative and effective nonexperimental antibiotic, chloramphenicol, was being administered free in the same hospital.

Jesse Gelsinger[14] suffered from a rare genetic disorder called ornithine transcarbamylase deficiency, which although requiring cumbersome treatment with diet and drugs, was not a life-threatening disorder for him. In 1999, he volunteered for a Phase I experimental gene therapy at the University of Pennsylvania; his personal goal, it is thought, was to help the treatment of babies with this disorder rather than to benefit himself. He was injected with corrective genes incorporated into an adenovirus vector, despite animal data suggesting toxicity of the vector. Three days later, he was dead from multiple organ failure, apparently due to an overwhelming inflammatory reaction to the vector, which had unexpectedly regained its virulence. Bioethical concerns raised afterwards included inadequacy of the informed consent (failure fully to reveal toxicity in previous animal experiments), bending of the rules (Jesse's ammonia levels exceeded the upper limits set by the protocol), and conflict of interest (one of the investigators had a significant financial interest in the study outcome).

In 2001, Ellen Roche, a volunteer in a Phase I study at Johns Hopkins University, died after an experimental inhalation of hexamethonium.[15] Two major ethical lapses have been suggested. First, the toxic nature of the inhalant had been underestimated by the clinical investigators, in spite of (admittedly decades old) literature demonstrating this toxicity. Second, the volunteer had been an employee in the laboratories of the same university, thus presenting a potential for coercion to take part in the study.

---

[12] http://facstaff.gpc.edu/~shale/humanities/composition/assignments/experiment/tuskegee.html; accessed April 15, 2010

[13] Sources include http://www.mindfully.org/Industry/Pfizer-Trovan-Nigerian-Suit.htm; accessed April 15, 2010

[14] Many sources, including http://www.gene.ch/gentech/1999/Dec/msg00005.html; accessed April 15, 2010

[15] Sources include http://www.ahrp.org/infomail/0701/19.php; accessed April 15, 2010

Allocation of resources

Resource allocation is a bioethical concern in all aspects of medicine, for instance, how limited resources should be allocated among different groups, and is a pivotal component of social justice (discussed above). It applies to the pharmaceutical industry and its allocation of funds for drug research and development. Such issues include the following:

- exotic therapies versus cheaper more widely useful therapies;
- therapies for old versus young, rich versus poor, one ethnic group versus another, and so on;
- public need versus profitability.

Allocation of scarce resources can be decided in a number of ways, for example by the principles of utilitarianism (such as by using medical criteria to select those most likely to benefit) or by random choice.

Ethics committees

Robert Pearlman, a bioethicist and physician at the University of Washington, asks a series of questions about hospital ethical committees and Institutional Review Boards (IRBs), which can be easily generalized to other settings (Perlman, 1997):

- *Membership:* Who should sit on an ethics committee?
- *Roles:* Advisory or mandatory?
- *Outcomes:* What to do if consensus is impossible?
- *Ethics education for committee members:* Content?
- *Hospital (or company) policies on ethics:* What should these be?
- *Quality assurance:* How to measure?

It is true that, in the hospital environment, such committees' activities may have greater scope than those of a clinical trial IRB. Robert Veatch, a bioethicist at Georgetown University, has pointed out that hospital ethics committees (Veatch, 1977)

- make specific patient-care decisions;
- make broad policy decisions;
- provide counseling and support;
- establish likely prognoses.

All of these can impinge, directly or indirectly, on the autonomy of patients, and deflect hospital care from the best principles of beneficence for each individual case. Furthermore, Bernard Lo, a physician and bioethicist at UCSF, discusses possible pitfalls of ethics committees (Lo, 1987): There can be excessive pressure to reach agreement, impairment rather than improvement of decision making, and the broader dangers of "group-think," that is, attraction toward consensus overcoming the voicing of independent, and possibly discordant, points of view.

Bioethicists in the pharmaceutical industry

Although it is true that most of the egregious violations of bioethics, in an investigational context, have resulted from the actions of governments and academic institutions, we should nonetheless ask a pivotal question: Is there now a need for formal recognition of bioethicists as an integral part of the pharmaceutical medicine "team"?

This question has many aspects. Who can be a bioethicist?—should it be only someone with a degree from one of the now numerous university departments of bioethics? Increasingly, bioethics awareness, training, and expertise is needed throughout the pharmaceutical industry and related regulatory and research areas. Or is the increasing use of data safety monitoring boards, together with their approval of the protocols they monitor, a better way to go?

These are unsettled questions, with able protagonists on all sides. We may hope that, in the future, there will be sufficient flexibility to adapt the necessary safeguards to the type of clinical study. A "one size fits all" approach is hardly likely to be useful.

References

Beecher HK. Ethics and clinical research. *N Engl J Med.* 1966; **274**(24):1354–1360; reprinted in *Bioethics: An Introduction to the History, Methods, and Practice,* Jecker, Jonsen, Pearlman (eds). Jones and Bartlett: Sudbury, UK; 1997.

Bentham J. First published c. 1820 in *An Introduction to the Principles of Morals and Legislation,* Section XVIII, and reprinted in *Bioethics: an Anthology,* Kuhse, Singer (eds). Blackwell Publishers: Oxford and Malden, UK; 1999.

Gilligan C. *In a Different Voice: Psychological Theory and Women's Development*. Harvard University Press: Cambridge, MA, USA, 1982.

Huth EJ. *Quantitative evidence for judgments on the efficacy of inoculation for the prevention of smallpox: England and New England in the 1700s*. The James Lind Library, 2005; http://www.jameslindlibrary.org/trial_records/17th_18th_Century/jurin/jurin_commentary.php; accessed April 15, 2010.

Kant I. Duties towards animals, from *Lectures on Ethics*, trans. Louis Infield. Harper and Row: New York, USA; 1963, and reprinted in *Bioethics: An Anthology*, Kuhse, Singer (eds). Blackwell Publishers: Oxford and Malden, UK; 1999 (written about 1790).

Lo, B. Behind closed doors: promises and pitfalls of ethical committees. *N Engl J Med* 1987; **317**: 46–50; reprinted in *Bioethics: An Introduction to the History, Methods, and Practice*, Jecker, Jonsen, Pearlman (eds). Jones and Bartlett: Sudbury, UK, 1997.

Pearlman RA. Introduction to the practice of bioethics, in *Bioethics: An Introduction to the History, Methods, and Practice*, Jecker, Jonsen, Pearlman (eds). Jones and Bartlett: Sudbury, UK; 1997; 259–272.

Sherwin Susan. Feminist and medical ethics: two different approaches to contextual ethics. *Hypatia* 1989; **4**(Summer):57–71; reprinted (abridged) in *Bioethics: An Introduction to the History, Methods, and Practice*, Jecker, Jonsen, Pearlman (eds). Jones and Bartlett: Sudbury, UK, 1997.

Singer P. *Philosophic Exchange*. 1974pp. 103–116, and reprinted in *Bioethics: An Anthology*, Kuhse, Singer (eds). Blackwell Publishers: Oxford and Malden, UK, 1999.

Veatch RM. Hospital ethics committees: is there a role? *Hastings Center Report* 1977 **7(3)**, 22–25; reprinted (abridged) in *Bioethics: An Introduction to the History, Methods, and Practice*, Jecker, Jonsen, Pearlman (eds). Jones and Bartlett: Sudbury, UK, 1997.

CHAPTER 51

Pharmaceutical Medicine and the Law

Sarah Croft[1]

Shook, Hardy & Bacon International LLP, London, UK

Introduction

In this chapter, I introduce basic legal principles and some of the legal concepts most relevant to the pharmaceutical physician. The central topics are introduced and then expanded upon in the following sections.

Individual or corporate responsibility?

The circumstances in which a pharmaceutical physician will personally be sued under the civil law are relatively infrequent. The individual doctor or pharmaceutical physician, who is usually an agent of the company, does not, under UK law, fall within the definition of a "producer" or "manufacturer," although a pharmaceutical company usually does. Therefore, the individual pharmaceutical physician is unlikely to have proceedings brought against him or her personally, except in rare circumstances.[2] It is much more likely that a company

will be a defendant to an action by an individual patient or by another company, whether in tort or in contract. The deeper pockets of the company, in comparison to the individual pharmaceutical physician, practically guarantee that this is also the case in the US. It is sometimes the case that the company and the pharmaceutical physician are sued in negligence, where the allegations include specific acts for which the pharmaceutical physician is responsible, such as the warnings in a data sheet or the reports from a clinical trial. Regardless of who might be held legally responsible, an understanding of the relevant legal framework is essential.

It is possible that criminal sanctions could be applied to the individual but such proceedings are not common. In the event of a death, pursuant to the UK Corporate Manslaughter and Corporate Homicide Act 2007, criminal proceedings could also be brought against a company. Further, as discussed elsewhere, both the UK and US regulations make it an offense for an applicant (i.e., a company) to give false information in connection with an application for a license for a pharmaceutical product. Most regulations, however, also provide that where a company makes a misrepresentation and it can also be shown that the misrepresentation was committed with the consent and connivance of, or attributable to the neglect of, any director, manager, or similar officer of the company, those individuals may also be personally liable. This may obviously affect the pharmaceutical physician who, if a director or equivalent in the company, may be the signatory to advertising materials.

---

[1] With thanks to E. Bolton in Shook, Hardy and Bacon International LLP London, and J. Stevenson in Shook, Hardy and Bacon LLP Kansas City

[2] See *Staples v. Merck & Co., Inc., et al.*, 270 F. Supp. 2d 833 (N.D. Tex. 2003) (consumers sued clinical researcher and research facility for strategic procedural purposes in lawsuit against manufacturer). Although originally sued, the clinical researcher and facility were eventually dismissed from the case

---

Principles and Practice of Pharmaceutical Medicine, 3rd edition.
Edited by L.D. Edwards, A.W. Fox, P.D. Stonier.
© 2011 Blackwell Publishing Ltd.

Criminal and civil law distinguished

A crime is an offense or wrongdoing against the state and is punishable by the state, whereas civil law concerns the breach of a private right or duty. Thus, in contrast to criminal cases, most civil actions are not brought by the state but by private individuals or other legal entities, such as corporations. In some instances, an individual's actions can give rise to both a criminal offense and a civil liability, for example, an assault can result in a prosecution by the state and a claim by the victim for damages for personal injury.

Another important distinction between criminal and civil cases is the threshold "burden of proof" that must be reached in order to prove the case against the defendant. Generally speaking, in a criminal case, the prosecutor for the state must prove its case "beyond a reasonable doubt." In civil actions, the plaintiff must prove his or her case "on a balance of probabilities." The standard of proof for criminal matters is higher, essentially because an individual's life or liberty may be at risk.

Criminal law

Fortunately, instances are rare in which pharmaceutical physicians face criminal prosecution. There are a number of specific ways, however, in which the criminal law can affect pharmaceutical companies and their physicians.

Statutory offenses may apply to the pharmaceutical physician in the regulatory context. This will, of course, vary from country to country but in the UK, for example, the Medicines Act of 1968 creates offenses, such as providing false information when applying to license a product.

Further, it is provided under the UK Corporate Manslaughter and Corporate Homicide Act 2007 that "an organization . . . is guilty of an offence if the way in which its activities are managed or organized a) causes a person's death, and b) amounts to a gross breach of a relevant duty of care owed by the organization to the deceased." Under the Act a "relevant duty of care" in relation to an organization means any of the duties owed by it under the law of negligence as listed in s.2(1)(a)–(d) and a "gross breach" is one which "falls far below" the standards expected in the circumstances. The Act is not limited such that it will cover all industries and a wide range of organizations.

In the US, the Food, Drug, and Cosmetics Act (FDCA)[3] also creates statutory offenses for certain actions or inactions. For example, it is not permissible to sell a misbranded drug or device. A drug is "misbranded," if among other things, its labeling is "false or misleading in any particular," or contains inadequate directions or warnings.[4] In addition, an adulterated product may not be introduced, such as one that has been modified from its intended use.[5]

The US Supreme Court has observed that an offense is committed "by all who do have such a responsible share in the furtherance of the transaction which the statute outlaws."[6] Furthermore, the Court has interpreted the FDCA as imposing "not only a positive duty to seek out and remedy violations when they occur but also, and primarily, a duty to implement measures that will ensure that violations will not occur."[7] The Prescription Drug Marketing Act of 1987 (PDMA, part of the FDCA) was enacted to address marketing practices that contribute to a second-hand market for drugs, such as distribution of free samples, coupons for reduced or free drugs, and deeply discounted drugs.[8] The PDMA makes it a crime knowingly to sell, purchase, or trade a prescription drug sample.[9] This Act also prohibits the re-sale of any prescription drug previously purchased by a healthcare entity.[10] The Anti-Kickback Statute, as the name suggests, prohibits knowingly and wilfully offering, paying,

---

[3] 21 USC Sections 301–393
[4] 21 USC Sections 352(a) and (f)
[5] 21 USC Section 331
[6] US v. Dotterweich, 320 US 277, 285 (1943) (finding president of company individually guilty for shipping misbranded and adulterated drugs)
[7] US v. Park, 421 US 658, 672 (1975)
[8] 21 USC Sections 331(t) and 333(b)
[9] 21 USC Section 353(c)(1)
[10] 21 USC Section 353(c)(3)(A)

soliciting, or receiving remuneration in order to induce business payable by a healthcare facility or program that is Federally funded (for example, through Medicaid).[11]

Another area where potential criminal liability may occasionally emerge is fraud or forgery during the course of a clinical trial. In the US, the Office of Research Integrity investigates allegations of scientific misconduct in Federally funded research.[12] Sanctions for research misconduct can be severe; in one case, a researcher was sentenced to 71 months of jail time and ordered to pay US$639,000 in restitution.[13] Pharmaceutical physicians, who are involved in designing and monitoring clinical trials, will be aware of the need to build in various safeguards to protect against the possibility of these offenses. Courts expect foresight and diligence from individuals who voluntarily assume positions of authority in enterprises that affect the health and well-being of the public.

The Federal Corrupt Practices Act (FCPA)[14] is another source of potential criminal liability. The FCPA prohibits bribery of foreign officials, and the Act broadly defines "foreign official."[15] Prosecutions of pharmaceutical companies under the FCPA have been rare; only one company has been prosecuted under the FCPA in the statute's history. In late 2009, however, officials at the US Department of Justice stated that FCPA violations by pharmaceutical companies will be a new focus of the department. The FCPA is of particular relevance to the pharmaceutical industry because health systems outside the US are often regulated and operated by government entities. Violations can result in significant fines and penalties. For example, a company can be fined up to US$2 million per violation of the anti-bribery provisions.[16] Individuals can face fines of up to US$100,000 and imprisonment for up to five years for willful violations.[17]

Civil law

The two main areas of civil law that may affect the pharmaceutical physician are the law of contract and the law of tort. Essentially, a contract is a legally binding agreement between individuals (or other legal entities such as corporations), where one of the parties assumes an obligation or makes a promise to the other. Usually, the parties to the contract have obligations and gain rights under the agreement. The law of contract regulates the enforceability of such agreements and the steps that can be taken if the contract is broken. Perhaps the most fundamental feature of contractual liability is that it is strict and not fault-based. This means, broadly speaking, that it does not matter whether a party to the contract acted reasonably or not; what matters is whether the contract has been broken.

The pharmaceutical physician will be very familiar with certain types of contracts, depending on his or her role within the company. Examples include agreements with contract research organizations, contracts for the sale of the finished pharmaceutical product, and licensing or distribution agreements.

Usually, there is no contract between a pharmaceutical company and the patient who is prescribed a product by a doctor. In the UK, it has been held that where a product is prescribed under a National Health Service scheme, it is not prescribed as a result of a contract between the pharmaceutical company and the patient because legislation exists that requires a pharmacist to supply the product on the production of a valid prescription.[18] For

---

[11] 42 USC Section 1320a–7b(b) (remuneration includes discounts, gifts, free supplies, equipment, or any item of value)

[12] See 42 CFR Part 93 "Public Health Service Policies on Research Misconduct" (2005)

[13] 71 Fed. Reg. 9555-56

[14] 15 USC Sections 78dd-1, *et seq*

[15] 15 USC Sections 78dd-1(f)(1)(A) ("The term 'foreign official' means any officer or employee of a foreign government or any department, agency, or instrumentality thereof, or of a public international organization, or any person acting in an official capacity for or on behalf of any such government or department, agency, or instrumentality, or for or on behalf of any such public international organization")

[16] 15 USC Sections 78dd-1(g)(1)

[17] 15 USC Sections 78dd-1(g)(2)

[18] *Pfizer Corp. v. Ministry of Health* (1965). 1 All ER 450, HL

non-prescription, "over-the-counter" (OTC) products, there is a contract between the retailer and the consumer who purchases the pharmaceutical product, but there is still usually no direct link in contractual terms to the manufacturer of the product. It may be, however, that the contract between the manufacturer and the retailer contains an indemnity provision. Then, in the event of a successful claim for breach of contract made against the retailer by the customer, the manufacturer may be required to reimburse the retailer for the amount ordered to be paid in compensation to the customer.

In the US, as in the UK, a contractual right of action generally exists only between parties to the contract. This is known as the rule of privity. Courts in the US have recognized that, in a mass-consumption society, there is little real privity between manufacturers and consumers: Manufacturers are remote to the ultimate consumer, sales are accomplished through intermediaries, and products are marketed through the use of advertising media. Some courts, however, have carved out an exception to the privity rule for contract claims, recognizing for example, that in certain circumstances consumers may bring breach of express warranty claims against pharmaceutical companies, based on statements made in the package insert as well as promotional literature and advertisements.[19]

For the individual pharmaceutical physician, an important contract will be his or her own contract of employment with the company. This is likely to contain terms, which if broken by the individual, could give rise to a claim being made against him or her and, of course, *vice versa*. The contract of employment may cover matters such as confidentiality and restrictive covenants, as well as defining the individual's role and responsibilities within the company.

Distinct from the law of contract, the law of tort serves to regulate standards of behavior, operating to deter conduct that may cause injury or damage and to remedy the consequences of such actions.[20] This area of law includes the tort of negligence. An important and well-known case in the development of the tort of negligence in the UK is the case of *Donoghue v. Stevenson*, which involved a woman, Mrs Donoghue, who was unfortunate enough to drink from a bottle of ginger beer containing the remains of a snail.[21] There was no contract between Mrs Donoghue and the manufacturer of the ginger beer, so she could not claim a breach of contract. The court held, however, that the company actually had a "duty of care" to the ultimate consumer of its product to take reasonable care in the manufacture of its product.[22] The main elements of negligence have been distilled from this statement in various UK cases over time. In order for a person (the "plaintiff" or "claimant") to prove negligence by another (the "defendant"), he or she must show:

- that the defendant owes the plaintiff a duty of care;
- the defendant has breached the duty of care; and
- the breach of duty caused damage that the plaintiff alleges he or she suffered.[23]

In order to succeed in a claim of negligence, a plaintiff must prove all three elements. It is not enough to show that the defendant had a duty of care and was in breach of it. There must be proof that the breach caused the plaintiff's alleged injury, which is often the most difficult task for a plaintiff, especially in claims concerning pharmaceutical products, where there may be other possible causes of the plaintiff's condition.

---

[19] See *Overstreet v. Norden Labs., Inc.*, 669 F.2d 1286, 1289–90 (6th Cir. 1982); *Morris v. Parke Davis & Co.*, 667 F. Supp. 1332, 1347–48 (CD Cal. 1987); *Tinnerholm v. Parke Davis & Co.*, 285 F. Supp. 432, 442–43 (SDNY 1968)

[20] See generally *Clerk and Lindsell on Torts*, London: Sweet & Maxwell, 19th edition. In French "tort" means "wrong"

[21] *Donoghue v. Stevenson* (1932). A.C. 562

[22] ". . . a manufacturer of products which he sells in such a form as to show that he intends them to reach the ultimate consumer in the form in which they left him, with no reasonable possibility of intermediate examination, and with the knowledge that the absence of reasonable care in the preparation or putting up of the products will result in an injury to the consumer's life or property, owes a duty to the consumer to take that reasonable care" (per Lord Atkin at p. 599)

[23] This is a simplification of a complex area of law for the purposes of this introductory chapter

In the law of tort, including negligence, liability is fault-based. It must be proved that the defendant was at fault in that he or she acted wrongfully and as a result violated a right of the plaintiff, causing harm to him or her. The requirement of fault differentiates a genuine accident from a negligent act for which the injured person can be compensated.

Liability can result under other laws in the US, such as the False Claims Act (FCA), which provides for civil proceedings to punish healthcare fraud when a person knowingly causes a false claim to be made to a government agency.[24] A lawsuit can be filed by the government or by a citizen, commonly referred to as a whistleblower, who then receives a portion of the monetary recovery.[25] In June 2009 the Fraud Enforcement and Recovery Act (FERA) was signed into law, which further expanded the scope of the FCA.[26] Under FERA, providers now face severe penalties for "knowingly and improperly avoid[ing] or decreas[ing] an obligation to pay or transmit money or property to the government."[27] Even before FERA, monetary recoveries for FCA violations had become quite large, leading to an increasing number of whistleblowers filing claims against pharmaceutical companies and physicians.

To complicate matters, in some countries, liability may also arise in tort without proof of fault. This is known as strict liability. An important example of strict liability for pharmaceutical companies is what is commonly referred to as the "European Products Liability Directive," which introduced a Europe-wide scheme of strict liability for defective products[28] (see Chapter 55 on "Pharmaceutical Product Liability"). As liability is strict, the defenses that are available in the legislation are most important. The relevant UK legislation, for example, includes

a "development risk defense" which means that it is a defense to a claim if the state of scientific knowledge was such that the producer could not have discovered the defect.[29]

The US has also adopted a theory of strict liability. This theory imposes liability on the seller of a product that is unreasonably dangerous because of a defect in its design, manufacture, or warnings. There are special provisions carved out for pharmaceutical products because of their value to society and the fact they are "unavoidably unsafe." Such products need to be accompanied by an adequate warning. Under strict liability, a pharmaceutical company is unquestionably subject to strict liability as a "seller" of a pharmaceutical product. A pharmaceutical physician, however, is generally not subject to this type of liability.

The legal framework for regulating pharmaceutical products

As any pharmaceutical physician is well aware, the development, manufacture, marketing, and safety of pharmaceutical products are subject to close governmental control in most countries through specific regulations on the sale of medicines and medical devices. Pharmaceutical physicians play a key role in ensuring that, at each stage in the life of a pharmaceutical product, the regulatory requirements have been met. As discussed above, there may be criminal implications if certain requirements are not fulfilled. In a negligence action against the pharmaceutical company, the failure by the company or by one or more individual employees to comply with the regulations may also be relevant to the question of whether or not a company has acted reasonably. Indeed, in the US, some courts have held that a company failing to comply with government regulations may be presumed to be negligent; known as "negligence-per-se," it essentially lessens the plaintiff's burden regarding the standard of care owed by the

---

[24] 31 USC Section 3729 *et seq*

[25] 31 USC Section 3730(d)(1)–(2)

[26] Fraud Enforcement and Recovery Act of 2009, Pub.L. No. 111-21, 123 Stat. 1617

[27] 31 U.S.C. § 3729(a)(1)(G). Fines for Section 3729(a) violations include US$5,500 to US$11,000 per violation plus three times the amount of damages which the Government sustains resulting from the false claim

[28] EC Directive 85/374/EEC

[29] Consumer Protection Act (1987) s.4(1)(e)

defendant.[30] Negligence-per-se focuses on the defendant's actions, whereas in strict liability, the focus is on the product and whether it was defective.[31]

In the UK, regulation is derived from the Medicines Act of 1968, which provides a comprehensive system of licensing affecting most aspects of the sale of medicinal products. It also contains provisions on related matters, such as pharmacovigilance and the requirements for the reporting of adverse events. The Medicines Act encompasses measures contained in European Community Directives, including the first on the control of medicines, introduced in 1965.[32] The Medicines Act led to the creation of various UK regulatory bodies to carry out the functions outlined in it, including the following:

• *The Licensing Authority,*[33] which decides whether licenses for medical products should be granted.

• *The Medicines and Healthcare Products Regulatory Agency (MHRA),* a government body set up in 2003 to ensure that medicines and medical devices work and are "acceptably safe".

• *The Commission on Human Medicines (CHM),* established under s.2(A) of the Medicines Act 1968 (as amended) and providing independent expert advice to the MHRA and the Licensing Authority.[34]

As well as domestic legislation, there is extensive European legislation governing member states. The European Community has over the years established measures to harmonize the regulation of medicines throughout Europe.[35] In 2001, all European Community Directives adopted between 1965 and 1999 on the regulation of medicines were consolidated into a "Community Code."[36] At the time, the Code could not incorporate the new Clinical Trials Directive harmonizing EU controls on the approval and conduct of clinical trials (i.e., Directive 2001/20/EC).[37] The Community Code has, however, since been amended to take into account the Directive's ethics.[38]

It was through this series of, now codified, Directives that a European-wide Committee for Proprietary Medicinal Products was created, now known as the Committee for Medicinal Products for Human Use (CHMP).[39] Its role is significant, because in conjunction with the European Medicines Agency (EMA) established in February 1995,[40] it is responsible for overseeing the procedures established for the regulatory harmonization of pharmaceutical products throughout Europe, namely:[41]

• The "centralized procedure," which involves one single application made to the EMA. This is now mandatory for certain products.[42]

---

[30] See *Ahles v. Tabor*, 34 P.3d 1076, 1078 (Idaho 2001)

[31] See, generally, Andrew E. Costa, "Negligence per se Theories in Pharmaceutical & Medical Device Litigation," 57 MELR 51 (2005)

[32] EC Directive 65/65/EEC now codified into "Community Code" EC Directive 2001/83/EC

[33] See ss. 1(1) and 6(1) of the Medicines Act 1968

[34] An amalgamation of two previously separate advisory bodies, The Medicines Commission and the Committee on the Safety of Medicines. Its duties are set out in s.3 (as amended by the Medicines (Advisory Bodies) Regulations 2005 SI 2005/1094)

[35] See, for example, "Community Code" 2001/83/EC and amending Directives 2003/63/EC (implemented in the UK by SI 2003/2321); 2004/27/EC (implemented in the UK by various statutory instruments); 2009/53/EC (providing that variations to all types of marketing authorizations will be subject to harmonized rules) and Council Reg. 1394/2007 (creating a single European authorization process for the authorization, supervision, and pharmacovigilance of advanced therapy medicinal products; see later footnote 42)

[36] EC Directive 2001/83/EC

[37] Implemented in the UK by the Medicines for Human Use (Clinical Trials) Regulations 2004 SI 2004/1031

[38] By EC Directive 2004/27/EC

[39] Council Reg. 726/2004

[40] By Council Reg. 2309/93 and formerly known as the European Agency for the Evaluation of Medicinal Products but shortened to the European Medicines Agency by Reg. 726/2004 (see following footnote).

[41] Council Reg. 2309/93 since replaced by Reg. 726/2004

[42] Annexed to Council Reg. 726/2004 are the products requiring authorization via the centralized procedure. This list now also includes "advanced therapy medicinal products" (ATMPs). These are defined as gene therapy medicinal products, somatic cell therapy products or tissue engineered products. A committee for advanced therapies (CAT) has been established by the EMA. The CAT will prepare a draft opinion which will be submitted

- The "mutual recognition" procedure (or the "decentralized procedure"), which is in essence a national registration recognized by the other member states for products that fall outside the scope of the centralized procedure.

In the centralized procedure, it is the CHMP that initially decides whether the new product should be authorized and gives its "opinion" to the EMA. Also, through the mutual recognition procedure, it is the CHMP that resolves any disputes. Thus, there are two ways in which a drug may be granted a license in the UK; *via* the EMA (be it through the centralized or mutual recognition procedure) or through its own MHRA.

The above procedures were re-evaluated in 2001 as required in the originating legislation.[43] The findings of the Commission plus the intervening introduction of the "Community Code" prompted the replacement of Regulation 2309/93 by Regulation 726/2004. The new regulation was drawn up to improve the previous version taking into account practical experience and to update all references to Directives since codified. The regulation also sets out the EMA's other tasks such as coordinating existing resources for the evaluation, supervision, and pharmacovigilance of medicinal products. Regulation 726/2004 will itself be reviewed "at least" every ten years.[44] In the meantime, it has been amended[45] and measures to strengthen its pharmacovigilance procedures were proposed in 2009.[46]

One of the new developments of the European legislation above is the introduction of financial penalties for failure to comply with obligations and the "naming and shaming" of offending companies.

The UK, Medicines Act (1968) places responsibility on the applicant for a license, which in most cases is a company, not on an individual within the company. The legal responsibility is thus that of the company (and those in positions of leadership and authority) to comply with the various regulations under the Act. Under certain circumstances, the regulatory authority (i.e., the government) may be sued if it was allegedly somehow at fault in granting or failing to withdraw a license for the product that supposedly caused harm.[47]

In the US, pharmaceutical products are the most heavily regulated of all consumer products. The Food and Drug Administration (FDA) is the primary regulatory agency and the FDCA[48] is the principal statute governing pharmaceutical products. The FDCA requires FDA approval of prescription medicines as "safe *and* effective" before they may be sold in the US (emphasis added).[49] Regulations relating to pharmaceutical products address the safety and efficacy of pharmaceuticals and range from initial testing of a drug to post-marketing surveillance. The law regarding the conflict or balance between state and Federal laws—called "pre-emption"—is convoluted and is the source of extensive legal debate (see Chapter 55).

In the US, as elsewhere, labeling is a crucial issue in litigation. The FDA's regulation on labeling covers all written materials attached to or accompanying the product or container, as well as journal, television, and radio advertising. The labeling used to inform physicians about the drug's uses and risks is a crucial element for the FDA's determination of drug approval.[50] The FDA regulates all such labeling, including "all written, printed, or graphic matter" used in advertising the drug.[51] After FDA approval, a manufacturer may sell and advertise the drug in accordance with the approved uses on

---

to the CHMP for final approval. The regulatory framework for ATMPs is established by Council Reg. 1394/2007 and its provisions applied from December 30, 2008. The UK legislation implementing these regulations is as yet to be laid before Parliament.

[43] Council Reg. 2309/93 Art. 71

[44] Art. 86

[45] See, for example, footnote 42

[46] See Community document "COM(2008) 664 Final" for the opinion of the European Economic and Social Committee on the Commission's proposals for a new Regulation. See also the European Data Protection Supervisor's opinion at footnote 60

[47] For example, in the UK the government was a defendant in actions brought by hemophiliacs alleging contamination with the HIV virus through use of blood products

[48] 21 USC Sections 301–393

[49] 21 USC Sections 355(d) and 393(b)(2)(B)

[50] 50 Federal Register 7452-01, 7470 (22 February 1985)

[51] 21 CFR Section 1.3(a)

the drug label. "Off-label" use is any use for the drug that is not approved by the FDA.

As in other countries, the US Federal regulation of a drug does not end with the approval of the drug and the company being granted a license for it. The FDA requires drug manufacturers to engage in post-market surveillance of the approved drugs and can include revisions to the labeling. A manufacturer must report to the FDA and investigate any adverse events (AERs) in accordance with FDA regulations. Further, FDA regulations require a manufacturer to issue subsequent warnings whenever there is "reasonable evidence of an association of a serious hazard with a drug; a causal relationship need not have been proved."[52] The US Supreme Court has held that "the manufacturer bears responsibility for the content of its label at all times. It is charged both with crafting an adequate label and with ensuring that its warnings remain adequate as long as the drug is on the market."[53] Pharmaceutical litigation in the US and elsewhere often centers on the manner in which clinical trial data and AERs are processed and reported and how such information is incorporated into labeling changes. The pharmaceutical physician will often be central to this process

Legal procedures

Although most legal procedures are not directly relevant to the work of the pharmaceutical physician, there are some procedural considerations worth acknowledging.[54] In the US and the UK, when pharmaceutical litigation ensues against a pharmaceutical manufacturer, the manufacturer has a legal obligation to preserve documents, including electronic correspondence, that is related to the litigation.[55] All employees should heed such notices

to preserve documents and email correspondence. Failure to do so may result in the company being sanctioned by the court. It is worth bearing in mind that memoranda, email, and other types of internal documents can become evidence in a lawsuit.

Data protection

An important area that will impact on a pharmaceutical company and its employees is the law as to data protection. Governed in the UK by the Data Protection Act of 1998 (enacted to comply with EC Directive 95/46/EEC), this wide-ranging piece of legislation was designed to allay privacy concerns as technology developed, allowing widespread availability of information relating to individuals. In the context of a pharmaceutical physician or company, the main concern will be data collection in clinical trials. The Act is based on eight "principles"[56] by which all "personal" data must be processed. Thus, the processing of personal data is not prohibited, provided these principles are adhered to and the Information Commissioner is notified.[57] Where data are considered "sensitive," however, extra safeguards are added.[58] The Act also establishes certain rights of the data subject.[59] On a practical level, the Clinical Trials Directive introduced "EudraCT," a European database for interventional clinical trials with the aim that information on clinical trials should be shared between all member states. Both this and the Health Service (Control of Patient Information) Regulations 2002, which apply to confidential patient information, expressly provide, however, that they should not be interpreted in a manner inconsistent with the 1998 Act.[60] It should be noted that breach of the Act could result in criminal penalties.

---

[52] 21 CFR Section 201.57(e)

[53] *Wyeth v. Levine*, 129 S.Ct. 1187, 1198 (US 2009)

[54] Zubulake v. UBS Warburg LLC, 220 F.R.D. 212 (S.D.N.Y. 2003); and *Stevenson v. Union Pacific Railroad Company*, 354 F.3d 739 (8th Cir. 2004)

[55] *Zubulake v. UBS Warburg LLC*, 220 F.R.D. 212 (S.D.N.Y. 2003); and *Stevenson v. Union Pacific Railroad Company*, 354 F.3d 739 (8th Cir. 2004)

[56] See Data Protection Act 1998, Schedule 1 Parts I and II

[57] See s.17 of Act for notification requirement

[58] For definition of "sensitive personal data", see s.2. The extra safeguards relating to the First Principle are contained in Schedule 3

[59] See Part II of Data Protection Act 1998 generally

[60] Article 17 of Directive 2001/20/EC; Schedule 1 Part 2 of the Medicines for Human Use (Clinical Trials) Regulations 2004 implementing the Directive, and the Health Service (Control of Patient Information) Regulations 2002 SI

In the US, Federal legislation—the Health Insurance Portability and Accountability Act of 1996 (HIPAA)—serves to make patient information more strictly protected than before.[61] Although most pharmaceutical companies have limited access to patient names and other health information, any patient information must be carefully guarded to avoid violation of HIPAA statutes, which address the use and disclosure of individuals' medical information by "covered entities," and set standards for individuals' rights to control the use of their medical information. Violations can result in fines and/or, in some instances, imprisonment.[62]

Pharmaceutical industry voluntary codes

In addition to the provisions of the UK Medicines Act (1968), European Directives, and other similar mandates, the pharmaceutical industry also carries out a measure of self-regulation through its industry bodies. In the UK, for example, the Association of the British Pharmaceutical Industry (ABPI) is the trade association for around 90 companies producing prescription medicines. The Association's Code of Practice for the Pharmaceutical Industry ('the Code") is operated by the Prescription Medicines Code of Practice Authority (PMCPA), which was

established by the ABPI as an independent authority. The Code applies to the promotion to UK health professionals and appropriate administrative staff of medicines for prescribing as well as to information made available to the general public and patients about such medicines. It does not cover the promotion of OTC medicines when the object is to encourage purchase by the public.[63]

Voluntary codes are not legally enforceable in the same way as a statute. It is a condition of membership of the ABPI, however, that the pharmaceutical companies abide by the Code. In addition, the Code contains a number of sanctions that may be imposed against member companies. Complaints are made to the PMCPA and, if it is decided that there has been a breach of the Code, the company concerned has five working days to provide a written undertaking to discontinue the promotional activity in question, with an "administrative charge" levied. The amount depends on the number of breaches. There are also other sanctions available to the PMCPA (and its Appeal Board), such as auditing the company in breach of its procedures to comply with the Code or reporting it to the Board of Management of the ABPI, which has the authority to reprimand the company publicly or revoke its membership to the ABPI. All complaints and their outcomes are reported by the PMCPA on a quarterly basis and also online. Details of ongoing cases can also be found online.

Some provisions of the Code are of particular importance to pharmaceutical physicians. Clause 14, for example, requires that promotional material be certified by two senior officials in the company, one of whom must be a registered medical practitioner. The other is usually a pharmacist. The promotion must be certified to be in accordance with the Code; it must confirm that the material is accurate, balanced, fair, objective, and unambiguous, is based on an up-to-date evaluation of all the evidence, and is in no way misleading. Certificate renewal is required every two years.

2002/1438. See also, however, the European Data Protection Supervisor's opinion 2009/C 229/04 on proposed amendments to Council Reg. 726/2004 and Directive 2001/83/EC in the context of pharmacovigilance and the risks for data protection

[61] See Health Insurance Portability and Accountability Act of 1996 (HIPAA)

[62] See Pub. L. 104-191; 42 USC Section1320d-5; Pub. L. 104-191; 42 USC Section 1320d-6. A person who knowingly obtains or discloses individually identifiable health information in violation of HIPAA faces a fine of US$50,000 and up to one-year imprisonment. The criminal penalties increase to US$100,000 and up to five years imprisonment if the wrongful conduct involves false pretences, and to US$250,000 and up to ten years imprisonment if the wrongful conduct involves the intent to sell, transfer, or use individually identifiable health information for commercial advantage, personal gain, or malicious harm. Criminal sanctions will be enforced by the Department of Justice

---

[63] See ABPI Code of Practice for the Pharmaceutical Industry 2008 and "Quick Guide to the Code for Health Professionals," published by the PMCPA July 2008

The US equivalent is the Pharmaceutical Research and Manufacturers of America (PhRMA), a trade association founded in 1958. PhRMA is a non-profit scientific and professional organization of more than 100 pharmaceutical manufacturers. In 2002, PhRMA published a voluntary Code entitled "Interactions with Health Care Professionals." The Code sought to ensure that interactions between healthcare providers and pharmaceutical companies meet the highest ethical standards. In 2009, the Code was strengthened due to concerns of policy makers and healthcare professionals that the earlier Code did not adequately cover questionable practices. The many large fines levied against companies—totaling billions of dollars—as well as the plea bargains, no admission of guilt settlements, and decree agreements with Federal and state authorities, all provided impetus for the 2009 revisions.

Among the changes made to the Code are to require full justification for selecting and paying retainers and honorariums to consultants on medical or marketing advisory panels, and full disclosure of speakers or consultants employed by the pharmaceutical industry who serve on formulary committees or clinical committees advising on therapeutic treatments and categories to be implemented. The Code also severely restricts the use of meals, gifts, and entertainments to health professionals. Gone are the plastic pens and other reminder gifts, as well as "Dish and Dash" free meals for practitioners and their office staff. Rigid criteria for restaurant "educational meals" are included. The Code also prohibits entertainment or recreational activities at meetings and resorts. In addition, the Code calls for the separation of funds for continuing medical education from marketing influence. Most firms have set up units independent of Marketing and under Medical Affairs to administer such grants and are not allowed to direct the program content. Finally, the Code requires that the Compliance Officer and the Chief Executive Officer of the member firms sign, on an annual basis, an attestation that the firm is in compliance with the Code.

PhRMA also issues guidelines and principles. Two of the most recent again focus on areas of controversy. In December 2008, revised "Guiding Principles on Direct to Consumer Advertisements About Prescription Medicines" were issued. The Guiding Principles address concerns about potentially misleading direct-to-consumer (DTC) advertisements by requiring that the advertisements comply with FDCA regulations and thereby educate consumers about prescription medications. The other, in force since October 2009, is "Principles on Conduct of Clinical Trials and Communication of Clinical Trial Results." The Principles were enacted in response to criticism from many sources—in particular the International Committee of Medical Journal Editors (ICMJE). The Principles focus on protecting research participants, conducting high-quality rigorous clinical research trials, ensuring objectivity in research, and providing full disclosure of information from clinical trials to healthcare professions in a timely manner, while respecting patient privacy.

Conclusion

Caution and compliance are bywords for pharmaceutical physicians. They must be knowledgeable about the many laws and regulations that directly affect pharmaceutical manufacturers and their employees. Sanctions for failing to comply with these requirements may be severe, both for the manufacturer and for the individual. Consequently, pharmaceutical corporations need to develop, implement, and maintain effective compliance programs and related training, and pharmaceutical physicians should stay informed of the regulations and laws relevant to the industry in order to ensure compliance. Regulatory compliance, and effective internal communication can avert potential problems and potential legal liability for both the manufacturer and its employees.

CHAPTER 52

Fraud and Misconduct in Clinical Research

Jane Barrett
Gawsworth, Cheshire, UK

Introduction

Research misconduct strikes at the very heart of scientific objectivity. Its very existence raises doubts about the integrity of the results and lessens our trust in the work of others. We must be able to believe in the reliability of scientific research.

There has been much published on the incidence, detection, and prosecution of publication fraud, rather less on fraud and misconduct in clinical research, but we should be equally concerned about research fraud. The Consensus Conference on Misconduct in Biomedical Research convened by the Faculty of Pharmaceutical Medicine and the Royal College of Physicians of Edinburgh in 1999 defined research misconduct as "behavior by a researcher, intentional or not, that falls short of good ethical and scientific standards" (Edinburgh Royal College of Physicians, 2000). Frank Wells, co-founder of MedicoLegal Investigations Ltd, the only specialist research fraud investigation company in Europe, prefers "the generation of false data with the intention to deceive." Both definitions have value, combining to highlight the deliberate and unacceptable practice of bad science and bad ethics.

How common is research fraud?

Carelessness is common, research fraud less so, but both are almost impossible to quantify. The US

Principles and Practice of Pharmaceutical Medicine, 3rd edition.
Edited by L.D. Edwards, A.W. Fox, P.D. Stonier.
© 2011 Blackwell Publishing Ltd.

Food and Drug Administration (FDA) has offered estimates of around 5% of clinical trials. Some authorities suggest a rate of 1%, some up to 7% (Ankier, 2004). My experience suggests a figure around the 3% mark. The number of clinical trials running at any one time must be in the hundreds of thousands, leaving potential for an unacceptable number of studies producing data that are unreliable or even fabricated. More than 70% of the audiences of two separate international clinical research conferences within the last few years agreed they had seen clinical research fraud. Most had done nothing about it.

Fraud or misconduct?

It is tempting to use the words fraud and misconduct almost interchangeably, but in most cases, they can be differentiated. In broad terms, research fraud is defined as willful behavior that breaches the principles of good practice in research. Fraud must have an element of deliberate action or recklessness: true fraud is not an accidental act. The definition of research malpractice provided by the Wellcome Trust is a useful starting point, and it makes clear the element of intent:

> The fabrication, falsification, plagiarism or deception in proposing, carrying out or reporting results of research or deliberate, dangerous or negligent deviations from accepted practices in carrying out research. It includes failure to follow established protocols if this failure results in unreasonable harm

or risk to humans, other vertebrates or the environment, and facilitating misconduct in research by collusion in, or concealment of, such actions by others. It also includes intentional, unauthorized use, disclosure or removal of or damage to research-related property of another including apparatus, materials, writings, data, hardware or software or any other substances or devices used in or produced by the conduct of research.

It does not include honest error or honest differences in the design, execution, interpretation or judgement in evaluating research methods or results, or misconduct unrelated to the research process. Similarly, it does not include poor research unless this encompasses the intention to deceive."[1]

Another method of differentiation relates to those affected. Others are always harmed by fraud, whereas in some cases of misconduct there may be no obvious victims. (Note the caveats; some cases of misconduct do indeed result in harm to others). Foremost among those harmed by fraud are patients or research subjects who may have received unnecessary treatment, not had full safety assessments while taking an experimental drug, or been entered into a study about which they knew nothing. Patient records may have been altered to show untrue diagnoses to make them appear eligible for the study: this often remains uncorrected.

Sponsoring pharmaceutical companies are harmed if they have paid for fraudulent data that they cannot subsequently use or if a drug is delayed in gaining a license, and the families of fraudulent doctors who lose their license to practice when prosecuted and found guilty also suffer financially. Journal editors who unknowingly publish the fraudulent results can be harmed, as happened to Professor Geoffrey Chamberlain in the Pearce case discussed later in this chapter.

All fraud is also misconduct by definition, but misconduct *per se* is not so clear-cut. It could be accidental, for example missing the due date for patient assessments, or carelessly completing case record forms, but the point where carelessness becomes misconduct and misconduct becomes fraud is indistinct. A safety assessment might be omitted because the research team forgot about it or the research subject did not present him- or herself to the laboratory to have the blood drawn. Equally, it might be because a researcher decided not to do it because of too much work or because he or she decided it was not important. Serious but nonfraudulent misconduct might be the inappropriate delegation of study tasks to an inexperienced member of the study team without input or supervision from the Principal Investigator. Distinction must be drawn between clinical research that is of poor quality and that which is fraudulent. Errors are common, represent lack of attention to detail, pressure of work and time, inadequate or overcomplicated case record forms, or plain carelessness. By contrast, immaculately completed record forms may prove to be too good to be true, very few researchers actually keeping perfect records.

What constitutes research fraud?

There are many types of research fraud,[2] and the following list is not exhaustive, but it is useful to consider the various categories.

Fabrication: the deliberate invention of research data/results, or the deliberate fabrication of laboratory analysis

An eminent UK gynecologist, Malcolm Pearce, published two papers in the *British Journal of Obstetrics and Gynaecology* in 1994, one claiming to have successfully reimplanted an ectopic fetus, the second being an extensive series of case studies in a syndrome so uncommon that a major referral center was seeing only one or two new cases a

---

[1] http://www.wellcome.ac.uk/stellent/groups/corporatesite/@policy_communications/documents/web_document/wtd002754.pdf; accessed June 15, 2009

[2] Definition of research misconduct, see http://www.bristol.ac.uk/secretary/studentrulesregs/researchmisc.html; accessed May 15, 2009

month. Over three years, Pearce reported on 191 women he claimed to have seen and on whom he had run a battery of complex tests, including karyotyping both the women and their partners. Pearce was an editor of the journal and the Editor in Chief, Professor Geoffrey Chamberlain, was his head of department and named as co-author of one of the papers. Chamberlain's role in the work is not known, but he was quoted by a newspaper as saying, "The head of department's name is always put on reports out of politeness. I was not part of this work, but I have always trusted Mr Pearce" (Sheikh, 2000). When the fraud was discovered, due only to the actions of a whistleblower, both men found their careers effectively ended.

The most commonly fabricated documents are consent forms and patient diary cards. The diary cards allegedly submitted by the patients of a general practitioner (GP) in northern England were all immaculately completed and in pristine condition. This marked them out from the cards collected from other investigational sites, which were dirty and showed signs of frequent handling. Additionally, the handwriting on all diary cards was very similar, and an idiosyncratic mark made by the investigator when he wrote was noted many times on the diary cards. The doctor was found guilty of fraud and his license to practice medicine was withdrawn.

Falsification: the deliberate distortion or omission of undesired data/results, including the dishonest misinterpretation of results

William McBride, an Australian obstetrician, wrote a letter to the *Lancet* in 1961 in which he suggested that the drug thalidomide, when given to pregnant women, was causing severe limb deformities in their babies (McBride, 1961). Nobody else had raised concerns at that time about the dangers of this newly marketed drug. McBride's hypothesis was based on limited anecdotal observations, but he was subsequently shown to be right and thalidomide was removed from the market. In 1982, he published research that showed that the active substance in Debendox, a drug for morning sickness of pregnancy, caused birth defects in rabbits (McBride, Vardy and French, 1982). The

manufacturers took the drug off the market, but no researchers could reproduce his work. It later transpired that McBride had altered research results, and Debendox had no teratogenic effects. Ten years later, McBride was found guilty of scientific fraud by a medical tribunal and removed from the Medical Register (Humphrey, 1994).

Manipulation of data is seen when attempts have been made to show larger differences between groups than really exist, to reduce the variability of results, or to invent extra data (Evans, 2001). In a double blind study in diabetic neuropathy, the results showed that there was significantly better pain relief with the active treatment than with placebo. However, at one site the patients worst affected by the disease all received active medication, while those least affected were apparently randomly allocated to placebo. Analysis of the patients at this site showed statistically significant improvement on the study drug, whereas analysis of the other sites excluding that one site did not. It was found that the investigator had a means of accessing the randomization code so that he could allocate the patients to what he had decided was the "correct" medication, thus skewing the data to support his hypothesis.

Plagiarism: the deliberate unacknowledged presentation/ exploitation of the work and ideas of others as one's own

The culture in schools and universities seems increasingly accepting of a certain amount of plagiarism. A survey some years ago in the United Kingdom showed that 16% of respondents had plagiarized work more than once and that a further 9% had plagiarized once, most commonly by copying material for essays from the Internet (Eaton, 2004). The detection rate was only 3%, despite the availability of software capable of detecting copied work. Although not actively condoned, plagiarism is not always dealt with as firmly as one might hope. Submitting another's essay as one's own work may well amount to fraud, and if it seems to have been accepted by those responsible for marking the work, one barrier to committing further fraud has been removed. Given the low rate of detection compared with the rate of plagiarism, it would seem that there needs to be significant attention paid to the education of tomorrow's researchers as to what constitutes good scientific and ethical behavior.

This is underlined by the fact that 24% of those students who replied to the survey claimed to have received no guidance as to what constituted plagiarism. Education of students and scientists as they enter their research career must, therefore, include the concept of research honesty and ethics, as well as trial design and methodology.

Deception: the deliberate concealment of a conflict of interest or inclusion of deliberately misleading statements in research funding proposals or other documents

Kimon Angelides ran a university laboratory in the United States when he was found to have intentionally falsified data in five grant applications submitted to the National Institutes of Health, seeking a total of US$4 million in research funds. Initial concerns were raised by his departmental head who noticed inconsistencies in grant applications. On being investigated, Angelides conceded that elements of his grant applications were false, but attempted to deflect responsibility by accusing two members of his laboratory (a graduate student and a postdoctoral fellow) of deceiving him by providing the falsified data. Other false information, particularly those appearing in the published papers, he claimed to be matters of data interpretation or simple errors.[3]

Recruiting and consenting patients without ethics approval

Independent ethical review of clinical research is central to the protection of the rights of patients. It can sometimes be a time-consuming process. Using

---

[3] http://ori.dhhs.gov/misconduct/ori_summary_angelides.shtml; accessed June 15, 2009

modern scanners and copying equipment, it is relatively easy to produce a document that appears to be ethics committee or Institutional Review Board approval to start a study. Studies may not start without ethical approval, and funding will not be forthcoming until it is given, and so time is probably the driving force behind this type of fraud.

One prolific triallist in the UK tried to justify not having sought ethics committee approval for a study by telling the sponsoring company that it was not needed because the trial was virtually the same as one he had completed the year before. The same doctor misled sponsors by using the same patients in different studies, subjecting them to tests, including brain scans, which had not been approved by an ethics committee.

Failure to document consent appropriately

Forged consent forms are one of the most common types of research fraud. A monitor from a Contract Research Organization (CRO) took the trouble to lay out all the patient consent forms at one site side by side. She noticed that the patients' signatures looked similar to each other and some of the letters resembled the handwriting of one of the study team. It transpired that none of the patients involved in the study had any knowledge of being in a trial. The study involved the women taking hormone replacement therapy (HRT) over several months, with a biopsy of their uterine lining being done before and after treatment. All had been supplied with the drug from the desk drawer of their GP, but none had given consent.

Misquotation or misrepresentation of the results of other researchers

This was how William McBride achieved the material for his infamous publication (described earlier in this chapter). Phil Vardy was a scientist working for McBride who discovered that the results of his experiments had been falsified by McBride. When he confronted McBride, he was sacked, and had to move away from the area to get another job, losing his marriage in the process. It was five years before Vardy was persuaded to publicize the fraud.

Noncompliance: the willful failure to comply with statutory and sponsor and professional body obligations

Investigation of one case can show several different fraudulent practices. John Anderton, an exemplary and highly respected physician in Edinburgh, came under suspicion when the trial monitor noticed that the signatures of some patients on the consent forms did not seem to match other signatures in their hospital notes. It was found that electrocardiograms (ECGs) and nuclear medicine investigations were apparently reported on forms that had been taken out of use some time before the start of the study. Records had been created documenting the effects of treatment before the patients were actually treated, and there were major discrepancies between the case record forms and the letters to patients' GPs. Hospital registers did not record patients' attendance for many of their stated visits, some patients were listed as attending hospital on public holidays when the outpatient department was closed, and 13 visit dates coincided with the investigator's own vacation. Some of the ECGs and X-rays had been tampered with to remove dates and patient identification. Perhaps the most damning evidence was that patients at this site showed an apparent rise in drug metabolite levels at a time point when all other sites recorded a fall, and they reported one-eighth of the number of adverse events of other sites. Anderton had his name erased from the Medical Register after being found guilty of serious professional misconduct.

Inappropriate attribution of authorship and gifted authorship on publications

Of all the abuses of scientific research, gift authorship is the most common and seemingly the most lightly regarded. This is nowhere better illustrated than in the Pearce/Chamberlain case described above.

Inciting others to be involved in research misconduct

Robert Fiddes was an eminent researcher in the US. In a lengthy and detailed fraud running over several years he changed patient notes to show that they had a specific false condition, and instructed his study staff to buy bacteria from a commercial supplier and send it to testing laboratories under the names of patients. He used cervical smears from other sources and entered the results into the patient notes, and used blood from employees, passing it off as being from patients. He made his staff wear Holter monitors and took ECGs from them, again claiming that they were taken from patients. Despite pharmaceutical company and FDA inspections, the fraud was only recognized when a former employee blew the whistle. Fiddes was sentenced to 15 months in prison, and fined almost US$1 million (Eichenwald and Kolata, 1999).

Collusion in or concealment of research misconduct by others

The General Medical Council (GMC), the United Kingdom's governing body for doctors, has made it clear that a doctor's failure to report suspicions, allegations, or evidence of scientific fraud and misconduct to the appropriate body will result in that doctor also facing disciplinary action. This happened to Professor Timothy Peters, who knew that a colleague, Dr Anjan Bannerjee, had fabricated data in a clinical trial and did not report it. Both men were found guilty of serious professional misconduct: Bannerjee was suspended and Peters received a severe reprimand. His punishment was less than it might have been because of his previous exemplary career and because the case was already ten years old.

However, it is not uncommon for those who expose the wrongdoing of others in any area to experience negative consequences, despite legislation to provide a framework and protection for them.[4] Damage to whistleblowers who act in good faith can usually be avoided, but it is essential that they are properly assessed and managed by someone experienced in the role. Perhaps this, in part, explains why more biomedical fraud is not exposed, even though it may have been recognized. For example, it took some years before Phil Vardy reluctantly blew the whistle on McBride.

---

[4] In the UK, the Public Interest Disclosure Act, 1988

Vardy was not the only whistleblower to become a victim. Dr David Edwards was a partner in Geoffrey Fairhurst's General Practice in the United Kingdom when he reported Fairhurst to the GMC for research misconduct (Edwards, 2001). There was a long wait for a hearing, during which Edwards' marriage came under extreme stress. After the guilty verdict on Fairhurst, Edwards had graffiti sprayed on his surgery door by angry patients, and was faced with possible financial ruin for some time.

Malicious unfounded accusation of misconduct against another

It is perhaps fear of being shown to be wrong that holds many back from making allegations of research fraud. The term of whistleblower does not have a good connotation and is being widely replaced by such euphemisms as "Open-Practice Policy." It is in an attempt to minimize risk both to those who report suspected fraud and to those accused of it that all National Health Service (NHS) Trusts and universities in the UK have published clear policies on such matters.

What is being done about handling research fraud?

Given the growing concern over research misconduct, a number of organizations have proposed that universities and other research institutions should safeguard public confidence in research by formulating good research practice guidelines and laying down clear and equitable procedures for investigating allegations of research misconduct. Increasingly, funding agencies are making it a condition of eligibility for research grants that institutions have in place agreed procedures for governing good research practice. Although the principles involved are not new, the presence and use of a published code of practice is widely regarded as the best preventative measure against research misconduct. Such policies have stepwise procedures describing how to proceed, including clarifying responsibilities at each stage and stressing the need for full documentation.

The United States

The United States was the first to take a stand on the detection and prosecution of research fraud. A national body was established in 1972 to ensure that research subjects had true protection. This organization became the Office for Human Research Protections (OHRP) in 2000. The OHRP, which falls under the jurisdiction of the Department of Health and Human Services (HHS), provides guidance, education, and clarification on human research subject protection. It has implemented a program to supervise compliance to the Code of Federal Regulations, the legislation surrounding clinical trials in human subjects in the US. Importantly, the OHRP reviews investigations undertaken by institutions of cases of alleged non-compliance with the regulations and determines with those institutions the action to be taken.

The United States has a second official body overseeing research and ensuring its probity: the Office of Research Integrity (ORI), which is part of the Office of Public Health and Science (OPHS). Its purpose is to promote integrity in biomedical and behavioral research projects supported by the Public Health Service (PHS) worldwide. It monitors institutional investigations of research, helps to develop policies, and provides training and support to researchers.

The FDA plays a major part in the prevention and detection of research fraud and misconduct. The FDA carries out two different types of reviews. Study-orientated audits are conducted on clinical trial data itself, in order to ensure patient eligibility, and investigator-orientated inspections can be carried out either routinely or because a sponsor has concerns. If the inspectors have reason to believe that a site has not complied with regulatory requirements or has engaged in fraudulent activity—for which the definition in the Federal Code[5] is very similar to that of the Wellcome Trust quoted earlier—they have the power to disqualify the investigator from taking part in

---

[5] "Fabrication, falsification, plagiarism, or other practices that seriously deviate from those that are commonly accepted within the scientific community for proposing, conducting, or reporting research" (42 CFR 50.102)

further research, or to severely restrict that person's activities. Such findings are widely publicized both within and outside the US on the so-called "Black List."

Europe

Although European countries take research fraud and misconduct seriously, most have no official sanctions in research fraud. The first research misconduct committees in the Nordic countries date from the early 1990s. Their roles may be both preventive and investigative, but they do not, for the most part, allow sanctions to be taken; that remains in the hands of the institutions.

Finland

The first such committee was the National Research Ethics Council of Finland, founded in 1991, under the auspices of the Department of Education. It does not itself investigate research fraud, but produces guidelines for the prevention, handling, and investigation of alleged scientific dishonesty. The responsibility for investigation and actions to be taken against those found guilty remains firmly with the universities and research institutes. All such cases are reported to the Council, which gives nonlegally binding advice.

Denmark

Denmark has had the Danish Committee on Scientific Dishonesty since 1992, chaired by a High Court Judge. This Committee was charged with investigating cases and giving a formal opinion. After 1999, the Committee was split into three, only one officially covering health and medical science, but the three groups often sit together to consider cases. The Committees do not have sanctions as such, but can recommend sanctions to be taken, or can decide to make a report to the police.

Norway

There has been a National Committee for the Evaluation of Dishonesty in Health Research in Norway since 1994, charged with preventing and investigating scientific dishonesty, based heavily on the Danish Committee model. The Committee reports findings to the institution and the involved parties, but again leaves any sanctions up to the employers.

Sweden

In Sweden, the relevant institutions conduct their own investigations, with an expert advisory group, founded in 1997 and linked to the Swedish Medical Research Council (MFR), providing guidance. It too follows the Danish model of investigations. There have been proposals recently for a central committee to take over some of the elements of the investigation.

Germany

The largest academic research-funding agency in Germany, the Deutsche Forschungsgemeinschaft (German Research Foundation, known as DFG), formulated "rules of good scientific practice" in 1999 after a major scandal in which 47 published papers came under suspicion, with the aim of advising and assisting researchers nationwide. Every institution in Germany also has its own committee to investigate and suggest actions in cases of suspected research misconduct, and the Federal Länder inspectors play a supportive role. The Committee of Inquiry on Allegations of Scientific Misconduct (Ausschuss zur Untersuchung von Vorwürfen wissenschaftlichen Fehlverhaltens) investigates allegations of scientific misconduct carried out by those who receive DFG funding and members of DFG bodies involved in consultation and decision-making processes. If scientific misconduct is established, the committee's findings are forwarded to the central steering Joint Committee with a recommendation.

France

The principal medical body in France established a group of experts in 1999, the Délégation à l'Intégrité Scientifique, to focus on both the prevention of research fraud and the sanctions to be taken against individuals or institutions, although there have been few official reports of fraud. There are detailed sequential procedures to be followed, and much use has been made of the experiences of other countries.

United Kingdom

In the UK, a Joint Consensus Conference on Misconduct in Biomedical Research was held in Edinburgh in 1999 with all major stakeholders and interested parties represented. The panel's main conclusion was that "a national panel should be established—with public representation—to provide advice and assistance on request" (Stonier *et al.*, 2001). The suggestions for the remit of this panel included the development of models of good practice, assistance with investigation of alleged misconduct, and the collection and publication of information on incidents of research fraud and misconduct. It was only in 2004 that a National Panel for Research Integrity (NPRI) received funding in a joint venture headed by UK Universities and the Department of Health/NHS. The UK Research Integrity Office (UKRIO) became operational in 2006, with potentially huge benefits to patients, the pharmaceutical industry, and the medical profession.

The stated remit was to produce a code of practice for staff working in the NHS, universities, and the health industry, to give support to whistleblowers, and to provide experts to ensure the quality of future research. UKRIO does not have a direct investigative function, which could have been a real deterrent to those who might be considering fraud, but seems to be more concerned with setting standards. Any mechanism aimed at unifying response to and actions taken against clinical research fraud will be a major step forward, although progress toward this has not been widely publicized. It is widely hoped that such a national body will restore the UK's position as a leading country in biomedical research (Farthing, 2004).

In the UK, some groups involved in biomedical research are already subject to disciplinary action by their professional bodies. Doctors answer to the GMC, the Statutory Body registering doctors to practice, charged with the responsibility of monitoring standards and protecting patients. Nurses, health visitors, and midwives are responsible to the UK Central Council. Almost 30 doctors in the UK have been reported to the GMC for research fraud in the last ten years. All but one were found guilty of serious professional misconduct, and most were suspended or erased from the Medical Register, thus losing their license to practice medicine. The GMC has made it clear that it regards research fraud as extremely serious and will punish it hard. Although other countries have official channels for its investigation, more cases have been reported in the UK, but there is no reason to suppose that the incidence of fraud here differs from other countries. There have been many criticisms of the slowness of the process of bringing doctors to the GMC to account for their activities, and accusations made that the process is not sufficiently transparent.

Why commit research fraud?

This is a difficult question to answer, and there is certainly more than one answer. The creation of fraudulent data probably takes as long—if not longer—than its legitimate counterpart. Money seems to be one motivator, others being vanity or arrogance and the need to achieve publications to further career aims. Peter Jay, co-founder with Frank Wells of MedicoLegal Investigations, lists greed, need, and breed as the main tempters. The first is self-explanatory, the second category includes addiction to drugs, alcohol, and gambling, and the third acknowledges the adrenaline buzz achieved by lying, cheating, and deceiving. (The GMC recognizes that "need" is better dealt with under its health procedures.)

What has been the impact of European legislation?

The European Union (EU) Clinical Trials Directive[6] came into force in May 2004, enshrining good clinical practice (GCP) in law, and giving for the

---

[6] Directive 2001/20/EC of the European Parliament and of the Council of April 4, 2001, on the approximation of the laws, regulations, and administrative provisions of the Member States relating to the implementation of good clinical practice in the conduct of clinical trials on medicinal products for human use. *Official Journal*, May 1, 2001

first time specific legal standing to research in human subjects. Under the new laws, compliance with GCP became a legal obligation, and providing false information to an ethics committee or the national competent authority issuing authority to carry out human research, therefore, by definition became an offense. Although the legislation does not specifically mention the investigation and prosecution of research fraud and misconduct, it does allow the "Competent Authorities"—the bodies established by each Member State to authorize clinical research—to undertake inspections of sponsors and investigational sites, thus bringing Europe more into line with the US and the FDA. There is, sadly, no evidence that the presence of a statutory framework for research has reduced the incidence of fraud.

Indeed, some people point to the higher incidence of research fraud and misconduct in the US, who has had its Federal Regulations, very similar to Europe's Directive, for many years. One wonders if that is because there is more fraud in the US *per se*, or because there are official bodies involved with proactive powers and roles to identify and investigate it.

What can be done to prevent fraud?

Research governance

In the UK, the Research Governance Framework for Health and Social Care (2000, second edition produced 2005)[7] laid down standards, delivery mechanisms, and monitoring requirements for all NHS research in England and Wales. The stress is on the rights and well-being of study participants, but it also actively promotes good quality research, which by definition excludes fraud. It puts stress on the need for the review of research at all stages, and this is seen as being a significant potential tool in the prevention of fraud.

---

[7] http://www.dh.gov.uk/en/Publicationsandstatistics/ Publications/PublicationsPolicyAndGuidance/DH_4108962; accessed June 15, 2009

Publications

The editors of scientific journals, vehemently expressing their abhorrence of research and publication fraud, established the Committee on Publication Ethics (COPE) in the UK in 1997. They recommend peer review and require all named authors to sign the letter of submission, coupled with clear declarations from all parties as to conflict of interest. Such procedures would have prevented Pearce's fraud because the paper on the reimplantation of the ectopic fetus had not undergone peer review, and the co-authors were not required to detail their involvement.

Standard operating procedures (SOPs)

Adherence to SOPs has a major protective effect in suspected research fraud and misconduct. First, it enables an organization to make clear the consequences of research fraud to the researcher at the start of the research, with the intent of preventing such dishonesty. Second, it gives a framework for the reporting and subsequent investigation of potential misconduct, and consequent legal protection for those following such guidelines, especially if the finding of the investigation is that there was no misconduct. SOPs should begin with an unequivocal statement that all cases of suspected misconduct and fraud will be vigorously investigated and, if indicated, prosecuted, and that failure to investigate is not acceptable. There should be a clearly described process for the reporting of suspicions within the hierarchy of the organization or sponsoring company, and detailed guidance for the investigation of such suspicions, including the recruitment of external agencies when so indicated.

But the best thought out, best written SOP is without value if all parties concerned do not receive training in its use, and so this must be a priority for all new staff joining an organization concerned with research, whether as researcher or sponsor. It should make clear that an employee of any organization who sees potential fraud and does not report it would him- or herself be guilty of misconduct.

What can be done if fraud is suspected?

In general, the role of national bodies involved in the investigation of research fraud and misconduct is merely to advise and support the relevant institutions, but it is for those institutions themselves to decide whether to take action against those found to have acted dishonestly. The situation in the US is somewhat different; the FDA can order the closure of institutions and circulates the names of wrongdoers on their "Black List." The ORI can recommend the withdrawal of Federal funding, and the French authorities, too, can take direct action. The system for dealing with doctors suspected of research crime in the United Kingdom revolves around the GMC, which stated in 1992 that their disciplinary committee would take a very serious view of proven clinical research fraud. The role of the GMC was discussed earlier in this chapter, but it can only investigate suspected fraud or misconduct after a formal complaint in the form of a Statutory Declaration is made, and there is no authority to deal with nonmedical research personnel. Nurses and midwives are responsible for their behavior to the UK Central Council, and other healthcare workers have their own governing bodies.

There are potential criminal sanctions against fraudulent researchers, but these are seldom, if ever, pursued. In most countries, there is no law specifically relating to fraud. One needs to draw elements from laws relating to deception, theft, offenses against the person, and forgery and counterfeiting. However, the police and judiciary would find it difficult to follow the intricacies of research fraud, and as the amount of money involved is usually relatively small, might not be particularly interested in following a case through. Perhaps, more importantly, the time that it would typically take for such a case to come before a criminal or civil court would allow even more fraud to be committed, and more patients to be put at risk.

The pharmaceutical industry has been extremely active in its efforts to prevent and detect research fraud and misconduct, and most companies are now comfortable taking action when appropriate. The Association of the British Pharmaceutical Industry (ABPI) has encouraged its member companies to do so and has provided much support and encouragement. The new European Directive on clinical trials and the International Conference on Harmonization (ICH) have both aided a growing understanding and awareness of the issue, and most pharmaceutical companies now have standard procedures for handling cases of suspected fraud. The interests of the industry lie partly in protecting patients, but also in protecting and maintaining the quality and integrity of clinical research. Many of the doctors brought before the GMC for research misconduct have been involved with more than one pharmaceutical company, and the Medical Director of the ABPI has a process to bring together two or more companies with suspicions about the same doctor to enable a joint case to be made. A similar process exists in Germany. Sadly, there are, as yet, no sanctions if a company refuses to cooperate or investigate.

Comment should also be made about the way whistleblowers—those raising concerns about suspected misconduct—are handled. Most countries have legislation in place to protect them, on condition that they raise their concerns within the organization, according to that organization's standard procedures, and are without malice. However, advice is rarely given in these guidance documents on how to proceed if the person suspected of misconduct is in a senior position within the organization, and the procedures often recommend whistleblowers to report their concerns to one person only, thus putting themselves into a potentially very vulnerable position. Whistleblowers should not be handled lightly or by the inexperienced.

Conclusions

Research fraud is a reality, but in the past healthcare professionals and academia have sometimes chosen to turn a blind eye, and pharmaceutical companies tacitly condoned it by choosing not to investigate fully or to bring prosecutions. The climate now is changing, driven by all those parties, but medical research is still vulnerable in the absence of any effective mechanism to combat and detect fraud. To pretend that fraud does not exist is effectively to condone it. To take no action when fraud is suspected or when blatant evidence is seen is not acceptable. The most vulnerable potential victims are the patients; whichever definition of fraud is used, the fact that patients have been exploited remains. This exploitation occurs when ethics committee authorization is not sought or is forged, denying patients the protection of review of the safety and ethics of the study. It occurs when safety data are not recorded or when patients are treated with inappropriate drugs. It occurs when drugs are licensed or withdrawn from the market using fraudulent data. It occurs when there are incorrect details on their patient notes.

The eradication of research fraud will not be easy. Research governance will be a significant step toward eradication, but only if everyone accepts the possibility for the existence of fraud and is alert to its presence. SOPs provide a framework within which it is easier to follow up suspicions of fraud and misconduct, but they only work if everyone concerned has been trained in their use and remembers to use them: their presence alone is not a safeguard against fraud. Ethics committees too have their place in the fight against fraud. Again, they need to be aware of the possibility of fraud, and need to have a mechanism whereby they can report concerns, for example, of an inappropriate number of studies running at one site.

Three elements are necessary to improve the situation. There must be official bodies in each country with real powers to investigate and prosecute clinical research fraud. There must be a widespread and unequivocal acceptance that failure to act on suspicions of fraud is itself serious misconduct. And finally there must be an acceptance of the application of the same rules, no matter who sponsors research, whether it be industry or academia. Most clinical researchers, like most members of the public, are honest. However, to pretend that clinical research fraud and misconduct do not exist is to allow bad medicine, bad science, and above all, abuse of patients.

References

Ankier S. Misconduct and fraud in clinical research. In *Medical Law and Research*. Ankier Associates, 2004; www.medreslaw.com; accessed April 15, 2010.

Eaton L. A quarter of UK students are guilty of plagiarism, survey shows. *BMJ* 2004; **329**:70.

Edinburgh Royal College of Physicians. *Supplement 7: Joint Consensus Conference on Misconduct in Biomedical Research*, 2000.

Edwards D. Whistleblower. In *Fraud and Misconduct in Biomedical Research*, third edition. S Lock, F Wells, M Farthing (eds). BMJ Books: London, UK, 2001.

Eichenwald K, Kolata G. A doctor's drug studies turn into fraud. *New York Times*, Section A, New York Edition, May 17, 1999.

Evans S. Statistical aspects of the detection of fraud. In *Fraud and Misconduct in Biomedical Research*, third edition. S Lock, F Wells, M Farthing (eds). BMJ Books: London, UK, 2001.

Farthing MJG. Publish, and be damned ... The road to research misconduct. *J R Coll Physicians Edinb* 2004; **34**:301–304.

Humphrey GF. Scientific fraud: the McBride case–judgment. *Med Sci Law* 1994; **34**(4):299–306.

McBride WG. Thalidomide and congenital abnormalities. *Lancet* 1961; **2**:1358.

McBride WG, Vardy PH, French J. Effects of scopolamine hydrobromide on the development of the chick and rabbit embryo. *Aust J Biol Sci* 1982; **35**(2):173–178.

Sheikh A. Publication ethics and the research assessment exercise: reflections on the troubled question of authorship. *J Med Ethics* 2000; **26**:422–426.

Stonier P, Lowe GDO, McInnes G, Murie J, Petrie J, Wells F. A national panel for research integrity: a proposed blueprint for the prevention and investigation of misconduct in biomedical research. *Proc R Coll Physicians Edinb* 2001; **31**:253–255.

SECTION VIII
Business Aspects

Introduction

Contrary to popular opinion, governments and health services develop almost no drugs and discover very few. In the developed world, almost all the therapeutic advances of the last half-century have been the result of the efforts of the pharmaceutical industry. This is actually also true in the developing parts of the world, although public health measures in those regions may also have greater scope for improving the human condition.

So how does the pharmaceutical industry do it? Compared with, say, the car manufacturing industry, drugs have long development cycles, huge development costs, high project failure rates, intense and regressive regulation, high compliance costs, shortened patent horizons, government-enforced price controls, numerous competitors, and great product liability issues when a product does make it to the marketplace. This set of conditions is highly unattractive for an industry that might want to borrow money and attract investors.

So it becomes a fact of life for large pharmaceutical companies that they must fund their research and development activities themselves. Not only that, but one way or another, they must also fund development candidates that emerge from small pharmaceutical or biotechnology companies, too. The latter cannot afford Phase III studies, and would find it impossible to recruit a sales force.

But research and develop we must. If we do not the industry will wither approximately at the rate of appearance of generic products. Such a withered industry will bring to an end almost all progress in medicine.

This section therefore concentrates on the financial aspects of pharmaceutical medicine. This may be an unattractive subject to the idealists. But Churchill once said: "Democracy is the worst form of government, except for all those other forms that have been tried from time to time." (House of Commons, November 11, 1947). Perhaps we should replace the words "democracy" and "government" with the terms "private enterprise" and "medical progress," respectively.

CHAPTER 53

The Multinational Corporations: Cultural Challenges, the Legal/Regulatory Framework and the Medico-commercial Environment

R. Drucker[1] & R. Graham Hughes[2]
[1]Technomark Life Sciences LLP, Durham, NC, USA
[2]Consultant in Pharmaceutical Development, Merlimont, France

Cultural challenges

"Culture" has been defined as the "totality of socially transmitted behavior patterns, arts, beliefs, institutions, and all other products of human work and thought typical of a population or community at a given time" (*Webster's Dictionary*, 1984). With respect to the multinational pharmaceutical corporation, culture can be thought of at three levels: (i) societal; (ii) medical; and (iii) corporate. At each level, culture has an omnipresent impact on drug development, prior to and after regulatory approval. Sensitivity to cultural considerations will help identify, conceive, present, and respond to issues in drug development. It may also help to identify sources of competitive advantage.

Societal culture

Societal culture describes those attributes of culture pervading a population or community inhabiting a given geographical area. Individuals from the same societal culture share common values. A multinational corporation has to deal with many societal cultures, even, sometimes, within a single nation. Differences in societal culture will result in different responses to key issues. Table 53.1 indicates a range of culturally determined responses to important questions.

One can apply the concepts in Table 53.1 to the pharmaceutical industry, for example, to management practices originating from one culture being applied in a different cultural setting. For example, companies in the United States tend to use control systems that exert more checks and balances on personnel than do European companies (a habit that may have historical origins in a Christian, nonconformist set of traditions emphasizing a belief that all people are intrinsically evil).

Similarly, companies with development programs involving contraceptive drugs have sometimes aroused criticisms among their personnel, depending on country, religious background, and personal beliefs.

Other cross-cultural differences revolve around the distinction between group goal seeking and individual goal seeking. Group goals are emphasized by those who see a lineal relationship of person to person as important; this contrasts with those cultures of an individualistic disposition that emphasize individual goals (Japan versus the US is a clear example of this dichotomy). Concern for the welfare of the extended family might result in the

Principles and Practice of Pharmaceutical Medicine, 3rd edition.
Edited by L.D. Edwards, A.W. Fox, P.D. Stonier.

Table 53.1 Cultural influences on life issues (modified from Kluckhohn and Strodtbeck, 1961): geographical contexts are an obvious oversimplification

	Alternative cultural presumptions		
	1	2	3
What is the character of human nature?	Humans are evil	Humans are a mixture of good and evil	Humans are good
What is the relationship of humans to nature?	Humans are subject to nature	Humans are in harmony with nature	Humans are master of nature
What is the temporal focus of life?	To the past	To the present	To the future
What is the modality of human activities?	Activity that gives spontaneous expression to impulse and desires	Activity that emphasizes as a goal the development of all aspects of the self	Activity that is motivated primarily toward measurable accomplishments
What is the relationship of human to human?	Lineal: group goals are primary and an important goal is continuity through time	Collateral: group goals are primary; well-regulated continuity of group relationships through time is not critical	Individual: the individual's goals are most important
Geographical contexts	Asia	Europe	North America

hiring of a close relative in one culture, but cause accusations of nepotism in another.

Medical culture

Differing perceptions of health and disease by patients, healthcare providers, and governing and regulatory bodies are the primary elements of medical culture (Riphagen, 1992). Aspects of medical culture of particular importance to the pharmaceutical industry are those affecting drug development, approval, and marketing, including those that may determine whether a drug should have prescription or over-the-counter status. Other aspects of concern are the type of healthcare funding favored by a particular culture: private insurance or public funding through taxation.

An attempted convergence of medical cultures is currently underway in the area of drug development and regulatory approval, under the auspices of the International Committee on Harmonization (ICH). Note that this regulatory harmonization will probably have no influence whatsoever on increasing the uniformity of prescribing behavior. Convergent thinking is also seen in a worldwide effort to

control healthcare expenditure. The various cost-cutting approaches have included the following:
- reduced prescribing volume;
- decreased price of medicines;
- decreased reimbursement for medicines;
- delisting of medicines from reimbursement lists;
- encouragement to parallel trade;
- control of overall company profitability;
- drug formularies and National Institute for Health and Clinical Excellence (NICE);
- encouragement of generic substitution;
- encouragement of therapeutic substitution;
- assignment of pharmaceutical budgets to institutions and individuals;
- encouragement of self-medication.

Despite the *prima facie* attraction of cultural convergence in medicine, there are not only major differences in the incidence and prevalence of many diseases between countries, but also in expectations of these different cultural groups of patients. Even in a relatively homogeneous region such as Western Europe, the incidence of adverse drug reactions to a standard therapy varies dramatically from country to country. The perception of the nature and significance of given disease states varies by country, and the trigger to seek professional assistance also varies. The ensuing doctor–patient relationships reflect not only the national medical culture, but also broader societal culture in such practical matters as the patient's "right to know," freedom of information, tendency to litigation for malpractice, and so on.

Corporate culture

In any company, the corporate culture permeates every aspect of the company's activities, affecting promotion prospects, risk propensity, and individual and group behaviors.

The principal concern of the multinational corporation is the extent to which corporate culture conflicts or fits in with the societal and medical culture(s) in each country where the company operates. Corporate culture is evidenced by shared values about the conduct of business, and may be strong or weak.

The most successful corporate culture is one that can foster leadership that is responsive to potential conflict arising in multinational operations from cultural diversity. Organizations with such a culture express a clear vision that is understood and supported internationally. Such organizations benefit from an alignment of business values among employees worldwide, despite varied national and cultural backgrounds. Even though it divested its pharmaceutical businesses in September 2009, Procter and Gamble is the classic example of a strong corporate culture that successfully crosses business and geographical boundaries.

Complexities can also arise when a multinational pharmaceutical company engages the services of another organization, such as a multinational contract research organization (CRO). They are bound to have different corporate cultures. In each country where the two multinationals need to collaborate, there is a need not only to reconcile those differences in corporate culture, but also to be jointly responsive to local societal and medical cultural considerations: Avoid a three-way culture clash!

Languages

A multinational corporation necessarily conducts its business in many different languages, presenting challenges of internal and external communications. Companies with a weak corporate culture are paradoxically more likely to cause local tensions by insisting on a rigid mode of operation. Companies with a strong corporate culture are more likely to operate according to local cultural norms under the guidance of local management. For example, the "or not," as in "would you like a drink or not," can be regarded as aggressive when spoken in English in England, and yet when spoken in English in Singapore is intended as a courtesy, indicating that the questioner truly is not trying to influence your decision.

Societal, medical, and corporate culture interplay

Figure 53.1 depicts how the cultural responsiveness of a company in a given country is determined by the overlap of its corporate culture with local societal and medical cultures. The more that the circle corresponding with corporate culture overlaps those of societal and medical culture, the more the area available for culturally appropriate behavior is increased. Figure 53.1 also provides a framework for comparing central with peripheral control of national affiliates. There are many determinants of the balance between the two. However, if a corporate culture is dissonant with the societal and medical cultural imperatives of a subsidiary or affiliate organization, yet is imposed upon that organization because of a policy of

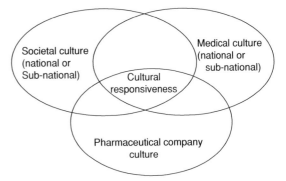

Figure 53.1 Venn diagram identifying area available for culturally appropriate behavior (with thanks to Andrew Fletcher).

"centralization," then a suboptimal outcome is likely. Conversely, a strong, responsive corporate culture that is consonant with local societal and medical values increases the likelihood of success. A locally responsive corporate culture favors neither centralization nor decentralization—this will depend on many other considerations (e.g., size of operations, in-country management capability, etc.). However, it facilitates an appropriate devolution of managerial power, which might otherwise be difficult or even impossible. The challenge to the multinational corporation, therefore, is to have a strong corporate culture that is compatible with diverse societal and medical cultures.

The legal/regulatory framework for drug development in Europe and the United States

The ICH document *General Considerations for Clinical Trials*, seeks to do the following:

• Describe the internationally accepted principles and practices in the conduct of both individual clinical trials and the overall development strategy for new medicinal products.

• Facilitate the evaluation and acceptance of foreign clinical trial data by promoting common understanding of general principles and approaches, and also the definition of relevant terms.

• Present an overview of the ICH clinical safety and efficacy documents and facilitate the user's access to guidance pertinent to clinical trials within these documents.

In Western Europe, in spite of the Clinical Trials Directive, there is still no uniformity in the documentation that is required to be submitted to the authorities (Table 53.2). Some countries require brief summaries of available information, whereas others require detailed information on the preclinical, pharmacy, chemistry, and other clinical data to be submitted.

All European countries require, in common with the US and in conformity with the Declaration of Helsinki, that ethics committees (the European version of Institutional Review Boards (IRBs) in

Table 53.2 European requirements for submissions to competent authorities to obtain clearance for initiation of clinical trials

	Protocol and supporting documents	EC (IRB) approval	Insurance certificate
Austria	×		
Belgium	×	×	
Denmark	×		×
Finland	×		
France	×	×	×
Germany	×	×	
Greece	×		×
Ireland	×		
Italy	×		
The Netherlands	×		
Norway	×	×	×
Portugal	×	×	
Spain	×		
Sweden	×		
UK	×		

the United States) review protocols from Phases I–IV and the general conduct of trials outside the formal protocol document. However, there is wide variation in Europe as to how this procedure is enacted.

In countries such as France, Spain, and Germany, there is a national system of ethics committees that duplicate similar work at a local level. In the United Kingdom, there are a wide variety of ethics committees, such as commercial committees, those set up by the Royal College of Physicians, and those run by local area health authorities or hospital trusts.

Similarly, in the US, both "local" and "central" IRBs exist. The latter can support multicenter studies and are more likely to be professional and fee-paying. It has been questioned whether an IRB in, say, Seattle can truly serve the needs of a Cuban–American patient in Miami.

Local medical and societal cultural factors impact on the ethics committee approvals, so that a study that is considered to be ethical in one country may be regarded as unethical in another. An example of this may be the unacceptability of the use of placebo control in depression studies in

Germany, whereas similar studies would be permitted elsewhere. Similarly, the common practice of extensive blood sampling in Belgium, especially in pediatric studies, would be regarded as excessive and hence unethical in other countries.

In the Central and Eastern Region (CEE) of Europe, the clinical trials approval system continues to evolve rapidly. In general, the regulations are converging towards the EU model of submission and approval, but local practices make interpretation at the national level a necessity for the expedient approval of any clinical trial project or program.

Irritatingly, there is no initiative in Europe to standardize clinical trial submissions, which would be preferable even if no bureaucracy gave up its peculiarity, and an accreted globally-acceptable submission was the result. For the present, all National Competent Authorities require the protocol and investigators' information. The ethics committee approval must be obtained in advance and submitted with the application in Belgium, France, Germany, Norway, and Portugal. An insurance certificate is needed in Denmark, France, Greece, and Norway. Newer members of the EU seem to be asking for inconsistent things that vary from application to application when they choose to delay the study.

Insurance practices again exhibit cross-cultural differences. The EU guidelines for patient protection lay down that there should be "sufficient" insurance provision. However, some countries have taken this requirement a step further by laying down the actual sums for which individual patients, or in the case of Germany, the total number of patients, must be covered. In the US, patients and volunteers are in general insured by the institution in which the study is conducted; the fees for this are not directly reimbursed by the sponsor but form part of the overall study cost.

Out of jurisdiction legal representation is another innovation. The European Medicines Agency (EMA) and many European national competent authorities will not accept clinical trial applications directly from sponsors outside the EU. Thus, these applications come from a within-EU legal representative, who in turn, must again provide the correct indemnities and hold the right insurances.

Apart from the administrative burdens and the financial implications of insurance, timing of the approval process is of the essence. There are wide variations from country to country, which depend not only on the approval times from the national competent authorities but also on the ethical committee approval times.

The Investigational New Drug (IND) application system in the US is often seen as more problematic for companies than the EU system. However, if the United States is a potential market for the product under investigation, there can be significant advantages to conducting studies under an IND, in parallel perhaps with other studies in Europe. An IND application is required in the US before any new medicinal product may be introduced into humans, or before any established product is used in an experimental or novel way. This applies not only to a commercial sponsor but also to independent physicians or academic departments wishing to conduct experimental therapy for their own purposes.

Unlike in Europe, the US IND generally requires the submission of full-length study reports whether clinical or preclinical studies, together with relevant summaries to guide the reviewer through the document. Although the writing involved in the preparation of an IND may be regarded as onerous, because the Food and Drug Administration (FDA) reviewing staff views the 1571 form as a totality, its preparation should not be regarded as a routine exercise. Rather, it should be an occasion for a critical internal appraisal of the data available and how they support the proposed protocol. Clearly, this is how the FDA views the document. The FDA peer review is thus not just an administrative hurdle to be jumped but also is often a useful, confidential third-party review of the drug development program, and once studies have received IND approval, further protocols can be added with little trouble. Of course, the IND lays down responsibilities for sponsors, which include minimum reporting times for adverse events and completion of qualification forms for investigators, and so on.

These steps add to the administrative load of the clinical drug development process. It is generally thought that it would be a bold company that submitted a New Drug Application (NDA) to the FDA without the FDA's prior involvement via an IND. However, this has been done successfully in the past and will probably occur again.

A very important cultural difference between Europe and the United States, which impacts on drug development, is indirectly expressed at the stage when the regulatory authority examines the final submitted product license-application dossier.

In the US, the FDA adopts a bottom-up stance, in which it looks at the basic raw data and sees what conclusions can be drawn from it, using its own criteria for analysis and interpretation. In Europe, the authorities tend to take the opposite approach: they look at the conclusions of all the studies, as manifested in the proposed labeling, patient leaflets, and summary of product information, and examine to what extent the data presented justify those conclusions. Hitherto, in Europe, considerable importance is placed on the role of independent experts, whose critical reports on the various sections of the dossier provide a sort of *vade mecum* for the reviewer. It is vitally important to understand in detail that the expert report required in Europe is not the same as the integrated summary required by the FDA.

In drug development, therefore, significant differences exist on a country-by-country basis in Europe as well as, to a far lesser extent, on a state-by-state basis in the US. These differences manifest themselves not only in the legal/regulatory framework but also in the commercial practices that surround the conduct of clinical trials by licensed medical practitioners.

The medico-commercial environment in the United States and Europe

One of the major differences between the United States and Europe, as regards the conduct of clinical trials, is the financing of medical care in the two regions. Throughout Europe, medical care is largely funded by governments. In the US (with some exceptions such as the State of California, the Commonwealth of Massachusetts, and military veterans nationwide), medical care is largely funded through private insurance, generally paid by the patient's employer. Coverage for many of those less able to pay, such as the indigent and the elderly, is provided by the Federal government through the Medicare and Medicaid programs, and these are likely to be revised in major ways during 2010.

In the USA, for patients without ready access to medical care, participation in a clinical trial may provide needed medical care. Note, however, that this can be an ethical issue when the free provision of clinical care becomes an inducement to signing the informed consent document.

CROs and site management organizations (SMOs) are organizations that run clinical trials, using physicians who are full-time, part-time, or contract employees. The companies employ regulatory staff, for IRB filing, adverse event notification, and so on, as well as site coordinators, nurses. and quality control personnel. SMOs might also recruit patients on behalf of their doctors, from databases built up over the years, or by press and radio/TV advertising, and even by direct telemarketing. Non-physician staff do initial screening of potential subjects on the telephone and in face-to-face interviews. Most SMOs exist in conventional treatment centers; others treat only patients who are enrolled into clinical studies, and have no other role than to run clinical trials, rather in the same way as Phase I units.

The advantages for the sponsor are several: recruitment by sites is rapid, they are used to dealing with IRBs, monitoring is straightforward, the quality of data is good, and the general service is cost-effective. For the patient, there is free medical care and medication, together with "compensation" for inconvenience, which can add up to an appreciable sum (in some cases a few hundreds of dollars per night of incarceration).

Some hospital units in Europe have recently become more commercially minded and have set themselves up as profit centers within their own hospitals. As financial pressures increase, with the increased cost of medical technology and the unfavorable demographics of an ageing population, we would expect to see more hospitals going along this route.

Differences in societal and medical cultures thus impact significantly on the development of novel drugs. The ICH process has, to a major extent, harmonized requirements but cannot and will not of itself influence how the data to fulfill these requirements are generated and collected. For the foreseeable future, the US will be seen as the more prescriptive, litigious society—suspicious of the results, building conclusions from the evidence. Europe, in so far as it can be regarded as a unity, even today, has yet to accept the ever-present lawyer in all public contexts, so that to the American observer it will continue to look *laissez-faire* and superficial in its regulation of drug development.

References

Kluckhohn F, Strodtbeck F. *Variations in Value Orientation*. Row, Peterson: Evanston, IL, USA, 1961.

Riphagen F. Different practices and perceptions from country to country. In *Conference Proceedings: How to Cope with Different Medical Cultures in Europe*. IBC: London, UK, 1992.

Webster's New Riverside University Dictionary II. Riverside Publishing Co.: Baltimore, MD, USA, 1984.

Further reading

Payer L. *Medicine and Culture: Notions of Health and Sickness*. Gollancz: London, UK, 1990.

CHAPTER 54

Advertising and Marketing

Jonathan Belsey

JB Medical Ltd, Sudbury, Suffolk, UK

The process of developing a new pharmaceutical product incurs both significant costs and risks. On average, only 1 in 5000 pharmaceutical products tested is eventually approved for patient use, and only 3 out of 10 approved drugs in the US generate enough revenue to meet or exceed average research and development (R&D) costs, which have been estimated at anything between US$500 million to US$2 billion per product (DiMasi *et al.*, 2003; Adams and Brantner, 2006). The average lead time between patenting a new chemical entity and achieving approval for marketing has fallen over recent years to 6.4 years (Keyhani, Diener-West, and Powe, 2006). With patent protection typically only lasting 15–18 years, this leaves only around 10 years of exclusive marketing to recoup R&D costs. Of course, patent protection does not guarantee market share; with around 90% of patented drugs having direct competitors (Australian Academy of Science, 1995) and an increasing requirement in many markets to demonstrate cost effectiveness versus active comparators, the opportunity to generate return on investment is severely limited.

Pharmaceutical companies in the US spent US$31.5 billion developing and testing new drugs in 2004, equivalent to about 10% of domestic sales (National Science Foundation (NSF), 2008). However, fewer than 30 new chemical entities (NCE) were introduced in 2003, compared to 53 in 1996. Of the 919 NCEs launched in the period 1982–2003, fewer than half (385) were launched across four or more G7 markets and could thus be considered global products (Grabowski and Wang, 2006), with the potential for making major returns on R&D development costs.

These factors combine to severely limit market exposure and consequently potential sales. Effective marketing strategies are therefore essential for the continued financial viability of new product development.

What is marketing?

Marketing is a process of identifying the needs, wants, and demands of customers and organizing the creation, offering, and exchange of ideas, products, and services of value to both the customer and the organization. Marketing requires a clear and specific focus on the market and the customer, so that all promotional activity can be tailored as appropriately as possible to each customer group or segment. Marketing is ubiquitous, pervasive, and extremely competitive. In the US, it has been suggested that the average person is exposed to several thousand promotional messages a day. Although this is probably an overestimate, the true value undoubtedly runs into the hundreds (AMIC, 2002; James, 2004).

Pharmaceuticals are different from other products

The pharmaceutical industry differs from other industries in that in many cases a third party is responsible for the decision to purchase and make

Principles and Practice of Pharmaceutical Medicine, 3rd edition.
Edited by L.D. Edwards, A.W. Fox, P.D. Stonier.
© 2011 Blackwell Publishing Ltd.

payment. These third parties include the prescribing health professional, who makes the decision about whether a prescription is required and, if so, what drug and in what quantity; the dispensing pharmacist, who may be actively encouraged to dispense alternative brands or generic equivalents of what was prescribed; pharmaceutical wholesalers, which prefer to purchase from cheap suppliers; and the organizations ultimately responsible for paying—governments, via state health providers such as the National Health Service in the UK or Medicaid and Medicare in the US, and health insurance organizations (Kanavos, 2001). This all combines to provide a complex market facing increasing cost-containment restrictions globally.

There are other unique facets of the pharmaceutical market. Pharmaceuticals are seen as life-saving interventions, therefore infinitely desirable, but with potentially serious side effects, leading to ethical dilemmas about their widespread use. This is particularly the case for anti-infective agents, where overuse leads to resistance to antibiotics. They can also be perceived as a tool for the unscrupulous manipulation of prescribers and patients by the multinational pharmaceutical industry. There are strict laws to control quality of the products and most countries have a national formulary on which all products must be included if they are to be prescribed in that country. Advertising of products by brand name to the final consumer, the patient, is prohibited in all countries except the US and New Zealand (James, 2004).

The pharmaceutical industry aims to produce effective drugs but it needs to do this while meeting its main objective of profitability in a competitive environment. This can lead to an uneasy conflict with governments that are trying to contain costs of healthcare, in particular of prescribing costs. The relationship between the pharmaceutical industry, government, and the NHS in the UK has been fairly stable, but initiatives such as the National Institute for Clinical Excellence (NICE), established in 1999 to promote cost-effective practice and prescribing, threaten this balance (Walley *et al.*, 2000). Although the approach seems to have been an effective means of reconciling prescribing expenditure with a profitable pharmaceutical industry

(Walley, Mrazek, and Mossialos, 2005), concerns regarding access to treatment and restriction of the market have been voiced by many (BMA, 2009).

All EU governments have taken measures to contain pharmaceutical spending, with an increasing demand for data on cost-effectiveness generally operating at the stage of re-imbursement negotiation (Kanavos, 2002). The World Health Organization also actively encourages development of drug policies based on the promotion of generic medicines. To date, however, there is little objective evidence that these strategies significantly impact on pharmaceutical spend. Although in England the total pharmaceutical spend grew at a much reduced rate from 2004–2008, compared to the period 1998–2003 (Department of Health, 2009), much of this was achieved by global price-cut negotiation with the pharmaceutical industry, rather than changes in prescribing behavior. Across the rest of Europe, pharmaceutical spend continues to grow. In 2003, the mean European annual spend per capita on pharmaceuticals was US$394 (PPP corrected): by 2007, this figure had risen to US$460 (OECD, 2009).

The pharmaceutical market is also very competitive. In England in 2008, 842.5 million prescription items were dispensed in the community, with a total net ingredient cost of over £8.3 billion (Department of Health, 2009). However, there were several hundred pharmaceutical manufacturers competing for a share in this market, with no single pharmaceutical company having more than 9.3% of the overall market; and globally, a similar picture emerges, with the largest single company commanding just 6.7% of the overall market.[1]

Product versus brand

The pharmaceutical industry relies on patent laws to maximize its income from a new product. However, patents were a late addition to

---

[1] Association of the British Pharmaceutical Industry (ABPI). Facts and statistics from the Pharmaceutical Industry; http://www.abpi.org.uk/statistics/intro.asp; accessed January 29, 2010)

pharmaceutical industry regulations, with many European countries only permitting patent protection once their industries had reached a degree of development—France in 1960, Germany in 1968, Japan in 1976, Switzerland in 1977, and Italy and Sweden in 1978 (Oxfam, 2001).

Generic drugs were introduced in the 1980s, as cheap equivalents to branded drugs that are no longer protected by patents. The R&D costs for generic products are much lower than for the original branded products, and unit production costs are very low. This means that once patent protection ceases and generic versions are on the market, sales of the more expensive branded product tend to fall. Pharmaceutical companies needed to develop strategies to cope with the limited timespan of patent protection (James, 2004).

One strategy to deal with the competition from cheap generic drugs is to promote the concept of brand rather than product. Branding was originally used to denote purity of product by the first pharmaceutical companies. Brand equity is the unique set of assets linked to the brand name that add value to brands and give customers a reason to prescribe and use them. The brand is now seen as the only tangible unit of value in the pharmaceutical company and its greatest asset. Brands are highly significant to patients as something in which to trust and of importance to their health (James, 2004).

Positioning is the process of establishing a brand in the mind of the target consumer so that the brand is seen to meet their needs. The attributes of the product are compared to the requirements of the consumer. Market leaders often show ideal positioning, when the product attributes are unique and highly relevant to customers (James, 2004).

The customers

Although the *consumers* of the product are the patients, *customers* include anyone who can make a decision about prescribing, spending money on, or taking a drug, and as such each group requires a different marketing strategy.

Prescribers can be classed according to how rapidly they change their practice when faced with information about a new product. Those most willing to try something new are known as *innovators* and *early adopters*, and in general account for 15% of the group. The next third are the *early majority*, followed by another third of the *late majority*, with the 16% least willing to change called *laggards* (James, 2004).

The product life cycle

Rapid penetration strategies around the launch of a new product tend to target early adopters and early majority prescribers. The next phase of the drug life cycle, the growth phase, is aimed at increasing perception of value and loyalty among users and recruiting new customers from nonusers. During the maturity phase the only new prescribers are laggards and sales begin to fall due to new competitors and brand saturation. Finally, the product loses its patent, which usually results in a significant drop in sales (James, 2004).

Regulations regarding marketing of prescription drugs

The United States and Canada

The Food and Drug Administration (FDA) has regulated advertising of prescription drugs in the US since 1962 under the Federal Food, Drug, and Cosmetic Act and related regulations. Advertising for other products, including over-the-counter (OTC) products, is controlled by the Federal Trade Commission under different rules. The FDA's Division of Drug Marketing, Advertising, and Communications oversees promotional labelling and advertising of prescription drugs (Rados, 2004). In the US, direct-to-consumer (DTC) advertising of prescription drugs is permitted, but controlled by regulations to make sure that all information is accurate and balanced with details of possible side effects as well as statements of benefits that could be expected. Details of how to access more detailed information must also be provided (US

Department of Health and Human Services, 1999). Canada has banned DTC advertising of prescription drugs since 1949, but Canadians living close to the US border have easy access to television and radio advertisements (Palumbo and Mullins, 2002).

The United Kingdom and Europe

Medicines cannot be promoted in the UK until they have been granted marketing authorization from the UK Medicines Control Agency or the European Medicines Agency (EMA). There are three categories of licensed medicines available in the UK: prescription-only (POM), pharmacy sale (P), and general sales medicines (GSL). The position of a medicine in one of these categories is on the decision of the Health Ministers on the advice of the Medicines Control Agency, the Committee on the Safety of Medicines, and the Medicines Commission, based on the product's possible use, any side effects, and risk of its misuse. POMs and certain pharmacy sales medicines must not be promoted to the general public, but can be marketed to the medical profession. The Association of the British Pharmaceutical Industry (ABPI) Code of Practice regulates promotional activities (ABPI, 2008a).

DTC advertising is prohibited within the EU, although general access to the Internet circumvents these regulations to an increasing extent (Palumbo and Mullins, 2002).

International patent laws

Patent laws were updated internationally via the World Trade Organization's Trade-Related Aspects of Intellectual Property Rights (TRIPS) Agreement. Adopted in 2001, this sets out minimal standards for the protection of intellectual property rights, which now lasts for at least 20 years from filing. The problem of developing countries being unable to afford necessary drugs, especially for HIV/AIDS, was addressed by the clause allowing countries to make or import generic versions of drugs under compulsory licensing, where the country's own pharmaceutical industry is allowed to manufacture generic versions of essential drugs still protected by patent, or parallel trade, where branded drugs made more cheaply in other countries are imported at lower cost ('t Hoen, 2003).

Marketing budgets

Reliable data on pharmaceutical marketing spend is limited. In 2004, the estimate of the amount spent in the US ranged from US$27.7–57.5 billion (Gagnon and Lexchin, 2008). This compares with R&D spend for the same year of US$31.5 billion, and represents approximately 9–18% of total sales value (NSF, 2008). Based on reported spends from both companies and physicians, distribution of the marketing spend was estimated as follows (Gagnon and Lexchin, 2008):

- 35.5% on detailing;
- 27.7% on product samples;
- 7% on DTC advertising;
- 3.5% on meetings;
- 0.9% on professional journal advertising;
- 0.5% on mailings, e-mailing etc;
- 25% on unmonitored spending.

In the UK, the Pharmaceutical Price Regulatory Scheme limits overall marketing spend to around 7–8% of sales turnover,[2] although secrecy regarding arrangements for each company make direct comparisons with the US market difficult to achieve. However, given that DTC advertising is not available and supply of product samples is of much lesser importance, it seems likely that the core marketing activities are broadly comparable in the two markets.

Strategies

For any product, there are a range of approaches for marketing. The most successful strategies are coordinated and clearly focused on the target audience and brand values.

Marketing strategy is the broad idea of how a company's strengths are used to achieve its objectives and how to allocate resources to best meet sales targets. It depends on an understanding of how the product compared favorably with its

---

[2] ABPI. Understanding the PPRS; http://www.abpi.org.uk/publications/publication_details/pprs/default.asp; accessed January 29, 2009

competitors, in terms of efficacy, safety, convenience, or cost. Increasingly, new products are modified older ones with greater efficacy or fewer side effects. However, selling branded products on the basis of cost is progressively more difficult with increased use of generics and cost-effectiveness strategies by prescribers. Pharmaceutical companies now tend to use either a highly focused clinical strategy showing the unique features of their brand that give it value to prescribers, or develop a unique set of conditions around a brand such as continuing medical education support or research funding, in order to create brand loyalty (James, 2004).

Marketing strategies have traditionally been built around the four Ps (James, 2004):

• *Product:* development of the brand concept, plus other services associated with the brand such as diagnostic, monitoring, drug delivery, and education support.

• *Price:* the only element to generate revenue; the crucial engine of market success and driver of profitability.

• *Place:* activities to ensure that the product is easily available and accessible to customers, including distribution channels and discount systems.

• *Promotion:* communicating customer benefits and building brand reputation and trust from customers.

Additionally, two new Ps are also relevant (James, 2004):

• *Political relationships* with organizations responsible for payment.

• *Patients*, who have increasing economic input into their care and access to information.

Although the strongest marketing strategies are focused on specific customer groups who are most likely to benefit from the product, many pharmaceutical companies adopt a "weak" marketing strategy, presenting the sales proposition to as wide an audience as possible. This is driven partly by a reluctance to niche the product, and thereby limit potential sales. Larger markets are easier to enter, but are also subject to more fierce competition, and therefore require greater marketing spend to achieve recognition. Despite frequent declarations of the demise of the pharmaceutical rep, marketing capability continues to be closely related to the size of the sales force. Although representative numbers

have now fallen from their peak, as the industry struggles to contain costs, the value of face-to-face contact as a tool to increase market share remains essentially unchallenged (Aasland and Forde, 2004; Prosser, Almond, and Walley, 2003; Sondergaard *et al.*, 2009; Vancelik *et al.*, 2007; Zipkin and Steinman, 2005).

Having said that, the potential for online marketing is strong, particularly where materials can be directly aimed at the consumer. One study of marketing activities for a branded drug in the US found that marketing efforts generated 22% of prescriptions. Of this, television generated 12%, details and face-to-face contacts generated 6%, print generated 3%, and online activities 1%. Online activities accounted for 3% of total media buy, but generated 7% of marketing-driven prescriptions and was more responsive than television or print. It required US$11.33 per incremental prescription, compared to US$17.12 for television and US$13.33 for print.[3]

Approaches to marketing

The range of potential marketing tactics is large, and includes the following:

• advertisements to prescribers in medical journals and other publications;
• detailing to prescribers (face-to-face visits);
• free samples and gifts to prescribers;
• medical education activities for prescribers;
• DTC advertising to patients via general publications, radio, and television;
• disease awareness campaigns, targeted at patients;
• Internet sites, targeting patients and prescribers;
• contributions to patient support groups;
• other activities.

Advertisements in medical journals

Advertising can be considered to be any representation by any means whatever for the purpose of

---

[3] DoubleClick Media Mix Modeling case study: Pharmaceutical, September 2002

promoting directly or indirectly the sale or disposal of any food, drug, cosmetic, or device. Promotion of a drug prior to market authorization is not permitted because the proposed indications have not yet been verified (Health Canada, 2005).

Advertising should be undertaken when it provides the kind of reach and presence among existing and potential customers that other promotional options cannot achieve. Advertising can be used to project a brand in the market, to reward and encourage customers, to establish a presence, and to give a personality or attitude to a brand. The campaign should be designed around the available marketing budget and needs a good, simple idea if it is to stand out from other messages and information.[4]

Many medical journals rely on advertising to survive and this gives pharmaceutical companies a degree of power over editorial content. US studies have shown that more frequent exposure of prescribers to advertisements heightened product and message awareness and increased prescriptions, as well as increased confidence in the claims made by the advertisements (Vitry, 1996). In Australia, a survey of antihypertensive advertising showed that the most heavily advertised products were the most frequently prescribed, while the least advertised products were prescribed least (Vitry and Lai, 2009). However, a UK study failed to show a clear association between the extent of advertising and subsequent prescribing by GPs (Jones, Greenfield, and Bradley, 1999). This may in part be due to a perception that claims made in drug advertisements may be misleading (Villanueva *et al.*, 2003).

GPs are increasingly using computers for accounting, prescribing, and medical records, and so screen advertising is an alternative to print. However, care must be taken that patients do not have access to the advertisements in countries where DTC advertising is prohibited (Nolan, 2000).

---

[4] Pharmaceutical Marketing Live. Practical Guide to advertising and branding; www.pmlive.com/documents/pdf_downloads/Practical_Guides/practical_guide_to_advertising_and_branding; (purchase required); accessed January 29, 2010

Detailing to prescribers

Face-to-face contact between pharmaceutical representatives and prescribers has long been the backbone of marketing and has taken the bulk of marketing budgets. Attitudes to representatives vary from individual to individual. Pharmaceutical sales reps have incentives to be overly positive when discussing their products with prescribers because they are interested in selling drugs not providing information (Rubin, 2004). At the same time, 20% of GPs are responsible for 80% of all prescriptions. It is estimated that 30–60% of GPs in the UK do not see reps regularly or frequently, and those who do see reps give them only a few minutes to promote their products. However, while rep numbers increased by 40% and their overall cost by 70%, face-to-face contacts increased by only 13% between 1994–2002 in the UK (Prosser and Walley, 2003). GPs in the UK who do see drug reps perceive these visits as a good way of accessing new drug information quickly, and many feel they have the necessary skills to appraise the information provided (Prosser and Walley, 2003).

A US study found that pharmaceutical representatives thought certain services they offered were valued more by target physicians than did the physicians themselves, in particular product detailing, provision of research details, expert consultant role, and recruiting physicians to participate in FDA approval drug studies. Physicians only valued free product samples and promotional meals as much as drug reps did (Gaedeke, Tootelian, and Sanders, 1999).

Regardless of these perceptions, evidence from a wide range of countries has demonstrated the efficacy of face-to-face approaches in increasing market share (Aasland and Forde, 2004; Prosser, Almond and Walley, 2003; Sondergaard *et al.*, 2009; Vancelik *et al.*, 2007; Zipkin and Steinman, 2005).

Free samples and gifts

Standard marketing practice internationally includes samples, gifts, printed information, and invitations in contacts with prescribers, based on the principle of reciprocity to influence prescribing (Roughead, Harvey, and Gilbert, 1998). Giving prescribers free samples of drugs for their own use or to pass on to patients is a more common practice in the US, where more patients have to purchase their medication at cost price than in the UK. Free sample availability has been shown to influence prescribing habits in the US (Boltri, Gordon, and Vogel, 2002).

The practice of giving free gifts to prescribers may also be viewed with suspicion by doctors and patients, and is subject to regulations. A survey of psychiatrists in Canada in the 1990s found that they had received a median of one personal meeting, ten drug lunches, two promotional items, and one drug sample in the past year, with a median value of gifts received of US$20. Fewer than half of the doctors thought they would maintain the current contact levels with drug reps if they did not receive promotional gifts. The more money and promotional items received, the more likely they were to believe that this did not influence their prescribing (Hodges, 1995). A survey of hospital doctors in the US found that even those who thought that sponsored lunches and pens were inappropriate gifts had accepted such items. 61% of doctors thought that industry promotions and contacts did not influence their own prescribing but only 16% thought that the prescribing of others was equally unaffected (Steiman, Shlipak, and McPhee, 2001).

Direct-to-consumer advertising

DTC advertising is the promotion of prescription medicines to the general public. The US and New Zealand are the only OECD countries that allow DTC promotion. However, *de facto* DTC advertising may occur in other countries such as in advertisements about a specific disease or condition that does not include a drug name but bears a pharmaceutical company logo or name (Vitry, 2004).

DTC advertising began in the US in 1981 with an ibuprofen product, available at the time by prescription only, being advertised in a consumer-oriented magazine. Other manufacturers followed,

leading to a moratorium from 1983–1985 imposed by the FDA. It was then decided that there was no evidence that DTC advertising was endangering consumers and the practice was allowed to continue without specific focused regulation. The first television DTC advertisement appeared in 1997 (Lee, 2001).

There are three types of DTC advertisements:
• Advertisements for specific prescription drugs are subject to strict regulations in the US. They must contain a summary of risks and benefits, as well as detailing how customers can access more information about the drug. They must be fair and balanced, with no false or misleading information and must not omit material facts.
• Disease awareness advertisements, which do not mention a specific drug, are not regulated by the FDA.
• Reminder advertisements, which just give the name of the product but not its uses, do not have to include risk information (Rados, 2004).

DTC advertising expenditure in the US increased from US$1.2 billion in 1998, to a peak of US$5.4 billion in 2006. Since then, however, spending has dropped significantly to an estimated US$4.8 billion in 2008 (TNS Media Intelligence, 2008). Of this, 60% was spent on television, 37% on print, and 3% on billboards and other media advertisements (Rosenthal *et al.*, 2002). Use of DTC advertising varies from one pharmaceutical company to another. In 2000, first quarter, both Merck and Glaxo Wellcome spent more on DTC than on professional advertising, while Eli Lilly and Novartis both spent less than one-tenth as much on DTC as on professional promotion (Matthews, 2001).

DTC advertising is also very effective. A study of the effects of DTC advertising in the US concluded that a 10% increase in DTC spending would be expected to yield a 1% increase in sales of drugs in that class. The figures for 1999–2000 show that an estimated 12% of the growth in total prescription drug spending at that time was attributable to DTC advertising, a yield of an additional US$4.20 in sales for every dollar spent on DTC advertising (Kaiser Family Foundation, 2003). Caution might be advised, however, because other researchers have suggested that DTC advertising increases sales for the drug class as a whole, rather than exclusively for the product being promoted (Atherly and Rubin, 2009).

Proponents of DTC advertising claim that, although it can encourage more drug consumption, this can lead to overall cost-cutting if it means other, more expensive treatments are not needed later (Matthews, 2001). In contrast, most physicians in the US have negative feelings about DTC advertising, especially feeling that they do not provide enough information on cost, alternative treatment options, or side effects. More than half thought that DTC ads increased consultation length and encouraged patients to ask for specific medication, and only 29% thought they could be a positive trend in healthcare (Robinson *et al.*, 2004).

Within the EU, member states are prohibited from allowing the advertising to the general public of medicinal products that are available on prescription only, and may prohibit such advertising where the product is eligible for reimbursement. However, non-prescription products may be advertised generally (European Commission, 2000; MHRA, 2005). Despite the restrictions on formal advertisement, it is nonetheless possible to get a disease-related marketing message across to the public in other ways. Patients in the UK can be targeted legitimately by public relations activities, disease area advertising, and patient support programmes. Additionally, since August 2003, the Medicines and Healthcare Products Regulatory Agency (MHRA) has specifically relaxed regulations to permit commercial sponsorship of disease awareness campaigns (MHRA, 2003).

Disease awareness campaigns

Although DTC ads are not permitted in most countries, disease awareness campaigns (DAC) are legal on the basis that they advance public health. In the UK, the Medicines Control Agency guidelines state that DACs must be aimed at increasing awareness of a disease and provide health education information on the disease and its management. It must not be used to promote or stimulate public demand for the use of a particular product or encourage patients to contact their doctors to ask for specific medication. Treatment options can be discussed as long as patients are not encouraged to ask for one of these in particular. DACs should raise awareness of symptoms and risk factors, in order to encourage early diagnosis and treatment and minimize progression and complications of the disease (MHRA, 2003).

DACs can be successful when the company can capture a major share of the increased prescribing market, such as where there are few competing treatment options; or where a change in prescribing practice can be caused by tackling consumer inertia. This second approach is less likely to lead to increased sales. Customers can be motivated to respond to a campaign if they believe they are susceptible, that the disease might be serious, and that it can be prevented. Mild fear can arouse interest but too much fear may lead to denial (Worah and Bimbrahw, 2003).

Internet marketing

The Internet can provide the in-depth content seen in print advertising, the real-time impact of television, the immediate response of direct mail, and the mass reach of outdoor advertising. It is estimated that about 25% of online information is related to health, over 50% of adults who use the Internet use it for healthcare information, and a quarter of patients who go to disease-specific websites ask their doctors for a specific brand of medication in the US (Matthews, 2001).

Online marketing includes the following:
- online advertising, via banner ads and e-mail;
- viral marketing, which disseminates marketing messages via "pass-along e-mail";
- direct marketing, offering more cost-effective sales to online customers;
- customer relationship management, which maps customer purchase histories and demographics to allow a more tailored marketing approach;
- search engine optimization, where companies leverage search engine listings;
- V-detailing: most widely used in the UK, the GP views a content-rich interactive presentation on a condition and treatment;

- live-remote detailing: a real-time online interaction with a company representative;
- direct links to pharmaceutical companies' websites and systems;
- messaging to GPs' hand-held computers (Worah and Bimbrahw, 2003).

The use of e-marketing in the pharmaceutical industry is still in its infancy and is subject to increasing regulations. In the UK, the ABPI code of practice requires that the website should be hosted in the UK, that content should comply with relevant guidance for written materials, and that access to product-specific materials should be effectively limited to professional users.[5] In practice, however, there is no bar to UK users accessing drug information hosted in other countries, where regulations are less restrictive. It is therefore debatable whether these restrictions have anything other than a nominal effect.

The use of the Internet for professional purposes has escalated rapidly. A 2009 report from the US suggests that mean internet usage among physicians now stands at 8 hours per week, up from 2.5 hours in 2002 (Manhattan Research, 2009). Explicit use of e-detailing has the potential to exploit this changing pattern in a cost-effective fashion. Although both e-detailing and traditional representative contact can influence prescribing practice, the costs associated with face-to-face detailing are nearly double those of electronic contacts (Gonul, Carter, and Wind, 2009).

The actual amount spent on e-detailing is difficult to estimate. In the US, the total annual spend on pharmaceutical advertising (prescription-only plus OTC drugs) in 2005 was around US$13.8 billion. Of this, around US$170 million was explicitly online (1.2%).[6] However, this spend does not capture activities such as search engine optimiza-

tion and live-remote detailing, and so the true figure is likely to be substantially higher. A recent judgement by the FDA, however, may substantially impact this figure: Following its decision to outlaw "click-through" advertising for product-related websites, a dramatic reduction in pharma online presence has been forecast (Thomaselli, 2009).

Internet-based campaigns now often run side-by-side with other media that can be used to promote websites. However, certain groups still have restricted access, and so conventional approaches are still needed. Websites may need to be different for prescribers and the public, with content checked constantly to make sure that the information is current, complete, and free of conflicts. All communications need to be consistent with the overall marketing message, however. Websites can also be used to coordinate activities prior to launch and ensure rapid spread of up-to-date materials and messages

Patient support groups

Many pharmaceutical companies provide funding for patient groups, either without specifying what the money should be used for, or to sponsor a specific product for which the company has no direct involvement. The ABPI Code of Practice reflects UK and EU legislation, which prohibits pharmaceutical companies from undertaking or sponsoring any activity deemed to be promoting a prescription-only product to the public. Patient groups are independent voluntary organizations that usually prefer not to be controlled by a sponsor; but at the same time they are charities that need to raise funds from a wide funding base. Companies must not sponsor any activity by patient groups that would breach the ABPI Code if they were to do so directly, and all funding arrangements must be transparent (ABPI, 2008b).

Medical education activities

Pharmaceutical companies can become involved with medical education activities via sponsored

---

[5] MHRA Advertising of medicines: guidance for consumer websites offering medical treatment services; http://www.mhra.gov.uk/home/groups/pl-a/documents/websiteresources/con031140.pdf; accessed January 29, 2010)

[6] TNS Media Intelligence. US Spending on Pharmaceutical Advertising; http://www.imediaconnection.com/content/10832.asp; accessed January 29, 2010

meetings and conferences, as well as paying for the authorship of reference texts and peer-reviewed journal articles (Health Canada, 2005).

In the US, activities performed by, or on behalf of, pharmaceutical companies that market relevant products are subject to FDA regulation, whereas activities supported by pharmaceutical companies but delivered by agencies otherwise independent from pharmaceutical industry promotional influences are not. This is so that constraints on advertising and labelling do not restrict freedom of speech of participants in scientific and educational activities, such as discussion about unapproved uses, which cannot occur in directly sponsored, promotional activities. However, it can be difficult to determine where the line is between these two levels of involvement of sponsors, especially when the industry has been taking a growing role in Continuing Medical Education (CME) activities (US Department of Health and Human Services, 1997).

The Pri-Med 2004 CME Insight survey of US physicians found that 22% of doctors see industry sponsorship of CME as a good thing and 64% see it as essential to making CME events accessible and available. Almost three-quarters of primary care physicians surveyed were unwilling to pay more than US$100 in fees to attend a CME event, and fewer than one-third would pay US$1,000 (Pri-Med, 2004).

There is increasing pressure in both the US and Europe to distance the provision of CME from pharmaceutical industry sponsorship.[7] A recent report from the American Medical Association's Council on Ethical and Judicial Affairs (CEJA) is calling for an end to almost all commercial support for professional education.[8] Although the report has yet to be adopted as policy by the American Medical Association as a whole, it seems inevitable

that some further degree of restriction will be placed on this type of marketing activity.

Conclusions

Effective marketing of pharmaceuticals is fundamental to achieving return on R&D investment. Increasing focus on the ethics of industry activity, coupled with a changing relationship between payers and prescribers, presents broad new challenges for the marketer. Although face-to-face sales activity will continue to have a central role in this process for many years to come, it is inevitable that the focus of activity will gradually shift away from traditional broad marketing strategies to a more targeted approach, addressing the needs of the budget holder as much as that of the clinician. Meeting the needs of this slow revolution will require closer integration of research and marketing agendas, coupled with a willingness to move away from some of the sacred cows of marketing doctrine. Existing marketing models have worked well for the past two decades but, as the experience of the financial markets has shown in recent years, past performance is not necessarily a good indicator of future performance.

References

Aasland OG, Forde R. [Physicians and drug industry: attitudes and practice]. *Tidsskr Nor Laegeforen* 2004; **124**:2603–2606.

Adams C, Brantner V. Estimating the cost of new drug development: is it really 802 million dollars? *Health Aff (Millwood)* 2006; **25**(2):420–428.

AMIC (Advertising Media Internet Center. *The Media Guru. 24/6/2002 #5375*, 2002; http://www.amic.com/guru/askguru.asp?year=2002; accessed January 29, 2010.

ABPI (Association of the British Pharmaceutical Industry). *Code of Practice for the Pharmaceutical Industry*, 2008a; http://www.pmcpa.org.uk/files/sitecontent/ABPI_Code_of_Practice_2008.pdf; accessed January 29, 2010.

ABPI (Association of the British Pharmaceutical Industry). *Guidance on working with patient organisations*, 2008b; http://www.pmcpa.org.uk/files/sitecontent/

---

[7] TNS Media Intelligence. US Spending on Pharmaceutical Advertising; http://www.imediaconnection.com/content/10832.asp; accessed January 29, 2010

[8] Council on Ethical and Judicial Affairs. Financial arrangements with industry in continuing medical education; http://policymed.typepad.com/files/ceja-report-on-cme-2-i-09.pdf; accessed January 29, 2010

20080714/patient_groups_and_pharma_working_together.pdf; accessed January 29, 2010.

Atherly A, Rubin PH. The cost-effectiveness of direct-to-consumer advertising for prescription drugs. *Med Care Res Rev* 2009; **66**(6):639–657.

Australian Academy of Science. *Submission to the Industry Commission inquiry into the pharmaceutical industry*, August 1995; http://www.science.org.au/reports/pharmsub.htm; accessed January 29, 2010.

Boltri JM, Gordon ER, Vogel RL. Effect of antihypertensive samples on physician prescribing patterns. *Fam Med* 2002; **34**:729–731.

BMA. Editorial: A model for NICE in the US. *BMJ* 2009; **338**:b2221.

Department of Health. *Prescriptions dispensed in the community, statistics for 1998 to 2008: England*, 2009; http://www.ic.nhs.uk/pubs/presdisp98-08; accessed January 29, 2010.

DiMasi J, Hansen R, Grabowski H. The price of innovation: new estimates of drug development costs. *J Health Econ* 2003; **22**(2):151–185.

European Commission. *Pharmaceuticals in the European Union*, 2000; http://ec.europa.eu/enterprise/sectors/pharmaceuticals/index_en.htm; accessed April 16, 2010.

Gaedeke RM, Tootelian DH, Sanders EE. Value of services provided by pharmaceutical companies: perceptions of physicians and pharmaceutical sales representatives. *Health Mark Q* 1999; **17**:23–31.

Gagnon MA, Lexchin J. The cost of pushing pills: a new estimate of pharmaceutical promotion expenditures in the United States. *PLoS Med* 2008; http://www.plosmedicine.org/article/fetchSingleRepresentation.action?uri=info:doi/10.1371/journal.pmed.0050001.sd003; accessed April 16, 2010

Gonul FF, Carter F, Wind J. What kind of patients and physicians value direct-to-consumer advertising of prescription drugs. *Health Care Manag Sci* 2000; **3**:215–226.

Grabowski HG, Wang YR. The quantity and quality of worldwide new drug introductions, 1982–2003. *Health Aff (Millwood)* 2006; **25**:452–460.

Health Canada. *The distinction between advertising and other activities*, updated 2005; http://www.hc-sc.gc.ca/dhp-mps/advert-publicit/pol/actv_promo_vs_info-eng.php; accessed January 29, 2010.

Hodges B. Interactions with the pharmaceutical industry: experiences and attitudes of psychiatry residents, interns and clerks. *CMAJ* 1995; **153**:553–559.

James B. *An introduction to pharmaceutical marketing*. Scrip reports 2004; http://www.pjbpubs.com/uploads/QZ1xik73rxirlre5hbfx.pdf; accessed January 29, 2010.

Jones M, Greenfield S, Bradley C. A survey of the advertising of nine new drugs in the general practice literature. *J Clin Pharm Ther* 1999; **24**:451–460.

Kaiser Family Foundation (2003). *Demand effects of recent changes in prescription drug promotion.* June 2003; http://www.kff.org/rxdrugs/upload/Demand-Effects-of-Recent-Changes-in-Prescription-Drug-Promotion-Report.pdf; accessed April 16, 2010.

Kanavos P. *Overview of pharmaceutical pricing and reimbursement regulation in Europe* (Working Paper). LSE Health: London, 2001.

Kanavos P. *Overview of pharmaceutical pricing and reimbursement in Europe*, 2002; http://ec.europa.eu/enterprise/phabiocom/docs/synthesis.pdf; accessed January 29, 2010.

Keyhani S, Diener-West M, Powe N. Are development times for pharmaceuticals increasing or decreasing? *Health Aff (Millwood)* 2006; **25**:461–468.

Lee R (2001). Direct-to-consumer advertising. *Orthopedic Technology Review* 2001; **3**.

Manhattan Research. *How digital is shaping the future of pharmaceutical marketing*, 2009; http://www.manhattanresearch.com/files/White_Papers/How_Digital_is_Shaping_the_Future_of_Pharma_Marketing.pdf; accessed January 29, 2010.

Matthews M. Who's afraid of pharmaceutical advertising? *Institute for Policy Innovation Policy report 155*, May 2001.

MHRA. *MHRA Guidance Note 23. Disease awareness campaigns guidelines*, 2003; http://www.mhra.gov.uk/home/idcplg?IdcService=GET_FILE&dDocName=CON007555&RevisionSelectionMethod=Latest; accessed January 29, 2010.

MHRA. *MHRA Guidance Note 23. The Blue Guide: Advertising and promotion of medicines in the UK*, 2005; http://www.mhra.gov.uk/home/idcplg?IdcService=GET_FILE&dDocName=CON007552&RevisionSelectionMethod=Latest; accessed January 29, 2010.

NSF (National Science Foundation). *Research and Development in Industry: 2004.* December 2008; http://www.nsf.gov/statistics/nsf09301/pdf/nsf09301.pdf; accessed January 29, 2010.

Nolan A. Pharmaceutical advertising in clinical software. *Aust Prescr* 2000; **23**:52–53.

OECD. *OECD Health Data 2009: Statistics and Indicators for 30 Countries*, 2009; http://www.oecd.org/document/30/0,3343,en_2649_34631_12968734_1_1_1_1,00.html; accessed January 29, 2010.

Oxfam. *Oxfam briefing paper 4. Priced out of reach. How WTO patent policies will reduce access to medicines in the developing world*, 2001; http://www.oxfam.org.uk/resources/policy/health/index.html; accessed April 16, 2010.

Palumbo FB, Mullins CD. The development of direct-to-consumer prescription drug advertising regulation. *Food and Drug Law Journal* 2002; **57**:423–443.

Pri-Med. *CME Insight survey*, 2004; http://www.primed.com/PMO/DocumentDisplay.aspx?id=478; accessed January 29, 2010.

Prosser H, Almond S, Walley T. Influences on GPs' decision to prescribe new drugs-the importance of who says what. *Fam Pract* 2003; **20**:61–68.

Prosser H, Walley T. Understanding why GPs see pharmaceutical representatives: a qualitative interview study. *Br J Gen Pract* 2003; **53**:305–311.

Rados C. *Truth in advertising: Rx drug ads come of age*. FDA Consumer July–August 2004. FDA: Washington, DC, USA, 2004.

Robinson AR, Hohmann KB, Rifkin JI, *et al.* Direct-to-consumer pharmaceutical advertising. *Arch Intern Med* 2004; **164**:427–432.

Rosenthal MB, Berndt ER, Donohue JM, *et al.* Promotion of prescription drugs to consumers. *N Engl J Med* 2002; **346**:498–505.

Roughead EE, Harvey KJ, Gilbert AL. Commercial detailing techniques used by pharmaceutical representatives to influence prescribing. *Aust NZ J Med* 1998; **28**:306–310.

Rubin PH. Pharmaceutical marketing: Medical and industry biases. *Journal of Pharmaceutical Finance, Economics & Policy* 2004; **13**:65–79

Sondergaard J, Vach K, Kragstrup J, Andersen M. Impact of pharmaceutical representative visits on GPs' drug preferences. *Fam Pract* 2009; **26**:204–209.

Steiman MA, Shlipak MG, McPhee SJ. Of principles and pens: attitudes and practices of medicine housestaff toward pharmaceutical industry promotions. *Am J Med* 2001; **110**:551–557.

't Hoen E. Patents, prices and patients. (Pharmaceuticals). UN Chronicle June–August 2003; http://www.findarticles.com/cf_dls/m1309/2_40/105657537/print.jhtml; accessed January 29, 2010.

Thomaselli R. Pharma drops search advertising after FDA warning. Advertising Age, October 6 2009; http://adage.com/article?article_id=139500 (requires registration); accessed January 29, 2010.

TNS Media Intelligence. Advertising investment trend report: Direct-to-consumer pharmaceutical industry, 2008; http://www.tns-mi.com/downloads/DTCPharmaReport.pdf; accessed April 16, 2010.

US Department of Health and Human Services. Food and Drug Administration. *Guidance for Industry. Industry-supported scientific and educational activities*. November 1997; http://www.fda.gov/downloads/Regulatory Information/Guidances/UCM125602.pdf; accessed January 29, 2010.

US Department of Health and Human Services. Food and Drug Administration, Center for Drug Evaluation and Research, Center for Biologics Evaluation and Research, Center for Veterinary Medicine. Guidance for Industry. *Consumer-directed broadcast advertisements*, August 1999.

Vancelik S, Beyhun NE, Acemoglu H, Calikoglu O. Impact of pharmaceutical promotion on prescribing decisions of general practitioners in Eastern Turkey. *BMC Public Health* 2007; **7**:122.

Villanueva P, Peiro S, Librero J, *et al.* Accuracy of pharmaceutical advertisements in medical journals. *Lancet* 2003; **361**:27–32

Vitry A. Drug advertising affects your prescribing. *Aust Prescr* 1996; **19**:103

Vitry A. Is Australia free from direct-to-consumer advertising? *Aust Prescr* 2004; **27**:4–6.

Vitry A, Lai YH. Advertising of antihypertensive medicines and prescription sales in Australia. *Intern Med J* 2009; **39**(11):728–732.

Walley T, Mrazek M, Mossialos E. Regulating pharmaceutical markets: improving efficiency and controlling costs in the UK. *Int J Health Plann Manage* 2005; **20**:375–398.

Walley T, Earl-Slater A, Haycox A, *et al.* An integrated national pharmaceutical policy for the United Kingdom? *BMJ* 2000; **321**:1523–1526.

Worah V, Bimbrahw N. Guide to DTC pharmaceutical advertising on the Internet. Owen Graduate School of Management at Vanderbilt University: Nashville, TN, USA, 2003.

Zipkin DA, Steinman MA. Interactions between pharmaceutical representatives and doctors in training. A thematic review. *J Gen Intern Med* 2005; **20**:777–786.

CHAPTER 55

Pharmaceutical Product Liability

Han W. Choi[1*] *& Jae Hong Lee*[2*]
[1]Oracle Investment Management, Inc., Greenwich, CT, USA
[2]Morrison & Foerster, L.L.P., San Diego, CA, USA

Product liability is one of the fastest growing and most economically significant applications of tort law. Product liability actions against pharmaceutical companies are among the most widely publicized classes of suits in the United States and Europe, prompting pharmaceutical companies to lobby vigorously for tort reform. (Nace *et al.*, 1997). The liability burden on pharmaceutical companies has been described as grossly disproportionate to their sales in comparison with other manufacturing industries (The Progress & Freedom Foundation, 1996, p. 101). Direct comparisons, however, are difficult because the market for pharmaceuticals is unlike the usual market situation, where con-

*The authors hereby certify that all of the views expressed in this chapter accurately reflect their personal views about the subject matter and any companies and their securities mentioned in this chapter. Readers should also be aware that the authors may at any given time be active investors in companies and their securities mentioned in this chapter. The authors may also at any given time also be working with specialists in the relevant securities and may at any given time have long or short positions in, act as principal in, and buy or sell, the securities or derivatives (including options and warrants) thereof of companies referred to in this chapter. The views expressed in this chapter are not offers to sell or the solicitations of an offer to buy any security in any jurisdiction where such an offer or solicitation would be illegal. It does not constitute a personal recommendation or take into account the particular investment objectives, financial situations, or needs of any individual reader.

Principles and Practice of Pharmaceutical Medicine, 3rd edition.
Edited by L.D. Edwards, A.W. Fox, P.D. Stonier.
© 2011 Blackwell Publishing Ltd.

sumers have options among competing products on the basis of quality and price. In the case of pharmaceuticals, a physician generally selects the specific drug, and the consumer bears only a fraction of the cost burden, because health insurance defrays a significant part of the cost (Mossialos *et al.*, 1994). The recent increase in product liability actions against pharmaceutical companies as well as healthcare professionals has also been described as having an impact on the practice of medicine itself (Pendell, 2003). This chapter will introduce the basic concepts of pharmaceutical product liability law, review recent developments and emerging trends among pharmaceutical companies and product liability lawyers, and discuss how they might impact the industry as a whole in the future.

Principles of product liability law

In general terms, "product liability" refers to the liability of a seller of a product which, because of a defect, causes damage to its purchaser, user, or sometimes a bystander. Responsibility for a product defect that causes damage lies with all sellers of the product who are in the distribution chain including the product manufacturer, manufacturers of component parts, wholesalers, and retail stores that sold the product to the consumer. Laws in most countries and jurisdictions require that a product meet the ordinary expectations of the ordinary consumer. When a product has an unexpected defect or danger, that product cannot be said to meet the expectations of the consumer. Product liability law is primarily based on case law that varies from jurisdiction to jurisdiction. In the US, there is no Federal product liability law *per se*. Typically, product liability claims are based on state laws and relevant commercial statutes, modeled on the Uniform Commercial Code (UCC), that pertain to warranty rules that govern manufacturers and their products. Early cases held that, for product liability to arise, at some point, the product must have been sold in the marketplace through a contractual relationship, known as "privity of contract," between the person injured and the supplier of the product. However, in most countries and jurisdictions today, the privity requirement no longer exists, and the injured person does not have to be the purchaser of the product in order to recover. Any person who foreseeably could have been injured by a defective product can recover in tort for his or her injuries, as long as the product was in the stream of commerce.

Product liability law, generally and as it pertains to pharmaceutical companies, is broadly based on legal principles involving contract law, tort law, and relevant statutory provisions of the country or jurisdiction where the action is brought (Jones, 1993). However, there are three fundamental legal principles under which a seller of a product can be liable for damages incurred from the use of that product: strict liability, warranty, and negligence.

Strict liability

Strict liability is a principle of both tort law and contract law, which provides that a seller of a product is liable without fault for damage caused by that product if it is sold in a defective condition that is unreasonably dangerous to the user or consumer. Thus, strict liability would mean that pharmaceutical companies would have to pay damages in some cases, even when they had impeccably researched their drugs (Hunter, 1993). Strict product liability similarly applies not only to the product's manufacturer but also to its retailer and to any other party in the distribution chain. However, a product would not give rise to strict liability if it is found to be "unavoidably unsafe." This has direct relevance to pharmaceutical companies, in that most courts have agreed that a product will not give rise to strict liability if it is unavoidably unsafe, as described by labeled descriptions of adverse events, and if

its benefits can outweigh its dangers. Furthermore, most courts have also held that the existence of "unreasonable danger" and "defectiveness" should be based on the state of scientific knowledge and technology at the time when the product is sold and not on the date when the resulting product liability case comes to trial. The courts have taken a similar approach to "failure to warn" claims in that if the state of scientific knowledge and technology at the time of manufacture is such that the defect or danger is neither known nor knowable, not only is the manufacturer protected from ordinary strict liability, but also the manufacturer is relieved of its duty to warn of the unknowable danger. The manufacturer, however, is held to the standard of an expert in the product in determining what was known or knowable.

Warranty

Warranty is a principle of both tort law and contract law that allows a purchaser of a product to bring a cause of action against the immediate seller of that product if the person can demonstrate that the seller expressly or implicitly made representations about the quality of the product that were ultimately false or misleading, without the need to demonstrate negligence on the part of the seller. Thus, the seller may have reasonably and honestly believed that his or her representations or warranties were true, and could not possibly have discovered the defect in the product, and yet the plaintiff may nonetheless recover. Many countries have enacted statutes that apply to such warranties and resulting product liability actions. For example, in the US, the UCC includes provisions regarding warranties and forms the legal basis for product liability actions brought under the principle of warranty. UCC Section 2-313 provides that an express warranty may be produced by an "affirmation of fact or promise" about a product by a description of that product or by the use of a sample or model. The existence of a warranty as to the quality of a product may also be inferred from the fact that the seller has offered the product for sale. The UCC also imposes several implied warranties as a matter of law. The most important of these is the warranty of merchantability under UCC Section

2-314, which states that the warranty that goods shall be merchantable is implied in a contract for their sale if the seller is a merchant with respect to goods of that kind. Similarly, a retailer who did not manufacture a product is nonetheless held to have impliedly warranted its merchantability by virtue of the fact that he or she has sold it, assuming that the person deals in goods of that kind. In addition, under UCC Section 2-315, a seller of goods may also implicitly warrant that goods are "fit for a particular purpose" if the seller knows that the purchaser wants the goods for a particular purpose, and the purchaser relies on the seller's judgment to purchase the goods in question.

Negligence

Negligence is a principle of tort law that may be defined as the breach of a duty of care owed by one party, the defendant, to another party, the plaintiff, the breach of which results in damage to the plaintiff. The concept of duty of care serves to define the interests protected by the tort of negligence by determining whether the type of damage suffered by the plaintiff is actionable. The plaintiff must also demonstrate that there is a sufficient causal connection between the defendant's negligence and the damage incurred. The damage in question may arise through malfeasance (a wrongful or illegal act) or nonfeasance (a wrongful or illegal failure to act) and may consist of personal injury or damage to property, categorized as pure economic loss under civil law. Manufacturers, retailers, bailers (e.g., those who distribute pharmaceutical products on behalf of drug manufacturers), and other suppliers may be liable to plaintiffs under the principles of negligence if they are found to have breached a duty of care.

Types of product defects

Under strict liability, a plaintiff in a product liability case must prove that the product that caused injury was defective, and that the defect made the product unreasonably dangerous. There are three types of defects that might cause injury and give rise to manufacturer or supplier liability: manufacturing defects, design defects, and failure-to-warn defects.

Manufacturing defects

Manufacturing defects involve a product where the particular item that causes damage to the plaintiff is different from the design intended to be manufactured by the defendant, and the difference is attributable to the manufacturing process for the item in question. However, very few pharmaceutical product liability claims allege manufacturing defects because quality control standards are closely regulated and have traditionally been extremely high in the pharmaceutical industry (European Federation of Pharmaceutical Industries and Associations, 1999).

Design defects

Design defects involve a product where all similar items manufactured by the defendant are the same, and they all bear a feature whose design is defective and unreasonably dangerous. These design defect claims often involve additional allegations of negligence on the part of the defendant even though they may be based on strict liability principles in that the plaintiff often alleges that the manufacturer should have been aware of the safety attributes of its design and, in failing to do so, breached its duty of care.

Failure to warn

Finally, failure-to-warn defects—also known as marketing defects—are flaws in the way a product is marketed, such as improper labeling, insufficient instructions, or inadequate safety warnings. Recently, these type of claims are more commonly referred to as "failure to warn" and simply refer to the legal premise that manufacturers and suppliers of products must give proper warnings of the dangers and risks of their products so that consumers can make informed decisions regarding whether to use them. However, the success of any such claim depends not just on the adequacy of the warning in question, but also on the plaintiff's own knowledge of the product. A negligent or intentional misrepresentation regarding a product may also give rise to a product liability claim.

Legal defenses in product liability cases

The defenses available to manufacturers in product liability actions vary, depending on the jurisdiction in which the action is filed. However, certain legal principles commonly constitute a full or partial defense to product liability actions. These broad legal principles, among others, are: disclaimers, contributory negligence, and learned intermediaries.

Disclaimers

With regard to product liability actions brought under the principles of warranty, a defendant may assert a defense based on a disclaimer from a warranty associated with the purchase or use of the product in question. For example, in the US under UCC Section 2-316(2), a seller of a product may make a written disclaimer of the warranty of merchantability if it is conspicuous. However, it should also be noted that the Magnuson–Moss Federal Trade Commission Improvement Act of 1974, 15 USC Section 2301, *et seq.*, provides that, if a written warranty is given to a consumer, there cannot be any disclaimer of any implied warranty.

Contributory negligence

A defense of contributory negligence asserts that a plaintiff who is him- or herself negligent in that he or she does not take reasonable care to protect him- or herself from damage, and whose negligence contributes proximately to his or her injuries, is either entitled only to reduced recovery from his or her damages, or in some countries and states, is totally barred from recovery (Heuston and Buckley, 1992). In these cases, the plaintiff is held to the same standard of care as the defendant, which is that of a reasonable party similarly situated.

Although a plaintiff's contributory negligence will be a defense in product liability actions brought under the principles of negligence, some courts have agreed that in most actions brought under the principles of warranty or strict liability, contributory negligence may not be a viable defense—but this varies from jurisdiction to jurisdiction. For example, if a plaintiff's contributory negligence lies in a failure to inspect the product or a failure to become aware of the danger from that product, virtually all courts agree that this is not a defense. However, if the plaintiff learns of the risk and voluntarily assumes the risk in purchasing and/or using the product, contributory negligence may be a defense to strict liability. Similarly, if the plaintiff's contributory negligence consists of his or her abnormal use or misuse of the product in question, this may be a defense to strict liability, depending on the degree of foreseeability of the abnormal use or misuse.

Learned intermediaries

Pharmaceutical manufacturers often rely on the "learned intermediary" defense, which asserts that if the manufacturer properly warned or instructed a physician (the "learned intermediary") who then prescribes the drug to a plaintiff, liability may not be imposed. However, liability may be imposed in circumstances such as "direct-to-consumer" advertising, which may be held to have diluted other warnings made by the manufacturer.

It should be noted that until 2009, regulatory compliance or "preemption" was frequently used by pharmaceutical manufacturers as a defense in product liability cases. In the US, the general rule had originally been that, unless Congress intended to preempt the states from requiring stricter or different warnings, the defendant's compliance with regulatory requirements did not preclude liability (McCartney and Rheingold, 1996). However, several states, such as New Jersey, enacted statutes that allowed regulatory compliance as a valid defense in pharmaceutical product liability actions (N.J. Code Section 2A:58C-4). A handful of other states also adopted modified versions of a regulatory compliance defense which, for example, barred punitive damages for drugs approved by the FDA or created a rebuttable presumption of nonliability in light of FDA approval (Lifton and Bufano, 2004). However, in a landmark decision handed down by the US Supreme Court in 2009, the Court held that the labeling approval by the FDA may not preempt state laws or shield companies from legal damages as part of liability claims (*Wyeth v. Levine*, 129 S. Ct. 1187 (2009)).

International issues

In recent years, pharmaceutical companies have faced increased litigation from overseas claimants because of the international differences in product liability laws that make them easier targets in the US. Such differences include the absence of discovery mechanisms, jury trials, legal contingency fees, and variations in the learned intermediary doctrines in many foreign jurisdictions. Lawsuits are also being filed in the US because foreign parties claim they cannot get justice or adequate compensation in their own country—for example, they may claim that they do not have a claim under their own nation's laws or that they are unable to have their case heard for many years. The concept of *forum non conveniens* developed in the US (and other so-called "common law" jurisdictions such as Australia and New Zealand[1]) as a device that permitted US courts to return cases to foreign jurisdictions when litigation in the US was determined to be inconvenient or a foreign jurisdiction was deemed to be a more appropriate forum.

The plaintiffs' bar also has become increasingly sophisticated in using global regulatory inconsistencies to their clients' advantage during discovery and at trial. During the course of litigation, pharmaceutical companies are now routinely faced with discovery requests, designed to identify documents and data relating to their dealings with foreign regulatory agencies. Plaintiffs' counsel regularly point to differences in labeling and product design resulting from pharmaceutical companies' compliance with foreign regulations as evidence of "defectiveness" in similar or identical products marketed in the US (Moore and Cullen, 1999). Thus, in overview, the global marketing of pharmaceuticals has had significant product liability impli-

cations resulting from jurisdictional issues, maintaining records for different regulatory agencies, and compliance or noncompliance with regulatory requirements in different marketing venues.

Landmark cases

In contrast to the ostensibly uniform framework of product liability law that defines drug-induced tort, the history of high-profile pharmaceutical injury litigation shows that the practical prosecution of drug-related injury claims is broadly varied as it reflects the many possible types of drug-induced injuries. Although the breadth of potential harms from the use of pharmaceuticals is, in theory, limitless, adverse drug effects generally fall into one of seven groups (Dukes, Mildred, and Swartz, 1998):

- toxic effects, where the drug causes an undesired pharmacologic effect on the body;
- allergic effects, where the drug has an unpredictably severe or harmful effect on hypersensitive individuals;
- dependence, where users of the drug develop a psychological or physiologic need for the drug;
- indirect injury, where the drug interferes with mental or physical functions, resulting in collateral injuries;
- interactions, where ingesting the drug in the context of other drugs or foods causes injury;
- inefficacy, where the drug fails to perform its intended function;
- socially adverse effects, where a drug (usually an antibiotic) is overused by a population of patients, resulting in the rise and spread of resistant microorganisms.

The following discussion of two high-profile product liability cases shows how plaintiffs, corporations, attorneys, and courts have applied product liability jurisprudence to varied types of pharmacological injury and the impact of product liability matters on the laws and regulations governing pharmaceutical products.

Thalidomide

The drug thalidomide caused one of the most vivid and widely publicized tragedies in the history of

---

[1] The concept of *forum non conveniens* is generally not recognized in most non-US jurisdictions that are based on "civil law"—e.g., many nations in the European Union

medicine (Bernstein, 1997).[2] Thalidomide was first synthesized in West Germany in 1953 by Ciba A.G., but it was initially abandoned after tests in laboratory animals revealed neither a beneficial nor a toxic effect. A few years later, chemists at another West German pharmaceutical company, Chemie Grunenthal A.G., deduced from thalidomide's chemical structure that it might have an anticonvulsant effect, and they experimented with giving thalidomide to epileptics. Ensuing studies revealed thalidomide to be ineffective anticonvulsant, but showed that it acted as a mild hypnotic or sedative. On the basis of these data, Chemie Grunenthal A.G. brought thalidomide to market under the trade name Contergan in October 1957 (Robertson, 1972). Thalidomide was an early success and the drug soon became a favorite sleeping tablet for over-the-counter consumers and in healthcare institutions. Promoted as a safe tranquilizer, suggested uses of thalidomide included mild depression, flu, stomach disorders, menstrual tensio, and even stage fright (Allen, 1997). Also an antiemetic, Contergan was commonly prescribed for the nausea of pregnancy (Sherman and Strauss, 1986; cf. Burley, 1986).

Although thalidomide had shown no toxicity to laboratory animals when tested by Ciba and Chemie Grunenthal A.G., potentially irreversible peripheral polyneuritis was soon identified in patients following long-term use of thalidomide (Crawford, 1994). Other reported toxicity symptoms included severe constipation, dizziness, hangover, loss of memory, and hypotension (D'Arcy, 1994). Chemie Grunenthal A.G. initially defended thalidomide as a safe product and attributed the reports to overdosage and prolonged use. A pharmacologist at the FDA, Dr Frances Kelsey, saw

reports of these adverse effects and requested more data from the drug's manufacturers to show that it was safe (see D'Arcy, 1994).[3] In what has been heralded as "one of the FDA's finest hours" (see D'Arcy, 1994), Dr Kelsey withheld FDA approval of thalidomide—a decision that was subsequently validated as the reports of neurotoxicity were confirmed and even more troubling reports arose concerning thalidomide's adverse effects on fetuses. In 1961, physicians in Germany realized with alarm that the growing number of otherwise rare severe congenital malformations, including phocomelia (defective development of limbs) and amelia (absence of limbs), could be attributed to the use by women of even a single dose of thalidomide during the critical first few weeks of their pregnancy (Wiedemann, 1961). In subsequent years, it became clear that thalidomide was one of the most potent teratogens in the medical pharmacopoeia. Almost 100% of women who took thalidomide during the sensitive period (days 21–36 of gestation) produced malformed infants (D'Arcy, 1994). The spectrum of malformations was also notable for its breadth. In addition to phocomelia and amelia, so-called "thalidomide babies" suffered from spinal cord defects, cleft lip or palate, absent or abnormal external ears, and heart, renal, gastrointestinal, or urogenital malformations (D'Arcy, 1994; see also US HHS, 1997). Before the epidemic ran its course, over 12,000 infants were born with deformities attributable to thalidomide (Flaherty, 1984; Sherman and Strauss, 1986; see also Szeinberg and Sheba, 1968[4]).

Not surprisingly, the thalidomide episode spawned numerous lawsuits based on strict product liability, defective design, negligence, and other theories of liability (Cook, Doyle, and Jabbari, 1991; Dworkin, 1979). Some of these cases settled for substantial sums of money

---

[2] Bernstein notes that thalidomide quickly entered the lexicon as a metaphor for poison and evil. "For years I have heard the word Wait!," wrote Martin Luther King Jr in his famous Letter from Birmingham City Jail (1963). "It rings in the ear of every Negro with a piercing familiarity. This 'Wait' has almost always meant 'Never.' It has been a tranquilizing *thalidomide*, relieving the emotional stress for a moment, only to give birth to an ill-formed infant of frustration." (emphasis added)

---

[3] Dr Kelsey was particularly conscious of the potentially harmful effects of drugs on fetuses after working on a malaria project during World War II in which quinine (another teratogen) was studied

[4] Szeinberg and Sheba (1968) estimates that 10,000 deformed babies were born in Germany, 1,000 in Japan, 400 in England, and 280 in Scandinavian countries

(Waterhouse, 1995). However, the true legal legacy of the thalidomide episode was to focus the attention of lawmakers and scientists on the potential risks of all medications. The thalidomide episode is generally credited with promoting the institution of stronger and more effective drug regulations worldwide. In the US, the thalidomide tragedy is credited with helping to win passage of the 1962 Kefauver-Harris Amendment to the Federal Food, Drug, and Cosmetic Act, which introduced or strengthened requirements for drug manufacturers to demonstrate the safety and efficacy of their drugs prior to market approval. The German Pharmaceutical Law of 1976 and the Japanese Drug Side-Effect Injury Relief Fund Act of 1979 were also indirect products of the thalidomide experience (Bernstein, 1997). Drug manufacturers in Sweden adopted voluntary regulations, and drug legislation in Canada was tightened in accordance with the stricter laws and regulations in the US. The experience with thalidomide resulted in a generally safer pharmaceutical market in many parts of the world.

Diethylstilbestrol (DES)

DES is a synthetic analog of estrogen, first manufactured in the United Kingdom in 1937. The inventor's altruistic decision not to patent DES led to the drug's manufacture by more than 300 companies (Ferguson, 1996), a fact that substantially impacted later legal actions. The therapeutic benefits of DES were largely theoretical at the time of its introduction, with few if any rigorous clinical trials performed to evaluate its efficacy. Nevertheless, physicians and industry began to promote the use of DES to prevent miscarriages and generally improve the outcomes of pregnancies. The FDA approved DES in 1947 for the prevention of early miscarriage. Despite early evidence that DES did not prevent miscarriage or other pregnancy complications (Schrager and Potter, 2004), DES came into wide use, due largely to support by physicians and industry, approval by the FDA, and low cost (partly attributable to the competition between many manufacturers). It is estimated that between 3 and 4 million women ingested DES in the US alone, with 20,000 to 100,000 fetuses

exposed to DES *in utero*, each year, for 20 years (Dutton, 1988).

Beginning approximately 15 years after the peak of DES use, doctors found that female children of mothers who had taken DES during their gestation tended to develop preneoplastic vaginal and cervical changes in adolescence or adulthood. An association between *in utero* DES exposure and vaginal clear cell adenocarcinoma was documented (Schrager and Potter, 2004). Male and female DES children also showed an increased incidence of fertility disturbances after puberty (Dukes, Mildred, and Swartz, 1998). In 1984, the World Health Organization estimated that hundreds of thousands of pregnancies, especially in the US and The Netherlands, were potentially affected (Buitendijk, 1984).

Since the early 1980s, thousands of pharmaceutical product liability cases have been brought against the manufacturers of DES. These plaintiffs had a stronger strict liability design defect claim than those for thalidomide because DES, marketed to prevent miscarriages, had no demonstrable clinical benefit. In *Barker v. Lull Engineering Co.* (1978), a California court adopted a "risk–benefit" test to assess whether a product was defective. This test for defectiveness required a court to weigh a drug's benefits against its potential risks, in light of evidence that the drug could have been designed more safely, or that other drugs were available that confer similar benefits with less risk. A drug with little or no demonstrable therapeutic benefit, like DES, was far more likely to be found defective in design under the *Barker* risk–benefit test.

An interesting aspect of the DES story has been the alleged impact of DES on multiple generations with a single exposure. Unlike thalidomide's teratogenicity, which affects only fetuses exposed during gestation, DES is thought by some potentially to affect three generations—the woman who originally took the DES, the daughter of that woman, and the granddaughter of that woman. Women who took DES while they were pregnant have a slightly elevated risk of developing breast cancer, which is more likely to occur after the age of 50 (Schrager and Potter, 2004). Their daughters who were exposed *in utero* have an increased risk of vaginal and cervical clear cell adenocarcinoma, which is more likely to develop between 17 to 22 years of age (Schrager and Potter, 2004). It has been asserted that the grandchildren of women who took DES are also at increased risk for certain conditions. In one case, *Enright v. Eli Lilly & Co.* (1991), the plaintiff claimed that her cerebral palsy resulted from deformities in the reproductive system of her mother, which had been caused by her grandmother's ingestion of DES during pregnancy. Stressing the need to limit manufacturers' exposure to tort liability, the New York State Court of Appeals decided that a cause of action could be brought only by those who ingested the drug or were exposed to it *in utero* (Brahams, 1991). Both the delayed manifestation of injuries possibly associated with DES exposure and the possible multigenerational effects have important legal implications, including statutes of limitation and other restrictions on liability.

Although the two-generation limitation excluded a few plaintiffs outright, a more important hurdle facing DES plaintiffs was establishing specific causation to prove that one specific manufacturer of DES produced the pills that were ingested by their mothers. This burden of proof was challenging to meet, in part because of the two- to three-decade delay between ingestion of DES by the mother and the manifestation of injury in the exposed child. The passage of time and the loss of medical and pharmacy records made it difficult in most cases for plaintiffs to determine the specific manufacturer that made their mothers' DES. Also, anecdotal evidence suggested that pharmacists commonly dispensed DES from different manufacturers fungibly (Schreiber and Hirsh, 1985).

A lasting legal legacy of the thousands of DES cases litigated in the US are novel approaches to causation that allow plaintiffs who cannot prove specific causation by a specific manufacturer to hold one or more of the manufacturers of DES liable for their injuries. Among these theories, the four most commonly and successfully invoked are the following:

- *alternative liability*, where a plaintiff sues all the manufacturers of DES and the court places the burden on the defendants to prove that they were not the manufacturer of the allegedly injuring drug;[5]
- *concerted action*, where the plaintiff shows express or implicit agreement among defendants to commit the tort, in which case all defendants are equally liable;[6]
- *market share liability*, where the plaintiff is required only to show that the defendants benefited from a substantial share of the drug market, to shift the burden to the defendants to show that they did not produce the particular injuring drug;[7]
- *Hymowitz theory*, where the court focuses on the assertion that all manufacturers of an injurious product increase the risk to the general public, and thus holds each defendant liable in proportion to its share of the drug's nationwide market, regardless of whether the defendant could prove that it did not make the actual preparation that injured the plaintiff.[8]

Recent cases and developments

Since the thalidomide and DES cases, a growing number of drugs have been the subject of product liability actions including Accutane (acne), Baycol (high cholesterol), Bextra (pain and inflammation), Crestor (high cholesterol), Celebrex (pain and inflammation), Fen-Phen (weight loss),

---

[5] Alternative liability originated in the landmark case *Summers v. Tice*, 1948, where the plaintiff was shot in the eye by one of two negligent hunters who had shot in his direction. The doctrine is now memorialized in the Second Restatement of Torts: "Where the conduct of two or more actors is tortious, and it is proved that harm has been caused to the plaintiff by only one of them, but there is uncertainty as to which one has caused it, the burden is upon each actor to prove that he has not caused the harm" (Second Restatement of Torts § 433 B (3)

[6] See, e.g., *Bichler v. Eli Lilly & Co.*, 1982; concert of action found among DES defendants who pooled information on the basic chemical formula and model package inserts

[7] See *Sindell v. Abbott Laboratories*, 1980; market share liability introduced by the California court specifically in response to the difficulties in proving causation faced by DES plaintiffs

[8] See *Hymowitz v. Eli Lilly & Co.*, 1989

Rezulin (Diabetes), Propulsid (acid reflux), Trovan (bacterial infections), Vioxx (pain and inflammation), and Zyprexa (schizophrenia). Among these, the cases that have developed most quickly and arguably have the greatest potential size, scope and visibility involve Baycol, Fen-Phen, and Vioxx.

In addition, the US Supreme Court addressed the issue of Federal preemption in pharmaceutical liability suits in the landmark *Wyeth v. Levine* case. These matters are briefly discussed below. It is important to note that litigation involving many of these drugs is ongoing, and new developments can occur on an ongoing basis, which may materially alter the landscape of other pharmaceutical product liability actions.

Baycol (cerivastatin)

Baycol (cerivastatin) was developed by Bayer A.G. and approved by the FDA for use in the US in 1997. It is a member of a class of cholesterol-lowering drugs that are commonly referred to as "statins." Statins such as Baycol lower cholesterol levels by blocking a specific enzyme in the body that is involved in the synthesis of cholesterol. Although all statins have been associated with very rare reports of rhabdomyolysis, a muscle disorder, cases of fatal rhabdomyolysis in association with the use of Baycol have been reported significantly more frequently than for other approved statins. On August 8, 2001, Bayer announced that it was voluntarily withdrawing Baycol from the US market because of reports of sometimes fatal rhabdomyolysis.

Since Baycol's withdrawal, lawsuits comprising over 9,000 cases have been filed against Bayer.[9] The actions in the US, which included many class action suits, have been based primarily on theories of product liability, consumer fraud, medical monitoring, predatory pricing, and unjust enrichment. These lawsuits sought remedies including compensatory and punitive damages, disgorgement

of funds received from the marketing and sales of Baycol, and the establishment of a trust fund to finance the medical monitoring of former Baycol users.

Since there were an extremely large number of Federal cases filed, the cases were considered for transfer to a single Federal court through a process known as "multidistrict litigation" or MDL. Transfer of cases to a single Federal court through the MDL process is intended to make pretrial proceedings (e.g., the discovery process) more efficient. The transfer of cases usually requires a finding that the cases share common questions of fact. The Federal Judicial Panel on Multidistrict Litigation determined that many of these cases did indeed involve common questions of fact and virtually all cases filed in Federal court were transferred to the US Federal court in the District of Minnesota in December 2001. That federal court then dealt with discovery and other pretrial matters. When cases were ready for trial, they were returned to their "home" Federal court for the actual trial. A number of cases remained in various state courts as well. The vast majority of cases did not go to trial. Many cases were dismissed and many were settled out of court. As of November 2008, the defendants and plaintiffs in the MDL proceedings jointly reported that 3,134 cases had been settled for a total sum of US$1,168,233,835. As of that time, only about 35 active cases remained and 141 cases had been submitted for mediation.[10] The Baycol matter is a good illustration of how mass pharmaceutical tort litigation is handled in the US, especially when it is impractical to take every case to trial.

Fen-Phen (pondimin/phentermine)

Until the late 1990s, fenfluramine and the other drug that made up the Fen-Phen regimen, phentermine, had been on the market in the US for over 20 years. Fenfluramine is an appetite suppressant that was sold by A.H. Robins Inc., and

---

[9] See the US District Court of the District of Minnesota's website on the Baycol Product Liability Litigation at: http://www.mnd.uscourts.gov/MDL-Baycol/index.shtml; accessed August 25, 2009

[10] *In re: Baycol Products Liability Litigation*, case no. 01-md-01431, Transcript of Status Conference on November 12, 2008, available at: http://www.mnd.uscourts.gov/MDL-Baycol/transcripts/111208bc.PDF; accessed on August 25, 2009

Wyeth-Ayerst Laboratories Co., divisions of American Home Products Corp. Phentermine is a type of amphetamine that has been sold under many names and made by many companies. Fenfluramine is thought to cause weight loss by increasing the levels of a brain chemical, serotonin, which suppresses appetite. Phentermine, which acts on another brain chemical, dopamine, increases the body's metabolism and is thought to have a role in reducing minor side effects caused by fenfluramine. Both drugs were approved by the FDA as short-term diet aids, but they were never approved for use together as part of a weight reduction regimen.

The Fen-Phen combination regimen started in 1992 after the publication of an article that showed dramatic weight loss when both drugs were taken together. In 1995, the FDA was asked to approve a new diet drug, dexfenfluramine or Redux. Developed by Interneuron Pharmaceuticals Inc., a Massachusetts company, Redux is a purified form of fenfluramine. However, prior reports had linked fenfluramine use with primary pulmonary hypertension (PPH), a rare but potentially fatal cardiopulmonary disease. The FDA finally approved fenfluramine and Redux went on the market in April 1996. In July 1997, the Mayo Clinic released results from a study that found 24 cases of heart valve damage in Fen-Phen users, all of whom were women. The FDA subsequently issued a warning about heart valve problems associated with the use of Redux and Pondimin (another brand of fenfluramine). The FDA warning and the publication of the Mayo Clinic study in the *New England Journal of Medicine*, led to the withdrawal of Pondimin and Redux from the market in September 1997.

Product liability litigation involving American Home Products (now called Wyeth, a part of Pfizer) has continued since then, with Wyeth being named as a defendant in numerous legal actions alleging that the use of Redux and/or Pondimin, independently or in combination with phentermine, caused certain serious conditions, including valvular heart disease and PPH. As large as the Baycol litigation was and is, it is dwarfed by the Fen-Phen litigation. For Fen-Phen litigation alone, Wyeth recorded litigation charges of US$4.5 billion in 2004, US$2 billion in 2003 and US$1.4 billion in 2002. Pay-

ments to the nationwide class action settlement funds, individual settlement payments, legal fees, and other items were US$850.2 million, US$434.2 million, and US$1.307 billion for 2004, 2003, and 2002, respectively. By 2008, the final value of the class action settlement—which did not actually settle all cases—was approximately US$6.44 billion. Plaintiffs' attorneys from approximately 70 firms who worked on the class action suit were awarded legal fees totaling more than US$567.67 million for 578,048 hours of work (roughly equivalent to 66 years of round-the-clock work), for an hourly rate of more than US$982.[11] These numbers in the Fen-Phen litigation provide a good example of the financial interests that play an immense role in driving mass pharmaceutical tort litigation.

Vioxx (rofecoxib)

Vioxx (rofecoxib) was developed by Merck & Co. Inc. (Merck) and approved by the FDA in May 1999, for the treatment of osteoarthritis, menstrual pain, and the management of acute pain in adults. Vioxx belongs to a class of non-steroidal anti-inflammatory drugs (NSAIDs) that block the enzyme, cyclooxygenase-2, commonly referred to as "Cox-2". On September 30, 2004, Merck announced that it was voluntarily withdrawing Vioxx from the market worldwide after results from a clinical trial indicated that Vioxx users may have an increased risk of suffering a heart attack, stroke, or other cardiovascular event. The risk–benefit profile of Vioxx and other Cox-2s has been widely debated since then. On February 16–18, 2005, the FDA held a joint meeting of the Arthritis Advisory Committee and the Drug Safety and Risk Management Advisory Committee. The committees discussed the overall benefit to risk considerations (including cardiovascular and gastrointestinal safety concerns) for Cox-2 selective NSAIDs and related agents. On February 18, 2005, the members of the committees were asked to

---

[11] Frankel A. US$982 an hour for Fen-Phen plaintiffs' lawyers. *American Lawyer*, 2008, available at: http:// www.law.com/jsp/tal/PubArticleTAL.jsp?id= 900005508457; accessed on August 25, 2009

vote on whether the overall risk versus benefit profile for Vioxx supported marketing in the US. The members of the committees voted 17 to 15 in support of the marketing of Vioxx in the US.

The FDA Advisory Committee meeting and vote, of course, had little effect on the filing of litigation. Federal and state product liability lawsuits involving individual claims, as well as several putative class actions, were filed against Merck with respect to Vioxx. As with other mass pharmaceutical tort actions, the cases filed in Federal court were consolidated into a single MDL action—in the US District Court for the Eastern District of Louisiana in February 2005—for more efficient handling of pretrial matters. To date, over 5,000 cases are currently pending before that Federal court as part of the MDL action. Many, if not most, of the cases were to be resolved through the Vioxx Resolution Program announced on November 9, 2007.[12] Under this Resolution Program, Merck was to pay approximately US$4.85 billion into a settlement fund. This was not a class action settlement. Instead, cases involving claims of myocardial infarction or stroke were to be evaluated on an individual basis.

Multiple cases have gone to trial in Federal and state courts. The experience from those trials permitted the judge handling the MDL action to outline very specifically what plaintiffs were required to show in order to prevail at trial. As in all pharmaceutical product liability suits involving personal injuries, the plaintiffs were required to prove both *general causation* (i.e., that Vioxx can cause the claimed injury) and *specific causation* (i.e., that Vioxx caused the specific injury claimed by the specific plaintiff). As Judge Eldon Fallon put it:

> In order to prevail, the plaintiff must show that Vioxx was problematic; that Merck knew at some time that it was problematic and continued either manufacturing or selling the drug and not alerting doctors to this. That's general causation. If that is successfully proved by the plaintiff, then the plaintiff

must prove special [i.e., specific] causation; namely, that they took Vioxx and received an injury as a result of Vioxx and didn't know of the risks while they were taking Vioxx.[13]

As seen in this quote, a plaintiff must always prove general causation first and must then prove specific causation. It is not possible to prove specific causation without proving general causation first.

An interesting corollary to this matter was the attention that the Vioxx litigation drew to all drugs in its class (the Cox-2 inhibitors). When the adverse events for Vioxx were reported, the FDA began examining data for all Cox-2 inhibitors and the even broader class of drugs known as NSAIDs to which Cox-2 inhibitors belong. Ultimately, the FDA required manufacturers of other Cox-2 inhibitors (e.g., Bextra and Celebrex) to include boxed warnings (aka "black box warnings") highlighting the increased risk of cardiovascular adverse events. NSAID manufacturers were asked to including more specific information regarding the potential cardiovascular and gastrointestinal risks of their products.[14] The Vioxx litigation shows how mass tort litigation for one member of a class or family of drugs can have a substantial impact on related products.

Federal preemption (Phenergan and *Wyeth v. Levine*)

In light of the enormous expense of litigating matters such as those involving Baycol, Fen-phen, and Vioxx, pharmaceutical companies and their attorneys explored ways to avoid altogether certain types of product liability claims. One approach that had gained momentum in recent years was to argue Federal preemption of failure-to-warn claims. The basic idea is straightforward. It was argued that

---

[12] *In re: Vioxx Products Liability Litigation*, MDL Docket No. 1657, Joint Report No. 49 of Plaintiffs' and Defendants' Liaison Counsel, available at: http://vioxx.laed.uscourts .gov/Reports/JointReport49.pdf; accessed on August 25, 2009

[13] *In re: Vioxx Products Liability Litigation*, MDL Docket No. 1657, Transcript of October 21, 2008 Video Conference Before the Honorable Eldon E. Fallon, United States District Judge, available at: http://vioxx.laed.uscourts.gov/Transcripts/October% 2021%20Transcript.pdf; accessed August 25, 2009
[14] See http://www.fda.gov/Drugs/DrugSafety/Postmarket-DrugSafetyInformationforPatientsandProviders/ UCM103420; accessed on August 25, 2009

since the FDA's approval was required for all pharmaceutical labeling, state laws and state tort actions could not penalize pharmaceutical marketers for claimed deficiencies in that labeling. This argument has its roots in the Supremacy Clause of the US Constitution (Article VI, paragraph 2), which established Federal laws as the "supreme Law of the Land." This argument for Federal preemption of failure-to-warn claims had a mixed reception in federal district courts around the country and was ripe for resolution by the US Supreme Court.

In pushing for Federal preemption, the pharmaceutical industry was hoping to replicate the success of the medical device industry in *Riegal v. Medtronic, Inc.* (128 S. Ct. 999 (2008)), where the US Supreme Court had granted medical device manufacturers some limited Federal protection from certain product liability claims based on state tort law. However, the Federal preemption issue considered in *Riegel* differed in a fundamentally important way. In *Riegal*, there was an argument made for *express* Federal preemption of certain state tort claims based on a provision of a Federal statute, the Medical Device Amendments of 1976, which prohibits states from establishing "any requirement . . . which is different from, or in addition to, any [Federal] requirement" and "which relates to the safety or effectiveness of the device."[15] The Supreme Court in *Riegal* interpreted this provision as an explicit expression of Congress's intent to preempt state law for certain safety-related requirements for medical devices. In contrast, there was no equivalent Federal statute extending such protection for pharmaceutical manufacturers. What the

pharmaceutical industry was advocating was an *implied* Federal preemption of state tort claims in situations where it was arguably impossible to comply with both Federal law (i.e., FDA mandates) and state law.

The US Supreme Court finally took up the issue in 2008 by hearing arguments in *Wyeth v. Levine* (129 S. Ct. 1187 (2009)). *Wyeth v. Levine* involved the drug Phenergan (promethazine hydrochloride), which is used to treat nausea. Phenergan can be administered either intramuscularly or intravenously. If the IV route is used, the drug may be given rapidly by the IV-push method or more slowly through an IV-drip. Phenergan is a "corrosive" drug that can cause gangrene if it enters a patient's artery, an event that is more likely to occur with the rapid IV-push method. The Plaintiff's injury resulted from an IV-push injection of Phenergan. The injected Phenergan entered her artery (due to the negligence of the physician assistant performing the injection) and Ms Levine eventually developed gangrene, requiring amputation of her right hand and forearm. This was a particularly devastating loss for Ms Levine because she was a professional musician. Ms Levine filed suit against Wyeth, basing her claims on Vermont state common-law negligence and strict liability tort theories.

In the Vermont state trial court, Ms Levine argued that Wyeth's labeling for Phenergan was defective because it failed to instruct clinicians to use the safer IV-drip method instead of the higher-risk IV push technique. She also alleged that Phenergan was not reasonably safe for intravenous administration because the foreseeable risks of gangrene and loss of limb are too great in relation to the drug's therapeutic benefits. Wyeth filed a motion for summary judgment, arguing that Ms Levine's failure-to-warn claims were preempted by Federal law. The trial court rejected Wyeth's preemption argument, finding no evidence that Wyeth had "earnestly attempted" to strengthen the intravenous injection warning and finding no evidence that the FDA had "specifically disallowed" stronger language in the Phenergan labeling concerning intra-articular injections. The trial court found no evidence that the FDA had established

---

[15] 21 U.S.C. § 360k(a). The provision reads:
"Except as provided in subsection (b) of this section, no State or political subdivision of a State may establish or continue in effect with respect to a device intended for human use any requirement—(1) which is different from, or in addition to, any requirement applicable under this chapter to the device, and (2) which relates to the safety or effectiveness of the device or to any other matter included in a requirement applicable to the device under this chapter"

a "ceiling" on the warnings that Wyeth could put into its labeling. In its instructions to the jury, the trial judge stated that compliance with FDA requirements did not establish that warnings in the Phenergan label were adequate. The trial judge also informed the jury that FDA regulations permit a drug manufacturer to change a product label to add or strengthen a warning without prior FDA approval so long as it later submits the revised warning for review and approval—a reference to Federal regulations permitting certain immediate labeling changes through a so-called "Changes-Being-Effected" (or "CBE") supplement.[16] The jury found Wyeth to be negligent and that Phenergan was a defective product because of inadequate warnings and instructions in the Phenergan label. The Vermont Supreme Court eventually affirmed the jury's decision and the US Supreme Court agreed to hear the appeal.

At the Supreme Court, Wyeth made two distinct preemption arguments. First, Wyeth argued that Ms Levine's state law claims were preempted because it was impossible to comply with both the state-law duties underlying her claims and the Federal labeling duties with which Wyeth was obligated to comply. The Supreme Court rejected this argument by noting that Wyeth could strengthen the warnings and instructions in the Phenergan label without prior FDA approval through a CBE supplement. The Court went further and asserted that it was always the pharmaceutical company, and not the FDA, who "bears responsibility for the content of its label at all times." The Supreme Court concluded that Wyeth had failed to demonstrate that it was "impossible" to comply with both Federal and state requirements.

Wyeth also argued the Ms Levine's state law claims were preempted because requiring Wyeth to comply with a state-law duty would interfere with "Congress's purpose to entrust an expert [Federal] agency [i.e., the FDA] to make drug labeling decisions." The Supreme Court also rejected this argument. The Court noted that Congress has never provided for a Federal remedy in the

Food, Drug, and Cosmetic Act for consumers who were harmed by unsafe or ineffective drugs. The Court also noted that Congress had not enacted a preemption provision like the one that protected medical device manufacturers for pharmaceutical products. In the Court's view, Congress did not intend FDA oversight to be the exclusive means for ensuring drug safety and effectiveness. The Court also rejected Wyeth's reliance on a preamble to a 2006 FDA regulation that governed the content and format of prescription drug labels. In that preamble, the FDA declared that the Food, Drug, and Cosmetic Act establishes both a "floor" and "ceiling" for drug regulation and that FDA approval of a label "preempts conflicting or contrary State law."[17] The Court determined that this statement from the FDA did not merit deference from the Court because it had been finalized without notice or opportunity for comment, was contrary to the apparent purposes of Congress, and reversed the FDA's own long-standing views regarding Federal preemption. The Supreme Court affirmed the Vermont Supreme Court's ruling in favor of Ms Levine.

In summary, it appears that Federal preemption of state tort law claims against pharmaceutical manufacturers—absent a specific warning submitted to the FDA that was rejected—is unlikely to be a viable option following the *Wyeth v. Levine* decision. The Supreme Court has firmly placed the ultimate responsibility for the content of pharmaceutical labels in the hands of the manufacturers, and it is now the responsibility of manufacturers to ensure that their drug labels comply with FDA regulations as well as the requirements of state law.

Conclusions

This chapter has provided a brief overview of the doctrinal framework of products liability law that is applied in pharmaceutical injury cases. Though a full explication of the theories, definitions and defenses involved with products liability law is quite complex, this chapter summarizes these

---

[16] See 21 C.F.R. § 314.70(c)(6)(iii)

[17] 71 Fed. Reg. 3922, 2006

elements as they most specifically relate to pharmaceuticals. Although the drug industry is heavily regulated in the US by the FDA and abroad by analogous agencies, products liability tort in the forms discussed here constitutes an increasingly prominent parallel regulatory means by which defective products can be removed from the market and negligent manufacturers can be censured. Despite the increase in products liability litigation, plaintiffs such as those who brought suits in the thalidomide and DES litigations frequently face unpredictable and difficult hurdles to recovery under existing legal theories. This makes the area of pharmaceutical products liability an especially productive area for new theories of liability and for defense from liability. Ultimately, it is the responsibility of courts to approve or disapprove of these novel theories and to strike the right balance between deterring irresponsible drug manufacturers and encouraging beneficial drug development.

References

Allen W. The return of thalidomide: are we ready to forget images like this and give the drug another chance? *St. Louis Post-Dispatch*: 28 September 1997; 01B.

Allen D, Bourne C, Holyoak J (eds) *Accident Compensation after Pearson*. Sweet & Maxwell: London, UK, 1979, Chapter 3, p. 161

Barker v. Lull Engineering. 20 Cal. 3d 413, 573 p. 2d 443, 143 Cal. Rptr. 225, 1978.

Bernstein S. Formed by thalidomide: mass torts as a false cure for toxic exposure. *Colum L Rev* 1997; **97**:2153.

Bichler v. Ru Lilly & Co. 79 App. Div. 2d 317, 436 N.Y.S. 2d 625 (App. Div. 1981); 55 N.Y. 2d 571, 450 N.Y.S. 2d 776, 436 N.E. 2d 182, 1982.

Brahams D. Diethylstilbestrol: [sic] third-generation injury claims. *Medico-Legal J* 1991; **59**:126.

Buitendijk S. DES—The Time Bomb Drug. In *Report of the 13th European Symposium on Clinical Pharmacological Evaluation in Drug Control*. World Health Organization: Regional Office for Europe, Copenhagen, Denmark, 1984.

Burley D. The decline and fall of thalidomide. In *Orphan Diseases and Orphan Drugs*, Scheinberg IH, Walshe JM (eds). Manchester University Press, in association with The Fulbright Commission: London, UK, 1986.

Cook T, Doyle C, Jabbari D. *Pharmaceuticals, Biotechnology and the Law*. Macmillan: Basingstoke, UK, 1991, 364.

Crawford CL. Use of thalidomide in leprosy. *Adverse Drug React Toxicol Rev* 1994; **13**:177.

D'Arcy PF. Thalidomide revisited. Thirteen adverse drug reactions. *Toxicol Rev* 1994; **13**:65.

Dukes G, Mildred M, Swartz B. *Responsibility for Drug-induced Injury: A Reference Book for Health Professions and Manufacturers*. IOS Press: Oxford, UK, 1998.

Dutton D. *Worse than the Disease: Pitfalls of Medical Progress*. Cambridge University Press: Cambridge, UK, 1988, 87.

Dworkin G. Pearson: implications for severely handicapped children and products liability. In *Accident Compensation after Pearson*, Allen D, Bourne C, Holyoak J (eds). Sweet & Maxwell: London, UK, 1979.

Enright v. Eli Lilly & Co. 77 N.Y. 2d 377, 570 N.E. 2d 198, (1991).

European Federation of Pharmaceutical Industries and Associations. Green Paper on Liability for Defective Products, 1999.

Ferguson PR. *Drug Injuries and the Pursuit of Compensation*. Sweet & Maxwell: London, UK, 1996.

Flaherty, FJ. Last thalidomide suits settle to end legal era. *Natl Law J* 1984; **6**:32.

Heuston RFV, Buckley RA. *Salmond & Heuston on the Law of Torts*, twentieth edition. Sweet & Maxwell: London, UK, 1992, 310–312.

Hunter R. Product liability: dangerous to development. *Int Corporate Law* 1993; **27**:27–28.

Hymowitz v. Eli Lilly & Co. 73 N.Y. 2d 487, 539 N.E. 2d 1069, 541 N.Y.S 2d 941, 1989.

Jones MA. *Textbook on Torts*, fourth edition. Blackstone: London, UK, 1993, 302–213.

Lifton DE, Bufano MM. A call for continued state law tort reform. *Pharmaceutical & Medical Device Law Bulletin* 2004; **4**(3).

McCartney TE, Rheingold PD. From prescription to over-the-counter: watered-down warnings. *Trial* 1996; **32**(34):24.

Moore TM, Cullen SA. Impact of global pharmaceutical regulations on US products liability exposure. *Defense Counsel J* 1999; **66**(1):101–108.

Mossialos E, Ranos C, Abel-Smith B. *Cost Containment, Pricing and Financing of Pharmaceuticals in the European Community: The Policy-Maker's View*. LSE Health and Pharmetrica: Athens, 1994, 18–19.

Nace BJ, Robb GC, Rogers JS, *et al*. Products liability: tips and tactics. *Trial* 1997; **33**(11):38.

Pendell J. *The Adverse Side Effects of Pharmaceutical Litigation*. AEI-Brookings Joint Center for Regulatory Studies: Washington, DC, USA, 2003.

Robertson G. Thalidomide revisited. *Okla St Med Assoc J* 1972; **65**:45.

Schrager S, Potter BE. Diethystilbestrol Exposure. *American Family Physician* 2004; **69**(10):2395–2400.

Schreiber L, Hirsh HL. Theories of liability applied to overcome the unique "identification problem" in DES cases. *Med Law* 1985; **4**:337.

Sherman M, Strauss S. Thalidomide: a twenty-five year perspective. *Food Drug Cosmetic Law J* 1986; **41**:458–466.

Sindell v. Abbott Laboratories (1980) 26 Cal. 3d 588, 607 p. 2d 924, 163 Cal. Rptr. 132.

Szeinberg A, Sheba C. Pharmacogenetics. *Israel J Med Sci* 1968; **4**(3):488.

The Progress & Freedom Foundation. *Advancing Medical Innovation: Health, Safety and the Role of Government in the 21st Century*. The Progress & Freedom Foundation: Washington, DC, USA, 1996.

Summers v. Tice. 33 Cal. 2d 80, 199 P. 2d 1, 1948.

US HHS. MIH will hold public scientific workshop on thalidomide—potential benefits and risks. August 9 1997, M2 Presswire.

Waterhouse R. Thalidomide victims given £3.75 million bail-out. *The Independent*, May 4, 1995; 2.

Wiedemann HR. Hinweis auf eine derzeitige Haufung hypo-und aplasticher Fehlbildungen der Gliedmassen. *Med Welt* 1961; **37**:1864.

Further reading

Ferguson P. Pharmaceutical products liability: 30 years of law reform? *Juridical Rev* 1992; **3**:226–39.

DeConinck J (1994) The impact of product liability on the marketing of prescription drugs. *Am Business Rev* **12**(1): 79–85.

Hamilton v. Fife Health Board (1993) 4 Med. L.R. 201; 1993 S.L.T. 624; 1993 S.C.L.R. 408.

Harris Interactive Inc. (1993) Pharmaceutical Liability Study commissioned by the U.S. Chamber Institute for Legal Reform: Washington, DC.

The Sunday Times (1973). *The Thalidomide Children and the Law*. Andre Deutsch: London.

CHAPTER 56

Patents

Gabriel Lopez
Basking Ridge, NJ, USA

The realities of modern international corporations and the international marketplace for pharmaceuticals demand a global view of patents and other forms of intellectual property. Because patents are territorial, that is, they only protect an invention within the borders of the issuing country, the inventor must think of protecting an invention in countries other than the home country. National patent applications are very frequently followed by applications in other countries, as we will see below. Therefore, although the following discussion concentrates on the USA, which is the largest and most profitable market for pharmaceutical products, this chapter will also reference international patent concepts.

Even if it were limited to US law, this chapter would not be intended as a learned treatise on patent law, given the enormity of the subject. Rather, it is designed to expose those in the pharmaceutical industry only to some general principles. It is biased toward pharmaceutical patent practice; meaning that issues totally different from those discussed herein might arise if the invention were a computer program, an electric switch, or a device for milking yaks. Also to be remembered is that, as in most fields of law, both the substantive and procedural aspects of the subject are always changing, by legislative act, judicial ruling, or international treaty. This constant change will make today's statements on substance and procedure, not necessarily obsolete, but certainly dated in the not too distant future.

As a simple example of these changes is the calculation of a patent's life span, which used to be 17 years, calculated from the *date of issue*. But US patents filed after June 7, 1995, last 20 years, calculated from the *date of filing* (which has been typical outside the US for many years). Also, a form of tax, known as a maintenance fee, is now imposed on US patents. If the patentee does not pay each fee as it becomes due, the patent lapses. Finally, US patents can be extended *via* two different mechanisms. Under the rules of Patent Term Restoration, certain patents, mostly pharmaceutical patents, can be extended for up to five years. The theory is that the patentee has suffered an injustice because the patentee was essentially denied a portion of the patent's life and not allowed to earn potential profit from the patented invention because of the need to first obtain regulatory (e.g., Food and Drug Administration (FDA)) approval before bringing the product to market. Under the rules of Patent Term Adjustment, extensions can also be obtained for certain procedural delays during the prosecution of a patent application. The actual term extension for each patent is determined by its specific facts. These two calculations are independent of one another. Patent Term Adjustment is not limited to pharmaceutical patents. "When does this US patent expire?" used to be, but no longer is, a trivial question to answer.

Intellectual property

Types of intellectual property

Patents are just one of a class of intellectual property rights; that is, rights to intangible property

Principles and Practice of Pharmaceutical Medicine, 3rd edition.
Edited by L.D. Edwards, A.W. Fox, P.D. Stonier.
© 2011 Blackwell Publishing Ltd.

(as contrasted to the right to real property, such as the deed to a house.) These intellectual property rights are Copyrights, Trademarks, Seed Protection, Trade Secrets, and Patents. Each "right" differs from the others primarily in the type of property it protects, how it is obtained, and the length of protection. Some of the characteristics of these rights are as follows:

• *Copyrights.* These protect the expression of an idea. Protection may be obtained by marking the work, as with the symbol ©. The term is typically for the life of the creator plus a number of years. Articles in medical journals are usually copyrighted.

• *Trademarks (and the related service marks).* These protect logos, company names, container shapes, color patterns, etc. Drug trade names are usually protected by trademarks.

• *Seed protection.* These protect agricultural seeds.

• *Trade secrets.* These protect information that is not publicly available and not divulged to anyone unless there is a confidentiality relationship therewith. Trade secret protection has no statutory life span; protection lasts as long as divulgation is prevented. Whether the divulgation occurs innocently or through intent, error, or malice is irrelevant; once the secret is out, it is out and protection ends. There may be monetary recovery through court action against a malicious or negligent divulger, who may also be punished under the penal codes if malicious. But this is usually small comfort to the previous trade secret owner.

• *Patents.* These protect designs, asexually produced plants, things, processes, and business methods. Pharmaceutical patents typically protect new chemical entities, synthetic processes, formulations, and methods of treatment. (Designs, plant patents, and business methods are not further discussed.) Protection is obtained by filing and then successfully prosecuting a patent application that discloses the invention. The patent term is typically 20 years from the filing date (see above).

Note that patents and trade Secrets are antithetical types of protection. To protect by trade secret, the invention must never be disclosed; whereas to protect by patent, disclosure at the time of filing is essential. The patent applicant receives a monopolistic right for a period of years in exchange for putting the invention in the hands of the public (for "public" read "competitor"). *This exchange of monopoly for divulgation is at the core of the patent concept.* Failure of the inventor fully to disclose an invention has led to patent invalidation.

Selecting the type of protection

Although the subject matter that is intended to be protected largely dictates what type of protection is available and/or preferable (for example, one could obtain copyright protection but not trademark protection for a new song), there can be overlaps. Probably most common is the overlap between patents and trade secrets. If an invention can be commercialized without divulging the invention and without risk of its being back-engineered, the innovator should seriously consider not seeking a patent at all, but rather keeping the invention secret. Possibly the longest kept such trade secret is the formula for Coca-Cola®, which to this day has not been stolen, divulged, or back-engineered. A patent for this formulation would have described this invention in detail and would have expired decades ago.

It is not always easy to make the correct decision among alternatives when seeking to protect inventions. The inventor who decides on trade secret protection may regret that decision in a few years when the secret is inadvertently or maliciously revealed or when some analytical tool is developed that allows back-engineering of the invention. In the area of pharmaceuticals, trade secret protection in not likely to be sought by the inventor because a new chemical entity is often the invention that needs protection and such an invention necessarily must be publicly divulged. Two types of pharmaceutical inventions, however, are often kept as trade secrets: manufacturing process improvements and screening assays.

Short history of patents

Patents are not a new concept. They were granted at least as far back as ancient Greece and Babylon. Nor are they the product of only one form of government. Essentially every country has some form of patent protection, albeit not necessarily as strong as that in the USA and the other industrialized countries. Patent laws have long existed even in noncapitalist systems, such as the former USSR. That intellectual property is a highly valued concept can be no better demonstrated than by the observation that there are only two rights (patents and copyrights) that are specifically mentioned in the US Constitution. (The much praised Bill of Rights was a group of ten amendments added to the basic document.) Sect. 8, para. 8 reads:

> To promote the progress of science and the useful arts by securing for limited times to authors and inventors the exclusive rights to their respective writings and discoveries.

Limitations on patent rights

Patents, however, are not free of their detractors. Since they are a form of monopoly and because monopolies have been subject to abuse (e.g., granting the king's cousin a monopoly on the local water well), anti-monopoly laws (e.g., restraint of trade, anti-trust, etc.) exist which can be used to limit a patentee's rights. Another limitation on patent rights is simply prohibiting the grant of patents on certain types of inventions, typically based on ethical or economic considerations. There are arguments against "patenting life," as a result of which some types of biotechnology inventions are unpatentable in many countries. Among these can be included patenting transgenic animals, pieces of the human genome, and of course, human clones. Many countries prohibit methods of treating humans. Another, older prohibition is that against granting patents to pharmaceuticals *per se*. Although their numbers are diminishing, many countries have allowed only limited patent protection on pharmaceuticals. Typically what can be patented in these countries is a process to synthesize the compounds but not on the compounds *per se*. These, so called, "process countries" are mostly nonindustrialized. They have argued that they would be at an economic disadvantage if they were to grant compound *per se* protection because they do not have the in-house infrastructure to invent/patent such compounds themselves.

All such patents would be granted to foreign, international pharmaceutical houses, as a consequence of which, moneys would always be flowing out of these countries to pay for vital pharmaceutical drugs. Many "process" countries have already amended or agreed to amend their laws to include compound *per se* protection. The subtleties of these ethical and economic debates are beyond the scope of this discussion.

Patent protection

Fundamental patent rights

A patent is a monopoly for a period of time that gives the patentee *the right to exclude others* from making, using, selling, or offering to sell the patented invention. Patents are limited geographically, temporally, and by the rights of others. Because others may have superior rights or because the invention may be illegal, a patent never gives the patentee a right to practice the invention. This is a basic concept that is often unappreciated by the non-practitioner.

Patent licensing

Thus, the oft-heard, "We just licensed in the right to make Compound X," when a patent license has been negotiated, is legally incorrect. It would imply that the right conveyed by the license is actually greater than that possessed by the licensor. However, the licensor does *not* have the right to make Compound X, only the right to deny that right to others. What is generally conveyed by a patent license, and depending on the wording thereof, is (i) protection from a patent infringement suit by the licensor and (ii) the right to sue others for patent infringement.

A relatively simple example explains this concept. Assume three pharmaceutical companies/patentees: (i) P1 has obtained a patent on a compound with a side-chain defined as an alkyl of 1–10 carbon atoms; (ii) P2 has obtained a patent on a compound within the scope of P1's patent, wherein the side-chain is limited to propyl (i.e., three carbon atoms); and (iii) P3 has obtained a patent on a combination of compounds, one of which is the P2 compound.

The P1 patent is said to "dominate" the P2 patent. P1 has the right to exclude others, including P2, from making a compound within the scope of P1's patent but cannot itself make the compound with a propyl side-chain, because this is the subject of the P2 patent. How can this matter be resolved, without costly court battles, if each wishes to benefit from its invention?

1. If P2's compound is a much more marketable product, it might be in both patentees' interests to cross-license their respective patents (a "freedom to operate" license), because neither patentee could sell the more desirable product without an accommodation with the other.

2. P2 could also buy P1's product, if it were being marketed, and then modify it to produce a propyl side-chain compound, because the sale exhausts P1's patent rights in the compound sold. However, P1 may have no interest in selling a suitable compound. Also, it may be economically unfeasible for P2 if the purchasing and modification costs would make the compound noncompetitive against other available pharmaceuticals.

The situation can quickly become more complicated if we now add P3. The license negotiated, as described above between the first and second patentees, does not affect P3, who is not a party to the license. If P3 attempts to sell its combination product, both P1 and P2 could sue for patent infringement under their respective patents, even though neither of them claimed a combination with other compounds. Again, if the combination product is of sufficient marketing interest, cross-licensing would be appropriate. In some technologies, multiple-party cross licenses and "freedom to operate" licenses are common. This is often the case in biotechnological inventions, where multiple synthesis-related inventions by different parties are involved.

Patentable subject matter

Patentable subject matter covers a very broad range of the terms "things" and "processes." These include compounds *per se* (i.e., new chemical entities), compositions (e.g., a chemical entity and a pharmaceutically acceptable carrier or two chemical entities), life forms (e.g., a purified, newly discovered microorganism, a constructed microorganism, or a region of DNA), devices (e.g., a surgical appliance), chemical syntheses, screening assays, and methods of using a compound or composition. Shorter than to define what is the patentable is to define what is legally unpatentable. Generally, unpatentable subject matter includes products of nature (i.e., naturally occurring articles), scientific principles, some biotechnology inventions, and some inventions related to atomic energy and nuclear material. The prohibitions against patents on methods of human treatment and compounds *per se* have been discussed above. In the "process countries" (defined above) patents can be obtained on a process to make a compound, but not on the chemical entity itself. Inherently, this is a more limited patent right, because (i) it may be very difficult to prove that a particular process is being infringed; and (ii) alternative manufacturing processes may be developed that do not infringe.

Criteria for obtaining a patent

There are three criteria for obtaining a patent. The claimed invention must be: (i) novel, (ii) unobvious, and (iii) useful or utile. There are somewhat subtle differences in what these concepts mean in different countries, which can lead to different outcomes when the inventor tries to obtain patent protection for the same invention in different countries. But generally these three criteria are universally accepted. Of these, novelty and utility are usually the easiest criteria to deal with.

Novelty

An invention is *novel* if it was not part of the "prior art" before the priority date (see below) of the patent application that claims the invention. The "prior art" comprises all oral or written information publicly available before the priority date of the application. This criterion is essentially absolute everywhere except in the USA, where there is a "grace period" of one year within which one can file a patent application even if the invention has been earlier divulged either by the inventor or by another. Novelty is fairly strictly interpreted; that is, the destruction of novelty requires a specific prior description of the invention being claimed. Thus, one can obtain a patent on a compound even if it is within the scope of the generic formula in an earlier publication that teaches multiple substituents on a core structure but which does not specifically show the now-claimed compound. To determine novelty one compares the date of invention (under US law) or priority filing date with the divulgation date of the supposed prior art. If the subject matter is the same and the divulgation date of the publication precedes the invention/filing date, the invention fails the first test and cannot be patented.

In the USA one further twist on divulgation dates is that a US patent is a reference as of its earliest US filing date. Since a US patent application used not to be publicly available until the patent issued and since the allowance of a patent could be delayed either by a prolonged prosecution in the Patent Office (which could include appealing an adverse determination by the Examiner both within the Patent Office and then to the courts) or by the filing of one or more continuation applications, a US patent could become a reference as of its earliest US filing date many, many years after said filing date. Such patents (sometimes referred to as "submarine patents") can be used as weapons in litigation to invalidate competitors' patents, the applications for which were filed after said earliest filing date. Now that the US has joined the rest of the world in publishing applications 18 months after filing, "submarine patents" are becoming much less of an issue.

Utility

An invention is *utile* if it has a practical end use. The requirement can be met by a statement of what the invention can be used for and how to use it; for example, "This compound is useful for the treatment of asthma when administered at a dose of 0.1–5.0 μg/kg/day." A more complete teaching would include modes of administration, dosage forms, delivery systems, etc. The utility must be currently available. Although commercial availability is not necessary, mere assertions such as "these

are therapeutic agents," or "they are for pharmaceutical purposes" are generally insufficient. If the asserted utility is believable on its face to persons skilled in the art in view of the state of the art as of the filing date, the burden is upon the Examiner to give adequate support for rejections for lack of utility. As stated by Commissioner. Lehman at a hearing on October 17, 1994: "In other words, if an applicant presents a scientifically plausible use for the claimed invention, it will be sufficient to satisfy the utility requirement." Two types of inventions that tend to fail the utility test are perpetual motion machines (the Patent Office wants to see working models of these) and "unbelievable" cures without supporting experimental data (e.g., a cure for AIDS).

Unobviousness

The third, and most difficult, criterion is *unobviousness*, or inventive step, as it is known outside the US. The process for deciding whether or not an invention is obvious was succinctly stated in a US court decision (the Deere case). According to the Deere decision the Patent Examiner should determine obviousness using a three-prong approach:

1. Determine the scope and content of the prior art.

2. Ascertain the differences between the prior art and the claims.

3. Resolve the level of ordinary skill in the pertinent art.

Although Deere is a US decision and is only binding therein, the principle enunciated is followed, more or less, by most patent offices worldwide.

Of course, this three-prong approach is much easier to enunciate than to practice. Consequently, much time and effort is typically spend during the prosecution of a patent application trying to convince the Examiner that the rejection of the claims on the basis of obviousness is incorrect because one or more of the Deere prongs has failed. Steps (1) and (2) of the Deere analysis tend to be fairly straightforward. However, it is in the third step that a judgment call must be made by the Examiner, which presents the most problems. Even if the applicant and Examiner agree on the first two steps, the conclusion to be drawn therefrom is rarely easily agreed upon. Obviousness, like beauty, appears to be more often than not in the eye of the Examiner-beholder.

The matter is made worse by the organization of patent applications, which are usually drafted by first stating the background of the invention, which may include a description of the closest prior art and some unresolved problem therewith, followed by a statement of the invention. It should not be too surprising that an Examiner, presented with both a statement of a problem and the solution to the problem, would respond by concluding that the solution is obvious. Most of us have probably had a similar response upon being shown the solution to a trivial geometric puzzle, which, of course, up to that moment had completely baffled us. Hindsight in deciding the question of obviousness, as in many other endeavors, is 20/20. (In Europe, the Examiner's approach to a determination of obviousness is based on "the problem to be solved." The problem/solution organization just described makes it easier for the European Examiner to find the claims "lacking in inventive step.")

The task then is to convince the Examiner to reconsider the obviousness rejection. Many approaches are possible. (In the following examples, the claimed invention is a compound and the prior art discloses structurally similar compounds. However, analogous arguments can be made for process claims, composition claims, etc.).

The simplest arguments are based on structural differences. For example, the reference compound contains an alkyl substituent at the position where the claimed compound contains an aryl group. The argument is that alkyl does not suggest aryl. Similarly, arguments can be made that "C" does not suggest "S"; "2-phenyl" does not suggest "3-phenyl"; "S" does not suggest "O"; "S" does not suggest "SO_2," and so on.

An argument based on structural differences becomes more compelling if related to physical properties, such as biological activity. For example, the reference compound had no activity, had a different activity, had the same but less activity, or had a side effect not exhibited by the claimed compound. Note that since the rejection is based on what is disclosed in the prior art, the applicant can use what is disclosed in the art to construct an argument. Thus, if the reference discloses that the compound has an ED_{50} of 100 µg/kg and the claimed compound has an ED_{50} of 10 µg/kg, an argument based the enhanced activity of the claimed compound can be made without actually having to generate data to determine the already disclosed ED_{50} of the reference compound.

Another argument may be that the prior art actually taught away from the invention; for example, the compounds were known to be toxic or unstable, or there was a progression in the references away from the invention (for example, the claimed compound contains a methyl substituent whereas the earliest of three references cited against the applicant teaches an alkyl group at the same position of 4–7 carbons, the second reference teaches 10–15 carbons, and the latest reference teaches 20–30 carbons).

Another, albeit weaker, approach is to argue from "secondary considerations." It brings in such secondary considerations as the commercial success of the invention, that there was a long-felt need in the art for a solution to some problem, the failed attempts of many others to solve whatever problem the invention solves, and so on.

It is often the case that the above arguments are made in combination with some limitations on the scope of the claimed subject matter. More often than not, the allowed claims are narrower in scope that those that were initially filed.

Failing to convince by mere argumentation, the applicant may choose to introduce tangible evidence, which is typically in the form of a signed declaration that presents the results of comparative testing, that is, a side-by-side comparison in some assay of the prior art and claimed compounds.

Short biography of a patent application

With the understanding that there really is no typical patent application, the following is an attempt to describe a typical and highly simplified patent application life span. The setting is an international pharmaceutical corporation.

The inventor prepares an Invention Disclosure describing the invention. The Disclosure is reviewed/approved by Research and forwarded to a Patent Committee for further review. If it is decided that the invention is worthy of patent protection, a patent application is drafted, finalized, and filed within several months after approval by the Committee. (In the US, patent applications can only be filed by inventors and patents are only granted to inventors. Outside the US, however, non-inventors can be applicants. These applicants are usually the organizations that hired the inventors, but they could be others.)

In about one year from filing, a Patent Examiner takes up the application and communicates (usually in the form of a Rejection) with the patent attorney handling the application. Issues of novelty, utility, and obviousness are argued back and forth and after about another year or two, the application is either allowed (in which case an Issue Fee is paid and the patent is granted) or the Examiner issues a Final Rejection, to which the response is an Appeal. Appeals are handled by a three-person Board, which reviews all the arguments presented by the applicant and the Examiner. Favorable decisions by the Board of Appeals result in an allowance. Unfavorable decisions can be appealed to the courts or simply result in abandonment of the application by the inventor. Board decisions are currently taking about two years from the time the Applicant's Brief and the Examiner's Answer are submitted to the Board. This process is what is meant by patent prosecution; that is, the give-and-take between the applicant (more typically, the applicant's agent or attorney) and the Patent Office, which results in granting or denying the grant of a patent.

In parallel with the above, about 9–10 months after filing the application, a decision must be made by the Patent Committee about if, where, and how to Foreign File the application, which must be done by one year from the filing date if the applicant is to claim the benefit of the Paris Convention (see below).

The foreign filing decision-making process varies from organization to organization (sometimes even differing from subsidiary to subsidiary within the same company) but is often in the form of a committee comprising members from Research, Marketing, and Patents, preferably armed with a tiered country list. An extremely potent new drug, marketable worldwide, with a high likelihood of being patented is a candidate for global foreign filings. An invention of lesser value might be filed on a more-limited basis (e.g., USA, EC, Canada, and Japan) while still protecting a significant amount of sales. An invention of very little continued interest might (i) be made publicly available as by allowing the application to publish at 18 months after the priority date, but then allowing the application to lapse by nonresponse to the next Patent Office letter, or (ii) not published at all as by expressly abandoning the pending application.

If it is decided to proceed with national filings, the application is sent to an agent in each country with instructions to file the application by the one-year anniversary date.

If a Patent Cooperation Treaty (PCT) (see below) filing is decided, the application can be filed by the applicant in the PCT Receiving Office of the US Patent Office. Decisions then have to be made shortly before 30 months after the initial filing date with regard to national filings, as described below in the section on "The Patent Cooperation Treaty."

National filings, whether directly or through the PCT, are handled by each country's Patent Office. There are a multitude of statutory, formalistic, and stylistic differences among all the Patent Offices, resolved with the help of the local patent agents. However, typically there is a review by an Examiner, amendments and arguments by the applicant, and either an Allowance or an Appeal (i.e., a procedural system similar to that in the US). In the European Patent Office (EPO), Japan, and many other countries, an Allowance does not automatically result in the granting of a patent. In these countries, when the Examiner decides there is patentable subject matter, the allowed claims are published for Opposition. During the Opposition period (6–9 months), anyone can protest the granting of the patent. Opponents present their written arguments, at which time the applicant is given the opportunity to rebut. If the matter is not resolved after a period of arguments and counter-arguments, the matter is orally argued before and decided by an Opposition Board. As with a US patent application involved in an Interference (see below), ultimate issuance of a patent may take years in the case of a vigorously contested Opposition.

Finally, after the patent has issued, it must be "maintained." Maintenance fees must be paid periodically to each country in order to keep the patent in force: Failure to pay results in a lapsed patent.

International treaties

Although patents are territorial, that is, they are granted by and enforced in individual countries, several international treaties have had a major impact on patent practice on a global scale. Although the lists of signatory countries are not identical for all treaties, essentially all major countries are signatories to all the treaties described herein (with the exception of the EPC, which is available only to EC countries).

The Paris Convention

The first and most important of these treaties is the Paris Convention for the Protection of Industrial Property of 1883. "The Convention" allows an applicant to file a patent application in any of the Convention countries and then, no more than one year after the filing, to file corresponding patent applications in any, or all, of the other Convention countries and to claim the benefit of the filing date of said earlier patent application.

The significance of the Paris Convention cannot be overstated. The first filing date, "the priority date," shuts off the prior art, not only in the country of original filing but also in all the other signatory countries. Since absolute novelty is the rule almost everywhere except the US, it is very advantageous to the applicant to be able to fix a date certain after which no later publicly available information can be cited as prior art, either by a Patent Examiner during prosecution of the application or by opposing counsel in litigation (i.e., in a courtroom) in any Convention country. (Actually, multiple related patent applications (typically, each

an expansion of and/or a more detailed version of a prior one) can be and often are filed within the "Convention Year." Each of these establishes a different priority date for whatever is newly disclosed therein. However, it is simpler, to confine the rest of discussion to a single priority filing and a single priority date.)

There is a great economic advantage to this arrangement, because the applicant need only file one application to stop the prior art. The applicant then has one year in which to evaluate the invention and decide if additional, that is "foreign," filings are warranted.

The European Patent Convention (EPC)

This is the treaty under which the European Community (EC) created the European Patent Office (EPO) to receive and prosecute patent applications with jurisdiction over the whole EC. Only EC countries can be signatories to the EPC. This system works in parallel with the European national patent offices, which have not been closed. In fact, on filing an EPO patent application, the applicant designates in which of the EC countries patent protection is sought. If the application is successfully prosecuted, the applicant is then granted a patent by each of the designated countries; that is, each signatory country has agreed to have the EPO determine patentable subject matter and then grants its own patents based on the EPO's favorable decisions.

If one wishes to file a patent application in Europe, there are three routes from which one must choose: (i) file nationally (i.e., country-by-country); (ii) file in the EPO; and (iii) simultaneously file nationally and in the EPO. (The third route is an expensive alternative and little used.) Unless the country list is very small, an EPO filing has several advantages. Procedurally, it is the simplest since there is only one filing, one prosecution, and one set of allowed claims. The entire proceeding can be handled in any one of the official languages (English, German, and French). The cost of translating into the non-official languages can be deferred until the end of prosecution. If there is an adverse decision, or if the application is abandoned because the subject matter is no longer of interest to the applicant, there are no translation costs. The EPO route does suffer from the "all your eggs in one basket" problem, which, of course, does not exist if one files nationally. This is not viewed by most applicants as a significant impediment.

The Patent Cooperation Treaty (PCT)

The PCT of 1970 created an extremely practical and economic mechanism for worldwide patent filing that has been steadily gaining in popularity. The treaty created the World Intellectual Property Organization (WIPO), which is headquartered in Geneva and which administers the provisions of the treaty. As with an EPO application, when filing a PCT application one initially designates those countries, or regional patent offices such as the EPO, in which patents are to be sought at a later date, during the "National Phase." The PCT application is itself not a patent application, in the sense that no "PCT patent" is ever granted. Instead, it reserves to the applicant the right to file national patent applications in the future in the one or more of the initially designated countries. A PCT filing comprises both an international phase and a national phase.

International phase

The PCT filing results in an International Search and the issuance of an International Search Report, a Written Opinion (which comments on the three aspects of patentability (novelty, obviousness, and utility) as they apply to the claims, and possibly comments on other matters as well), and an International Preliminary Examination Report (IPER). The WIPO will also publish the patent application 18 months after the priority date. The designation "WO..." in the upper right-hand of what many incorrectly call a "patent" actually indicates that the document is only a published PCT patent application, not a patent. The PCT patent application is itself never prosecuted to allowance. The filing allows an applicant to defer further action (and cost) until 30 months from the priority date, giving the applicant some time to consider both (i) the value of the invention (does it work? is it marketable?) and (ii) the contents of the Search Report,

Written Opinion, and International Preliminary Examination Report (how close is the prior art and how likely is it that it can be overcome?). There is clearly a great advantage both in time and cost (no national filing fees, agents' fees, or translation costs) resulting from deferring national filing until 30 months after the priority date.

National phase

Mechanically, this means filing a patent application (through one's patent agents) in each of those countries initially designated, and still of interest, and advising each national Patent Office that the national application is based on the PCT filing. It is the WIPO's responsibility to forward all the documents from the international phase to these national offices. Prosecution of each application is then handled by each country independently of what any other country may be doing with a corresponding application. Since each national patent office must act in conformity with the patent laws of that country, the Written Opinion and IPER cannot control and there may be a broad range of reactions from the national patent offices to the Written Opinion/IPER during the national prosecution stage. Some offices appear to totally abdicate responsibility and incorporate the results reached during the international phase into their own decisions, whereas others appear to disregard them in whole or in part. In any case, the applicant is in a much more desirable position if a favorable and well reasoned decision was reached during the international phase. Ultimate allowance or rejection proceeds on a country-by-country basis.

The Budapest Treaty on the International Recognition of the Deposit of Microorganisms for the Purposes of Patent Procedure

There is an inherent problem with many biotech inventions, which was eloquently, if somewhat presciently, stated by Mr Joyce Kilmer: "...But only God can make a tree." This is not a theological argument against "patenting life" but rather recognition that present-day science has its limitations. Until the better microscope is built (and patented), we simply cannot describe every atom in very complex organic structures, for example, an *E. coli* cell, and thus cannot teach how to make one. If an invention requires such a cell, the applicant cannot meet the obligation to disclose the invention in a patent specification; that is, there is no way to put the invention in the hands of the public without also giving the cell to the public. However, the cell is likely to be a valuable asset and the applicant will probably not wish to divulge it unless a patent has issued.

One solution to this problem is to make a restricted deposit of the cell in a public depository, which provides a unique accession number identifying the deposit. By agreement with the depository, the restriction is lifted in the future, for example, when a patent issues referring to the cell. The applicant can then meet the disclosure requirement by providing the deposit's accession number in the specification. This approach works best if only one country is involved but does not work as well with multiple international filings because the patent office in each country may have its own rules as to what constitutes an acceptable depository, acceptable restrictions on access to the public, and so on.

The Budapest Treaty resolves these issues by providing a list of approved depositories throughout the world and one set of deposit conditions, which include *restricted* access to a deposit by the public *prior to* patent grant. The inventor need make only one deposit under one set of rules to enable the invention and the public gets disclosure of the invention under certain restricted conditions prior to patent grant.

General Agreement on Tariffs and Trades (GATT)

GATT is one of the latest attempts at global patent harmonization, that is, amending patent laws everywhere so that they are more or less alike, mostly more. For example, as a result of GATT, many "process countries" have agreed to grant compound *per se* patents. This somewhat recent (1994) treaty has had significant impacts on US patent practice, most of which are procedural and too arcane for discussion herein.

It was GATT that brought about the change in US patent terms. As discussed above, prior to June 8, 1995, US patents lasted 17 years from grant. Now the US has adopted the worldwide standard and US patent last 20 years from first USA filing. According to US Patent Office figures the average chemical patent application is pending slightly less than two years. Therefore, the new 20-year patent has a slightly longer patent life than the old 17-year patent. However, this computation ignores the practical reality that many pharmaceutical patent applications are rarely simply just filed and then granted in two years. Rather, many initial pharmaceutical patent applications are the first of a string of related filings, the last of which may occur many years after the first. Under the new rules, patents issued from these later-filed applications all expire 20 years from first the filing date. This results in a considerably reduced patent life versus a comparable 17-year patent.

GATT did not remove one peculiarity of US patent law: interference practice (see the next section). However, it did bring about one change, concerning the place of invention. Prior to GATT, one could only prove the date of invention by reference to acts committed in the USA. Non-US inventors had long complained about the favoritism of this rule since it gave US inventors a clear advantage, for example, in deciding the earlier inventor during an interference. Under GATT, non-US acts can now be used as part of the proof of the date of invention, thus, somewhat leveling the international playing field.

Interference practice

Unlike the rest of the world, US patent practice is a "first-to-invent" rather than "first-to-file" system, the argument being that the US Constitutional basis for the patent system was to secure rights for inventors not for hasty filers. This occasionally leads to a quasi-judicial proceeding known as an interference.

An interference arises when two (or more, but this complicates matters even further) patent applications are filed in the US Patent Office at about the same time and much the same subject matter is determined by the Examiner to be allowable in each application. (In the first-to-file countries, the second application is simply rejected over the first. This ends the matter unless the second applicant can successfully argue that the Examiner has misunderstood either of the inventions, i.e., that in fact there is no overlapping subject matter, or that there is some fundamental error in the first application, e.g., that the first application does not actually teach what it appears to teach.) Usually the determination of overlapping subject matter occurs while both of the applications are still in prosecution, but it can also occur if one has already been granted and a patent has issued.

The declaration of an interference can either be the result of an internal check at the US Patent Office of pending applications or as the result of provocation by an applicant. This occurs when the applicant sees a patent issue with overlapping subject matter based on an application filed by another within certain time limits. There does not have to a complete overlap in allowable subject matter, merely some overlap. The applicant then "copies claims" from the patent for purposes of having an interference declared. Since the Examiner must first determine that the applications contain otherwise allowable subject matter, interferences take place only at the end of the prosecution stage.

The interference is referred to as quasi-judicial because, as in a trial, two opposing sides argue against each other and present evidence either in support of their own side or to contradict the other side. The US Patent Office sets up a schedule for exchanging proofs, calling witnesses, and so on. Ultimately, a decision is made by a panel of Administrative Patent Judges as to which party is the first to invent and is be to granted a patent. This decision is binding on both parties; however, it can be appealed to the civil courts.

Interference practice is defended by many as the only way to ensure that the true (read "first") inventor is granted a patent in accord with the US Constitutional intent. It is also attacked by many as a costly and time-consuming proceeding that serves no real purpose since "inventor" can just as easily be defined as the one who files first,

independently of when the invention was actually is made. Interestingly, most decisions are rendered in favor of the first applicant, and so the outcome is often the same as if the US were to convert to the first-to-file system. There is pressure from the international community for the US to adopt a first-to-file system but, for now, interferences will continue.

Biotechnology

Biotechnology (hereinafter, biotech) can loosely be defined as the science of very large and very complicated living molecules. The patent concepts that have developed over the decades to deal with a myriad of inventions covering organic compounds (i.e., "small molecules") can generally be, and have been, adapted to cover biotech inventions. However, biotech inventions have two basic types of problems: one technological, the other societal.

Technological

One of the issues on the technological side is the question of enablement. This has been discussed in part in the section dealing with The Budapest Treaty (see above). But even if the inventor tries to put the invention or a precursor of the invention in the hands of the public as by a Budapest deposit, the public may still not be able to reproduce the invention; for example, because of an inherent instability in the deposited material.

Another technological question is how fully to describe the invention. Analogously to a description of a piece of real property (i.e., land) found in a deed, the "metes and bounds" of the invention must be described in a patent application in such clear and concise terms that a potential infringer would be able to figure out what acts are infringing and which are not. In the biotech area it is often not easy to describe fully the thing that has been invented. The stick formulas used to describe classical pharmaceutical compounds are rarely of any value because a precise structure is rarely known. The physical properties of biotech inventions are often "fuzzy." A descriptive expression such as

"... having a molecular weight of 75–95 kD" may be the best the inventor can provide but it is not very precise. Each type of biotech invention presents its own technological difficulties, which must be resolved using whatever tools are available when preparing a patent application.

Societal

On the societal side there is the understandable concern about "patenting life." This is another example of the difficulties that arise when technology races ahead of society's capacity to even understand that there is a potential new problem. Although plant patents and other protections for agricultural inventions (all of which were known to be living organisms) had been granted for many years, patent offices had simultaneously refused to grant patents for inventions of living, nonplant organisms. This all began to change with the 1980 US Supreme Court decision in the Chakrabarty case, where the invention was a modified microorganism. The issue before the Court was whether an invention could be denied patent protection solely because the claimed material was alive. The Court said "no" and the biotech industry exploded onto the scene.

No one today complains about patenting microbes. However, the intensity of the debate is understandable when the inventions involve human DNA, because these are seen by some as endangering our humanity. Today, the major issues relate to patenting transgenic mammals, pieces of the human genome, and human clones. Tomorrow, the great issue of the day may be patenting cyborgs; that is, organisms comprising synthetic and human components. Undoubtedly, some of these issues will be resolved soon and some will be hotly debated for a long time; at least, until a hotter issue emerges.

The value of patents

Patents are clearly of great economic value to the patentee because they can be used to block competition, because they can be licensed-out, thus producing a revenue stream even if the patentee has no interest in actually selling the patented product, or because they can be bargaining chips in cross-licensing arrangements, just to name a few advantages. For a start-up company the mere granting of a patent can add tens of millions of dollars to the value of the enterprise, somewhat independently of what the patent actually covers. This converts into more-ready access to additional funding from venture capitalists and increased value in the price of the company's stock when a public offering is made.

Patents may be of value for only a few years in rapidly developing technological areas; that is, until the next "big thing" makes the patented technology obsolete. Patents are also arguably of lesser value than a well-recognized trademark, which does not expire in 20 years.

Pharmaceutical patents in particular have come under attack in recent years, largely due to the perceived high costs of medicines. Thus, in the US there is pressure to allow the importation of foreign-purchased drugs, even though a US patent exists that would normally be expected to bar such importation. In the EC there is no barrier to the free movement of goods within the EC. So, if a drug is not covered by a patent in a first EC country, it can be purchased there (presumably at a cheaper price) and moved to a second EC country, even though there is a patent in the second country that covers the drug. The ability of the patentee to bar these importations at the border has been eliminated.

Another diminution in the value of patents in the US is the result of the Hatch–Waxman Act. This law provides a significant economic incentive to generics companies to attack the validity of US patents. (See Chapter 32 (on Generics) for a more complete discussion on this subject.)

In the current economic climate, with its emphasis on controlling the ever-rising cost of healthcare, it is not unreasonable to believe that efforts will be made to limit the cost of pharmaceuticals and other health-related inventions. Placing limits on the monopolistic aspects of patents cannot be ruled out. One example of such measures is compulsory licensing, a practice already in effect in some other countries. Under such a scheme, the patentee would be forced to license the invention to a competitor at a "reasonable" royalty rate, as determined by an administrative body. The patentee would continue to profit from the patent, but clearly at a lower rate than if it were allowed to market the invention without the license.

Whether or not any or some cost-containing measures are in the best interest of the society is a point of contention. If one believes that the pharmaceutical companies' profits are not only unjustifiable but also put at risk the health of many in the general population who would benefit from but cannot afford the "exorbitant" cost of available treatments, then cost control is fully justifiable. However, if one believes that the best guarantee of a continuing supply of new medicines and other health-related inventions is a market where the innovator can profit from the invention and that these profits are justified by the vast monetary investments typically required to produce these and future beneficial inventions, then government attempts to restrain these profits may ultimately prove injurious.

CHAPTER 57

Outsourcing Clinical Drug Development Activities to Contract Research Organizations (CROs): Critical Success Factors

John R. Vogel

John R. Vogel Associates Inc., Kihei, HI, USA

The most dramatic change in the last four decades of clinical drug development is the trend toward extensive outsourcing to contract research organizations (CROs) and niche providers. Between 1994 and 2007, the pharmaceutical industry eliminated more than 40,000 jobs, many in R&D. The global economic downturn in 2008 has resulted in nearly doubling that number. The task of developing new products with dramatically smaller in-house staffs has led pharmaceutical companies to increase their reliance on CROs. It was previously estimated that more than 60% of all clinical studies involved significant outsourcing (Getz, 2006a, b). That number might easily reach 80% during 2010.

As pharmaceutical companies strive to increase productivity and decrease costs, they must improve their skills in dealing with CROs. This chapter examines the challenges of outsourcing clinical drug development activities and identifies critical success factors for working with CROs.

Principles and Practice of Pharmaceutical Medicine, 3rd edition.
Edited by L.D. Edwards, A.W. Fox, P.D. Stonier.
© 2011 Blackwell Publishing Ltd.

Pharmaceutical industry views of CROs

"Traditional" view of a CRO

The view that working with a CRO involves unacceptable risk was often expressed by pharmaceutical industry personnel. One project leader who had successfully developed several drugs commented: "There is significant risk in relying on CROs. I would rather use my own personnel." The characteristics of this "traditional" view of working with a CRO are shown in Table 57.1.

In-house staffing is based on long-term workload projections, which focus on the peaks rather than the valleys. The CRO is used as a back-up, when the workload exceeds projections or when staffing levels fall due to a hiring freeze. The CRO is treated as an extension of in-house staff and may be asked to relocate its personnel to the sponsor's site. In order to minimize risk, the sponsor contracts the minimum range of services and retains the critical activities for its own staff. The decision to use a CRO is delayed until all other options are exhausted. CRO evaluation and selection occurs at the eleventh hour in a "crisis" atmosphere, where time is the major concern, rather than quality or cost.

Using a CRO in such a way often leads to disappointing results. Outsourcing failures can usually be traced to one of three causes:

Table 57.1 "Traditional" view of a CRO

In-house staffing is based on expected workload

A CRO is used when in-house resources become inadequate

A crisis management atmosphere exists

The CRO is viewed as an extension of in-house staff

The scope of services is limited

Time is a major concern

Table 57.2 "Modern" view of a CRO

In-house staffing is based on "core" needs

CROs are included in resource planning

CROs are prequalified, based on therapeutic expertise, range of services, and compatibility with the sponsor

Personnel are trained in CRO skills

Quality and cost are the major concerns

- The sponsor selects the wrong CRO.
- The sponsor does not articulate its needs clearly.
- The sponsor does not manage the project.

"Modern" view of a CRO

The value of outsourcing is becoming more evident. For example, *The January/February 2006 Tufts CSDD Impact Report* (Tufts Center for the Study of Drug Development, 2006) reported that clinical trials conducted by CROs are completed up to 30% more quickly than those conducted in-house. At the same time economic and political pressures are forcing the pharmaceutical industry to redefine itself. As Elliott Sigal, president of research and development at Bristol-Myers Squibb, put it (Sigal, 2008): "We wonder whether the traditionally do-it-all, own-it-all from every part of the value chain is sustainable. It's certainly a risky and costly model."

The modern view of outsourcing distinguishes between "core" and "non-core" activities. Core activities are those that the sponsor can perform at a faster pace, lower cost, or superior quality in-house. Non-core activities are candidates for outsourcing where a CRO or niche provider can offer an advantage in timing or cost with equivalent quality. The modern drug development plan includes an analysis of which activities will be conducted in-house and which will be outsourced. A list of "prequalified" CROs is developed by matching the sponsor's anticipated needs with the range of services and therapeutic area expertise various CROs provide. The role of the sponsor's personnel is redefined from conducting the project to managing the CRO. The sponsor's staff receives training on how to work with CROs. Advance planning and training enables the sponsor to direct its attention

to ensuring the timing, cost, and quality of CRO services. The characteristics of the "modern" view of working with a CRO are shown in Table 57.2.

The role of CROs in drug development

Surveys of pharmaceutical industry use of CROs (Vogel, 1993; Getz and Vogel, 1995; Vogel and Getz, 2005; Getz and Vogel, 2009), and the balance sheets of publically-quoted CRO corporations, provide ample evidence that outsourcing is expanding. Since 2001, outsourcing has grown at a faster rate (13.4 versus 9.1%) than R&D spending (Muken and Cherny, 2009). The disparity in growth rates is evidence that sponsors are shifting activities away from in-house staff toward external providers.

As sponsors become more experienced using CROs they are modifying the mix of services used. In 1992, sponsors were most likely to contract out site recruitment and study monitoring, whereas other activities were conducted in-house. By 1994, sponsors reported large increases in the use of CROs for data management, statistical analysis, and medical writing. Results of a recent sponsor survey (Getz and Vogel, 2009) show a decline in reported use of CROs for study monitoring, data collection, and patient recruitment. This may be due to the emergence of niche providers offering these services in competition with CROs.

Deciding when to use a CRO

Strategies for using CROs typically fall into three categories:
- transactional outsourcing;
- functional outsourcing;
- outsourcing alliances.

Transactional outsourcing

These are essentially "one-off" relationships in which the sponsor outsources a single task or a single project with little or no expectation of using that CRO or outsourcing those activities in the future. This often occurs with the "traditional" view of outsourcing. A sponsor maintains in-house staff levels capable of performing the projected work-load. Individual studies or selected activities within a study are contracted to a CRO only when in-house resources become inadequate because of an unforeseen study or a reduction in staff.

Claimed advantages to transactional outsourcing are that the sponsor can exert maximum control over the project. Risk may be limited by outsourcing a minimum scope of services (e.g., study monitoring but not data management and analysis). Many sponsors believe it is less costly to use in-house resources, although Hill (1994) suggests that the costs of contracting out are roughly equivalent. A further advantage is that the sponsor maintains in-house drug development expertise.

However, transactional outsourcing has significant disadvantages that result from the absence of a long-range outsourcing strategy. It is likely that a fully staffed in-house organization will exceed needs from time to time or that development of a poorly performing drug may be terminated. Both instances may lead to layoffs, severance payments, and relocation costs. A project in a new therapeutic area may require the addition of new personnel with knowledge and experience in that area. Staffing up for large Phase III studies, which typically involve thousands of patients, is expensive and time-consuming. Minimizing the work contracted to CROs provides little opportunity for the sponsor's staff to acquire the necessary skills to work with CROs when they are needed. If the sponsor delays the decision to use a CRO until the last minute, finding and contracting with the CRO may delay the study and the New Drug Application (NDA) or Marketing Authorization Application (MAA). The pressure to select a CRO provides inadequate opportunity to define the sponsor's needs and select the right CRO.

Functional outsourcing

With this strategy, the sponsor outsources nearly all the company's work in a specific functional area (e.g., data management or study monitoring) to a single provider.

This strategy has the advantage of minimizing start-up activities. As each new project arises, the existing "functional provider" assumes responsibility for the target activity. This eliminates the need for evaluating, selecting, and contracting with a provider for each new project. The sponsor and provider also enjoy the efficiency that results from being familiar with each other's practices and corporate culture. However, there are disadvantages to functional outsourcing. The sponsor is essentially putting "all its eggs in one basket." A problem within the functional provider (e.g., financial instability) or between the sponsor and provider could affect a wide range of projects. The sponsor is also betting that the provider can accommodate future growth in the need for services in the designated functional area. The existence of a functional agreement in one area may impact outsourcing opportunities in other areas. For example, eliminating a potentially lucrative service may make the rest of the project less attractive to a full-service CRO. And finally, the sponsor must manage interactions between the functional provider and CROs involved in the projects and ensure seamless integration of data between the two.

Outsourcing alliances

The sponsor and its CRO partner define a range of services that the sponsor has committed to assign to the CRO for a full-scale project or several projects in a portfolio. The emphasis is on a long-term commitment.

This strategy eliminates the need to contract each new phase of a project. It is assumed that the sponsor and CRO will become progressively more efficient in working together. In return for guaranteed business the CRO may be willing to discount its rates. The sponsor may offer incentives for work completed ahead of schedule. The creation of a sponsor-CRO alliance requires a great deal of groundwork. The sponsor must carefully evaluate the ability of the CRO to accommodate its needs across a range of studies and, perhaps, multiple therapeutic indications. The CRO must assess the sponsor's pipeline and determine the risk of candidates failing to meet go-no-go criteria resulting in project cancellations.

Current sponsor practices

A survey of nearly 400 pharmaceutical company respondents (Getz and Vogel, 2009) revealed a mix of outsourcing relationships. The functional outsourcing model may be gaining in popularity (45% of respondents reported using it) while transactional outsourcing appears to have declined (35%). Of respondents, 20% said that they had formed outsourcing alliances with CROs.

Frequent causes of sponsor/CRO problems

People working in pharmaceutical companies are often unprepared for their new role of working with a CRO. Pharmaceutical drug development staff consist of highly skilled technical people, for example, physicians, clinical research associates (CRAs), data managers, statisticians, and medical writers, who joined the industry to use their skills. Those jobs are increasingly located in the CRO industry. The new job—managing other people who are performing these tasks—is one for which few, if any, people have been formally trained.

Problems with contracted studies can often be traced to one of three causes:

• *The wrong CRO is selected.* Sponsors often make the mistake of assuming that a CRO that has performed well on one study will be equally capable of conducting a study in a different therapeutic area. Some sponsors mistakenly assume that all CROs are the same, and that it is not possible to determine which one will be most capable of performing a specific planned study.

• *The sponsor fails to articulate its needs clearly.* Sponsors sometimes issue a request for proposal (RFP) with little more than a protocol outline, and expect CROs to guess what services and resources are required. The result of inadequate information is that CROs underestimate the sponsor's needs, assigning insufficient numbers of personnel, or inadequately trained staff to the study. This can result in errors, delays, and cost overruns.

• *The sponsor fails to manage the study.* Sponsors sometimes make the mistake of assuming that in-house resources are not needed once the study is outsourced. In most cases, the sponsor should continue to play a critical role in a contracted study, providing guidance to the CRO and ensuring that agreed standards and timelines are achieved. There is no such thing as a "turn-key" project managed by a CRO.

Three critical steps to ensure success with a CRO

In order to ensure successful outsourcing, the sponsor should focus on three critical steps:

1. Determine accurate study specifications.
2. Select the right CRO.
3. Manage the study.

The remainder of this chapter outlines the benefits of these steps and describes specific activities that sponsors should carry out to ensure successful outsourcing.

Determine study specifications

Study specifications are a list of activities required to initiate, conduct, analyze, and report the results of a clinical study. They include tasks that will be performed in-house and those to be contracted out to one or more CROs (Vogel and Nelson, 1993).

Importance of accurate study specifications

Accurate study specifications are a critical tool for planning a study. They assign responsibility to the various disciplines involved in the study (e.g., clinical research, regulatory affairs, data management, clinical manufacturing, programming, statistics, and medical writing). By comparing study specifications with internal capabilities, the sponsor can identify activities that must be contracted out.

This analysis also provides useful criteria for selecting the right type of CRO: a niche provider or full service CRO.

Study specifications also enable the sponsor to make more accurate projections of study costs and timing. Study specifications are an essential element of the sponsor's RFP and the CRO's proposal. Study specifications should be included in the RFP in order to familiarize CROs with the sponsor's project and goals. Study specifications enable the CRO to break down the individual tasks and materials on which it is asked to quote cost and timing, and provides a useful format for the budget proposal. Accurate study specifications enable the CRO to perform a "reality check" on the sponsor's expectations. Often, CROs add items to the study specifications (e.g., activities or materials to be provided by the sponsor or other CRO services) that the sponsor may have overlooked. Moreover, CROs can and do decline to submit a proposal because they believe the sponsor's study specifications describe an unachievable study plan (especially with small companies).

The study specifications also enable the sponsor to conduct a "reality check" on the CRO's understanding of the study and to determine that the proposal covers the project scope. Study specifications facilitate comparison of proposals from different CROs and help ensure that the sponsor's attention is focused on the resources the CRO will provide, as well as on the proposed budget.

Study specifications are also an important tool for managing the study. They help define the various in-house disciplines that will be interacting with the CRO and to project the level of sponsor involvement required. They help focus the sponsor's attention on the deliverables and provide milestones and timelines to assist the sponsor in measuring study progress. Accurate study specifications promote a thorough evaluation of the CRO's performance during, and on completion of, the study.

The study specifications worksheet

An example of a *study specifications worksheet* is shown in Figure 57.1. The first page of the worksheet, entitled Study Details, is designed to provide an overview of the study and includes information on key parameters, such as the number of patients, number of visits, expected enrollment rate, and number of sites. It also includes information on the healthcare setting (e.g., academic medical center, private practice, or managed care) and the regulatory status of the product. The Materials and Actions section of the worksheet is divided into 21 categories, chosen after consultation with several CROs and designed to be consistent with activities on which CROs base their bids.

In order to facilitate the process, sponsors should use the suggested categories. Within each category are several specific activities listed as examples. The sponsor may list as many specific activities as appropriate for the study. For each activity, the sponsor should indicate whether that activity will be the sponsor's responsibility or the CRO's responsibility by placing a check in the appropriate column. In those cases where the sponsor feels that the activity will be shared with the CRO, sponsors should examine the activity to determine whether it could be broken down into more discrete items. This will minimize confusion over who actually is responsible for the activity. The last section of the study specifications worksheet is entitled Project Timeline. It contains the sponsor's projected dates for completion of study milestones. Dauntingly, 26 suggested milestones are listed; the sponsor may wish to modify the list according to its own milestones. However, attention to these milestones at the beginning of a study will pay ample dividends later.

Preparing study specifications

Study specifications are typically prepared by the sponsor's project team or the project leader. Small companies may hire a drug development consultant or CRO to help prepare study specifications. Ideally, preparation of study specifications should begin four to six months before the study begins. Details of all activities may not be available at this point, but sufficient lead time must be given for identifying the necessary services, evaluating in-house capability, and selecting a CRO. Details can be added as they are identified.

STUDY SPECIFICATIONS WORKSHEET

Study details

1. Project leader:

2. Product name:

3. Dose form:

4. Indication

5. Study objective:

6. Study design:

7. Total number of patients:

8. Age range:

9. Sex:

10. Number of visits (run-in phase):

11. Number of visits (treatment phase):

12. Number of visits (follow-up phase):

13. Expected enrollment rate:

14. Number of study sites:

15. Minimum number of patients/site:

16. Healthcare setting:

_____ Academic

_____ Managed care

_____ Private practice

_____ Other (specify)

17. Regulatory status:

_____ New IND

_____ Phase II

_____ Phase III

_____ Phase IIIb

_____ Phase IV

_____ Other (specify):

Figure 57.1 Study specifications worksheet (reproduced with permission from Vogel and Nelson, 1993).

STUDY SPECIFICATIONS WORKSHEET

Materials and actions		
Activity	Sponsor's responsibility	CRO's responsibility
1. IND reporting		
A. Prepare IND updates		
B. Submit IND updates to regulatory agencies		
2. Protocol preparation		
A. Design study		
B. Write protocol		
C. Draft informed consent		
3. Case report form preparation		
A. Design case report forms		
B. Print case report forms		
4. Pre-study preparation		
A. Propose study sites		
B. Provide site evaluation reports		
C. Select investigators		
D. Provide central IRB		
E. Negotiate site budgets		
5. Investigator meeting		
A. Plan investigator meeting		
B. Conduct investigator meeting		
6. Study initiation		
A. Validate pre-study documents		
B. Set up investigator files		
C. Conduct initiation visit at each site		

Figure 57.1 (*Continued*)

STUDY SPECIFICATIONS WORKSHEET

Materials and actions

Activity	Sponsor's responsibility	CRO's responsibility
7. Site monitoring		
A. Conduct monitoring visits (at intervals of __ weeks)		
B. Maintain telephone contacts with study sites (at intervals of __ weeks)		
C. Provide written monitoring reports to sponsor (at intervals of __ weeks)		
D. Communicate with sponsor via electronic mail		
8. Site closeout		
A. Perform drug accountability audit		
B. Dispose of unused clinical supplies		
C. Provide closeout report		
9. Regulatory auditing		
A. Audit study sites		
B. Provide audit report		
10. Serious adverse event (SAE) reporting		
Submit SAE reports to sponsor		
11. Site management		
A. Negotiate investigator grants/contracts		
B. Manage investigator payments		
C. Provide project status reports to sponsor at intervals of __ weeks)		
12. Project management		
A. Conduct project management meetings		
B. Provide minutes of meetings		
C. Provide project status reports		
D. Provide data management reports		
13. Database design and validation		
A. Design database		
B. Set up data-entry program		
C. Create database		

Figure 57.1 (*Continued*)

STUDY SPECIFICATIONS WORKSHEET

Materials and actions

Activity	Sponsor's responsibility	CRO's responsibility
14. Data cleanup		
A. Write data management guidelines and edit specifications		
B. Run edit checks		
C. Clean up case report forms		
D. Perform Q.C. on __ % of CRFs		
15. Data entry		
A. Enter CRFs		
B. Code adverse events and concomitant medications		
16. Generation and review of tables		
A. Prepare tables and listings		
B. Perform Q.C. on __ % of tables		
17. Statistical plan and analysis		
A. Generate statistical plan		
B. Prepare shell tables and listings		
C. Perform analysis		
D. Write statistical methods		
18. Integrated clinical and statistical report		
A. Prepare integrated tables		
B. Write statistical methods		
C. Provide discussion of the significance of results		
19. Manuscript preparation		
A. Prepare draft manuscript		
B. Prepare up to __ revisions		
C. Prepare abstract		
20. Drug packaging and distribution		
A. Formulate and package drugs		
B. Create randomization schedule		

Figure 57.1 (*Continued*)

STUDY SPECIFICATIONS WORKSHEET

Materials and actions			
	Activity	Sponsor's responsibility	CRO's responsibility
21.	Regulatory submissions		
	A. Prepare NDA/PLA		
	B. Prepare SNDA		
	C. Prepare CANDA/CAPLA		
	D. Prepare IND/NDA annual report		
	E. Prepare 120-day safety updates		

Figure 57.1 (*Continued*)

Selecting the right CRO

The three Cs of CRO selection

The three most important criteria for selecting a CRO are as follows:

1. capability
2. compatibility
3. cost.

The most important criterion is *capability*. Can the CRO provide the needed services? Are the CRO's personnel well qualified, and do they have experience in the therapeutic area? If the CRO is not capable of performing the study, it is likely to fail to meet the sponsor's expectations. A disastrous outcome could delay product development, have a negative impact on the sponsor's economic well-being, and harm the careers of sponsor staff.

The second most important criterion is *compatibility*. Are the CRO's procedures and practices compatible with the sponsor's? Is the chemistry between the CRO and sponsor good? The sponsor should examine the CRO's standard operating procedures (SOPs) and talk with CRO staff to determine not only whether the CRO is meeting the requirements of good clinical practices (GLP), but also whether its practices closely parallel the sponsor's. CROs sometimes claim they can work "according to the sponsor's SOPs," but the results are likely to be disappointing if the two companies have vastly different approaches or use incompatible technologies.

The third important factor is *cost*. Equally important are the business terms. The sponsor must ensure that the CRO's price and terms of agreement are acceptable. Sponsors are sceptical of low bids because they may result from the CRO underestimating the resources required to complete the project. High bids, however, may indicate that the CRO overvalues its services. Demands for large advance payment and imposition of severe penalties for cancellation should not be accepted.

Prequalifying CROs

Selecting a CRO requires effort by all sponsor disciplines involved in the study. Evaluating a large number of CROs is costly, time consuming, and in the short-term, unproductive. A more practical approach is to prequalify CROs to identify the most appropriate candidates for in-depth evaluation. This approach has several advantages. Not all CROs can perform the same range of services. Different CROs are experienced in particular therapeutic areas. Some CROs have more recent experience in conducting studies similar to that planned by the sponsor, or staff with special expertise. Promotional material received from CROs is often

STUDY SPECIFICATIONS WORKSHEET		
Project timeline		
	Milestone	Date
1.	Sign contract	
2.	Submit list of proposed study sites	
3.	Submit draft protocol	
4.	Enroll investigators	
5.	Protocol approval	
6.	Case report forms/MOPs approval	
7.	Hold multi-investigator meeting	
8.	Complete IRB approvals	
9.	Ship drugs/CRFs	
10.	First patient enrolled	
11.	Data management guidelines approved	
12.	25% of valid patients completed	
13.	50% of valid patients completed	
14.	75% of valid patients completed	
15.	Last valid patient completed	
16.	Submission of first CRF to data management	
17.	Submission of last CRF to data management	
18.	Lock database	
19.	Transfer database to sponsor	
20.	Analysis plan and shell tables/listings	
21.	Draft statistical tables and listings available	
22.	Final statistical tables and listings available	
23.	Draft integrated study report	
24.	Final study report	
25.	NDA/PLA; SNDA; CANDA/CAPLA	
26.	Publication	
27.	Other (specify):	

Figure 57.1 (*Continued*)

not very informative. Most CRO brochures look similar, make similar claims, and do not enable the sponsor to differentiate among the large number of candidates. It is important for a sponsor to distinguish between "can do" and "have done." CROs are prone to claim they "can do" whatever the sponsor wants. The sponsor should focus on what the CRO "has done" and make its own predictions about what the CRO can do.

The automobile industry sets out an interesting model for the pharmaceutical industry to consider. Automobile manufacturers are essentially becoming design houses. The automobile industry has become highly adept at prequalifying suppliers of major components, while no longer putting out to bid each component for each assembly. Rather, they create specifications for major components, such as transmissions or braking systems, and then turn to a small group of prequalified "first-tier" suppliers to design, build, and supply those components. Those on the cutting edge of drug development are moving in an analogous direction in their relationships with CROs.

The request for information (RFI)

This approach was first described by Vogel and Resnick in 1996:

1. From an in-house database, one of the various commercial directories of CROs, or a consultant's database, the sponsor should select those CROs that offer the desired range of services and claim to have experience in the target therapeutic area.

2. The sponsor should contact each CRO and request the details of experience in the target therapeutic area. The CRO's response should describe specific studies completed. For each study, the CRO should provide information on the range of services provided, the number of study sites, project enrolment, actual number of patients completed, and the number of months required to complete the study. The CRO should also describe the expertise of personnel who are likely to be involved in the project.

3. The sponsor should review the responses from the CROs and select several of the most qualified ones for on-site visits.

Leveraging CRO experience

There are several advantages to prequalifying CROs and placing emphasis on the CRO's expertise in the target therapeutic area. A CRO with such expertise may be able to provide valuable input to the study plan and should have a ready list of qualified investigators, which can save the sponsor's time. The CRO will be able to make more accurate predictions of patient enrollment if those estimates are based on recent experience rather than optimistic projections from study sites. In addition, experienced CRO staff will likely be more efficient at study monitoring, problem solving, data clean-up, and report writing.

It may be possible to leverage the skills of a number of different CROs with competencies in specific areas to create a "virtual" drug development process. Ideally, highly specialized, narrowly focused companies provide their services along the value chain of drug development, leaving the sponsor's role as one of initial discovery of the chemical entity, and then management of the drug development process and the value chain. Today, most sponsors contract with full-service CROs and closely manage the project, but some are exploring the advantages of using multiple "niche providers" as a "virtual" CRO (Lightfoot and Vogel, 1996).

Requesting and evaluating proposals from CROs

After conducting on-site visits to prequalified CROs, a sponsor should select three to five CROs who will be invited to submit a proposal.

Contents of the RFP

The RFP consists of a cover letter, detailed instructions to proposers, a copy of the study protocol, the completed study specifications worksheet, a resource allocations worksheet, and a copy of the sponsor's standard CRO agreement. The cover letter should briefly describe the study goal, provide an overview of the clinical plan, specify the proposal due date, indicate that the CRO may be invited to present its proposal orally to the sponsor, and specify the timing for the sponsor's reply. The

Table 57.3 Instructions to bidders

General requirements:
Confidentiality
Discrepancies and omissions
Preparation costs
Form of proposal
Modification and withdrawal
Contract award
Return of documents
Subcontracting
CRO's qualifications:
Capabilities
Experience
Key personnel
Study plan
Investigator recruitment plan
Availability of patients
Project management
Communication with sponsor
Business terms
Insurance
CRO's services and fees:
Activities to be performed by the sponsor
Services to be provided by the bidder
Resource allocations
Service fees
Estimated pass-through costs

CRO should be given approximately two weeks to prepare a proposal, and the sponsor should expect to reply to the proposals within two weeks.

Instructions to bidders

Subjects to be covered in the instructions to bidders are listed in Table 57.3. Under the general requirements section, the sponsor should specify the following:

1. *Confidentiality:* The CRO must treat all information in the RFP as confidential.

2. *Discrepancies and omissions:* The CRO is responsible for bringing these to the sponsor's attention.

3. *Preparation costs:* The CRO bears the cost of preparing and submitting the proposal.

4. *Form of proposal:* The proposal must be in the format prescribed by the sponsor and must address all areas of the RFP.

5. *Modification and withdrawal:* The responder may modify or withdraw the proposal if the sponsor receives notice prior to the proposal due date.

6. *Contract award:* The sponsor has the right to select the successful proposal or not to award the contract.

7. *Return of documents:* The CRO must return the RFP if requested.

8. *Subcontracting:* The CRO may not subcontract services without the sponsor's permission.

The sponsor has the right to evaluate and approve the subcontractor. In the section on CRO qualifications, the sponsor should ask the CRO to address the following aspects:

9. *Capabilities:* Provide a brief description of the services offered and how they relate to the activities requested.

10. *Experience:* Summarize experience in the therapeutic area, including the number of prior studies conducted by personnel who are still on staff (for each study, include number of study sites, number of subjects, study duration, and range of services), and cite the relevant experience gained by staff while in previous academic, industry, or external positions.

11. *Key personnel:* Briefly describe the training and experience required for key positions that will be involved in the present study (e.g., project manager, medical director, CRA, data administration manager, database administrator, programmer, statistician, medical writer, and regulatory affairs manager) and provide résumés (CVs) of typical personnel in these positions.

12. *Study plan:* An overview of the study design and plan for implementation.

13. *Investigator recruitment plan:* How qualified investigators will be identified (e.g., database, previous study), and evaluate their appropriateness for the study.

14. *Availability of subjects:* How subjects will be recruited (e.g., subject database, advertising), and predict the enrolment rate.

15. *Project management:* An overview of the plan to coordinate sites and manage study initiation, execution, data cleanup, analysis, report preparation, and regulatory services.

16. *Communication with sponsor:* The frequency and formats for periodic progress/status reports, ability to establish specific electronic links with the sponsor (e.g., email, secure website), and meetings with the sponsor.

17. *Payment terms:* Terms and milestones for sponsor payments.

18. *Insurance:* A copy of insurance certificates for clinical trials insurance and forms of mutual indemnity.

The section on CRO services and fees should instruct the CRO to describe the following:

19. *Activities to be performed by the sponsor:* This is a list of the materials and activities the CRO expects the sponsor to provide.

20. *Services to be provided by the CRO:* This is a list of the materials and services the CRO will provide.

21. *Resource allocations:* This is a list of the types of personnel to be involved in the study, the estimated number of hours/FTEs for each skill level, and the fee charged for each skill level (see the resource allocations worksheet described in the following section.

22. *Service fees:* Identification of the cost for each category of service listed in the study specifications.

23. *Estimated pass-through costs:* Estimates for costs that will not be subjected to mark-up (e.g., travel, central laboratory, central IRB, investigator grants).

The resource allocations worksheet

The principal criterion for selecting a CRO, *capability*, is determined largely by what skill levels and amount of effort (hours/FTEs) the CRO proposes to use to conduct the study. Cost, which is another important selection criterion, is determined by the rates charged for each skill level. CROs should be required to summarize these data in a *resource allocations worksheet* (see Figure 57.2; Vogel and Resnick, 1996).

The worksheet lists the same 21 service categories addressed by the sponsor in the study specifications worksheet. For each category, the bidder should list the types of personnel who will be involved in performing that service. For each type of personnel, the CRO should define the number of hours/FTEs, the rate charged per unit of time and the total cost for that person to perform that service.

Figure 57.3 shows two examples of resource allocations for protocol preparation. On the bottom, the CRO proposes a team, consisting of a project physician, project manager, statistician, CRA, medical writer, and secretary, with a total cost of US$39,120. The top shows another proposal for the same activity, where the task of writing the protocol is assigned to a physician, who will be billed at US$200/h, with a total cost of US$52,000.

The resource allocations enable the sponsor to make a more critical evaluation of a proposal than if the cost of each service was simply listed. In both these examples, the cost of writing a protocol is about US$52,000. However, most sponsors would agree that the "team approach" is highly preferable to assigning the task to an individual physician. Without the resource allocations data, the sponsor would not have been able to differentiate between the two proposals.

The sponsor should circulate the proposals to staff who represent the disciplines for which the CRO will be expected to provide services. Each staff member should review the proposals and prepare written evaluations. A convenient way to compare several proposals is to use an evaluation form, such as that proposed by Vogel and Schober (1993), seen here as Figure 57.4.

After evaluating the proposals, the sponsor may decide to invite two or three CROs for a face-to-face meeting or a conference call, to provide an opportunity for each to present its proposal and answer questions (Vogel and Resnick, 1996).

Managing the sponsor–CRO relationship

Defining accurate study specifications and selecting the right CRO are critical to achieving success in an outsourced study. However, careful attention must also be paid to managing the study and the sponsor–CRO relationship. The sponsor may mistakenly assume that, once the study is contracted, its staff can be fully allocated to other projects. In fact, a significant in-house effort is needed to manage the project. Most sponsors report that managing an outsourced project requires at least

RESOURCE ALLOCATIONS WORKSHEET - (Part A)

ACTIVITY	PERSONNEL	EFFORT	RATE	TOTAL	ASSUMPTIONS
1. IND reporting					
2. Protocol preparation					
3. Case report form preparation					
4. Pre-study preparation					
5. Investigator meeting					
6. Study initiation					
7. Site monitoring					
8. Site closeout					
9. Regulatory auditing					
10. Serious adverse event (SAE) reporting					
11. Site management					
12. Project management					

Figure 57.2 Resource allocations worksheet (reproduced with permission from Vogel and Resnick, 1996).

RESOURCE ALLOCATIONS WORKSHEET - (Part B)

ACTIVITY	PERSONNEL	EFFORT	RATE	TOTAL	ASSUMPTIONS
13. Database design and validation					
14. Data cleanup					
15. Data entry					
16. Generation and review of tables					
17. Statistical plan and analysis					
18. Integrated clinical and statistical report					
19. Manuscript preparation					
20. Drug packaging and distribution					
21. Regulatory submissions					

Figure 57.2 (*Continued*)

RESOURCE ALLOCATIONS EXAMPLES

ACTIVITY	PERSONNEL	EFFORT	RATE	TOTAL	ASSUMPTIONS
EXAMPLE A Protocol preparation	Project physician	260	150	39 000	Total = $39 000
EXAMPLE B Protocol preparation	Project physician	80	150	12 000	
	Project manager	24	80	1920	
	Statistician	48	100	4800	
	CRA	120	80	9600	
	Medical writer	160	50	8000	
	Secretary	80	35	2800	Total = $39 120

Figure 57.3 Resource allocations examples (reproduced with permission from Vogel and Resnick, 1996).

CONTRACT RESEARCH ORGANIZATION BID EVALUATION FORM

Selection parameter	CROs (Score 1–5)			
	CRO A	CRO B	CRO C	CRO D
1. *Bidder's qualifications*—is it likely that the bidder will be able to provide the services required by the study?				
2. *Experience*—does the bidder have adequate experience in the therapeutic area?				
3. *Key personnel*—do the personnel in key positions have adequate training and experience for these positions?				
4. *Study plan*—do the bidder's overview of the study design and plan for its implementation accurately reflect the sponsor's needs?				
5. *Investigator recruitment plan*—has the bidder presented a convincing plan (e.g. investigator database, list from recent study) for recruiting qualified investigators?				
6. *Availability of patients*—does the bidder have a reasonable strategy (e.g. patient database, advertising) for recruiting patients and is the projected enrollment rate realistic?				
7. *Project management*—Has the bidder described an appropriate plan for coordinating sites and managing the study?				
8. *Communication with the sponsor*—are the proposed frequency and formats of written and telephone reports acceptable?				
9. *Activities to be performed by the sponsor*—is the list of the sponsor's obligations accurate?				
10. *Services to be provided by the bidder*—does the list of materials and services to be provided by the bidder agree with the sponsor's study specifications?				
11. *Resource allocations*—for each activity to be performed by the CRO, are the types of personnel appropriate and are the estimated workloads (FTEs) realistic?				
12. *Costs*—are the estimated costs reasonable?				
TOTAL SCORE:				

Figure 57.4 Contract research organization bid evaluation form (reproduced with permission from Vogel and Schober, 1993).

20% of the resources that would have been needed to conduct the same project in-house. The sponsor should follow three principles for managing an outsourced project:

- Clarify the roles and responsibilities of the sponsor and CRO.
- Define and use "performance metrics" to measure study progress.
- Ensure efficient communication between the sponsor and CRO.

Sponsor roles and responsibilities

It is the sponsor's responsibility to design the study, determine which materials and actions it provides, and define the services it requires from the CRO. Accurate study specifications communicate this to CROs. The sponsor must also ensure that the CRO understands and agrees to its expectations. Evaluation of proposals by a multidisciplinary sponsor team, with special attention paid to proposed resource allocations, helps the sponsor verify that CROs understand its needs and provide a reasonable plan to meet them.

The study specifications and the contract with a selected CRO identify key study milestones and timelines. These help ensure that the study is completed on schedule. However, in practice, the intervals between milestones are too long to enable the sponsor and CRO to make mid-course corrections and keep the study on target. The sponsor needs to monitor CRO accomplishments using objective outcome measures (see discussion in the "Performance metrics" section, below). The sponsor must recognize red flags that signal the need for corrective action. If requested by the CRO, the sponsor should assist in resolving problems by providing needed information and, if appropriate, making amendments to the study protocol. Such assistance should be provided in timely fashion and involve the appropriate level of authority at the sponsor.

Despite the sponsor and CRO's best efforts to predict all aspects of the study, there often arise occasions on which the study requires CRO services that exceed expectations. In these cases, the sponsor must be prepared to negotiate a "change order agreement" to cover the expenses of additional CRO services. In certain cases, the sponsor may

Table 57.4 Roles and responsibilities of the sponsor

Define the study specifications
Provide information to the CRO
Monitor results
Recognize "red flags"
Resolve problems
Approve changes in "scope"

approve a change order that amends the study timeline. Sponsor roles and responsibilities are summarized in Table 57.4.

CRO roles and responsibilities

The CRO should evaluate the feasibility of the sponsor's study plan. If the sponsor has provided detailed study specifications and the CRO is experienced in the target therapeutic area, it will be possible for the CRO to compare its past experiences with the sponsor's projections and to identify any inconsistencies. If the CRO believes it cannot achieve the sponsor's expectation (e.g., enrol three patients/month at each site in an arrhythmia study), it is important to bring it to the sponsor's attention and negotiate a more realistic goal.

The CRO has a responsibility to staff the study with adequate numbers of competent, well managed personnel. This can present a challenge, especially in areas prone to high turnover, such as CRAs. The CRO must have an adequate training and evaluation program to ensure staff performance and must not promote inexperienced personnel to critical positions, such as project manager. It is the CRO's responsibility to conduct the study activities as prescribed in the study specifications and the sponsor–CRO agreement.

Despite the CRO's best efforts, problems will arise. Too often a CRO tries to solve a problem without bringing it to the sponsor's attention. Valuable time may be lost if the sponsor, which could have provided useful information to the CRO, is not consulted. When a problem cannot be readily resolved, the CRO should bring it to the sponsor's attention and present proposed solutions. The CRO should also ensure that proposed solutions are practical and cost-effective. The CRO's experience

Table 57.5 Roles and responsibilities of the CRO

Evaluate feasibility

Provide adequate, competent, well-managed staff

Conduct study activities

Manage processes

Bring problems and proposed solutions to the sponsor's attention

Ensure that solutions are cost-effective

with similar studies may be an asset in solving the problem. CRO roles and responsibilities are summarized in Table 57.5.

Performance metrics

Identification and communication of problems requires that the two parties agree on what constitutes a true problem. Often a sponsor identifies what it believes to be a significant variance, yet the CRO fails to respond because experience tells it that the variance will not have an impact on the end result. The result of this miscommunication is that the sponsor loses trust in the CRO, and the relationship is harmed. Performance metrics allow the sponsor and CRO to measure the same thing.

Performance metrics are systematic and objective measures of CRO and sponsor performance. Their validity is established by demonstrating that they are related to achieving quality, ensuring timeliness and managing cost. Performance metrics should be negotiated between the sponsor and CRO prior to the study.

They can be established for the qualifications of CRO personnel (e.g., a senior CRA must have at least two years of clinical research experience); timing and content of reports (e.g., the CRA's monitoring report must follow the format of the example given, and a copy of the report must be received by the sponsor within two weeks of the monitoring visit); patient enrolment (e.g., each site must enroll a minimum of ten patients/month for the first four months of the study); cycle times (e.g., questions on case report form content, "queries," must be generated within one week of receipt of the data by the CRO); database accuracy (e.g., the error

rate as determined by comparing actual case report forms with the CRO database must be no more than 0.01); billing practices (e.g., the CRO will invoice the sponsor for the exact amount paid to investigators without a mark-up); and compliance audits (e.g., the CRO must have written, detailed, SOPs, for various activities and must be able to demonstrate that its staff routinely complies with the SOPs).

Performance metrics enable the sponsor to focus on the outcome (managing the CRO) rather than the process (micromanaging the CRO). Micromanaging the CRO by analyzing and monitoring its internal processes is disruptive and conveys a message of mistrust. Performance metrics help distinguish between the sponsor's role, to verify that the CRO is achieving the agreed-upon standards and timelines, and the CRO's role, to select the most appropriate processes to achieve these objectives. When performance metrics demonstrate that the CRO is failing to meet the objective, the sponsor and CRO have a shared responsibility to examine the process and agree on an appropriate solution. After corrective actions have been taken, the performance metrics help demonstrate that the desired effect has been achieved.

The sponsor–CRO communication/ decision-making model

The CRO's team members are expected to carry out the study activities, whereas the sponsor's team functions as a resource to the CRO. Most interactions between the sponsor and the CRO will take place between the individual team members and their technical counterparts. Discussions between sponsor and CRO technical staff should focus on information exchange and issue identification. Team members should inform their respective project managers of all communications between sponsor and CRO personnel. The benefit of informing the project manager of all issues is that the project manager can compare input from different team members, relay information to other team members as necessary, and detect issues that may not yet be apparent to the team.

Project managers are responsible for ensuring that their respective teams perform as expected.

This may require them to negotiate with functional department heads to acquire needed resources, or to resolve a performance problem. Like any other human interaction, when a problem arises between the sponsor and CRO, project managers with a good relationship are most likely to negotiate a mutually acceptable solution and document the same in a change order, when appropriate. Technical team members should not independently negotiate changes with their counterparts.

Sponsor–CRO study initiation meeting

The sponsor and CRO teams should hold a "kick-off" meeting prior to initiation of the study. The goals of the meeting are listed as follows:

1. To promote camaraderie and ownership of the study among team members.

2. To clarify the roles and responsibilities of the sponsor and CRO.

3. To identify the primary sponsor and CRO contacts.

4. To present the agreed performance metrics and audit procedures.

5. To define the approach to problem resolution.

6. To define those changes that can be agreed upon informally and those that require a formal change order.

The meeting should begin with introductions of team members and their respective project managers. It is recommended that both sponsor and CRO senior managers make brief presentations, underscoring the importance of the study and reinforcing that the project managers have "bottom line" responsibility. Additional activities include a review of the performance metrics, explanation of the responsibilities of the sponsor and CRO project managers, review of the responsibilities of the sponsor and CRO teams, description of the communication/decision-making process, and discussion of problem-solving procedures.

The meeting should include exercises designed to teach team members how to recognize behaviors that enhance and impair sponsor–CRO relationships. Participants should also engage in role-playing designed to teach efficient problem-solving techniques. In order to be most effective, the role-plays should be based on scenarios that are likely to occur in the planned study. Down-time (e.g.,

pre-meeting dinner and socialization in the hotel bar) can be invaluable in the long run.

Sponsor–CRO periodic oversight meetings

The sponsor and CRO should meet formally at an agreed frequency, and certainly not less than once every three months. The attendees should include the project managers and their respective team members, as determined by the status of the study and the topics to be discussed. The goals of periodic oversight meetings are listed as follows:

1. To review the status of the study milestones and timelines.

2. To review the budget in terms of cost-to-date, change orders executed, and the latest projection for total cost.

3. To identify ways in which the sponsor and CRO have each significantly advanced the study.

4. To identify opportunities for improvement.

Lessons learned exercises

Maintaining an efficient outsourcing relationship requires ongoing and accurate assessments of sponsor and CRO performance. The "lessons learned" exercise as described by Blankstein (2004) is a nonconfrontational approach to measuring and improving sponsor–CRO team performance. Lessons learned can be conducted at major milestones throughout the project. The objective is to collect, share, and evaluate information on how well the sponsor and CRO teams are performing a variety of critical tasks.

Quantitative and narrative questions are circulated to sponsor and team members (see Tables 57.6 and 57.7) and the results are collected without attribution. A popular approach is to use a secure website to circulate questionnaires and collect data. The combined sponsor–CRO team meets to review the lessons learned results, celebrate strengths, and discuss ways of improving on weaknesses. It is beneficial to have a "facilitator" (who is not a team member) present the results and lead the discussion. This helps to ensure balanced participation by the sponsor and CRO and maintains a focus on positive actions. Similarly, it is recommended that the meeting be restricted to operational team

Table 57.6 Examples of quantitative questions (rate between 1–10, with 1 being the lowest and 10 the highest)

- Leadership of the sponsor team
- Leadership of the CRO team
- Communication between sponsor team members
- Communication between CRO team members
- Coordination between sponsor and CRO functional groups
- Problem solving by the combined team
- Clarity of team member roles and responsibilities
- Meeting management (clear agendas, starts and ends on-time, worthwhile attending, etc.)
- Change order management (timely communication and ability to reach timely agreement)
- Ability to trust team members

members and that management not be invited to participate.

The facilitator shows the mean score and range for each question. A mean <5 or a wide range of scores signals weakness. A mean >8 or a narrow range indicates strength. Negative narratives point to weaknesses. Positive comments indicate strengths.

The combined team agrees on actions to remedy weaknesses and maintain strengths. Action steps are written on a flip chart for all to see and buy into. At the next milestone a new lessons learned exercise can be used to verify improvement.

Identifying and resolving problems

Problems during the study always occur. The goal is to identify them an early stage, so that they

Table 57.7 Examples of narrative questions

- What three words describe what it was like to be a member of this team?
- Did everyone know what was expected of her/him? Did you know what was expected of you?
- What went well? What went poorly?
- What is the one thing that we should not repeat if we have another project like this?
- What training should take place prior to beginning a project like this again?

have minimal impact on study cost, timing, and quality. It is also important to address problems when they are small enough to be easily resolved. Earliest detection of problems will likely take place at the technical level. Members of the sponsor and CRO teams will readily perceive issues in their individual technical areas. It is important for a team member to inform the project manager of any issue before attempting to resolve it. This information will enable the project manager to determine whether the problem is an isolated case, which can be resolved at the technical level, or if it is part of a larger problem that needs to be addressed with the corresponding project manager.

Ten "red flags"

Red flags are early warnings that may not require immediate action, but should be evaluated to determine whether a significant underlying problem exists. Each team member may wish to prepare a list of red flags for his or her individual technical area. Ten typical red flags and the possible significant underlying problems are as follows:

1. *Selection of inexperienced investigators by the CRO:* The CRO monitoring staff may be inexperienced.

2. *Questions from the study site directed to the sponsor:* The CRO may not have provided adequate training to site personnel.

3. *Inadequate monitoring reports from the CRO:* The CRO monitoring staff may not be receiving adequate training and supervision.

4. *Enrollment of patients who do not fit the study criteria:* The investigator may not understand the study protocol.

5. *A higher screening-to-enrollment ratio at one site than at others:* The investigator may be "padding the budget" by performing unnecessary screening procedures.

6. *Failure of the CRO to submit monitoring reports promptly after completing visits:* The CRO may not have adequately staffed this study.

7. *Frequent rescheduling of meetings and reports by the CRO:* The CRO staff may be carrying excessive workloads.

8. *Delays in cleaning up case record forms (CRFs):* The CRO may be processing CRFs in batches, which can hide monitoring problems and delay study completion.

9. *Changes in CRO personnel:* The CRO may be experiencing labour problems.

10. *Unscheduled request for payment by the CRO:* The CRO may be experiencing financial problems.

Sponsor–CRO end-of-study meeting

The sponsor and the CRO should hold a formal meeting at the end of the study. The goals of this meeting are listed as follows:

1. To review the actual budget and timeline as compared to the sponsor's and the CRO's expectations.

2. To characterize the quality and timing of materials and activities performed by the sponsor and of the services performed by the CRO.

3. To discuss follow-up of any unresolved issues (e.g., cost overruns, incomplete services).

Conclusions

In summary, more effective contracting of clinical drug-development activities to CROs can be achieved by applying the following methods:

1. Choose the outsourcing strategy (transactional, functional, or alliance) that best fits your needs and corporate culture. Use a strategic approach to outsourcing.

2. Follow the three principles for achieving success with CROs: define accurate study specifications, select the right CRO, and manage the study.

3. Select CROs according to the three Cs: capability, compatibility, and cost.

4. Evaluate the CRO's resource allocations.

5. Define the performance metrics.

6. Ensure efficient communication with the CRO.

7. Conduct periodic "lessons-learned" exercises.

It is important to recognize that the roles and the responsibilities of the sponsor and the CRO are complementary. Dedication and skill are required of both the sponsor and the CRO team members to achieve successful outsourcing.

References

Blankstein, L. Implementation of a lessons learned process to improve clinical project team performance. *American Pharmaceutical Outsourcing* 2004; **5**(4):8–15.

Getz KA. CRO contribution to drug development is substantial and growing globally. *Tufts CSDD Impact Report* 2006a; **8**(1):2.

Getz KA. The impact of outsourcing. *Scrip Reports* 2006b; April(155):39–41.

Getz KA, Vogel JR. Achieving results with contract research organizations: their evolving role in clinical development. *Appl Clin Trials* 1995; **4**(4):32–38.

Getz KA, Vogel JR. Successful outsourcing: Tracking global CRO usage. *Applied Clinical Trials* 2009; **18**(6):42–50.

Hill T. Calculating the cost of clinical research. *Scrip Mag* 1994; **3**:28–30.

Lightfoot GD, Vogel JR. Contracting CROs into your organization: new strategies for new challenges. In *The Drug Development Process: Increasing Efficiency and Cost-effectiveness*, Welling PG, Lasagna L, Banakar UV (eds). Marcel Dekker: New York, USA, 1996, 317–335.

Muken R, Cherny M. CRO 101: From Skeptics to Saviors, *Deutsche Bank, Global Markets Report* 2009; May **12**:29–32.

Sigal, E. Keynote address. *IBC 13th Annual World Congress, Drug Discovery and Development of Innovative Therapeutics,* Boston, MA, USA, August 6, 2008.

Tufts Center for the Study of Drug Development. *The January/February 2006 Tufts CSDD Impact Report,* 2006; available from http://csdd.tufts.edu/reports (subscription necessary); general website accessed April 27, 2010.

Vogel JR. Achieving results with contract research organizations: pharmaceutical industry views. *Appl Clin Trials* 1993; **2**(1):44–49.

Vogel JR, Getz KA. Successful outsourcing: tracking the evolving use of full-service and niche-service CROs. *Appl Clin Trials* 2005; **14**(6):54–60.

Vogel JR, Nelson SR. Achieving results with contract research organizations: determining the study specifications. *Appl Clin Trials* 1993; **2**(5):70–76.

Vogel JR, Resnick N. Achieving results with contract research organizations: a case study in evaluating and selecting a CRO. *Appl Clin Trials* 1996; **5**(6):30–36.

Vogel JR, Schober RA. Achieving results with contract research organizations: requesting and evaluating proposals from CROs. *Appl Clin Trials* 1993; **2**(12):32–41.

CHAPTER 58

The Impact of Managed Care on the US Pharmaceutical Industry

Robert J. Chaponis,[1] Christine Hanson-Divers[2], & Marilyn J. Wells[3]

[1]Novartis, Parsippany, NJ, USA
[2]AstraZeneca, Cary, NC, USA
[3]East Stroudsburg University, East Stroudsburg, PA, USA

After rising sharply during the 1970s and 1980s, overall healthcare costs in the United States leveled in the 1990s, only to start soaring again in 2000 and rising faster than the average annual growth rate of the economy overall, with projections to rise to unsustainable levels in future years. The control of healthcare costs during the 1990s has been attributed to the dramatic growth of managed care with tight cost management procedures. In fact, health plan premium increases were at a record low from 1994 to 1998. Conversely, health benefit costs increased nearly 15% in 2002, while inflation was around 2% (PricewaterhouseCoopers, 2002). The paradigm shift from a largely fee-for-service (FFS) to a managed care environment in the late 1980s and early 1990s affected every aspect of the healthcare system, including the pharmaceutical industry. Managed care organizations (MCOs) brought healthcare costs under control through a variety of strategies, including controlled access to healthcare providers, health plan benefit limitations and restrictions, including pharmacy benefits and products, and capitated reimbursement systems. However, as health benefit costs have been escalating by double-digits over the past five years, employers and health plans have shifted health benefit costs to their workers by reducing contribution levels, eliminating benefits completely, or moving to higher deductible plan designs (Main *et al.*, 2009). Despite these cost-shifting programs, health benefit costs are now rising 6–8% per year, with forecasts to continue at this rate through 2018 (Center for Medicare & Medicaid Services, 2009).

Although satisfied with the results of slowed increases in healthcare costs, purchasers and consumers were less satisfied with restricted access to providers and benefit limitations and restrictions. This criticism received much media attention. As a result, purchasers and consumers pressured MCOs to abandon procedures that worked in the 1990s, moving from tightly managed health benefit plans to more conventional indemnity plans. As a result, the rapid departure of managed care principles contributed to a return of rising costs. Other factors that have been attributed to rising healthcare costs include drugs and medical advances; profit margins on healthcare products and services, provider expenses; government mandates and regulation; litigation and risk management; general inflation; and other miscellaneous factors such as fraud and abuse (PricewaterhouseCoopers, 2002). Foremost among these cost drivers were drugs, medical devices, and other medical advances, accounting for 22% of the overall increase, or US$15 billion of the increase in premiums (PricewaterhouseCoopers, 2002).

Compounding the cost situation, the deep economic recession in 2008 is impacting the managed care industry. The employer-sponsored health benefits marketplace is contracting, as employers cut

Principles and Practice of Pharmaceutical Medicine, 3rd edition.
Edited by L.D. Edwards, A.W. Fox, P.D. Stonier.
© 2011 Blackwell Publishing Ltd.

jobs, exit the health benefits market, reduce coverage and financial sponsorship, and employees opt out of or become ineligible for benefits (Main *et al.*, 2009). Ripple effects include decreasing revenues among medical practices, decelerating growth in hospital spending, slowing growth in physician and clinical services spending, and decreasing growth in the demand for prescription drugs, as consumers fill fewer prescriptions or are increasingly receptive to switching to lower-cost generic drugs (Centers for Medicare & Medicaid Services, 2009; Bendix, 2009). The American Recovery and Reinvestment Act mitigated the impact of the recession through extension of benefits, subsidies, and additional Medicaid funding (Main *et al.*, 2009). Prescription drug spending is projected to rebound as accelerations in Medicare and Medicaid offset private drug spending growth (Centers for Medicare & Medicaid Services, 2009).

Also as a result of rising healthcare costs and the deep economic recession with an uncertain recovery, employer-sponsored health benefit plans in 2010 are expected to reflect higher premiums and new trends in benefit packages, including changes in prescription drug benefits. For example, some companies are introducing 100% coverage for preventive medications or zero co-pays on prescription drug therapies shown to reduce hospitalizations and lower health costs (Miller, 2009). Conversely, as in past recessions, employees may use more medical services and drugs due to concern over loss of jobs, and consequently, health benefits. Further, an ageing population and use of expensive new drugs are driving pharmaceutical costs for MCOs. According to national health expenditure projections, prescription drug expenditures are projected to increase from 4% of national health expenditures in 2010 to 8.6% in 2018 (Centers for Medicare & Medicaid Services, 2009).

With prescription medications continuing to account for an increasing proportion of total medical costs, MCOs are being forced to continue to design and implement new drug benefit management techniques. Traditionally, managed care impacted pharmaceutical products after reaching the market through pharmacy benefit restrictions, limitations, and product formularies. More recently, managed care has influenced pharmaceuticals much earlier in the product life cycle; in many cases, before a product even enters the market. The recent economic recession, combined with unsustainable rising costs, and proposed healthcare reform, are current priorities for managed care and the pharmaceutical industry. However, MCOs continue to be a major customer to the pharmaceutical industry, with increasing leveraging and purchasing power. Therefore, MCOs have a profound impact on how the pharmaceutical industry develops, markets, distributes, and generates revenue for products. This impact will only increase in the future. This chapter introduces basic concepts in managed care, discusses the impact of managed care on the pharmaceutical industry, and concludes with a discussion of emerging trends in managed care and how they may impact the pharmaceutical industry in the future.

The concepts of managed care

The basic concepts of managed care have evolved and are continuing to evolve over time. To understand this evolution, a brief historical perspective is presented first, followed by discussions of the language and principles of managed care.

Historical perspectives

Surpassing traditional indemnity, or FFS health insurance policies, managed care health plans now represent the largest and fastest growing type of coverage for health and medical care in the US. From a rather slow initial growth period, which began in 1929 with the establishment of the first prepaid group practice plan, managed healthcare has grown substantially over the last 30 years (Health Insurance Association of America, 1996). By the mid-1970s, approximately five million people were enrolled in prepaid group practice plans (MacLeod, 1993). As of 2009, over 126 million people were enrolled in some type of managed healthcare organization (Managed Care National Statistics, 2009). According to the Health Confidence Survey (Employee Benefit Research Institute, 2007), of the 82.8% of the US population who were insured, approximately 92% of employees participating in employment-based health plans were enrolled in a managed care plan, up from 48% in 1992.

Concern over rapidly rising healthcare costs has been the driving force behind the rapid growth of managed care. Inherently, a FFS system, where reimbursement and compensation for services are directly related to delivery or utilization of services, has the potential to promote over utilization and drive costs upward. Alternatively, a managed care system, where payment for healthcare is typically prepaid or capitated, has more control over the utilization of services, and thereby costs. The potential for managed care to control healthcare costs successfully has long been recognized and supported by the government, starting with the Health Maintenance Organization (HMO) Act of 1973 to more recent healthcare reform initiatives, including the introduction, in 1998, of a Medicare Prospective Payment System (PPS) for nursing facilities.

In the managed care system, there are three major market segments—consumers, payers, and providers—each with their own distinct groups. Individual health plan members or patients represent the consumer segment. Payers, who are largely defined by their purchasing power, include employer groups (e.g., larger employers, small employers, small business coalitions, cooperative purchasing arrangements, etc.), the government (e.g., government agencies, public insurance programs such as Medicare and Medicaid, etc.), and MCOs (e.g., HMOs, preferred provider organizations (PPOs), etc.). Providers include healthcare organizations (e.g., accredited hospitals, ambulatory care centers, behavioral healthcare facilities, etc.), healthcare professionals (e.g., physicians, pharmacists, nurses, etc.), and depending on their business model, may include MCOs.

Although each of these market segments and groups has unique concerns, they also share common goals, through which their collective actions are defining managed care. For example, managed care systems have an intrinsic conflict between prepayment for healthcare and under-utilization of needed benefits and services. This conflict has given rise to a greater demand by consumers and providers for managed care to demonstrate quality of care, patient satisfaction, and cost-effectiveness of selected services.

The language of managed care

To further explore the principles of managed care, an accurate knowledge of managed care terminology is essential. As managed care is an evolving paradigm, with new systems and models emerging continually, no single, universal definition exists for many of even the most basic managed care terms. Certain elements and characteristics, however, are commonly associated with each, in spite of variations in definition and interpretation by the various market segments.

A MCO is any type of system that integrates the financing and delivery of healthcare to voluntarily enrolled plan members. Common distinguishing characteristics of MCOs include the following:

- arrangements with selected providers to deliver a comprehensive package of health plan benefits to enrollees;
- clear standards for selection of healthcare providers;
- a focus on wellness, preventive care, and disease management to keep plan members healthy, and thereby reduce medical costs;
- formal quality improvement and utilization review programs.

Based upon how these healthcare delivery and financial management strategies are designed and implemented, MCOs are classified into different types or models: HMOs, PPOs, point-of-service (POS) plans, and integrated service networks. In addition, pharmacy benefit management (PBM) and behavioral health (BH) organizations provide specialized services to managed care.

A HMO is a type of MCO that offers comprehensive healthcare to voluntarily enrolled members, who prepay a fixed amount of money in exchange for access to a clearly defined package of health plan benefits. Generally, HMOs receive a fixed fee from members, regardless of whether healthcare services are used or not, that is, they are prepaid on a capitated basis. A primary distinguishing characteristic of HMOs is that, upon enrollment, members are required to select a primary care physician (PCP), who not only delivers comprehensive care but also serves as the gatekeeper to specialty services, such as seeing a physician specialist. If a member seeks nonemergency services from an HMO provider without a referral from his or her PCP, or seeks services from a provider who is not affiliated with the HMO, those services typically will not be covered by the health plan. With these two characteristics in common, HMOs are further characterized into basic models.

A *staff model* HMO owns its healthcare facilities and employs physicians and other providers to provide the healthcare services to its membership. All premiums and revenues accrue to the HMO, which compensates providers by salary and incentive programs. Alternatively, a *group model* HMO contracts with a group of physicians and other providers, who are organized as a partnership or professional corporation. The health plan compensates the medical group for contracted services at a negotiated rate, and then the group is responsible for compensating its physicians and contracting with hospitals and other providers for care of their patients.

A *network model* HMO is a health plan that contracts with many large physician groups and community pharmacies to provide care to its members. As with group model HMOs, network HMOs do not own their own facilities and typically compensate each provider group at a negotiated, capitated rate. Finally, an *individual practice association* (IPA) is an HMO model that contracts with independent physicians, pharmacies, and providers in their own practice settings to provide medical services to its enrollees.

Recently surpassing HMOs as the most common type of MCO is the PPO. A PPO is an organization that contracts with providers to deliver healthcare services at a negotiated discount off of their standard fees or the usual and customary rate (UCR), which is the standard for those services in that geographical region. The PPO then encourages plan members to select providers from this network of preferred providers; however, it does not limit members to this closed panel of providers. By selecting network providers, plan members pay lower co-payments and deductibles than if they were to select a non-network provider. Also, unlike HMOs, plan members are not required to select a PCP. Typically, they may seek care from any network provider without penalty.

Another type of MCO is a POS plan, which is a hybrid between an HMO and PPO. Like HMOs, POS plans typically use PCPs to deliver the comprehensive set of health benefits and to serve as gatekeepers to control access or referrals to specialists. Like PPOs, POS plans also allow health plan members to use non-participating or non-network providers at a reduced level of benefits (e.g., higher co-payments, higher deductibles, etc.). POS plans have emerged in response to needs and desires in both the consumer and payer market segments. Dissatisfied with both restricted access to providers in HMOs and higher premium costs associated with PPOs, consumers have responded favorably to the emergence of POS plans that blend the flexibility of PPOs with the lower costs of HMOs. HMOs have willingly developed such plans to gain competitive advantage over PPO plans.

A gradually increasing trend in managed care is the emergence of integrated services networks (ISNs). ISNs are large integrated organizations that incorporate facilities, providers, and payers. These organizations provide patients with an array of healthcare services through providers who are affiliated under a single payment structure.

Recent trends in managed care indicate increasing numbers of PPO, POS, and IPA plans. This movement represents a shift from the more restrictive staff and group model HMO plans to the less restrictive types of managed care plans with open-ended coverage. According to the Managed Care National Statistics (2009) about 50% of managed care enrollees reported enrollment in the less restrictive PPO-type plans.

According to 1997 statistics, 92% of HMOs engage a pharmaceutical benefit manager (PBM): that is, a company to administer all or part of their pharmaceutical benefits and services (Hoechst Marion Roussel, 1998). Some of the basic functions provided by PBMs include dispensing, formulary management, mail-order drug dispensing, drug utilization reviews (DURs), prescription claims processing, and academic or counter-detailing.

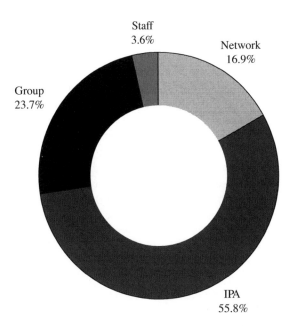

Staff
3.6%

Network
16.9%

Group
23.7%

IPA
55.8%

Figure 58.1 1997 health maintenance organization (HMO) enrollment by model type (adapted from Hoechst Marion Roussel, 1998).

Academic detailing supports formulary adherence through the use of educational interventions, such as telephone calls or letters, to prescribers. Among HMOs, over 90% of IPA and network models contract with PBMs, in contrast to 69% of staff model HMOs (Hoechst Marion Roussel, 1998). Overall, 86.9% of all managed care plans contract with PBMs for their prescription drug benefit claims processing services (Hoechst Marion Roussel, 1998) (see Figure 58.1).

Key principles of managed care

Successful managed care systems deliver high quality healthcare to their members, while maintaining low operating costs through effective application of basic principles of managed care. Three key issues addressed by these managed care principles include provider compensation, cost containment, and quality of care.

Provider compensation includes the methods by which MCOs financially compensate or pay their providers. Provider compensation varies with the nature of the relationship between the MCO and

the provider (e.g., employer–employee, contractual agreements, strategic partnerships, joint ventures, etc.).

Typically, payments are negotiated and may include a variety of methods, including the following:

• *Capitation:* The MCO negotiates with the provider, who agrees to provide a clearly defined set of healthcare services to plan members for a fixed amount per member per month (PMPM), regardless of the amount of services delivered.

• *Discounted FFS:* The MCO negotiates with the provider, who agrees to provide services to enrollees at a discount from their UCRs for FFS patients.

• *Per diem:* The MCO negotiates with a provider organization (e.g., accredited hospitals, ambulatory care centers, etc.), who agrees to deliver care for a fixed rate per day that an enrollee receives care.

• *Per case*: The MCO negotiates with the provider, who agrees to deliver care for a fixed amount or rate of compensation per case for a specified illness or condition.

• *Risk-sh*aring: The MCO negotiates with the provider, who agrees to deliver effective, efficient, and high-quality care to all enrollees with some degree of financial risk.

• *Pay-for-performance:* The MCO negotiates with the provider to be rewarded for achievement of agreed upon performance measures (e.g., percentage of patients reaching treatment goal, decrease in hospitalization rates, increase enrollment of patients in disease management programs).

Integral to these payment methods are their administrative methods. For example, two specialized approaches to assessing payment methods are carve-out and global costs. With *carve-outs*, the MCO negotiates with a specialized provider or service organization, such as a PBM, to provide a narrowly defined set of specific services. Reimbursement for these carve-out services, however, is usually on a capitated basis. With *global costs*, an MCO allocates all healthcare costs under one budget. Some MCOs may even negotiate with providers and healthcare facilities, who agree to receive a global fee for all professional services and institutional expenses for a particular episode of care or diagnosis, except optional benefits, such as medications. Typically, this global fee is capitated.

Although provider compensation methods are effective in controlling a significant proportion of managed care costs, they cannot work alone, because there are other priority issues that continually challenge managed care's ability to deliver high-quality services, and yet control healthcare costs. Cost containment issues that influence business decisions in managed care include medical loss ratios (MLRs), member costs, and pharmacoeconomic and outcomes data.

The MLR is a cost:revenue ratio. It is calculated by dividing the total costs of delivering the health and medical care covered by plan benefits (i.e., total costs) by the total revenues received from members in the form of dues or premium payments (i.e., total revenues), and then multiplying by 100%:

Medical loss ratio

= Total costs/Total revenue × 100%

From a business perspective, MCOs aim for low costs and high revenues, resulting in a small MLR. Managed care executives, however, must continually balance the demands of their various constituents to achieve an acceptable MLR; for example, members want unlimited access to providers and the very best medical treatments with zero-to-low annual premium increases, while shareholders and investors want operating costs (e.g., medical costs, provider compensation, etc.) held to a minimum with annual premium increases. According to industry experts, these forces can be significant, as indicated by the sizable differences in MLRs for indemnity health insurance companies versus HMOs. For indemnity health insurance, the MLR is usually in excess of 90%. For cost-efficient HMOs, it is usually less than 80–85%.

Another way in which MCOs evaluate their costs is by assessing Per Member Per Month (PMPM) costs: the total monthly costs divided by the total number of members. Most MCOs track the PMPM costs to determine trends, evaluate intervention programs, estimate future costs, determine capitation fees, and identify poorly-managed diseases.

When available, MCOs can use pharmacoeconomic and outcomes information to drive the choice for cost-efficient therapeutic alternatives. For this reason, pharmacoeconomic and outcomes data are becoming increasingly important to MCO decision-makers, including formulary decision-makers. Pharmacoeconomic and outcomes data tend to have the greatest impact on unmanaged care decisions when the novel product or drug under consideration produces positive patient outcomes, or yields substantial cost savings within the first 6–12 months of initiation of therapy, as compared to older, less expensive therapies. If positive pharmacoeconomic or patient outcomes are not seen until 2–5 years after initiating drug therapy, the economic information tends to have a lesser impact on the MCO's pharmaceutical benefit or drug therapy decisions.

The increasing importance for pharmacoeconomics data is directly reflected by the emergence of comparative effectiveness research (CER). CER is the comparison of a healthcare intervention to other healthcare interventions with the same treatment outcome goal. The focus is on real-world effectiveness and not clinical efficacy that is established through randomized controlled trials. Additional information regarding CER is included in the "Emerging trends in managed care and their impact on the pharmaceutical industry," section later in this chapter.

Intrinsic to the principles of managed care is the conflict between the desire to control costs and the desire to promote quality of care. Two common measures of quality of care are health plan member satisfaction and health plan accreditation. Member satisfaction surveys assess the extent to which a managed care plan is able to satisfy the diverse needs of its members. Increasingly, member satisfaction is an important measure for MCOs, because it can impact the ability of the plan to attract and retain new members, reduce turnover rates, and achieve accreditation.

Accreditation of managed care plans is a relatively new process, driven by consumer demand for improved quality of care. In recent years, several non-profit entities have developed mechanisms for evaluating and accrediting MCOs. The

National Committee for Quality Assurance (NCQA) has emerged as the most recognized and respected among these. NCQA's accreditation process is designed to assess, measure, and report on the quality of care provided by managed care plans. To receive accreditation, a managed care plan must demonstrate the ability to provide consumers with protections required by the accrediting agency, and continuously to monitor and improve the quality of care for its members. One section of the NCQA accreditation process requires the MCOs to report on quality measures called the Health Plan Employer Data and Information Set (HEDIS), which requires plans to follow the specific guidelines to report these quality measures to NCQA. These HEDIS scores allow for comparisons among plans because they are a standardized set of quality measures. It is important to note that accreditation status is not an absolute guarantee of the quality of care that an individual plan member may receive, or that a network provider may deliver. As competition in the managed care market continues to stiffen, accreditation is becoming increasingly important to MCOs.

The impact of managed care on the pharmaceutical industry

In the late 1970s, pharmaceutical companies developed and marketed new products to physicians with minimal, if any, interference from third-party insurers and payers. Even in the mid-1980s, the pharmaceutical industry paid little attention to group- and staff-model HMOs because they imposed restrictions on sales representatives and demanded price concessions (Pollard, 1990). Over the last two decades, however, managed care plans have experienced sustained growth and consolidation and, in the process, demonstrated their ability to impact the pharmaceutical industry. For example, managed care plans have driven pharmaceutical costs down by demanding economic proof of a product's cost-effectiveness, by measuring the impact of products on health status (e.g., patient outcomes, quality of life, etc.) and by integrating drug utilization into standard treatment

protocols. Managed care plans represent a major customer base of the pharmaceutical industry and advancements in pharmacotherapy have had a profound impact on how pharmaceutical manufacturers develop and market products to MCOs.

To understand more fully the impact of managed care on the pharmaceutical industry, a look at managed care's cost-containment strategies and continued movement toward multiple payers will be presented first, followed by the influential market dynamics of increased competition and changing demographics. Concluding the section will be a discussion of how these factors have impacted the pharmaceutical industry's research and development priorities and product life cycles.

Managed care cost-containment strategies

According to current managed care industry estimates, prescription medications account for up to 15% of total medical costs for some managed care plans (Meyer, 1998). In addition, prescription drug costs are rising by 15–20% each year, much faster than other components of healthcare, for many managed care plans (Meyer, 1998). Furthermore, as the pharmaceutical industry introduces a rush of innovative and expensive drugs, MCOs are mounting defensive strategies to control prescription costs and yet maintain quality of care for their members. Managed care plans that have implemented integrated formulary and disease management programs, outcomes assessment, and risk-sharing contracts, have been more successful at controlling pharmaceutical costs than plans without such strategies.

Formulary management is the most common strategy used by managed care plans for controlling increasing drug costs and access to prescription medications. A formulary is a list of drug products that have been reviewed and approved for use in a particular medical setting. Typically, normal prescribing is restricted to drugs listed in the formulary. In general, drug products are classified into one of three categories: generic, preferred, or non-preferred. A cost-containment strategy used by many MCOs is to encourage drug utilization of generic and preferred drug products only. A formulary system is a method of drug-use control that involves a systematic approach to evaluating drug products, providing guidelines for utilization, informing appropriate parties of current formulary status and policies, enforcing adherence to those policies, and implementing the system.

Responsibility for developing, maintaining, and enforcing formulary systems in managed care lies with the pharmacy and therapeutics (P&T) committee, which normally comprises health plan physicians and clinical pharmacists. Additional responsibilities of a managed care P&T committee may include development, implementation, or maintenance of drug utilization policies, DUR programs, prescribing protocols, generic drug substitution policies, and educational programs.

The formulary approval process for a new drug is a two-step process in managed care. Reimbursement status is determined in the first step; formulary inclusion in the second step. The decision for reimbursement usually occurs 0–6 months postlaunch, and its purpose is to determine whether or not a product will be covered by the plan. Typically, this decision is made before the product is evaluated for formulary acceptance. A MCO will then determine whether or not the product will be included on the formulary by routing the new product through the plan's formulary evaluation and decision process, which usually occurs 6–12 months after launch. This committee evaluates the new product and generally classifies it as either preferred or non-preferred. Therefore, under a managed care plan, the US Food and Drug Administration (FDA) approval of a new product is no longer a guarantee of unrestricted access to the product, because evidence of a drug product's economic value is typically required prior to formulary acceptance.

In general, MCOs with formulary programs use a variety of methods to enforce formulary adherence to their preferred agents (i.e., generic and preferred drug products). These methods vary in their restrictions, and typically include financial incentives for both prescribers and patients. Table 58.1 lists and defines typical restriction methods, such as prior authorization and treatment limitations. Table 58.2 lists commonly used enforcement strategies and financial incentives, including switch programs, differentiated/tiered copayments, and education programs. Of particular interest is the multi-tiered formulary with increasing differentials among the various product tiers. Tiered formulary benefits typically have three tiers with increasing patient co-payments. For example, generics may have a US$5–10, preferred drug products a US$20–30, and non-preferred agents a US$40–50 co-payment. Depending on the product category, patients are responsible for paying the corresponding co-payment fee when purchasing their prescription. This cost-sharing system was designed to combat rapidly growing expenditures and to make consumers more accountable and involved in their healthcare decisions.

Some major insurance companies are now offering plans that include a fourth tier option to cover expensive biologic agents. Rather than

Table 58.1 Drug utilization restrictions used by managed care organizations

Restriction	Definition
Prior authorization	A physician or patient must receive authorization by the plan before the drug will be covered
Quantity limitations	The amount of medications prescribed/dispensed is limited to a prespecified quantity (usually a monthly limit)
Specialist-only	Only specialists are allowed to prescribe medication
Treatment limitations	Treatments are limited on a per-member or per-year basis
Step protocols	Treatments are restricted to a specific step in a protocol (i.e. a second- or third-line treatment in a protocol)
Patient criterion	Patient must qualify for treatment by meeting specific criteria (usually used in conjunction with a prior authorization program)

Table 58.2 Formulary enforcement policies used by managed care organizations

Enforcement policy	Definition
Switch programs	Whereby physicians are called and asked to switch to a specific formulary product
Risk sharing	Policies whereby the physician (usually the primary care provider (PCP)) is placed at financial risk for providing services (including prescription drugs) to the patients
Financial penalties	Physicians are financially penalized for prescribing non-formulary products
Differential/tiered co-payments	Member's prescription co-payments are higher for non-formulary products
Out-of-pocket payments	Members pay for non-formulary drugs (either a fixed amount/co-payment or the fee-for-service (FFS) cost of the prescription)
Education programs	Education programs for physicians (usually the PCP) to educate physicians on formulary products and selection criteria
Report cards/performance records	Monthly or quarterly reports comparing and evaluating physicians' prescribing patterns are generated and distributed to all participating physicians
Intervention programs	Telephone calls and/or letters are sent to physicians prescribing non-formulary drugs

a fixed co-pay, the model incorporates a co-insurance approach in which patients are charged a percentage—typically 20–30%—of the drug's cost (Lee *et al.*, 2008). The harsh reality is that for most patients, the out-of-pocket expenses usually far exceed what their budgets can bear, which can amount to thousands of dollars a month. Tier 4 systems have now been incorporated into 86% of Medicare drug plans and 10% of private commercial plans that include drug benefits (Kolata, 2008). With patient out-of-pocket drug costs rising and co-pay differences between tiers widening, the pharmaceutical industry can expect more patients to raise financial questions about branded products that their physicians prescribe. Accordingly, health plan members will increasingly be forced to make choices as financial priorities affect the traditional doctor–patient relationship (Studin, 2004).

An emerging trend in formulary management is the decline in the utilization of enforcement and restriction strategies such as switch and prior authorization programs (Litton *et al.*, 2000). These programs typically have high administrative and internal resource costs, significant time consumption, limited success on drug utilization, and dissatisfaction among patients and providers (Olson, 2002). Instead, MCOs are expanding their use of multi-tiered co-payment systems, and increasing the co-pay differentials between the

tiers. When multi-tier systems were first developed, generally only a few dollars differentiated each level of tiers. Currently, it is not uncommon to see US$15–30 differences between single-tier levels (Fendrick *et al.*, 2001). With the exception of the tier 4 model, where patients are charged a percentage of the drug cost, the benefits of using this type of system over switch or prior authorization programs are multifaceted in that the multi-tiered system is simple and economical to administer, offers patients a choice in making decisions without restrictive access to medications, and provides a reasonable level of satisfaction compared with other programs (Olson, 2002).

In addition to the use of multi-tiered co-payment systems to control costs, MCOs are frequently using generic incentives and mail-order delivery systems. Typical generic incentives are financially based, either being the lowest tier in a tiered system or having coupons offered to cover the co-payment for a one-month utilization. Audit reports have demonstrated that a mere 1% increase in generic utilization can result in a multimillion dollar savings to the plan (Olson, 2002). Mail-order service is another cost containment strategy that MCOs use, including PBMs. Mail service pharmacy covers maintenance medications for up to a 90-day supply of medications at a reduced co-payment. Advantages of mail-order services include discounts on dispensing fees compared to retail pharmacies/networks, home delivery convenience for patients, and the opportunity to manage cost and compliance (Pharmacy Benefit Management Institute, 2000).

With individual health plan members in a unique position to make independent purchasing decisions, the cumulative impact of increasing cost differences between product tiers and the availability of a broad array of generic products presents a marketing challenge to the branded pharmaceutical industry. Accordingly, the managed care business units of pharmaceutical manufacturers may need to address consumer–member marketing if they are to realize market share success and sustained product growth at the plan level (Studin, 2004).

The pharmaceutical industry has long challenged the necessity of formularies and related enforcement policies that restrict a prescriber's choice. In response, pharmaceutical companies have engaged a number of their own strategies to counter managed care's cost-containment practices. For example, they are funding pharmacoeconomic, quality-of-life, and other outcome studies to demonstrate the economic and societal value of a drug product, and thereby influence formulary acceptance by managed care decision makers. In general, MCOs view pharmaceutical industry sponsored economic evaluations as useful in comparing therapeutically similar products; however, sponsor bias and applicability of study results to a plan's population are major concerns (Luce *et al.*, 1996). Out of all the research conducted by MCOs, economic studies have the greatest potential to guide formulary decisions.

Another increasingly important strategy for the pharmaceutical industry is assessing whether a new product's therapeutic category is on the MCO's "radar screen." Criteria for inclusion of a product's therapeutic category on an MCO's radar include the following:
- the current budget and resources allocated for patients with the target disease;
- the ability of the plan to realize a significant return on investment if the disease is managed (i.e., cost-effectiveness) appropriately;

- the ability of the plan to provide staff for development and implementation of disease management programs;
- the ability of the plan to measure effectively the impact of a disease management program.

Because of increased difficulty in getting a new drug on an MCO's formulary, it is now common for pharmaceutical companies to collaborate with managed care decision-makers in "round table" or "advisory board" meetings. These discussions, which normally occur before product launch or as early as Phases II and III of clinical development, are helpful in determining reimbursement status and identifying potential barriers and restrictions that may be placed on the product, once approved. To facilitate these types of discussions, many major pharmaceutical companies have created separate field-based medical groups, as an extension of their medical science liaison (MSL) function, which focus exclusively on MCOs through the scientific exchange of clinical and economic data to justify preferential tier placement of a new drug on the formulary.

Providing support to disease management programs represents another pharmaceutical industry strategy to counter managed care cost-containment efforts. Disease management is "a collaborative process which assesses, plans, implements, coordinates, monitors, and evaluates options and services to meet an individual's health needs through communication and available resources to promote quality cost-effective outcomes" (Care Management Society of America, 1995). Resources needed to support these programs include patient education materials/programs, physician education, patient adherence programs, case manager training, and evaluation expertise. MCOs are increasingly adopting disease management programs to provide comprehensive medical care and improve patient outcomes at a lower cost (Schulman *et al.*, 1996). Today, virtually all managed care plans offer a disease management program for asthma to prevent costly emergency department visits and hospitalizations. Some MCOs have even forged partnerships with pharmaceutical manufactures to assist in evaluating a disease management program's effectiveness and to access scientific and financial support for the program.

Risk-sharing contracts between the MCO and the pharmaceutical company, through which both parties share in the financial risks and rewards of doing business, are a common business strategy. Package pricing (i.e., special discount on a product line) and rebate programs that reward an MCO for achieving a certain market share of the product are two other contracting strategies that have been adopted by the pharmaceutical industry.

In addition to integrated formulary and disease management programs, outcomes assessment, and risk sharing contracts, MCOs are implementing a variety of other value-added services and programs to minimize costs, modify provider behavior, enhance patient outcomes, and differentiate themselves in the marketplace. The pharmaceutical industry has responded to its managed care customer base needs by offering a variety of innovative, value added services, including medication compliance programs, patient education programs, and call center services.

Multiple payer influence in managed care

In addition to cost-containment strategies, managed care is impacting the pharmaceutical industry through a continued movement toward multiple payers of healthcare. The make-up of the payer market is changing as increasing numbers of MCOs are doing business with the government and large employers. These payer market segments are exerting a greater influence on the scope of their health plan benefits and treatment decisions.

Both the Federal government and state agencies are moving increasing numbers of Medicare and Medicaid recipients, respectively, into managed care plans, to control healthcare expenditures, including drug costs. Clearly, the impetus has been the ability of managed care plans to reduce healthcare expenditures, which is accomplished by shifting the focus of healthcare away from incident-driven delivery to preventive and coordinated care. State Medicaid agencies have actively promoted managed care plans to recipients. Likewise, Medicare actively encouraged enrollees participation in

Medicare managed care plans, resulting in steady increases in the 1990s. Although some MCOs initially offered prescription drug benefits as an incentive to attract Medicare enrollees, drug benefits were often capped or eliminated due to escalating costs, and traditionally, prescription drugs have not been covered on an outpatient basis under Medicare. To fill this gap, from January 1, 2006 outpatient prescription drugs are covered under Part D of Medicare, as enacted by the Medicare Prescription Drug, Improvement and Modernization Act of 2003.

Under the Part D Prescription Drug Benefit, Medicare beneficiaries will be able to obtain a prescription drug benefit by one of three means: a traditional Medicare FFS plan with a separate prescription drug plan (PDP), an enhanced FFS plan that provides an integrated PDP, or a Medicare Advantage plan (the program that replaced Medicare + Choice from January 1, 2006). HMOs that offer a Medicare Advantage plan must ensure that their drug benefits at least match those of the standard package (Grubert et al., 2004). Prior to the Part D Prescription Drug Benefit, Medicare-endorsed drug discount cards were available during a transitional phase from 2004 to 2006. Accordingly, MCOs that have already established the capacity to administer pharmacy benefits over a broad area have a significant advantage in negotiating for PDP contracts to cover Medicare beneficiaries. Those MCOs with experience in Medicare risk-contracting, marketing and brand strength, and pharmacy management capabilities are in the best position to take advantage of the new Medicare reforms (Grubert et al., 2004).

Although the effect of employers on the pharmaceutical industry continues to evolve, employers are significant purchasers of managed care health plans and, as such, in a position to impact significantly the pharmaceutical industry. Driven by cost-sharing motives, the shift to tiered co-insurance with consumers financing a portion of the cost will enable employers to better estimate member costs and budget more appropriately. Market dynamics indicate that in the future, large employers or employer groups will work directly with buyers and providers of healthcare, thereby challenging managed care for contracts with employers. In addition, employers may require MCOs to use fewer carve-out services, like PBMs, to encourage a more global perspective in caring for their employees. Responding to the needs of both payers—employers and MCOs—the pharmaceutical industry is positioned to sponsor wellness and preventive care programs to help differentiate MCOs from their competitors and facilitate contracts with employers. Finally, the influence of employers in improving quality standards, patient safety, and affordability of healthcare is gaining momentum through initiatives such as The Leap-Frog Group, a national consortium of Fortune 500 companies, and other large private and public employer healthcare purchasers.

One of the most unprecedented strategies by an MCO to reduce drug costs involved the switch of the non-sedating antihistamine loratadine (Claritin) to over-the-counter (OTC) status. Traditionally, pharmaceutical companies have petitioned the US FDA to switch their products from RX to OTC to extend patent life and create new markets for their products, thus increasing revenue. In 1998, Wellpoint (one of nation's largest health insurers) petitioned the FDA to switch second-generation antihistamines from RX to OTC status (Food & Drug Letter, 2002). In its petition, Wellpoint argued that second-generation antihistamines were safer and more effective than traditional sedating antihistamines currently sold OTC. Further, by making the class available OTC, Wellpoint would save about US$90 million: US$45 million from prescription costs and US$45 million for co-pays (Food & Drug Letter, 2002). Faced with competition from other manufacturers to launch generic versions of OTC Claritin and an FDA Advisory Committee's overwhelming recommendation supporting the OTC switch, the manufacturer agreed to file a supplemental New Drug Application (NDA) to move their product to OTC status. For the first time, a party other than a pharmaceutical company petitioned the FDA for OTC switch approval (Food & Drug Letter, 2002). At the time of the loratadine RX-to-OTC switch, some PBMs shifted existing second-generation antihistamines to a more expensive tier to further discourage prescription antihistamine

use and reduce cost, thus requiring a higher co-payment by the patient.

Although RX-to-OTC switches result in preferential cost-savings for payers, most members face increased out-of-pocket costs. As more drugs move from prescription to OTC availability, many insurers have directed plan members to the switched products, and some MCOs have even begun providing coverage for selected OTC drugs to encourage their use. With the co-payment for a third tier non-preferred brand averaging US$40–50 per month, the lower price of OTC drugs compared with similar prescription products in a given therapeutic class has persuaded some health plans to add certain switched products to their formularies. For these switched products, eligible members are charged a nominal co-payment of around US$5 (Sipkoff, 2008), with most plans requiring a prescription for the OTC product or generic equivalent to take advantage of the benefit. For example, Blue Cross Blue Shield of Michigan covers the OTC heartburn medication omeprazole (Prilosec) in an effort to move patients off prescription esomeprazole (Nexium). The insurer has estimated that the switch could save eligible members more than US$9 million a year in out-of-pocket costs (Blue Cross Blue Shield of Michigan website, 2007). Coverage by MCOs of effective OTC products that were once prescription drugs provides two benefits: (i) reducing healthcare costs by maintaining quality of care; and (ii) the ability of an MCO to continue to monitor member use of medications.

Finally, consumers, or individual health plan members, represent another payer group within managed care. Consumers pay for healthcare through health plan premiums, deductibles, and benefit-specific co-payments, including prescription drug co-payments. To address consumer needs, as well as to expand market share, many pharmaceutical companies have invested significant resources in direct-to-consumer advertising (DTCA) campaigns. Furthermore, because the FDA relaxed advertising regulations in 1997, pharmaceutical companies can now make product-specific health claims and link it to treatment of the indicated disease, as long as they disclose the major risks and side effects of the product. As a result, spending by the pharmaceutical industry on DTCA in the United States has steadily increased over the last several years from US$1.2 billion in 1998 (IMS Health website, 1999) to US$4.2 billion in 2004 (NOP World Health, 2005).

Consumer advocate groups contend that DTCA has the potential to alert patients to potentially serious medical conditions and available drug therapies. Within the pharmaceutical industry, drug product managers see increased use of their product by better-informed consumers. MCOs have responded less enthusiastically to DTCA, due to its potential to increase drug costs through overuse of prescription medications. In support of this position, a recent Yankelovic patient awareness survey found that 15% of consumers discussed an advertised drug with their physicians, and 8% visited a doctor specifically to discuss an advertised product (Headden and Melton, 1998). Critics further contend that DTCA increases the overall costs of medical care, therapeutic alternatives and side effects of the medication are often inadequately presented, and information may be misleading (Gandy, 1992). Despite the resistance, DTCA is a powerful tool that the pharmaceutical industry continues to use to increase product awareness and market share in a multiple-payer managed care system.

Managed care market competition

A managed care market dynamic that has impacted the pharmaceutical industry is increased competition. With the managed care market becoming increasingly competitive due to market saturation, many MCOs are employing innovative strategies to recruit and retain members. One such strategy is to offer enrollees multiple products and expanded health plan benefits. In a US national survey of managed care health plans, Gold and Hurley (1997) found that MCOs are providing a selection of benefit offerings in response to customer interests and to ease the transition to more traditional managed care, especially in consumer markets with low managed care penetration; 71% of the plans in their sample offered at least two products, and a majority of plans with multiple products offered three or more options.

One such benefit design is Consumer Driven Health Care (CDHC). CDHC is an insurance benefit design where patient costs are determined by free market variables and patient choice of a service(s) that each individual patient decides to use. A patient has the option to use Health Savings Accounts (as tax benefit) to pay for healthcare. CDHC theoretically assumes that only necessary services will be sought out and paid for by patients in order to reduce costs. Decision-making remains largely in the patient's hands and CDHC health benefits are typically described as having high deductibles for both the medical and pharmacy benefits. This means that individuals would have to pay out-of-pocket the medical deductible (typically US$2,000) before their medical insurance begins to pay for the services. Separately, individuals must pay their pharmacy deductible (typically US$500) before their pharmacy benefit begins to pay for their prescriptions. Often, once the deductible is met, a patient then becomes eligible for nominal co-pay. CDHC has caused the emergence of a new benefit model called Value Based Insurance Design (VBID) or Value Based Benefit Design (VBBD).

In highly penetrated managed care markets, health plans are strategically expanding benefits and services to foster loyalty and improve member retention, largely in response to the realization that it costs five to seven times more to recruit a new health plan member than to keep one (Edlin, 1998). Health Net, based in Woodland Hills, California, and a subsidiary of Foundation Health Systems, automatically enrolls members in their WellRewards program, which offers discounts of 20–50% on quality health-related products and services, including vitamins and supplements, sports and fitness equipment, veterinary services, pet care supplies, and medically supervised weight management (Edlin, 1998). Prudential HealthCare of South Florida offers members nicotine patches at a discount through its smoking cessation program, Committed Quitters, and bicycle helmets for US$10 through its bike helmet program for members and nonmembers (Edlin, 1998).

This expansion of health plan benefits and availability of multiple product offerings has created new opportunities for the pharmaceutical industry: for example, pharmaceutical manufacturers with drug products in therapeutic areas not traditionally covered by managed care, such as smoking cessation, weight loss, and infertility, are now targeting plans with expanded benefits in those areas to promote their products. Another strategy employed by the pharmaceutical industry is to offer a portfolio of value-added services associated with a product, rather than promoting the therapeutic benefits of an individual drug, to help managed health plans achieve market differentiation and a competitive advantage.

Within the managed care industry, increased market competition has led to the emergence of the sales and marketing director and the benefits director as key decision-makers, with increasing influence on medical decisions, including pharmacy benefits and formulary coverage. To communicate with and sell to these stakeholders effectively, the pharmaceutical industry has developed specialized sales teams, and expanded the responsibility of the managed care sales force to identify and target these directors for selected sales promotions.

Industry-wide consolidations, acquisitions, and mergers are also affecting managed care market competition. Since the early-1990s, mergers and acquisitions among MCOs and insurers have occurred at a record pace. In late 1998, Aetna US Healthcare, formed by an US$8.9 billion acquisition of US Healthcare by Aetna in 1996, announced plans to acquire Prudential Healthcare for US$1 billion, making the combined entity the largest managed care company in the United States with 18.9 million members (Aetna US Healthcare website, 2009). One evident outcome of consolidation among MCOs and insurers is that the pharmaceutical industry is now dealing with fewer, larger customers, who are gatekeepers for member services. As managed care market consolidation continues, it will become increasingly important for the pharmaceutical industry to identify and understand the role of the gatekeeper in formulary decisions, monitor product utilization through provider pharmacies and health systems, and develop strategies to link inpatient and outpatient drug use to coordinate pharmaceutical care.

In response to consolidations throughout the entire healthcare industry, as well as to increasing drug-development costs, the pharmaceutical industry has also experienced a series of mergers and acquisitions in the last decade. Since the late 1990s and through the new millennium, horizontal integration in the pharmaceutical industry produced giant drug conglomerations, such as AstraZeneca, Sanofi-Aventis, GlaxoSmithKline, and Pfizer (comprising legacy companies Warner-Lambert and Pharmacia). As of this writing, Pfizer has announced its acquisition of rival Wyeth and Merck intends to merge with Schering-Plough to continue the trend of horizontal integration. These transactions enable economies of scale in research and marketing to better compete with rival firms. In addition, merging companies claim they will benefit from enhanced research and development capacity and better access to global markets (Bond and Weissman, 1997).

Since the 1990s, another aspect of market competition that caused even greater concern to MCOs and payers than pharmaceutical manufacturer consolidations was the pharmaceutical industry's trend toward vertical integration through the acquisition of PBMs. Because they manage drug benefits for approximately half of the US population, PBMs have significant buying power, and therefore represented a real threat to a pharmaceutical company's market share and profits (Bond and Weissman, 1997). In 1993, Merck & Co. paid a record US$6.6 billion to purchase Medco, and less than one year later, SmithKline Beecham acquired Diversified Pharmaceutical Services (DPS) and Eli Lilly bought PCS Health Systems. Despite allegations from consumer advocate groups that the transactions were made to preserve each acquirer's market share and profits from brand name products, the pharmaceutical companies contended that vertical integration of a PBM has enabled each to deliver integrated pharmaceutical care and compete more effectively in the managed care arena.

While the Merck–Medco alignment generated robust sales for Merck products that might otherwise have been spent on competitors' products, Lilly struggled to increase its market share of brand name products on the PCS formulary. In the fall of

1998, Lilly announced that it was leaving the PBM business and selling PCS to Rite Aid, one of the nation's largest pharmacy chains. In 1999, SmithKline Beecham announced the divestiture of its PBM subsidiary DPS to sharpen its focus on pharmaceuticals and consumer healthcare. Although Merck had a successful run of the PBM market for nine years, it too followed suit in 2002 by divesting its Medco subsidiary to concentrate on its core business strategy of discovering, developing, and marketing pharmaceuticals. Departing from the trend of pharmaceutical companies acquiring PBMs, in March 2007, CVS Corporation and Caremark Rx, Inc. merged to form CVS/Caremark Corporation, creating an unprecedented retail model by integrating pharmacy services with the largest US drug store chain and the second largest PBM.

Finally, with increased consolidation in the managed care and pharmaceutical industries, as well as throughout the healthcare industry, comprehensive, integrated data management systems will be needed to enable industry partners to collect, manage, analyze, and disseminate medical and utilization information in a comprehensive and standardized manner. Integrated data management systems are critical for healthcare consumers, payers, and providers, because they enable each group to evaluate treatment selections or use decisions, identify substandard utilization patterns, provide comprehensive and accessible medical records for plan providers, and identify risk factors for chronic and expensive urgent-driven healthcare needs. A complete, integrated management system allows pharmaceutical companies to demonstrate how prescription medications may decrease costs and optimize the quality of care provided to an MCO's members.

Population and managed care market demographics

The US population and managed care market demographics are changing significantly, largely due to increased life expectancies and an ageing "baby boom" generation (i.e., individuals born during 1946–1964). As this generation reaches retirement age, there will be a larger geriatric market than ever before, as an estimated 10,065 Americans turn 50 years old each day, according to US census data.

The 2000 Census counted nearly 35 million people in the US who were 65 years of age or older, about one of every eight Americans. By 2030, demographics estimate that one in every five Americans will be aged 65 or older. Those aged 85 or older, the "oldest-old," are the fastest growing segment of the elderly population. This latter group is of special interest to healthcare planners because those 85 or older are more than likely to require health services (Himes, 2001).

Although Medicare beneficiaries have not enrolled in managed care plans at rates seen in the employer market, trends have mirrored the employer market. Enrollment in Medicare managed care increased steadily in the 1990s, and has continued to increase in the past decade, from 6.3 million enrollees in 2000 to 10 million in 2008, representing a 23% share of membership (Kaiser Family Foundation, 2004; Main *et al.*, 2009). Cost management and oversight will become increasingly important in this expanding senior market, due to the expanded benefits created under the Medicare Prescription Drug, Improvement, and Modernization Act (MMA) of 2003, including prescription drug coverage, low-income assistance, and preventive benefits. Since 2006, more than 40 million elderly and disabled Americans have had an opportunity to enroll in a Medicare Part D prescription drug plan. An assessment of evidence from 2006 to 2009 indicates that Medicare Part D has reduced the number who lacked prescription drug coverage and Federal spending has been lower than initially projected, Medicare spending accounts for a growing proportion of the Federal budget (Neuman and Cubanski, 2009). Thus, policymakers could face pressure to deal aggressively with pharmaceutical costs, particularly as broader health policy discussions look to Medicare as a key lever in controlling the growth of healthcare costs (Newman and Cubanski, 2009). Amidst focus on economic recovery and healthcare reform, expectations are that Medicare Part D is more likely to be fine-tuned than overhauled. According to Neuman and Cubanski (2009), issues considered by the 111th Congress may include improving coverage, simplifying choices, closing the coverage gap, improving coverage for low-income beneficiaries, and lowering prices and spending.

Additionally, as growing numbers of people move into the senior care market, increasing incidence of chronic diseases, including Alzheimer's disease, arthritis and, osteoporosis, will influence healthcare markets and managed care plan dynamics. Sloane *et al*. (2002) predicted no "less than a threefold rise in the total number of persons with Alzheimer's disease between 2000 and 2050." Riggs and Melton (1995) estimated a fourfold increase in the global fracture rate over the next 50 years, reaching 6.25 million hip fractures by 2050. Exemplifying the influence of chronic diseases on healthcare and managed care, a one-time "Welcome to Medicare" physical exam, cardiovascular screening, and bone mass measurements are among the new and current preventive services available to beneficiaries covered under Medicare. New Medicare Specialty Plans provide more focused heathcare to manage a specific disease or condition. Both this growing geriatric population and managed care plans with significant numbers of Medicare enrollees will continue to drive the demand for better treatment options.

The pharmaceutical industry has started to respond to the increasing geriatric market with increased research and development for products for the treatment of chronic diseases. Some pharmaceutical firms have even established geriatric focused research departments to identify and address the special needs of the elderly.

Pharmaceutical research and development

In addition to the influence of a growing geriatric market segment on pharmaceutical industry research and development, each of the other managed care and market influences—cost-containment strategies, multiple payers, and market competition—have collectively impacted pharmaceutical research and development. The pharmaceutical industry is highly competitive and heavily invested in research and development. For example, recent consolidations among pharmaceutical companies are due, in part, to the enormous

risk and expense in bringing a new drug to market and the desire to spread development costs over a larger revenue base (Pollard, 1990). Increased global competition has also influenced pharmaceutical industry research and development. Finally, MCOs and PBMs, focused on cost-containment strategies, are resisting expensive drugs that lack explicit advantages over older, less expensive therapies. They are forcing the pharmaceutical industry to focus on drug candidates with the largest potential for financial return, a move that has raised concerns about which drugs get developed. Therefore, there is increasing concern that clinical research in the US is being threatened by the proliferation of managed care.

One indication of this concern over pharmaceutical research and development is that pharmaceutical manufacturers are shifting clinical investigations from costly academic medical centers (AMCs) to less expensive private study centers and third-party contract research organizations (CROs), to reduce both drug development time and costs. In 1988, AMCs accounted for 80% of investigators and ten years later, that percentage had dropped to 46% (Lightfoot *et al*., 1999). Some MCOs are reluctant to refer members to AMC-conducted trials, even if the research is pharmaceutical industry-sponsored, due to concerns of higher patient-care costs and litigation over unexpected adverse events. Critics contend that the managed care practice of restricting patient access to AMCs for specialized care has accelerated declining physician revenues, which directly affects the ability of an AMC to engage in clinical research (Burnett, 1996). Furthermore, declining AMC patient-care revenues and the pharmaceutical industry's cost-saving strategy of shifting studies to CROs are contributing to a lack of funding for training future research investigators.

Despite MCO concerns over patient costs and liability issues, the number of research studies is steadily increasing in the managed care setting. Many investigators believe that the managed care setting is ideal for conducting clinical research, because care is standardized and easier to control, potential study patients can be easily identified through centralized databases, and the population is representative of the real world, especially for post-marketing and safety surveillance studies. In fact, most MCOs are more interested in establishing the effectiveness of a product—that is, how well the drug performs under real-world conditions—than in determining a product's efficacy through rigorously-controlled clinical trials. Although rare, some firms will halt development of a compound as early as Phase II trials if there appears to be no perceived economic value. Conversely, pharmaceutical companies with favorable outcomes and pharmacoeconomic (i.e., cost-effectiveness) data at the launch of a new product have assisted MCOs in their formulary decision processes and have had successful launch campaigns. Indeed, prelaunch research participation may help a MCO to gain a competitive edge, by integrating experimental care into clinical practice and offering new treatment options to their members.

Pharmaceutical product life cycles

In addition to its influence on pharmaceutical industry research and development, managed care has significantly impacted product life cycles. Drugs identified as preferred products by managed care health plans have a steeper, or faster, uptake and initial growth period (as shown in Figure 58.2) than products that are covered non-formulary. MCO-preferred products reach their sales peak earlier and experience a longer, sustained maturation phase. Covered, non-formulary products never reach as high a maturation peak as preferred products. However, once a preferred product's patent expires, there is a rapid decline in sales, because most

health plans routinely switch the formulary choice to a generic equivalent. In addition to identifying preferred products for reimbursement, MCOs are implementing disease management programs to foster increased utilization of the preferred product over similar, but competitive, products.

Pharmaceutical companies are adopting a number of strategies to maximize market share of a new product in a managed care environment. Achieving formulary acceptance by MCOs is the first step for ensuring a successful life cycle for a prescription product, as shown in Figure 58.3. To influence positively formulary decisions and gain preferred product status, pharmaceutical companies are generating pharmacoeconomic and outcomes data. Once accepted by the managed care health plan's P&T Committee, pharmaceutical companies may invest in pull-through programs to increase market share and appropriate utilization of the product. Pull-through programs may involve special contracting agreements or comprehensive disease management initiatives to highlight the clinical and economic value of a specific product. In addition to pull-through programs and value-added services, such as patient education materials, pharmaceutical companies are discounting targeted prescription drug products or entire product lines where competition is fierce.

The value of evidence-based medicine as the new "gold standard" for clinical practice is poised to play a greater role in driving the market share success of pharmaceuticals, particularly in the managed care and Medicare environments. Although the pharmaceutical industry agrees that

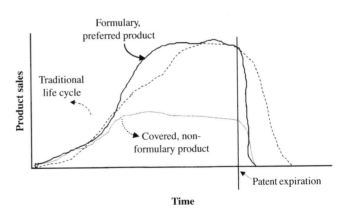

Figure 58.2 Impact of managed care on
pharmaceutical product life cycle.

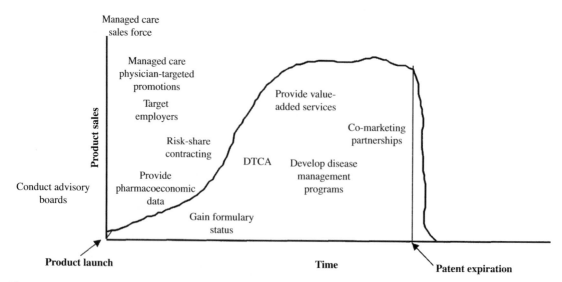

Figure 58.3 Pharmaceutical industry strategic initiatives during the product life cycle.

evidence-based medicine improves quality in medical practice, critics contend that it tends to commodify products by holistically categorizing them based on class effect and product interchangeability, thereby minimizing individual product differences (Studin, 2004). To address an emerging evidence-based commodity environment, it is suggested that the pharmaceutical industry promotes the adoption of consensus guidelines and protocols to standardize treatment approaches. The new horizon for managed care marketing will be defined by increased product commodification justified not by cost but by quality. Accordingly, pharmaceutical manufacturers will need to address quality-driven commodification imperatives (Studin, 2004).

Equally as important as optimizing patient outcomes through the appropriate use of pharmaceuticals is ensuring that patients take their drugs on time in the dosages prescribed. The consequences of noncompliance (nonadherence) and its impact of disease management can be dangerous and costly in the short and long-term. Studies have shown than nonadherence to prescribed medications causes approximately 125,000 deaths annually in the US (Burrell and Levy, 1984), and leads to 10% of hospital and 23% of nursing home admissions (National Pharmaceutical Council, 1992).

Patient adherence with chronic medications in the US averages only 50% (Haynes *et al.*, 2000). For chronic conditions, such as diabetes, adherence to prescribed medication regimens plays a critical role in achieving improved health outcomes, thus reducing disease progression and healthcare costs (Hunt *et al.*, 2009). Complicating this challenge is the effect that high out-of-pocket costs can have on medication adherence, even among patients with prescription drug insurance (Briesacher *et al.*, 2009). With the advent of comparative effectiveness research, which strives to determine the healthcare interventions that work best for a given patient, the pharmaceutical industry is in a unique position to partner with MCOs to assess important determinants of real world effectiveness, including medical adherence through the conduct of practical clinical trials (PCTs). Although the incentives for pharmaceutical companies to sponsor such research initiatives fully may be unclear, because of time, cost, and potential misalignment with marketing objectives, the advantages are evident to MCOs in establishing a drug's real world effectiveness and cost-effectiveness separately from the traditional randomized controlled trial (RCT) used for registration purposes (Luce *et al.*, 2008).

Finally, to maintain a healthy product life cycle until patent expiration, pharmaceutical companies are engaging business strategies, including risk-sharing contracts, DTCA, and co-marketing partnerships. Pharmaceutical companies are developing co-marketing partnerships in record numbers to achieve maximum global market penetration, by leveraging research and marketing strengths in key therapeutic areas. Co-marketing partnerships are being formed through joint ventures, licensing agreements, strategic alliances, traditional mergers, and acquisitions (Kaniecki and Goldberg-Arnold, 1993).

Emerging trends in managed care and their impact on the pharmaceutical industry

Diverse factors will continue to influence managed care in the future, and subsequently impact the pharmaceutical industry. Managed care consumers, payers, and providers will continue to be the key facilitators of change. Key areas in which these distinct but interconnected market segments will drive change include the recent trends in the employer segment, an increased need for comparative effectiveness research, and the US healthcare reform efforts.

Employer segment

The employer segment has long been recognized as an important payer in the MCO market. However, until recently, employers have not been a priority customer segment to the pharmaceutical industry. Many recent activities have elevated this segment as a pivotal customer to manufacturers.

Employer coalitions

The healthcare market has undergone consolidation and within the employer segment this trend is also apparent. Employer coalitions formed by aggregations of employers across the country, including three major coalition types: (i) informational, which are those that serve as forums for the sharing of information among employers and representation of payer interests in healthcare

debate; (ii) purchasing, which are those that additionally engage in purchasing activity and strategy for members; and (iii) combination of informational and purchasing. Regardless of what type, most employer coalitions are frequently involved in matters of quality assessment of care and influencing healthcare matters in the policy development arena.

Recently, purchasing coalitions formed by large and medium-sized employers have received a great deal of attention. These coalitions are seen by some as an embodiment of the concept of "managed competition," under which consumers would be organized into large group purchasing pools in local markets and thus are increasingly important healthcare decision-makers.

An example of a coalition's influence in the pharmaceutical environment is their ability to develop and direct the implementation of benefit designs that may limit branded pharmaceutical agents to second-line treatments (e.g., a generic-only or generic-first formulary). PBMs have long recognized the importance of the employer segment and include coalition representation on formulary P&T committees, drive utilization of mail-order services through benefit design, and offer value-added services. The consolidation of decision-making power via coalitions has made them an important customer segment to the pharmaceutical industry.

Value Based Insurance Design (VBID)

Employers are shifting their view of health benefits from that of a necessary expense to a critical investment in the health management of their employees. This shift is reflected in the emergence of VBID (or VBBD) benefits. VBID is a benefit design strategy whereby patient costs are determined by a group of decision-makers based on the likely value of a service to that individual patient type. This benefit model assumes that patients have knowledge gaps and are not equipped to act optimally on a full benefit; thereby, rejecting CDHC economic theory that higher co-pays cause patients to select clinical services correctly to optimize quality and cost. VBID models vary a great deal because they may be either disease-focused or behaviorally-focused. For example, one type

VBID model may offer increased access (i.e., lower copays) for specific chronic diseases, while another model may offer incentives (e.g., lower copays) for members who demonstrate adherence to treatments. VBID's premise is that low co-pays will lead to improved adherence leading to better outcomes and overall lowered costs. The development of the VBID models is based on scientific evidence, thus promoting evidence-based treatments. Negatively, VBID typically results in higher monthly insurance premiums for employers. Therefore, the employer segment and the pharmaceutical industry are very interested in expanding the science base necessary to develop and evaluate the impact of this type of benefit on overall quality and cost of healthcare.

Increased requirements for comparative effectiveness research

Comparative effectiveness research (CER) it the comparison of one diagnostic or treatment option to one or more with the same treatment outcome. In CER studies, real-world effectiveness is the primary objective, not clinical efficacy. To plan and implement successful launch campaigns, the pharmaceutical industry will increasingly have to meet payers need for CER to assist in formulary decision-making processes, implementing disease management strategies, selection of treatment algorithms, and improving quality of healthcare.

Another indicator of the rising importance of CER is that for the first time, the US Congress provided substantial amounts of money toward comparing the effectiveness of different treatments for the same illness. The American Recovery and Reinvestment Act (ARRA) of 2009 contained millions of dollars for CEA. The funds provided by the ARRA are to support research assessing the comparative effectiveness of healthcare treatments and strategies, through efforts that

• conduct, support, or synthesize research that compares the clinical outcomes, effectiveness, and appropriateness of items, services, and procedures that are used to prevent, diagnose, or treat diseases, disorders, and other health conditions;
• encourage the development and use of clinical registries, clinical data networks, and other forms of electronic health data that can be used to generate or obtain outcomes data.

Additionally, within the healthcare reform discussions, CER has been identified as being essential for clinicians and patients to decide on the best treatment and to improve the health of communities and the performance of the health system.

Healthcare reform

In the United States, healthcare reform has become a priority issue due to the increasing number of under- and non-insured people and the increasing costs of healthcare. The basic premises of healthcare reform include the following:
• broaden the population that receives healthcare coverage through either public sector insurance programs or private sector insurance companies;
• expand the array of healthcare providers from which consumers may choose;
• improve the access to healthcare;
• improve the quality of healthcare;
• decrease the cost of healthcare.

The draft legislation being considered by the US Congress has the potential to impact pharmaceutical companies in four ways:
• *Redistribution of the payer mix:* Although the effect on pharmaceutical utilization by a large number of previously uninsured individuals who will now have access to healthcare may seem to provide a huge opportunity for manufacturers, the impact of this group on marketplace will be tempered by the payer type groups in which these individuals will fall. Government payers require manufacturers to pay significantly more rebates than a private payer. Therefore, the outcome of a large shift from the private (employer) payer to the government payer would result in a reduction in profitability.
• *Utilization of pharmaceutical products:* Again the impact of a large group into the marketplace will have both a positive and negative effect. There will be more individuals who will be treated with pharmaceutical products, but most reform efforts will drive increased use of generics.
• *Reimbursement, pricing, and rebates of pharmaceuticals:* Most healthcare reform proposals directly address reimbursement, pricing, and rebates issues. Proposed cuts in reimbursement to provider and

manufacturers and introduction of competitive pricing may directly impact profitability of pharmaceutical manufactures.

• *Comparative effectiveness research:* As mentioned in the preceding section, CER has been identified by Congress as being essential for clinicians and patients to decide on the best treatment and to improve the health of communities and the performance of the health system.

Healthcare reform is a very complex issue that may impact the pharmaceutical industry in a variety of ways. Additionally, the impact of the reform will not be uniform across products within a company's portfolio. Pharmaceutical companies are actively evaluating the impact of healthcare reform on their portfolio and making strategic changes to their current pricing, reimbursement, research (CER), pipeline, and managed market strategies.

Summary

Managed care has surpassed traditional indemnity or FFS health insurance to become the predominant form of coverage for health and medical care in the United States. Concern over rapidly rising healthcare costs has been the driving force behind the rapid growth of managed care in recent decades. Through effective application of key managed care principles of restricted access to healthcare providers, defined health plan benefits and services, and capitated reimbursement, MCOs have demonstrated their ability to control healthcare costs. In the process, managed care has affected every aspect of the healthcare industry, including the pharmaceutical industry.

With medications accounting for an increasing proportion of total medical costs, MCOs have been forced to implement cost-containment strategies to managed pharmacy benefits, including integrated formulary and disease management programs, comparative effectiveness research, and risk-sharing contracts. In addition, MCOs have become a major customer base to the pharmaceutical industry, with increasing leveraging and purchasing power. Therefore, managed care has had a significant impact on the way the pharmaceutical industry develops, markets, distributes, and generates revenue. Two aspects of the pharmaceutical industry that have been impacted the greatest are pharmaceutical research and development and product life cycles.

Finally, diverse factors will continue to influence managed care into the future, and subsequently, the pharmaceutical industry. Emerging trends include the importance of the employer segment, increasing demand for comparative effectiveness research, and the United States healthcare reform efforts. Therefore, the pharmaceutical industry must be positioned to maximize sales of targeted products and services and return on investment in an increasingly complex managed healthcare system.

References

Aetna US Healthcare website. Aetna to acquire Prudential Healthcare for $1 billion, 2009. http://www.aetna.com/about-aetna-insurance/aetna-corporate-profile/aetna-history/index.html; accessed April 20, 2010.

Bendix J. Doctors, administrators grapple with impact of recession, June 26, 2009; http://www.modernmedicine.com/modernmedicine/Modern+Medicine+Now/Doctors-administrators-grapple-with-impact-of-rece/ArticleStandard/Article/detail/606806; accessed April 20, 2010.

Blue Cross Blue Shield of Michigan website. Blue Cross Blue Shield of Michigan now covers Prilosec OTC—Switching from Nexium could save eligible members more than $9 million in out-of-pockets costs, 2007; http://www.bcbsm.com/pr/pr_09-05-2007_96933.shtml; accessed April 20, 2010.

Bond P, Weissman R. The cost of mergers and acquisitions in the US healthcare sector. *Int J Health Serv* 1997; **27**(1):77–87.

Briesacher BA, Andrade SE, Fouayzi H, *et al.* Medication adherence and use of generic drug therapies. *Am J Manag Care* 2009; **15**(7):450–456.

Burnett DA. Evolving market will change clinical research. *Health Affairs* 1996; **15**(3):90–92.

Burrell CD, Levy RA. Therapeutic consequences of noncompliance. Improving medication compliance. *Proceedings of a symposium. National Pharmaceutical Council: Washington, DC, USA,* 1984, 7–16.

Care Management Society of America. *Standards of practice for case management.* Care Management Society of America: Little Rock, AR, USA, 1995.

Center for Medicare & Medicaid Services, Office of the Actuary. National health expenditure projections 2008–2018; 2009; http://www.cms.hhs.gov/National HealthExpendData/downloads/proj2008.pdf; accessed April 20, 2010.

Edlin M. Fostering member loyalty. *Healthplan* 1998; **39**(5):73–78.

Employee Benefit Research Institute. Managed care confusion. Health Confidence Survey, 2007; http://www.ebri.org/pdf/notespdf/EBRI_Notes_11a-20071 .pdf: accessed April 20, 2010.

Fendrick AM, Smith DG, Cherew ME, Shah SN. A benefit-based copay for prescription drugs: patient contribution based on total benefits, not drug acquisition cost. *Am. J. MC* 2001; **7**(9):861–867.

Food & Drug Letter. Claritin approval marks significant shift in Rx-to-OTC Switches. *Food Drug Lett* 2002, (FDANews.com, 666).

Gandy W. Advertising badly to the public. *N Engl J Med* 1992; **326**:350.

Gold M, Hurley R. The role of managed care "products" in managed care plans. *Inquiry* 1997; **34**:29–37.

Grubert N, Hamer R, Waller R. Medicare reform–potential impact on the pharmaceutical and managed care industries, physicians, and patients. Spectrum– Pharmacoeconomics, Pricing, and Reimbursement, Decision Resources, *Medicare Reform*; 2004; 1–13.

Haynes R *et al.* Interventions for helping patients to follow prescriptions for medications. *Cochrane Database of Systematic Review* 2000; 2.

Headden S, Melton M. Madison Ave. loves drug ads: Cures for ulcers, toe fungus, even fleas. US News World Rep 1998; **20**:56–57.

Health Insurance Association of America. *Managed Care: Integrating the Delivery and Financing of Health Care,* second edition. Health Insurance Association of America: Washington, DC, USA, 1996.

Himes CL. Elderly Americans. *Popul Bull* 2001; **56**(4):2–8.

Hoechst Marion Roussel. *Managed Care Digest Series.* Hoechst Marion Roussel: Kansas City, MO, USA, 1998.

Hunt J, Rozenfeld Y, Shenolikar R. Effect of patient medication cost share on adherence and glycemic control. *Manag Care* 2009; **18**(7):47–53.

IMS Health website. Prescription drug ad spending in US exceeds $1.2 billion through November 1998, 1999. Available at http://www.IMSHealth.com/html/news_arc/02_09_1999_145.htm.

Kaiser Family Foundation. Trends and indicators in the changing health care marketplace. Trends & Indicators Chartbook, 2004; http://www.kff.org/insurance/7031/ti2004-2-17.cfm; accessed April 20, 2010.

Kaniecki DJ, Goldberg-Arnold RJ. Integrating worldwide marketing needs and clinical research. *J Clin Pharmacol* 1993; **33**(10):989–992.

Kolata G. Co-payments go way up for drugs with high prices. *New York Times,* April 14, 2008.

Lee TH, Emanuel EJ. Tier 4 drugs and the fraying of the social compact. *N Engl J. Med* 2008; **359**:333–335.

Lightfoot GD, Sanford SM, Shefrin A. Can investigator certification improve the quality of clinical research? *Qual Manag Health Care* 1999; **7**(3):31–36.

Litton LM, Sisk FA, Akins ME. Managing drug costs: the perception of managed care pharmacy directors. *Am J Manag Care* 2000; **6**(7):805–814.

Luce BR, Lyles CA, Rentz AM. The view from managed care pharmacy. *Health Affairs* 1996; **15**(4):168–176.

Luce BR, Paramore LC, Parasuraman B, *et al.* Can managed care organizations partner with manufacturers for comparative effectiveness research? *Am J Manag Care* 2008; **14**(3):149–156.

MacLeod GK. An overview of managed healthcare. In *The Managed Health Care Handbook,* second edition. Aspen: Gaithersburg, MD, USA, 1993.

Main T, Bernene C, Morsfall J. The recession: US managed care's mandate for change, 2009; http://www.oliverwyman.com/de/pdf-files/OW_EN_HLS_2009_Recession-final.pdf; accessed April 20, 2010.

Managed Care National Statistics. 2009; http://www.mcareol.com/factshts/factnati.htm.; accessed April 20, 2010.

Meyer H. The pills that ate your profits. *Hospitals Health Networks* 1998; **2**:19–22.

Miller S. Open enrolment: Six benefit trends for 2010, 2009; http://www.shrm.org/hrdisciplines/benefits/Articles/Pages/SixBenefitTrends.aspx; accessed April 20, 2010.

National Pharmaceutical Council. *Noncompliance with medication regimens. An economic tragedy. Emerging issues in pharmaceutical cost-containing.* National Pharmaceutical Council: Washington, DC, USA, 1992, 1–16.

Neuman P, Cubanski J. Medicare Part D update: Lessons learned and unfinished business. *NEJM* 2009; **361**:406–414.

NOP World Health. How DTC advertising fared in 2004. *Drug Topics* 2005; **149**(7):34.

Olson BM. Approaches to pharmacy benefit management and the impact of consumer cost sharing. *Clin Ther* 2002; **15**:250–272.

Pharmacy Benefit Management Institute. *Wyeth-Ayerst prescription drug benefit cost and plan design survey report.* Wellman Publishing, Inc.: Albuquerque, NM, USA, 2000.

Pollard MR. Managed care and a changing pharmaceutical industry. *Health Affairs* 1990; **9**(3):55–65.

PricewaterhouseCoopers. *The Factors Fueling Rising Healthcare Costs.* PricewaterhouseCoopers: Washington, DC, USA, April, 2002.

Riggs BL, Melton LJ III. The worldwide problem of osteoporosis: Insights afforded by epidemiology. *Bone* 1995; **17**(5 Suppl):505S–511S.

Schulman KA, Rubenstein LE, Abernethy DR, *et al.* The effect of pharmaceutical benefit managers: Is it being evaluated? *Ann Intern Med* 1996; **124**(10):906–913.

Sipkoff M. Insurers increasingly direct members toward OTC products, 2008; http://www.managedcaremag.com/archives/0804/0804.medmgmt.html; accessed April 20, 2010.

Sloane PD, Zimmerman S, Suchindran C, *et al.* The public health impact of Alzheimer's disease, 2000–2050: Potential implication of treatment advances. *Ann Rev Public Health*, 2002; **23**:213–231.

Studin I. New horizons in pharmaceutical managed-care marketing. *Pharm Executive* 2004; **24**(10):100–112.

APPENDIX
Useful Web Links

Since our textbook's earlier editions, the World Wide Web has continued to expand exponentially, and the plethora of websites of relevance to pharmaceutical medicine has grown commensurately.

Although websites change constantly and the options are enormous, the following collection is again offered as a list of sites that the editors have found useful. Note that many of these websites offer links to still more sites. Although great care has been taken, please accept our apologies for choices with which you disagree and for any outdated links.

Regulatory links

Australia—Therapeutic Goods Administration: www.tga.gov.au

Canada—Health Protection Branch (HPB): www.hc-sc.gc.ca

European Medicines Agency (EMA): www.ema.europa.eu

European Confederation of Medical Devices Associations: www.eucomed.be

International Conference on Harmonization of Technical Requirements for Registration of Pharmaceuticals for Human Use (ICH): www.ich.org

International Federation of Pharmaceutical Manufacturers & Associations (IFPMA): www.ifpma.org

Japan—Ministry of Health and Welfare (Koseisho): http://www.mhlw.go.jp/english

RAPS (Regulatory Affairs Professional Society): www.raps.org

US Code of Federal Regulations: http://www.gpoaccess.gov/cfr/ or with better layout: http://www.law.cornell.edu/cfr/

US Code of Federal Regulations, Title 21: Food and Drugs: http://www4.law.cornell.edu/cfr/21cfr.htm#start

US Food and Drug Administration (FDA): www.fda.gov

US Food and Drug Administration Center for Biologics Evaluation and Research (CBER): http://www.fda.gov/BiologicsBloodVaccines/default.htm

Worldwide Regulatory Affairs Information: www.rainfo.com

Pharmaceutical-related societies

Academy of Pharmaceutical Physicians and Investigators (APPI): www.appinet.org

Drug Information Association (DIA): www.diahome.org

Faculty of Pharmaceutical Medicine of the Royal Colleges of Physicians of the United Kingdom: www.fpm.org.uk

International Federation of Associations of Pharmaceutical Physicians (IFAPP): www.IFAPP.org

International Federation of Pharmaceutical Manufacturers Associations (IFPMA): www.ifpma.org

Links for national associations of pharmaceutical physicians

International Federation of Associations of Pharmaceutical Physicians (IFAPP): http://www.ifapp.org/home/join-us/members

Pharmaceutical Research and Manufacturers of America (PhRMA): http://www.phrma.org/

Principles and Practice of Pharmaceutical Medicine, 3rd edition.
Edited by L.D. Edwards, A.W. Fox, P.D. Stonier.
© 2011 Blackwell Publishing Ltd.

Other medical societies and organizations

American Medical Association (AMA): www.ama-assn.org

Association of American Medical Colleges (AAMC): www.aamc.org

Centers for Disease Control and Prevention (CDC): www.cdc.gov

National Institutes of Health (NIH): www.nih.gov

WHO—World Health Organization: www.who.int/en

Pharmaceutical companies

Pharmaceutical Company Directory, Worldwide: http://www.medilexicon.com/pharmaceutical companies.php

Contract research organizations

Listing of CROs: http://secure.ibpaalliance.org/assets/usrdocs/contract-research-companies.html

Ethics in clinical research

Belmont Report: http://ohsr.od.nih.gov/guidelines/belmont.html

Bioethics information: www.bioethics.net

Code of Federal Regulations, Protection of Human Subjects: http://ohsr.od.nih.gov/guidelines/45cfr46.html

Guidelines for the Conduct of Research Involving Human Subjects at the National Institutes of Health: http://ohsr.od.nih.gov/guidelines/Gray Booklet82404.pdf

ICH Guideline for Good Clinical Practice: http://www.ich.org/LOB/media/MEDIA482.pdf

Multiple Bioethics Links (provided by the New Jersey law firm of Sherman, Silverstein, Kohl, Rose & Podolsky): http://www.sskrplaw.com/ lawyer-attorney-1472325.html

Nuremberg Code: http://ohsr.od.nih.gov/guidelines/nuremberg.html

Office of Human Subjects Research: http://ohsr.od.nih.gov/

World Medical Association Declaration of Helsinki (2004 update): http://ohsr.od.nih.gov/guidelines/helsinki.html

Miscellaneous

Cochrane Collaboration: www.cochrane.org

E-Medicine (general clinical medicine): www.emedicine.com

General Information for Pharmaceutical Medicine Professionals: www.medilexicon.com

PERI Pharmaceutical Medicine Certificate Program: http://www.peri.org/pharm_courses.cfm

Pharmacy Information on the Internet: www.pharmweb.net

Post-Graduate Programme in Pharmacology and Pharmaceutical Medicine: http://www.ulb.ac.be/medecine/pharmed/PROGRAMME/programme.htm

Rx-List (general drug and labeling information): www.rxlist.com

Science Daily (breaking medical news and many other aspects of science, updated several times daily): www.sciencedaily.com

The Merck Manuals (general clinical medicine): www.merckmanuals.com

Index

Page numbers in *italics* represent figures, those in **bold** represent tables.

Printed and bound by CPI Group (UK) Ltd, Croydon, CR0 4YY